CLEMENTE · ANATOMY

W9-BZD-219

FROM THE PREFACE TO THE FIRST EDITION

Twenty-five years ago, while a student at the University of Pennsylvania, I marvelled at the clarity, completeness, and boldness of the anatomical illustrations of the original German editions of Professor Johannes Sobotta's Atlas and their excellent three-volume, English counterparts, the recent editions of which were authored by the late Professor Frank H. J. Figge. It is a matter of record that before World War II these atlases were the most popular ones consulted by American medical students. In the United States, with the advent of other anatomical atlases, the shortening of courses of anatomy in the medical schools, and the increase in publishing cost, the excellent but larger editions of the Sobotta atlases have become virtually unknown to a full generation of students. During the past 20 years of teaching Gross Anatomy at the University of California at Los Angeles, I have found only a handful of students who are familiar with the beautiful and still unexcelled Sobotta illustration.

This volume introduces several departures from the former Sobotta atlases. It is the first English edition that represents the Sobotta plates in a regional sequence – the pectoral region and upper extremity, the thorax, the abdomen, the pelvis and perineum, the lower extremity, the back, vertebral column and spinal cord, and finally, the neck and head. This sequence is consistent with that followed in many courses presented in the United States and Canada and one which should be useful to students in other countries.

Several illustrations never before published are presented in this atlas. These have been drawn by Jill Penkhus, who for a number of years has been the resident medical artist in the Anatomy Department at the UCLA School of Medicine.

Many have contributed to bringing this Atlas to fruition. I thank Dr. David S. Maxwell, Professor and Vice Chairman for Gross Anatomy and my colleague at UCLA, for his encouragement and suggestions. I also wish to express my appreciation to Caroline Belz and Louise Campbell, who spent many hours proofreading and typing the original text. I especially wish to thank Mary Mansor for constructing the index – a most laborious task. I am grateful to Barbara Robins for her assistance in typing some of the early parts of the manuscript, and above all, to her sister Julie, who is my wife and who makes all of my efforts worthwhile through her encouragement and devotion.

Los Angeles, California, January, 1975   CARMINE D. CLEMENTE

PREFACE TO THE FOURTH EDITION

It is a pleasure once again to offer a new edition of this atlas for students studying Anatomy in medical, dental, and other health professional schools. Additionally, many residents in postgraduate training have told me that they still refer to copies of former editions of this atlas during their residency years. The continuing popularity of this book has encouraged me to make this edition even better than previous ones.

There are many changes in this edition. In fact, almost every plate and its accompanying notes have been altered. A larger type size and clearer leader lines, easier to follow, have replaced previous ones on most of the figures. Many of the notes have been rewritten and changes suggested by students here at UCLA and other students in the United States and abroad have been incorporated.

There are 135 more figures in this edition than in the third edition, representing an increase of nearly 17%. These have helped to make the various sections of the book more complete. About half of the additional figures (68) have been added to the sections on the Abdomen, Pelvis and Perineum, regions which students have asked for additional information. Most of these figures (44) were added to the section on the Pelvis and Perineum. The remainder of the new figures (67) have been distributed throughout other parts of the book, with the Lower Limb (additional 29 figures) and Neck and Head (additional 18 figures) sections receiving the most. More figures on Surface Anatomy and new Charts for each of the Muscle Groups have been included for the convenience of students. These figures and charts list simplified Origins, Insertions, Innervations, and Actions of the individual muscles. One additional feature in this edition is the detailed listing of the figures in front of each part of the Atlas. These can be used as a logical study guide sequentially consistent with the instruction in most Anatomy courses.

Students will find a more spacious organization of figures on many plates in this edition in comparison to those in the third edition. This was especially emphasized in the sections on the limbs. As in previous editions, I have tried to maintain the **accuracy** of the labels and notes, a feature which numerous students have remarked was characteristic of this Atlas. I wish to encourage all students and anyone else who find misspellings or errors to write to me so that these can be changed in future printings.

Most of the figures of this edition have come from the 3rd Edition of this Atlas or from the 20th German Edition of Sobotta, edited by Professor Reinhard Putz, Director of the Institute of Anatomy in Munich and Professor Reinhard Pabst from the University of Hannover in Germany. I am most grateful to them for their elegant anatomical figures. Also I am greatly indebted to Dr. Lothar Wicke for figures from his *Atlas of Radiographic Anatomy*. Additionally, a number of illustrations have been used from the classic Pernkopf textbook, *Atlas of Topographic and Applied Human Anatomy* and still others have come from the Benninghoff-Goerttler textbooks and from earlier editions of the Sobotta Atlas edited by Professors Helmut Ferner and Jochen Staubesand. I also wish to acknowledge with appreciation Professor Gene Colborn from the Medical College of Georgia in Augusta, Georgia, USA, for producing six line drawings.

Many of the drawings in this edition are new and many others are exact redrawings of figures used previously. I am especially grateful to the publishers both in Baltimore and Munich for allowing me to enlarge the Atlas, to enhance the clarity of the figures and to reset all of the plates and notes. Special thanks are extended to Dr. Michael Urban and Timothy S. Satterfield and to Renate Hausdorf, Dorle Matussek, Raymond Reter and Crystal Taylor for their enormous help in bringing this book to completion. I am also grateful to Deborah Tourtlotte for compiling the index. In Los Angeles, I thank Drs. Charles H. Sawyer and Anthony M. Adinolfi for their support and suggestions through the years. Finally, and most importantly, I dedicate this volume to my wife, Julie, for her love and unending kindness through the decades.

Los Angeles, California. July, 1996   CARMINE D. CLEMENTE

Editor: Jane Velker
Managing Editor: Crystal Taylor
Production Coordinator: Raymond E. Reter
Production: Renate Hausdorf
Cover Designer: Dieter Vollendorf
Typesetter: Typodata GmbH
Printer: Neue Stalling
Digitized Illustrations: Typodata GmbH
Binder: Neue Stalling

351 West Camden Street
Baltimore, Maryland 21201-2436 USA

Rose Tree Corporate Center
1400 North Providence Road
Building II, Suite 5025
Media, Pennsylvania 19063-2043 USA

The pictures on the end leaves of the present volume show reproductions of the work of "Andreas Vesalii de corporis humani fabrica libri septem," which appeared in Basel in 1542. Andreas Vesalius (Brussels 1514, 1574) urged and practiced the dissection of human bodies and may be considered to be the founder of Modern Anatomy.

The illustrations in this atlas have been published in recent editions of:
Sobotta, Atlas der Anatomie des Menschen, 20. Auflage, Edited by R. Putz and R. Pabst, Urban & Schwarzenberg.
Sobotta, Atlas der Anatomie des Menschen, 19. Auflage, Edited by H. Ferner and J. Staubesand, Urban & Schwarzenberg.
Pernkopf, Eduard, Atlas of Topographical and Applied Human Anatomy, 3rd Edition, Edited by W. Platzer, Urban & Schwarzenberg.
Benninghoff/Goerttler, Lehrbuch der Anatomie des Menschen, Edited by H. Ferner and J. Staubesand, Urban & Schwarzenberg.
Wicke, Lothar, Atlas of Radiographic Anatomy, 4th and 5th Editions, Urban & Schwarzenberg.
Clemente, Carmine D., Anatomy: A Regional Atlas of the Human Body, 3rd Edition, Urban & Schwarzenberg.
Figures 7, 27, 28, 41, 191, and 693 were drawn under the direction of Dr. Gene L. Colborn, Medical College of Georgia, Augusta, Georgia, USA.

Printed in Germany
The first edition of this atlas was published in 1975 by Urban & Schwarzenberg (ISBN 3-541-07141-9) and copublished in North America by Lea & Febiger, Philadelphia (ISBN 0-8121-0496-X).

Library of Congress Cataloging-in-Publication Data

Clemente, Carmine D.
    Anatomy, a regional atlas of the human body / Carmine D. Clemente.
  -- 4th ed.
      p.   cm.
    Includes bibliographical references and index.
    ISBN 0-683-30305-8
    1. Anatomy, Surgical and topographical--Atlases.   I. Title.
  [DNLM: 1. Anatomy, Regional--atlases.   QS 17 C626a 1997]
  QM531.C57   1997
  611'.0022'2--dc21
  DNLM/DLC
  for Library of Congress   96-47623

To purchase additional copies of this book, call our customer service department at **(8 00) 6 38-06 72** or fax orders to **(8 00) 4 47-84 38**. For other book services, including chapter reprints and large quantity sales, ask for the Special Sales department.

Canadian customers should call **(8 00) 6 65-11 48**, or fax **(8 00) 6 65-01 03**. For all other calls originating outside of the United States, please call **(410) 5 28-42 23** or fax us at **(410) 5 28-85 50**.

Visit Williams & Wilkins on the Internet: **http://www.wwilkins.com** or contact our customer service department at **custserv@wwilkins.com.** Williams & Wilkins customer service representatives are available from 8:30 am to 6:00 pm, EST, Monday through Friday, for telephone access.

97 98 99 00 01
1   2   3   4   5   6   7   8   9 10

Anatomy

A Regional Atlas of the Human Body

Carmine D. Clemente

Professor of Anatomy and Cell Biology and
Professor of Neurobiology, Emeritus (Recalled)
University of California at Los Angeles School of Medicine;

Professor of Surgery (Anatomy)
Charles R. Drew University of Medicine and Science
Los Angeles, California

4th Edition

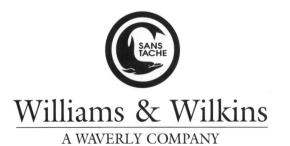

Williams & Wilkins
A WAVERLY COMPANY

BALTIMORE • PHILADELPHIA • LONDON • PARIS • BANGKOK
BUENOS AIRES • HONG KONG • MUNICH • SYDNEY • TOKYO • WROCLAW

FROM THE PREFACE TO THE THIRD EDITION

Once again, my primary objective in the preparation of this edition has been to facilitate the task of the learning of anatomy by students in the medical, dental, and other health professions. Because of the popularity and acceptance of the two previous editions, this edition has expanded the coverage of certain regions of the body that were treated more thinly in the 1975 and 1981 editions. I extend my appreciation to the publisher for allowing me this freedom. It is sometimes said that if a book used in the teaching of a major professional field ever achieves a third edition, there is a possibility that it has finally reached maturity. I hope that this is the case with this atlas. There are 96 new figures included in this edition while six figures from the 2nd edition have been eliminated. This net increase of 90 figures represents a 13% enlargement of the atlas over the previous edition. Of the new figures, a total of 34 (35%) were added to the sections on the thorax, abdomen and pelvis, 37 (39%) were added to the limbs and 25 (26%) were added to the sections on neck and head. More specifically, for the thorax some of the figures added depict the bony thoracic cage, the position of the heart within the chest, the coronary arteries, the sympathetic trunks and the fetal heart. Four new cross-sections at various levels of the abdomen along with additional figures on the anterior abdominal wall, the female inguinal region, lymphatics of the stomach, the appendix and its blood supply, the posterior abdominal wall, and the female perineum have been included. In the sections on the upper and lower extremities there is an additional coverage of the shoulder and elbow joints and especially the knee joint. Other figures illustrating the surface anatomy and cutaneous innervation of the limbs, as well as arteriograms and other x-rays have also been included. The section on neck and head has been enhanced by 10 new figures on the eye, 6 on the oral cavity, and 4 on the ear. Five other figures on the neck and dura mater have also been added.

One of the more significant features of this edition is the fact that over 225 of the figures used in this book are precise repaintings of the older illustrations used in former editions. Further, a number of other figures that were black and white illustrations in previous editions now are presented in full color. This new art is, for the most part, brighter and more vivid in color than the old, and my many thanks go to the several artists who produced these new works because their creations strictly adhered to the older illustrations and resulted in meticulously perfect reproductions. At Urban & Schwarzenberg, I thank Mr. Michael Urban and Wulf J. Dietrich in Munich and Mr. Braxton Mitchell and Norman W. Och in Baltimore for their continuing support in this effort to create an atlas that best meets the needs of students. Finally and most importantly, I want to thank my wife, Julie, for her patience and for her compassionate and generous spirit in support of my writing efforts.

Los Angeles, California, December, 1986   CARMINE D. CLEMENTE

CONTENTS

Contents continued

PLATES CONTAINING MUSCLE CHARTS

PART I
PECTORAL REGION; AXILLA; SHOULDER AND UPPER LIMB

(PLATES 1–90 – FIGURES 1–144)

PART I PECTORAL REGION; AXILLA; SHOULDER and UPPER LIMB

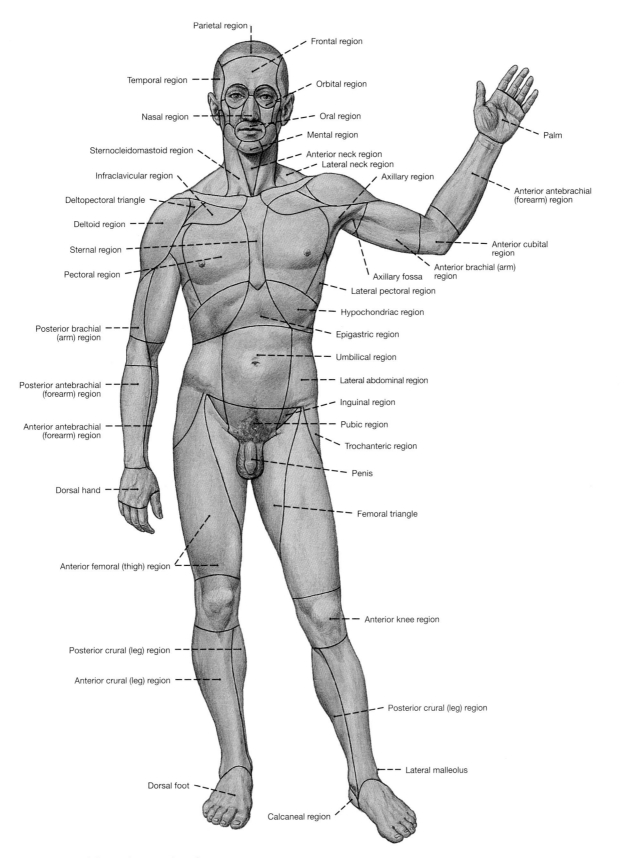

Parietal region
Frontal region
Temporal region
Orbital region
Nasal region
Oral region
Mental region
Sternocleidomastoid region
Anterior neck region
Lateral neck region
Infraclavicular region
Axillary region
Deltopectoral triangle
Deltoid region
Sternal region
Pectoral region
Posterior brachial (arm) region
Posterior antebrachial (forearm) region
Anterior antebrachial (forearm) region
Dorsal hand
Anterior femoral (thigh) region
Posterior crural (leg) region
Anterior crural (leg) region
Dorsal foot
Calcaneal region

Palm
Anterior antebrachial (forearm) region
Anterior cubital region
Anterior brachial (arm) region
Axillary fossa
Lateral pectoral region
Hypochondriac region
Epigastric region
Umbilical region
Lateral abdominal region
Inguinal region
Pubic region
Trochanteric region
Penis
Femoral triangle
Anterior knee region
Posterior crural (leg) region
Lateral malleolus

Fig. 1: Regions of the Body: Anterior View

NOTE: 1) surface areas are identified by specific names to describe the location of structures and symptoms precisely.

2) some regions are named after bones (sternal, parietal, infraclavicular, etc.), others for muscles (deltoid, pectoral, sternocleidomastoid), and still others for specialized anatomical structures (umbilical, oral, nasal, etc.).

3) the principal regions of the body include the pectoral region and upper extremity, the thorax, abdomen, pelvis and perineum, lower extremity, back and spinal column and the neck and head.

Fig. 1   I

PLATE 2   **Surface Anatomy of the Male Thorax**

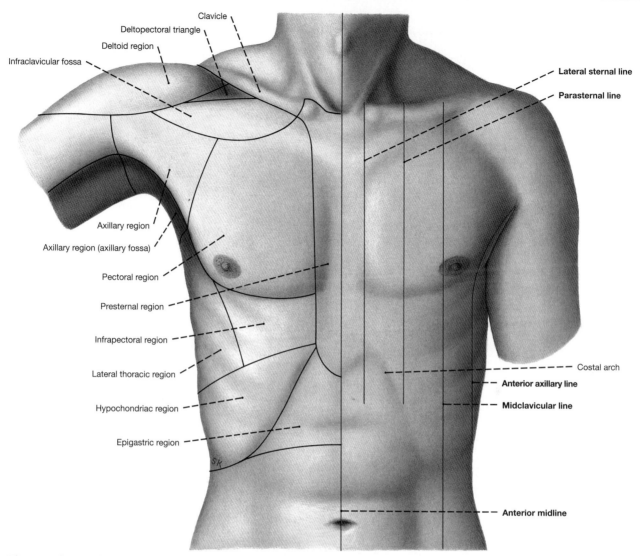

Clavicle
Deltopectoral triangle
Deltoid region
Infraclavicular fossa

Lateral sternal line
Parasternal line

Axillary region
Axillary region (axillary fossa)
Pectoral region
Presternal region
Infrapectoral region
Lateral thoracic region
Hypochondriac region
Epigastric region

Costal arch
Anterior axillary line
Midclavicular line

Anterior midline

Fig. 2: Regions and Longitudinal Lines on the Anterior Surface of the Male Thorax
NOTE: 1) the lateral sternal line descends along the lateral border of the sternum.
 2) other lines parallel to this are called parasternal lines.
 3) the male nipple lies near the midclavicular line.
 4) the anterior axillary line descends from the anterior axillary fold.

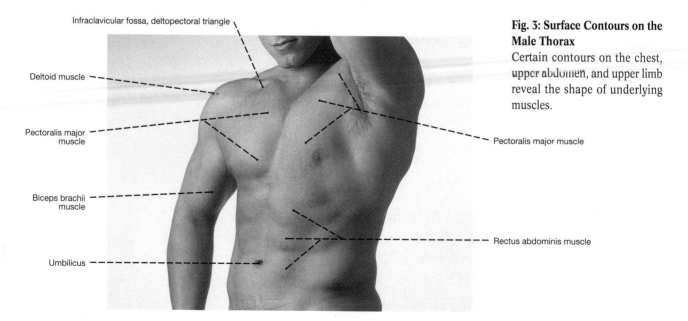

Infraclavicular fossa, deltopectoral triangle

Deltoid muscle

Pectoralis major muscle

Biceps brachii muscle

Umbilicus

Pectoralis major muscle

Rectus abdominis muscle

Fig. 3: Surface Contours on the Male Thorax
Certain contours on the chest, upper abdomen, and upper limb reveal the shape of underlying muscles.

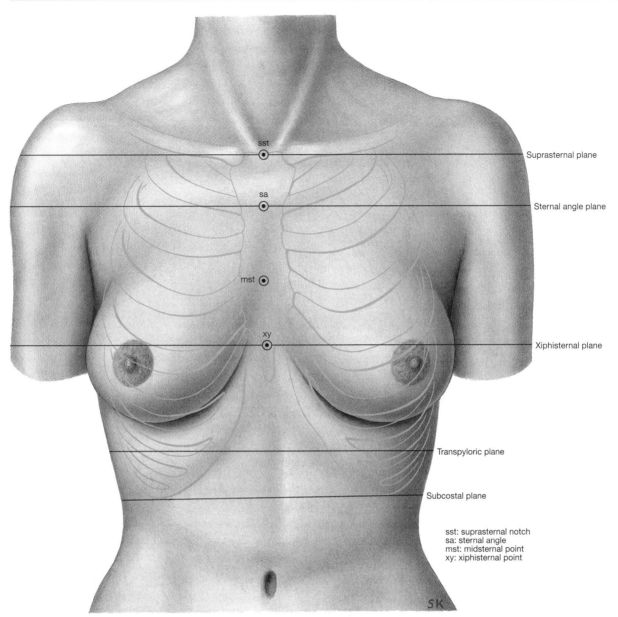

Fig. 4: Transverse Planes Shown on the Surface of the Female Thorax

NOTE: 1) the suprasternal plane projects back to the T2 vertebra, the sternal angle to T4, the xiphisternal junction to T9, and the transpyloric plane to L1.

      2) the subcostal plane, below the 10th rib anteriorly, projects back to L2.

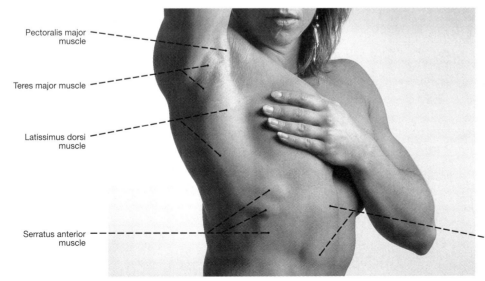

Fig. 5: Surface Contours on the Lateral Thorax of a Young Woman
Note the contours of well-developed latissimus dorsi, pectoralis major, teres major, and serratus anterior muscles.

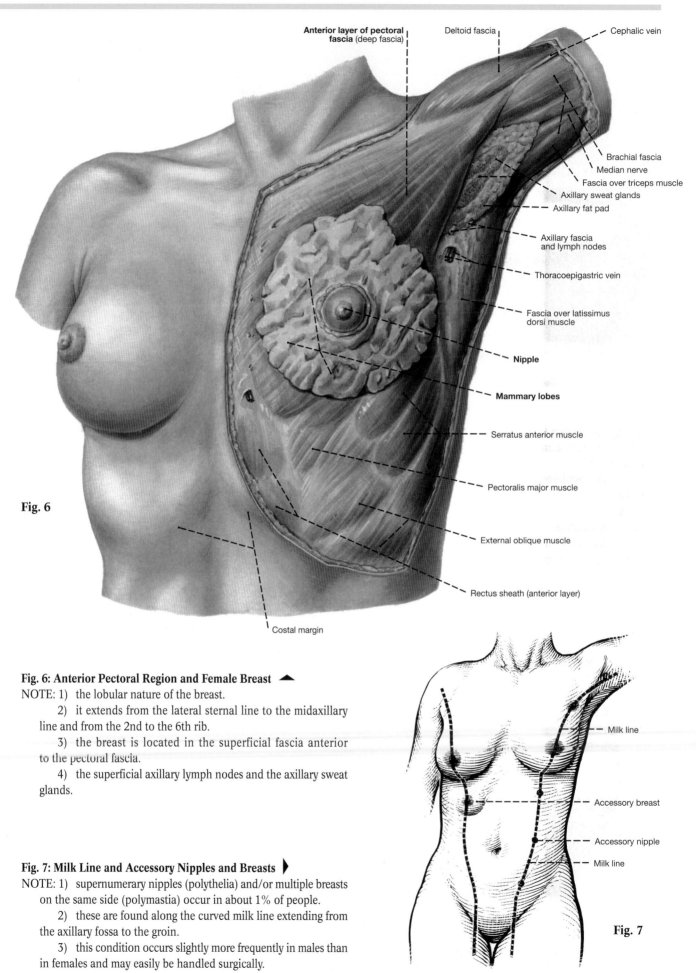

Anterior layer of pectoral fascia (deep fascia)

Deltoid fascia

Cephalic vein

Brachial fascia

Median nerve

Fascia over triceps muscle

Axillary sweat glands

Axillary fat pad

Axillary fascia and lymph nodes

Thoracoepigastric vein

Fascia over latissimus dorsi muscle

Nipple

Mammary lobes

Serratus anterior muscle

Pectoralis major muscle

External oblique muscle

Rectus sheath (anterior layer)

Costal margin

Fig. 6

Milk line

Accessory breast

Accessory nipple

Milk line

Fig. 7

Fig. 6: Anterior Pectoral Region and Female Breast ▲

NOTE: 1) the lobular nature of the breast.

2) it extends from the lateral sternal line to the midaxillary line and from the 2nd to the 6th rib.

3) the breast is located in the superficial fascia anterior to the pectoral fascia.

4) the superficial axillary lymph nodes and the axillary sweat glands.

Fig. 7: Milk Line and Accessory Nipples and Breasts ▶

NOTE: 1) supernumerary nipples (polythelia) and/or multiple breasts on the same side (polymastia) occur in about 1% of people.

2) these are found along the curved milk line extending from the axillary fossa to the groin.

3) this condition occurs slightly more frequently in males than in females and may easily be handled surgically.

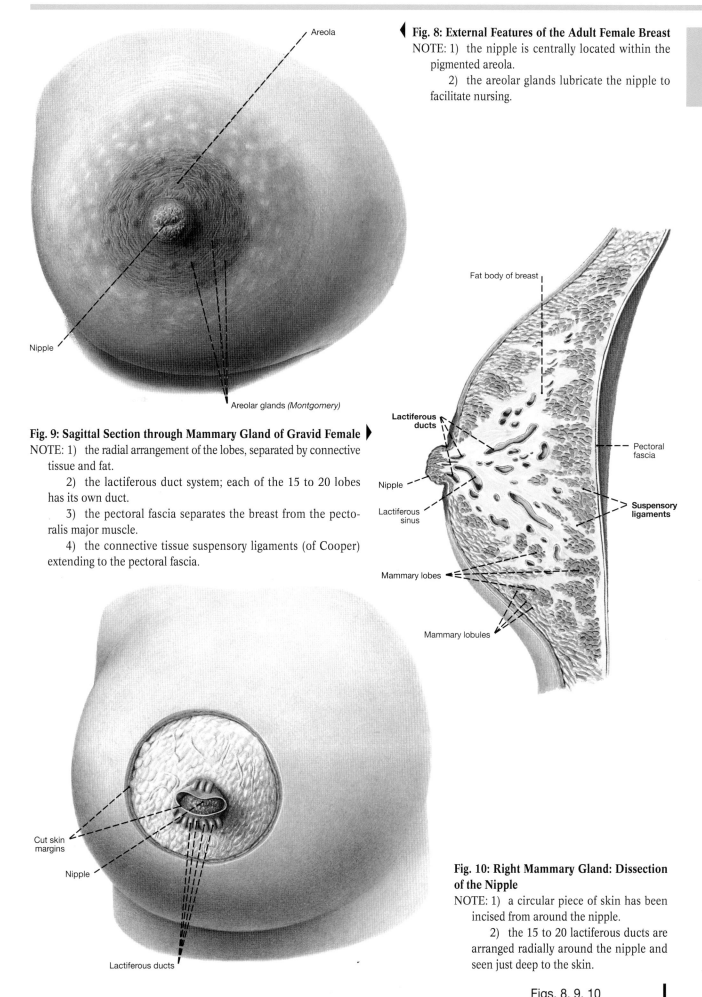

Fig. 8: External Features of the Adult Female Breast
NOTE: 1) the nipple is centrally located within the pigmented areola.

2) the areolar glands lubricate the nipple to facilitate nursing.

Fig. 9: Sagittal Section through Mammary Gland of Gravid Female ▶
NOTE: 1) the radial arrangement of the lobes, separated by connective tissue and fat.

2) the lactiferous duct system; each of the 15 to 20 lobes has its own duct.

3) the pectoral fascia separates the breast from the pectoralis major muscle.

4) the connective tissue suspensory ligaments (of Cooper) extending to the pectoral fascia.

Fig. 10: Right Mammary Gland: Dissection of the Nipple
NOTE: 1) a circular piece of skin has been incised from around the nipple.

2) the 15 to 20 lactiferous ducts are arranged radially around the nipple and seen just deep to the skin.

Figs. 8, 9, 10

PLATE 6   Lymphatic Drainage of the Breast; Lymphangiogram of Axilla

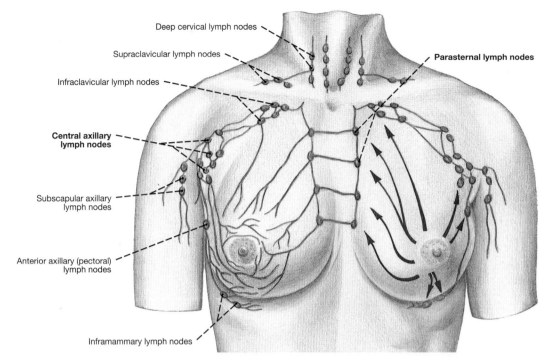

Fig. 11: Lymphatic Drainage from the Adult Female Breast
NOTE: 1) numerous lymph vessels in the breast communicate in a subareolar plexus deep to and around the nipple.
  2) about 75% of the lymph from the breast courses laterally and upward to axillary and infraclavicular nodes.
  3) most of the remaining lymph passes medially to parasternal nodes along the internal thoracic vessels.
  4) some lymph vessels drain downward to upper abdominal nodes and some go to the opposite breast.

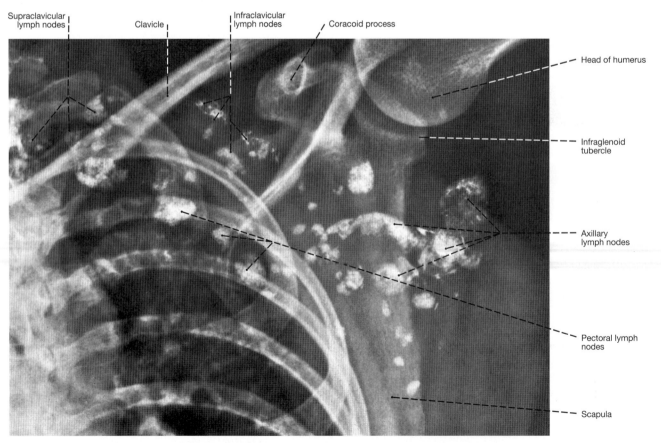

Fig. 12: Lymphangiogram of the Pectoral and Axillary Lymph Nodes
(From: Wicke, L., *Atlas of Radiologic Anatomy,* 4th Edition, Urban & Schwarzenberg, Baltimore, 1987).

Figs. 11, 12

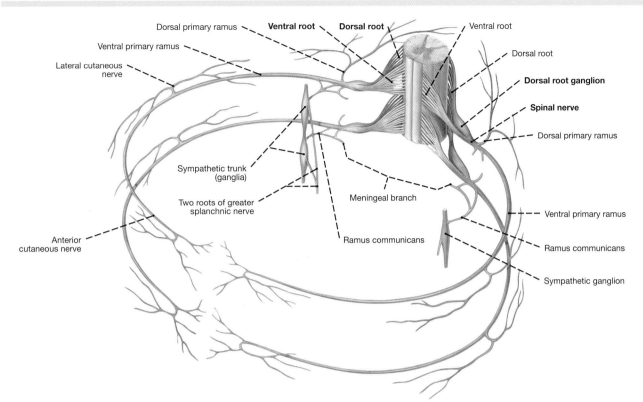

Fig. 13: Two Typical Spinal Nerves: Their Origin, Branches, and Connections to the Sympathetic Trunk

NOTE: 1) each spinal nerve attaches to the spinal cord by a dorsal (sensory) root and a ventral (motor) root.

   2) each dorsal root contains a spinal ganglion where the cell bodies of sensory neurons are found.

   3) the dorsal and ventral roots of the same segment join to form a spinal nerve, which soon divides into dorsal and ventral primary rami.

   4) the dorsal primary ramus supplies the back; the ventral primary ramus supplies the lateral and anterior walls of the trunk.

   5) spinal nerves communicate with the sympathetic trunk by way of rami communicantes.

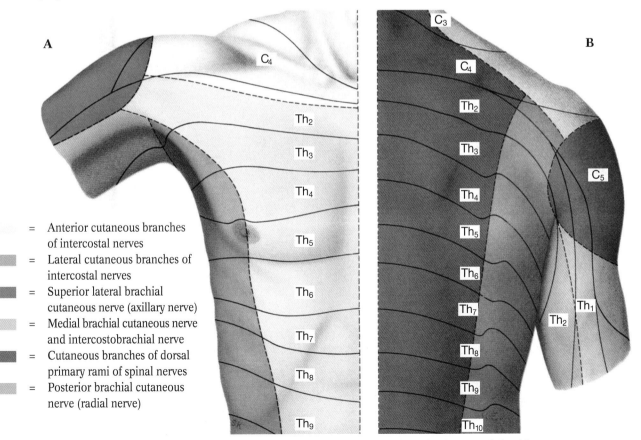

= Anterior cutaneous branches of intercostal nerves

= Lateral cutaneous branches of intercostal nerves

= Superior lateral brachial cutaneous nerve (axillary nerve)

= Medial brachial cutaneous nerve and intercostobrachial nerve

= Cutaneous branches of dorsal primary rami of spinal nerves

= Posterior brachial cutaneous nerve (radial nerve)

Fig. 14: Innervation Fields of Cutaneous Nerves. A, Anterior thorax and axilla; **B,** Posterior thorax and shoulder.

PLATE 8   Superficial Vessels and Nerves of the Anterior Trunk

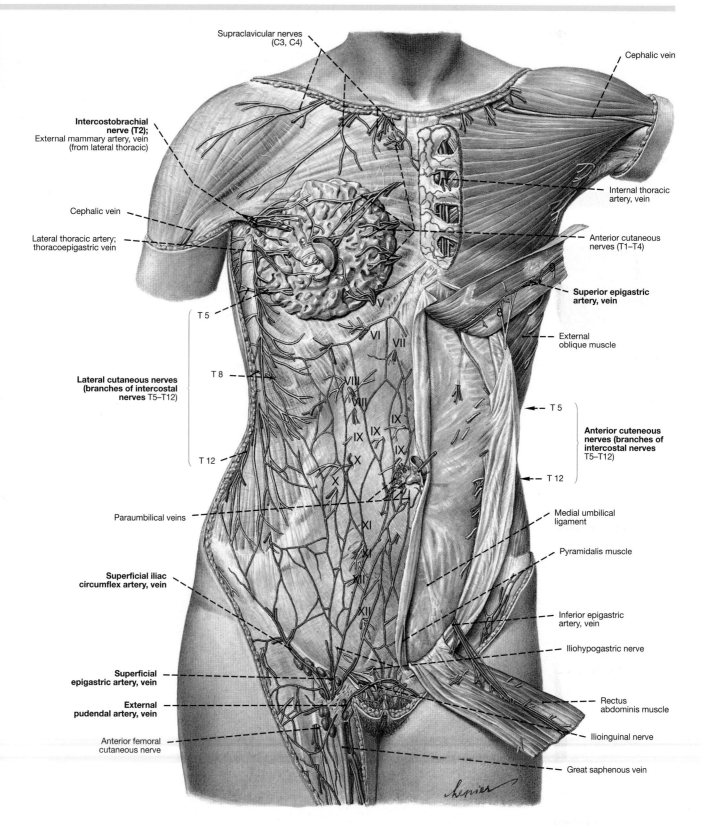

Supraclavicular nerves (C3, C4)

Cephalic vein

Intercostobrachial nerve (T2); External mammary artery, vein (from lateral thoracic)

Internal thoracic artery, vein

Cephalic vein

Lateral thoracic artery; thoracoepigastric vein

Anterior cutaneous nerves (T1–T4)

Superior epigastric artery, vein

External oblique muscle

T 5

VI VII

Lateral cutaneous nerves (branches of intercostal nerves T5–T12)

T 8

VIII

VII

T 5

IX

IX IX

IX

Anterior cuteneous nerves (branches of intercostal nerves T5–T12)

T 12

X

T 12

X

Medial umbilical ligament

Paraumbilical veins

XI

Pyramidalis muscle

XII

Superficial iliac circumflex artery, vein

Inferior epigastric artery, vein

Iliohypogastric nerve

Superficial epigastric artery, vein

Rectus abdominis muscle

External pudendal artery, vein

Ilioinguinal nerve

Anterior femoral cutaneous nerve

Great saphenous vein

Fig. 15: Superficial Vessels and Nerves of the Ventral Trunk: Pectoral Region and Anterior Abdominal Wall

NOTE: 1) cutaneous innervation of the trunk: supraclavicular nerves (C3, C4), intercostal nerves (T1–T12), and the ilioinguinal and iliohypogastric branches of L1.

2) the intercostal nerves give off lateral and anterior cutaneous branches.

3) anastomoses between the thoracoepigastric vein above and the superficial iliac circumflex and inferior epigastric veins below.

4) the breast; its innervation: T2 to T6 intercostal nerves,
                its blood supply: internal thoracic artery, lateral thoracic artery, intercostal arteries.

5) the nipple at the level of T4 and the umbilicus at the level of T10.

Fig. 15

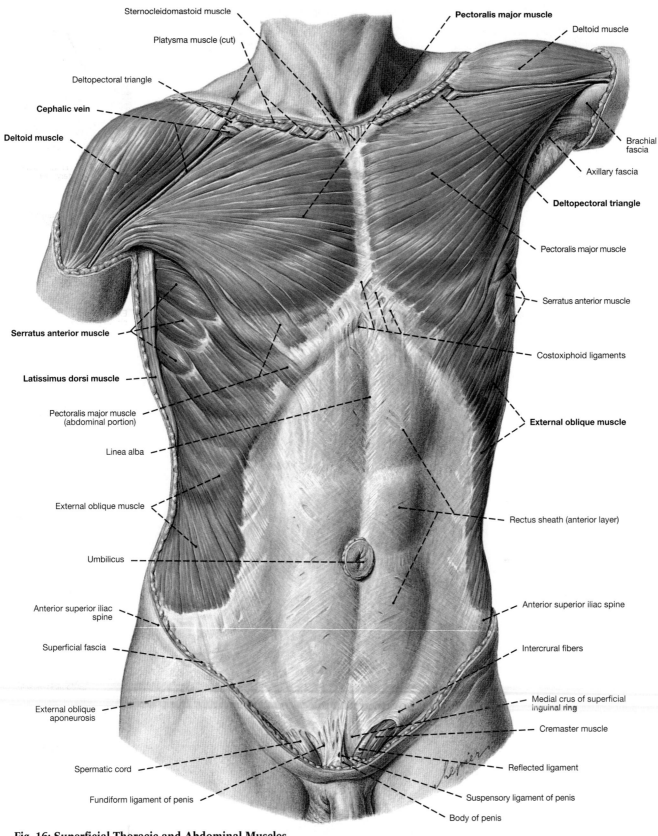

Sternocleidomastoid muscle

Platysma muscle (cut)

Deltopectoral triangle

Cephalic vein

Deltoid muscle

Serratus anterior muscle

Latissimus dorsi muscle

Pectoralis major muscle (abdominal portion)

Linea alba

External oblique muscle

Umbilicus

Anterior superior iliac spine

Superficial fascia

External oblique aponeurosis

Spermatic cord

Fundiform ligament of penis

Pectoralis major muscle

Deltoid muscle

Brachial fascia

Axillary fascia

Deltopectoral triangle

Pectoralis major muscle

Serratus anterior muscle

Costoxiphoid ligaments

External oblique muscle

Rectus sheath (anterior layer)

Anterior superior iliac spine

Intercrural fibers

Medial crus of superficial inguinal ring

Cremaster muscle

Reflected ligament

Suspensory ligament of penis

Body of penis

Fig. 16: Superficial Thoracic and Abdominal Muscles

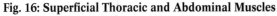

Muscle	Origin	Insertion	Innervation	Action
Pectoralis Major	Medial ½ of clavicle; 2nd to 6th ribs; costal margin of sternum; aponeurosis of external oblique	Humerus, lateral lip of intertubercular sulcus	Lateral (C5, 6, 7) and medial (C8, T1) pectoral nerves	Adducts and rotates arm medially; **sternal part:** helps extend humerus **clavicular part:** helps flex humerus

Fig. 16

PLATE 10   Pectoral Region: Superficial Vessels and Cutaneous Nerves

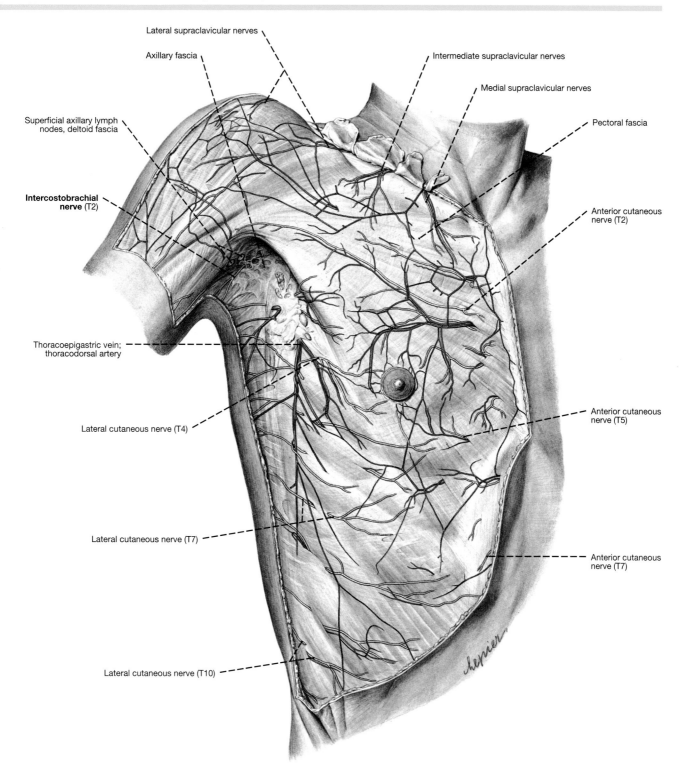

Fig. 17: Anterior Thoracic Wall; Superficial Dissection in the Male

NOTE: 1)   the skin and superficial fascia have been removed, but the cutaneous vessels and nerves have been retained.

2)   the cutaneous neurovascular structures penetrate through the deep fascia (pectoral fascia) to get to the superficial fascia and skin.

3)   most of the cutaneous vessels and nerves are anterior vend lateral cutaneous branches of the intercostal nerves.

4)   the supraclavicular nerves derived from C3 and C4.

5)   the intercostobrachial nerve (T2). It joins the medial brachial cutaneous nerve to supply the skin of the axillary fossa and upper medial arm.

Fig. 17

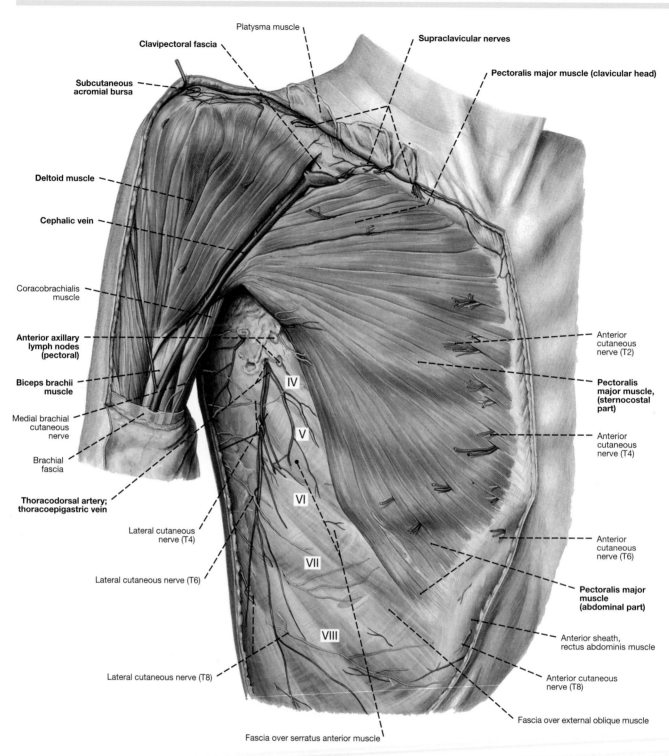

Platysma muscle

Clavipectoral fascia

Subcutaneous acromial bursa

Deltoid muscle

Cephalic vein

Coracobrachialis muscle

Anterior axillary lymph nodes (pectoral)

Biceps brachii muscle

Medial brachial cutaneous nerve

Brachial fascia

Thoracodorsal artery; thoracoepigastric vein

Lateral cutaneous nerve (T4)

Lateral cutaneous nerve (T6)

Lateral cutaneous nerve (T8)

Fascia over serratus anterior muscle

Supraclavicular nerves

Pectoralis major muscle (clavicular head)

Anterior cutaneous nerve (T2)

Pectoralis major muscle, (sternocostal part)

Anterior cutaneous nerve (T4)

Anterior cutaneous nerve (T6)

Pectoralis major muscle (abdominal part)

Anterior sheath, rectus abdominis muscle

Anterior cutaneous nerve (T8)

Fascia over external oblique muscle

IV V VI VII VIII

Fig. 18: Pectoralis Major and Deltoid Muscles, Anterior View

NOTE: 1) the anterior layer of the pectoral fascia and the deltoid fascia as seen in Fig. 17 have been removed.

2) the lateral cutaneous vessels and nerves penetrating through the intercostal spaces in the midaxillary line.

3) the anterior cutaneous vessels and nerves piercing the pectoralis major muscle along the lateral border of the sternum.

4) the **clavicular** fibers of this muscle course obliquely downward and laterally, the upper **sternocostal** fibers are directed nearly horizontally and the lower sternocostal and abdominal fibers ascend nearly vertically to the humerus.

5) the natural cleft between the clavicular and sternocostal heads. Detaching the clavicular head uncovers some of the vessels and nerves that supply this muscle (Fig. 20).

6) the 4th to the 8th ribs are labelled sequentially with Roman numerals.

Fig. 18

PLATE 12   Lateral Thoracic Wall and Superficial Axilla

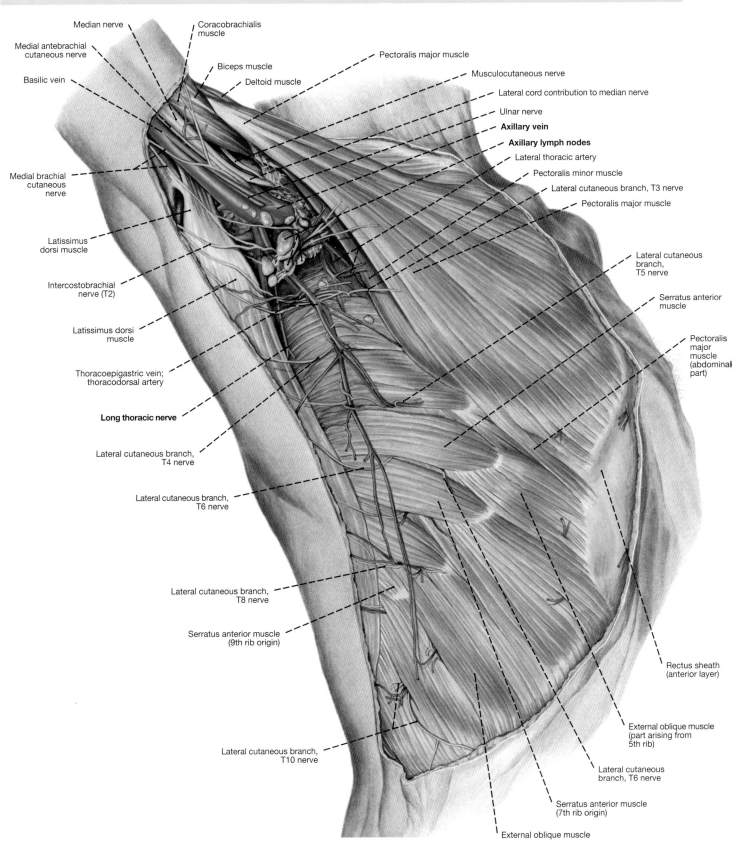

Median nerve

Medial antebrachial cutaneous nerve

Basilic vein

Coracobrachialis muscle

Biceps muscle

Deltoid muscle

Pectoralis major muscle

Musculocutaneous nerve

Lateral cord contribution to median nerve

Ulnar nerve

Axillary vein

Axillary lymph nodes

Lateral thoracic artery

Pectoralis minor muscle

Lateral cutaneous branch, T3 nerve

Pectoralis major muscle

Medial brachial cutaneous nerve

Latissimus dorsi muscle

Intercostobrachial nerve (T2)

Latissimus dorsi muscle

Thoracoepigastric vein; thoracodorsal artery

Long thoracic nerve

Lateral cutaneous branch, T4 nerve

Lateral cutaneous branch, T6 nerve

Lateral cutaneous branch, T8 nerve

Serratus anterior muscle (9th rib origin)

Lateral cutaneous branch, T10 nerve

Lateral cutaneous branch, T5 nerve

Serratus anterior muscle

Pectoralis major muscle (abdominal part)

Rectus sheath (anterior layer)

External oblique muscle (part arising from 5th rib)

Lateral cutaneous branch, T6 nerve

Serratus anterior muscle (7th rib origin)

External oblique muscle

Fig. 19: Lateral Aspect of the Upper Right Thoracic Wall and the Superficial Axillary Structures

Muscle	Origin	Insertion	Innervation	Action
Pectoralis Minor	Coracoid process of scapula	Ribs 2 to 5	Medial pectoral nerve (C8, T1)	Protracts scapula; elevates ribs
Serratus Anterior	Fleshy slips from upper 9 ribs	Medial border of scapula	Long thoracic nerve (C5, C6, C7)	Protracts and rotates scapula; holds scapula close to thoracic wall

Fig. 19

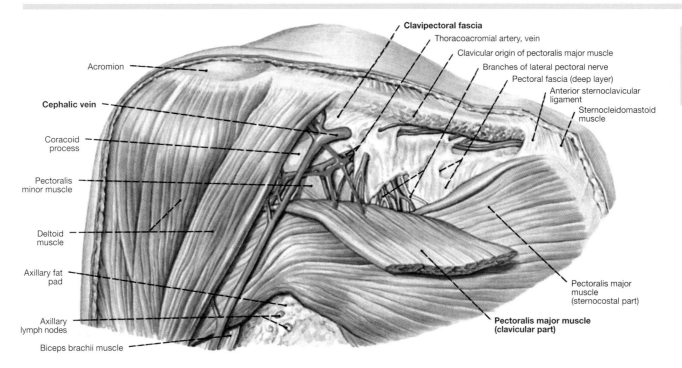

Clavipectoral fascia
Thoracoacromial artery, vein
Clavicular origin of pectoralis major muscle
Branches of lateral pectoral nerve
Pectoral fascia (deep layer)
Anterior sternoclavicular ligament
Sternocleidomastoid muscle
Acromion
Cephalic vein
Coracoid process
Pectoralis minor muscle
Deltoid muscle
Axillary fat pad
Axillary lymph nodes
Biceps brachii muscle
Pectoralis major muscle (sternocostal part)
Pectoralis major muscle (clavicular part)

Fig. 20: Deltopectoral Triangle (Right)

NOTE: 1)   the clavicular head of the pectoralis major has been severed and reflected downward.

2)   the investing layer of deep fascia covering the deep surface of the pectoralis major muscle and the **clavipectoral fascia,** which extends between the clavicle and the medial border of the pectoralis minor muscle, are exposed.

3)   the **cephalic vein** pierces the clavipectoral fascia to join the axillary vein.

4)   the **thoracoacromial artery** (from the axillary artery) and the **lateral pectoral nerve** (from the lateral cord of the brachial plexus) pierce through the fascia from below to supply blood to the region and to innervate the pectoralis major.

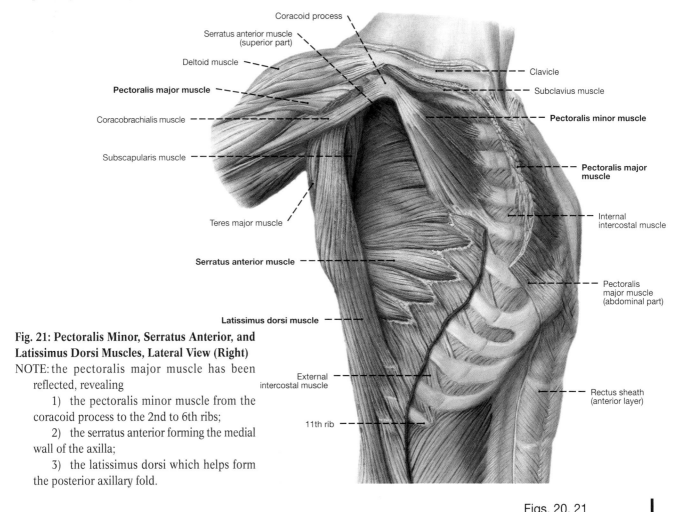

Coracoid process
Serratus anterior muscle (superior part)
Deltoid muscle
Pectoralis major muscle
Coracobrachialis muscle
Subscapularis muscle
Teres major muscle
Serratus anterior muscle
Latissimus dorsi muscle
External intercostal muscle
11th rib
Clavicle
Subclavius muscle
Pectoralis minor muscle
Pectoralis major muscle
Internal intercostal muscle
Pectoralis major muscle (abdominal part)
Rectus sheath (anterior layer)

Fig. 21: Pectoralis Minor, Serratus Anterior, and Latissimus Dorsi Muscles, Lateral View (Right)

NOTE: the pectoralis major muscle has been reflected, revealing

1)   the pectoralis minor muscle from the coracoid process to the 2nd to 6th ribs;

2)   the serratus anterior forming the medial wall of the axilla;

3)   the latissimus dorsi which helps form the posterior axillary fold.

PLATE 14   Axillary Vessels

1. Axillary vein
2. Basilic vein
3. Cephalic vein
4. Lateral border of the scapula
5. Lateral border of the latissimus dorsi
6. Head of humerus
7. Acromion
8. Venous valve
9. Brachial vein

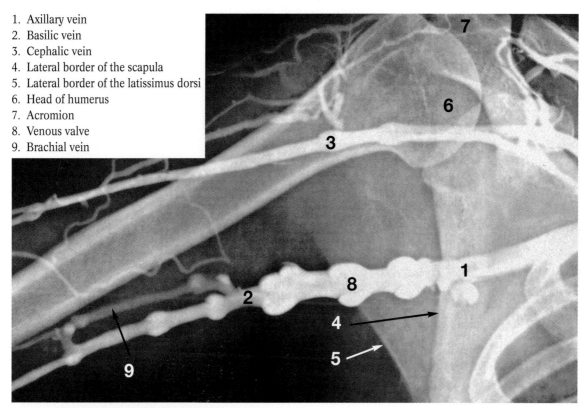

Fig. 22: Radiograph of Veins in the Axillary Region
NOTE: 1) the basilic vein (2) becomes the axillary vein (1).

2) one of the brachial veins (9) also flows into the axillary vein as does the cephalic vein (3), the junction of which is medial to the field shown here.

3) the venous valves (8) along the course of the axillary vein. These are shown schematically in Figure 25.

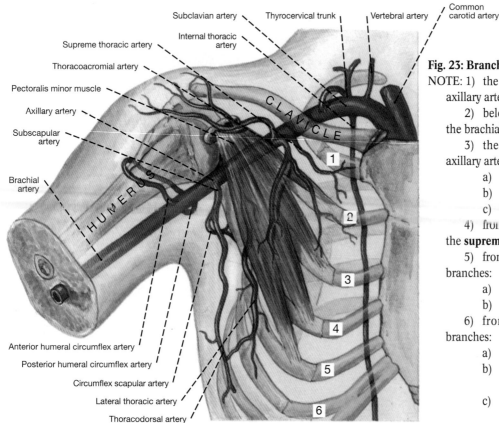

Subclavian artery   Thyrocervical trunk   Vertebral artery   Common carotid artery

Supreme thoracic artery

Internal thoracic artery

Thoracoacromial artery

Pectoralis minor muscle

Axillary artery

Subscapular artery

Brachial artery

Anterior humeral circumflex artery

Posterior humeral circumflex artery

Circumflex scapular artery

Lateral thoracic artery

Thoracodorsal artery

Fig. 23: Branches of the Axillary Artery
NOTE: 1) the subclavian artery becomes the axillary artery distal to the clavicle.

2) below the teres major, it becomes the brachial artery.

3) the pectoralis minor crosses the axillary artery, dividing it into three parts:
   a) medial to the muscle
   b) beneath the muscle
   c) lateral to the muscle

4) from the 1st part there is one branch, the **supreme thoracic artery.**

5) from the 2nd part are derived two branches:
   a) the **thoracoacromial artery**
   b) the **lateral thoracic artery**

6) from the 3rd part come three branches:
   a) the **subscapular artery**
   b) the **anterior humeral circumflex artery,**
   c) the **posterior humeral circumflex artery**

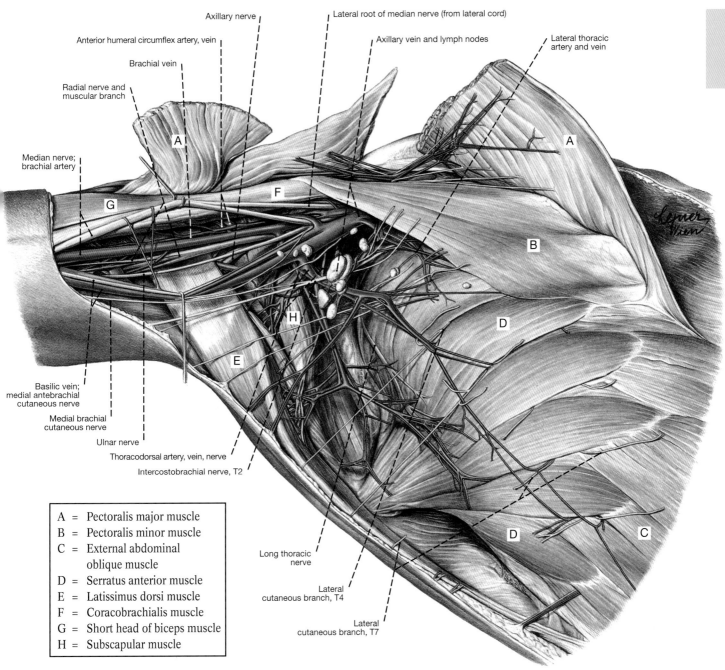

Axillary nerve

Anterior humeral circumflex artery, vein

Brachial vein

Radial nerve and muscular branch

Median nerve; brachial artery

Lateral root of median nerve (from lateral cord)

Axillary vein and lymph nodes

Lateral thoracic artery and vein

Basilic vein; medial antebrachial cutaneous nerve

Medial brachial cutaneous nerve

Ulnar nerve

Thoracodorsal artery, vein, nerve

Intercostobrachial nerve, T2

Long thoracic nerve

Lateral cutaneous branch, T4

Lateral cutaneous branch, T7

A = Pectoralis major muscle
B = Pectoralis minor muscle
C = External abdominal oblique muscle
D = Serratus anterior muscle
E = Latissimus dorsi muscle
F = Coracobrachialis muscle
G = Short head of biceps muscle
H = Subscapular muscle

Fig. 24: Neurovascular Structures in the Axillary Fossa and Upper Brachium

NOTE: 1) the pectoralis major has been cut and reflected.

2) the median nerve and its contributions from the lateral and medial cords of the brachial plexus have been elevated away from the brachial artery.

3) the basilic (and brachial) vein and the medial antebrachial cutaneous nerves have been deflected downward to expose the radial and ulnar nerves.

Fig. 25: Valves Visible in an Opened Segment of Vein ▶

NOTE: 1) venous valves are bicuspid semilunar folds.

2) in this figure, normal blood flow is from left to right.

3) reversed blood flow closes the valve because blood becomes trapped in the sinuses.

4) incompetent valves are the cause of varicosed veins.

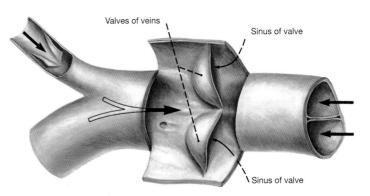

Valves of veins

Sinus of valve

Sinus of valve

PLATE 16   Brachial Plexus: Roots of Origin and General Schema

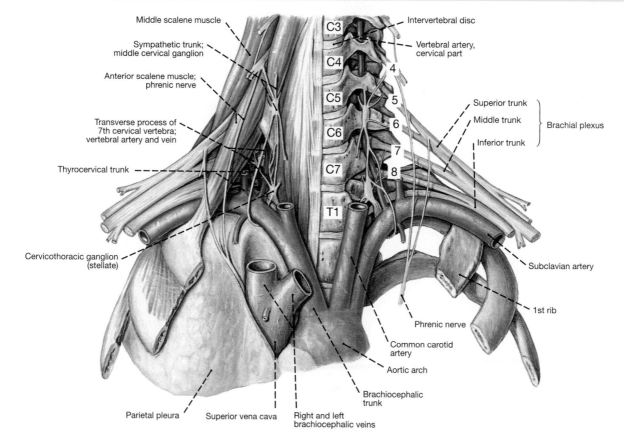

Fig. 26: Roots of Origin of the Brachial Plexus in the Posterior Lateral Neck Region

NOTE: 1) the roots of C5, C6, C7, C8, and T1 emerge from the vertebral column and form the upper, middle, and lower trunks of the brachial plexus.

2) C5 and C6 join to form the upper trunk, C7 forms the middle trunk, and C8 and T1 join to form the lower trunk.

3) crossing the first rib under the clavicle with the subclavian artery, each trunk splits into anterior and posterior divisions. The divisions then reassemble to form three cords: **lateral, medial,** and **posterior.** Now study Fig. 27 and read its NOTE.

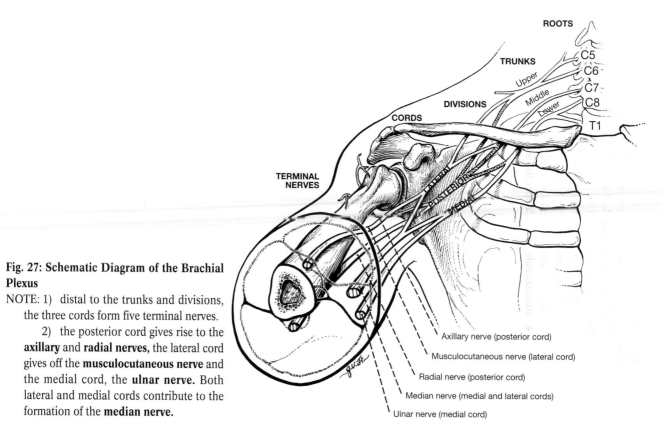

Fig. 27: Schematic Diagram of the Brachial Plexus

NOTE: 1) distal to the trunks and divisions, the three cords form five terminal nerves.

2) the posterior cord gives rise to the **axillary** and **radial nerves,** the lateral cord gives off the **musculocutaneous nerve** and the medial cord, the **ulnar nerve.** Both lateral and medial cords contribute to the formation of the **median nerve.**

Fig. 28: Complete Brachial Plexus

NOTE: in addition to the 5 terminal nerves discussed in the NOTES of Figs. 29 and 30, the brachial plexus gives rise to 11 other nerves. These are:

1. long thoracic nerve (roots C5, 6, 7)
2. dorsal scapular nerve (C5 root)
3. nerve to subclavius muscle (upper trunk)
4. suprascapular nerve (upper trunk)
5. lateral pectoral nerve (lateral cord)
6. medial pectoral nerve (medial cord)
7. medial brachial cutaneous nerve (medial cord)
8. medial antebrachial cutaneous nerve (medial cord)
9. upper subscapular nerve (posterior cord)
10. thoracodorsal nerve (posterior cord)
11. lower subscapular nerve (posterior cord)

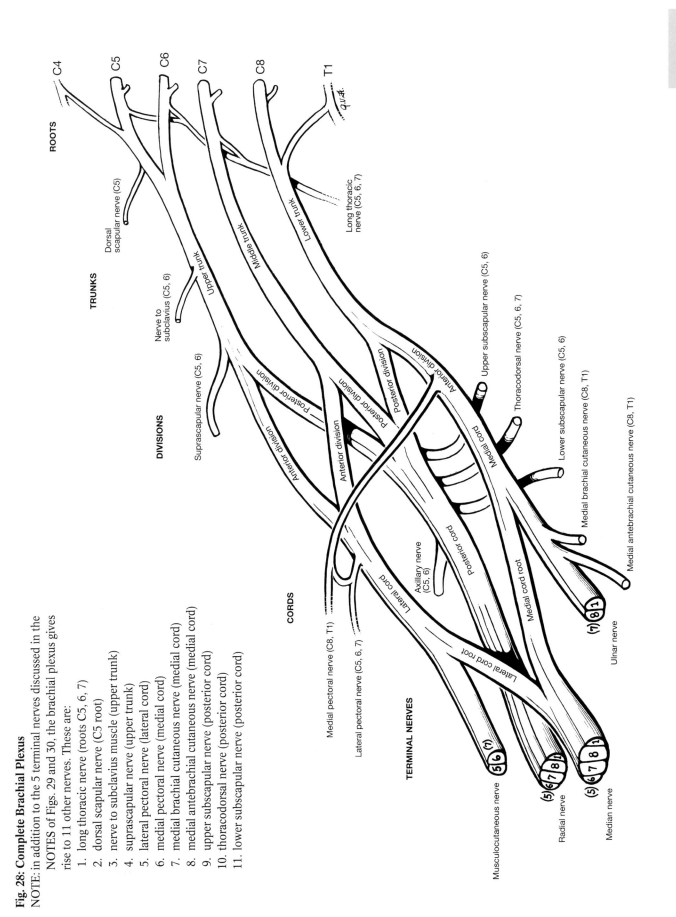

ROOTS

C4
C5
C6
C7
C8
T1

Dorsal scapular nerve (C5)

Long thoracic nerve (C5, 6, 7)

TRUNKS

Nerve to subclavius (C5, 6)

Upper trunk

Middle trunk

Lower trunk

Suprascapular nerve (C5, 6)

DIVISIONS

Posterior division

Anterior division

Posterior division

Anterior division

Posterior division

Anterior division

Upper subscapular nerve (C5, 6)

Thoracodorsal nerve (C5, 6, 7)

Lower subscapular nerve (C8, T1)

Medial brachial cutaneous nerve (C8, T1)

Medial antebrachial cutaneous nerve (C8, T1)

Medial cord

CORDS

Axillary nerve (C5, 6)

Posterior cord

Medial cord root

Lateral cord

Medial pectoral nerve (C8, T1)

Lateral pectoral nerve (C5, 6, 7)

Lateral cord root

TERMINAL NERVES

Musculocutaneous nerve

Radial nerve

Median nerve

Ulnar nerve

Fig. 28

PLATE 18   Dissection of Axilla: Superficial Vessels and Nerves

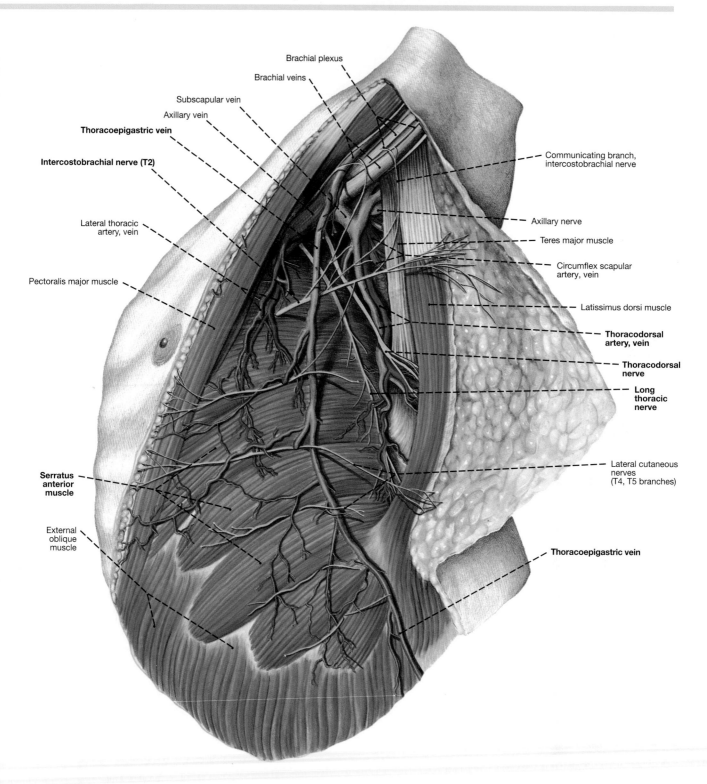

Brachial plexus

Brachial veins

Subscapular vein

Axillary vein

Thoracoepigastric vein

Intercostobrachial nerve (T2)

Lateral thoracic artery, vein

Pectoralis major muscle

Serratus anterior muscle

External oblique muscle

Communicating branch, intercostobrachial nerve

Axillary nerve

Teres major muscle

Circumflex scapular artery, vein

Latissimus dorsi muscle

Thoracodorsal artery, vein

Thoracodorsal nerve

Long thoracic nerve

Lateral cutaneous nerves (T4, T5 branches)

Thoracoepigastric vein

Fig. 29: Axilla: Superficial Vessels and Nerves (left)

NOTE: 1) the boundaries of the axilla are:

  a) **anteriorly,** the pectoralis major muscle

  b) **posteriorly,** the subscapularis, teres major, and latissimus dorsi muscles

  c) **medially,** the serratus anterior muscle covering the 2nd to the 6th ribs

  d) **laterally,** the bicipital groove of the humerus.

  2) the lower part of the serratus anterior muscle arises from the lower ribs as fleshy interdigitations with the external oblique muscle.

  3) the serratus anterior is innervated by the long thoracic nerve, and the latissimus dorsi by the thoracodorsal nerve.

  4) the axillary vein lies medial to the axillary artery and the brachial plexus.

  5) the descending course of the thoracoepigastric vein and the lateral thoracic vessels.

Fig. 29

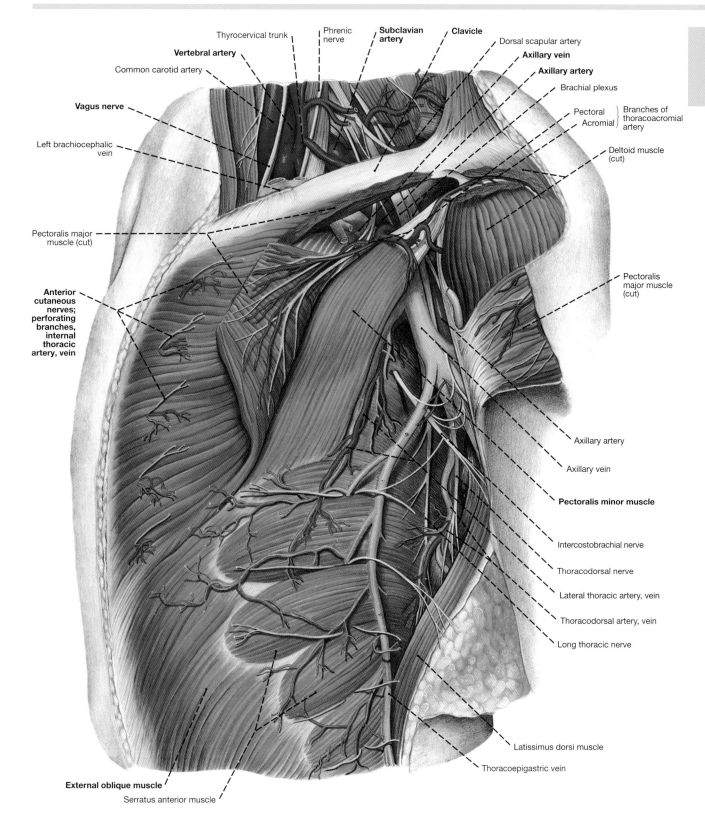

Fig. 30: Axilla (left): Deep Vessels and Nerves

NOTE: 1) the subclavian artery becomes the axillary artery distal to the clavicle.

2) the pectoralis minor muscle is capable of elevating the ribs if the coracoid attachment is fixed or of protracting the scapula if the costal attachment is fixed.

3) the axillary artery is surrounded by the three cords of the brachial plexus.

4) the thoracoacromial artery divides into **pectoral, acromial, deltoid** and small **clavicular** branches.

5) the intercostobrachial nerve (T2) pierces the 2nd intercostal space in its course toward the axilla and arm, and it communicates with the medial brachial cutaneous nerve.

Fig. 30

PLATE 20   Shoulder Region, Anterior Aspect: Muscles

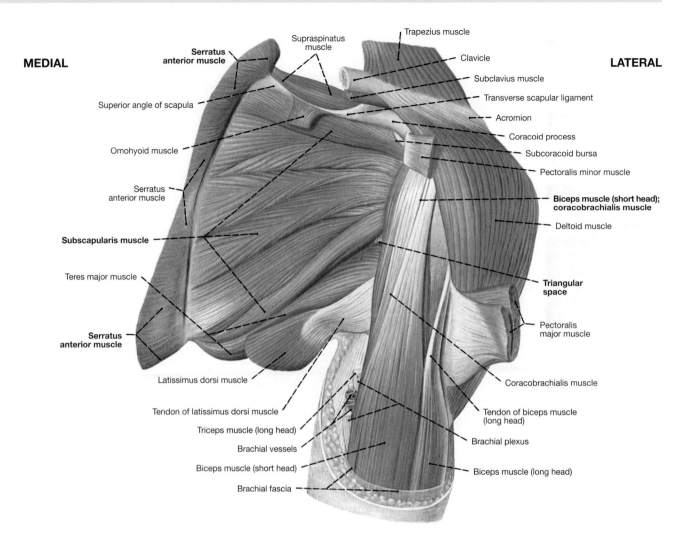

MEDIAL

LATERAL

Supraspinatus muscle

Trapezius muscle

Serratus anterior muscle

Clavicle

Superior angle of scapula

Subclavius muscle

Omohyoid muscle

Transverse scapular ligament

Serratus anterior muscle

Acromion

Subscapularis muscle

Coracoid process

Teres major muscle

Subcoracoid bursa

Serratus anterior muscle

Pectoralis minor muscle

Latissimus dorsi muscle

Biceps muscle (short head); coracobrachialis muscle

Tendon of latissimus dorsi muscle

Deltoid muscle

Triceps muscle (long head)

Triangular space

Brachial vessels

Pectoralis major muscle

Biceps muscle (short head)

Coracobrachialis muscle

Brachial fascia

Tendon of biceps muscle (long head)

Brachial plexus

Biceps muscle (long head)

Fig. 31: Muscles of Ventral Aspect of the Shoulder (left)

NOTE: 1) the large triangular mass of the subscapularis muscle occupying the concave subscapular fossa. From this broad origin, its fibers converge toward the humerus where it inserts on the lesser tuberosity.

2) the subscapularis along with the other muscles that constitute the "rotator cuff" (supraspinatus, infraspinatus and teres minor) help to stabilize the shoulder joint by keeping the head of the humerus in the glenoid fossa.

3) both the short head of the biceps and the coracobrachialis have a common origin from the coracoid process.

Muscle	Origin	Insertion	Innervation	Action
Subscapularis	Subscapular fossa of the scapula	Lesser tubercle of the humerus	Upper and lower subscapular nerves (C5, C6) from posterior cord of brachial plexus	Medial rotation of the humerus
Latissimus dorsi	Thoracolumbar fascia; Spinous processes of lower 6 thoracic and lumbar vertebrae, and the sacrum	Bottom of the intertubercular sulcus of the humerus	Thoracodorsal nerve (C6, C7, C8) from posterior cord of brachial plexus	Extends, adducts, and medially rotates the humerus

Fig. 31

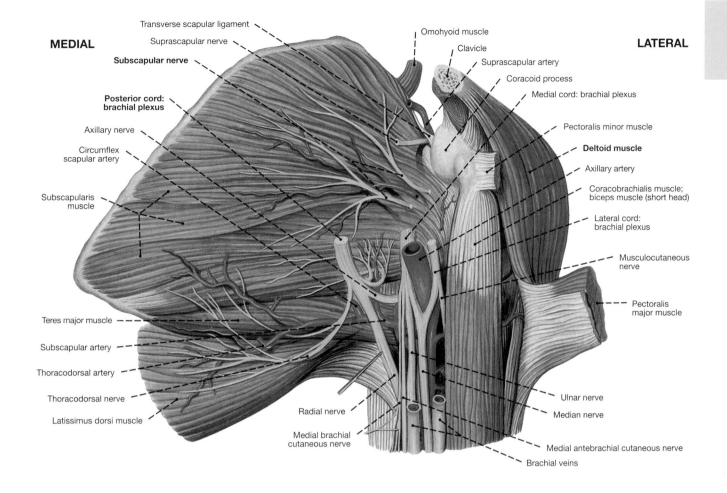

MEDIAL

LATERAL

- Transverse scapular ligament
- Suprascapular nerve
- **Subscapular nerve**
- **Posterior cord: brachial plexus**
- Axillary nerve
- Circumflex scapular artery
- Subscapularis muscle
- Teres major muscle
- Subscapular artery
- Thoracodorsal artery
- Thoracodorsal nerve
- Latissimus dorsi muscle
- Radial nerve
- Medial brachial cutaneous nerve

- Omohyoid muscle
- Clavicle
- Suprascapular artery
- Coracoid process
- Medial cord: brachial plexus
- Pectoralis minor muscle
- **Deltoid muscle**
- Axillary artery
- Coracobrachialis muscle; biceps muscle (short head)
- Lateral cord: brachial plexus
- Musculocutaneous nerve
- Pectoralis major muscle
- Ulnar nerve
- Median nerve
- Medial antebrachial cutaneous nerve
- Brachial veins

Fig. 32: Nerves and Vessels of Ventral Aspect of the Shoulder (left)

NOTE: 1) the relationships of the medial, lateral, and posterior cords of the brachial plexus to the axillary artery.

2) the posterior cord and its axillary and radial terminal nerves have been pulled medially from behind the axillary artery in this dissection.

3) the median nerve formed by contributions from the lateral and medial cords. Observe that the median nerve, its two roots of origin and the ulnar and musculocutaneous nerves outline an **M** formation on the anterior aspect of the axillary artery.

Muscle	Origin	Insertion	Innervation	Action
Deltoid	Lateral ⅓rd of clavicle; the acromion; spine of the scapula	Deltoid tubercle on lateral surface of humerus	Axillary nerve (C5, 6) from posterior cord of brachial plexus	Abduction of the humerus; anterior fibers assist in flexion and posterior fibers in extension of the humerus

Fig. 32

PLATE 22   Shoulder Region, Posterior Aspect: Muscles

LATERAL   **MEDIAL**

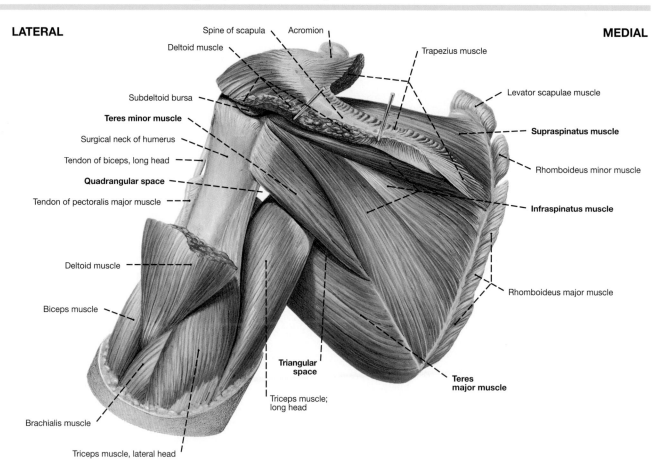

Spine of scapula — Acromion

Deltoid muscle

Trapezius muscle

Subdeltoid bursa

Levator scapulae muscle

Teres minor muscle

Surgical neck of humerus

Supraspinatus muscle

Tendon of biceps, long head

Rhomboideus minor muscle

Quadrangular space

Tendon of pectoralis major muscle

Infraspinatus muscle

Deltoid muscle

Rhomboideus major muscle

Biceps muscle

Triangular space

Teres major muscle

Brachialis muscle

Triceps muscle; long head

Triceps muscle, lateral head

Fig. 33: Dorsal Scapular Muscles (left)

NOTE: 1) the supraspinatus, infraspinatus, and teres minor all course laterally from the dorsal scapula and all are considered "rotator cuff" muscles.

2) these three muscles insert in sequence from above downward on the greater tubercle of the humerus.

3) the long head of the triceps intersects a space between the teres major and teres minor, forming a **quadrangular space** laterally and a **triangular space** medially.

4) through the quadrangular space pass the posterior humeral circumflex artery and the axillary nerve (see Fig. 57).

5) the circumflex scapular branch of the subscapular artery passes through the triangular space (see Fig. 57).

6) since the lateral border of the quadrangular space is the surgical neck of the humerus, the axillary nerve and posterior humeral circumflex artery are in danger if the bone is fractured at this site.

Muscle	Origin	Insertion	Innervation	Action
Supraspinatus	Supraspinatus fossa of the scapula	Highest facet of the greater tubercle of the humerus	Suprascapular nerve (C5)	Initiates abduction of the arm; rotates the humerus laterally
Infraspinatus	Infraspinatus fossa of the scapula	Middle part of greater tubercle of humerus	Suprascapular nerve (C5, 6)	Rotates the humerus laterally

Fig. 33

LATERAL   **MEDIAL**

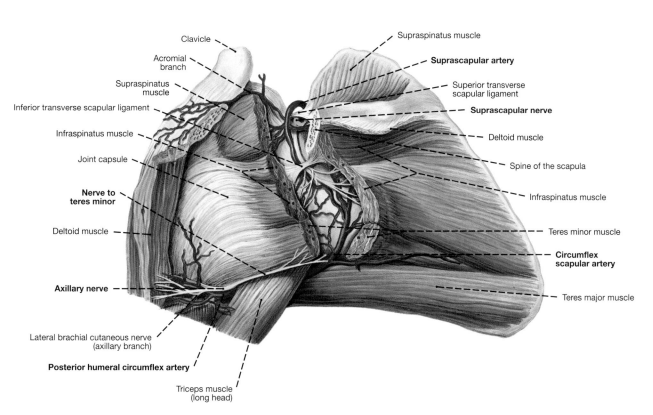

Clavicle

Acromial branch

Supraspinatus muscle

Inferior transverse scapular ligament

Infraspinatus muscle

Joint capsule

Nerve to teres minor

Deltoid muscle

Axillary nerve

Lateral brachial cutaneous nerve (axillary branch)

Posterior humeral circumflex artery

Triceps muscle (long head)

Supraspinatus muscle

Suprascapular artery

Superior transverse scapular ligament

Suprascapular nerve

Deltoid muscle

Spine of the scapula

Infraspinatus muscle

Teres minor muscle

Circumflex scapular artery

Teres major muscle

Fig. 34: Nerves and Vessels of Dorsal Scapular Region (left)

NOTE: 1)   the **superior** transverse scapular ligament bridges the scapular notch and the suprascapular nerve passes beneath the ligament while the suprascapular artery usually passes above it to reach the supraspinatus fossa.

2)   both the suprascapular nerve and artery pass beneath the **inferior** transverse scapular ligament to reach the infraspinatus fossa.

3)   the axillary nerve supplies four structures: a) the teres minor muscle, b) the deltoid muscle, c) the capsule of the shoulder joint, and d) the skin over the shoulder joint.

4)   the axillary nerve and posterior humeral circumflex artery from the dorsal view. These two structures have passed through the quadrangular space, whereas the circumflex scapular artery reaches the infraspinatus fossa through the triangular space.

Muscle	Origin	Insertion	Innervation	Action
Teres Major	Lower lateral border and inferior angle of the scapula	Crest of lesser tubercle and medial lip of intertubercular sulcus of humerus	Lower subscapular nerve (C5, 6)	Adducts and medially rotates the humerus; assists in extension of the arm
Teres Minor	Upper part of the lateral border of the scapula	Lower part of the greater tubercle of the humerus	Axillary nerve (C5)	Rotates humerus laterally; it weakly adducts humerus

Fig. 34   ▌

PLATE 24   Dermatomes of the Upper Limb

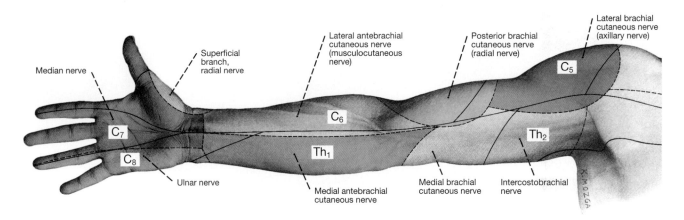

Fig. 35: Cutaneous Innervation and Dermatomes of the Upper Limb, Ventral Aspect

NOTE: 1) an area of skin surface that receives innervation from any single spinal nerve is called a **dermatome.**

2) the solid lines on this figure and on Fig. 36 are the boundaries between dermatomes, whereas the dashed lines are the fields of innervation of the various sensory nerves. The boundary between C5 and C6 laterally and T1 and T2 medially is called the **anterior axial line.**

3) the dermatomes on the anterior aspect of the limb commence over the anterior lateral surface of the brachium with the C5 dermatome.

4) continuing down laterally in the forearm is the C6 dermatome, the palmar and radial hand is C7, the ulnar aspect of the hand is C8, and then sequentially up the medial surface of the forearm and hand are the T1 and T2 dermatomes.

5) although there is overlap between adjacent dermatomes (such as between C5 and C6), **there is no overlap across the axial line** (such as between C6 and T1). This has important clinical significance, because differences in sensation across the axial line might help localize a problem in the spinal cord.

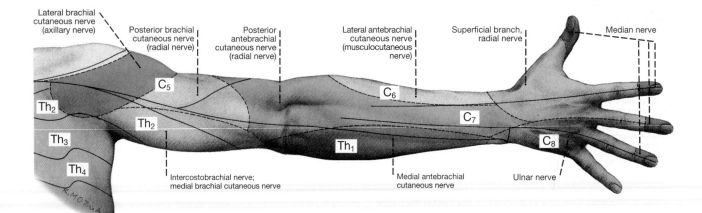

Fig. 36: Cutaneous Innervation and Dermatomes of the Upper Limb, Posterior Aspect

NOTE: 1) dermatomes on the dorsal surface of the upper limb start at the proximal lateral region of the arm with the C5 dermatome.

2) the C6 dermatome continues down the radial aspect of the forearm and hand, it includes the dorsal thumb and the radial part of the index finger.

3) the C7 dermatome includes the dorsal aspect of the middle finger and the adjacent halves of the index and ring fingers, as well as a strip of skin over the intermediate parts of the dorsal hand and forearm.

4) the C8 dermatome includes the little finger and the adjacent part of the ring finger and the ulnar part of the hand, along with a thin region of forearm skin.

5) continuing sequentially up the dorsal aspect of the medial (ulnar) side of the forearm and arm are the T1 and T2 dermatomes.

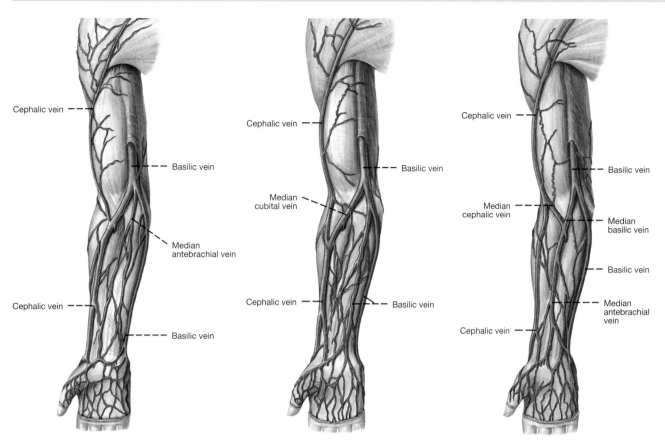

Fig. 37: Variations in the Venous Pattern of the Upper Extremity

NOTE: superficial veins are variable and are of significance clinically. The median cubital vein is often used for the withdrawal of blood and the injection of fluids into the vascular system. Care must be taken not to injure the median nerve or puncture the brachial artery, which lie deep to the median cubital vein and the underlying bicipital aponeurosis.

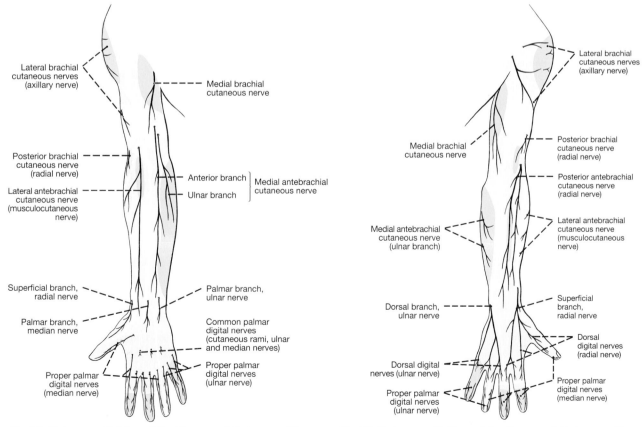

Fig. 38: Cutaneous Fields and the Courses of Cutaneous Nerves in the Superficial Fascia: Anterior Aspect of the Upper Limb

Fig. 39: Cutaneous Fields and the Courses of Cutaneous Nerves in the Superficial Fascia: Posterior Aspect of the Upper Limb

Fig. 37, 38, 39

PLATE 26   Surface and Skeletal Anatomy of the Upper Limb

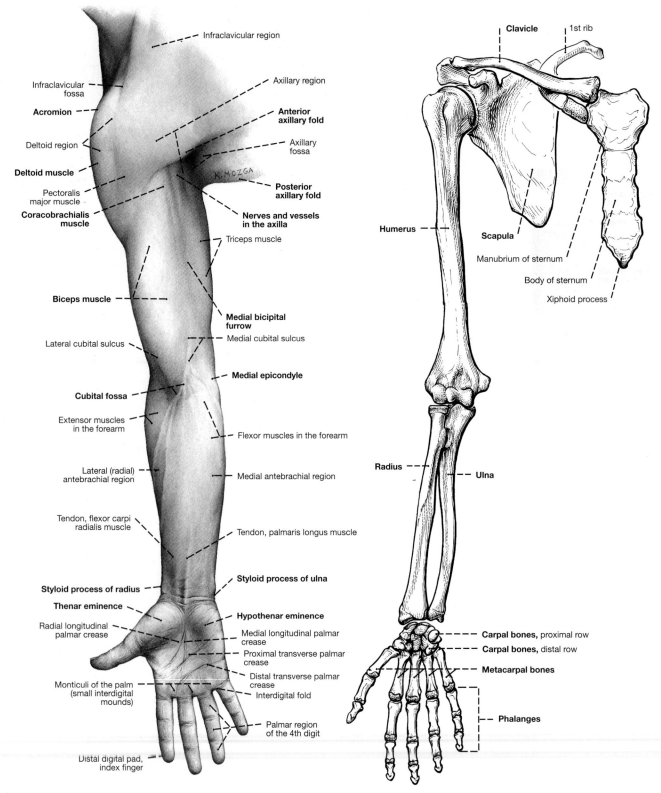

Infraclavicular region

Infraclavicular fossa

Acromion

Deltoid region

Deltoid muscle

Pectoralis major muscle

Coracobrachialis muscle

Biceps muscle

Lateral cubital sulcus

Cubital fossa

Extensor muscles in the forearm

Lateral (radial) antebrachial region

Tendon, flexor carpi radialis muscle

Styloid process of radius

Thenar eminence

Radial longitudinal palmar crease

Monticuli of the palm (small interdigital mounds)

Distal digital pad, index finger

Axillary region

Anterior axillary fold

Axillary fossa

Posterior axillary fold

Nerves and vessels in the axilla

Triceps muscle

Medial bicipital furrow

Medial cubital sulcus

Medial epicondyle

Flexor muscles in the forearm

Medial antebrachial region

Tendon, palmaris longus muscle

Styloid process of ulna

Hypothenar eminence

Medial longitudinal palmar crease

Proximal transverse palmar crease

Distal transverse palmar crease

Interdigital fold

Palmar region of the 4th digit

Clavicle   1st rib

Humerus

Radius

Scapula

Manubrium of sternum

Body of sternum

Xiphoid process

Ulna

Carpal bones, proximal row

Carpal bones, distal row

Metacarpal bones

Phalanges

Fig. 40: Surface Anatomy of the Right Upper Extremity, Anterior Aspect

NOTE: 1)   the vertically oriented medial bicipital furrow along the arm. The basilic vein and medial antebrachial cutaneous nerve course beneath the skin along this furrow. More deeply are found the brachial artery and vein and the median and ulnar nerves.

2)   the cubital fossa in front of the elbow joint, between the bellies of the flexor and extensor muscles in the upper forearm.

Fig. 41: Bones of the Upper Limb and Pectoral Girdle

NOTE: the pectoral girdle includes the clavicle and the bones to which it is attached; these are the manubrium of the sternum and the scapula.

Fig. 40, 41

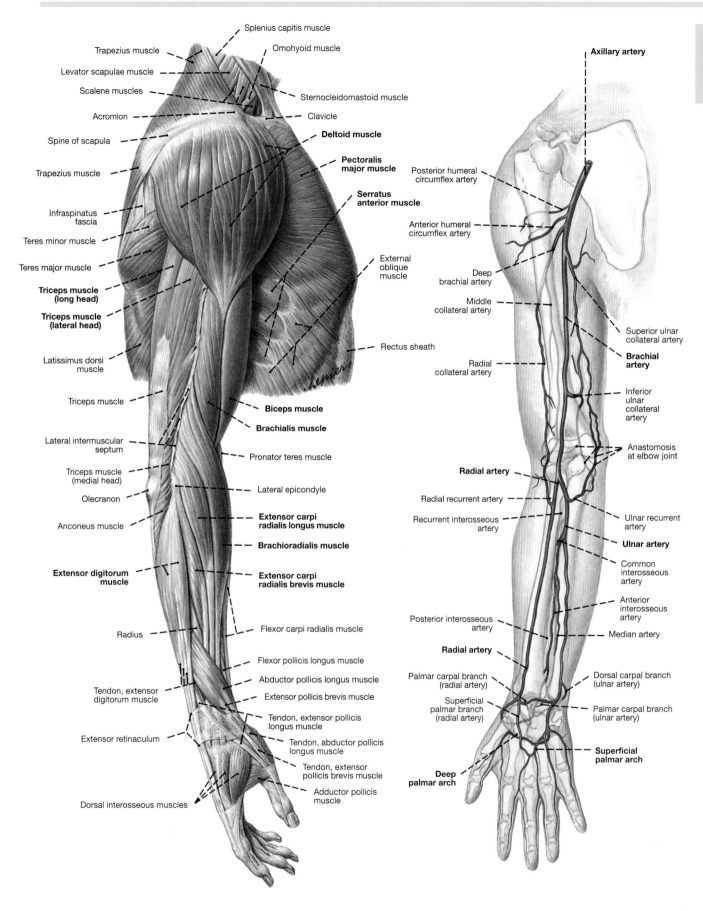

Fig. 42: Muscles of the Thorax and Right Upper Extremity, Lateral View

Fig. 43: Arteries of the Upper Extremity (Schematic Representation)

PLATE 28   Superficial Dissection of the Arm: Anterior View

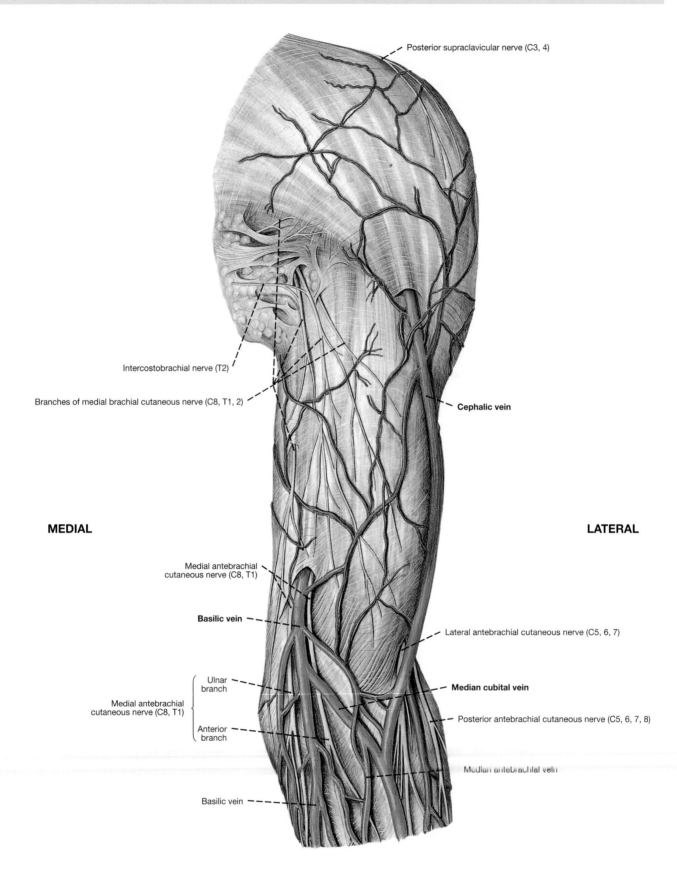

Posterior supraclavicular nerve (C3, 4)

Intercostobrachial nerve (T2)

Branches of medial brachial cutaneous nerve (C8, T1, 2)

Cephalic vein

MEDIAL

LATERAL

Medial antebrachial
cutaneous nerve (C8, T1)

Basilic vein

Lateral antebrachial cutaneous nerve (C5, 6, 7)

Ulnar
branch

Median cubital vein

Medial antebrachial
cutaneous nerve (C8, T1)

Anterior
branch

Posterior antebrachial cutaneous nerve (C5, 6, 7, 8)

Median antebrachial vein

Basilic vein

Fig. 44: Arm; Superficial Veins and Cutaneous Nerves of the Left Upper Limb (Anterior Surface)

NOTE: 1) the **basilic vein** ascends on the medial (ulnar) aspect of the arm, pierces the deep fascia and, at the lower border of the teres major, joins the brachial vein to form the axillary vein.

2) in contrast, the **cephalic vein** ascends along the lateral aspect of the arm toward the axillary vein, which it joins deep to the deltopectoral triangle.

3) the principal sensory nerves of the anterior arm region are the **medial brachial cutaneous** and **intercostobrachial nerves.**

Fig. 44

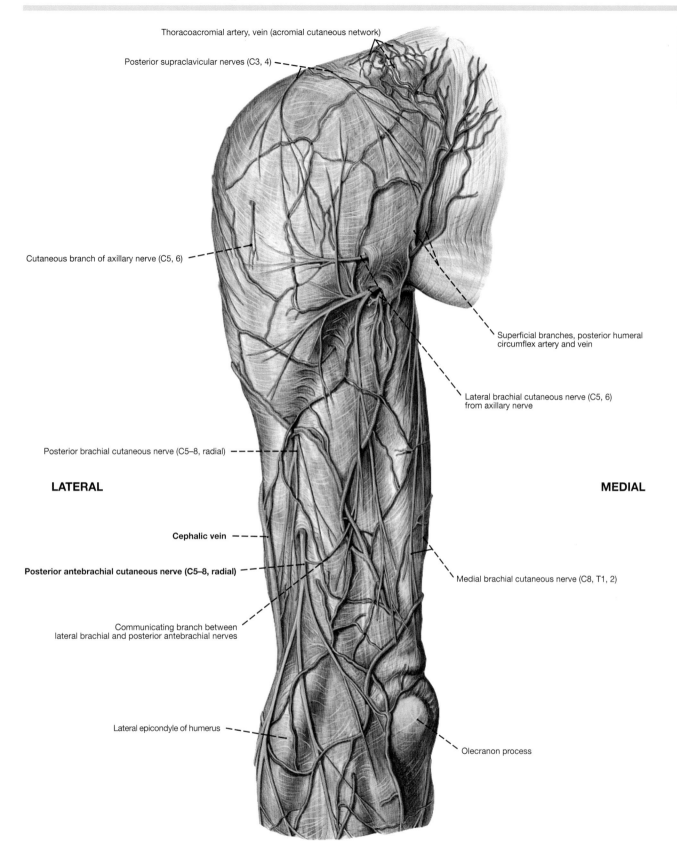

Thoracoacromial artery, vein (acromial cutaneous network)

Posterior supraclavicular nerves (C3, 4)

Cutaneous branch of axillary nerve (C5, 6)

Superficial branches, posterior humeral circumflex artery and vein

Lateral brachial cutaneous nerve (C5, 6) from axillary nerve

Posterior brachial cutaneous nerve (C5–8, radial)

LATERAL

MEDIAL

Cephalic vein

Posterior antebrachial cutaneous nerve (C5–8, radial)

Medial brachial cutaneous nerve (C8, T1, 2)

Communicating branch between lateral brachial and posterior antebrachial nerves

Lateral epicondyle of humerus

Olecranon process

Fig. 45: Arm; Superficial Veins and Cutaneous Nerves of Left Upper Limb (Posterior Surface)

NOTE: 1) the posterior arm region receives cutaneous innervation from the **radial** (posterior brachial cutaneous nerve) and **axillary** (lateral brachial cutaneous nerve) nerves. Both are derived from the posterior cord of the brachial plexus.

2) the **posterior antebrachial cutaneous nerve** (from the radial nerve) perforates the lateral head of the triceps about 5 cm above the elbow. Upon piercing the superficial fascia, it sends cutaneous branches to the dorsal surface of the forearm, as well as a communicating branch to cutaneous rami of the axillary nerve.

Fig. 45

PLATE 30   Anterior Dissection of the Shoulder and Arm: Muscles

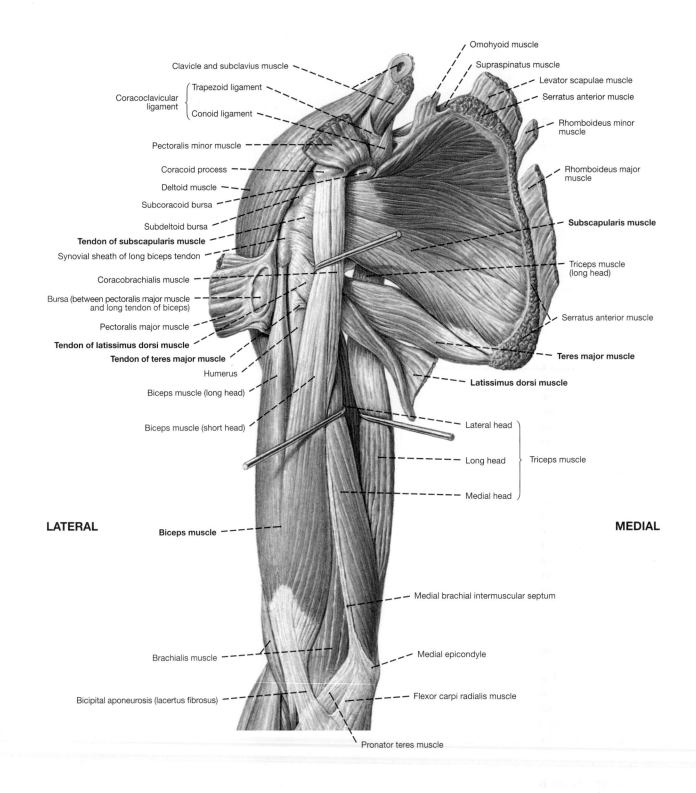

Omohyoid muscle

Clavicle and subclavius muscle

Supraspinatus muscle

Coracoclavicular ligament { Trapezoid ligament

Levator scapulae muscle

Serratus anterior muscle

Conoid ligament

Rhomboideus minor muscle

Pectoralis minor muscle

Coracoid process

Rhomboideus major muscle

Deltoid muscle

Subcoracoid bursa

Subdeltoid bursa

Subscapularis muscle

Tendon of subscapularis muscle

Synovial sheath of long biceps tendon

Triceps muscle (long head)

Coracobrachialis muscle

Bursa (between pectoralis major muscle and long tendon of biceps)

Serratus anterior muscle

Pectoralis major muscle

Tendon of latissimus dorsi muscle

Teres major muscle

Tendon of teres major muscle

Latissimus dorsi muscle

Humerus

Biceps muscle (long head)

Lateral head

Biceps muscle (short head)

Long head

Triceps muscle

Medial head

LATERAL

MEDIAL

Biceps muscle

Medial brachial intermuscular septum

Brachialis muscle

Medial epicondyle

Bicipital aponeurosis (lacertus fibrosus)

Flexor carpi radialis muscle

Pronator teres muscle

Fig. 46: Muscles of the Right Shoulder and Arm (Anterior View)

NOTE: 1)   the insertion of the subscapularis muscle on the lesser tubercle of the humerus. Distal to this, from medial to lateral, insert the teres major, latissimus dorsi, and pectoralis major muscles.

2)   the pectoralis minor, coracobrachialis, and the short head of the biceps all attach to the coracoid process.

3)   the tendon of insertion of the pectoralis major muscle and the long tendon of the biceps muscle are usually separated by a bursa.

4)   from its origin on the coracoid process, the short head of the biceps courses inferiorly and laterally across the tendons of the subscapularis and latissimus dorsi to join the belly of the long head.

5)   the biceps is a very powerful supinator of the forearm and it is an efficient flexor of the forearm, especially when the forearm is supinated.

Fig. 46

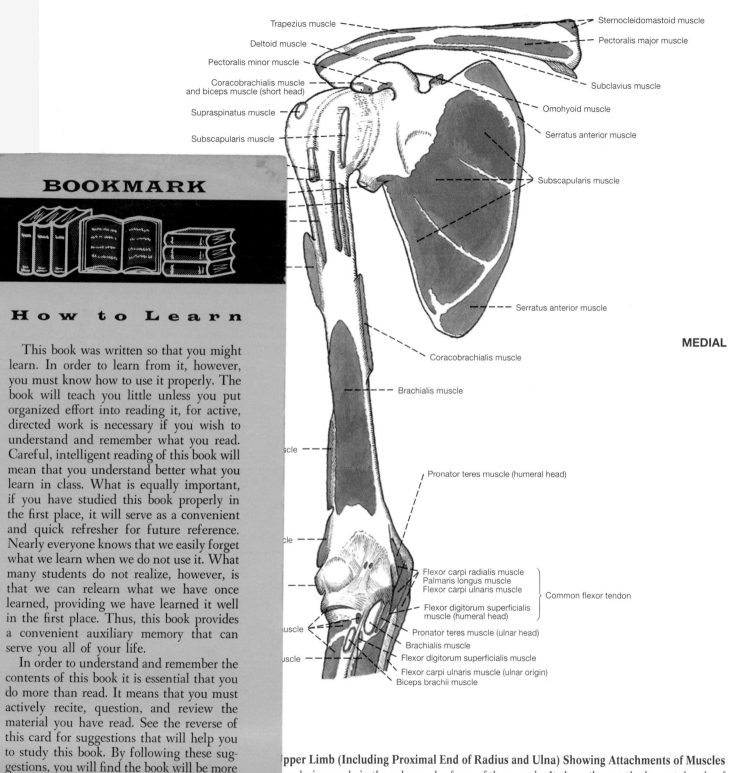

Trapezius muscle

Deltoid muscle

Pectoralis minor muscle

Coracobrachialis muscle
and biceps muscle (short head)

Supraspinatus muscle

Subscapularis muscle

Sternocleidomastoid muscle

Pectoralis major muscle

Subclavius muscle

Omohyoid muscle

Serratus anterior muscle

Subscapularis muscle

Serratus anterior muscle

MEDIAL

Coracobrachialis muscle

Brachialis muscle

...scle

Pronator teres muscle (humeral head)

...cle

...uscle

...uscle

Flexor carpi radialis muscle
Palmaris longus muscle
Flexor carpi ulnaris muscle

Flexor digitorum superficialis
muscle (humeral head)

Pronator teres muscle (ulnar head)

Brachialis muscle

Flexor digitorum superficialis muscle

Flexor carpi ulnaris muscle (ulnar origin)

Biceps brachii muscle

Common flexor tendon

pper Limb (Including Proximal End of Radius and Ulna) Showing Attachments of Muscles
...apularis muscle in the subscapular fossa of the scapula. Its **insertion** on the lesser tubercle of ...ions of the latissimus dorsi and teres major muscles.

...cross both the shoulder and elbow joints, but the coracobrachialis muscle crosses only the

...of the biceps commences within the capsule of the shoulder joint and immediately becomes ...he synovial membrane of the joint.

...t capsule, the tendon of the long head of the biceps descends in the intertubercular sulcus (bicipital groove). Inflammation of the synovial sheath of this tendon within the sulcus can be exceedingly painful because the tendon is closely bound to bone in this region.

5) the latissimus dorsi and teres major insert on the humerus medial to the tendon of the long head of the biceps, whereas the pectoralis major inserts lateral to it.

Fig. 47

PLATE 32   Muscles of the Anterior Arm; Superficial Dissection

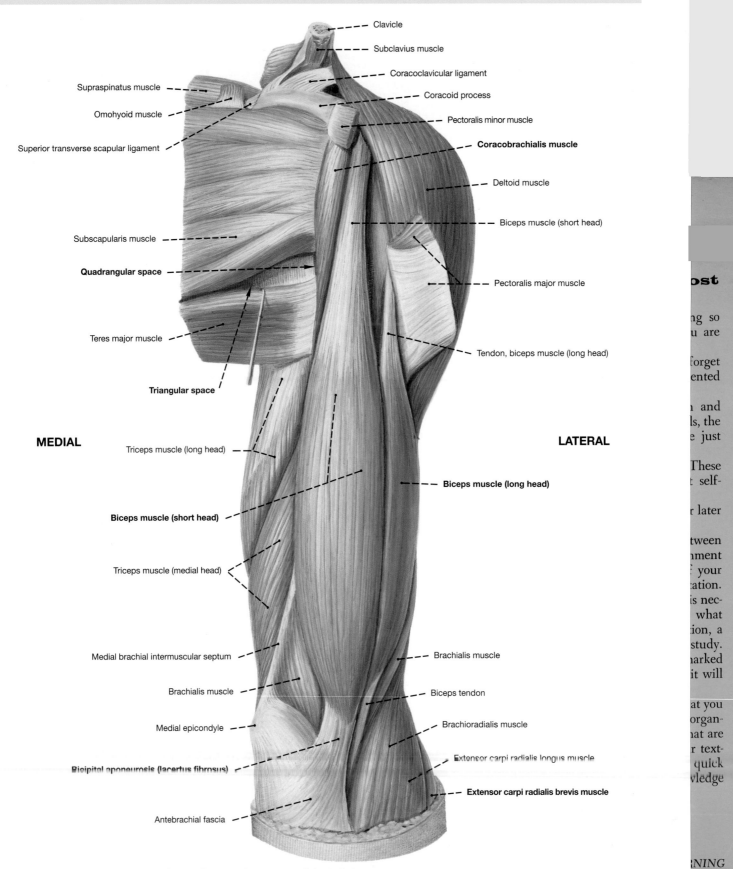

Clavicle

Subclavius muscle

Coracoclavicular ligament

Coracoid process

Pectoralis minor muscle

Coracobrachialis muscle

Deltoid muscle

Biceps muscle (short head)

Pectoralis major muscle

Tendon, biceps muscle (long head)

Supraspinatus muscle

Omohyoid muscle

Superior transverse scapular ligament

Subscapularis muscle

Quadrangular space

Teres major muscle

Triangular space

MEDIAL

LATERAL

Triceps muscle (long head)

Biceps muscle (long head)

Biceps muscle (short head)

Triceps muscle (medial head)

Medial brachial intermuscular septum

Brachialis muscle

Brachialis muscle

Biceps tendon

Medial epicondyle

Brachioradialis muscle

Extensor carpi radialis longus muscle

Bicipital aponeurosis (lacertus fibrosus)

Extensor carpi radialis brevis muscle

Antebrachial fascia

Fig. 48: Superficial View of Muscles on the Anterior Aspect of the Left Arm

	Muscle	Origin	Insertion	Innervation	Action
Biceps Brachii	Long Head	Supraglenoid tubercle of the scapula	Tuberosity of the radius and the bicipital aponeurosis	Musculocutaneous nerve (C5, C6)	Flexes and supinates the forearm. Long head can also assist in flexing the humerus
	Short Head	Coracoid process of the scapula			

Fig. 48

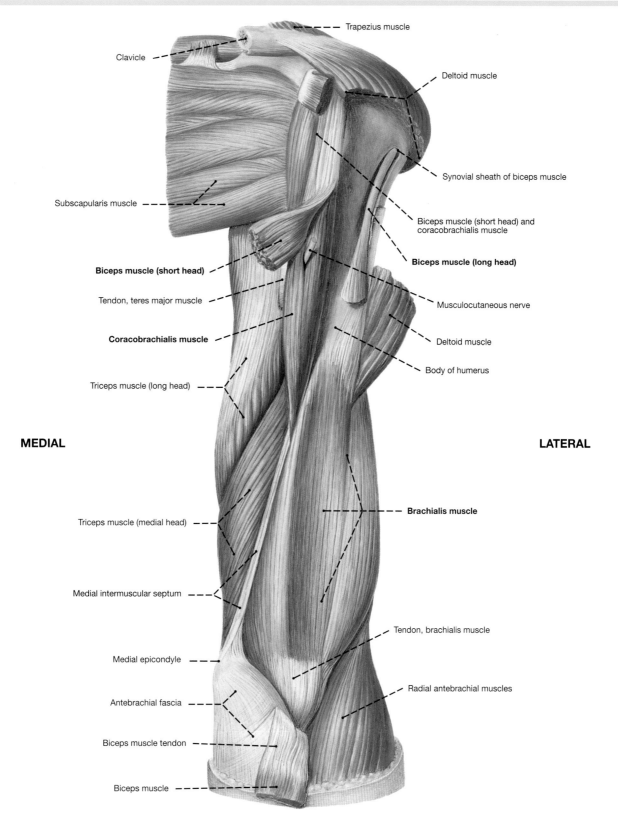

Trapezius muscle

Clavicle

Deltoid muscle

Subscapularis muscle

Synovial sheath of biceps muscle

Biceps muscle (short head) and coracobrachialis muscle

Biceps muscle (short head)

Tendon, teres major muscle

Biceps muscle (long head)

Coracobrachialis muscle

Musculocutaneous nerve

Triceps muscle (long head)

Deltoid muscle

Body of humerus

MEDIAL

LATERAL

Triceps muscle (medial head)

Brachialis muscle

Medial intermuscular septum

Medial epicondyle

Tendon, brachialis muscle

Antebrachial fascia

Radial antebrachial muscles

Biceps muscle tendon

Biceps muscle

Fig. 49: Deep View of Muscles on the Anterior Aspect of the Left Arm

Muscle	Origin	Insertion	Innervation	Action
Brachialis	Distal half of anterior surface of the humerus	Tuberosity of the ulna, and the anterior surface of the coronoid process	Musculocutaneous nerve and often a small branch of the radial nerve (C5, C6)	Powerful flexor of the forearm
Coracobrachialis	Coracoid process of the scapula	Along the medial surface of the humerus near its middle	Musculocutaneous nerve (C6, C7)	Flexes and adducts the arm

Fig. 49   I

PLATE 34   Brachial Artery and the Median and Ulnar Nerves in the Arm

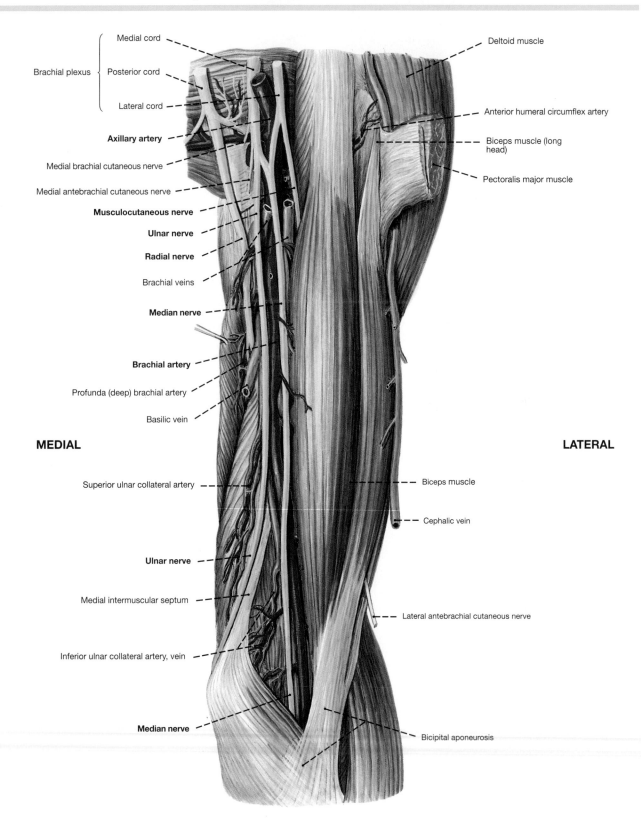

Medial cord

Brachial plexus { Posterior cord

Lateral cord

Axillary artery

Medial brachial cutaneous nerve

Medial antebrachial cutaneous nerve

Musculocutaneous nerve

Ulnar nerve

Radial nerve

Brachial veins

Median nerve

Brachial artery

Profunda (deep) brachial artery

Basilic vein

Deltoid muscle

Anterior humeral circumflex artery

Biceps muscle (long head)

Pectoralis major muscle

MEDIAL

LATERAL

Superior ulnar collateral artery

Biceps muscle

Cephalic vein

Ulnar nerve

Medial intermuscular septum

Lateral antebrachial cutaneous nerve

Inferior ulnar collateral artery, vein

Median nerve

Bicipital aponeurosis

Fig. 50: Vessels and Nerves of the Anterior Arm (left)

NOTE: 1) the **median nerve** crosses the brachial artery anteriorly from lateral to medial just above the cubital fossa.

2) the median nerve arises by two roots, one each from the medial and lateral cords of the brachial plexus. The lateral cord then continues downward as the **musculocutaneous nerve**, whereas the medial cord becomes the **ulnar nerve** distal to the axilla.

3) at the origin of the median nerve, its two roots and the musculocutaneous and ulnar nerves combine to form an outline that resembles the letter M.

4) neither the ulnar nor median nerve gives off branches in the arm region.

Fig. 50

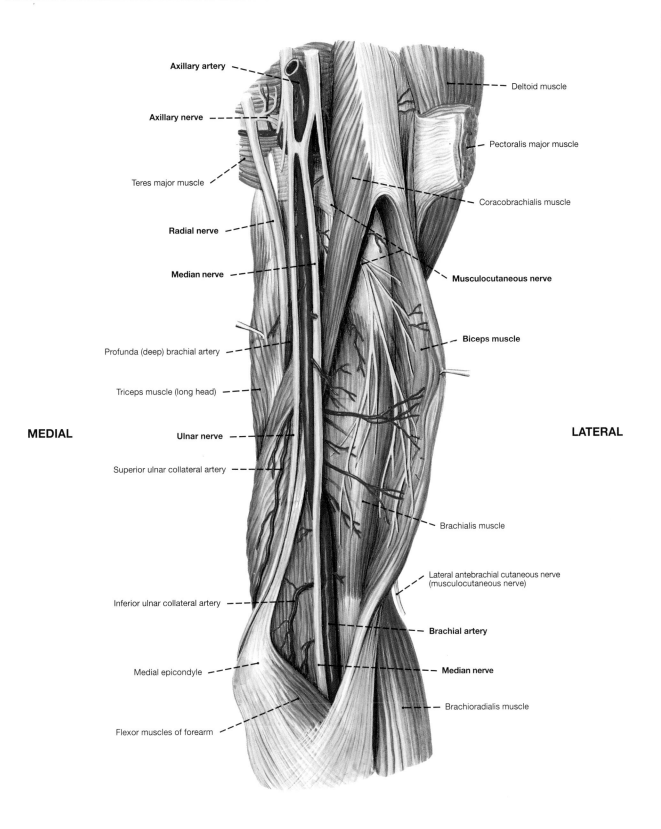

Axillary artery

Axillary nerve

Teres major muscle

Radial nerve

Median nerve

Profunda (deep) brachial artery

Triceps muscle (long head)

MEDIAL

Ulnar nerve

Superior ulnar collateral artery

Inferior ulnar collateral artery

Medial epicondyle

Flexor muscles of forearm

Deltoid muscle

Pectoralis major muscle

Coracobrachialis muscle

Musculocutaneous nerve

Biceps muscle

LATERAL

Brachialis muscle

Lateral antebrachial cutaneous nerve (musculocutaneous nerve)

Brachial artery

Median nerve

Brachioradialis muscle

Fig. 51: Nerves and Arteries of the Anterior Left Arm (Deep Dissection)

NOTE: 1) the musculocutaneous nerve descends from the lateral cord and perforates the coracobrachialis muscle, which it supplies.

2) the short head of the biceps muscle has been pulled aside to reveal the musculocutaneous nerve more deeply between the biceps and brachialis muscles, both of which it supplies. This nerve continues into the forearm as the **lateral antebrachial cutaneous nerve.**

3) the superficial course of the brachial artery in the arm. Its branches include the profunda (deep) brachial artery and the superior and inferior ulnar collateral arteries, in addition to its muscular branches.

Fig. 51

PLATE 36   Posterior Dissection of Shoulder and Arm: Muscles

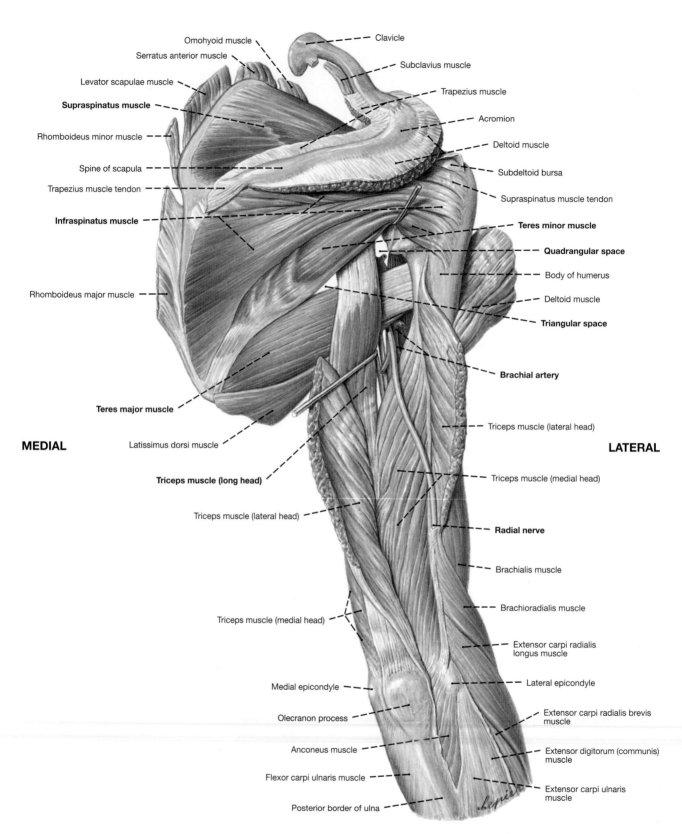

Omohyoid muscle

Serratus anterior muscle

Levator scapulae muscle

Supraspinatus muscle

Rhomboideus minor muscle

Spine of scapula

Trapezius muscle tendon

Infraspinatus muscle

Rhomboideus major muscle

Teres major muscle

MEDIAL

Latissimus dorsi muscle

Triceps muscle (long head)

Triceps muscle (lateral head)

Triceps muscle (medial head)

Medial epicondyle

Olecranon process

Anconeus muscle

Flexor carpi ulnaris muscle

Posterior border of ulna

Clavicle

Subclavius muscle

Trapezius muscle

Acromion

Deltoid muscle

Subdeltoid bursa

Supraspinatus muscle tendon

Teres minor muscle

Quadrangular space

Body of humerus

Deltoid muscle

Triangular space

Brachial artery

Triceps muscle (lateral head)

LATERAL

Triceps muscle (medial head)

Radial nerve

Brachialis muscle

Brachioradialis muscle

Extensor carpi radialis longus muscle

Lateral epicondyle

Extensor carpi radialis brevis muscle

Extensor digitorum (communis) muscle

Extensor carpi ulnaris muscle

Fig. 52: Muscles of the Shoulder and Deep Arm (Posterior View)

NOTE: 1) the deltoid muscle and the lateral head of the triceps have been severed, thereby exposing the course of the radial nerve in the upper arm.

2) the sequential insertions of the supraspinatus, infraspinatus, and teres minor on the greater tubercle of the humerus.

3) the boundaries of the quadrangular space: **medial,** long head of triceps; **lateral,** the humerus; **superior,** teres minor; **inferior,** teres major. Through the space course the axillary nerve and posterior humeral circumflex vessels.

4) the boundaries of the triangular space: **superior,** teres minor; **inferior,** teres major; **lateral,** long head of triceps. Through the space course the circumflex scapular vessels.

Fig. 52

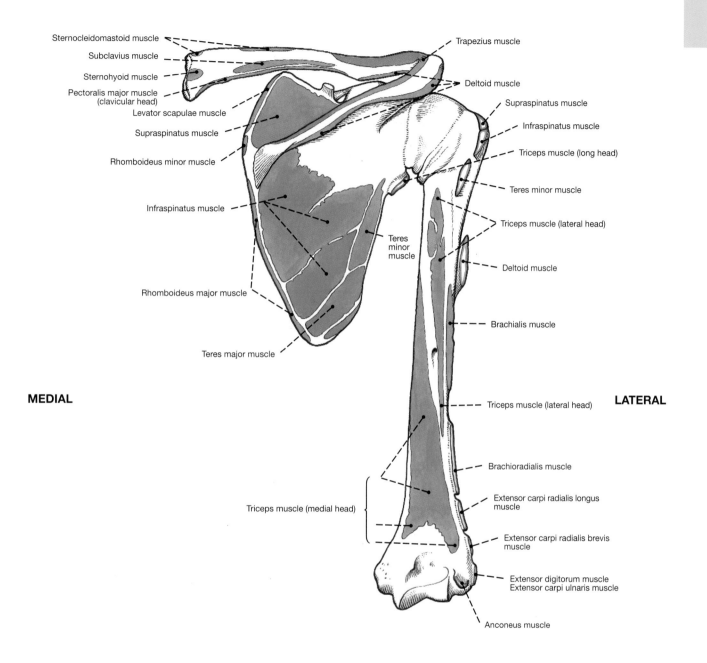

Sternocleidomastoid muscle
Subclavius muscle
Sternohyoid muscle
Pectoralis major muscle (clavicular head)
Levator scapulae muscle
Supraspinatus muscle
Rhomboideus minor muscle
Infraspinatus muscle
Rhomboideus major muscle
Teres major muscle

Trapezius muscle
Deltoid muscle
Supraspinatus muscle
Infraspinatus muscle
Triceps muscle (long head)
Teres minor muscle
Triceps muscle (lateral head)
Deltoid muscle
Brachialis muscle
Triceps muscle (lateral head)
Brachioradialis muscle
Extensor carpi radialis longus muscle
Extensor carpi radialis brevis muscle
Extensor digitorum muscle
Extensor carpi ulnaris muscle
Anconeus muscle

Teres minor muscle
Triceps muscle (medial head)

MEDIAL   **LATERAL**

Fig. 53: Posterior View of the Clavicle, Scapula, and Humerus Showing Muscle Attachments

Muscle	Origin	Insertion	Innervation	Action
Triceps Brachii	LONG HEAD Infraglenoid tubercle of the scapula LATERAL HEAD Posterior surface and lateral border of the humerus and the lateral intermuscular septum MEDIAL HEAD Posterior surface and medial border of the humerus and the medial intermuscular septum	Posterior part of the olecranon process of the ulna and the deep fascia of the dorsal forearm	Radial nerve (C7, C8)	All three heads extend the forearm at the elbow joint; the long head also extends the humerus at the shoulder joint

Fig. 53

PLATE 38   Muscles on the Lateral and Posterior Aspect of the Arm

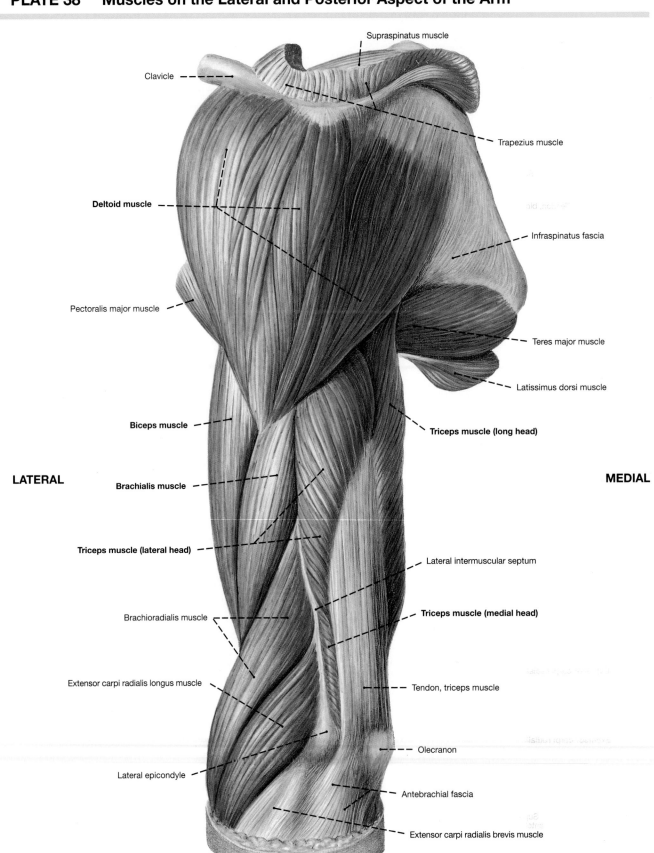

Supraspinatus muscle

Clavicle

Trapezius muscle

Deltoid muscle

Infraspinatus fascia

Pectoralis major muscle

Teres major muscle

Latissimus dorsi muscle

Biceps muscle

Triceps muscle (long head)

LATERAL

MEDIAL

Brachialis muscle

Triceps muscle (lateral head)

Lateral intermuscular septum

Triceps muscle (medial head)

Brachioradialis muscle

Extensor carpi radialis longus muscle

Tendon, triceps muscle

Olecranon

Lateral epicondyle

Antebrachial fascia

Extensor carpi radialis brevis muscle

Fig. 54: Muscles of the Arm (Lateral View)

NOTE: 1) the deltoid muscle acting as a whole abducts the arm. The clavicular portion flexes and medially rotates the arm, whereas the scapular part extends and laterally rotates the arm.

    2) the lateral intermuscular septum separates the anterior muscular compartment from the posterior muscular compartment.

    3) the sequential origin of the brachioradialis and extensor carpi radialis longus from the humerus above the lateral epicondyle, whereas the extensor carpi radialis brevis arises directly from the lateral epicondyle.

Fig. 54

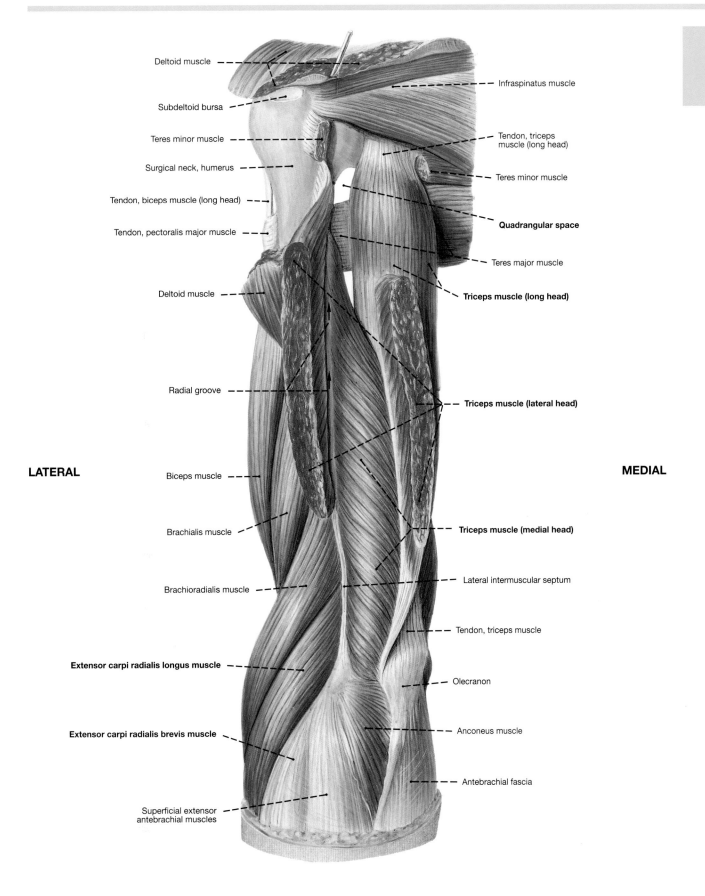

Deltoid muscle

Subdeltoid bursa

Teres minor muscle

Surgical neck, humerus

Tendon, biceps muscle (long head)

Tendon, pectoralis major muscle

Deltoid muscle

Radial groove

LATERAL

Biceps muscle

Brachialis muscle

Brachioradialis muscle

Extensor carpi radialis longus muscle

Extensor carpi radialis brevis muscle

Superficial extensor
antebrachial muscles

Infraspinatus muscle

Tendon, triceps
muscle (long head)

Teres minor muscle

Quadrangular space

Teres major muscle

Triceps muscle (long head)

Triceps muscle (lateral head)

MEDIAL

Triceps muscle (medial head)

Lateral intermuscular septum

Tendon, triceps muscle

Olecranon

Anconeus muscle

Antebrachial fascia

Fig. 55: Deep Muscles of the Arm and Shoulder, Posterior View

NOTE: 1) much of the deltoid and teres minor muscles has been removed in this dissection, and the lateral head of the triceps muscle
was transected and reflected. Observe the radial groove between the medial and lateral heads of the triceps.

2) the broad origin of the medial and lateral heads of the triceps from the posterior surface of the humerus (see Fig. 53).

Fig. 55   **I**

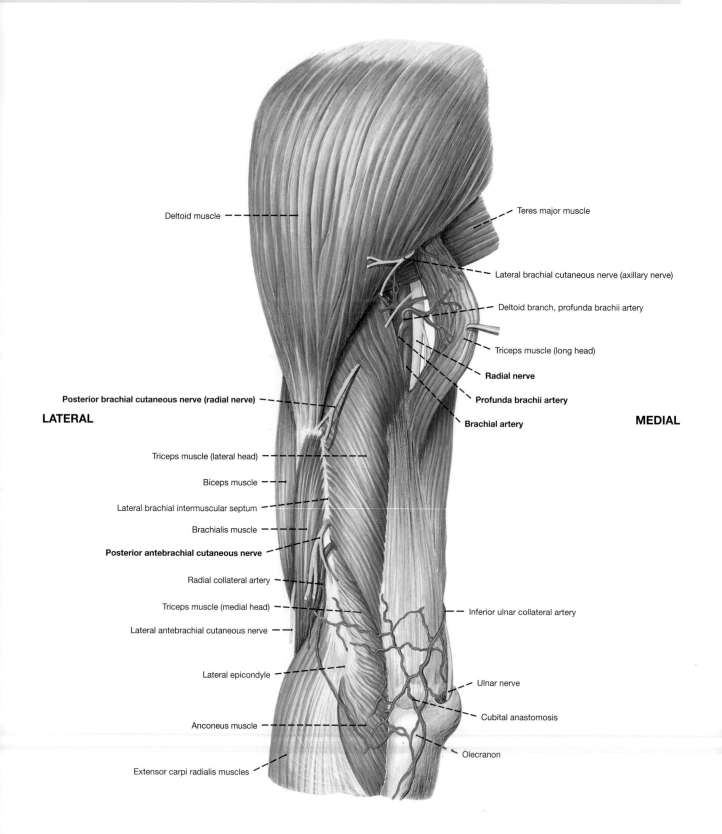

Deltoid muscle

Teres major muscle

Lateral brachial cutaneous nerve (axillary nerve)

Deltoid branch, profunda brachii artery

Triceps muscle (long head)

Radial nerve

Posterior brachial cutaneous nerve (radial nerve)

Profunda brachii artery

LATERAL

Brachial artery

MEDIAL

Triceps muscle (lateral head)

Biceps muscle

Lateral brachial intermuscular septum

Brachialis muscle

Posterior antebrachial cutaneous nerve

Radial collateral artery

Triceps muscle (medial head)

Inferior ulnar collateral artery

Lateral antebrachial cutaneous nerve

Lateral epicondyle

Ulnar nerve

Cubital anastomosis

Anconeus muscle

Olecranon

Extensor carpi radialis muscles

Fig. 56: Nerves and Arteries of the Left Posterior Arm (Superficial Branches)

NOTE: 1)   the origin of the profunda brachii artery from the brachial artery and its relationship to the radial nerve. The long head of the triceps has been pulled medially.

     2)   the relationship of the ulnar nerve to the olecranon process and the vascular anastomosis around the elbow.

     3)   both the posterior brachial and posterior antebrachial nerves of the radial nerve perforate the lateral head of the triceps muscle to reach the superficial fascia and skin.

     4)   the site of attachment of the deltoid muscle on the humerus, and the relationship of this attachment to the uppermost fibers of the brachialis muscle, the lateral intermuscular septum and the lateral head of the triceps muscle (see Fig. 53).

Fig. 56

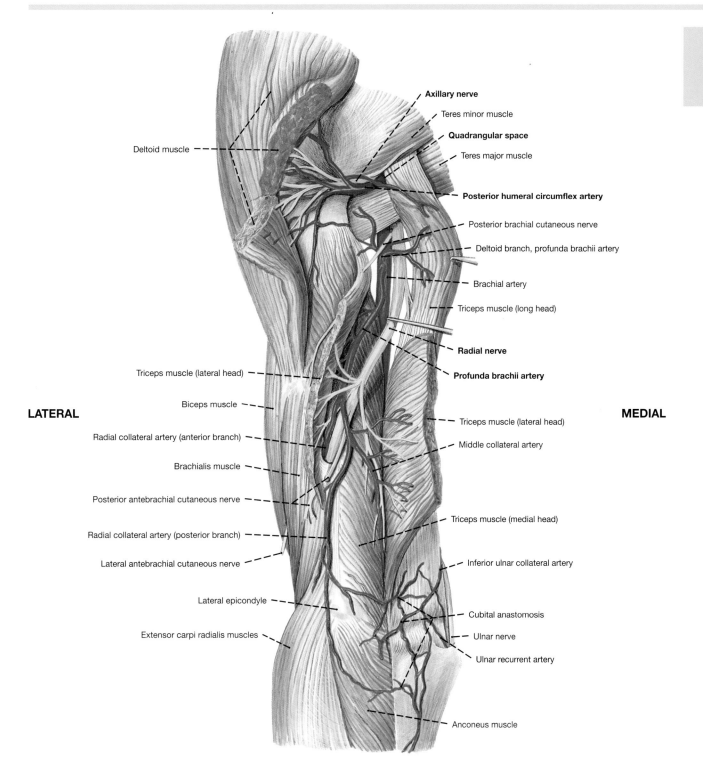

Axillary nerve

Teres minor muscle

Quadrangular space

Teres major muscle

Posterior humeral circumflex artery

Posterior brachial cutaneous nerve

Deltoid branch, profunda brachii artery

Brachial artery

Triceps muscle (long head)

Radial nerve

Profunda brachii artery

Triceps muscle (lateral head)

Middle collateral artery

Triceps muscle (medial head)

Inferior ulnar collateral artery

Cubital anastomosis

Ulnar nerve

Ulnar recurrent artery

Anconeus muscle

Deltoid muscle

Triceps muscle (lateral head)

Biceps muscle

LATERAL

Radial collateral artery (anterior branch)

Brachialis muscle

Posterior antebrachial cutaneous nerve

Radial collateral artery (posterior branch)

Lateral antebrachial cutaneous nerve

Lateral epicondyle

Extensor carpi radialis muscles

MEDIAL

Fig. 57: Deep Nerves and Arteries of the Posterior Arm

NOTE: 1)   the course of the axillary nerve and posterior humeral circumflex artery through the quadrangular space to reach the deltoid and dorsal shoulder region.

2)   the course of the radial nerve and profunda brachii artery along the musculospiral groove to the posterior brachial region. This groove lies along the body of the humerus between the origins of the lateral and medial heads of the triceps muscle.

3)   the common insertion of the three heads of the triceps muscle onto the olecranon process of the ulna.

4)   in addition to a **deltoid branch**, which anastomoses with the posterior humeral circumflex artery and helps supply the long head of the triceps along with the deltoid muscle, the profunda brachii artery gives off the **middle and radial collateral arteries.**

5)   these latter two vessels and the **superior and inferior ulnar collateral** branches of the brachial artery are the four descending vessels that participate in the anastomosis around the elbow joint (see Fig. 43).

Fig. 57

PLATE 42   **Superficial Dissection of the Anterior Forearm**

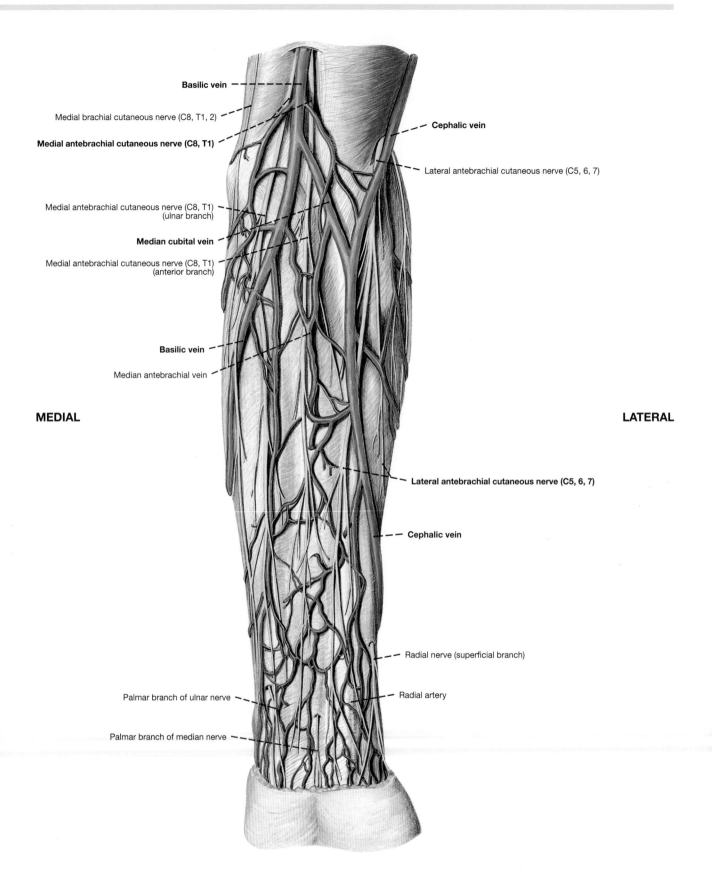

Basilic vein

Medial brachial cutaneous nerve (C8, T1, 2)

Medial antebrachial cutaneous nerve (C8, T1)

Medial antebrachial cutaneous nerve (C8, T1) (ulnar branch)

Median cubital vein

Medial antebrachial cutaneous nerve (C8, T1) (anterior branch)

Basilic vein

Median antebrachial vein

Cephalic vein

Lateral antebrachial cutaneous nerve (C5, 6, 7)

Lateral antebrachial cutaneous nerve (C5, 6, 7)

Cephalic vein

Radial nerve (superficial branch)

Radial artery

Palmar branch of ulnar nerve

Palmar branch of median nerve

MEDIAL

LATERAL

Fig. 58: Forearm; Superficial Veins, and Cutaneous Nerves of Left Upper Limb (Anterior Surface)
NOTE: 1)   the median cubital vein joins the cephalic and basilic veins in the cubital fossa.

2)   the main sessory nerves of the anterior forearm are the medial antebrachial cutaneous nerve (derived from the medial cord of the brachial plexus) and the lateral antebrachial cutaneous nerve, which is a continuation of the musculocutaneous nerve.

3)   the medial antebrachial cutaneous nerve courses with the basilic vein, while the lateral antebrachial cutaneous nerve lies next to the cephalic vein at the elbow.

Fig. 58

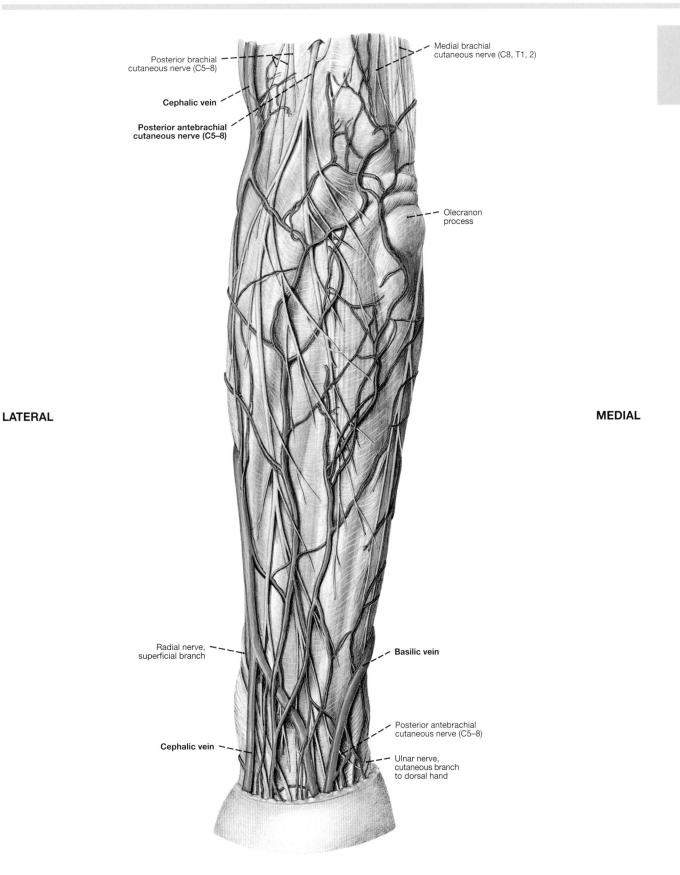

Posterior brachial
cutaneous nerve (C5–8)

Cephalic vein

**Posterior antebrachial
cutaneous nerve (C5–8)**

Medial brachial
cutaneous nerve (C8, T1, 2)

Olecranon
process

LATERAL

MEDIAL

Radial nerve,
superficial branch

Basilic vein

Cephalic vein

Posterior antebrachial
cutaneous nerve (C5–8)

Ulnar nerve,
cutaneous branch
to dorsal hand

Fig. 59: Forearm; Superficial Veins and Cutaneous Nerves of the Left Upper Limb (Posterior Surface)

NOTE: 1) branches of the radial nerve (posterior antebrachial cutaneous and superficial radial) contribute the principal innervation to the skin on the posterior aspect of the forearm.

2) at the wrist, the dorsal branch of the ulnar nerve passes backward onto the dorsal surface of the wrist and hand.

3) the basilic vein arises on the ulnar (or medial) side of the dorsum of the hand and wrist, while the cephalic vein arises on the radial (lateral) side.

Fig. 59   **I**

PLATE 44   Anterior Forearm: Superficial Muscles

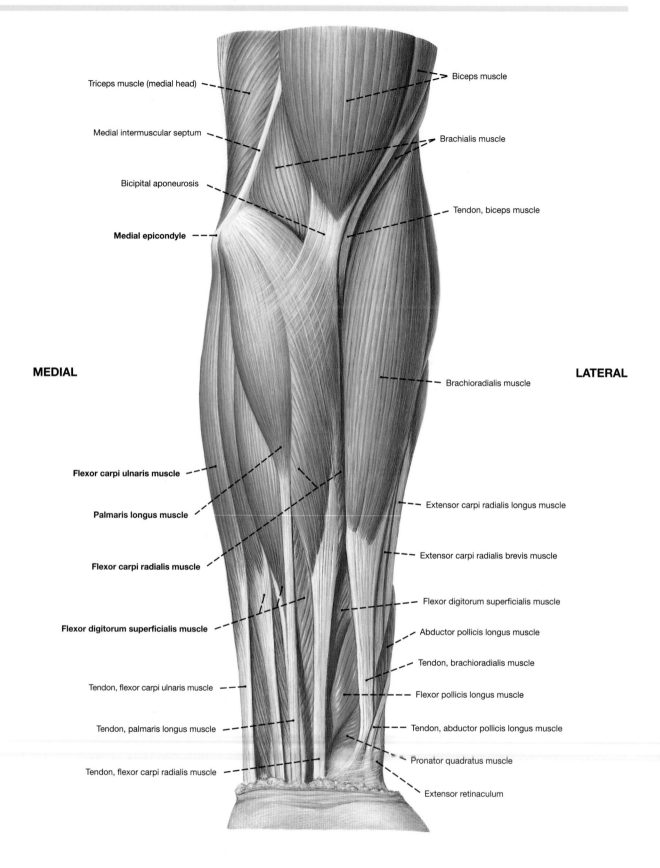

Triceps muscle (medial head)

Medial intermuscular septum

Bicipital aponeurosis

Medial epicondyle

MEDIAL

Flexor carpi ulnaris muscle

Palmaris longus muscle

Flexor carpi radialis muscle

Flexor digitorum superficialis muscle

Tendon, flexor carpi ulnaris muscle

Tendon, palmaris longus muscle

Tendon, flexor carpi radialis muscle

Biceps muscle

Brachialis muscle

Tendon, biceps muscle

LATERAL

Brachioradialis muscle

Extensor carpi radialis longus muscle

Extensor carpi radialis brevis muscle

Flexor digitorum superficialis muscle

Abductor pollicis longus muscle

Tendon, brachioradialis muscle

Flexor pollicis longus muscle

Tendon, abductor pollicis longus muscle

Pronator quadratus muscle

Extensor retinaculum

Fig. 60: Left Anterior Forearm Muscles, Superficial Group
NOTE: 1) the brachioradialis muscle is studied with the posterior forearm muscles and is not included with the flexor muscles of the anterior forearm.

2) the anterior forearm muscles arise from the medial epicondyle of the humerus and include the **pronator teres** (not labelled, see Fig. 61), **flexor carpi radialis, palmaris longus,** and **flexor carpi ulnaris.** Beneath these is the **flexor digitorum superficialis.**

Fig. 60

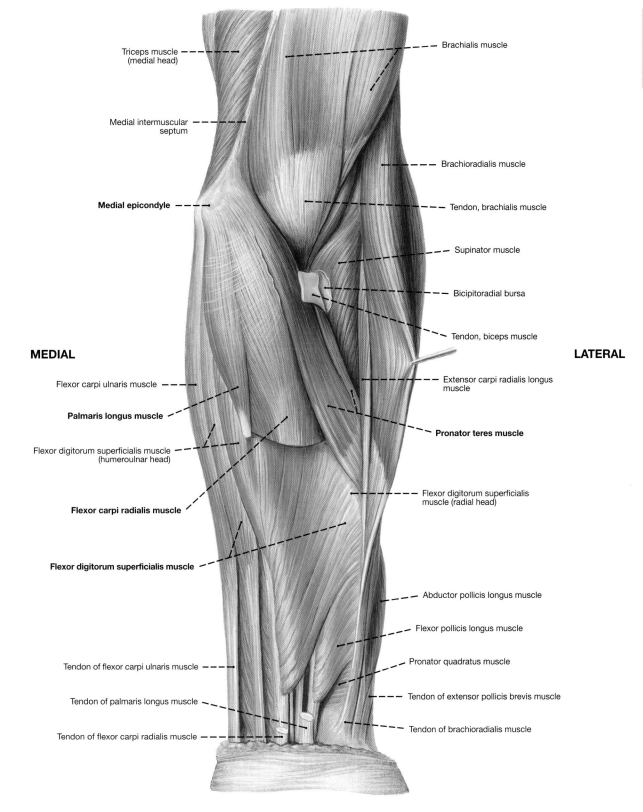

Triceps muscle
(medial head)

Brachialis muscle

Medial intermuscular
septum

Brachioradialis muscle

Medial epicondyle

Tendon, brachialis muscle

Supinator muscle

Bicipitoradial bursa

Tendon, biceps muscle

MEDIAL

LATERAL

Flexor carpi ulnaris muscle

Extensor carpi radialis longus
muscle

Palmaris longus muscle

Pronator teres muscle

Flexor digitorum superficialis muscle
(humeroulnar head)

Flexor carpi radialis muscle

Flexor digitorum superficialis
muscle (radial head)

Flexor digitorum superficialis muscle

Abductor pollicis longus muscle

Flexor pollicis longus muscle

Pronator quadratus muscle

Tendon of flexor carpi ulnaris muscle

Tendon of palmaris longus muscle

Tendon of extensor pollicis brevis muscle

Tendon of flexor carpi radialis muscle

Tendon of brachioradialis muscle

Fig. 61: Flexor Digitorum Superficialis Muscle and Related Muscles (Left)

NOTE: 1) the palmaris longus, flexor carpi radialis and insertion of the biceps have been cut to reveal the flexor digitorum superficialis and pronator teres.

2) the triangular cubital fossa is bounded medially by the superficial flexors and laterally by the extensors. Its floor is the brachialis muscle.

3) the pronator teres arises by two heads: a larger **humeral head** from the medial epicondyle, and a much smaller **ulnar head** from the coronoid process. It crosses the forearm obliquely to insert on the shaft of the radius.

4) the flexor digitorum superficialis arises broadly from the humerus and ulna medially (humeral-ulnar head) and from the anterior border of the radius laterally (radial head).

Fig. 61   I

PLATE 46 **Anterior Forearm: Deep Muscles**

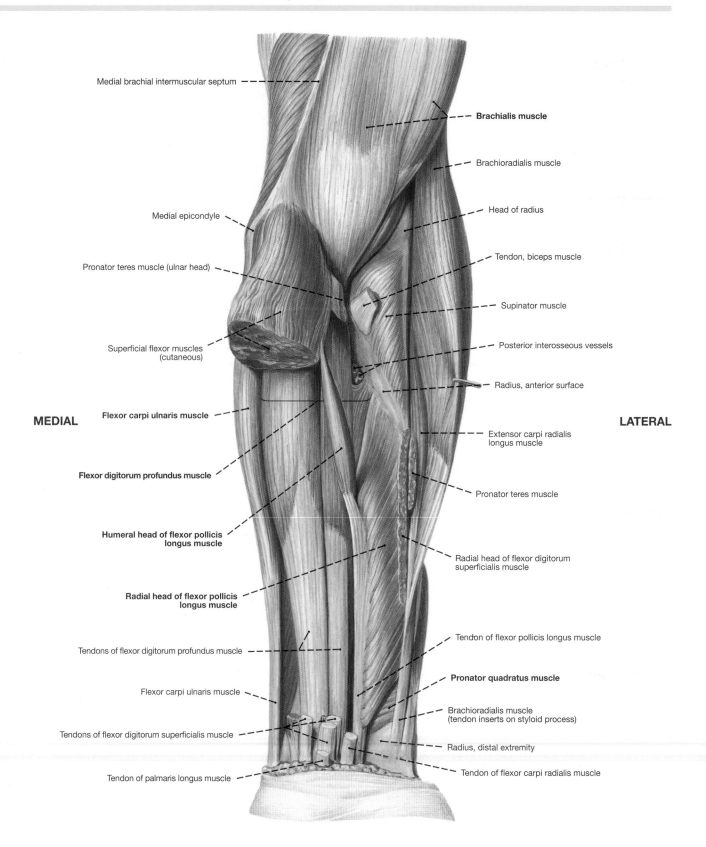

Medial brachial intermuscular septum

Brachialis muscle

Brachioradialis muscle

Head of radius

Medial epicondyle

Tendon, biceps muscle

Pronator teres muscle (ulnar head)

Supinator muscle

Posterior interosseous vessels

Superficial flexor muscles (cutaneous)

Radius, anterior surface

MEDIAL

LATERAL

Flexor carpi ulnaris muscle

Extensor carpi radialis longus muscle

Flexor digitorum profundus muscle

Pronator teres muscle

Humeral head of flexor pollicis longus muscle

Radial head of flexor digitorum superficialis muscle

Radial head of flexor pollicis longus muscle

Tendon of flexor pollicis longus muscle

Tendons of flexor digitorum profundus muscle

Pronator quadratus muscle

Flexor carpi ulnaris muscle

Brachioradialis muscle (tendon inserts on styloid process)

Tendons of flexor digitorum superficialis muscle

Radius, distal extremity

Tendon of palmaris longus muscle

Tendon of flexor carpi radialis muscle

Fig. 62: Left Anterior Forearm Muscles, Deep Group

NOTE: 1) the superficial anterior forearm muscles have been removed to reveal the three muscles of the deep group. These include the flexor digitorum profundus, the flexor pollicis longus, and the pronator quadratus.

2) the pronator quadratus is a small quadrangular muscle situated at the distal end of the forearm beneath the tendons of the flexor digitorum profundus and flexor pollicis longus. It is partially shown in this dissection and can better be seen in Fig. 83.

3) in this drawing, the tendons of the flexor digitorum profundus to the ring and little fingers and those to the middle and index fingers appear fused at the wrist, as if they were two structures rather than four.

Fig. 62

Flexor Muscles of Forearm: Superficial Group

Muscle	Origin	Insertion	Innervation	Action
Pronator Teres	HUMERAL HEAD Medial epicondyle of humerus ULNAR HEAD Coronoid process of ulna	Midway along the lateral surface of the radius	Median nerve (C6, C7) (enters the forearm by passing between the two heads)	Pronates and flexes the forearm
Flexor Carpi Radialis	Medial epicondyle of humerus	Base of the 2nd metacarpal bone	Median nerve (C6, C7)	Flexes the hand at the wrist joint; abducts the hand (radial flexes the hand)
Palmaris Longus	Medial epicondyle of humerus	Anterior flexor retinaculum and the palmar aponeurosis	Median nerve (C6, C7)	Flexes the hand at the wrist and tenses the palmar aponeurosis
Flexor Digitorum Superficialis	HUMEROULNAR HEAD Medial epicondyle of humerus and the coronoid process of ulna RADIAL HEAD Anterior surface of the radius below the radial tuberosity	By four long tendons onto the sides of the middle phalanx of the four medial fingers	Median nerve (C7, C8, T1)	Flexes the middle and proximal phalanges of the four medial fingers, also flexes the wrist
Flexor Carpi Ulnaris	HUMERAL HEAD Medial epicondyle of the humerus ULNAR HEAD Medial margin of the olecranon, and upper posterior border of the ulna	Pisiform bone and by ligaments to the hamate and 5th metacarpal bone	Ulnar nerve (C7, C8)	Flexes the hand at the wrist joint; adducts the hand (ulnar flexes the hand)

Flexor Muscles of the Forearm: Deep Group

Muscle	Origin	Insertion	Innervation	Action
Flexor Digitorum Profundus	Upper ¾ths of the anterior and medial aspects of the ulna and the ulnar half of the interosseous membrane	Anterior surface of the base of the distal phalanx of the four medial fingers	Median nerve by its interosseous branch; and the ulnar nerve (C8, T1)	Flexes the distal phalanx of the 4 medial fingers; also flexes the hand at the wrist
Flexor Pollicis Longus	RADIAL HEAD Anterior surface of radius and the adjacent part of the interosseous membrane HUMERAL HEAD Medial epicondyle of humerus or the coronoid process of the ulna	Base of the distal phalanx of the thumb	Median nerve by its interosseous branch (C8, T1)	Flexes the distal phalanx and helps in flexing the proximal phalanx of the thumb
Pronator Quadratus	Distal ¼ of anterior surface of the ulna	Distal ¼ of anterior surface of the radius	Median nerve by its interosseous branch (C8, T1)	Pronates the hand

PLATE 48   Anterior Forearm Vessels and Nerves: Superficial Dissection

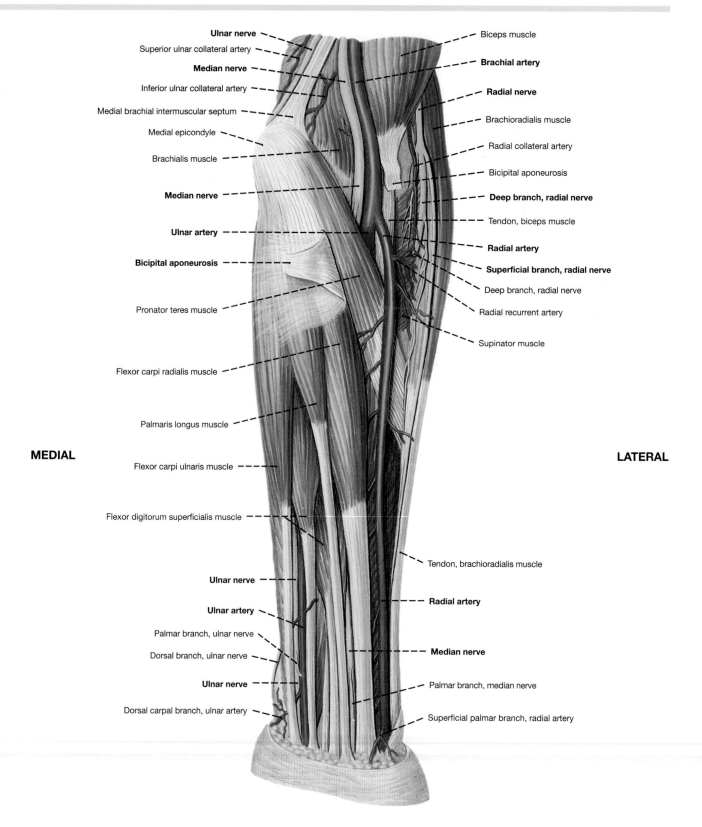

Ulnar nerve

Superior ulnar collateral artery

Median nerve

Inferior ulnar collateral artery

Medial brachial intermuscular septum

Medial epicondyle

Brachialis muscle

Median nerve

Ulnar artery

Bicipital aponeurosis

Pronator teres muscle

Flexor carpi radialis muscle

Palmaris longus muscle

MEDIAL

Flexor carpi ulnaris muscle

Flexor digitorum superficialis muscle

Ulnar nerve

Ulnar artery

Palmar branch, ulnar nerve

Dorsal branch, ulnar nerve

Ulnar nerve

Dorsal carpal branch, ulnar artery

Biceps muscle

Brachial artery

Radial nerve

Brachioradialis muscle

Radial collateral artery

Bicipital aponeurosis

Deep branch, radial nerve

Tendon, biceps muscle

Radial artery

Superficial branch, radial nerve

Deep branch, radial nerve

Radial recurrent artery

Supinator muscle

LATERAL

Tendon, brachioradialis muscle

Radial artery

Median nerve

Palmar branch, median nerve

Superficial palmar branch, radial artery

Fig. 63: Anterior Dissection of the Left Forearm Vessels and Nerves, Stage I

NOTE: 1) the bicipital aponeurosis has been reflected to reveal the underlying median nerve, brachial artery, and tendon of insertion of the biceps brachii muscle.

2) the brachioradialis muscle has been pulled laterally (toward the radial side) to expose the course of the radial artery and the division of the radial nerve into its superficial and deep branches.

3) the radial artery, as it descends in the forearm, courses anterior to the biceps brachii muscle, the supinator muscle, the tendon of insertion of the pronator teres, and the belly of the flexor pollicis longus (the latter is not labelled in this figure, but can be seen in Fig. 64).

Fig. 63

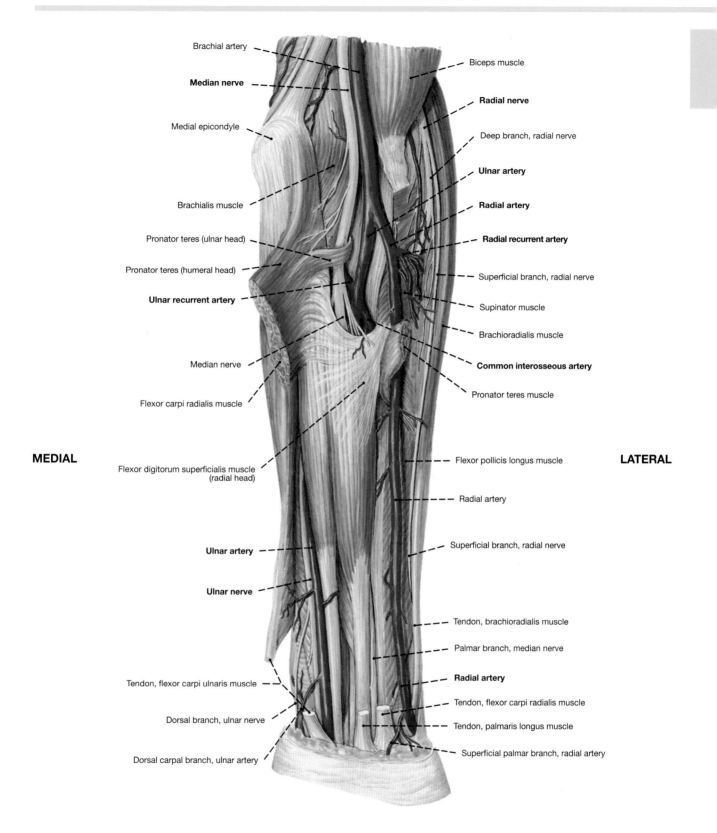

Brachial artery

Median nerve

Medial epicondyle

Brachialis muscle

Pronator teres (ulnar head)

Pronator teres (humeral head)

Ulnar recurrent artery

Median nerve

Flexor carpi radialis muscle

MEDIAL

Flexor digitorum superficialis muscle
(radial head)

Ulnar artery

Ulnar nerve

Tendon, flexor carpi ulnaris muscle

Dorsal branch, ulnar nerve

Dorsal carpal branch, ulnar artery

Biceps muscle

Radial nerve

Deep branch, radial nerve

Ulnar artery

Radial artery

Radial recurrent artery

Superficial branch, radial nerve

Supinator muscle

Brachioradialis muscle

Common interosseous artery

Pronator teres muscle

Flexor pollicis longus muscle

LATERAL

Radial artery

Superficial branch, radial nerve

Tendon, brachioradialis muscle

Palmar branch, median nerve

Radial artery

Tendon, flexor carpi radialis muscle

Tendon, palmaris longus muscle

Superficial palmar branch, radial artery

Fig. 64: Anterior Dissection of the Left Forearm Vessels and Nerves, Stage 2
NOTE: 1)   the pronator teres and flexor carpi radialis muscles are reflected just below the cubital fossa to show the bifurcation of the brachial artery into the ulnar and radial arteries.

2)   at the wrist, the tendon of the flexor carpi ulnaris muscle is severed and pulled aside to expose the ulnar nerve pland artery.

3)   the median nerve lies deep to the flexor digitorum superficialis muscle along much of its course in the forearm, but just above the wrist it usually becomes visible between the tendons. Observe that the tendons of the flexor pollicis longus and flexor carpi radialis are on its **radial side** and the tendons of the palmaris longus and flexor digitorum superficialis are on its **ulnar side.**

Fig. 64

PLATE 50   Anterior Forearm Vessels and Nerves: Deep Dissection

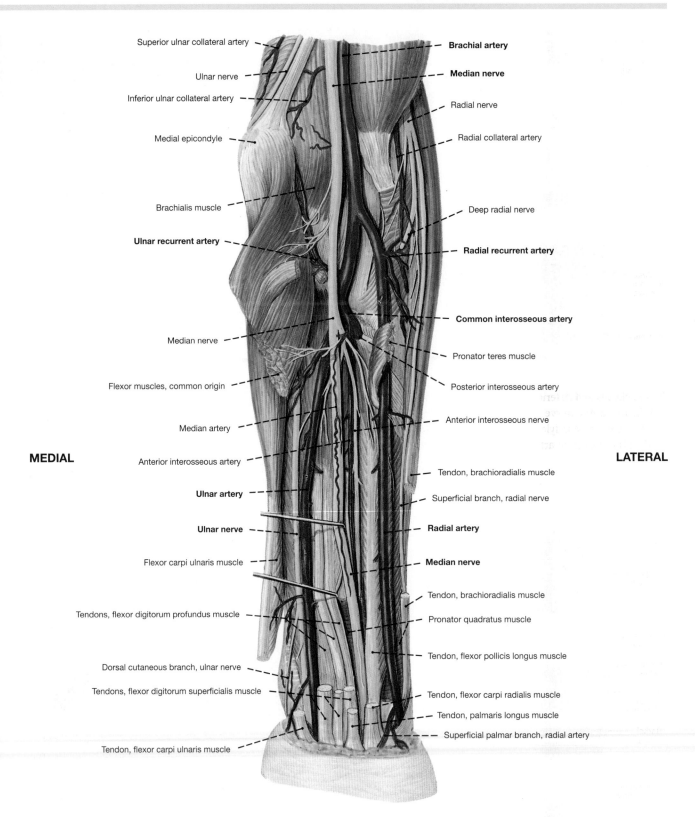

Superior ulnar collateral artery

Ulnar nerve

Inferior ulnar collateral artery

Medial epicondyle

Brachialis muscle

Ulnar recurrent artery

Median nerve

Flexor muscles, common origin

Median artery

Anterior interosseous artery

Ulnar artery

Ulnar nerve

Flexor carpi ulnaris muscle

Tendons, flexor digitorum profundus muscle

Dorsal cutaneous branch, ulnar nerve

Tendons, flexor digitorum superficialis muscle

Tendon, flexor carpi ulnaris muscle

Brachial artery

Median nerve

Radial nerve

Radial collateral artery

Deep radial nerve

Radial recurrent artery

Common interosseous artery

Pronator teres muscle

Posterior interosseous artery

Anterior interosseous nerve

Tendon, brachioradialis muscle

Superficial branch, radial nerve

Radial artery

Median nerve

Tendon, brachioradialis muscle

Pronator quadratus muscle

Tendon, flexor pollicis longus muscle

Tendon, flexor carpi radialis muscle

Tendon, palmaris longus muscle

Superficial palmar branch, radial artery

MEDIAL

LATERAL

Fig. 65: Anterior Dissection of the Left Forearm Vessels and Nerves, Stage 3
NOTE: 1) the division of the **brachial artery** into the **radial** and **ulnar arteries** at the lower end of the cubital fossa.

2) the **common interosseous artery** branches from the **ulnar artery** and divides almost immediately into the **anterior and posterior interosseous arteries.**

3) the courses of the ulnar and median nerves. In the lower half of the forearm, the **ulnar nerve** descends with the ulnar artery, whereas the **median nerve** descends in front of the anterior interosseous nerve and artery.

Fig. 65

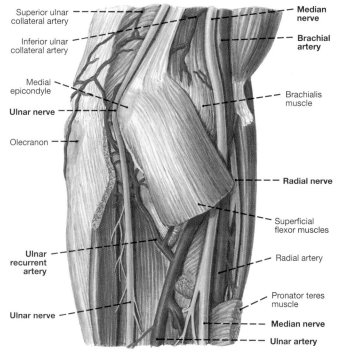

Fig. 66: Nerves and Arteries at the Elbow (Medial View)

NOTE: the **ulnar nerve** enters the forearm directly behind
the medial epicondyle, and at this site is closely related to
the **ulnar recurrent artery.**

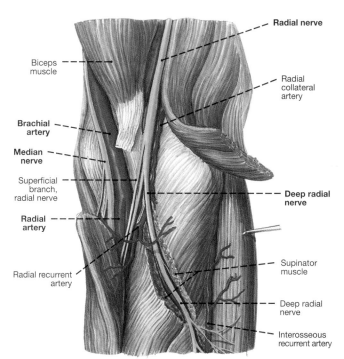

Fig. 67: Nerves and Arteries at the Elbow (Lateral View)

NOTE: the **deep radial nerve** passes into the forearm in front of
the lateral part of the elbow joint. It then courses dorsally
through the supinator muscle to supply the posterior forearm
muscles.

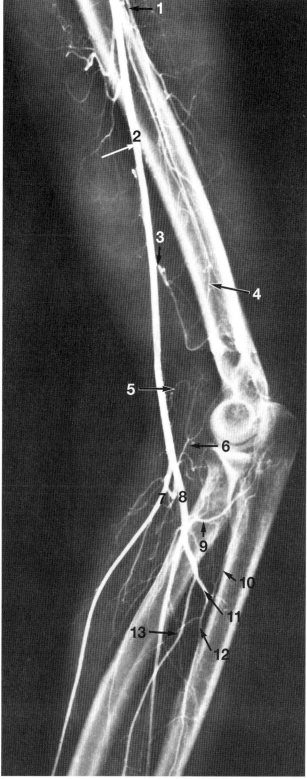

Fig. 68: A Brachial Arteriogram Showing the Origins of the
Vessels that Supply the Elbow and Forearm

1. Profunda brachii artery
2. Brachial artery
3. Superior ulnar
   collateral artery
4. Radial collateral artery
5. Inferior ulnar collateral artery
6. Radial recurrent artery
7. Radial artery
8. Ulnar artery
9. Ulnar recurrent artery
10. Recurrent interosseous artery
11. Common interosseous artery
12. Posterior interosseous
    artery
13. Anterior interosseous
    artery

Fig. 66, 67, 68   I

PLATE 52   **Superficial Extensor Muscles of Forearm: Posterior View**

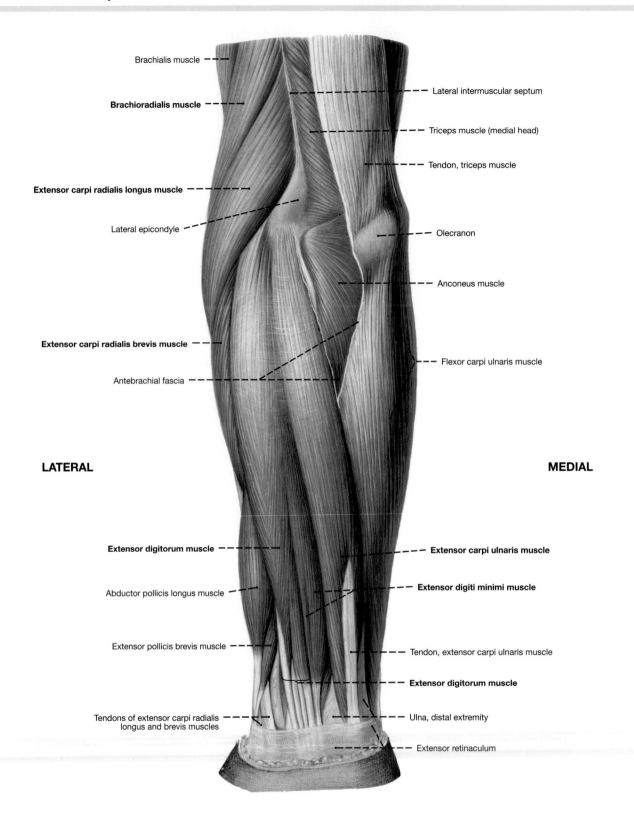

Brachialis muscle

Brachioradialis muscle

Extensor carpi radialis longus muscle

Lateral epicondyle

Extensor carpi radialis brevis muscle

Antebrachial fascia

Lateral intermuscular septum

Triceps muscle (medial head)

Tendon, triceps muscle

Olecranon

Anconeus muscle

Flexor carpi ulnaris muscle

LATERAL

MEDIAL

Extensor digitorum muscle

Abductor pollicis longus muscle

Extensor pollicis brevis muscle

Tendons of extensor carpi radialis longus and brevis muscles

Extensor carpi ulnaris muscle

Extensor digiti minimi muscle

Tendon, extensor carpi ulnaris muscle

Extensor digitorum muscle

Ulna, distal extremity

Extensor retinaculum

Fig. 69: Posterior Muscles of the Left Forearm, Superficial Group (Posterior View)
NOTE: the superficial radial group of extensor muscles of the forearm include the **brachioradialis muscle** and the **extensors carpi radialis longus and brevis.**

Muscle	Origin	Insertion	Innervation	Action
Brachioradialis	Upper ²⁄₃rds of lateral supracondylar ridge of humerus	Lateral aspect of the base of the styloid process of the radius	Radial nerve (C5, C6)	**Flexes** the forearm when the forearm is semipronated

Fig. 69

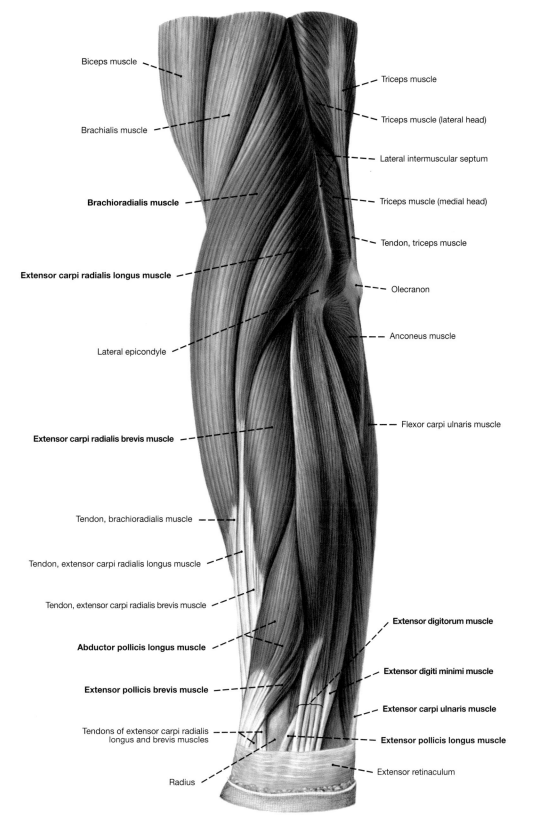

Biceps muscle

Brachialis muscle

Brachioradialis muscle

Extensor carpi radialis longus muscle

Lateral epicondyle

Extensor carpi radialis brevis muscle

Tendon, brachioradialis muscle

Tendon, extensor carpi radialis longus muscle

Tendon, extensor carpi radialis brevis muscle

Abductor pollicis longus muscle

Extensor pollicis brevis muscle

Tendons of extensor carpi radialis longus and brevis muscles

Radius

Triceps muscle

Triceps muscle (lateral head)

Lateral intermuscular septum

Triceps muscle (medial head)

Tendon, triceps muscle

Olecranon

Anconeus muscle

Flexor carpi ulnaris muscle

Extensor digitorum muscle

Extensor digiti minimi muscle

Extensor carpi ulnaris muscle

Extensor pollicis longus muscle

Extensor retinaculum

Fig. 70: Posterior Muscles of the Left Forearm, Superficial Group (Lateral View)

Muscle	Origin	Insertion	Innervation	Action
Extensor Carpi Radialis Longus	Lower 1/3rd of lateral supracondylar ridge of humerus	Dorsal surface of the base of the 2nd metacarpal bone	Radial nerve (C6, C7)	Extends the hand; abducts the hand at the wrist (radial flexion)
Extensor Carpi Radialis Brevis	Lateral epicondyle of humerus	Dorsal surface of the base of the 3rd metacarpal bone	Radial nerve (C6, C7)	Extends the hand; abducts the hand at the wrist (radial flexion)

Fig. 70 |

PLATE 54 Deep Extensor Muscles of the Forearm, Stage 1

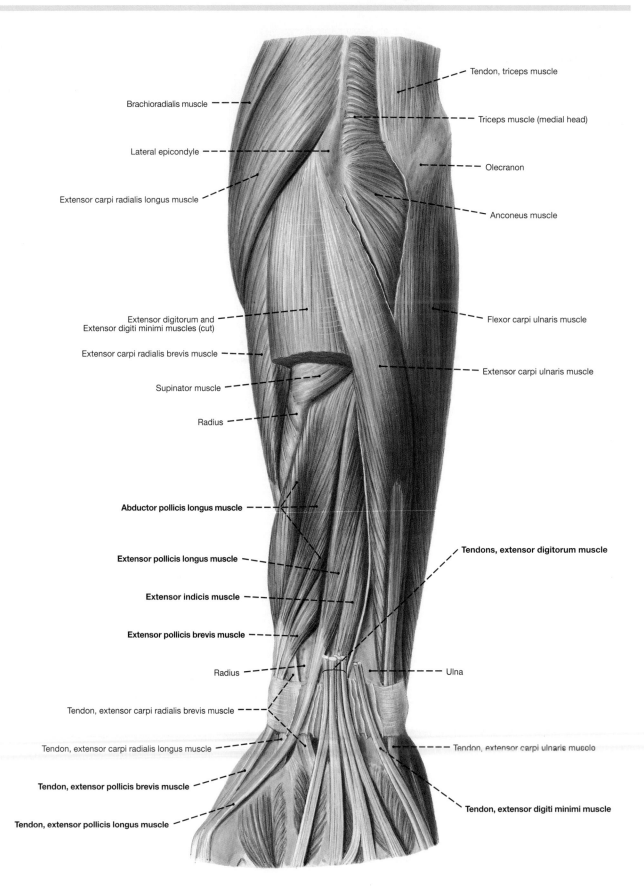

Tendon, triceps muscle

Brachioradialis muscle

Triceps muscle (medial head)

Lateral epicondyle

Olecranon

Extensor carpi radialis longus muscle

Anconeus muscle

Extensor digitorum and
Extensor digiti minimi muscles (cut)

Flexor carpi ulnaris muscle

Extensor carpi radialis brevis muscle

Extensor carpi ulnaris muscle

Supinator muscle

Radius

Abductor pollicis longus muscle

Tendons, extensor digitorum muscle

Extensor pollicis longus muscle

Extensor indicis muscle

Extensor pollicis brevis muscle

Radius

Ulna

Tendon, extensor carpi radialis brevis muscle

Tendon, extensor carpi radialis longus muscle

Tendon, extensor carpi ulnaris muscle

Tendon, extensor pollicis brevis muscle

Tendon, extensor pollicis longus muscle

Tendon, extensor digiti minimi muscle

Fig. 71: Thumb Muscles of the Left Posterior Forearm
NOTE: four other muscles complete the **superficial** extensor muscles on the posterior aspect of the forearm. These are the **extensor digitorum, extensor digiti minimi, extensor carpi ulnaris,** and the **anconeus.** There are also five **deep** extensor muscles: the **abductor pollicis longus, extensor pollicis longus** and **brevis, extensor indicis,** and the **supinator** muscle.

Fig. 71

Superficial Extensor Forearm Muscles (cont.)

Muscle	Origin	Insertion	Innervation	Action
Extensor Digitorum	Lateral epicondyle of humerus	Dorsum of middle and distal phalanges of the 4 fingers	Posterior interosseous branch of the radial nerve (C7, C8)	Extends the fingers and the hand
Extensor Digiti Minimi	Lateral epicondyle of humerus	Dorsal digital expansion of little finger	Posterior interosseous branch of the radial nerve (C7, C8)	Extends the little finger and the hand
Extensor Carpi Ulnaris	Lateral epicondyle of humerus	Medial side of the base of the 5th metacarpal bone	Posterior interosseous branch of the radial nerve (C7, C8)	Extends and adducts the hand (ulnar flexes hand)
Anconeus	Lateral epicondyle of humerus	Lateral side of olecranon and shaft of ulna	Radial nerve (C7, C8, T1)	Helps to extend the forearm at the elbow joint

Deep Extensor Forearm Muscles

Muscle	Origin	Insertion	Innervation	Action
Extensor Pollicis Longus	Posterior shaft of ulna and interosseous membrane	Base of the distal phalanx of the thumb	Posterior interosseous branch of the radial nerve (C7, C8)	Extends the thumb, and to a minor extent, the hand
Extensor Pollicis Brevis	Posterior surface of radius and interosseous membrane	Base of the proximal phalanx of the thumb	Posterior interosseous branch of the radial nerve (C7, C8)	Extends the proximal phalanx and metacarpal bone of thumb
Abductor Pollicis Longus	Posterior surfaces of both radius and ulna and interosseous membrane	Radial side of base of the 1st metacarpal bone, and on the trapezoid bone	Posterior interosseous branch of the radial nerve (C7, C8)	Abducts and assists in extending the thumb
Extensor Indicis	Posterior surface of the ulna and interosseous membrane	Into the extensor hood of the index finger	Posterior interosseous branch of the radial nerve (C7, C8)	Extends the index finger and helps extend the hand
Supinator	Lateral epicondyle of humerus; radial collateral ligament; supinator crest of ulna	Lateral surface of the proximal $\frac{1}{3}$rd of the radius	Posterior interosseous branch of the radial nerve (C6)	Rotates the radius to supinate the hand and forearm

PLATE 56   Deep Extensor Muscles of the Forearm

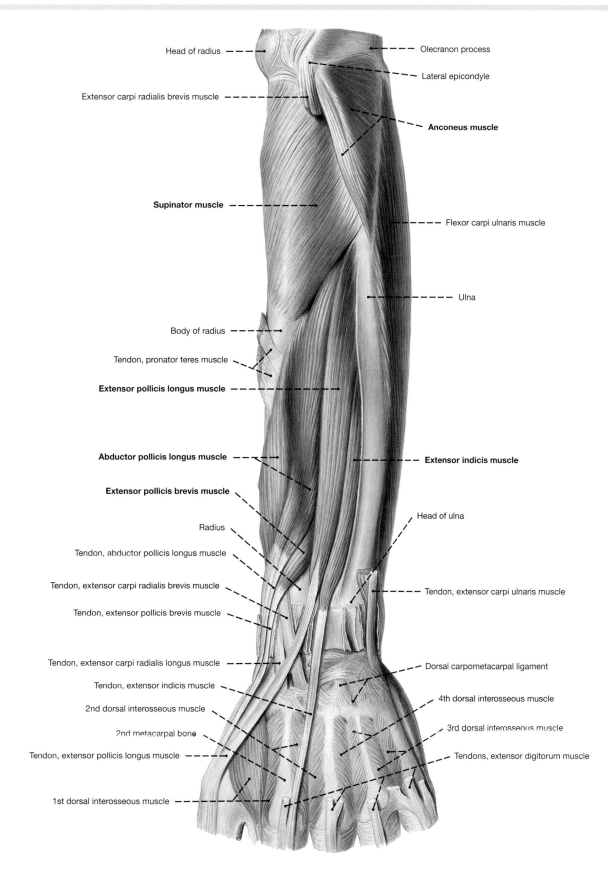

Head of radius

Olecranon process

Lateral epicondyle

Extensor carpi radialis brevis muscle

Anconeus muscle

Supinator muscle

Flexor carpi ulnaris muscle

Ulna

Body of radius

Tendon, pronator teres muscle

Extensor pollicis longus muscle

Abductor pollicis longus muscle

Extensor indicis muscle

Extensor pollicis brevis muscle

Radius

Head of ulna

Tendon, abductor pollicis longus muscle

Tendon, extensor carpi radialis brevis muscle

Tendon, extensor pollicis brevis muscle

Tendon, extensor carpi ulnaris muscle

Tendon, extensor carpi radialis longus muscle

Dorsal carpometacarpal ligament

Tendon, extensor indicis muscle

4th dorsal interosseous muscle

2nd dorsal interosseous muscle

3rd dorsal interosseous muscle

2nd metacarpal bone

Tendon, extensor pollicis longus muscle

Tendons, extensor digitorum muscle

1st dorsal interosseous muscle

Fig. 72: Left Posterior Forearm Muscles, Deep Group

NOTE: 1)   the three thumb muscles (abductor pollicis longus, and extensors pollicis brevis and longus) are exposed when the extensor digitorum, extensor digiti minimi, and extensor carpi ulnaris are removed.

2)   the extensor indicis courses to the index finger and the supinator is a broad muscle that stretches across the upper forearm from the humerus and ulna to the upper $\frac{1}{3}$rd of the radius.

Fig. 72

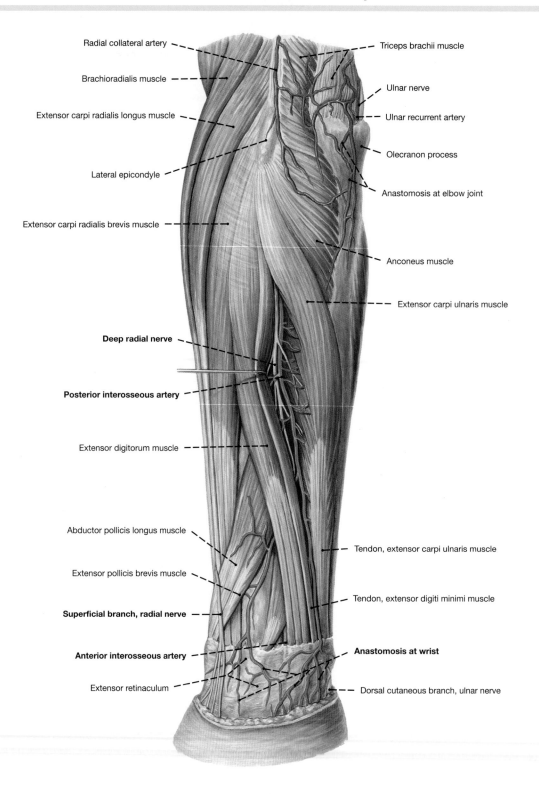

Radial collateral artery

Brachioradialis muscle

Extensor carpi radialis longus muscle

Lateral epicondyle

Extensor carpi radialis brevis muscle

Deep radial nerve

Posterior interosseous artery

Extensor digitorum muscle

Abductor pollicis longus muscle

Extensor pollicis brevis muscle

Superficial branch, radial nerve

Anterior interosseous artery

Extensor retinaculum

Triceps brachii muscle

Ulnar nerve

Ulnar recurrent artery

Olecranon process

Anastomosis at elbow joint

Anconeus muscle

Extensor carpi ulnaris muscle

Tendon, extensor carpi ulnaris muscle

Tendon, extensor digiti minimi muscle

Anastomosis at wrist

Dorsal cutaneous branch, ulnar nerve

Fig. 73: Nerves and Arteries of the Left Posterior Forearm

NOTE: 1) the extensor digiti minimi and extensor digitorum have been separated from the extensor carpi ulnaris to expose the **posterior interosseous artery** and the **deep radial nerve.**

    2) the posterior interosseous artery is derived in the anterior compartment of the forearm from the common interosseous artery, a branch of the ulnar artery, which divides into anterior and posterior interosseous branches (see Fig. 43).

    3) the posterior interosseous branch passes over the proximal border of the interosseous membrane to achieve the posterior compartment and it descends with the deep radial nerve between the superficial and deep extensor forearm muscles.

    4) in the distal forearm, the posterior interosseous artery anastomoses with terminal branches of the anterior interosseous artery to help form the carpal anastomosis at the wrist.

Fig. 73   I

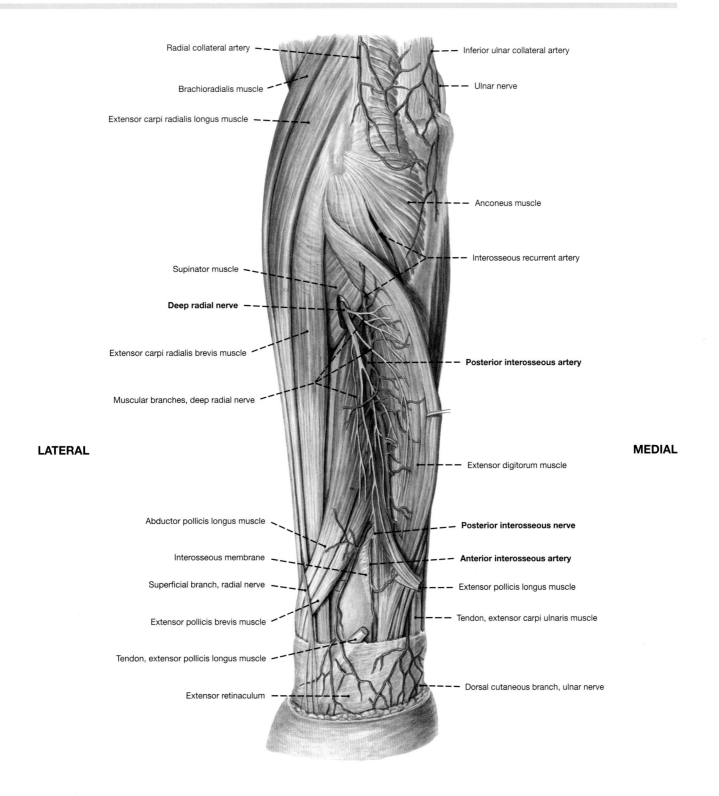

Radial collateral artery

Brachioradialis muscle

Extensor carpi radialis longus muscle

Supinator muscle

Deep radial nerve

Extensor carpi radialis brevis muscle

Muscular branches, deep radial nerve

LATERAL

Abductor pollicis longus muscle

Interosseous membrane

Superficial branch, radial nerve

Extensor pollicis brevis muscle

Tendon, extensor pollicis longus muscle

Extensor retinaculum

Inferior ulnar collateral artery

Ulnar nerve

Anconeus muscle

Interosseous recurrent artery

Posterior interosseous artery

MEDIAL

Extensor digitorum muscle

Posterior interosseous nerve

Anterior interosseous artery

Extensor pollicis longus muscle

Tendon, extensor carpi ulnaris muscle

Dorsal cutaneous branch, ulnar nerve

Fig. 74: Nerves and Arteries of the Left Posterior Forearm (Deep Dissection)

NOTE: 1)   the extensor digitorum muscle is separated from the extensor carpi radialis brevis and pulled medially to reveal the **posterior interosseous artery** and **deep radial nerve.**

2)   after the radial nerve leaves the radial groove of the humerus in the lower brachium, it divides into superficial and deep branches.

3)   the **superficial branch** descends along the lateral side of the forearm under cover of the brachioradialis muscle and becomes a sensory nerve to the dorsum of the hand.

4)   the **deep branch** enters the posterior forearm by piercing through the supinator muscle and, coursing along the dorsum of the interosseous membrane, is called the **posterior interosseous nerve.** It supplies all of the deep posterior forearm muscles and descends deep to the extensor pollicis longus muscle, which has been cut in this dissection.

Fig. 74

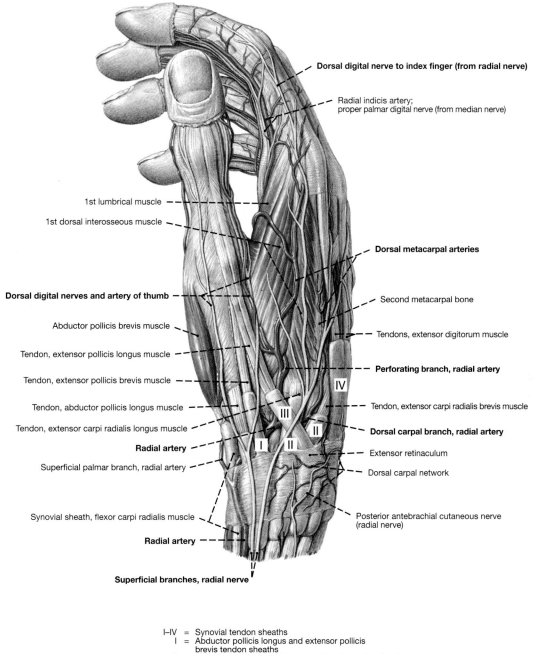

Dorsal digital nerve to index finger (from radial nerve)

Radial indicis artery;
proper palmar digital nerve (from median nerve)

1st lumbrical muscle

1st dorsal interosseous muscle

Dorsal metacarpal arteries

Dorsal digital nerves and artery of thumb

Second metacarpal bone

Abductor pollicis brevis muscle

Tendons, extensor digitorum muscle

Tendon, extensor pollicis longus muscle

Perforating branch, radial artery

Tendon, extensor pollicis brevis muscle

Tendon, abductor pollicis longus muscle

Tendon, extensor carpi radialis brevis muscle

Tendon, extensor carpi radialis longus muscle

Dorsal carpal branch, radial artery

Radial artery

Extensor retinaculum

Superficial palmar branch, radial artery

Dorsal carpal network

Synovial sheath, flexor carpi radialis muscle

Posterior antebrachial cutaneous nerve
(radial nerve)

Radial artery

Superficial branches, radial nerve

I–IV = Synovial tendon sheaths
  I = Abductor pollicis longus and extensor pollicis
      brevis tendon sheaths
  II = Extensor carpi radialis longus and brevis tendon sheaths
  III = Extensor pollicis longus tendon sheath
  IV = Extensor digitorum and extensor indicis tendon sheath

Fig. 75: Superficial Nerves, Arteries, and Tendons on the Radial Aspect of the Right Hand

NOTE: 1) only the skin and superficial fascia have been removed in this dissection, and the cutaneous nerves and superficial arteries to the thumb, radial side of the index finger, and dorsum of the hand have been retained.

2) the **superficial branches of the radial nerve** to the hand (see Figs. 58, 74, and 76). These supply the dorsum of the thumb, nearly to the tip, as well as the lateral (radial) half of the dorsum of the hand.

3) the radial nerve also supplies the proximal part of the dorsum of the index, middle, and lateral half of the ring fingers, as far as the proximal interphalangeal joint because the median nerve sends branches around the digits to supply the more distal parts of the fingers.

4) the distribution of the radial artery to the thumb and dorsum of the hand (see Figs. 78 and 79). Observe:

a) the **dorsal digital branch** to the thumb

b) the **radial indicis branch** to the index finger

c) the **perforating branch** that penetrates between the two heads of the first dorsal interosseous muscle

d) the **dorsal carpal branch** from which the dorsal metacarpal arteries arise

Fig. 75

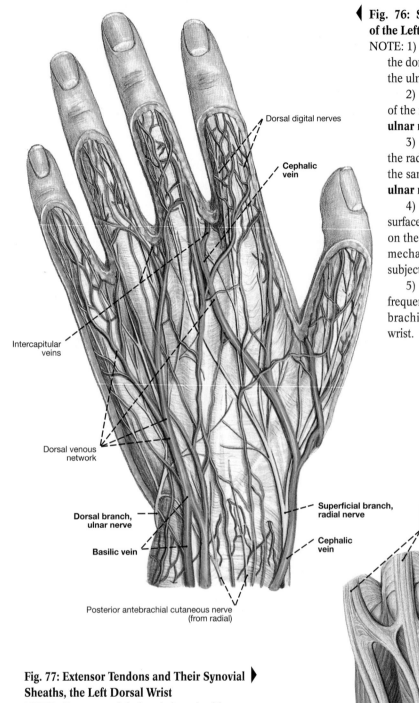

Dorsal digital nerves

Cephalic vein

Intercapitular veins

Dorsal venous network

Dorsal branch, ulnar nerve

Basilic vein

Superficial branch, radial nerve

Cephalic vein

Posterior antebrachial cutaneous nerve (from radial)

Fig. 76: Superficial Veins and Nerves of the Dorsum of the Left Hand

NOTE: 1) the **cephalic vein** originates on the radial side of the dorsum of the hand, whereas the **basilic vein** arises on the ulnar side.

2) the **superficial radial nerve** supplies the dorsum of the radial 3 ½ digits, whereas the **dorsal branch of the ulnar nerve** supplies the dorsum of the ulnar 1½ digits.

3) the dorsum of the distal phalanx (not dissected) of the radial 3 ½ digits is supplied by the **median nerve,** but the same region on the ulnar 1½ digits is supplied by the **ulnar nerve.**

4) there is a profuse venous plexus on the dorsal surface of the hand, but very few and small superficial veins on the palmar surface. This is beneficial because frequent mechanical pressures to which the palmar surface is subjected could injure surface vessels.

5) adjacent branches of the radial and ulnar nerve frequently communicate. Observe that the posterior antebrachial cutaneous branches usually terminate at the wrist.

Fig. 77: Extensor Tendons and Their Synovial Sheaths, the Left Dorsal Wrist

NOTE: 1) a synovial sheath is a double meso-thelial-lined envelope that surrounds a tendon, allowing it to move more freely beneath the retinaculum.

2) there are six synovial compartments on the dorsum of the wrist. From radial to ulnar these contain the tendons of:

    a) extensor pollicis brevis and abductor pollicis longus

    b) extensor carpi radialis longus and brevis

    c) extensor pollicis longus

    d) extensor digitorum and extensor indicis

    e) extensor digiti minimi

    f) extensor carpi ulnaris.

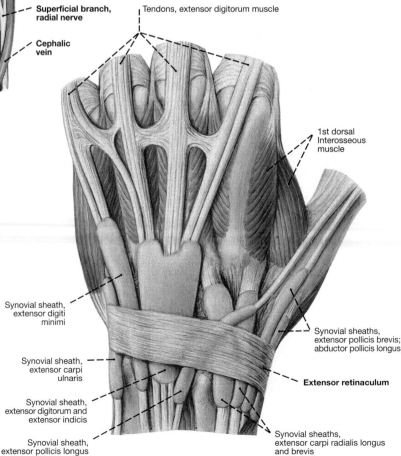

Tendons, extensor digitorum muscle

1st dorsal Interosseous muscle

Synovial sheath, extensor digiti minimi

Synovial sheaths, extensor pollicis brevis; abductor pollicis longus

Synovial sheath, extensor carpi ulnaris

Extensor retinaculum

Synovial sheath, extensor digitorum and extensor indicis

Synovial sheath, extensor pollicis longus

Synovial sheaths, extensor carpi radialis longus and brevis

Fig. 78: Arteries of the Left Dorsal Wrist and Hand, Deep View

NOTE: 1) the transverse course of the dorsal carpal branch of the radial artery.

2) the princeps pollicis branch of the radial artery coursing deep to the 1st dorsal interosseous muscle.

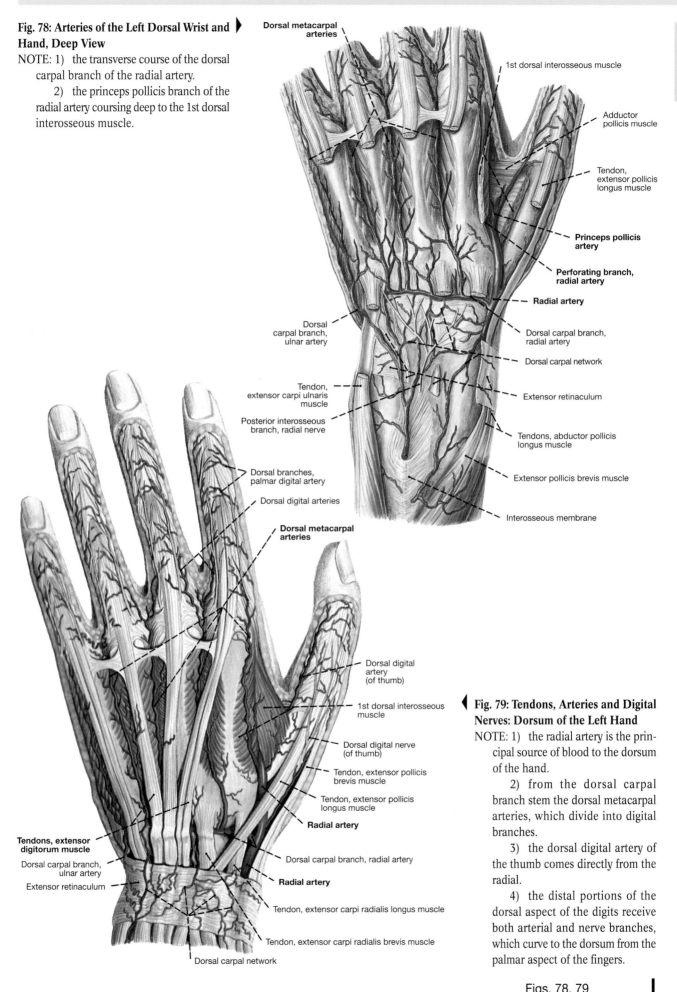

Dorsal metacarpal arteries

1st dorsal interosseous muscle

Adductor pollicis muscle

Tendon, extensor pollicis longus muscle

Princeps pollicis artery

Perforating branch, radial artery

Radial artery

Dorsal carpal branch, ulnar artery

Dorsal carpal branch, radial artery

Dorsal carpal network

Extensor retinaculum

Tendon, extensor carpi ulnaris muscle

Posterior interosseous branch, radial nerve

Tendons, abductor pollicis longus muscle

Extensor pollicis brevis muscle

Interosseous membrane

Dorsal branches, palmar digital artery

Dorsal digital arteries

Dorsal metacarpal arteries

Dorsal digital artery (of thumb)

1st dorsal interosseous muscle

Dorsal digital nerve (of thumb)

Tendon, extensor pollicis brevis muscle

Tendon, extensor pollicis longus muscle

Radial artery

Dorsal carpal branch, radial artery

Radial artery

Tendon, extensor carpi radialis longus muscle

Tendons, extensor digitorum muscle

Dorsal carpal branch, ulnar artery

Extensor retinaculum

Tendon, extensor carpi radialis brevis muscle

Dorsal carpal network

Fig. 79: Tendons, Arteries and Digital Nerves: Dorsum of the Left Hand

NOTE: 1) the radial artery is the principal source of blood to the dorsum of the hand.

2) from the dorsal carpal branch stem the dorsal metacarpal arteries, which divide into digital branches.

3) the dorsal digital artery of the thumb comes directly from the radial.

4) the distal portions of the dorsal aspect of the digits receive both arterial and nerve branches, which curve to the dorsum from the palmar aspect of the fingers.

Figs. 78, 79

PLATE 62   Palm of the Hand: Superficial Vessels and Nerves

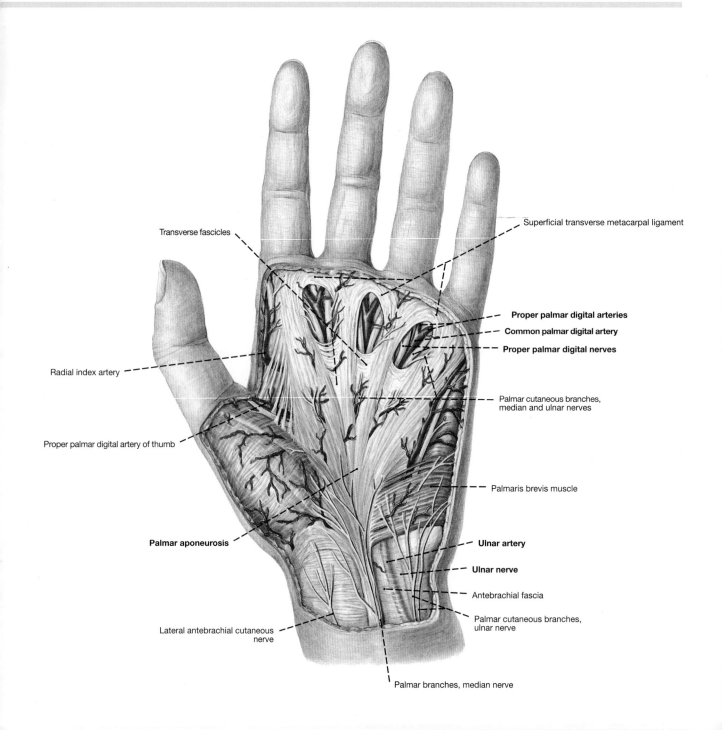

Transverse fascicles

Superficial transverse metacarpal ligament

Proper palmar digital arteries

Common palmar digital artery

Proper palmar digital nerves

Radial index artery

Palmar cutaneous branches, median and ulnar nerves

Proper palmar digital artery of thumb

Palmaris brevis muscle

Palmar aponeurosis

Ulnar artery

Ulnar nerve

Antebrachial fascia

Palmar cutaneous branches, ulnar nerve

Lateral antebrachial cutaneous nerve

Palmar branches, median nerve

Fig. 80: Superficial Nerves and Arteries of the Palm of the Left Hand
NOTE: 1) the thick fibrous palmar aponeurosis, which protects the palmar vessels and nerves and strengthens the midportion of the palm.

2) the radial $^2/_3$ rds of the palm is innervated by the median nerve, whereas the ulnar $^1/_3$ rd is supplied by the ulnar nerve.

3) the superficial exposure of vessels and nerves in the distal palm where the palmar aponeurosis is deficient.

Thenar (Thumb) Muscles of Hand

Muscle	Origin	Insertion	Innervation	Action
Abductor Pollicis Brevis	Flexor retinaculum and the tubercle of the trapezium	Base of proximal phalanx of thumb, dorsal digital expansion of thumb	Median nerve (C8, T1)	Abducts thumb
Opponens Pollicis	Flexor retinaculum and the tubercles of the scaphoid and trapezium bones	Whole length of lateral border of metacarpal bone of the thumb	Median nerve (C8, T1) and often a small branch of deep ulnar nerve	Opposes the thumb to the other fingers

Fig. 80

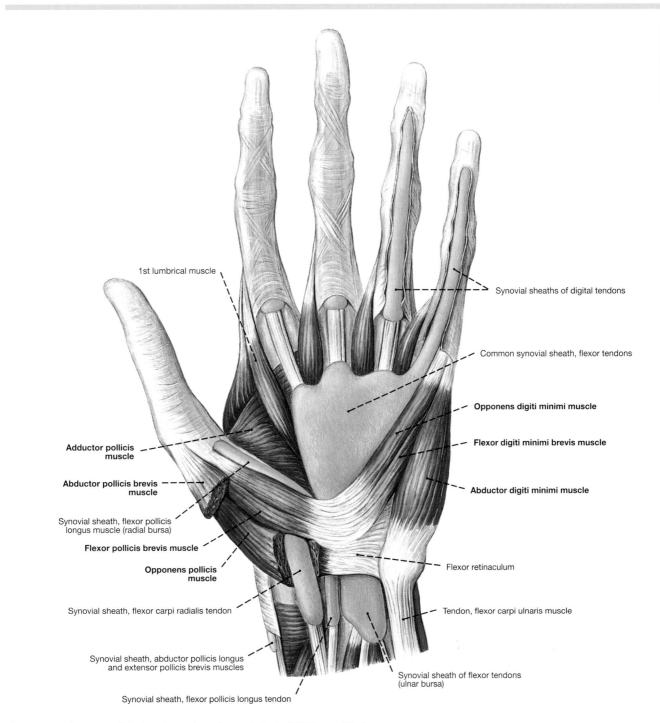

1st lumbrical muscle

Synovial sheaths of digital tendons

Common synovial sheath, flexor tendons

Opponens digiti minimi muscle

Flexor digiti minimi brevis muscle

Abductor digiti minimi muscle

Adductor pollicis muscle

Abductor pollicis brevis muscle

Synovial sheath, flexor pollicis longus muscle (radial bursa)

Flexor pollicis brevis muscle

Opponens pollicis muscle

Flexor retinaculum

Synovial sheath, flexor carpi radialis tendon

Tendon, flexor carpi ulnaris muscle

Synovial sheath, abductor pollicis longus and extensor pollicis brevis muscles

Synovial sheath of flexor tendons (ulnar bursa)

Synovial sheath, flexor pollicis longus tendon

Fig. 81: Muscles, Synovial Sheaths and Tendons of the Left Wrist and Palm

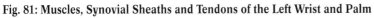

Thenar Muscles (cont.)

Muscle	Origin	Insertion	Innervation	Action
Flexor Pollicis Brevis	SUPERFICIAL HEAD Flexor retinaculum and tubercle of the trapezium DEEP HEAD Trapezoid and capitate bones	Radial side of base of the proximal phalanx of the thumb	SUPERFICIAL HEAD Median nerve (C8, T1) DEEP HEAD Deep branch of ulnar nerve (C8, T1)	Flexes proximal phalanx of thumb, flexes metacarpal bone and rotates it medially
Adductor Pollicis	OBLIQUE HEAD Capitate bone and bases of 2nd and 3rd metacarpal bones TRANSVERSE HEAD Palmar surface of 3rd metacarpal bone	Ulnar side of base of proximal phalanx of thumb	Deep branch of ulnar nerve (C8, T1)	Adducts the thumb

Fig. 81

PLATE 64   Palm of the Hand: Muscles and Flexor Tendon Insertions

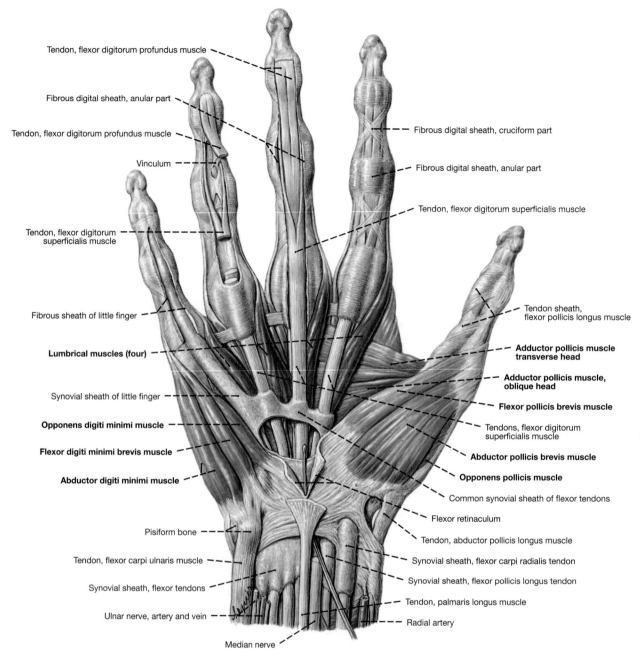

Tendon, flexor digitorum profundus muscle

Fibrous digital sheath, anular part

Tendon, flexor digitorum profundus muscle

Vinculum

Tendon, flexor digitorum superficialis muscle

Fibrous sheath of little finger

Lumbrical muscles (four)

Synovial sheath of little finger

Opponens digiti minimi muscle

Flexor digiti minimi brevis muscle

Abductor digiti minimi muscle

Pisiform bone

Tendon, flexor carpi ulnaris muscle

Synovial sheath, flexor tendons

Ulnar nerve, artery and vein

Median nerve

Fibrous digital sheath, cruciform part

Fibrous digital sheath, anular part

Tendon, flexor digitorum superficialis muscle

Tendon sheath, flexor pollicis longus muscle

Adductor pollicis muscle transverse head

Adductor pollicis muscle, oblique head

Flexor pollicis brevis muscle

Tendons, flexor digitorum superficialis muscle

Abductor pollicis brevis muscle

Opponens pollicis muscle

Common synovial sheath of flexor tendons

Flexor retinaculum

Tendon, abductor pollicis longus muscle

Synovial sheath, flexor carpi radialis tendon

Synovial sheath, flexor pollicis longus tendon

Tendon, palmaris longus muscle

Radial artery

Fig. 82: Muscles of the Right Hand

Hypothenar (Little Finger) Muscles of Hand

Muscle	Origin	Insertion	Innervation	Action
Palmaris Brevis (see Fig. 80)	Palmar aponeurosis and the flexor retinaculum	Into the dermis on the ulnar side of the hand	Ulnar nerve, superficial branch (C8, T1)	Helps tense the skin over the hypothenar muscles
Abductor Digiti Minimi	Pisiform bone and tendon of flexor carpi ulnaris	Base of proximal phalanx and dorsal aponeurosis of little finger	Ulnar nerve, deep branch (C8, T1)	Abducts the little finger
Flexor Digiti Minimi	Hamulus of the hamate bone and flexor retinaculum	Base of proximal phalanx of the little finger	Ulnar nerve, deep branch (C8, T1)	Flexes the little finger at metacarpophalangeal joint
Opponens Digiti Minimi	Hamulus of the hamate bone and flexor retinaculum	Ulnar side of 5th metacarpal bone	Ulnar nerve, deep branch (C8, T1)	Brings the little finger into opposition with the thumb

Fig. 82

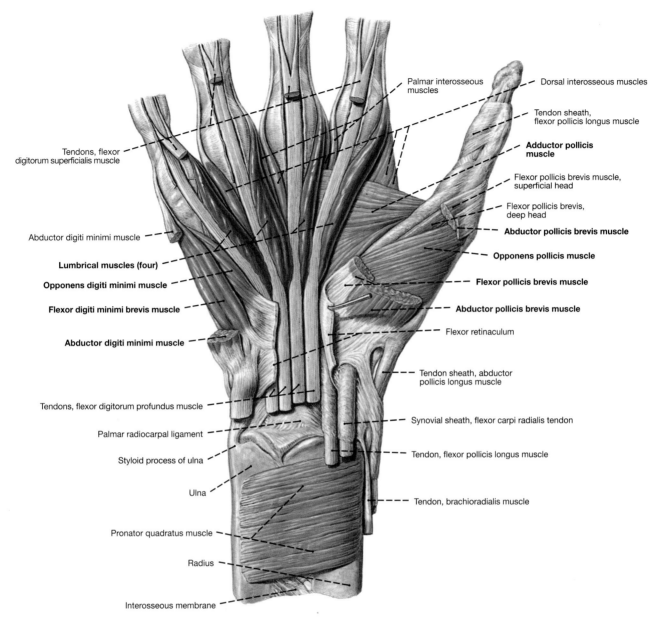

Palmar interosseous muscles

Dorsal interosseous muscles

Tendon sheath, flexor pollicis longus muscle

Adductor pollicis muscle

Flexor pollicis brevis muscle, superficial head

Flexor pollicis brevis, deep head

Abductor pollicis brevis muscle

Opponens pollicis muscle

Flexor pollicis brevis muscle

Abductor pollicis brevis muscle

Flexor retinaculum

Tendon sheath, abductor pollicis longus muscle

Synovial sheath, flexor carpi radialis tendon

Tendon, flexor pollicis longus muscle

Tendon, brachioradialis muscle

Tendons, flexor digitorum superficialis muscle

Abductor digiti minimi muscle

Lumbrical muscles (four)

Opponens digiti minimi muscle

Flexor digiti minimi brevis muscle

Abductor digiti minimi muscle

Tendons, flexor digitorum profundus muscle

Palmar radiocarpal ligament

Styloid process of ulna

Ulna

Pronator quadratus muscle

Radius

Interosseous membrane

Fig. 83: Deep Muscles of the Right Hand, Palmar View

NOTE: 1) the tendon of the flexor digitorum superficialis divides into two slips and allows the flexor digitorum profundus to pass and insert onto the distal phalanx.

2) in the fingers the tendons are encased in a synovial sheath and then bound by both crossed and transverse (cruciform and anular) fibrous sheaths (see Fig. 82).

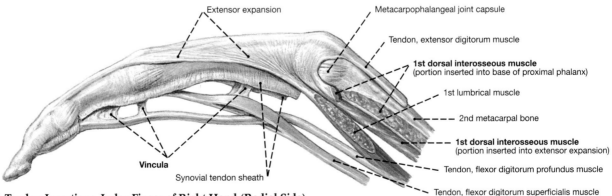

Extensor expansion

Metacarpophalangeal joint capsule

Tendon, extensor digitorum muscle

1st dorsal interosseous muscle (portion inserted into base of proximal phalanx)

1st lumbrical muscle

2nd metacarpal bone

1st dorsal interosseous muscle (portion inserted into extensor expansion)

Tendon, flexor digitorum profundus muscle

Tendon, flexor digitorum superficialis muscle

Vincula

Synovial tendon sheath

Fig. 84: Tendon Insertions, Index Finger of Right Hand (Radial Side)

NOTE: 1) the dorsal interosseous and lumbrical muscles join fibers from the extensor tendon in the formation of the dorsal extensor expansion.

2) the vincula are remnants of mesotendons and attach both superficial and deep tendons to the digital sheath.

PLATE 66   Palm of the Hand: Lumbrical and Interosseous Muscles

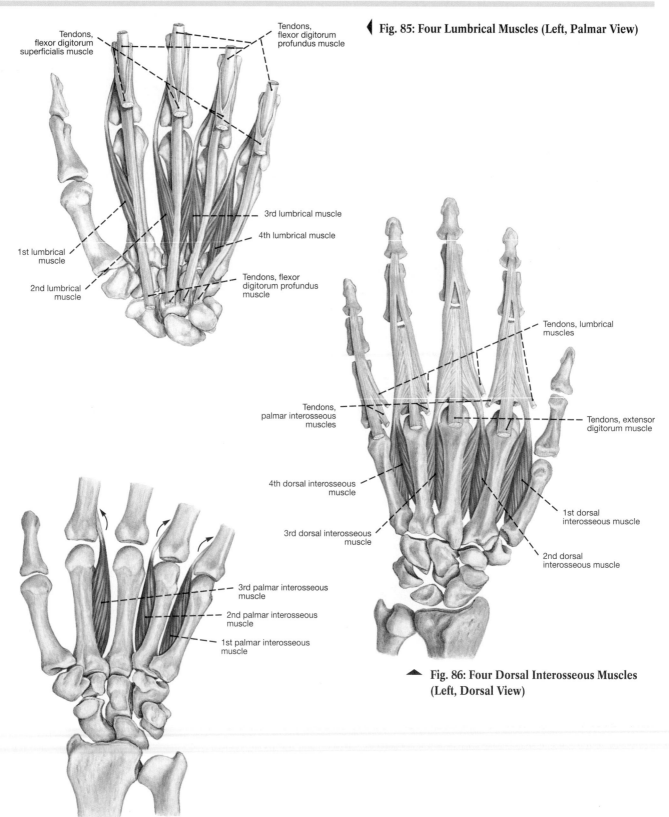

Tendons, flexor digitorum superficialis muscle

Tendons, flexor digitorum profundus muscle

◀ Fig. 85: Four Lumbrical Muscles (Left, Palmar View)

3rd lumbrical muscle

4th lumbrical muscle

1st lumbrical muscle

2nd lumbrical muscle

Tendons, flexor digitorum profundus muscle

Tendons, lumbrical muscles

Tendons, palmar interosseous muscles

Tendons, extensor digitorum muscle

4th dorsal interosseous muscle

3rd dorsal interosseous muscle

1st dorsal interosseous muscle

2nd dorsal interosseous muscle

▲ Fig. 86: Four Dorsal Interosseous Muscles (Left, Dorsal View)

3rd palmar interosseous muscle

2nd palmar interosseous muscle

1st palmar interosseous muscle

▲ Fig. 87: Three Palmar Interosseous Muscles (Left, Palmar View)

Lumbrical Muscles (Figs. 82–85)

Muscle	Origin	Insertion	Innervation	Action
Lumbrical Muscles (four)	Four tendons of flexor digitorum profundus muscle	Radial side of dorsal digital expansion, 2nd, 3rd, 4th, and 5th digits	Radial two lumbricals (1st and 2nd): median nerve Ulnar two lumbricals (3rd and 4th): ulnar nerve	Flex metacarpophalangeal joints; extend interphalangeal joints

Figs. 85, 86, 87

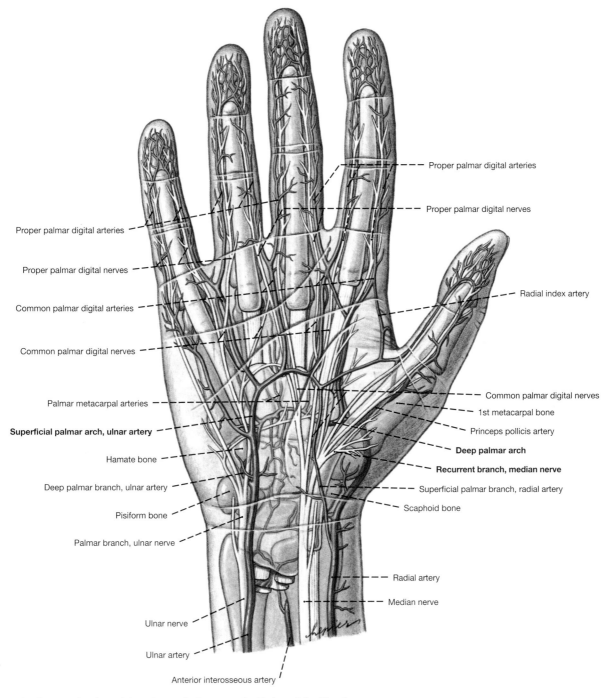

Proper palmar digital arteries

Proper palmar digital nerves

Proper palmar digital arteries

Proper palmar digital nerves

Common palmar digital arteries

Radial index artery

Common palmar digital nerves

Palmar metacarpal arteries

Common palmar digital nerves

1st metacarpal bone

Superficial palmar arch, ulnar artery

Princeps pollicis artery

Hamate bone

Deep palmar arch

Deep palmar branch, ulnar artery

Recurrent branch, median nerve

Pisiform bone

Superficial palmar branch, radial artery

Palmar branch, ulnar nerve

Scaphoid bone

Radial artery

Median nerve

Ulnar nerve

Ulnar artery

Anterior interosseous artery

Fig. 88: Surface Projection of Arteries and Nerves to the Palm of the Hand

Interosseous Muscles (Figs. 86, 87)

Muscle	Origin	Insertion	Innervation	Action
Dorsal Interossei (four)	Each arises by two heads from the adjacent sides of metacarpal bones	Bases of the proximal phalanges and the dorsal expansions of the 2nd, 3rd, and 4th fingers	Ulnar nerve, deep palmar branch (C8, T1)	Abduct fingers; flex at metacarpophalangeal joints and extend at interphalangeal joints
Palmar Interossei (three)	Each arises by one head from the 2nd, 4th and 5th metacarpal bones	Dorsal digital expansions of the 2nd, 4th and 5th fingers	Ulnar nerve, deep palmar branch (C8, T1)	Adduct fingers; flex at metacarpophalangeal joints and extend at interphalangeal joints

Fig. 88

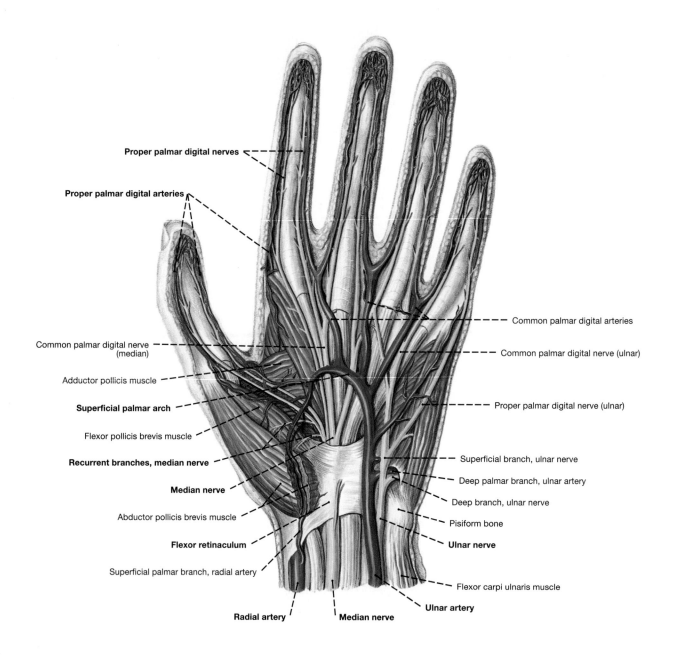

Proper palmar digital nerves

Proper palmar digital arteries

Common palmar digital nerve (median)

Adductor pollicis muscle

Superficial palmar arch

Flexor pollicis brevis muscle

Recurrent branches, median nerve

Median nerve

Abductor pollicis brevis muscle

Flexor retinaculum

Superficial palmar branch, radial artery

Radial artery

Median nerve

Common palmar digital arteries

Common palmar digital nerve (ulnar)

Proper palmar digital nerve (ulnar)

Superficial branch, ulnar nerve

Deep palmar branch, ulnar artery

Deep branch, ulnar nerve

Pisiform bone

Ulnar nerve

Flexor carpi ulnaris muscle

Ulnar artery

Fig. 89: Nerves and Arteries of the Left Palm, Superficial Palmar Arch

NOTE: 1) the **median nerve** enters the palm beneath the flexor retinaculum and supplies the muscles of the thenar eminence: abductor pollicis brevis, opponens pollicis, and the superficial head of the flexor pollicis brevis.

2) the **median nerve** also supplies the radial (lateral) two lumbrical muscles as well as the palmar surface of the lateral hand and lateral 3 ½ fingers.

3) the superficial location of the **recurrent branches of the median nerve,** which supply the thenar muscles. Just deep to the superficial fascia, these branches are easily injured.

4) the **ulnar nerve** enters the palm superficial to the flexor retinaculum, and it supplies the ulnar 1½ fingers and **all** the remaining muscles in the hand.

5) the **superficial palmar arterial arch** is derived principally from the ulnar artery. The arch is completed by the **palmar branch of the radial artery.** From the arch three or four **common palmar digital arteries** course distally and divide into **proper palmar digital arteries.** These accompany the corresponding digital nerves along the fingers.

Fig. 89

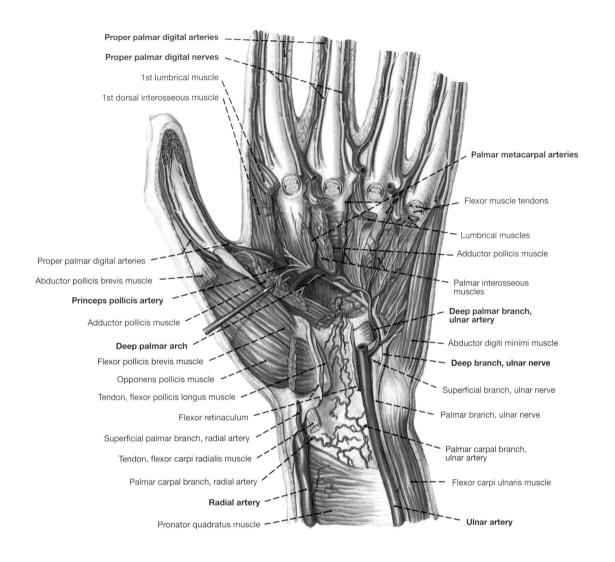

Proper palmar digital arteries

Proper palmar digital nerves

1st lumbrical muscle

1st dorsal interosseous muscle

Palmar metacarpal arteries

Flexor muscle tendons

Lumbrical muscles

Adductor pollicis muscle

Palmar interosseous muscles

Deep palmar branch, ulnar artery

Abductor digiti minimi muscle

Deep branch, ulnar nerve

Superficial branch, ulnar nerve

Palmar branch, ulnar nerve

Palmar carpal branch, ulnar artery

Flexor carpi ulnaris muscle

Ulnar artery

Proper palmar digital arteries

Abductor pollicis brevis muscle

Princeps pollicis artery

Adductor pollicis muscle

Deep palmar arch

Flexor pollicis brevis muscle

Opponens pollicis muscle

Tendon, flexor pollicis longus muscle

Flexor retinaculum

Superficial palmar branch, radial artery

Tendon, flexor carpi radialis muscle

Palmar carpal branch, radial artery

Radial artery

Pronator quadratus muscle

Fig. 90: Nerves and Arteries of the Left Palm, Deep Palmar Arch

NOTE: 1) the **radial artery** at the wrist enters the hand dorsally through the "anatomical snuff box" (see Figs. 78 and 79) and then passes distally, perforates the two heads of 1st dorsal interosseous muscle, and reaches the palm of the hand.

2) in the palm the radial artery forms the **deep palmar arch,** uniting medially with the **deep palmar branch** of the ulnar artery.

3) from the deep arch arise the **palmar metacarpal arteries** as well as the **princeps pollicis artery.**

4) the **deep branch of the ulnar nerve** courses with the deep palmar arterial arch. It supplies all the muscles in the deep palm.

5) there is a rich anastomosis between the superficial and deep arches and between the ulnar and radial arteries.

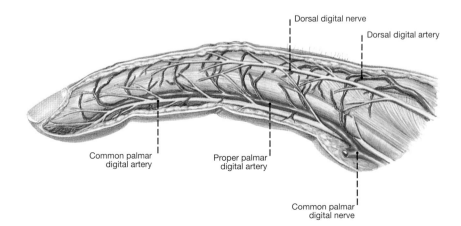

Dorsal digital nerve

Dorsal digital artery

Common palmar digital artery

Proper palmar digital artery

Common palmar digital nerve

Fig. 91: Nerves and Arteries of the Index Finger

NOTE: the **dorsal digital nerve and artery** extend only ²/₃rds the length of the finger. The distal ¹/₃rd is supplied by the **palmar digital nerve and artery,** which also supplies the entire palmar surface.

PLATE 70   Skeleton of the Thorax; Scapula

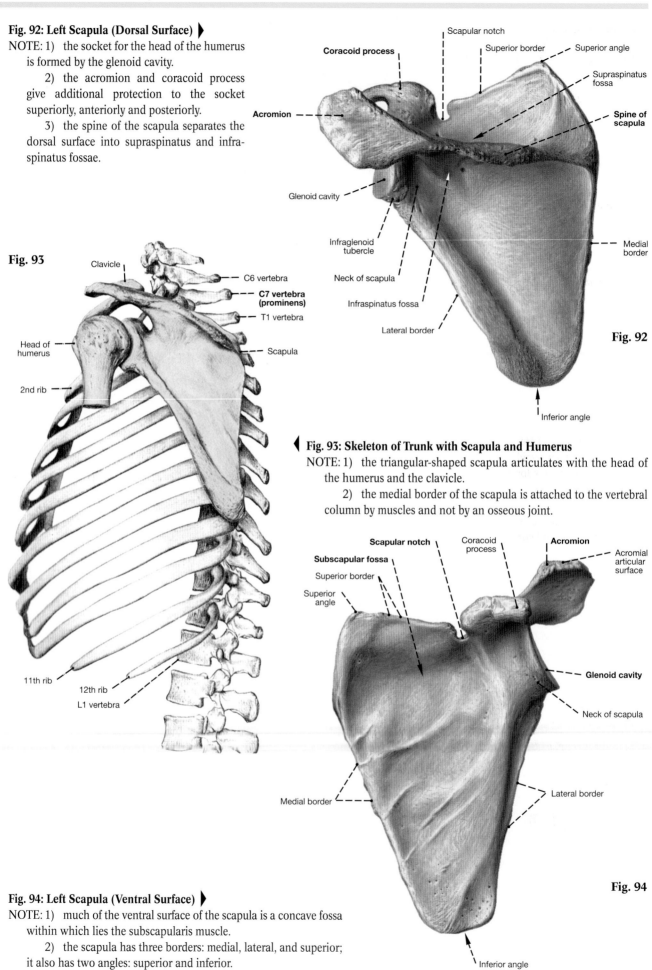

Fig. 92: Left Scapula (Dorsal Surface) ▶

NOTE: 1)   the socket for the head of the humerus
is formed by the glenoid cavity.

2)   the acromion and coracoid process
give additional protection to the socket
superiorly, anteriorly and posteriorly.

3)   the spine of the scapula separates the
dorsal surface into supraspinatus and infraspinatus fossae.

Scapular notch

Coracoid process

Superior border

Superior angle

Supraspinatus fossa

Acromion

Spine of scapula

Glenoid cavity

Infraglenoid tubercle

Medial border

Neck of scapula

Infraspinatus fossa

Lateral border

Fig. 92

Inferior angle

Fig. 93

Clavicle

C6 vertebra

C7 vertebra (prominens)

T1 vertebra

Head of humerus

Scapula

2nd rib

11th rib

12th rib

L1 vertebra

◀ **Fig. 93: Skeleton of Trunk with Scapula and Humerus**

NOTE: 1)   the triangular-shaped scapula articulates with the head of
the humerus and the clavicle.

2)   the medial border of the scapula is attached to the vertebral
column by muscles and not by an osseous joint.

Scapular notch

Coracoid process

Acromion

Acromial articular surface

Subscapular fossa

Superior border

Superior angle

Glenoid cavity

Neck of scapula

Medial border

Lateral border

Fig. 94

Fig. 94: Left Scapula (Ventral Surface) ▶

NOTE: 1)   much of the ventral surface of the scapula is a concave fossa
within which lies the subscapularis muscle.

2)   the scapula has three borders: medial, lateral, and superior;
it also has two angles: superior and inferior.

Inferior angle

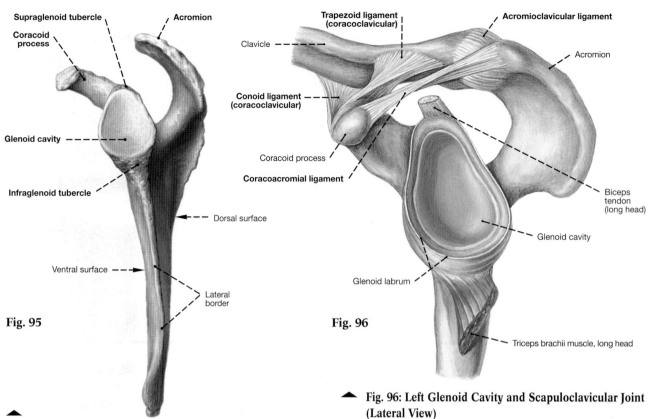

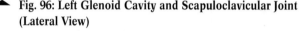

Fig. 95: Left Scapula, Lateral View

NOTE: 1) the supraglenoid and infraglenoid tubercles from which arise the long heads of the biceps and triceps muscles (see Fig. 39).

2) the anteriorly projecting coracoid process to which are attached the pectoralis minor, short head of biceps, and coracobrachialis muscles.

Fig. 96: Left Glenoid Cavity and Scapuloclavicular Joint (Lateral View)

NOTE: 1) the glenoid cavity was exposed by removing the articular capsule at the glenoid labrum.

2) the attachments at the supraglenoid (long head of biceps) and infraglenoid (long head of triceps) tubercles have been left intact.

3) the shallowness of the glenoid cavity is somewhat deepened (3 to 6 mm) by the glenoid labrum.

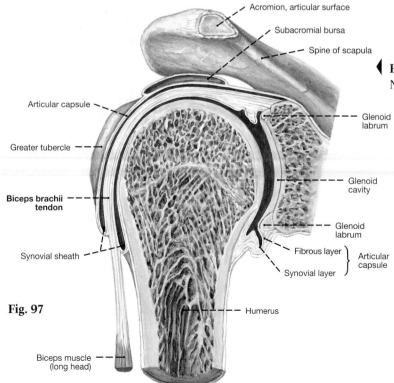

Fig. 97: Frontal Section Through Right Shoulder Joint

NOTE: 1) the tendon of the long head of the biceps is enclosed by a synovial sheath. Although the tendon passes through the joint, it is not within the synovial cavity.

2) the capsule of the joint is composed of a dense outer fibrous layer and a thin synovial inner layer.

3) a bursa is a sac lined by a synovial-like membrane. They are found at sites subjected to friction and usually do not communicate with the joint cavity.

4) in the shoulder, bursae are found between the capsule and muscle tendons such as the subscapularis, infraspinatus, and deltoid. The **subacromial bursa** lies deep to the coracoid and acromial processes.

PLATE 72   Acromioclavicular and Shoulder Joints

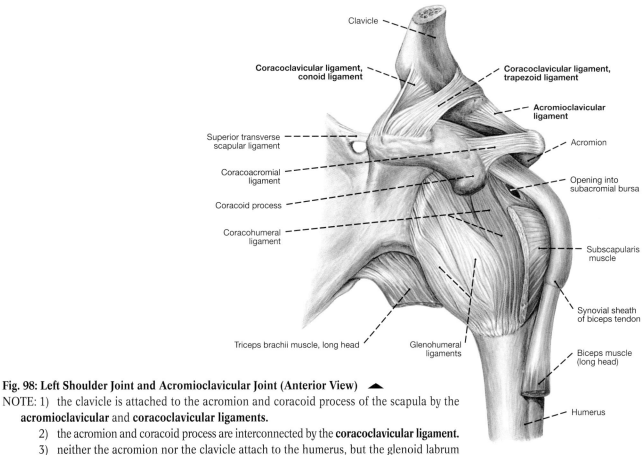

Clavicle

Coracoclavicular ligament, conoid ligament

Coracoclavicular ligament, trapezoid ligament

Acromioclavicular ligament

Superior transverse scapular ligament

Acromion

Coracoacromial ligament

Opening into subacromial bursa

Coracoid process

Coracohumeral ligament

Subscapularis muscle

Synovial sheath of biceps tendon

Triceps brachii muscle, long head

Glenohumeral ligaments

Biceps muscle (long head)

Humerus

Fig. 98: Left Shoulder Joint and Acromioclavicular Joint (Anterior View) ▲

NOTE: 1) the clavicle is attached to the acromion and coracoid process of the scapula by the **acromioclavicular** and **coracoclavicular ligaments.**

2)   the acromion and coracoid process are interconnected by the **coracoclavicular ligament.**

3)   neither the acromion nor the clavicle attach to the humerus, but the glenoid labrum and the coracoid process do.

4)   the acromion, coracoid process, and clavicle protect the shoulder from above. The joint is weakest inferiorly and anteriorly, directions where most dislocations occur.

5)   the **glenohumeral ligaments** are thickened bands that tend to strengthen the joint capsule anteriorly.

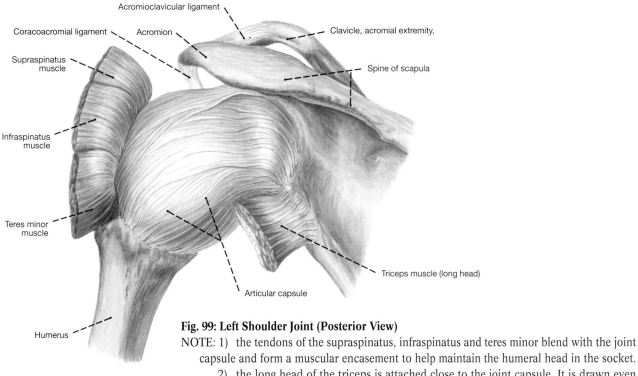

Acromioclavicular ligament

Coracoacromial ligament

Acromion

Clavicle, acromial extremity,

Supraspinatus muscle

Spine of scapula

Infraspinatus muscle

Teres minor muscle

Triceps muscle (long head)

Humerus

Articular capsule

Fig. 99: Left Shoulder Joint (Posterior View)

NOTE: 1) the tendons of the supraspinatus, infraspinatus and teres minor blend with the joint capsule and form a muscular encasement to help maintain the humeral head in the socket.

2)   the long head of the triceps is attached close to the joint capsule. It is drawn even closer in abduction of the arm and helps prevent dislocation.

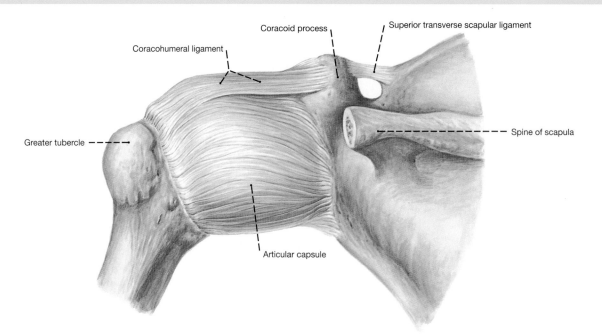

Fig. 100: Capsule of Left Shoulder Joint (Posterior View)

NOTE: 1) the articular capsule completely surrounds the joint. It is attached beyond the glenoid cavity on the scapula above and to the anatomical neck of the humerus below.

2) the superior part of the capsule is further strengthened by the coracohumeral ligament.

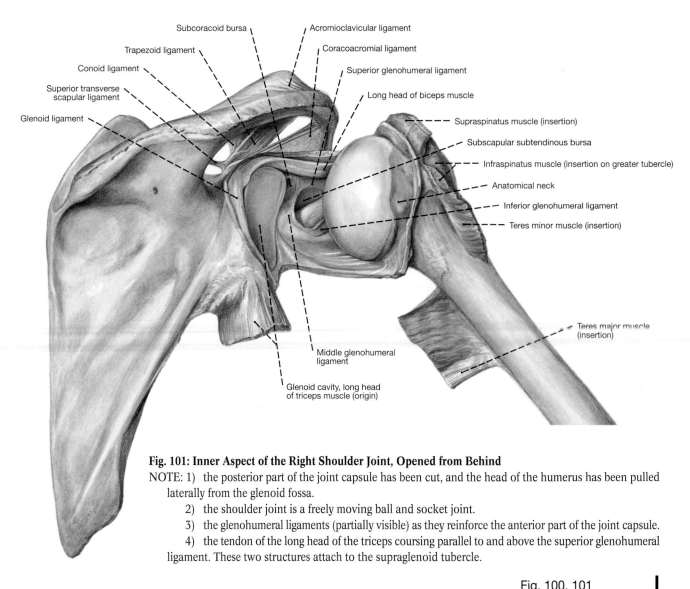

Fig. 101: Inner Aspect of the Right Shoulder Joint, Opened from Behind

NOTE: 1) the posterior part of the joint capsule has been cut, and the head of the humerus has been pulled laterally from the glenoid fossa.

2) the shoulder joint is a freely moving ball and socket joint.

3) the glenohumeral ligaments (partially visible) as they reinforce the anterior part of the joint capsule.

4) the tendon of the long head of the triceps coursing parallel to and above the superior glenohumeral ligament. These two structures attach to the supraglenoid tubercle.

PLATE 74   **Interior of the Shoulder Joint**

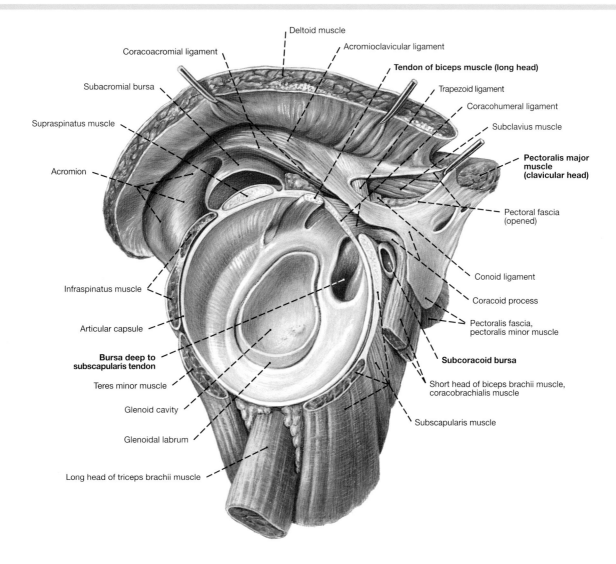

Deltoid muscle

Coracoacromial ligament

Acromioclavicular ligament

Tendon of biceps muscle (long head)

Subacromial bursa

Trapezoid ligament

Coracohumeral ligament

Supraspinatus muscle

Subclavius muscle

Acromion

Pectoralis major muscle (clavicular head)

Pectoral fascia (opened)

Infraspinatus muscle

Conoid ligament

Coracoid process

Articular capsule

Pectoralis fascia, pectoralis minor muscle

Bursa deep to subscapularis tendon

Subcoracoid bursa

Teres minor muscle

Short head of biceps brachii muscle, coracobrachialis muscle

Glenoid cavity

Subscapularis muscle

Glenoidal labrum

Long head of triceps brachii muscle

Fig. 102: Opened Socket of the Right Shoulder Joint

NOTE: 1) the head of the humerus has been removed from the glenoid fossa to reveal the glenoid labrum and the interior of the joint cavity.

2) the capsule of the joint is surrounded by muscles, the bellies or tendons of which are sectioned in this dissection. Sequentially these muscles include:

    a) the **supraspinatus** (tendon), **infraspinatus,** and **teres minor,** posteriorly

    b) the **long head of the triceps,** inferiorly, and

    c) the broad **subscapularis** muscle, anteriorly.

3) the entire joint is covered by the deltoid muscle, which arises from the clavicle, the acromion, and the spine of the scapula, and inserts on the deltoid tuberosity of the humerus.

4) the supraspinatus tendon and those of the infraspinatus, teres minor, and subscapularis muscles form the "rotator cuff". The first three tendons insert from above downward successively onto the greater tubercle, whereas the subscapularis inserts more anteriorly on the lesser tubercle. The "rotator cuff" helps hold the head of the humerus in the glenoid cavity of the scapula.

Fig. 102

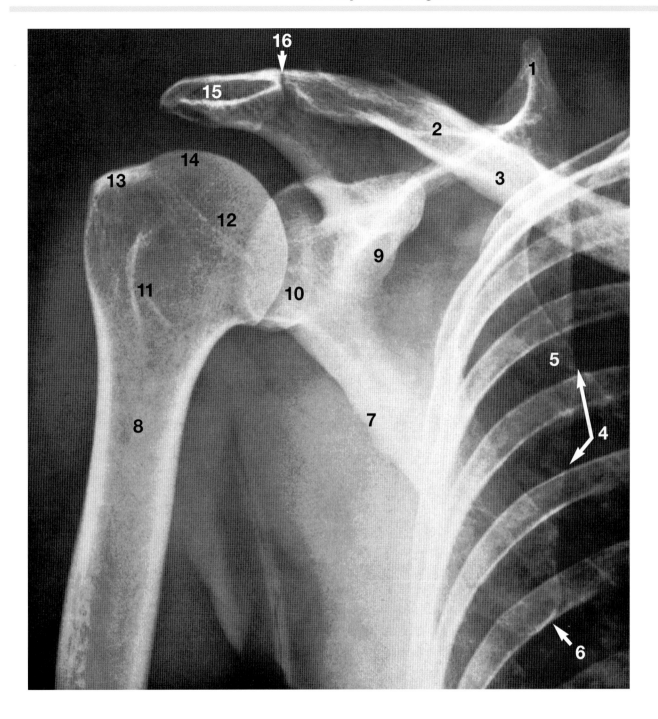

Fig 103· Radiograph of the Right Shoulder Region

1. Superior angle of scapula	5. Second rib	9. Coracoid process	13. Greater tubercle
2. Spine of scapula	6. Inferior angle of scapula	10. Glenoid cavity	14. Head of humerus
3. Clavicle	7. Lateral margin of scapula	11. Lesser tubercle	15. Acromion
4. Medial margin of scapula	8. Surgical neck of humerus	12. Anatomical neck of humerus	16. Acromioclavicular joint

NOTE: 1) the clavicle, scapula, and humerus are involved in the radiography of the shoulder region. The acromioclavicular joint is a **planar** type formed by the lateral end of the clavicle and the medial border of the acromion.

2) the glenohumeral, or shoulder, joint is remarkably loose and provides a free range of movement. Observe the wide separation between the humeral head and the glenoid cavity.

3) inferior **dislocations** of the head of the humerus are common because of minimal protection below. **A shoulder separation** results form a dislocation of the acromion under the lateral edge of the clavicle due to a strong blow to the lateral side of the joint.

4) the hemispheric smooth surface of the humeral head. Covered with hyalin cartilage, the head of the humerus is slightly constricted at the anatomical neck, where a line separates the articular part superomedially from the greater and lesser tubercles below.

5) below these tubercles, the humerus shows another constriction, called the surgical neck, where fractures frequently occur. (From Wicke L. Atlas of Radiologic Anatomy, 3rd Edition. Baltimore, Urban & Schwarzenberg, 1982).

Fig. 103   I

PLATE 76   Bones of the Upper Limb: Humerus

Figs. 104 and 105: Left Humerus

NOTE: 1) the hemispheric head of the humerus articulates with the glenoid cavity of the scapula.

2) the surgical neck of the humerus is frequently a site of fractures.

3) on the greater tubercle insert the supraspinatus, infraspinatus, and teres minor in that order. On the lesser tubercle inserts the subscapularis. These muscles form the **rotator cuff.**

4) within the intertubercular sulcus passes the tendon of the long head of the biceps.

5) adjacent to the **radial groove** courses the radial **nerve,** which is endangered by fractures of the humerus.

6) injury to the radial nerve in the arm results in a condition called **wrist drop,** because innervation to the extensors of the wrist and fingers is lost.

7) the distal extremity of the humerus articulates with the radius and ulna, the **capitulum** with the head of the radius, and the **trochlea** with the trochlear notch of the ulna.

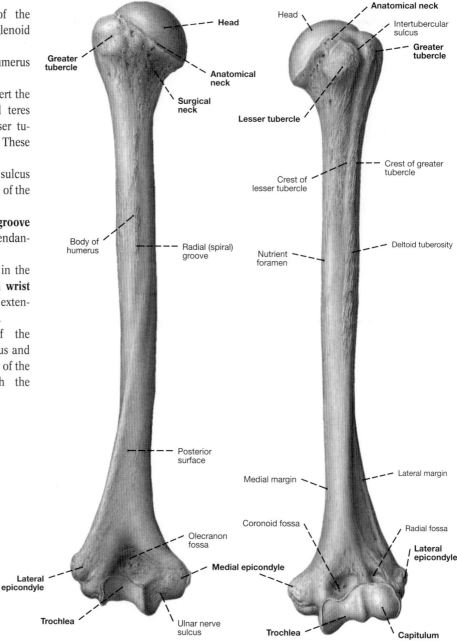

Fig. 104: Posterior View

Fig. 105: Anterior View

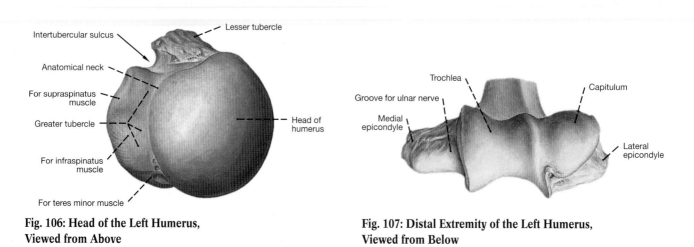

Fig. 106: Head of the Left Humerus, Viewed from Above

Fig. 107: Distal Extremity of the Left Humerus, Viewed from Below

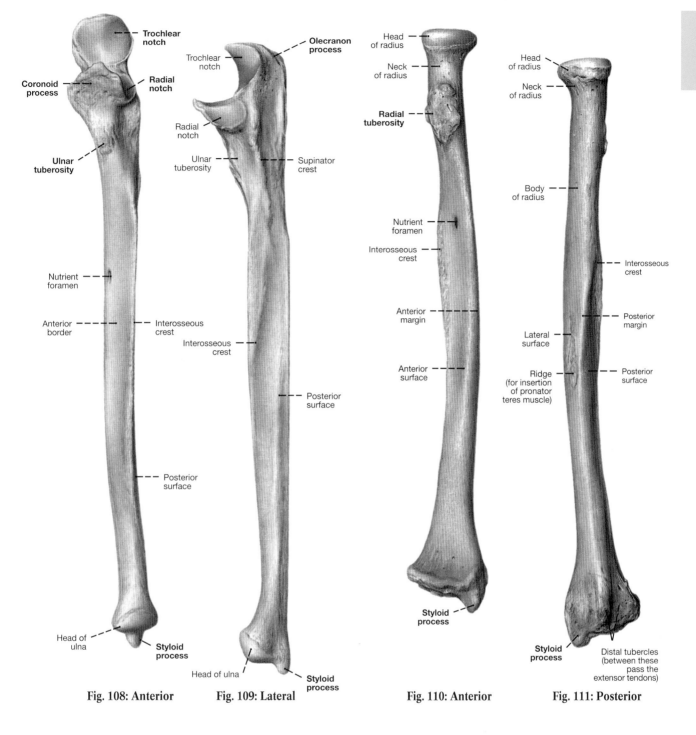

Fig. 108: Anterior   Fig. 109: Lateral   Fig. 110: Anterior   Fig. 111: Posterior

Left Ulna (Figs. 108 and 109)

NOTE: 1) the ulna is the medial bone of forearm. It has a superior extremity, a body or shaft, and an inferior extremity.

2) the **superior extremity** contains the **olecranon** and **coronoid processes** and two cavities, the **radial notch** for articulation with the radius and the **trochlear notch** for the trochlea of the humerus.

3) the brachialis muscle inserts on tuberosity of the ulna.

4) along the **body** of the ulna attaches the interosseous membrane.

5) the **distal extremity** is marked by the **ulnar head** laterally and the **styloid process** posteromedially.

Left Radius (Figs. 110 and 111)

NOTE: 1) the radius is situated lateral to the ulna, and it has a body and two extremities. Proximally, it attaches to both the humerus and ulna. Distally, it articulates with the carpal bones (scaphoid, lunate, and triquetrum) and with the ulna.

2) the **proximal extremity** contains a cylindrical head that articulates with both the **capitulum** of the humerus and the **radial notch** of the ulna.

3) onto the **radial tuberosity** inserts the tendon of the biceps brachii.

4) onto the **styloid process** attaches the brachioradialis muscle and the radial collateral ligament of the radiocarpal joint.

PLATE 78   Bones of the Wrist and Hand, Palmar Aspect

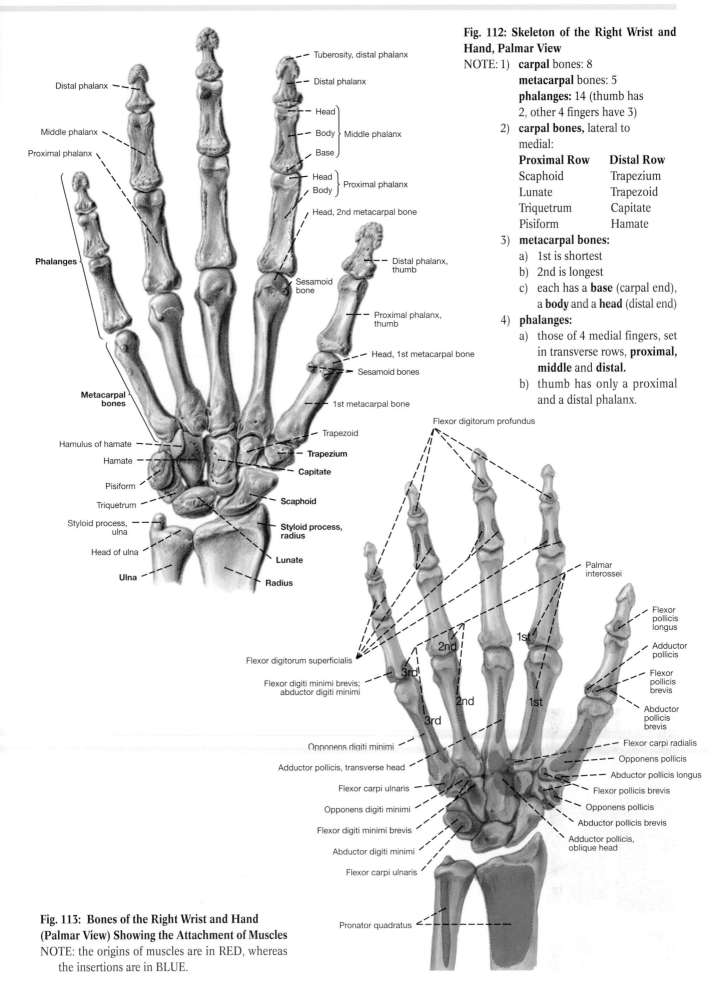

Tuberosity, distal phalanx

Distal phalanx

Distal phalanx

Middle phalanx

Head
Body } Middle phalanx
Base

Proximal phalanx

Head
Body } Proximal phalanx

Head, 2nd metacarpal bone

Phalanges

Distal phalanx, thumb

Sesamoid bone

Proximal phalanx, thumb

Metacarpal bones

Head, 1st metacarpal bone

Sesamoid bones

1st metacarpal bone

Hamulus of hamate

Trapezoid

Hamate

Trapezium

Pisiform

Capitate

Triquetrum

Scaphoid

Styloid process, ulna

Styloid process, radius

Head of ulna

Lunate

Ulna

Radius

Fig. 112: Skeleton of the Right Wrist and Hand, Palmar View

NOTE: 1) **carpal** bones: 8
metacarpal bones: 5
phalanges: 14 (thumb has 2, other 4 fingers have 3)

2) **carpal bones,** lateral to medial:

Proximal Row	Distal Row
Scaphoid	Trapezium
Lunate	Trapezoid
Triquetrum	Capitate
Pisiform	Hamate

3) **metacarpal bones:**
a) 1st is shortest
b) 2nd is longest
c) each has a **base** (carpal end), a **body** and a **head** (distal end)

4) **phalanges:**
a) those of 4 medial fingers, set in transverse rows, **proximal, middle** and **distal.**
b) thumb has only a proximal and a distal phalanx.

Flexor digitorum profundus

Palmar interossei

Flexor pollicis longus

Adductor pollicis

Flexor pollicis brevis

1st

2nd

1st

Abductor pollicis brevis

Flexor digitorum superficialis

3rd

2nd

1st

Flexor digiti minimi brevis; abductor digiti minimi

3rd

Flexor carpi radialis

Opponens digiti minimi

Opponens pollicis

Adductor pollicis, transverse head

Abductor pollicis longus

Flexor carpi ulnaris

Flexor pollicis brevis

Opponens digiti minimi

Opponens pollicis

Flexor digiti minimi brevis

Abductor pollicis brevis

Abductor digiti minimi

Adductor pollicis, oblique head

Flexor carpi ulnaris

Fig. 113: Bones of the Right Wrist and Hand (Palmar View) Showing the Attachment of Muscles
NOTE: the origins of muscles are in RED, whereas the insertions are in BLUE.

Pronator quadratus

Figs. 112, 113

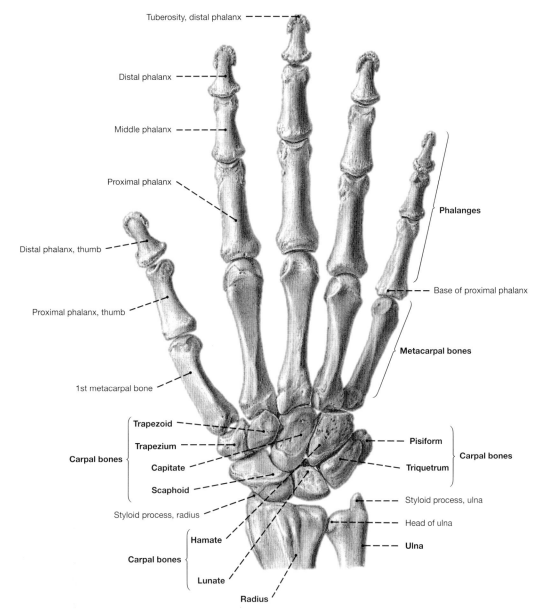

Tuberosity, distal phalanx

Distal phalanx

Middle phalanx

Proximal phalanx

Distal phalanx, thumb

Proximal phalanx, thumb

1st metacarpal bone

Phalanges

Base of proximal phalanx

Metacarpal bones

Trapezoid

Trapezium

Carpal bones

Capitate

Scaphoid

Styloid process, radius

Pisiform

Carpal bones

Triquetrum

Styloid process, ulna

Head of ulna

Ulna

Hamate

Carpal bones

Lunate

Radius

Fig. 114: Skeleton of the Right Wrist and Hand, Dorsal View

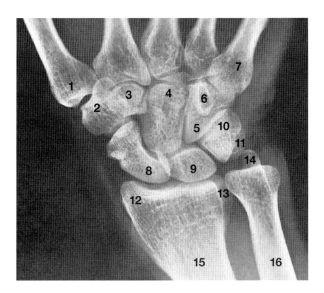

Fig. 115: X-ray of the Right Wrist, Dorso-ventral Projection
NOTE: following numbered structures:
1. Base of 1st metacarpal bone (thumb)
2. Trapezium bone
3. Trapezoid bone
4. Capitate bone
5. Hamate bone
6. Hamulus of hamate bone
7. Base of 5th metacarpal bone (little finger)
8. Scaphoid bone
9. Lunate bone
10. Triquetral bone
11. Pisiform bone
12. Styloid process of radius
13. Ulnar notch (distal radioulnar joint)
14. Styloid process of ulna
15. Radius
16. Ulna

(From Wicke L. Atlas of Radiologic Anatomy, 3rd Edition.
Baltimore, Urban & Schwarzenberg, 1982).

PLATE 80   Elbow and Radioulnar Joints, Ligaments

Fig. 116: Left Elbow Joint, Anterior View ▼

NOTE: 1) the elbow joint is a hinge or ginglymus joint.

2) the **trochlea** of the humerus is received in the trochlear notch of the ulna.

3) the **capitulum** of the humerus articulates with the head of the radius.

4) the articular capsule is loose, and it is thickened medially by the **ulnar collateral ligament** and laterally by the **radial collateral ligament.**

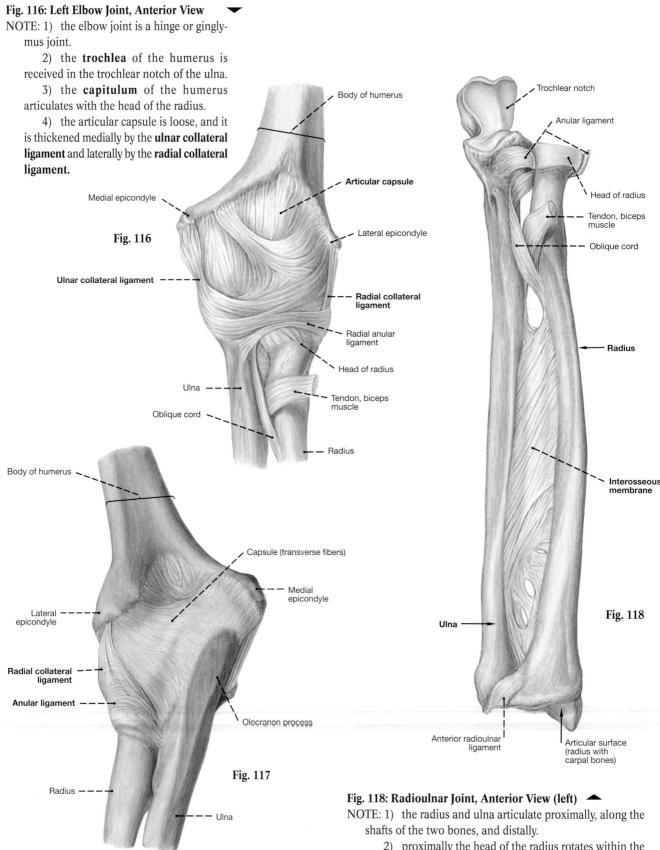

Fig. 116

Fig. 117: Left Elbow Joint, Posterolateral View ▲

NOTE: 1) the fan-shaped **radial collateral ligament** attaches above to the lateral epicondyle and blends with the capsule.

2) the upper border of the **radial anular ligament** also blends with the joint capsule.

Fig. 117

Fig. 118: Radioulnar Joint, Anterior View (left) ▲

NOTE: 1) the radius and ulna articulate proximally, along the shafts of the two bones, and distally.

2) proximally the head of the radius rotates within the radial notch of the ulna (pivot or trochoid joint).

3) the **anular ligament,** attached at both ends to the ulna, encircles the head of the radius, protecting the joint.

4) the interosseous membrane extends obliquely between the shafts of the two bones, whereas distally the head of the ulna attaches to the ulnar notch of the radius.

Fig. 118

Fig. 116, 117, 188

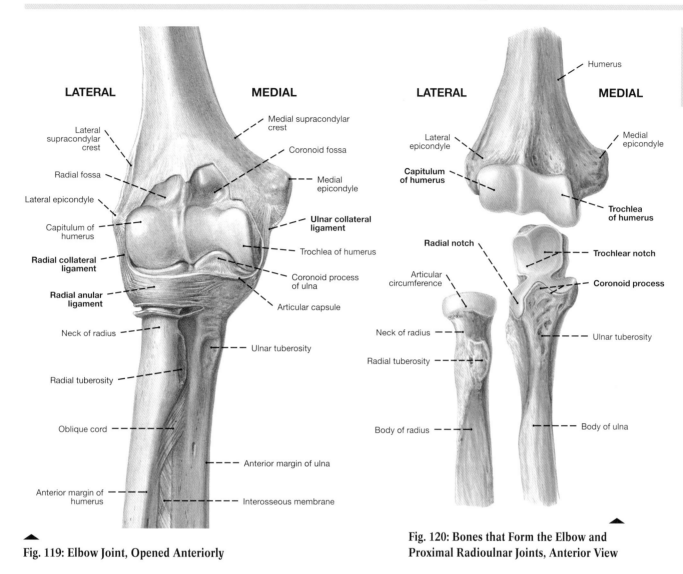

Fig. 119: Elbow Joint, Opened Anteriorly

Fig. 120: Bones that Form the Elbow and Proximal Radioulnar Joints, Anterior View

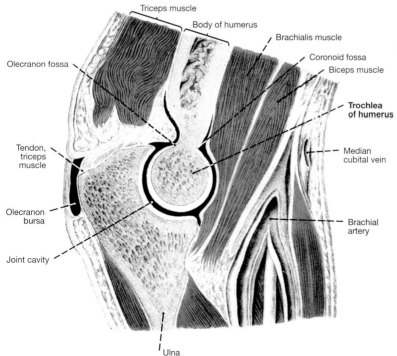

◀ **Fig. 121: Sagittal Section of the Left Elbow Joint**

NOTE: 1) the adaptation of the trochlea of the humerus with the trochlear notch of the ulna only allows flexion and extension and not lateral displacement.

2) the posterior surface of the olecranon is separated from the skin by a subcutaneous bursa and the insertion of the triceps.

3) **fractures** of the distal end of the humerus occur most often from falls on the outstretched hand, because the force is transmitted through the bones of the forearm to the humerus.

4) **fractures** of the olecranon result from direct trauma to the bone by a fall on the point of the elbow.

5) **posterior dislocation** of the ulna and attached radius is the most common dislocation at the elbow joint, again from falls on the outstretched and abducted hand.

Fig. 119, 120, 121 **I**

PLATE 82   Elbow Joint: Radiographs, Adult and Child

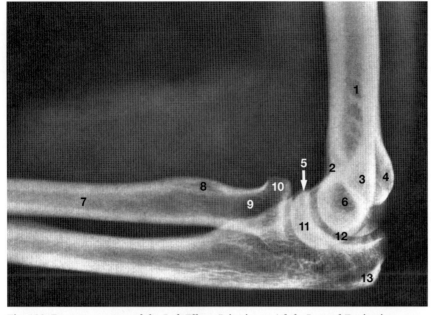

NOTE the following bony structures:

1. Body of humerus
2. Radial fossa
3. Olecranon fossa
4. Medial epicondyle
5. Coronoid process of ulna
6. Trochlea of humerus
7. Body of radius
8. Radial tuberosity
9. Neck of radius
10. Head of radius
11. Capitulum of humerus
12. Trochlear notch
13. Olecranon

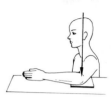

Fig. 122: Roentgenogram of the Left Elbow Joint in an Adult, Lateral Projection ▲

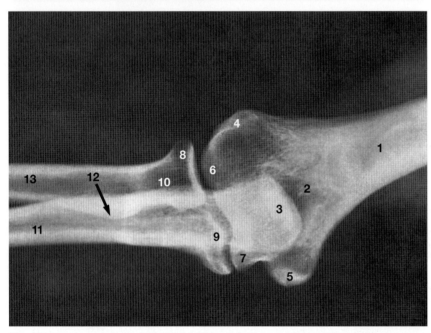

NOTE the following bony structures:

1. Body of humerus
2. Olecranon fossa
3. Olecranon
4. Lateral epicondyle
5. Medial epicondyle
6. Capitulum of humerus
7. Trochlea of humerus
8. Head of radius
9. Coronoid process of ulna
10. Neck of radius
11. Ulna
12. Radial tuberosity
13. Body of radius

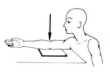

(Figures 96 and 97 from Wicke L. Atlas of Radiologic Anatomy, 4th Edition. Baltimore, Urban & Schwarzenberg, 1987).

Fig. 123: Roentgenogram of the Right Elbow Joint in an Adult (AP Projection) ▲

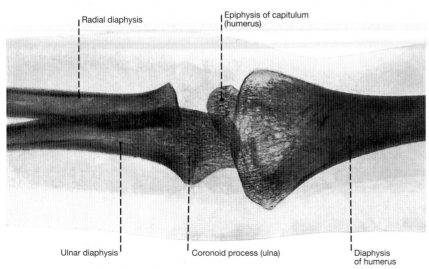

Radial diaphysis | Epiphysis of capitulum (humerus)

Ulnar diaphysis | Coronoid process (ulna) | Diaphysis of humerus

Fig. 124: Roentgenogram of the Elbow Joint in a 5½-Year-Old Boy

NOTE: 1) the shaft of a long bone is called the **diaphysis,** whereas a center of ossification, distinct from the shaft and usually at the end of a long bone, is called an **epiphysis.**

2) the epiphysis of the head of the radius is as yet not formed in the 5½-year-old child, whereas ossification has started in the humeral capitulum.

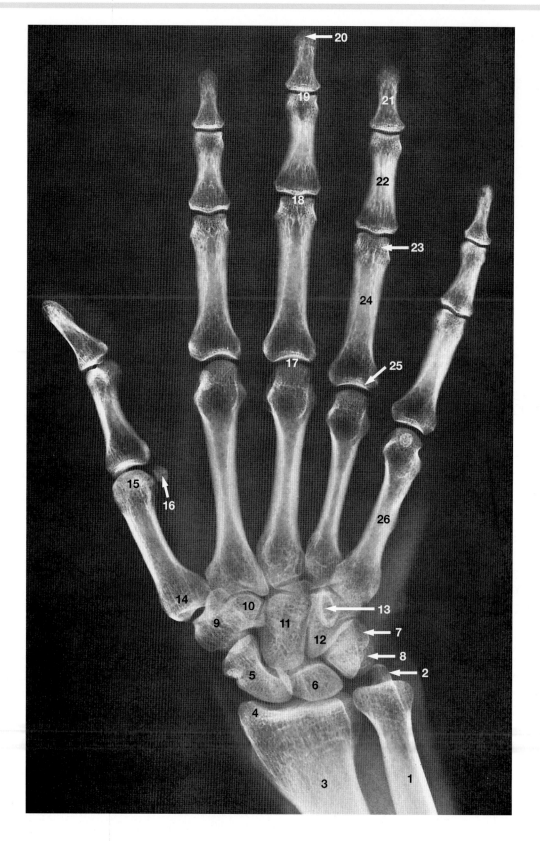

Fig. 125: X-ray of the Right Wrist and Hand, Dorsopalmar View

1.	Ulna	10.	Trapezoid	19.	Distal interphalangeal joint
2.	Styloid process of ulna	11.	Capitate	20.	Tuberosity of distal phalanx
3.	Radius	12.	Hamate	21.	Distal phalanx
4.	Styloid process of radius	13.	Hamulus of hamate	22.	Middle phalanx
5.	Scaphoid	14.	Base of 1st metacarpal bone		
6.	Lunate	15.	Head of 1st metacarpal bone		
7.	Triquetral	16.	Sesamoid bone		
8.	Pisiform	17.	Metacarpophalangeal joint		
9.	Trapezium	18.	Proximal interphalangeal joint		

23.	Head of phalanx
24.	Proximal phalanx
25.	Base of phalanx
26.	5th metacarpal bone

(From Wicke L. Atlas of Radiologic Anatomy, 4th Edition. Baltimore, Urban & Schwarzenberg, 1987).

Fig. 125   **I**

PLATE 84   **Wrist and Hand: Ligaments and Joints**

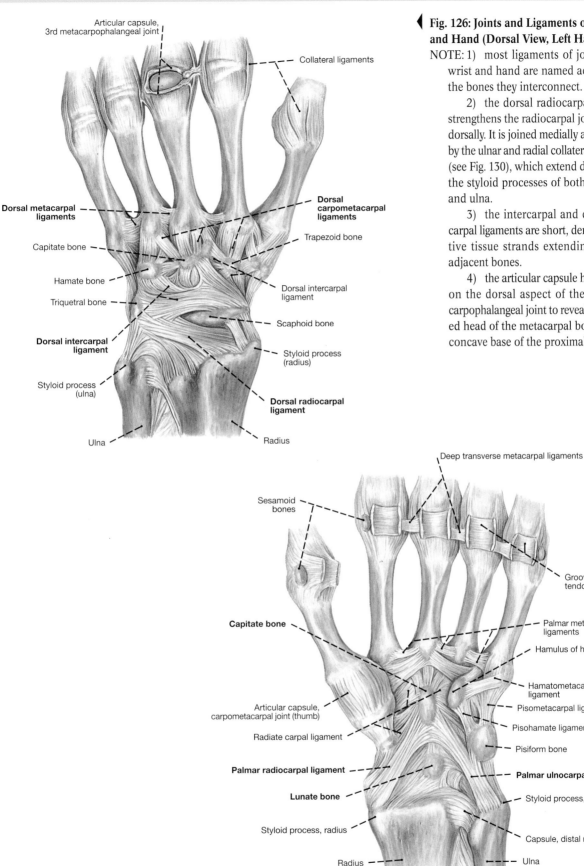

Articular capsule,
3rd metacarpophalangeal joint

Collateral ligaments

Dorsal metacarpal ligaments

Dorsal carpometacarpal ligaments

Capitate bone

Trapezoid bone

Hamate bone

Dorsal intercarpal ligament

Triquetral bone

Scaphoid bone

Dorsal intercarpal ligament

Styloid process (radius)

Styloid process (ulna)

Dorsal radiocarpal ligament

Ulna

Radius

Fig. 126: Joints and Ligaments of the Wrist and Hand (Dorsal View, Left Hand)

NOTE: 1) most ligaments of joints in the wrist and hand are named according to the bones they interconnect.

    2) the dorsal radiocarpal ligament strengthens the radiocarpal joint capsule dorsally. It is joined medially and laterally by the ulnar and radial collateral ligaments (see Fig. 130), which extend distally from the styloid processes of both the radius and ulna.

    3) the intercarpal and carpometacarpal ligaments are short, dense connective tissue strands extending between adjacent bones.

    4) the articular capsule has been cut on the dorsal aspect of the 3rd metacarpophalangeal joint to reveal the rounded head of the metacarpal bone and the concave base of the proximal phalanx.

Deep transverse metacarpal ligaments

Sesamoid bones

Grooves for flexor tendons

Capitate bone

Palmar metacarpal ligaments

Hamulus of hamate bone

Hamatometacarpal ligament

Articular capsule, carpometacarpal joint (thumb)

Pisometacarpal ligament

Pisohamate ligament

Radiate carpal ligament

Pisiform bone

Palmar radiocarpal ligament

Palmar ulnocarpal ligament

Lunate bone

Styloid process, ulna

Styloid process, radius

Capsule, distal radioulnar joint

Radius

Ulna

Fig. 127: Joints and Ligaments of the Wrist and Hand (Palmar View, Left Hand)

NOTE: 1) several strong ligaments in the palmar hand: the radiate ligament surrounding the capitate bone as well as pisohamate and pisometacarpal ligaments.

    2) the bases of the metacarpal bones are joined by the palmar metacarpal ligaments and the distal heads by the deep transverse metacarpal ligament.

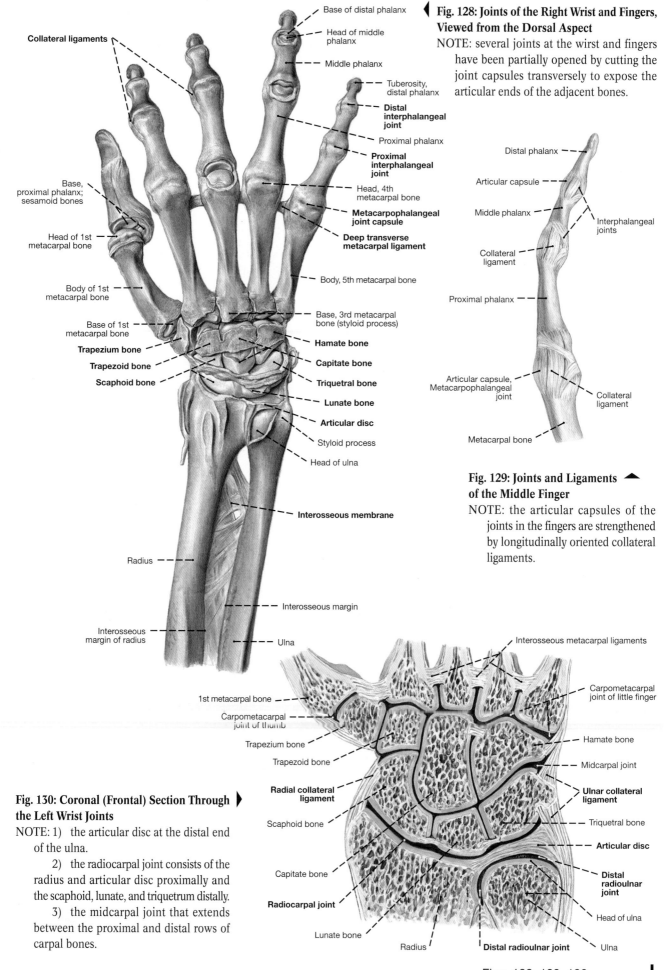

Collateral ligaments

Base of distal phalanx

Head of middle phalanx

Middle phalanx

Tuberosity, distal phalanx

Distal interphalangeal joint

Proximal phalanx

Proximal interphalangeal joint

Head, 4th metacarpal bone

Metacarpophalangeal joint capsule

Deep transverse metacarpal ligament

Base, proximal phalanx; sesamoid bones

Head of 1st metacarpal bone

Body of 1st metacarpal bone

Body, 5th metacarpal bone

Base of 1st metacarpal bone

Base, 3rd metacarpal bone (styloid process)

Trapezium bone

Hamate bone

Trapezoid bone

Capitate bone

Scaphoid bone

Triquetral bone

Lunate bone

Articular disc

Styloid process

Head of ulna

Interosseous membrane

Radius

Interosseous margin

Interosseous margin of radius

Ulna

Fig. 128: Joints of the Right Wrist and Fingers, Viewed from the Dorsal Aspect

NOTE: several joints at the wirst and fingers have been partially opened by cutting the joint capsules transversely to expose the articular ends of the adjacent bones.

Distal phalanx

Articular capsule

Middle phalanx

Interphalangeal joints

Collateral ligament

Proximal phalanx

Articular capsule, Metacarpophalangeal joint

Collateral ligament

Metacarpal bone

Fig. 129: Joints and Ligaments of the Middle Finger

NOTE: the articular capsules of the joints in the fingers are strengthened by longitudinally oriented collateral ligaments.

Interosseous metacarpal ligaments

1st metacarpal bone

Carpometacarpal joint of little finger

Carpometacarpal joint of thumb

Trapezium bone

Hamate bone

Trapezoid bone

Midcarpal joint

Radial collateral ligament

Ulnar collateral ligament

Scaphoid bone

Triquetral bone

Articular disc

Capitate bone

Distal radioulnar joint

Radiocarpal joint

Head of ulna

Lunate bone

Radius

Distal radioulnar joint

Ulna

Fig. 130: Coronal (Frontal) Section Through the Left Wrist Joints

NOTE: 1) the articular disc at the distal end of the ulna.

2) the radiocarpal joint consists of the radius and articular disc proximally and the scaphoid, lunate, and triquetrum distally.

3) the midcarpal joint that extends between the proximal and distal rows of carpal bones.

Figs. 128, 129, 130

PLATE 86   Cross-sections of the Upper Limb: Arm

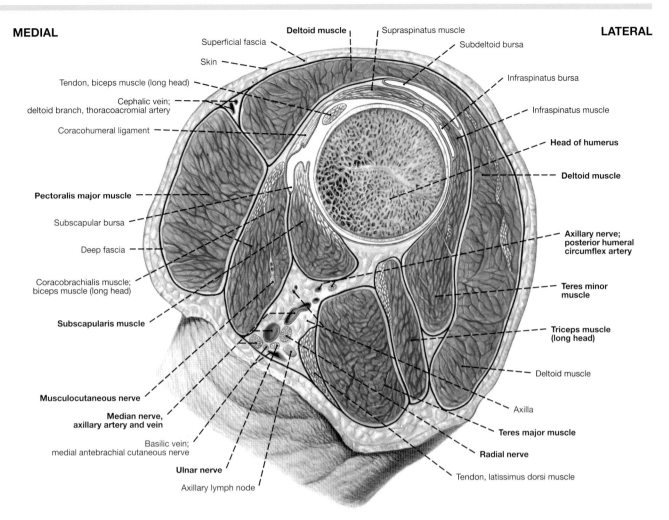

Fig. 131: Cross-section of the Right Upper Extremity Through the Head of the Humerus, Viewed from Above

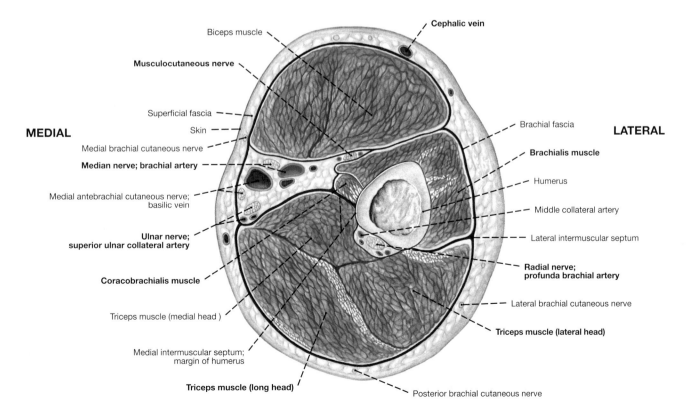

Fig. 132: Cross-section of the Right Upper Extremity Through the Middle of the Humerus, Viewed from Above

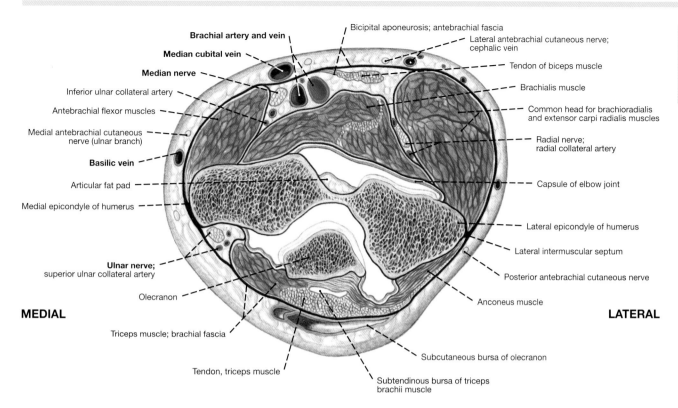

Fig. 133: Cross-section Through the Right Upper Extremity at the Level of the Elbow Joint

NOTE: 1) the ulnar nerve and superior ulnar collateral artery lie behind the medial epicondyle of the humerus, medial to the olecranon of the ulna.

2) the median nerve lies to the ulnar (medial) side of the brachial vein and artery in the cubital fossa, and all three structures lie deep to the cubital fascia and median cubital vein.

3) at this level, the radial nerve and radial collateral artery lie between the common origins of the extensor muscles **and** the deeply located brachialis muscle.

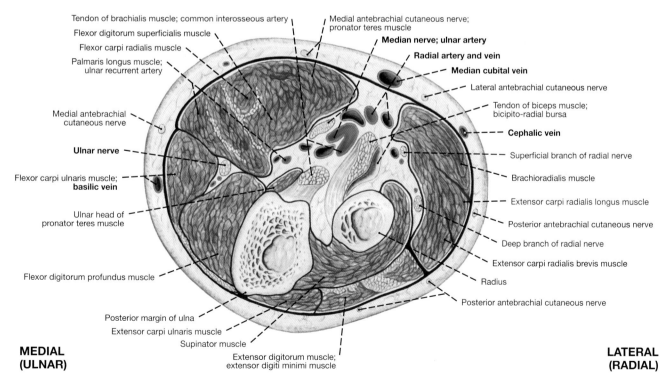

Fig. 134: Cross-section Through the Proximal Third of the Right Forearm

NOTE: 1) the common interosseous artery branching from the ulnar artery and the insertions of the biceps brachii and brachialis muscles to the radius and ulna, respectively.

2) the radial nerve has already divided into its superficial and deep branches.

PLATE 88   **Cross-sections of the Upper Limb: Middle and Distal Forearm**

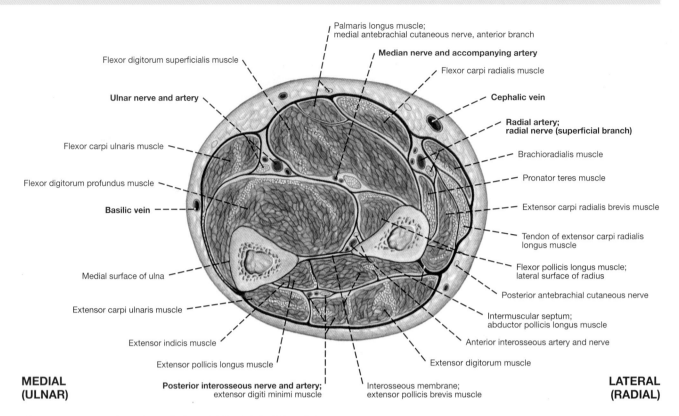

Palmaris longus muscle;
medial antebrachial cutaneous nerve, anterior branch

Median nerve and accompanying artery

Flexor carpi radialis muscle

Flexor digitorum superficialis muscle

Ulnar nerve and artery

Cephalic vein

**Radial artery;
radial nerve (superficial branch)**

Flexor carpi ulnaris muscle

Brachioradialis muscle

Flexor digitorum profundus muscle

Pronator teres muscle

Extensor carpi radialis brevis muscle

Basilic vein

Tendon of extensor carpi radialis
longus muscle

Flexor pollicis longus muscle;
lateral surface of radius

Medial surface of ulna

Posterior antebrachial cutaneous nerve

Extensor carpi ulnaris muscle

Intermuscular septum;
abductor pollicis longus muscle

Extensor indicis muscle

Anterior interosseous artery and nerve

Extensor pollicis longus muscle

Extensor digitorum muscle

**MEDIAL
(ULNAR)**

Posterior interosseous nerve and artery;
extensor digiti minimi muscle

Interosseous membrane;
extensor pollicis brevis muscle

**LATERAL
(RADIAL)**

Fig. 135: Cross-section Through the Middle Third of the Right Forearm
NOTE: 1)   at this level, the ulna, radius, interosseous membrane, and intermuscular septum clearly delineate the **posterior compartment,**
extending dorsally and laterally, from the **anterior compartment** located anteriorly and medially.
  2)   the **median nerve** coursing down the forearm deep to the flexor digitorum superficialis and anterior to the flexor digitorum
profundus and flexor pollicis longus.

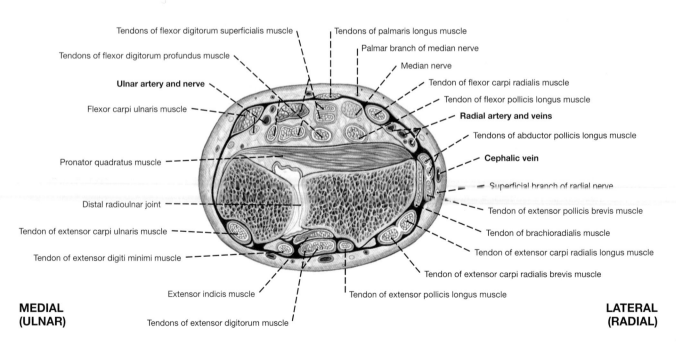

Tendons of flexor digitorum superficialis muscle

Tendons of palmaris longus muscle

Palmar branch of median nerve

Tendons of flexor digitorum profundus muscle

Median nerve

Ulnar artery and nerve

Tendon of flexor carpi radialis muscle

Tendon of flexor pollicis longus muscle

Flexor carpi ulnaris muscle

Radial artery and veins

Pronator quadratus muscle

Tendons of abductor pollicis longus muscle

Cephalic vein

Superficial branch of radial nerve

Distal radioulnar joint

Tendon of extensor pollicis brevis muscle

Tendon of extensor carpi ulnaris muscle

Tendon of brachioradialis muscle

Tendon of extensor digiti minimi muscle

Tendon of extensor carpi radialis longus muscle

Tendon of extensor carpi radialis brevis muscle

Extensor indicis muscle

Tendon of extensor pollicis longus muscle

**MEDIAL
(ULNAR)**

Tendons of extensor digitorum muscle

**LATERAL
(RADIAL)**

Fig. 136: Cross-section Through the Distal Third of the Right Forearm
NOTE 1)   in the distal forearm, the **ulnar nerve** has given off its dorsal branch, which supplies the ulnar part of the dorsum of the hand
and the dorsal surfaces of the little finger and half of the ring finger.
  2)   the extreme vulnerability of the ulnar nerve and artery, median nerve, radial artery, as well as all of the flexor tendons on
the anterior aspect of the wrist, and the extensor tendons and cephalic vein dorsally.

Fig. 135, 136

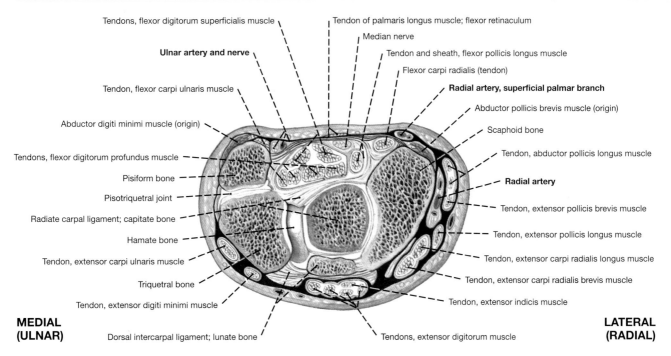

Tendons, flexor digitorum superficialis muscle
Tendon of palmaris longus muscle; flexor retinaculum
Median nerve
Ulnar artery and nerve
Tendon and sheath, flexor pollicis longus muscle
Flexor carpi radialis (tendon)
Tendon, flexor carpi ulnaris muscle
Radial artery, superficial palmar branch
Abductor digiti minimi muscle (origin)
Abductor pollicis brevis muscle (origin)
Scaphoid bone
Tendons, flexor digitorum profundus muscle
Tendon, abductor pollicis longus muscle
Pisiform bone
Radial artery
Pisotriquetral joint
Radiate carpal ligament; capitate bone
Tendon, extensor pollicis brevis muscle
Hamate bone
Tendon, extensor pollicis longus muscle
Tendon, extensor carpi ulnaris muscle
Tendon, extensor carpi radialis longus muscle
Triquetral bone
Tendon, extensor carpi radialis brevis muscle
Tendon, extensor digiti minimi muscle
Tendon, extensor indicis muscle

MEDIAL (ULNAR)
LATERAL (RADIAL)
Dorsal intercarpal ligament; lunate bone
Tendons, extensor digitorum muscle

Fig. 137: Cross-section Through the Hand at the Level of the First Row of Carpal Bones

NOTE: 1) the median nerve and the tendons of the flexors digitorum superficialis and profundus and the tendon of the flexor pollicis longus course deep to the **flexor retinaculum** into the hand through a space called the **carpal tunnel** (not labelled).

2) the carpal tunnel is a common site for compression of the median nerve resulting in a palsy called the carpal tunnel syndrome.

3) the ulnar nerve and artery course into the hand superficial to the flexor retinaculum.

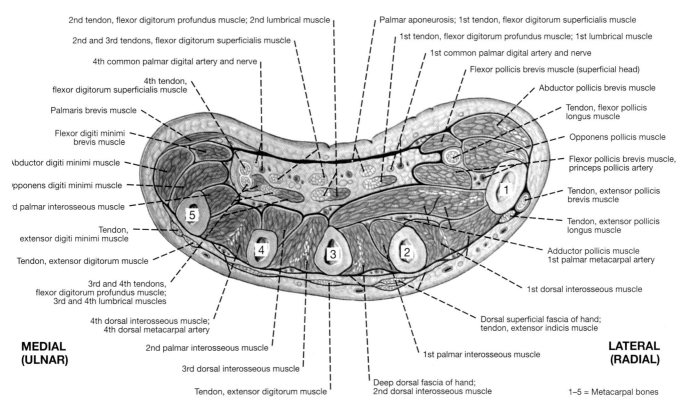

2nd tendon, flexor digitorum profundus muscle; 2nd lumbrical muscle
Palmar aponeurosis; 1st tendon, flexor digitorum superficialis muscle
2nd and 3rd tendons, flexor digitorum superficialis muscle
1st tendon, flexor digitorum profundus muscle; 1st lumbrical muscle
4th common palmar digital artery and nerve
1st common palmar digital artery and nerve
4th tendon, flexor digitorum superficialis muscle
Flexor pollicis brevis muscle (superficial head)
Palmaris brevis muscle
Abductor pollicis brevis muscle
Flexor digiti minimi brevis muscle
Tendon, flexor pollicis longus muscle
Abductor digiti minimi muscle
Opponens pollicis muscle
Opponens digiti minimi muscle
Flexor pollicis brevis muscle, princeps pollicis artery
3rd palmar interosseous muscle
Tendon, extensor pollicis brevis muscle
Tendon, extensor digiti minimi muscle
Tendon, extensor pollicis longus muscle
Tendon, extensor digitorum muscle
Adductor pollicis muscle 1st palmar metacarpal artery
3rd and 4th tendons, flexor digitorum profundus muscle; 3rd and 4th lumbrical muscles
1st dorsal interosseous muscle
4th dorsal interosseous muscle; 4th dorsal metacarpal artery
Dorsal superficial fascia of hand; tendon, extensor indicis muscle

MEDIAL (ULNAR)
2nd palmar interosseous muscle
1st palmar interosseous muscle
LATERAL (RADIAL)
3rd dorsal interosseous muscle
Deep dorsal fascia of hand; 2nd dorsal interosseous muscle
Tendon, extensor digitorum muscle
1–5 = Metacarpal bones

Fig. 138: Cross-section of the Right Hand Through the Metacarpal Bones

NOTE: 1) the four **dorsal interosseous muscles** that act as abductors of the fingers and fill the intervals between the metacarpal bones.

2) the three **palmar interosseous muscles** that serve as adductors of the fingers.

3) the **thenar muscles** on the radial side of the hand, and the **hypothenar muscles** on the ulnar side.

PLATE 90   Section of Fingers: Cross and Longitudinal; Fingernails

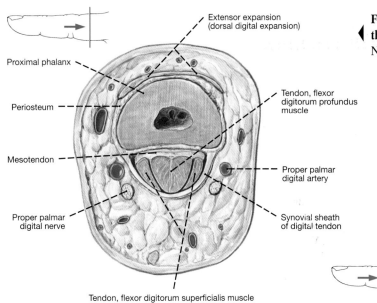

Proximal phalanx

Periosteum

Mesotendon

Proper palmar digital nerve

Extensor expansion (dorsal digital expansion)

Tendon, flexor digitorum profundus muscle

Proper palmar digital artery

Synovial sheath of digital tendon

Tendon, flexor digitorum superficialis muscle

Fig. 139: Cross-section of the Middle Finger Through the Proximal Phalanx

NOTE: 1) the extensor expansion (or extensor hood) over the dorsal aspect of the proximal phalanx and part of the middle phalanx.

2) into the extensor expansion blend the tendon of the extensor digitorum and the tendons of insertion of the adjacent interosseous and lumbrical muscles.

3) the synovial sheath on the palmar side of the phalanx, which surrounds the superficial and deep flexor tendons of the digit.

Fig. 140: Cross-section of the Middle Finger Through the Middle Phalanx

NOTE: 1) the location of the proper digital arteries and nerves within the subcutaneous tissue on the sides of the deep flexor tendon.

2) knowing the location of these neurovascular structures is important both for the application of local anesthesia to the digit and for the cessation of severe bleeding.

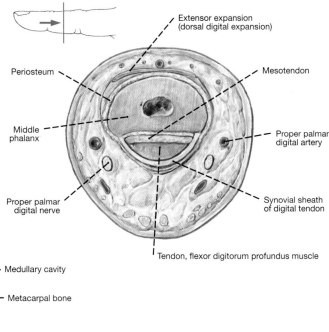

Extensor expansion (dorsal digital expansion)

Periosteum

Mesotendon

Middle phalanx

Proper palmar digital artery

Proper palmar digital nerve

Synovial sheath of digital tendon

Tendon, flexor digitorum profundus muscle

Articular capsule, metacarpophalangeal joint

Articular cartilage

Proximal phalanx

Tendon, periosteum

Head of phalanx

Articular capsule, interphalangeal joint

Base of middle phalanx

Medullary cavity

Metacarpal bone

Articular capsule, metacarpophalangeal joint

Distal phalanx

Middle phalanx

Fig. 141: Longitudinal Section Through a Flexed Finger

NOTE: the location of the flexion creases in relation to the corresponding joints.

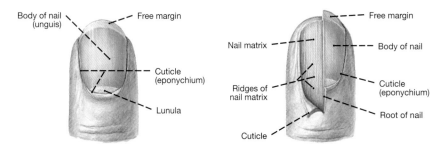

Body of nail (unguis)

Free margin

Cuticle (eponychium)

Lunula

Nail matrix

Ridges of nail matrix

Cuticle

Free margin

Body of nail

Cuticle (eponychium)

Root of nail

Free margin

Body of nail

Lateral margin

Lunula

Hidden margin

Root of nail

Fig. 142: Finger Nail, Normal Position (Dorsal View)

Fig. 143: Left Half of Finger Nailbed Exposed

Fig. 144: Body of Fingernail Removed From the Nailbed

Fig. 139–144

PART II
THE THORAX

(PLATES 91–158 – FIGURES 145–245)

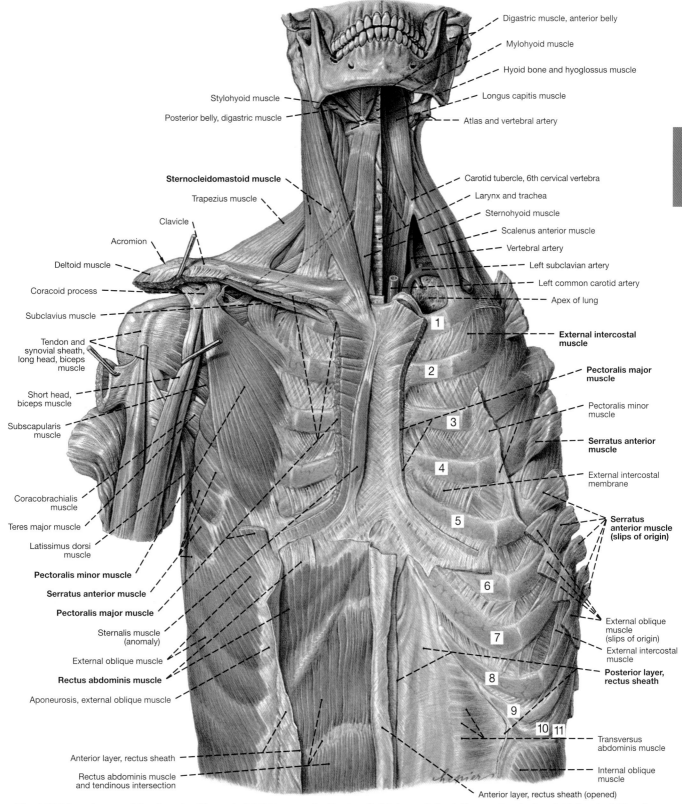

Digastric muscle, anterior belly

Mylohyoid muscle

Hyoid bone and hyoglossus muscle

Longus capitis muscle

Atlas and vertebral artery

Stylohyoid muscle

Posterior belly, digastric muscle

Carotid tubercle, 6th cervical vertebra

Larynx and trachea

Sternohyoid muscle

Scalenus anterior muscle

Vertebral artery

Left subclavian artery

Left common carotid artery

Apex of lung

Sternocleidomastoid muscle

Trapezius muscle

Clavicle

Acromion

Deltoid muscle

Coracoid process

Subclavius muscle

Tendon and synovial sheath, long head, biceps muscle

Short head, biceps muscle

Subscapularis muscle

Coracobrachialis muscle

Teres major muscle

Latissimus dorsi muscle

Pectoralis minor muscle

Serratus anterior muscle

Pectoralis major muscle

Sternalis muscle (anomaly)

External oblique muscle

Rectus abdominis muscle

Aponeurosis, external oblique muscle

Anterior layer, rectus sheath

Rectus abdominis muscle and tendinous intersection

External intercostal muscle

Pectoralis major muscle

Pectoralis minor muscle

Serratus anterior muscle

External intercostal membrane

Serratus anterior muscle (slips of origin)

External oblique muscle (slips of origin)

External intercostal muscle

Posterior layer, rectus sheath

Transversus abdominis muscle

Internal oblique muscle

Anterior layer, rectus sheath (opened)

1 2 3 4 5 6 7 8 9 10 11

Fig. 145: Musculature of the Anterior Thoracic Wall Deep to the Pectoralis Major and the Adjacent Cervical and Abdominal Muscles
NOTE: 1)   on the right side (reader's left), the anterior thoracic wall and upper arm are shown after removal of the pectoralis major muscle.

2)   on the left (reader's right), the upper limb and the superficial trunk and cervical muscles have been removed, exposing the ribs and intercostal tissues.

Muscle	Origin	Insertion	Innervation	Action
Subclavius	1st rib and its cartilage at their junction	Groove on the lower surface of middle ⅓rd of clavicle	Nerve to subclavius from upper trunk of brachial plexus (C5,C6)	Depresses and pulls clavicle forward

Fig. 145   II

PLATE 92   Anterior Thoracic Wall: Vessels and Nerves

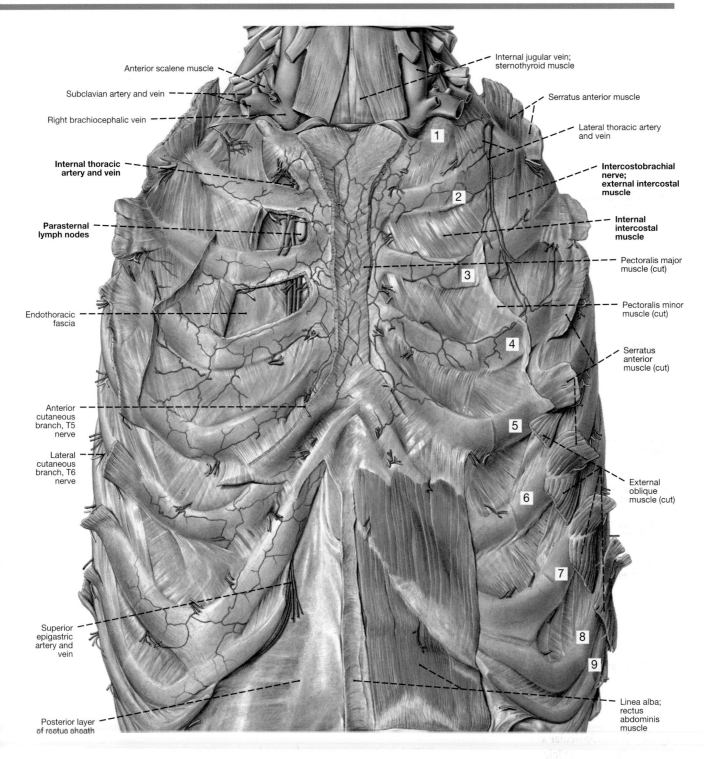

Anterior scalene muscle

Subclavian artery and vein

Right brachiocephalic vein

Internal thoracic artery and vein

Parasternal lymph nodes

Endothoracic fascia

Anterior cutaneous branch, T5 nerve

Lateral cutaneous branch, T6 nerve

Superior epigastric artery and vein

Posterior layer of rectus sheath

Internal jugular vein; sternothyroid muscle

Serratus anterior muscle

Lateral thoracic artery and vein

Intercostobrachial nerve; external intercostal muscle

Internal intercostal muscle

Pectoralis major muscle (cut)

Pectoralis minor muscle (cut)

Serratus anterior muscle (cut)

External oblique muscle (cut)

Linea alba; rectus abdominis muscle

Fig. 146: Anterior Thoracic Wall: Deep Vessels and Nerves

Muscle	Origin	Insertion	Innervation	Action
External Intercostal (11 muscles)	The lower border of a rib	Upper border of the rib below	Intercostal nerves	Elevate the ribs; active during normal inspiration
	Within intercostal space, each extends from the tubercle of the rib dorsally to the cartilage of the rib ventrally			
Internal Intercostal (11 muscles)	Ridge on the inner surface near lower border of rib	Upper border of the rib below	Intercostal nerves	Elevate the ribs; active during inspiration and expiration
	Within intercostal space, each extends from the sternum ventrally to the angle of the rib dorsally			

Fig. 146

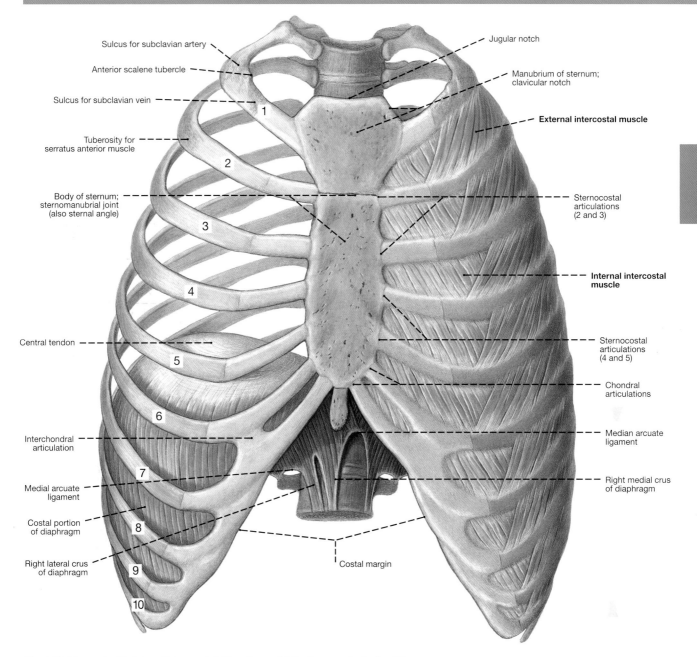

Sulcus for subclavian artery

Anterior scalene tubercle

Sulcus for subclavian vein

Tuberosity for serratus anterior muscle

Body of sternum; sternomanubrial joint (also sternal angle)

Central tendon

Interchondral articulation

Medial arcuate ligament

Costal portion of diaphragm

Right lateral crus of diaphragm

Jugular notch

Manubrium of sternum; clavicular notch

External intercostal muscle

Sternocostal articulations (2 and 3)

Internal intercostal muscle

Sternocostal articulations (4 and 5)

Chondral articulations

Median arcuate ligament

Right medial crus of diaphragm

Costal margin

Fig. 147: Thoracic Skeleton, Intercostal Muscles and Diaphragm, Anterior View

Fig. 148: Sternoclavicular and the First Two Sternocostal Joints

NOTE: 1) the sternoclavicular joint is formed by the junction of the clavicle with a) the upper lateral aspect of the manubrium and b) the cartilage of the first rib.

2) an articular disc is interposed between the clavicle and sternum and an articular capsule and fibrous ligamentous bands protect the joint.

3) the cartilages of the 2nd to the 7th ribs (see Fig. 147) articulate with the sternum by movable (diarthrodial) joints. The cartilage of the 1st rib, however, directly joins the sternum and, without a joint cavity, forms an immovable joint (synarthrosis).

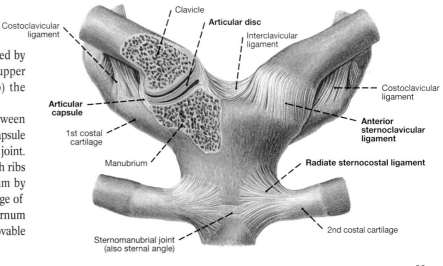

Costoclavicular ligament

Clavicle

Articular disc

Interclavicular ligament

Costoclavicular ligament

Anterior sternoclavicular ligament

Radiate sternocostal ligament

Articular capsule

1st costal cartilage

Manubrium

2nd costal cartilage

Sternomanubrial joint (also sternal angle)

PLATE 94   Thoracic Cage, Anterior View; Clavicle

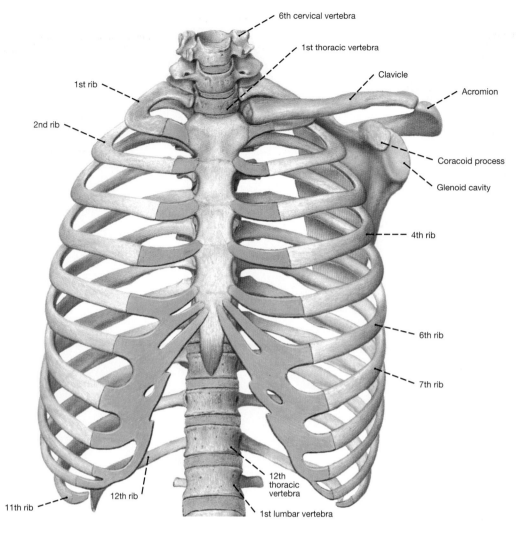

6th cervical vertebra

1st thoracic vertebra

Clavicle

Acromion

1st rib

2nd rib

Coracoid process

Glenoid cavity

4th rib

6th rib

7th rib

12th thoracic vertebra

11th rib

12th rib

1st lumbar vertebra

Fig. 149: Thoracic Skeleton, Anterior View

Left clavicle and scapula in yellow; costal cartilages and intervertebral discs are blue.

NOTE: 1) the skeleton of the thorax protects the thoracic organs. It is formed by 12 pairs of ribs that articulate posteriorly with the 12 thoracic vertebrae. Anteriorly the bony parts of the ribs are continued as cartilages, the upper 7 pairs of which are attached directly to the sternum.

2) the bony parts of the ribs fall progressively more lateral to the sternum from above downward, resulting in longer costal cartilages in lower ribs than in higher ones.

3) the thoracic cage is narrow superiorly at its inlet, but more broad inferiorly where it is in relationship to abdominal structures.

Fig. 150: Left Clavicle, Inferior View ▼

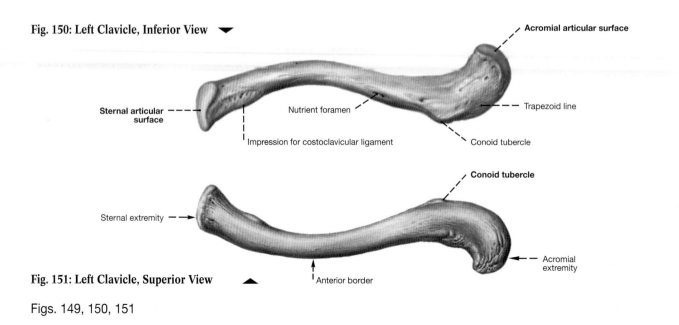

Acromial articular surface

Sternal articular surface

Nutrient foramen

Trapezoid line

Impression for costoclavicular ligament

Conoid tubercle

Conoid tubercle

Sternal extremity

Acromial extremity

Fig. 151: Left Clavicle, Superior View ▲

Anterior border

Figs. 149, 150, 151

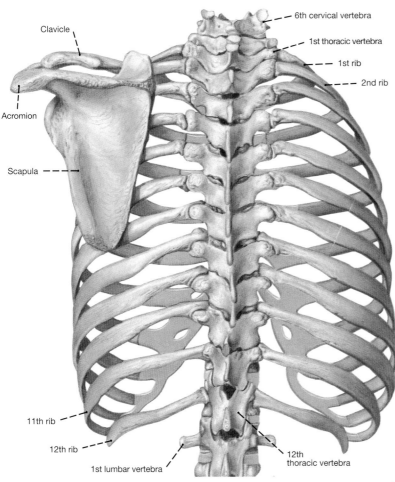

Clavicle

Acromion

Scapula

6th cervical vertebra

1st thoracic vertebra

1st rib

2nd rib

11th rib

12th rib

1st lumbar vertebra

12th thoracic vertebra

Fig. 152: Thoracic Skeleton, Posterior View
Left clavicle and scapula are shown in yellow.
NOTE: 1) the posterior skeleton of the thoracic cage consists of 12 thoracic vertebrae and the posterior parts of 12 pairs of ribs.

2) the extremity on the head of typical ribs possesses two articular facets separated by a crest (see Fig. 155: 8th rib).

3) these two facets articulate with the bodies of two adjacent vertebrae, whereas the crest is attached to the intervertebral disc. The lower facet articulates with the vertebra that corresponds with the rib, whereas the upper facet articulates with the adjacent vertebra above.

4) the crest between the facets articulates with the intervertebral disc.

5) the scapula affords some bony protection posteriorly to the upper lateral aspect of the thoracic cage.

Fig. 153: Sternum, Anterior View
NOTE: 1) the sternum consists of the manubrium, the body, and the xiphoid process and forms the middle portion of the anterior thoracic wall.

2) the manubrium articulates with the body at the **sternal angle.** The xiphoid process is thin and often cartilaginous.

3) the concave jugular notch, two clavicular notches and the 1st costal notches on the manubrium.

Fig. 154: Sternum, Lateral View
NOTE: 1) the clavicle and the 1st rib articulate with the manubrium. The 2nd rib articulates at the sternal angle. The 3rd to the 6th ribs articulate with the body of the sternum, whereas the 7th rib joins the sternum at the junction of the xiphoid process.

2) a line projected backward through the sternal angle crosses at the 4th thoracic level, whereas the xiphisternal junction lies at T9.

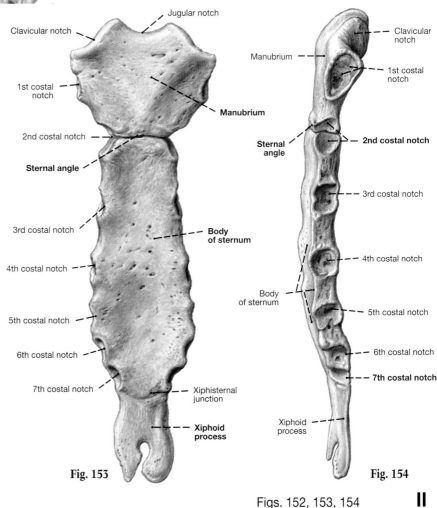

Jugular notch

Clavicular notch

1st costal notch

Manubrium

2nd costal notch

Sternal angle

3rd costal notch

4th costal notch

5th costal notch

6th costal notch

7th costal notch

Manubrium

Sternal angle

Body of sternum

Xiphisternal junction

Xiphoid process

Clavicular notch

Manubrium

1st costal notch

Sternal angle

2nd costal notch

3rd costal notch

Body of sternum

4th costal notch

5th costal notch

6th costal notch

7th costal notch

Xiphoid process

Fig. 153

Fig. 154

Figs. 152, 153, 154   **II**

PLATE 96   Thoracic Cage: Ribs

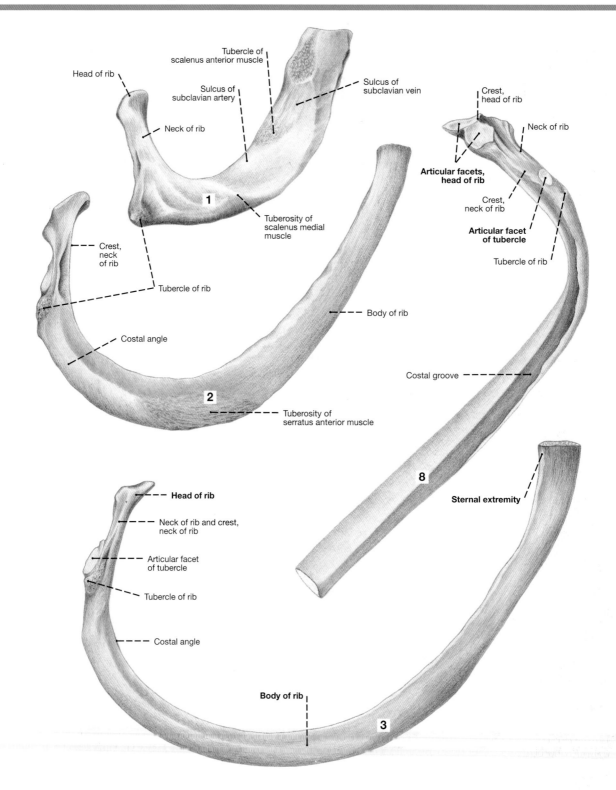

Fig. 155: 1st, 2nd, 3rd, and 8th Right Ribs

NOTE: 1) the superior surfaces of the 1st, 2nd, and 3rd ribs are illustrated in this figure, whereas the inferior surface of the 8th rib is shown.

2) each rib has a vertebral extremity directed posteriorly and a sternal extremity directed anteriorly. The body of the rib is the shaft that stretches between the extremities.

3) the vertebral end is marked by a **head,** a **neck,** and a **tubercle.** The head contains two facets for articulation with the bodies of the thoracic vertebrae, whereas the tubercle has a nonarticular roughened elevation and an articular facet, which attaches to the transverse process of thoracic vertebrae.

4) the 1st, 2nd, 10th, 11th and 12th ribs present certain structural differences from the 3rd through the 9th ribs. The 1st rib is the most curved, and the 2nd is shaped similar to the 1st, but it is longer. The 10th, 11th, and 12th ribs also have only a single facet on the rib-head.

Fig. 155

Fig. 156: Sternocostal Articulations, Frontal Section, ▶
Posterior View

NOTE: 1) the articulations of the first pair of ribs do not have joint
cavities but are directly cartilaginous unions (synchondroses),
similar to the joint between the manubrium and body of the
sternum.

2) each of the other sternocostal joints contains a true joint
cavity surrounded by a capsule. Intraarticular sternocostal ligaments
also attach the rib cartilage to the sternum. These are most frequently
found at the junctions of the 2nd and 3rd cartilages with the
sternum, but also may be seen in lower sternocostal joints.

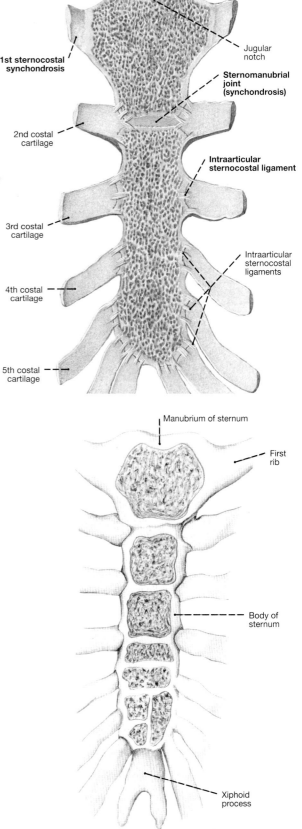

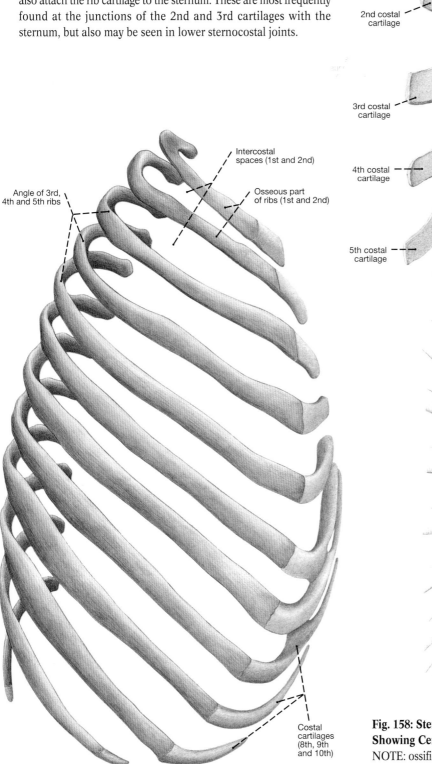

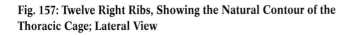

**Fig. 157: Twelve Right Ribs, Showing the Natural Contour of the
Thoracic Cage; Lateral View**

Fig. 158: Sternum of an 11-Year-Old Child, ▲
Showing Centers of Ossification

NOTE: ossification in the sternum starts in the manubrium
during the 5th or 6th prenatal month.

Other centers develop in the sternal body between the
7th month and the end of the 1st postnatal year.

PLATE 98   Thoracic Cage: Radiograph of the Chest

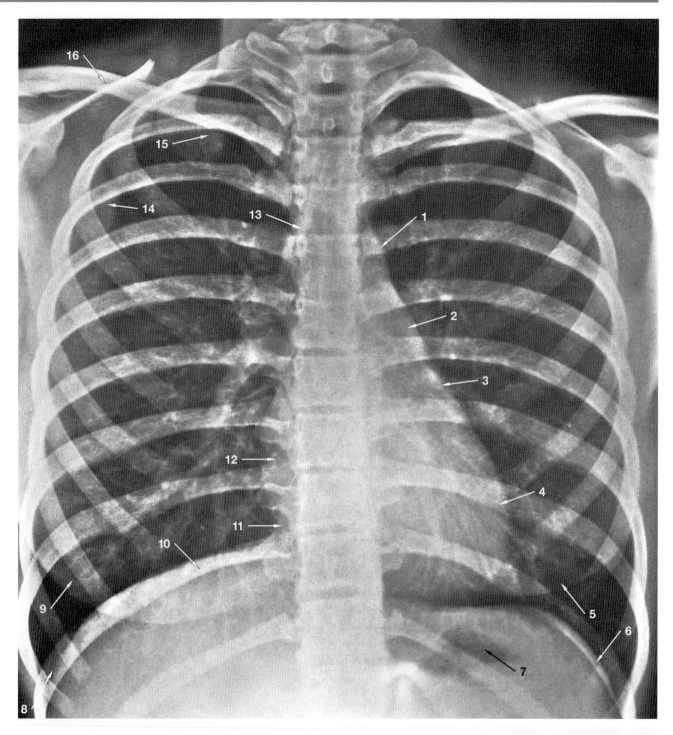

Fig. 159: Posterior-Anterior Radiograph of the Thorax Showing the Heart and Lungs

NOTE: 1) the contour of the heart and great vessels: arch of aorta (1), pulmonary trunk (2), inferior vena cava (11), and superior vena cava (13), and the relationship of these structures to the vertebral column.

2) the left margin of the heart is formed by the left auricle (3) and left ventricle (4), and it slopes toward the apex, which usually lies about 9 cm to the left of the midsternal line, deep to the 5th intercostal space.

3) the right margin of the heart (12) projects as a curved line slightly to the right of the vertebral column (and sternum). Observe that the heart rests on the diaphragm (6) and note the contours of the left (5) and right (9) breasts.

(From Wicke L. Atlas of Radiographic Anatomy, 4th Edition. Baltimore, Urban and Schwarzenberg, 1985).

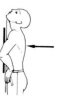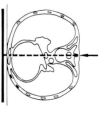

1. Arch of aorta	5. Contour of left breast	9. Contour of right breast	13. Superior vena cava
2. Pulmonary trunk	6. Diaphragm	10. Diaphragm	14. Medial border of scapula
3. Left auricle	7. Air in fundus of stomach	11. Inferior vena cava	15. First rib
4. Left ventricle	8. Costodiaphragmatic recess	12. Right atrium	16. Right clavicle

Fig. 159

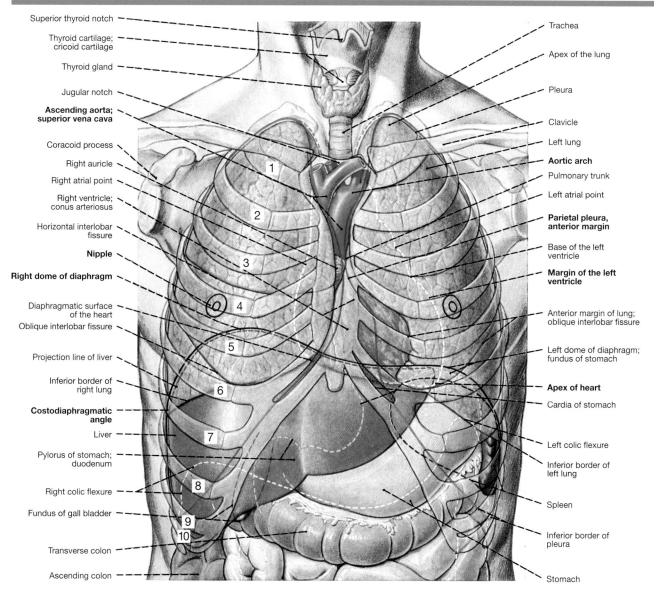

Superior thyroid notch
Thyroid cartilage; cricoid cartilage
Thyroid gland
Jugular notch
Ascending aorta; superior vena cava
Coracoid process
Right auricle
Right atrial point
Right ventricle; conus arteriosus
Horizontal interlobar fissure
Nipple
Right dome of diaphragm
Diaphragmatic surface of the heart
Oblique interlobar fissure
Projection line of liver
Inferior border of right lung
Costodiaphragmatic angle
Liver
Pylorus of stomach; duodenum
Right colic flexure
Fundus of gall bladder
Transverse colon
Ascending colon

Trachea
Apex of the lung
Pleura
Clavicle
Left lung
Aortic arch
Pulmonary trunk
Left atrial point
Parietal pleura, anterior margin
Base of the left ventricle
Margin of the left ventricle
Anterior margin of lung; oblique interlobar fissure
Left dome of diaphragm; fundus of stomach
Apex of heart
Cardia of stomach
Left colic flexure
Inferior border of left lung
Spleen
Inferior border of pleura
Stomach

Fig. 160: Thoracic and Upper Abdominal Viscera Projected onto the Anterior Surface of the Body

NOTE: 1) the outline of the heart and great vessels (white broken line) deep to the anterior border of the lungs.

2) the liver, lying below the diaphragm, extends upward as high as the 4th interspace on the right, and to the 5th interspace on the left (red broken line).

3) the superficial location of the superior vena cava and ascending aorta just deep to the manubrium of the sternum.

4) a triangular region containing the great vessels above and a lower triangular region over the heart (area of superficial cardiac dullness) are not covered by pleura.

5) the reflections of the pleura over the lungs. Observe that the anterior margins of the lung and pleura on the left side are indented to form the cardiac notch.

6) the position of the nipple over the 4th rib (or 4th intercostal space) in the male and in the young female. Observe also the apex of the heart deep to the 5th interspace.

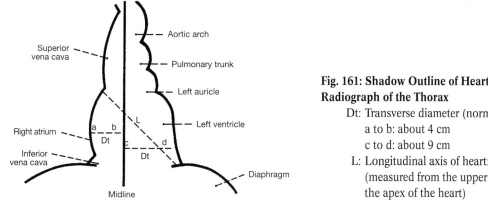

Superior vena cava
Right atrium
Inferior vena cava
Midline

Aortic arch
Pulmonary trunk
Left auricle
Left ventricle
Diaphragm

Fig. 161: Shadow Outline of Heart and Great Vessels in Radiograph of the Thorax

Dt: Transverse diameter (normal)
   a to b: about 4 cm
   c to d: about 9 cm
L: Longitudinal axis of heart: 15 to 16 cm
   (measured from the upper end of the right atrial shadow to the apex of the heart)

PLATE 100   **Anterior Thoracic and Abdominal Wall: Inner Surface**

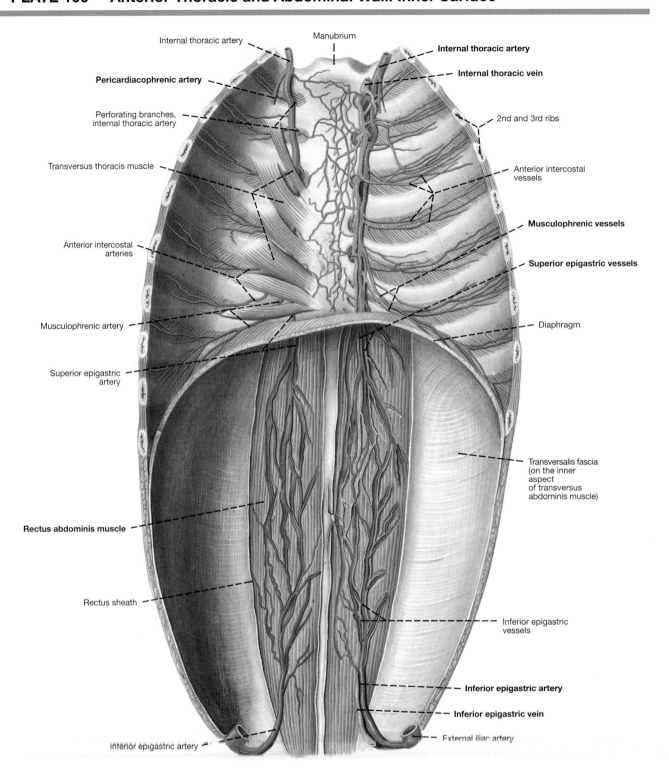

Internal thoracic artery
Manubrium
Internal thoracic artery
Pericardiacophrenic artery
Internal thoracic vein
Perforating branches, internal thoracic artery
2nd and 3rd ribs
Transversus thoracis muscle
Anterior intercostal vessels
Musculophrenic vessels
Anterior intercostal arteries
Superior epigastric vessels
Musculophrenic artery
Diaphragm
Superior epigastric artery
Transversalis fascia (on the inner aspect of transversus abdominis muscle)
Rectus abdominis muscle
Rectus sheath
Inferior epigastric vessels
Inferior epigastric artery
Inferior epigastric vein
External iliac artery
Inferior epigastric artery

Fig. 162: Muscles and Blood Vessels of the Thoracic and Abdominal Wall, Viewed from the Inside
NOTE: 1) the principal vessels dissected include the **internal thoracic** and **inferior epigastric** arteries and veins and their terminal branches.

2) the internal thoracic artery is a branch of the subclavian artery, and it descends behind the costal cartilages along the inner surface of the anterior thoracic wall in front of the transverse thoracis muscle and parallel to the margin of the sternum.

3) the internal thoracic artery gives rise to (a) the pericardiacophrenic artery, (b) small vessels to the thymus and to bronchial structures, (c) perforating branches to the chest wall, (d) anterior intercostal branches and finally it terminates as (e) the **musculophrenic** and **superior epigastric arteries.**

4) the superior epigastric artery anastomoses with the **inferior epigastric artery,** a branch of the external iliac artery. The anastomosis occurs within the rectus abdominis muscle.

Fig. 162

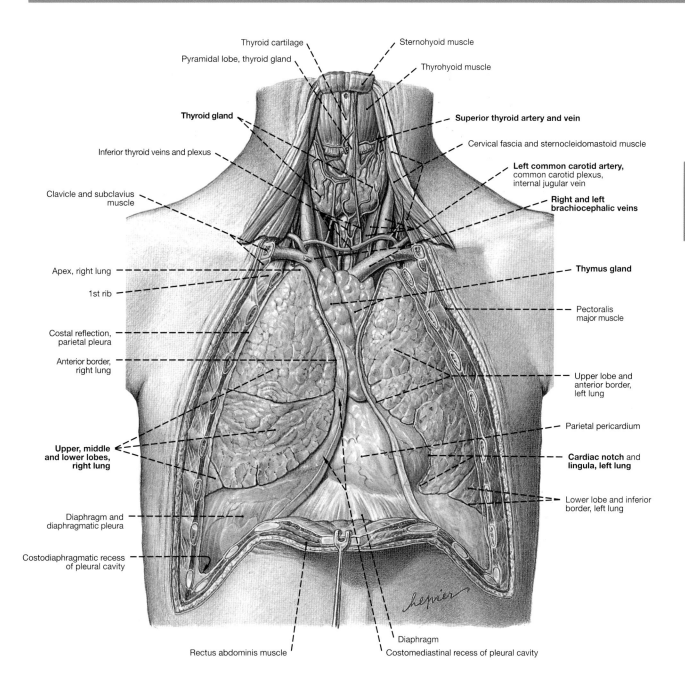

Thyroid cartilage

Pyramidal lobe, thyroid gland

Sternohyoid muscle

Thyrohyoid muscle

Thyroid gland

Inferior thyroid veins and plexus

Clavicle and subclavius muscle

Apex, right lung

1st rib

Costal reflection, parietal pleura

Anterior border, right lung

Upper, middle and lower lobes, right lung

Diaphragm and diaphragmatic pleura

Costodiaphragmatic recess of pleural cavity

Superior thyroid artery and vein

Cervical fascia and sternocleidomastoid muscle

Left common carotid artery, common carotid plexus, internal jugular vein

Right and left brachiocephalic veins

Thymus gland

Pectoralis major muscle

Upper lobe and anterior border, left lung

Parietal pericardium

Cardiac notch and **lingula, left lung**

Lower lobe and inferior border, left lung

Rectus abdominis muscle

Diaphragm

Costomediastinal recess of pleural cavity

Fig. 163: Thoracic Viscera and the Root of the Neck, Anterior Exposure

NOTE 1)   the anterior thoracic wall has been removed along with the medial parts of both clavicles to reveal the normal position of the heart, lungs, thymus, and thyroid gland. The great vessels in the superior aperture of the thorax are also exposed.

2)   the parietal pleura has been removed anteriorly. The thymus is situated between the two lungs superiorly, whereas inferiorly is found the bare area of the heart. Observe the **cardiac notch** along the anterior border of the left lung adjacent to the heart.

3)   the basal surface of both lungs and the inferior aspect of the heart rest on the diaphragm, whereas the apex of each lung extends superiorly above the level of the first rib.

4)   the rather transverse course in the superior mediastinum of the left brachiocephalic vein in contrast to the nearly vertical course of the right brachiocephalic vein. The two brachiocephalic veins join, deep to the thymus, to form the superior vena cava.

Fig. 163   **II**

PLATE 102   Reflections of Pleura: Anterior and Posterior Views

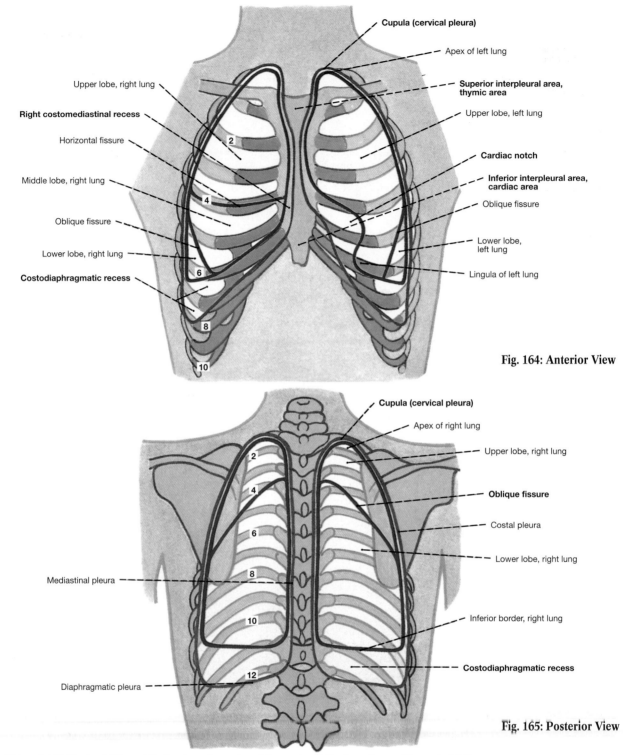

Cupula (cervical pleura)

Apex of left lung

Upper lobe, right lung

Superior interpleural area, thymic area

Right costomediastinal recess

Upper lobe, left lung

Horizontal fissure

2

Cardiac notch

Middle lobe, right lung

Inferior interpleural area, cardiac area

4

Oblique fissure

Oblique fissure

Lower lobe,
left lung

Lower lobe, right lung

6

Lingula of left lung

Costodiaphragmatic recess

8

10

Fig. 164: Anterior View

Cupula (cervical pleura)

Apex of right lung

2

Upper lobe, right lung

4

Oblique fissure

Costal pleura

6

Lower lobe, right lung

8

Mediastinal pleura

10

Inferior border, right lung

Costodiaphragmatic recess

12

Diaphragmatic pleura

Fig. 165: Posterior View

Figs. 164 and 165: Parietal Pleural Reflections (green) and Lungs (red) Projected onto Thoracic Wall

NOTE: 1)   each lung is invested by two layers of pleura that are continuous at the hilum of the lung, and thereby form an invaginated sac.

2)   the **parietal layer of pleura** (shown in green) is the outermost of the two layers and lines the inner surface of the thoracic wall and the superior surface of the diaphragm. The **visceral layer of pleura** closely invests and adheres to the surfaces of the lungs (in red).

3)   the potential space between the two pleural layers is called the **pleural cavity** and contains only a small amount of serous fluid in the healthy person, but it may contain considerable fluid and blood in pathological conditions.

4)   the parietal pleura is a continuous sheet, but parts of it are named in relation to their adjacent surfaces. Lining the inner surface of the ribs is the **costal pleura,** while the **diaphragmatic** and **mediastinal pleurae** are found on the surfaces of the diaphragm and mediastinum. Overlying the apex of each lung is the **cupula** or **cervical pleura.**

5)   due to the curvature of the diaphragm, a narrow recess is formed around its periphery into which the lung (visceral pleura) does not extend. An important potential space lies between the costal and diaphragmatic pleurae called the **costodiaphragmatic recess**, which may be punctured and drained of fluid without damage to the lung tissue.

Fig. 164, 165

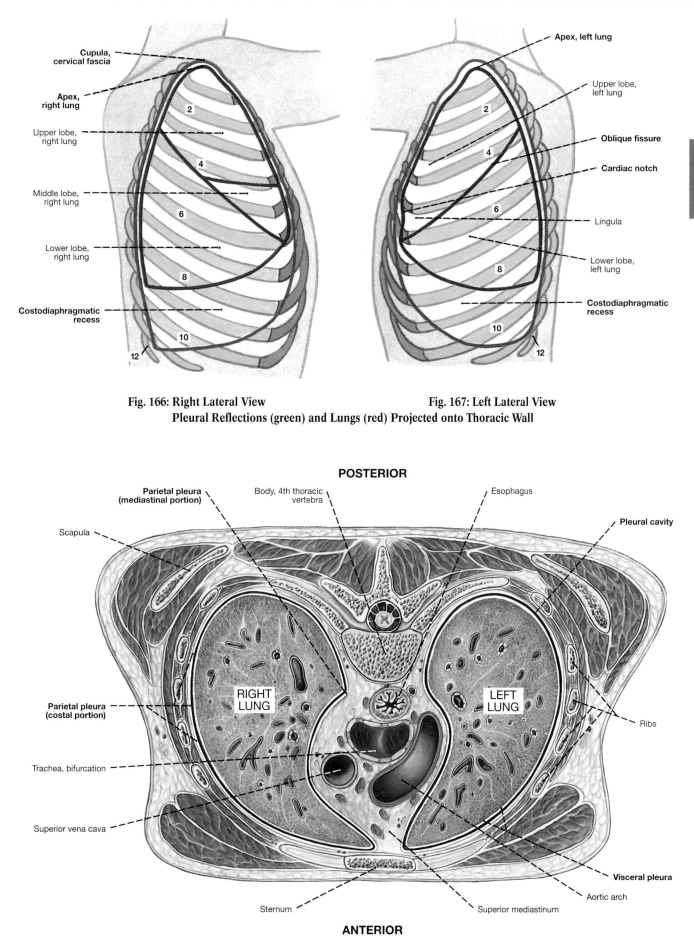

Fig. 166: Right Lateral View   **Fig. 167: Left Lateral View**
Pleural Reflections (green) and Lungs (red) Projected onto Thoracic Wall

Fig. 168: Cross-section of Thorax at the Level of the Tracheal Bifurcation and the 4th Thoracic Vertebra (Pleura Is Shown in White)

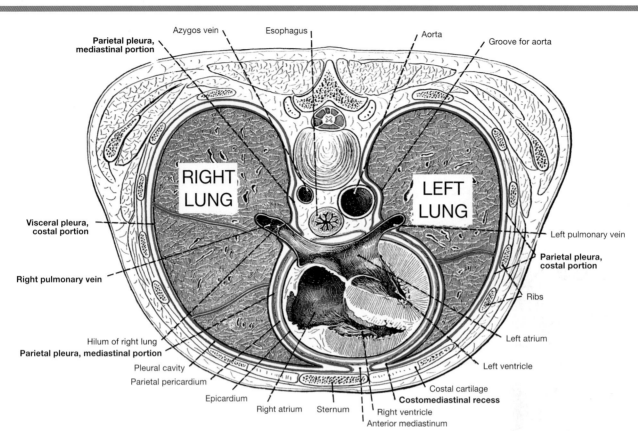

Fig. 169: Cross-section of Thorax Through the Hilum of the Lung at the Level of the Pulmonary Vein (Pleura in Red, Pericardium in Blue)

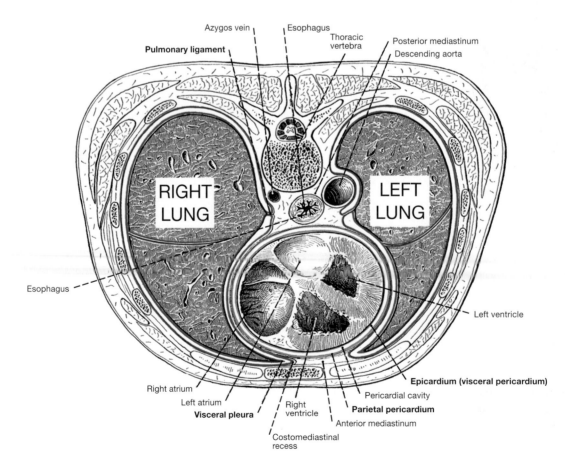

Fig. 170: Cross-section of the Thorax Inferior to Hilum at the Level of the Pulmonary Ligament (Pleura in Red, Pericardium in Blue)

Figs. 169, 170

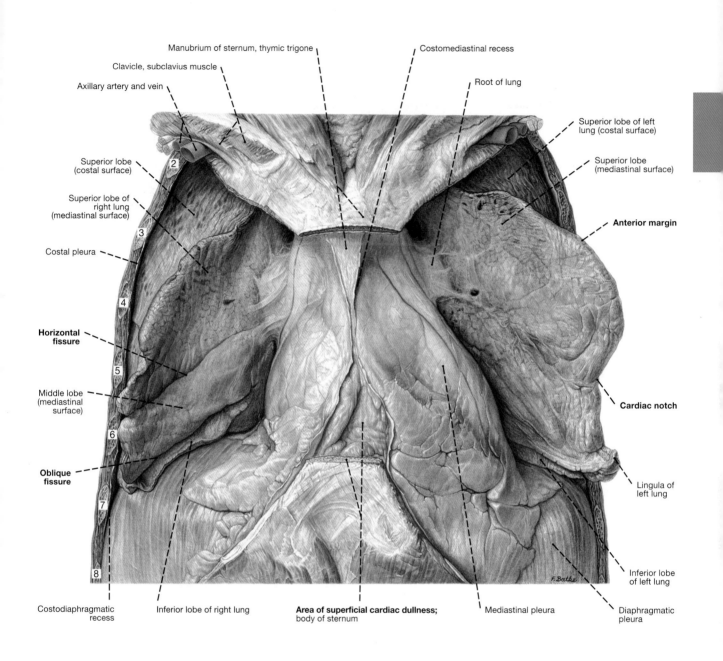

Manubrium of sternum, thymic trigone

Clavicle, subclavius muscle

Axillary artery and vein

Costomediastinal recess

Root of lung

Superior lobe of left lung (costal surface)

Superior lobe (costal surface)

Superior lobe (mediastinal surface)

Superior lobe of right lung (mediastinal surface)

Anterior margin

Costal pleura

Horizontal fissure

Middle lobe (mediastinal surface)

Cardiac notch

Oblique fissure

Lingula of left lung

Inferior lobe of left lung

Costodiaphragmatic recess

Inferior lobe of right lung

Area of superficial cardiac dullness; body of sternum

Mediastinal pleura

Diaphragmatic pleura

2 3 4 5 6 7 8

F. Bathe

Fig. 171: Thoracic Viscera, Anterior View

NOTE: 1) the anterior thoracic wall and most of the sternum has been removed upon opening the chest and exposing the pleura, lungs, pericardium, and heart.

2) additionally, the anterior borders of the two lungs have been retracted laterally revealing the pericardium and heart situated between the lungs in the middle mediastinum.

3) the transition from visceral pleura on the lung surface to mediastinal (parietal) pleura at the **hilum** of each lung.

4) the **right costodiaphragmatic recess** (on reader's lower left) which is a narrow potential space where the costal and diaphragmatic reflections of parietal pleura are separated from the visceral pleura that adheres to the lung surface.

5) the **costomediastinal recess** between the costal and mediastinal parietal pleura line of reflection and the anterior border of the lung just deep to the sternum. At this site, lung tissue does not reach the costomediastinal line of reflection thereby forming the recess between parietal and visceral pleurae.

Fig. 171   **II**

PLATE 106   Lungs: Lateral (Sternocostal) View

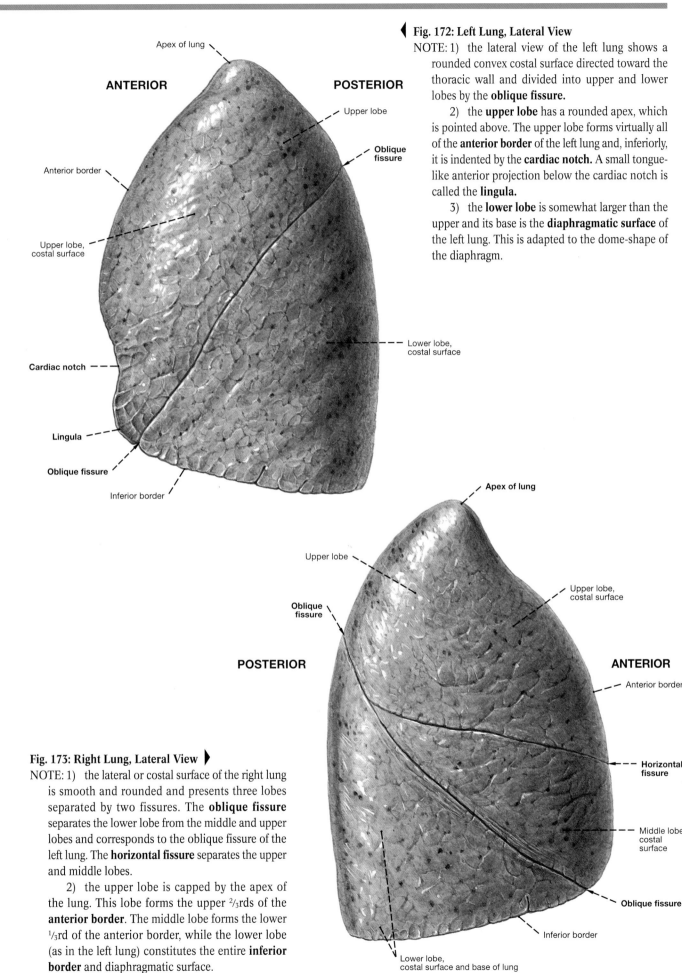

Apex of lung

ANTERIOR

POSTERIOR

Upper lobe

Oblique fissure

Anterior border

Upper lobe, costal surface

Cardiac notch

Lower lobe, costal surface

Lingula

Oblique fissure

Inferior border

◀ Fig. 172: Left Lung, Lateral View

NOTE: 1) the lateral view of the left lung shows a rounded convex costal surface directed toward the thoracic wall and divided into upper and lower lobes by the **oblique fissure.**

2) the **upper lobe** has a rounded apex, which is pointed above. The upper lobe forms virtually all of the **anterior border** of the left lung and, inferiorly, it is indented by the **cardiac notch.** A small tongue-like anterior projection below the cardiac notch is called the **lingula.**

3) the **lower lobe** is somewhat larger than the upper and its base is the **diaphragmatic surface** of the left lung. This is adapted to the dome-shape of the diaphragm.

Apex of lung

Upper lobe

Upper lobe, costal surface

Oblique fissure

POSTERIOR

ANTERIOR

Anterior border

Horizontal fissure

Fig. 173: Right Lung, Lateral View ▶

NOTE: 1) the lateral or costal surface of the right lung is smooth and rounded and presents three lobes separated by two fissures. The **oblique fissure** separates the lower lobe from the middle and upper lobes and corresponds to the oblique fissure of the left lung. The **horizontal fissure** separates the upper and middle lobes.

2) the upper lobe is capped by the apex of the lung. This lobe forms the upper 2/3rds of the **anterior border**. The middle lobe forms the lower 1/3rd of the anterior border, while the lower lobe (as in the left lung) constitutes the entire **inferior border** and diaphragmatic surface.

Middle lobe, costal surface

Oblique fissure

Inferior border

Lower lobe, costal surface and base of lung

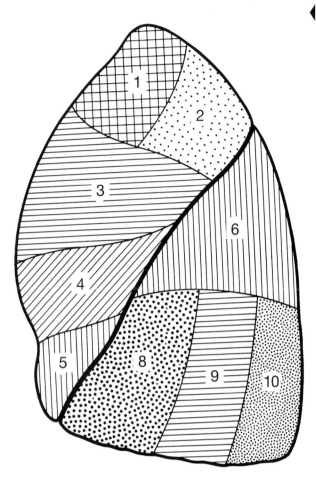

NOTE: 1) bronchopulmonary segments are anatomical subdivisions of the lung, each supplied by its own segmental (tertiary) bronchus and artery, and drained by intersegmental veins.

2) the trachea divides into two primary bronchi, each of which serves an entire lung. The primary bronchi divide into secondary or lobar bronchi. There are two lobar bronchi on the left and three on the right, each supplying a separate lobe.

3) secondary bronchi divide into segmental or tertiary bronchi, distributed to the bronchopulmonary segments. Usual descriptions of the bronchopulmonary segments define 8 to 10 segments in the left lung.

4) in the left lung, the segments are numbered and named as follows:

Upper lobe
1	Apical	
2	Posterior	Frequently considered as a single segment
3	Anterior	
4	Superior	Lingular
5	Inferior	

Lower lobe
6	Superior	
7	Medial basal	Usually considered as a single segment;
8	Anterior basal	medial basal cannot be seen from lateral view.
9	Lateral basal	
10	Posterior basal	

5) in the left lower lobe the medial basal bronchus arises separate from the anterior basal in only about 13% of humans studied.

Fig. 175: Right Lung, Bronchopulmonary Segments, ▶ Lateral View

NOTE: 1) subdivision of the lungs into functional bronchopulmonary segments allows the surgeon to determine whether segments of lung might be resected in operations in preference to entire lobes.

2) although minor variations exist in the division of the bronchial tree, a consistency has become accepted in the naming of bronchopulmonary segmentation. The nomenclature used here was published by Jackson and Huber (Dis Chest 1943; 9: 319–326) and is now used because it is the simplest and most straightforward of those suggested.

3) the bronchopulmonary segments of the right lung are numbered and named as follows:

Upper lobe		**Middle lobe**	
1	Apical	4	Lateral
2	Posterior	5	Medial
3	Anterior		

Lower lobe
6	Superior
7	Medial basal (cannot be seen from lateral view)
8	Anterior basal
9	Lateral basal
10	Posterior basal

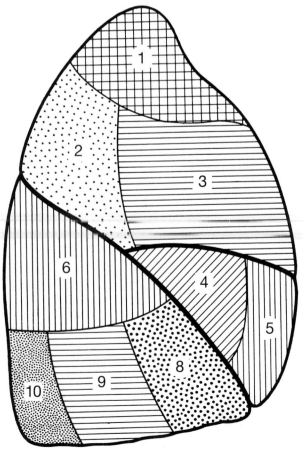

PLATE 108   Lungs: Medial (Mediastinal) View

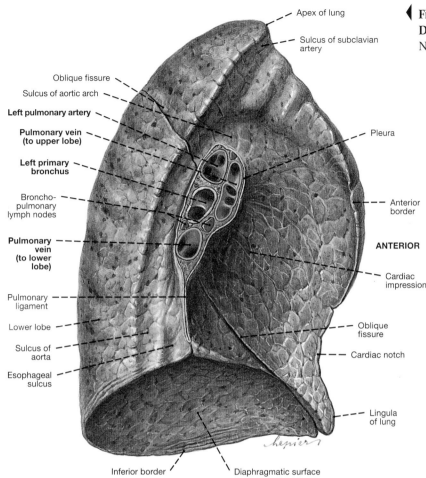

Fig. 176: Left Lung, Mediastinal and Diaphragmatic Surfaces

NOTE: 1) the concave diaphragmatic surface on the left lung covers most of the convex dome of the diaphragm, which is completely covered by parietal diaphragmatic pleura.

2) the mediastinal (or medial) surface of the left lung is also concave and presents the contours of the organs of the mediastinum. The large anterior concavity is the cardiac impression. Observe the grooves for the aortic arch, the aorta, and the subclavian artery as well as the esophagus inferiorly.

3) the structures at the hilum of the left lung include the **left pulmonary artery,** found superiorly, and below this the **left bronchus.** The **left pulmonary veins** lie anterior and inferior to the artery and bronchus. The **oblique fissure** completely divides the lung into two lobes.

Fig. 177: Right Lung, Mediastinal and Diaphragmatic Surfaces

NOTE: 1) the **diaphragmatic surface** of the right lung, similar to the left, is shaped to the contour of the diaphragm, while the **mediastinal surface** shows grooves for the superior vena cava and subclavian artery.

2) above the **hilum** of the right lung is the arched sulcus for the azygos vein which continues inferiorly behind the hilum of the lung. The cardiac impression on the right lung is more shallow than on the left.

3) the right bronchus frequently branches before the right pulmonary artery. Thus, often the most superior structure at the hilum of the right lung is the bronchus to the upper lobe (eparterial bronchus). The pulmonary artery lies anterior to the bronchus, while the pulmonary veins are located anterior and inferior to these structures.

4) the hilum of the lung is ensheathed by parietal pleura, the layers of which come into contact below to form the **pulmonary ligament.** This extends from the inferior border of the hilum to a point just above the diaphragm.

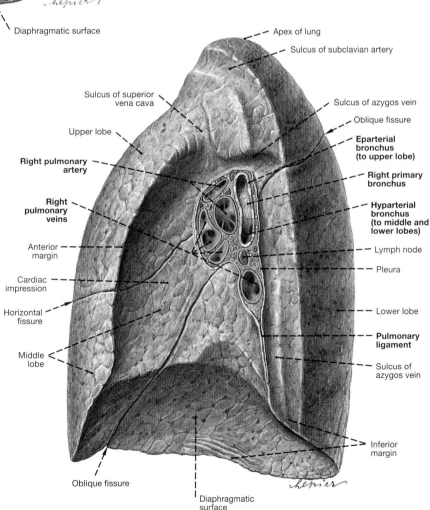

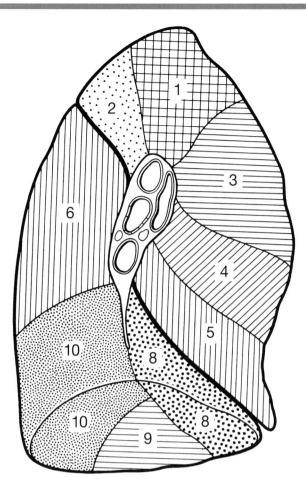

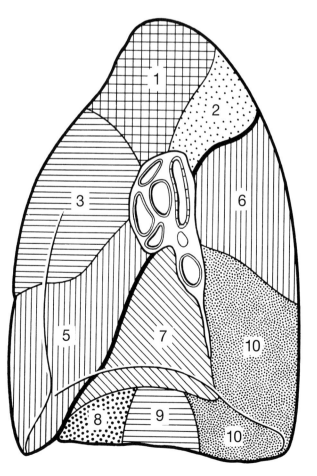

◀ **Fig. 178: Left Lung, Bronchopulmonary Segments, Medial View**

NOTE: the bronchopulmonary segments of the left lung are identified as follows:

Upper lobe		Lower lobe
1 Apical	⎫ Frequently	6 Superior
2 Posterior	⎬ considered as	7 Medial basal*
3 Anterior	⎭ one segment	8 Anterior basal*
4 Superior	⎫	9 Lateral basal
5 Inferior	⎬ Lingular	10 Posterior basal

* The medial basal and anterior basal segments were at one time frequently considered as a single bronchopulmonary segment. Today, however, they have been recognized as separate segments in a majority of left lungs. Therefore, on this figure that portion of segment 8 just inferior to the oblique fissure should be marked 7 and identified as medial basal.

Fig. 179: Right Lung, Bronchopulmonary Segments, ▶
Medial View

NOTE: the bronchopulmonary segments of the right lung are identified as follows:

Upper lobe
1 Apical
2 Posterior
3 Anterior

Middle lobe
4 Lateral (not seen from this view)
5 Medial

Lower lobe
6 Superior
7 Medial basal
8 Anterior basal
9 Lateral basal
10 Posterior basal

PLATE 110   Trachea and Bronchi

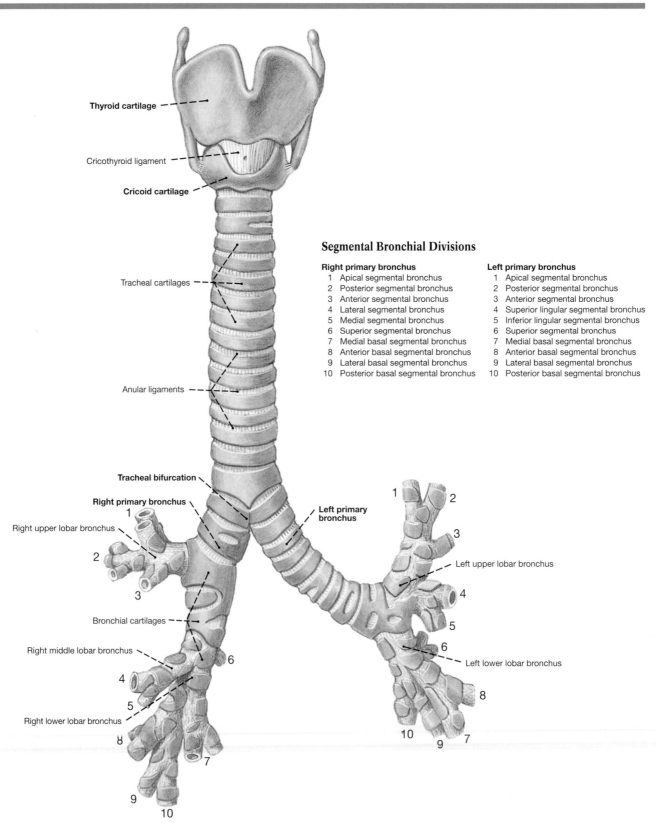

Thyroid cartilage

Cricothyroid ligament

Cricoid cartilage

Tracheal cartilages

Anular ligaments

Tracheal bifurcation

Right primary bronchus

Right upper lobar bronchus

Bronchial cartilages

Right middle lobar bronchus

Right lower lobar bronchus

Left primary bronchus

Left upper lobar bronchus

Left lower lobar bronchus

Segmental Bronchial Divisions

Right primary bronchus
1   Apical segmental bronchus
2   Posterior segmental bronchus
3   Anterior segmental bronchus
4   Lateral segmental bronchus
5   Medial segmental bronchus
6   Superior segmental bronchus
7   Medial basal segmental bronchus
8   Anterior basal segmental bronchus
9   Lateral basal segmental bronchus
10 Posterior basal segmental bronchus

Left primary bronchus
1   Apical segmental bronchus
2   Posterior segmental bronchus
3   Anterior segmental bronchus
4   Superior lingular segmental bronchus
5   Inferior lingular segmental bronchus
6   Superior segmental bronchus
7   Medial basal segmental bronchus
8   Anterior basal segmental bronchus
9   Lateral basal segmental bronchus
10 Posterior basal segmental bronchus

Fig. 180: Anterior Aspect of Larynx, Trachea, and Bronchi

NOTE: 1)   the **trachea** bifurcates into two **principal** (primary) **bronchi.** These then divide into **lobar** (secondary) **bronchi** which give rise to **segmental** (tertiary) **bronchi.**

2)   the larynx is located in the anterior aspect of the neck, and its thyroid and cricoid cartilages can be felt through the skin.

3)   the **thyroid cartilage,** projected posteriorly, lies at the level of the 4th and 5th cervical vertebrae, while the **cricoid cartilage** is at the 6th cervical level.

4)   the trachea commences at the lower end of the cricoid cartilage and extends slightly more than 4 inches before bifurcating into the two primary bronchi at the level of T4. Two inches of the trachea lie above the suprasternal notch in the neck, and about 2 inches of trachea are within the thorax above the tracheal bifurcation.

Fig. 180

RIGHT LUNG   LEFT LUNG

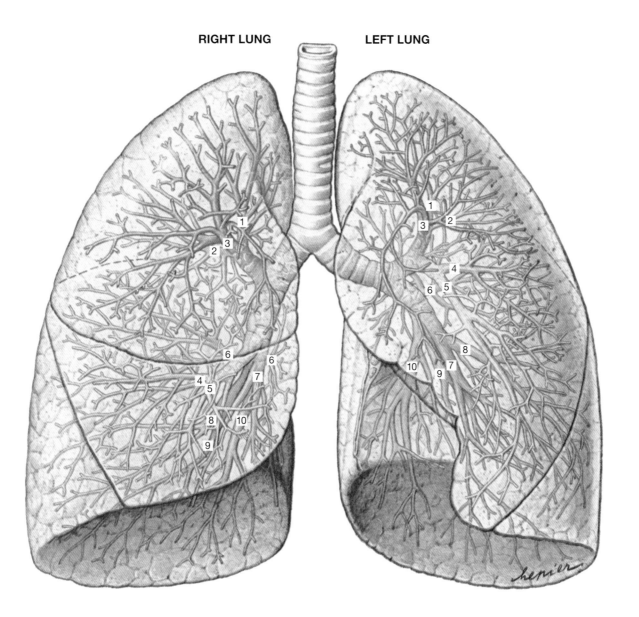

Fig. 181: Bronchial Tree and its Lobar and Bronchopulmonary Divisions, Anterior View

NOTE: 1)   as the trachea divides, the **left primary bronchus** diverges at a greater angle than the **right primary bronchus** to reach the left lung. The left bronchus, therefore, is directed more transversely and the right bronchus more inferiorly.

2)   **on the right side** the upper lobar bronchus branches from the primary bronchus almost immediately, even above the pulmonary artery (eparterial), while the bronchus directed toward the middle and lower lobes branches below the main stem of the pulmonary artery (hyparterial).

3)   **on the left side** the initial lobar bronchus, branching from the primary bronchus, is directed upward and lateral to the upper lobe segments and its lingular segments. The remaining lobar bronchus is directed inferiorly and soon divides into the segmental bronchi of the lower lobe.

4)   the segmental bronchi numbered in the figure above are as follows:

Right lung			Left lung		
1 Apical	6	Superior	1 Apical	6	Superior
2 Posterior	7	Medial basal	2 Posterior	7	Medial basal
3 Anterior	8	Anterior basal	3 Anterior	8	Anterior basal
4 Lateral	9	Lateral basal	4 Superior lingular	9	Lateral basal
5 Medial	10	Posterior basal	5 Inferior lingular	10	Posterior basal

Fig. 181   **II**

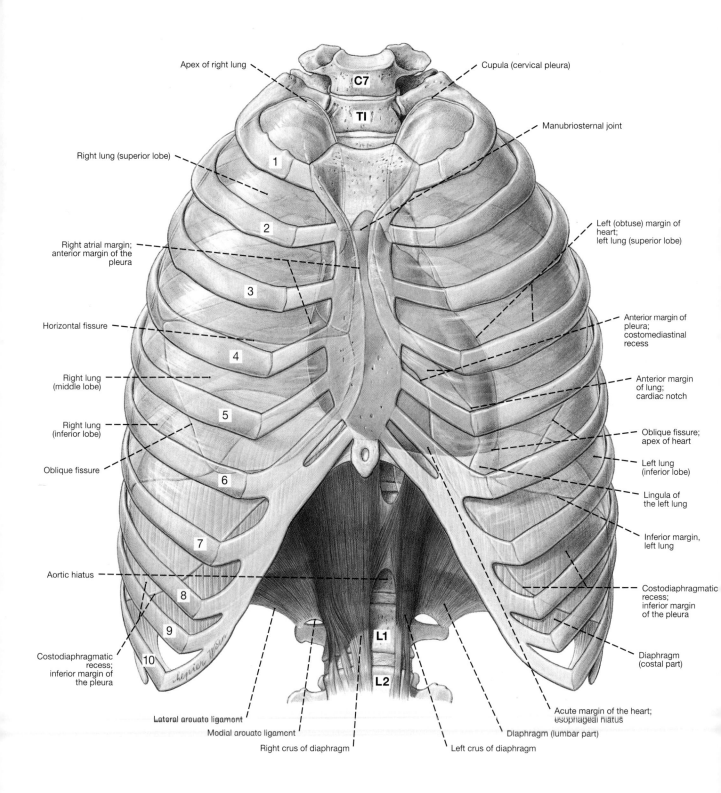

Apex of right lung

Cupula (cervical pleura)

C7

TI

Manubriosternal joint

Right lung (superior lobe)

1

2

Left (obtuse) margin of heart; left lung (superior lobe)

Right atrial margin; anterior margin of the pleura

3

Horizontal fissure

Anterior margin of pleura; costomediastinal recess

4

Right lung (middle lobe)

Anterior margin of lung; cardiac notch

5

Right lung (inferior lobe)

Oblique fissure; apex of heart

Left lung (inferior lobe)

Oblique fissure

6

Lingula of the left lung

Inferior margin, left lung

7

Aortic hiatus

8

Costodiaphragmatic recess; inferior margin of the pleura

9

L1

10

Diaphragm (costal part)

Costodiaphragmatic recess; inferior margin of the pleura

L2

Acute margin of the heart; esophageal hiatus

Lateral arcuate ligament

Medial arcuate ligament

Diaphragm (lumbar part)

Right crus of diaphragm

Left crus of diaphragm

Fig. 182: Position of the Heart Within the Thorax, Anterior View

NOTE: 1)   through the translucently drawn pleural sacs can be seen the interlobar fissures and the subpleural part of the heart. Part of the heart is overlaid by the anterior margins of the lungs and part is directly deep to the sternum.

     2)   the location of the heart is in the middle mediastinum in relationship to the overlying ribs and sternum. Compare this figure with Fig. 183, which, additionally, projects the positions of the cardiac valves with respect to the thoracic cage.

     3)   the diaphragm extends upward about one rib level higher on the right (4th interspace) than on the left (5th interspace).

Fig. 182

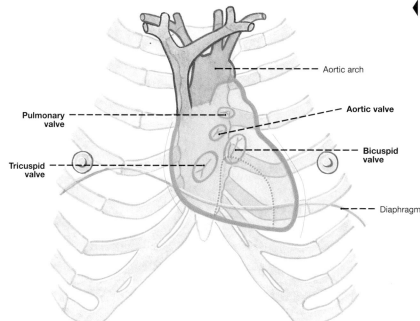

Aortic arch

Aortic valve

Pulmonary valve

Bicuspid valve

Tricuspid valve

Diaphragm

◀ **Fig. 183: Projection of the Heart and its Valves onto Anterior Thoracic Wall**

NOTE: 1) the **pulmonary valve** lies behind the sternal end of the 3rd left costal cartilage. The **aortic valve** is behind the sternum at the level of the 3rd intercostal space. The **mitral valve** (bicuspid) lies behind the 4th left sternocostal joint, and the **tricuspid valve** lies posterior to the middle of the sternum at the level of the 4th intercostal space.

2) the unbroken blue line indicates the **area of deep cardiac dullness** which produces a dull resonance by percussion. Lung tissue covers this area, but does not cover the area limited by the blue dotted line from which a less resonant **superficial cardiac** dullness is obtained.

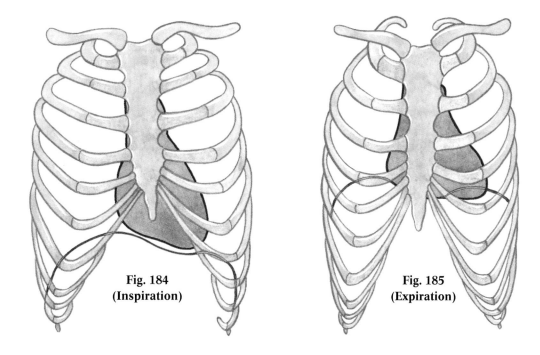

Fig. 184
(Inspiration)

Fig. 185
(Expiration)

Figs. 184 and 185: Positions of the Heart During Full Inspiration (Fig. 184) and During Full Expiration (Fig. 185)

NOTE: 1) during **full inspiration** (Fig. 184):

  (a) the thorax is enlarged by a lowering of the diaphragm due to contraction of its muscle fibers and by elevation and expansion of the thorax (ribs and sternum).

  (b) the chest expands anteroposteriorly, transversely, and vertically resulting in the heart becoming more oblong (i.e., its transverse diameter is decreased), and its apex and diaphragmatic surface are lowered.

  (c) inspiration is accompanied by relaxation of the anterior abdominal wall muscles, protrusion of the abdomen and a lowering of abdominal viscera.

2) during **full expiration** (Fig. 185):

  (a) the diaphragm is elevated because its muscle fibers relax and because the ribs and sternum contract the size of the thorax.

  (b) with the capacity of the thoracic cage diminished, there is an elevation of the diaphragmatic surface of the heart and the apex of the heart. This results in an increase in the transverse diameter of the heart.

  (c) expiration is accompanied by contraction of the anterior abdominal wall muscles and an elevation of the abdominal viscera, which also pushes the relaxed diaphragm upward.

PLATE 114   Mediastinum: Right Side, Pleura Intact

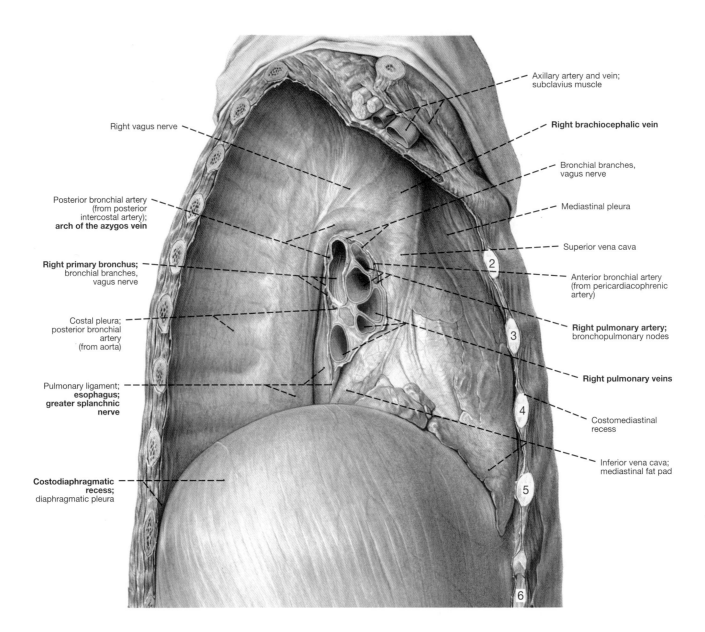

Axillary artery and vein;
subclavius muscle

Right brachiocephalic vein

Bronchial branches,
vagus nerve

Mediastinal pleura

Superior vena cava

Anterior bronchial artery
(from pericardiacophrenic
artery)

Right pulmonary artery;
bronchopulmonary nodes

Right pulmonary veins

Costomediastinal
recess

Inferior vena cava;
mediastinal fat pad

Right vagus nerve

Posterior bronchial artery
(from posterior
intercostal artery);
arch of the azygos vein

Right primary bronchus;
bronchial branches,
vagus nerve

Costal pleura;
posterior bronchial
artery
(from aorta)

Pulmonary ligament;
**esophagus;
greater splanchnic
nerve**

**Costodiaphragmatic
recess;**
diaphragmatic pleura

Fig. 186: Right Side of the Mediastinum: Mediastinal and Costal Pleurae Intact

NOTE: 1) with the right lung removed and the structures at the pulmonary hilum transected, the organs of the mediastinum can be seen under cover of the mediastinal pleura and the posterior part of the costal pleura.

2) the **pulmonary ligament** descending from the inferior end of the hilum. It is formed by the fusion of the anterior and posterior leaves of the mediastinal pleura just before its transition to becoming visceral pleura.

3) folds of mediastinal fat can be seen overlying the pericardium.

4) the **bronchial arteries.** Three bronchial arteries are observed in this dissection:

  a) one arises from the 2nd right posterior intercostal artery

  b) a second branches directly from the thoracic aorta

  c) the third arises from the pericardiacophrenic artery.

5) compare the projections made in the mediastinal pleura by the underlying organs in this figure with organs themselves seen in Fig. 187.

Fig. 186

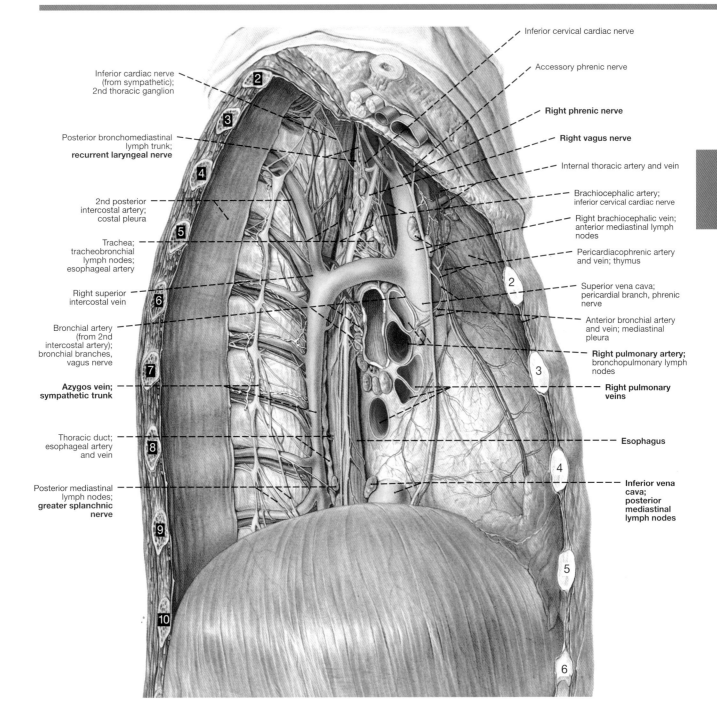

Inferior cervical cardiac nerve

Accessory phrenic nerve

Right phrenic nerve

Right vagus nerve

Internal thoracic artery and vein

Brachiocephalic artery; inferior cervical cardiac nerve

Right brachiocephalic vein; anterior mediastinal lymph nodes

Pericardiacophrenic artery and vein; thymus

Superior vena cava; pericardial branch, phrenic nerve

Anterior bronchial artery and vein; mediastinal pleura

Right pulmonary artery; bronchopulmonary lymph nodes

Right pulmonary veins

Esophagus

Inferior vena cava; posterior mediastinal lymph nodes

Inferior cardiac nerve (from sympathetic); 2nd thoracic ganglion

Posterior bronchomediastinal lymph trunk; **recurrent laryngeal nerve**

2nd posterior intercostal artery; costal pleura

Trachea; tracheobronchial lymph nodes; esophageal artery

Right superior intercostal vein

Bronchial artery (from 2nd intercostal artery); bronchial branches, vagus nerve

Azygos vein; sympathetic trunk

Thoracic duct; esophageal artery and vein

Posterior mediastinal lymph nodes; **greater splanchnic nerve**

Fig. 187: Right Side of the Mediastinum with the Mediastinal Pleura and Some Costal Pleura Removed

NOTE: 1) the lung has been removed, the structures at the hilum transected and the mediastinal pleura stripped away. This exposes the organs of the mediastinum and their right lateral surface is presented.

2) the right side of the heart covered by pericardium and the course of the **phrenic nerve** and **pericardiacophrenic vessels** are visible.

3) the ascending course of the **azygos vein,** its arch, and its junction with the superior vena cava.

4) the **right vagus nerve** descends in the thorax behind the root of the right lung to form the **posterior pulmonary plexus.** It then helps form the **esophageal plexus** and leaves the thorax on the posterior aspect of the esophagus.

5) the **dome of the diaphragm** on the right side as it takes the rounded form of the underlying liver. The inferior (diaphragmatic) surface of the heart rests on the diaphragm.

6) the position of the thoracic **sympathetic chain** of ganglia coursing longitudinally along the inner surface of the thoracic wall. Observe the **greater splanchnic nerve.**

Fig. 187   **II**

PLATE 116   Mediastinum: Left Side, Pleura Intact

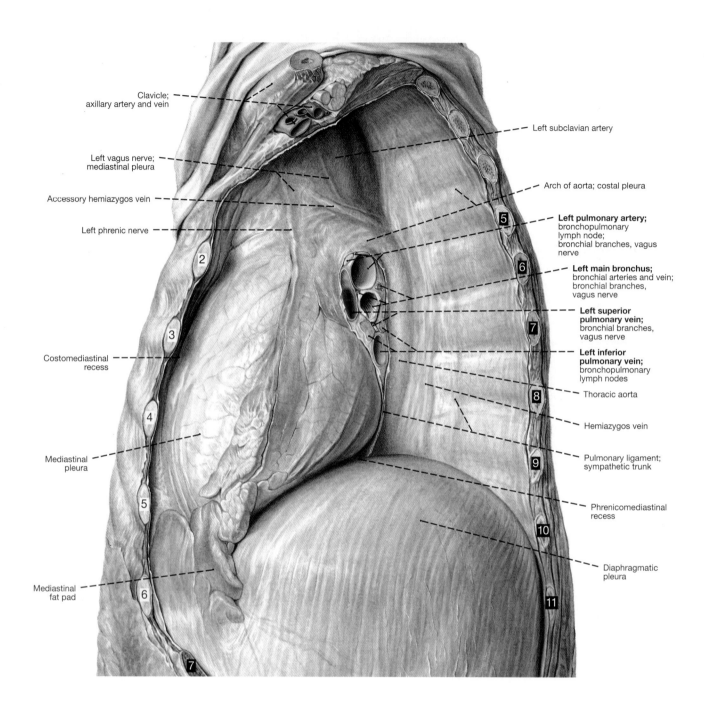

Clavicle;
axillary artery and vein

Left subclavian artery

Left vagus nerve;
mediastinal pleura

Arch of aorta; costal pleura

Accessory hemiazygos vein

Left pulmonary artery;
bronchopulmonary
lymph node;
bronchial branches, vagus
nerve

Left phrenic nerve

Left main bronchus;
bronchial arteries and vein;
bronchial branches,
vagus nerve

**Left superior
pulmonary vein;**
bronchial branches,
vagus nerve

**Left inferior
pulmonary vein;**
bronchopulmonary
lymph nodes

Costomediastinal
recess

Thoracic aorta

Hemiazygos vein

Mediastinal
pleura

Pulmonary ligament;
sympathetic trunk

Phrenicomediastinal
recess

Diaphragmatic
pleura

Mediastinal
fat pad

Fig. 188: Left Side of the Mediastinum: Mediastinal and Costal Pleura Intact

NOTE: 1) with the left lung removed and the hilar structures transected, the left side of the pericardium and certain organs in the
posterior mediastinum can be identified as they project into the overlying mediastinal and costal pleurae.

2) at the hilum, the **pulmonary artery** is superior and the **pulmonary veins** are anterior and inferior. The **primary bronchus**
lies between these and normally is more posterior.

3) the protrusion through the pleura of the **arch of the aorta** as well as the descending **thoracic aorta.** Posterior to these,
observe the bulges for the **hemiazygos vein** and the **sympathetic trunk** and its **ganglia.**

4) compare this figure with Figure 189 where much of the pleura has been removed.

Fig. 188

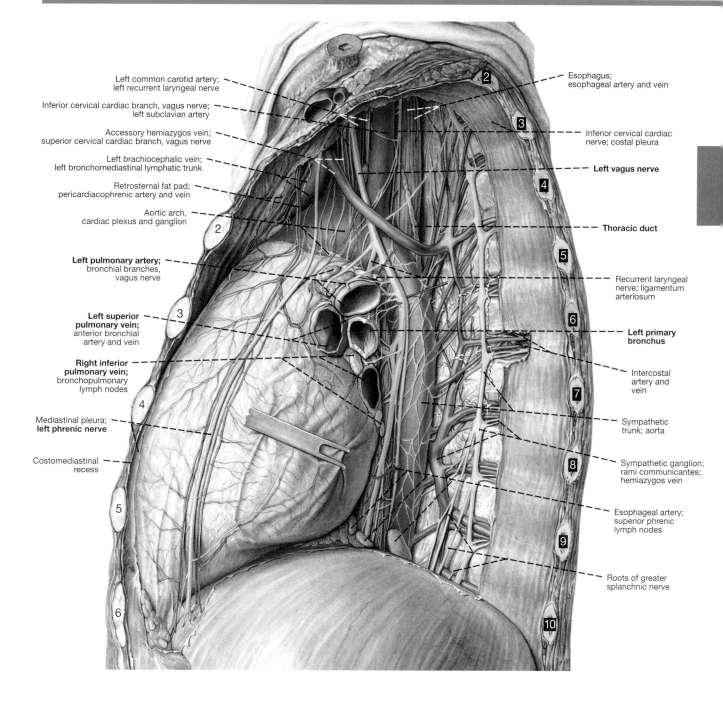

Left common carotid artery; left recurrent laryngeal nerve

Inferior cervical cardiac branch, vagus nerve; left subclavian artery

Accessory hemiazygos vein; superior cervical cardiac branch, vagus nerve

Left brachiocephalic vein; left bronchomediastinal lymphatic trunk

Retrosternal fat pad; pericardiacophrenic artery and vein

Aortic arch, cardiac plexus and ganglion

Left pulmonary artery; bronchial branches, vagus nerve

Left superior pulmonary vein; anterior bronchial artery and vein

Right inferior pulmonary vein; bronchopulmonary lymph nodes

Mediastinal pleura; **left phrenic nerve**

Costomediastinal recess

Esophagus; esophageal artery and vein

Inferior cervical cardiac nerve; costal pleura

Left vagus nerve

Thoracic duct

Recurrent laryngeal nerve; ligamentum arteriosum

Left primary bronchus

Intercostal artery and vein

Sympathetic trunk; aorta

Sympathetic ganglion; rami communicantes; hemiazygos vein

Esophageal artery; superior phrenic lymph nodes

Roots of greater splanchnic nerve

Fig. 189: Left Side of the Mediastinum with the Mediastinal Pleura and Some Costal Pleura Removed

NOTE: 1)   with the left lung removed along with most of the mediastinal pleura, the structures of the mediastinum are observed from their left side.

2)   the **left phrenic nerve** and **pericardiacophrenic vessels** course to the diaphragm along the pericardial covering over the left side of the heart.

3)   the **aorta** ascends about 2 inches before it arches posteriorly and to the left of the vertebral column.

4)   the descending **thoracic aorta,** which commences at about the level of the 4th thoracic vertebra. As it descends, it comes to lie anterior to the vertebral column.

5)   the **intercostal arteries** branch directly from the thoracic aorta. The typical intercostal artery and vein course along the inferior border of their respective rib. Because the superior border of the ribs is free of vessels and nerves, it is a safer site for injection or drainage of the thorax.

6)   the **left vagus nerve** lies lateral to the aortic arch and gives off the **recurrent laryngeal branch,** which passes inferior to the **ligamentum arteriosum.** The main trunk then continues to descend, contributes to the esophageal plexus, and enters the abdomen on the anterior aspect of the esophagus.

Fig. 189   II

PLATE 118   Mediastinum: Great Vessels; Subdivisions of Mediastinum

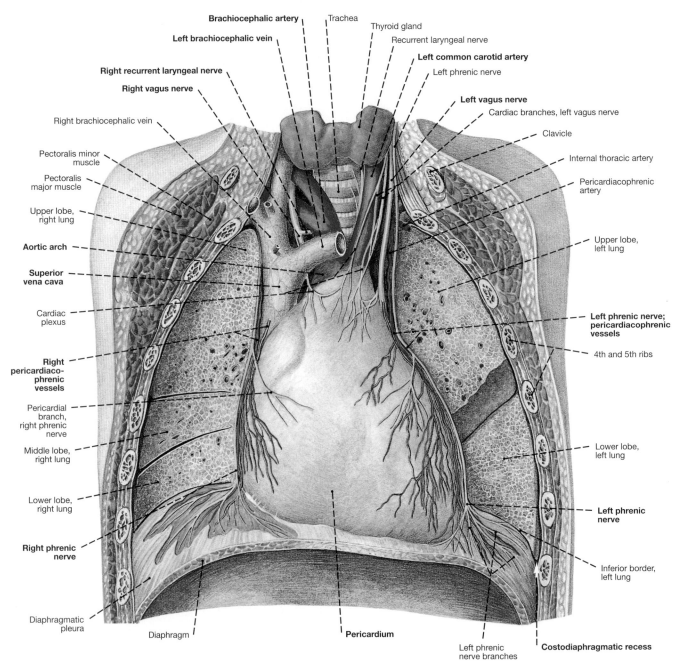

Brachiocephalic artery
Trachea
Thyroid gland
Recurrent laryngeal nerve
Left brachiocephalic vein
Left common carotid artery
Right recurrent laryngeal nerve
Left phrenic nerve
Right vagus nerve
Left vagus nerve
Cardiac branches, left vagus nerve
Right brachiocephalic vein
Clavicle
Pectoralis minor muscle
Internal thoracic artery
Pectoralis major muscle
Pericardiacophrenic artery
Upper lobe, right lung
Aortic arch
Upper lobe, left lung
Superior vena cava
Cardiac plexus
Left phrenic nerve; pericardiacophrenic vessels
Right pericardiaco-phrenic vessels
4th and 5th ribs
Pericardial branch, right phrenic nerve
Middle lobe, right lung
Lower lobe, left lung
Lower lobe, right lung
Right phrenic nerve
Left phrenic nerve
Inferior border, left lung
Diaphragmatic pleura
Diaphragm
Pericardium
Costodiaphragmatic recess
Left phrenic nerve branches

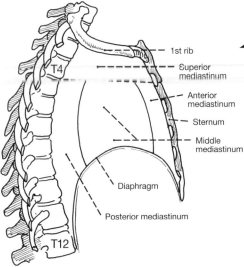

1st rib
Superior mediastinum
Anterior mediastinum
Sternum
Middle mediastinum
Diaphragm
Posterior mediastinum
T4
T12

▲ Fig. 191: Subdivisions of the Mediastinum

▲ Fig. 190: Adult Heart, Pericardium, and Superior Mediastinum, Anterior View
NOTE: 1) in this frontal section, the anterior thoracic wall and the anterior part of the lungs and diaphragm have been removed, leaving the **pericardium** and its vessels and nerves intact. The **vagus nerves** and some of their branches are also shown.

2) the **phrenic nerves** form in the neck (C3, 4, 5) and descend with the pericardiacophrenic vessels to innervate the diaphragm, but they also send some sensory fibers to the pericardium.

3) the pericardium is formed by an outer **fibrous layer**, which is lined by an inner serous sac. As the heart develops, it invaginates into the serous sac and becomes covered by a **visceral layer of serous pericardium** (epicardium) and a **parietal layer of serous pericardium.**

4) the visceral layer clings closely to the heart, while the parietal layer lines the inner surface of the fibrous pericardium. The potential space between the visceral and parietal layers contains a little serous fluid and is called the **pericardial cavity.**

Figs. 190, 191

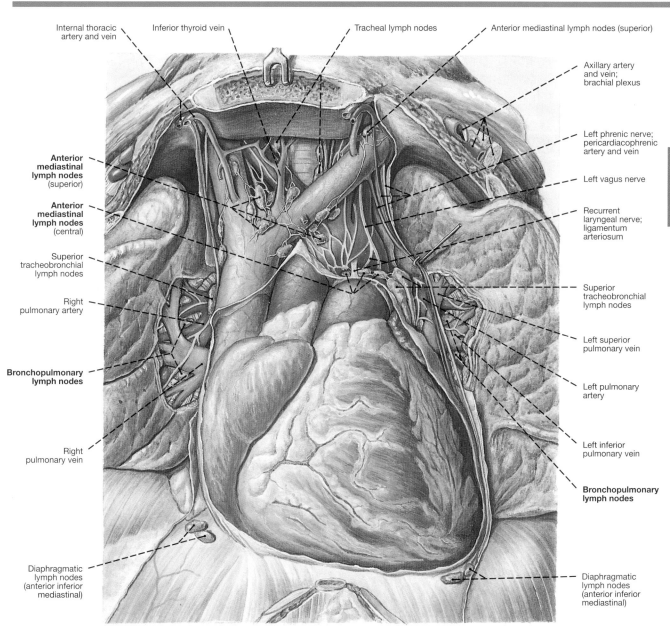

Internal thoracic artery and vein

Inferior thyroid vein

Tracheal lymph nodes

Anterior mediastinal lymph nodes (superior)

Axillary artery and vein; brachial plexus

Anterior mediastinal lymph nodes (superior)

Anterior mediastinal lymph nodes (central)

Superior tracheobronchial lymph nodes

Right pulmonary artery

Bronchopulmonary lymph nodes

Right pulmonary vein

Diaphragmatic lymph nodes (anterior inferior mediastinal)

Left phrenic nerve; pericardiacophrenic artery and vein

Left vagus nerve

Recurrent laryngeal nerve; ligamentum arteriosum

Superior tracheobronchial lymph nodes

Left superior pulmonary vein

Left pulmonary artery

Left inferior pulmonary vein

Bronchopulmonary lymph nodes

Diaphragmatic lymph nodes (anterior inferior mediastinal)

Fig. 192: Lymphatics of the Thorax, Anterior Aspect

NOTE: 1) the anterior thoracic wall was removed along with the ventral portion of the fibrous pericardium. The anterior borders of the lungs have been pulled laterally to reveal the lymph nodes at the roots of the lungs.

2) removal of the thymus and its related fat and reflection of the manubrium superiorly, exposes the organs at the thoracic inlet and their associated lymphatics.

3) lymph nodes in the anterior part of the thorax may be divided into those associated with the thoracic cage (parietal) and those associated with the organs (visceral). Probably all the nodes indicated in this figure are visceral nodes.

4) situated ventrally are the **anterior mediastinal nodes**, which include a superior group, which lies ventral to the brachiocephalic veins and a more centrally located group that lies ventral to the arch of the aorta. Inferiorly, anterior diaphragmatic nodes are sometimes also classified as part of the anterior mediastinal nodes.

5) large numbers of lymph nodes are associated with the trachea, the bronchi and the other structures at the root of the lung. These nodes have been aptly named **tracheal, tracheobronchial, bronchopulmonary**, and **pulmonary.**

Fig. 192   **II**

PLATE 120   Heart and Great Vessels with the Pericardium Opened

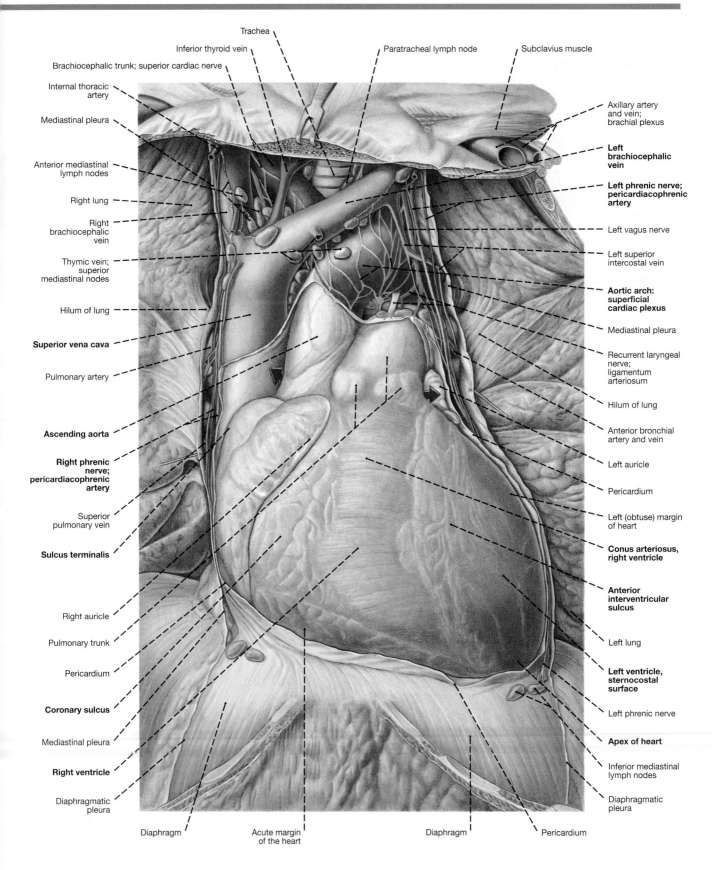

Trachea

Inferior thyroid vein

Paratracheal lymph node

Subclavius muscle

Brachiocephalic trunk; superior cardiac nerve

Internal thoracic artery

Mediastinal pleura

Anterior mediastinal lymph nodes

Right lung

Right brachiocephalic vein

Thymic vein; superior mediastinal nodes

Hilum of lung

Superior vena cava

Pulmonary artery

Ascending aorta

Right phrenic nerve; pericardiacophrenic artery

Superior pulmonary vein

Sulcus terminalis

Right auricle

Pulmonary trunk

Pericardium

Coronary sulcus

Mediastinal pleura

Right ventricle

Diaphragmatic pleura

Axillary artery and vein; brachial plexus

Left brachiocephalic vein

Left phrenic nerve; pericardiacophrenic artery

Left vagus nerve

Left superior intercostal vein

Aortic arch: superficial cardiac plexus

Mediastinal pleura

Recurrent laryngeal nerve; ligamentum arteriosum

Hilum of lung

Anterior bronchial artery and vein

Left auricle

Pericardium

Left (obtuse) margin of heart

Conus arteriosus, right ventricle

Anterior interventricular sulcus

Left lung

Left ventricle, sternocostal surface

Left phrenic nerve

Apex of heart

Inferior mediastinal lymph nodes

Diaphragmatic pleura

Diaphragm

Acute margin of the heart

Diaphragm

Pericardium

Fig. 193: Heart and Great Vessels, Anterior View

NOTE: 1)   the anterior portion of the pericardium has been removed along with remnants of the thymus to reveal the heart in its normal position within the middle mediastinum. The black arrow is in the **transverse pericardial sinus.**

2)   the **superior vena cava** formed by the junction of the **right** and **left brachiocephalic veins,** and the **aorta** overarching the **pulmonary trunk.**

Fig. 193

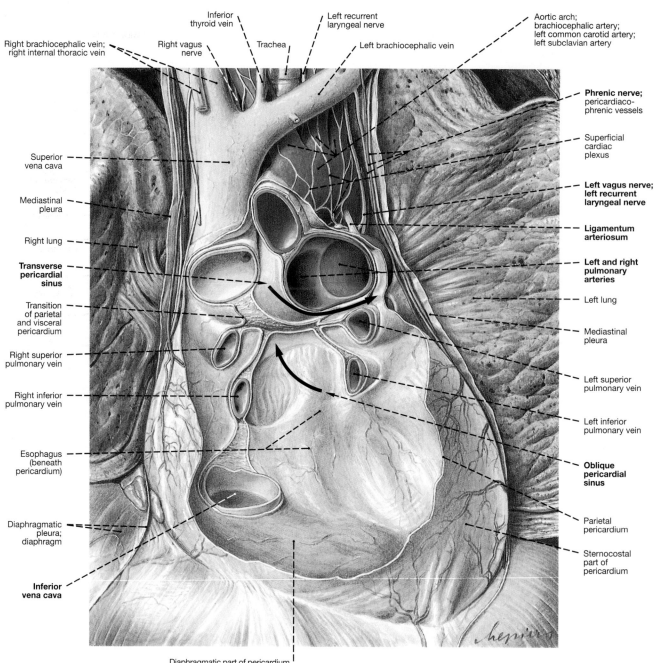

Inferior thyroid vein

Left recurrent laryngeal nerve

Aortic arch; brachiocephalic artery; left common carotid artery; left subclavian artery

Right brachiocephalic vein; right internal thoracic vein

Right vagus nerve

Trachea

Left brachiocephalic vein

Phrenic nerve; pericardiaco-phrenic vessels

Superior vena cava

Superficial cardiac plexus

Mediastinal pleura

Left vagus nerve; left recurrent laryngeal nerve

Right lung

Ligamentum arteriosum

Transverse pericardial sinus

Left and right pulmonary arteries

Transition of parietal and visceral pericardium

Left lung

Right superior pulmonary vein

Mediastinal pleura

Right inferior pulmonary vein

Left superior pulmonary vein

Esophagus (beneath pericardium)

Left inferior pulmonary vein

Oblique pericardial sinus

Diaphragmatic pleura; diaphragm

Parietal pericardium

Sternocostal part of pericardium

Inferior vena cava

Diaphragmatic part of pericardium

Fig. 194: Interior of the Pericardium, Anterior View

NOTE: 1) the pericardium has been opened anteriorly, and the heart has been severed from its attachment to the great vessels and removed. Eight vessels have been cut: the superior and inferior venae cavae, the four pulmonary veins, the pulmonary artery, and the aorta.

2) the **oblique pericardial sinus** is located in the central portion of the posterior wall of the pericardium and is bounded by the pericardial reflections over the pulmonary veins and the venae cavae (venous mesocardium).

3) with the heart in place and the pericardium opened anteriorly, the oblique pericardial sinus may be palpated by inserting several fingers behind the heart and probing superiorly until the blind pouch (cul de sac) of the sinus is felt.

4) the **transverse pericardial sinus** lies behind the pericardial reflection surrounding the aorta and pulmonary artery (arterial mesocardium). It may be located by probing from right to left with the index finger immediately behind the pulmonary trunk.

5) the site of bifurcation of the pulmonary trunk beneath the arch of the aorta and the course of the **left recurrent laryngeal nerve** beneath the **ligamentum arteriosum.**

Fig. 194   II

PLATE 122   Heart, Blood Supply: Anterior and Superior Surfaces

Fig. 195: Coronary Vessels, Anterior View

NOTE: 1) both the left and right coronary arteries arise from the ascending aorta. The **left coronary** is directed toward the left and soon divides into an **anterior interventricular branch,** which descends toward the apex and a **circumflex branch,** which passes posteriorly to the back of the heart.

2) the **right coronary** is directed toward the right and passes to the posterior heart within the coronary sulcus. In its course, branches from the right coronary supply the anterior surface of the right side (anterior cardiac artery). Its largest branch is the **posterior interventricular artery,** which courses toward the apex on the posterior or diaphragmatic surface of the heart.

3) the principal veins of the heart drain into the **coronary sinus** which flows into the right atrium. The distribution and course of the veins is similar to the arteries (see Figs. 197 and 198).

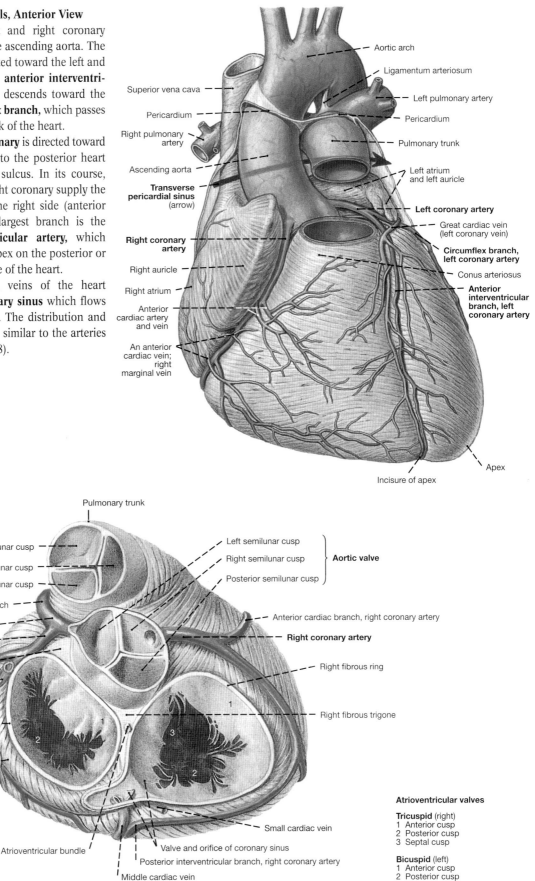

Fig. 196: Valves of the Heart and the Origin of the Coronary Vessels, Superior View

NOTE: the left coronary artery arises from the aortic wall in the aortic sinus behind the left semilunar cusp, and the right coronary stems from the aorta behind the right aortic sinus and right semilunar cusp.

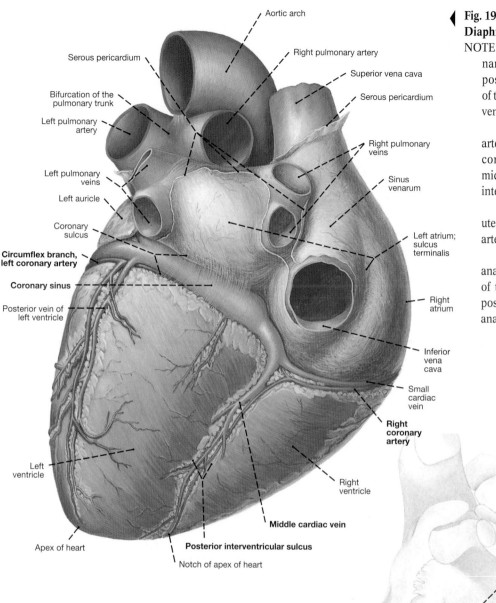

Aortic arch

Serous pericardium

Right pulmonary artery

Superior vena cava

Serous pericardium

Bifurcation of the pulmonary trunk

Left pulmonary artery

Right pulmonary veins

Left pulmonary veins

Sinus venarum

Left auricle

Coronary sulcus

Circumflex branch, left coronary artery

Left atrium; sulcus terminalis

Coronary sinus

Posterior vein of left ventricle

Right atrium

Inferior vena cava

Small cardiac vein

Right coronary artery

Left ventricle

Right ventricle

Apex of heart

Middle cardiac vein

Posterior interventricular sulcus

Notch of apex of heart

Fig. 197: Coronary Vessels, Diaphragmatic Surface of the Heart

NOTE: 1) both the left and right coronary arteries course around to the posterior or diaphragmatic surface of the heart to supply the left and right ventricles in that region.

2) the posterior interventricular artery is usually a branch of the right coronary, and it courses with the middle cardiac vein in the posterior interventricular sulcus.

3) the left coronary artery contributes one or more posterior ventricular arteries.

4) the two coronary arteries anastomose on this posterior surface of the heart, and their anterior and posterior interventricular branches anastomose at the apex.

Fig. 198: Venous Drainage of the Ventricles: Coronary Sinus

NOTE: 1) the left side and left margin of the heart are oriented forward such that the anterior interventricular vein is seen on the left and the middle cardiac vein is seen on the right.

2) the anterior **interventricular vein** becomes the **great cardiac vein.** As the great cardiac vein courses in the coronary sulcus, it gradually enlarges to form the **coronary sinus** and receives the **posterior vein of the left ventricle.** The **middle cardiac vein,** which runs in the posterior interventricular sulcus, also drains directly into the coronary sinus.

3) the coronary sinus opens into the right atrium.

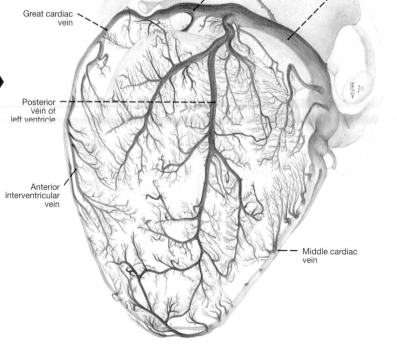

Great cardiac vein

Coronary sinus

Great cardiac vein

Posterior vein of left ventricle

Anterior interventricular vein

Middle cardiac vein

PLATE 124 **Heart and Great Vessels, Anterior View**

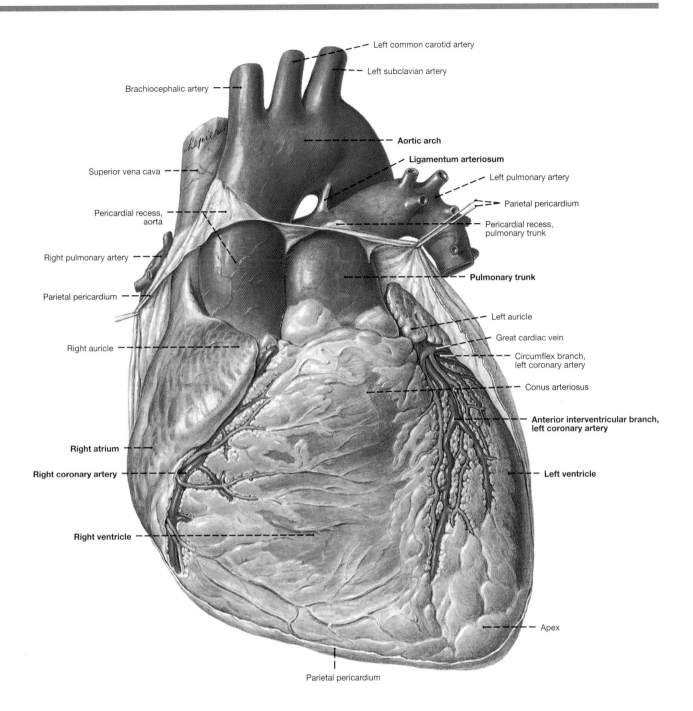

Left common carotid artery

Left subclavian artery

Brachiocephalic artery

Aortic arch

Ligamentum arteriosum

Superior vena cava

Left pulmonary artery

Parietal pericardium

Pericardial recess,
aorta

Pericardial recess,
pulmonary trunk

Right pulmonary artery

Pulmonary trunk

Parietal pericardium

Left auricle

Great cardiac vein

Right auricle

Circumflex branch,
left coronary artery

Conus arteriosus

**Anterior interventricular branch,
left coronary artery**

Right atrium

Right coronary artery

Left ventricle

Right ventricle

Apex

Parietal pericardium

Fig. 199: Ventral View of the Heart and Great Vessels
NOTE: 1) the heart is a muscular organ in the middle mediastinum and its **apex** points inferiorly, to the left and slightly anteriorly.
The **base** of the heart is opposite to the apex and is directed superiorly and to the right.

2) the great vessels attach to the heart at its base, and the pericardium is reflected over these vessels at their origin.

3) the anterior surface of the heart is its **sternocostal surface.** The auricular portion of the **right atrium** and much of the **right
ventricle** is seen from this anterior view; also a small part of the **left ventricle** is visible along the left border.

4) the **pulmonary trunk** originates from the right ventricle. To its right can be seen the **aorta** which arises from the left
ventricle. The **superior vena cava** can be seen opening into the upper aspect of the right atrium.

5) the **ligamentum arteriosum.** This fibrous structure between the left pulmonary artery and the aorta, is the remnant of
the fetal **ductus arteriosus** which, before birth, served to shunt blood directed to the lungs back into the aorta for systemic
distribution.

Fig. 199

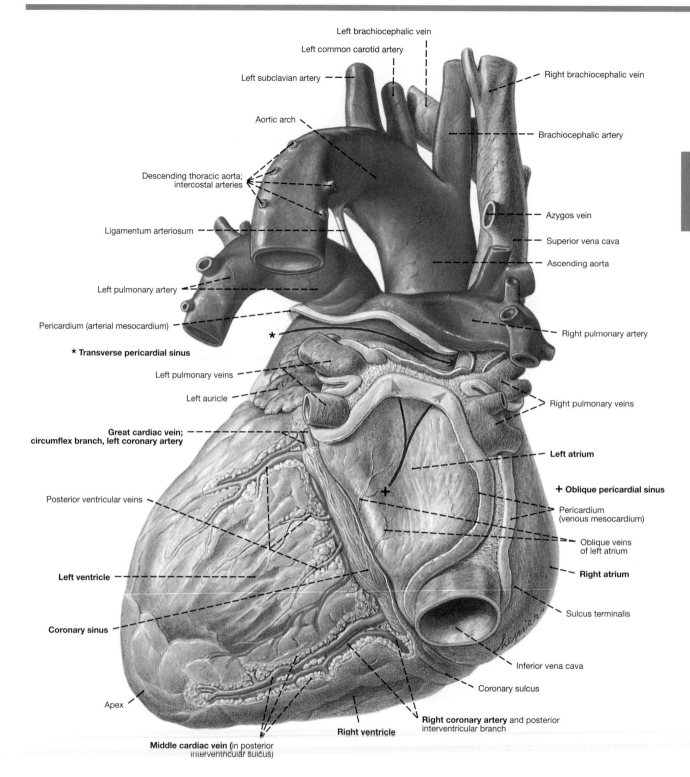

Left brachiocephalic vein

Left common carotid artery

Left subclavian artery

Right brachiocephalic vein

Aortic arch

Brachiocephalic artery

Descending thoracic aorta;
intercostal arteries

Azygos vein

Ligamentum arteriosum

Superior vena cava

Ascending aorta

Left pulmonary artery

Pericardium (arterial mesocardium)

Right pulmonary artery

* Transverse pericardial sinus

*

Left pulmonary veins

Left auricle

Right pulmonary veins

**Great cardiac vein;
circumflex branch, left coronary artery**

Left atrium

+ Oblique pericardial sinus

Posterior ventricular veins

+

Pericardium
(venous mesocardium)

Oblique veins
of left atrium

Left ventricle

Right atrium

Sulcus terminalis

Coronary sinus

Inferior vena cava

Coronary sulcus

Apex

Right coronary artery and posterior
interventricular branch

Right ventricle

Middle cardiac vein (in posterior
interventricular sulcus)

Fig. 200: Posterior View of the Heart and Great Vessels

NOTE: 1) the two pericardial sinuses. The black horizontal arrow indicates the **transverse pericardial sinus** which lies between the arterial mesocardium and the venous mesocardium. The vertical diverging double arrows lie in the **oblique pericardial sinus,** the boundary of which is limited by the pericardial reflections around the pulmonary veins.

2) the transverse sinus can be identified by placing your index finger behind the pulmonary artery and aorta with the heart in place. The oblique sinus is open inferiorly and can be felt by cupping your fingers behind the heart and pushing upward; superiorly this sinus forms a closed cul-de-sac.

3) the **coronary sinus** is a large vein and it separates the posterior atrial and ventricular surfaces. The posterior atrial surface consists principally of the left atrium, into which flow the pulmonary veins, but also note the right atrium and its superior vena cava below and to the right.

4) the posterior ventricular surface is formed principally by the left ventricle and this surface lies over the diaphragm.

Fig. 200   II

PLATE 126 Heart: Coronary Arteries

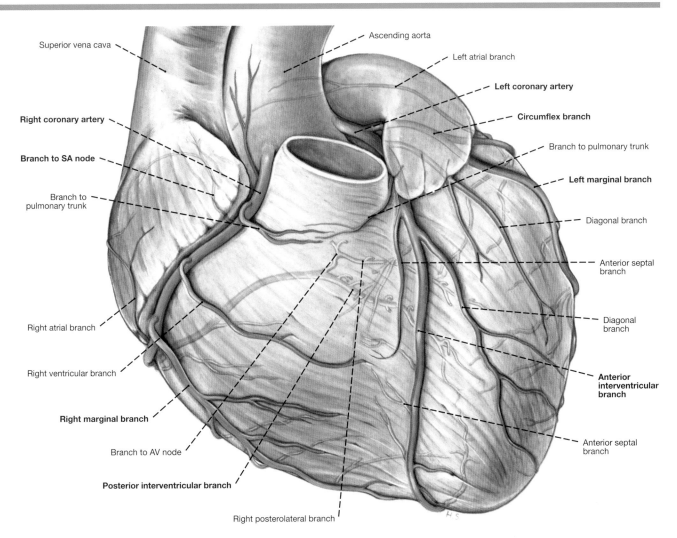

Superior vena cava

Right coronary artery

Branch to SA node

Branch to pulmonary trunk

Right atrial branch

Right ventricular branch

Right marginal branch

Branch to AV node

Posterior interventricular branch

Right posterolateral branch

Ascending aorta

Left atrial branch

Left coronary artery

Circumflex branch

Branch to pulmonary trunk

Left marginal branch

Diagonal branch

Anterior septal branch

Diagonal branch

Anterior interventricular branch

Anterior septal branch

Fig. 201: Complete Coronary Arterial System ▲

NOTE: 1) anastomoses between branches from the left and right coronary arteries (LCA and RCA) are visible in the substance of the posterior wall of the heart. These occur between the posterior interventricular branch of the RCA and the anterior interventricular branch of the LCA which continues around the apex of the heart to the posterior wall.

2) vessels from the circumflex and left marginal branches of the LCA also anastomose with branches from the RCA in the posterior wall.

3) branches supplying the sinoatrial (SA) node and the atrioventricular (AV) node arise from the RCA. In about 35% of cases, however, the artery to the SA node comes from the circumflex branch of the LCA. Similarly, in about 20% of specimens, the vessel to the AV node is derived from the circumflex branch of the LCA. (From a drawing by Professor Helmut Ferner at the University of Vienna).

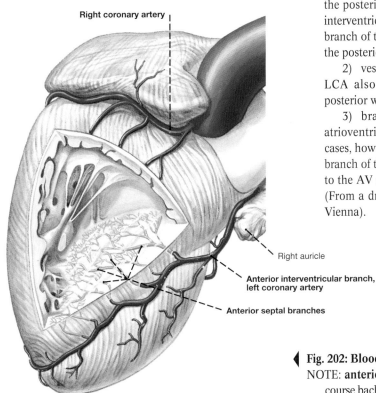

Right coronary artery

Right auricle

Anterior interventricular branch, left coronary artery

Anterior septal branches

◀ **Fig. 202: Blood Supply to the Interventricular Septum**

NOTE: **anterior septal branches** of the anterior interventricular artery course backward and downward to supply the interventricular septum.

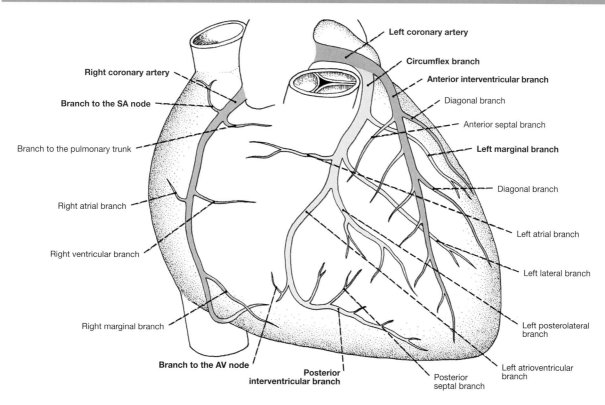

Fig. 203: Dominant Distribution to the Heart Wall from the Left Coronary Artery

NOTE: in hearts containing a dominant left coronary artery, there is very little contribution from the right coronary artery to the posterior wall of the left ventricle. In these cases, the posterior interventricular artery arises from the left coronary artery as a continuation of the enlarged circumflex branch.

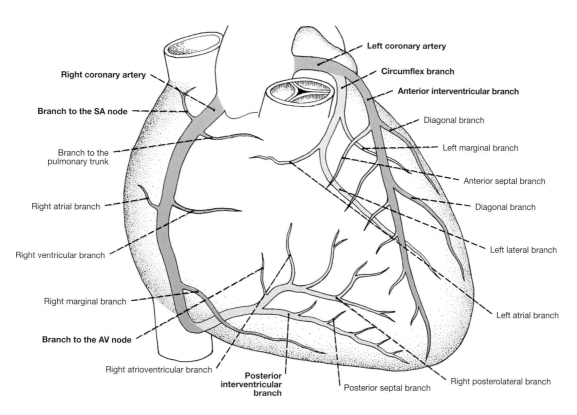

Fig. 204: Dominant Distribution to the Heart Wall from the Right Coronary Artery

NOTE: in hearts containing a dominant right coronary artery, the posterior wall of the left ventricle receives a larger share of its blood from the right coronary artery when compared with a left dominant coronary heart. In these instances the posterior interventricular artery arises from the right coronary, and the circumflex and marginal branches of the left coronary are relatively smaller.

PLATE 128   Heart: Arteriogram of the Left Coronary Artery

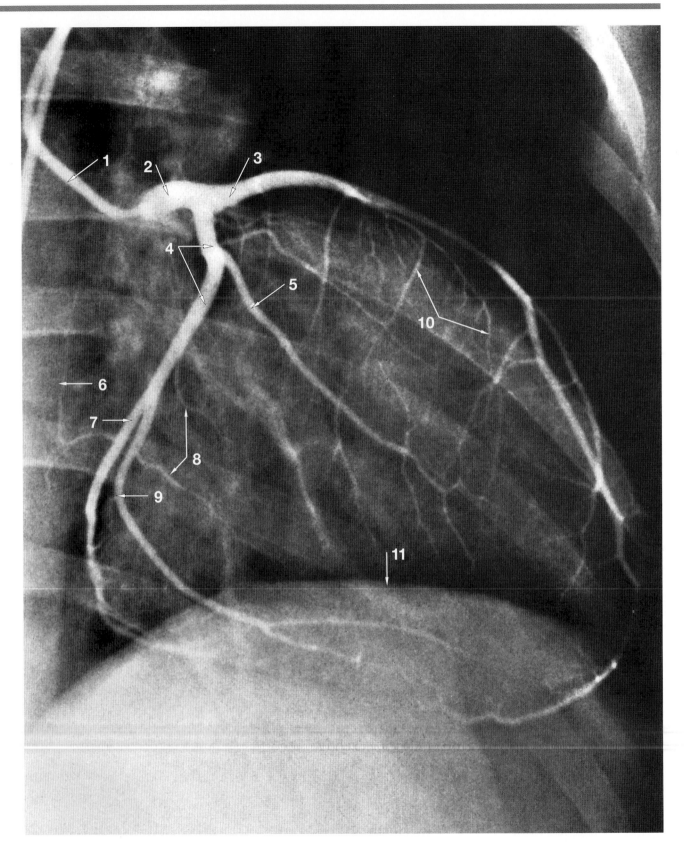

Fig. 205: Left Coronary Arteriogram

NOTE: this arteriogram of the left coronary artery is viewed from a right anterior oblique direction (From Wicke L. Atlas of Radiographic Anatomy, 4th Edition. Baltimore, Urban & Schwarzenberg, 1987).

1	Catheter	4	Circumflex branch	7	Left posterolateral branch of circumflex
2	Left coronary artery	5	Left marginal branch of circumflex	8	Posterior ventricular branches
3	Anterior interventricular branch	6	Posterior atrial branch	9	Posterior interventricular branch

10 Septal branches
11 Diaphragm

Fig. 205

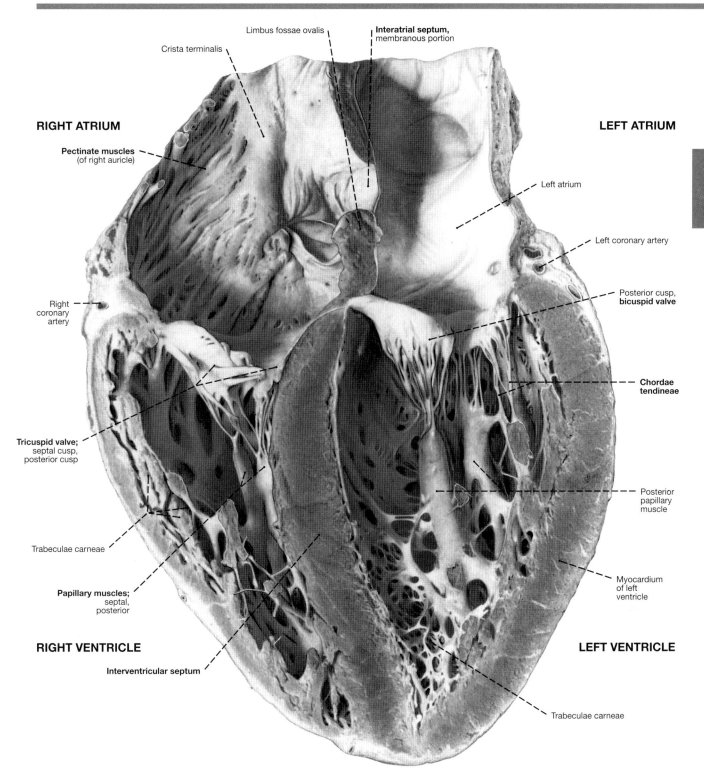

Crista terminalis
Limbus fossae ovalis
Interatrial septum, membranous portion

RIGHT ATRIUM

LEFT ATRIUM

Pectinate muscles (of right auricle)

Left atrium

Left coronary artery

Right coronary artery

Posterior cusp, **bicuspid valve**

Chordae tendineae

Tricuspid valve; septal cusp, posterior cusp

Posterior papillary muscle

Trabeculae carneae

Myocardium of left ventricle

Papillary muscles; septal, posterior

RIGHT VENTRICLE

LEFT VENTRICLE

Interventricular septum

Trabeculae carneae

Fig. 206: Frontal Section Through the Heart, Showing Dorsal Half of Heart

NOTE: 1)   the human heart is a four-chambered muscular organ and consists of an **atrium** and a **ventricle** on each side. The walls of the ventricles are thicker than those of the atria. The two atrial chambers are separated by an **interatrial septum,** which is continuous with the **interventricular septum** that divides the two ventricles.

2)   blood passes simultaneously from the two atria into their respective ventricles through the **tricuspid** and **bicuspid** or **atrioventricular** (AV) **valves.**

3)   on the right side, the AV valve consists of three cusps (tricuspid) and on the left side the AV valve has two cusps (bicuspid). The bicuspid valve is also called the **mitral valve.**

4)   the surfaces of the atria are smooth except for the **pectinate muscles.** The ventricles have muscular elevations called **trabeculae carneae** and **papillary muscles** that attach the heart wall to the cusps of the valves by way of **chordae tendineae.**

Fig. 206   II

PLATE 130   Heart: Right Atrium and Ventricle

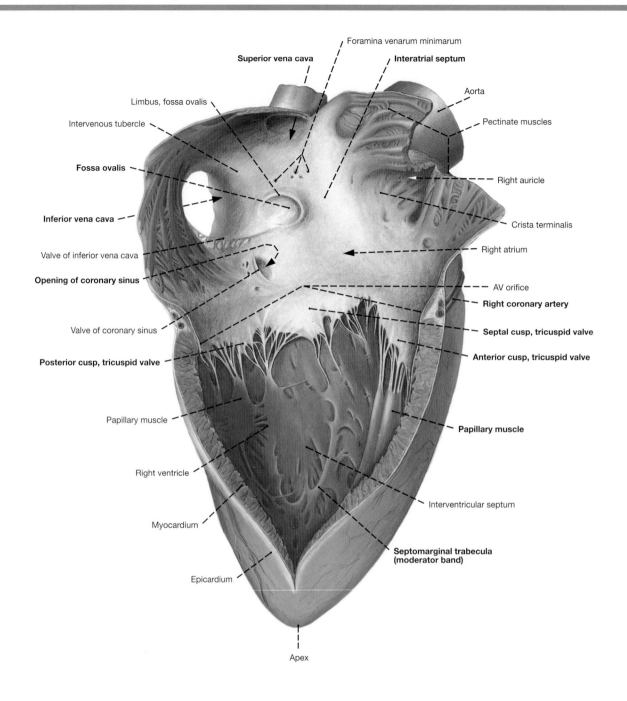

Fig. 207: Right Atrium and Right Ventricle

NOTE: 1) the right atrium consists of (a) a smooth area (at times called the **sinus venarum**) located between the openings of the superior vena cava and inferior vena cava and (b) the **right auricle,** which is marked by parallel muscle ridges called the **pectinate muscles.**

2) opening into the right atrium are the **superior vena cava,** the **inferior vena cava,** the **coronary sinus,** and the small **venarum minimarum** (Thebesian veins).

3) crescent-shaped valves are found at the right atrial openings of both the inferior vena cava and the coronary sinus.

4) the right atrioventricular (AV) opening is surrounded by the three cusps of the **tricuspid valve.** These are called the **anterior, posterior,** and **septal** cusps, and they are attached to the heart wall by way of the **chordae tendineae** and **papillary muscles.**

5) the thickness of the right ventricular wall (4 to 5 mm) is about one-third that of the left ventricle (see Fig. 206). Normal right ventricular systolic blood pressure ranges between 25 and 30 mm Hg, and it is also much less than normal left ventricular systolic pressure, which ranges between 120 and 140 mm Hg.

6) the **septomarginal trabecula** (moderator band) within which courses the right crus or branch of the **atrioventricular bundle** (of His).

Fig. 207

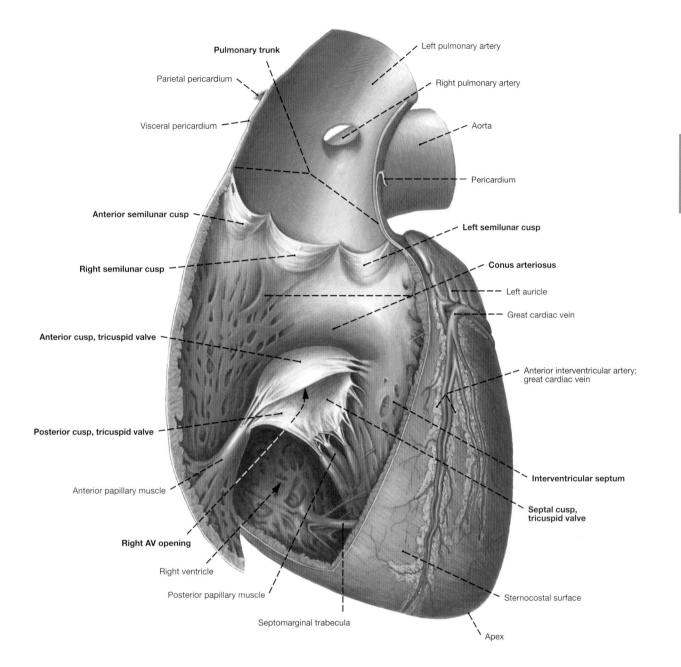

Pulmonary trunk

Parietal pericardium

Visceral pericardium

Anterior semilunar cusp

Right semilunar cusp

Anterior cusp, tricuspid valve

Posterior cusp, tricuspid valve

Anterior papillary muscle

Right AV opening

Right ventricle

Posterior papillary muscle

Septomarginal trabecula

Left pulmonary artery

Right pulmonary artery

Aorta

Pericardium

Left semilunar cusp

Conus arteriosus

Left auricle

Great cardiac vein

Anterior interventricular artery; great cardiac vein

Interventricular septum

Septal cusp, tricuspid valve

Sternocostal surface

Apex

Fig. 208: Right Ventricle and Pulmonary Trunk

NOTE: 1) the musculature of the right ventricle has been cut along a V-shaped incision, thereby forming a flap in the anterior wall of the ventricle. As the flap is reflected to the right, the origin of the **pulmonary trunk** and the cusps of its valve are exposed.

2) the three semilunar pulmonary cusps, which are interposed between the right ventricle and the pulmonary artery. They are called the **right, left,** and **anterior** semilunar pulmonary cusps and together they comprise the **pulmonary valve.**

3) the **septal, anterior,** and **posterior cusps** that form the **right atrioventricular** (AV) or **tricuspid valve.** Also note their attachments to the papillary muscles.

4) the smooth surface of the right ventricular wall at the site of origin of the pulmonary trunk. This is called the **conus arteriosus** of the right ventricle.

5) the attachment and shape of the tricuspid valve allow the cusps to open into the right ventricle when blood pressure in the atrium exceeds that in the ventricle. At some point during the cardiac cycle, ventricular pressure exceeds atrial pressure and the cusps close. Blood is prevented from regurgitating into the atrium because the perimeter of the cusps is secured to the heart wall and the free edges of the cusps are attached to the papillary muscles in the ventricle below.

Fig. 208   **II**

PLATE 132   Heart: Left Atrium and Ventricle

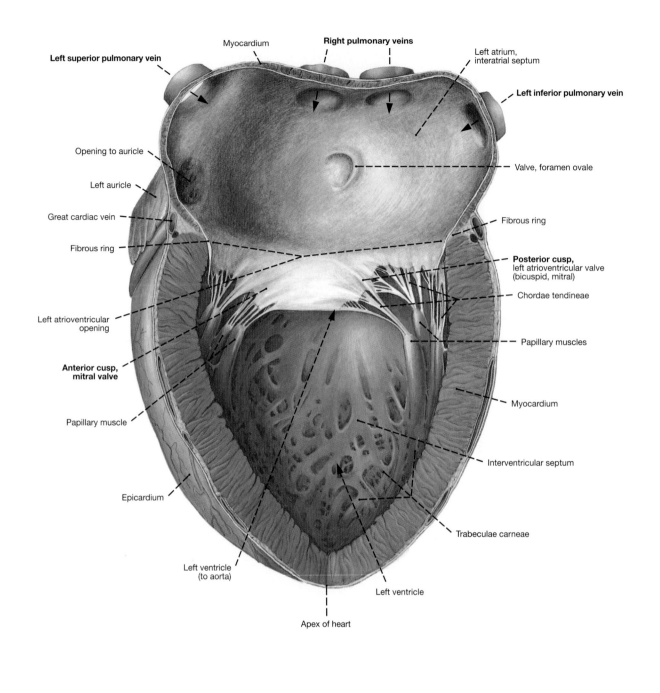

Myocardium

Right pulmonary veins

Left atrium, interatrial septum

Left superior pulmonary vein

Left inferior pulmonary vein

Opening to auricle

Valve, foramen ovale

Left auricle

Great cardiac vein

Fibrous ring

Fibrous ring

Posterior cusp, left atrioventricular valve (bicuspid, mitral)

Chordae tendineae

Left atrioventricular opening

Papillary muscles

Anterior cusp, mitral valve

Myocardium

Papillary muscle

Interventricular septum

Epicardium

Trabeculae carneae

Left ventricle (to aorta)

Left ventricle

Apex of heart

Fig. 209: Left Atrium and Left Ventricle, Internal Surface

NOTE: 1)   in this specimen, the heart has been opened to expose the inner surface of the left atrium and left ventricle. Likewise the left atrioventricular opening has been cut behind the **posterior cusp of the mitral valve,** thereby making that cusp visible.

2)   the left atrium receives the four **pulmonary veins** (two from each lung), while the left ventricle leads into the aorta (see arrow).

3)   the **interatrial septum** on the left side is marked by the valve of the foramen ovale (falx septi), which represents the remnant of the **septum primum** during the development of the interatrial septum. The crescent-shaped structure around the border of the valve is the limbus of the fossa ovalis and is the remnant of the **septum secundum.**

4)   the mitral valve consists of **anterior and posterior cusps** (only the posterior is seen in this figure). The cusps are attached to the left ventricular wall by means of chordae tendineae and papillary muscles in a manner similar to that seen in the right ventricle.

Fig. 207

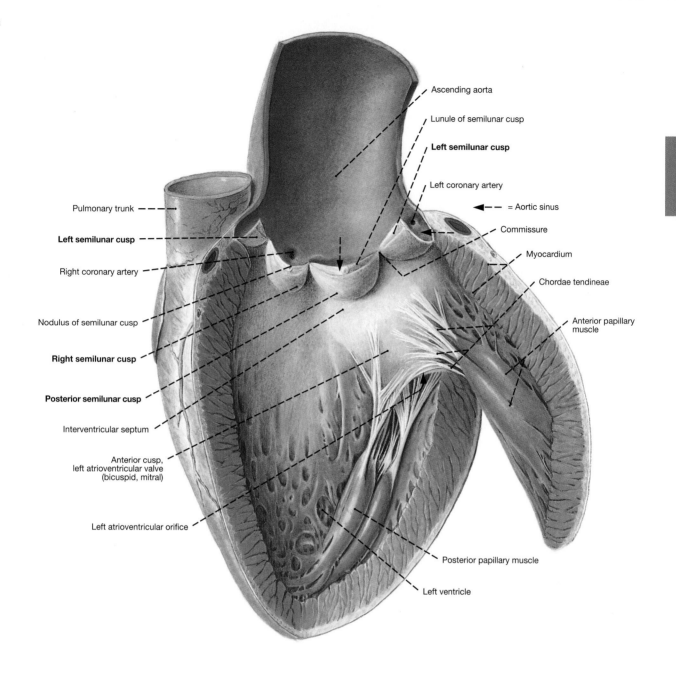

Fig. 210: Opened Left Ventricle and Aorta

NOTE: 1) in this dissection, the left ventricle was opened first to show the anterior and posterior papillary muscles that are related to the cusps of the left AV valve. A second cut was then made in the wall of the left ventricle (near the interventricular septum) that extends through the aortic opening to show the cusps of the **aortic valve.**

2) the opening of the left coronary artery in the aortic wall behind the (cut) **left semilunar cusp.** Also see the opening of the right coronary artery behind the **right semilunar cusp.** The **posterior cusp** of the aortic valve is the non-coronary cusp.

3) between the cusps and the wall of the aorta are pockets called the **aortic sinuses.** These trap blood during the cardiac cycle, thereby closing the valve.

4) each cusp is marked by a thickened fibrocartilaginous **nodule** at the center of its free margin. Extending out from the nodule on each side of the cusp are clear crescenteric areas of thinning of the free edges called **lunules,** while the points at which two adjacent cusps come together are called **commissures.**

Fig. 210   **II**

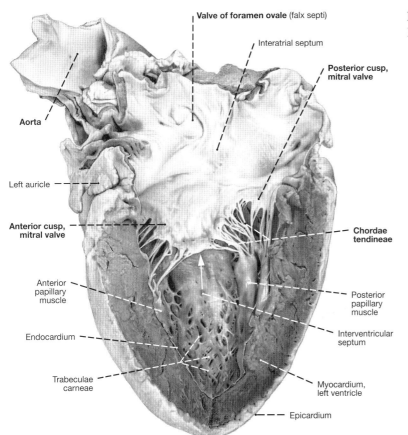

Valve of foramen ovale (falx septi)

Interatrial septum

Posterior cusp, mitral valve

Aorta

Left auricle

Anterior cusp, mitral valve

Chordae tendineae

Anterior papillary muscle

Posterior papillary muscle

Endocardium

Interventricular septum

Trabeculae carneae

Myocardium, left ventricle

Epicardium

Fig. 211: Left Atrium and Left Ventricle

NOTE: 1) this photograph shows the left side of the heart. A longitudinal section has been made through the heart to expose the smooth-walled left atrium above and the thick-walled left ventricle below. It should be compared with the drawing in Figure 209.

2) the left atrium receives the four pulmonary veins (two from each lung) and passes the oxygenated blood into the left ventricle.

3) the white arrow indicates the direction of blood flow from the left ventricle to the aorta.

4) the mitral or bicuspid valve, its anterior and posterior cusps and their papillary muscles and chordae tendineae.

5) a) the inner lining of the heart is the **endocardium;**
   b) the muscular layer is the **myocardium;**
   c) the outer covering is the **epicardium** (visceral pericardium).

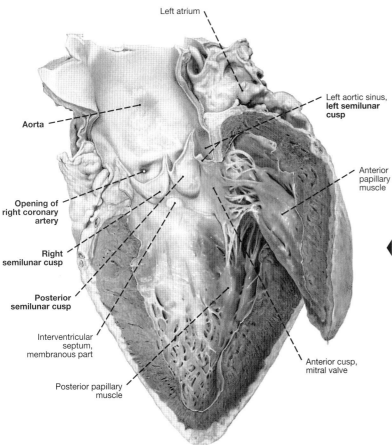

Left atrium

Aorta

Left aortic sinus, **left semilunar cusp**

Anterior papillary muscle

Opening of right coronary artery

Right semilunar cusp

Posterior semilunar cusp

Interventricular septum, membranous part

Anterior cusp, mitral valve

Posterior papillary muscle

◀ Fig. 212: Left Ventricle and Ascending Aorta

NOTE: 1) this photograph shows a longitudinal section of the heart that exposes the left ventricular cavity leading into the ascending aorta. Compare this figure with Figure 210.

2) during ventricular contraction, blood pressure in the left ventricle is elevated over that in the aorta and causes the aortic valve to open. As blood passes into the aorta, aortic pressure increases, and at some point exceeds ventricular pressure. Then, blood rushes back toward the ventricle and becomes trapped in the aortic sinuses, thereby closing the valve.

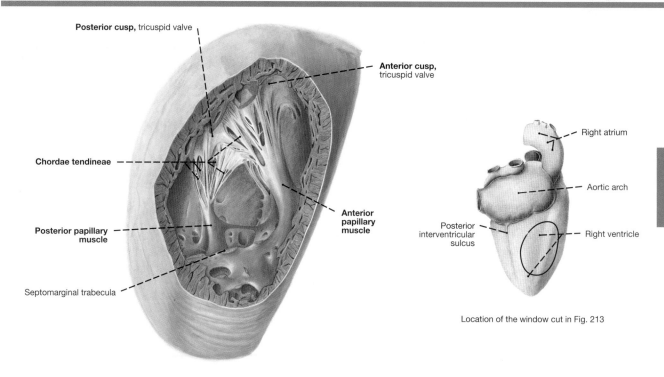

Location of the window cut in Fig. 213

Fig. 213: Right Ventricle: View of the Tricuspid Valve
NOTE: 1) a portion of the wall of the right ventricle has been removed (see sketch to the right). This exposes two of the three cusps (anterior and posterior) of the tricuspid valve and their attached papillary muscles.

2) the **anterior papillary muscle** arises from the anterior and septal walls. It is usually larger than the posterior and its chordae tendineae attach to both the anterior and posterior cusps. The **posterior papillary muscle** arises from the posterior wall and its chordae tendineae attach to the posterior and septal cusps. Small septal papillary muscles are also often seen.

3) the **septomarginal trabecula,** or moderator band, containing the atrioventricular bundle has been severed close to the ventricular wall.

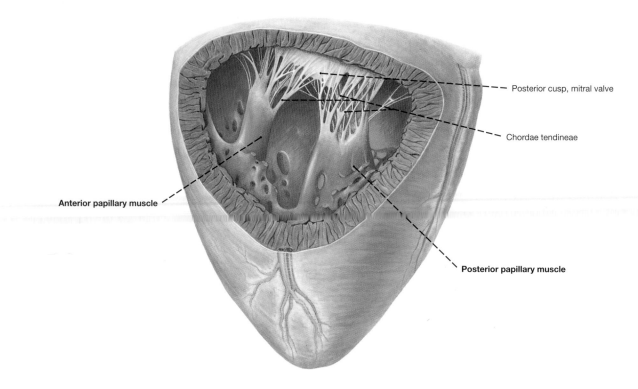

Fig. 214: Left Ventricle: View of the Mitral Valve
NOTE: a window has been cut through the myocardium on the posterior surface of the heart to show the **posterior and anterior papillary muscles** and their chordae tendineae that attach to the cusps of the mitral valve.

PLATE 136   Heart: Conduction System, Photographs

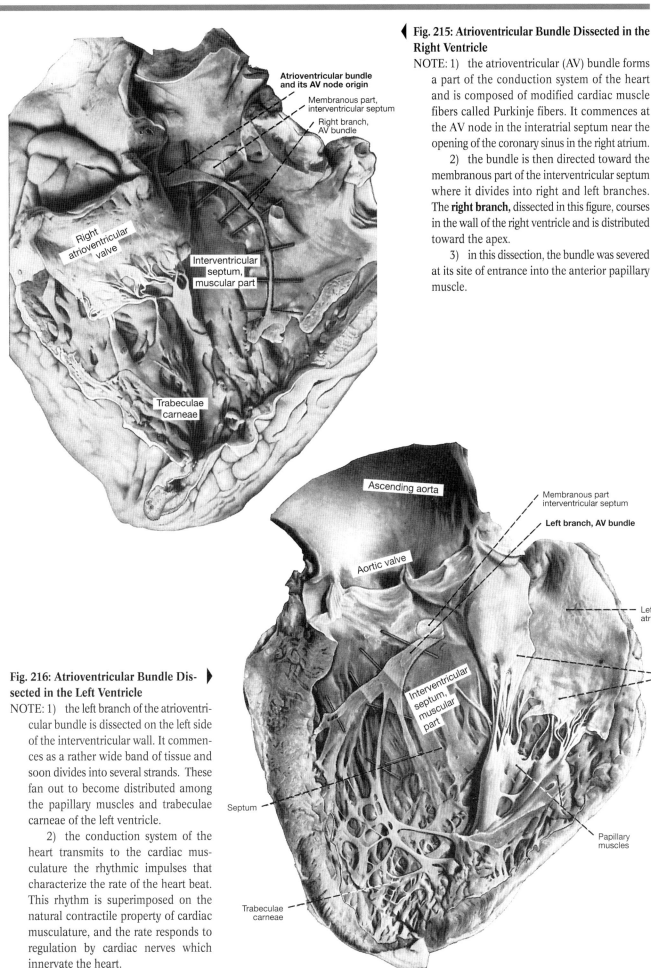

Fig. 215: Atrioventricular Bundle Dissected in the Right Ventricle

NOTE: 1) the atrioventricular (AV) bundle forms a part of the conduction system of the heart and is composed of modified cardiac muscle fibers called Purkinje fibers. It commences at the AV node in the interatrial septum near the opening of the coronary sinus in the right atrium.

2) the bundle is then directed toward the membranous part of the interventricular septum where it divides into right and left branches. The **right branch,** dissected in this figure, courses in the wall of the right ventricle and is distributed toward the apex.

3) in this dissection, the bundle was severed at its site of entrance into the anterior papillary muscle.

Labels (Fig. 215):
Atrioventricular bundle and its AV node origin
Membranous part, interventricular septum
Right branch, AV bundle
Right atrioventricular valve
Interventricular septum, muscular part
Trabeculae carneae

Fig. 216: Atrioventricular Bundle Dissected in the Left Ventricle

NOTE: 1) the left branch of the atrioventricular bundle is dissected on the left side of the interventricular wall. It commences as a rather wide band of tissue and soon divides into several strands. These fan out to become distributed among the papillary muscles and trabeculae carneae of the left ventricle.

2) the conduction system of the heart transmits to the cardiac musculature the rhythmic impulses that characterize the rate of the heart beat. This rhythm is superimposed on the natural contractile property of cardiac musculature, and the rate responds to regulation by cardiac nerves which innervate the heart.

Labels (Fig. 216):
Ascending aorta
Membranous part interventricular septum
Left branch, AV bundle
Aortic valve
Left atrium
Mitral valve
Interventricular septum, muscular part
Septum
Papillary muscles
Trabeculae carneae

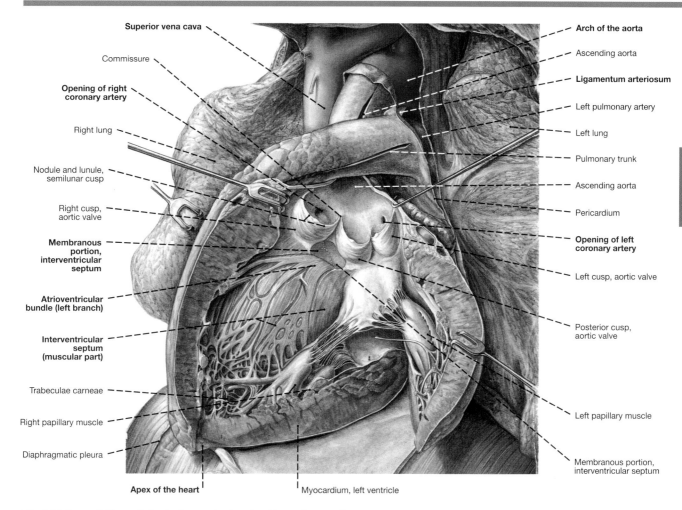

Superior vena cava

Commissure

Opening of right
coronary artery

Right lung

Nodule and lunule,
semilunar cusp

Right cusp,
aortic valve

Membranous
portion,
interventricular
septum

Atrioventricular
bundle (left branch)

Interventricular
septum
(muscular part)

Trabeculae carneae

Right papillary muscle

Diaphragmatic pleura

Apex of the heart

Myocardium, left ventricle

Arch of the aorta

Ascending aorta

Ligamentum arteriosum

Left pulmonary artery

Left lung

Pulmonary trunk

Ascending aorta

Pericardium

Opening of left
coronary artery

Left cusp, aortic valve

Posterior cusp,
aortic valve

Left papillary muscle

Membranous portion,
interventricular septum

Fig. 217: Lateral View of the Atrioventricular Bundle (Left Branch)
NOTE: the left branch of the AV bundle has been dissected (and shown in yellow) in its course along the left side of the interventricular septum. It is observed from within the opened left ventricle (compare with Fig. 216), as are the cusps of the mitral and aortic valves.

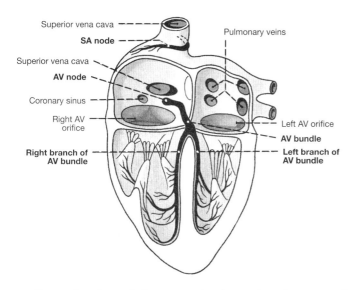

Superior vena cava

SA node

Superior vena cava

AV node

Coronary sinus

Right AV
orifice

Right branch of
AV bundle

Pulmonary veins

Left AV orifice

AV bundle

Left branch of
AV bundle

Fig. 218: Diagram of the Conduction System of the Heart
NOTE: 1) the cardiac cycle begins at the SA (sinoatrial) node located in the sulcus terminalis between the superior vena cava and the right atrium.

2) from this pacemaker, a wave of negativity (excitation) spreads over both atria and initiates atrial contraction, thereby increasing atrial blood pressure.

3) when atrial pressure exceeds ventricular pressure, both AV valves open and blood rushes into both ventricles. Soon the impulse reaches the AV node and is passed along the AV bundle to the two ventricles, causing them to contract.

4) when ventricular pressure exceeds atrial pressure, the AV valves close, and this can be heard with a stethoscope as the first of the two heart sounds of the heart beat.

5) continued ventricular contraction forces the pulmonary and aortic valves to open and blood rushes simultaneously into the pulmonary artery and aorta.

6) when the pressure in these vessels exceeds ventricular pressure, blood tends to rush back into the ventricles but gets trapped in the sinuses behind the semilunar cusps. This closes both the pulmonary and aortic valves resulting in the second of the two heart sounds heard with the stethoscope.

PLATE 138   Heart and Thymus in the Newborn Child

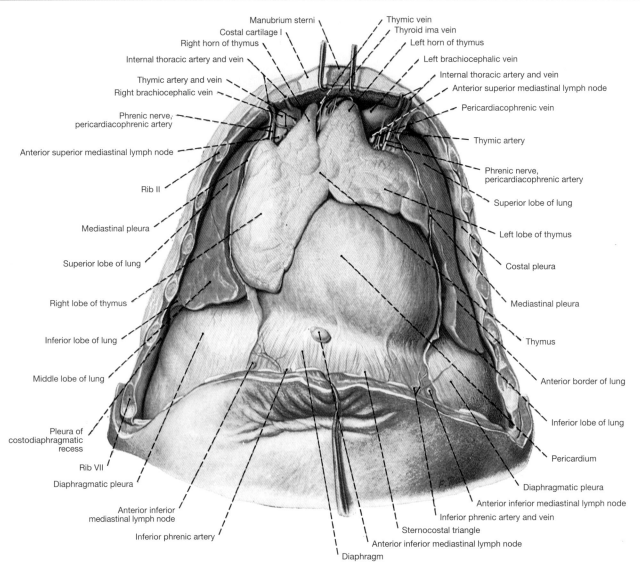

Manubrium sterni
Costal cartilage I
Right horn of thymus
Internal thoracic artery and vein
Thymic artery and vein
Right brachiocephalic vein
Phrenic nerve,
pericardiacophrenic artery
Anterior superior mediastinal lymph node
Rib II
Mediastinal pleura
Superior lobe of lung
Right lobe of thymus
Inferior lobe of lung
Middle lobe of lung
Pleura of
costodiaphragmatic
recess
Rib VII
Diaphragmatic pleura
Anterior inferior
mediastinal lymph node
Inferior phrenic artery

Thymic vein
Thyroid ima vein
Left horn of thymus
Left brachiocephalic vein
Internal thoracic artery and vein
Anterior superior mediastinal lymph node
Pericardiacophrenic vein
Thymic artery
Phrenic nerve,
pericardiacophrenic artery
Superior lobe of lung
Left lobe of thymus
Costal pleura
Mediastinal pleura
Thymus
Anterior border of lung
Inferior lobe of lung
Pericardium
Diaphragmatic pleura
Anterior inferior mediastinal lymph node
Inferior phrenic artery and vein
Sternocostal triangle
Anterior inferior mediastinal lymph node
Diaphragm

Fig. 219: Anterior View of the Pericardial Sac and Thymus in the Newborn Child
NOTE: in the newborn child, the great vessels of the superior mediastinum and the parietal pericardium over the base of the heart are covered by the thymus gland. This gland also extends into the root of the neck in the neonate.

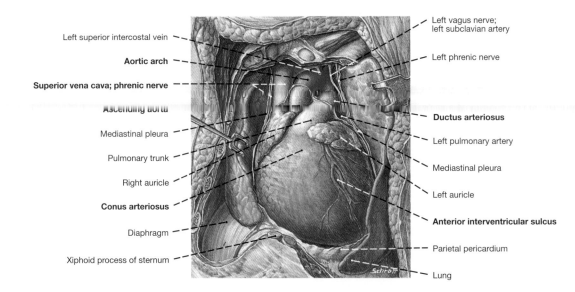

Left superior intercostal vein
Aortic arch
Superior vena cava; phrenic nerve
Ascending aorta
Mediastinal pleura
Pulmonary trunk
Right auricle
Conus arteriosus
Diaphragm
Xiphoid process of sternum

Left vagus nerve;
left subclavian artery
Left phrenic nerve
Ductus arteriosus
Left pulmonary artery
Mediastinal pleura
Left auricle
Anterior interventricular sulcus
Parietal pericardium
Lung

Fig. 220: Anterior View of the Heart and Great Vessels of a Newborn Child After Removal of the Thymus
NOTE: the **ductus arteriosus** is still an enlarged structure immediately after birth. It regresses in size during the first week of life.

Figs. 219, 220

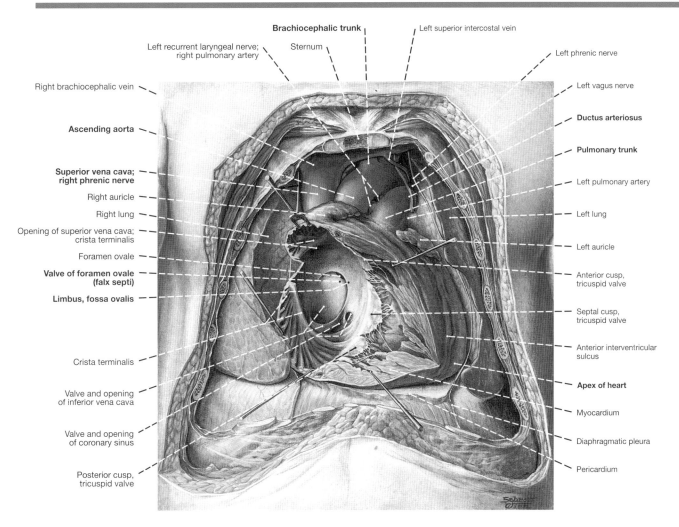

Brachiocephalic trunk

Left recurrent laryngeal nerve; right pulmonary artery

Sternum

Left superior intercostal vein

Left phrenic nerve

Right brachiocephalic vein

Left vagus nerve

Ascending aorta

Ductus arteriosus

Superior vena cava; right phrenic nerve

Pulmonary trunk

Right auricle

Left pulmonary artery

Right lung

Left lung

Opening of superior vena cava; crista terminalis

Left auricle

Foramen ovale

Anterior cusp, tricuspid valve

Valve of foramen ovale (falx septi)

Septal cusp, tricuspid valve

Limbus, fossa ovalis

Anterior interventricular sulcus

Crista terminalis

Apex of heart

Valve and opening of inferior vena cava

Myocardium

Valve and opening of coronary sinus

Diaphragmatic pleura

Pericardium

Posterior cusp, tricuspid valve

Fig. 221: Heart of Newborn Child: View of Right Atrium and Ventricle, Fossa Ovalis and Tricuspid Valve

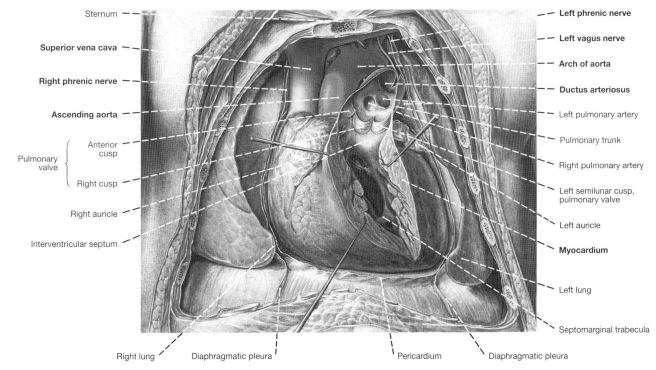

Sternum

Left phrenic nerve

Superior vena cava

Left vagus nerve

Right phrenic nerve

Arch of aorta

Ascending aorta

Ductus arteriosus

Pulmonary valve — Anterior cusp

Left pulmonary artery

Pulmonary trunk

Right cusp

Right pulmonary artery

Right auricle

Left semilunar cusp, pulmonary valve

Interventricular septum

Left auricle

Myocardium

Left lung

Septomarginal trabecula

Right lung   Diaphragmatic pleura   Pericardium   Diaphragmatic pleura

Fig. 222: Heart of Newborn Child: View of Pulmonary Trunk and Opened Right Ventricle

PLATE 140 Circulation of Blood in the Fetus

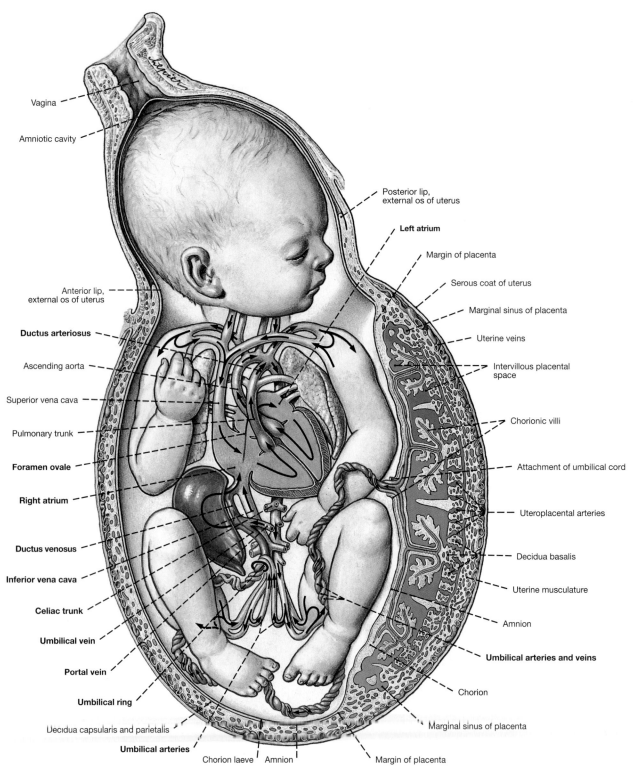

Vagina

Amniotic cavity

Anterior lip,
external os of uterus

Ductus arteriosus

Ascending aorta

Superior vena cava

Pulmonary trunk

Foramen ovale

Right atrium

Ductus venosus

Inferior vena cava

Celiac trunk

Umbilical vein

Portal vein

Umbilical ring

Decidua capsularis and parietalis

Umbilical arteries

Chorion laeve   Amnion

Posterior lip,
external os of uterus

Left atrium

Margin of placenta

Serous coat of uterus

Marginal sinus of placenta

Uterine veins

Intervillous placental
space

Chorionic villi

Attachment of umbilical cord

Uteroplacental arteries

Decidua basalis

Uterine musculature

Amnion

Umbilical arteries and veins

Chorion

Marginal sinus of placenta

Margin of placenta

Fig. 223: Circulation in the Fetus as Seen in Utero
NOTE: In the fetus:

1) deoxygenated blood courses to the placenta by way of the **umbilical arteries.** It is then both nourished and oxygenated and leaves the placenta by way of the **umbilical vein.**

2) much of the oxygenated blood bypasses the liver, coursing from the umbilical vein, through the **ductus venosus,** to reach the inferior vena cava.

3) from the inferior vena cava, blood enters the right atrium as does blood from the superior vena cava. Right atrial blood bypasses the lungs by means of two routes:

   a) across to the left atrium through the **foramen ovale,** then to the left ventricle and out the aorta to the rest of the fetal body, and

   b) to the right ventricle, out the pulmonary artery and through the **ductus arteriosus** to reach the aorta, and then to the rest of the fetal body (also see Fig. 224).

Fig. 223

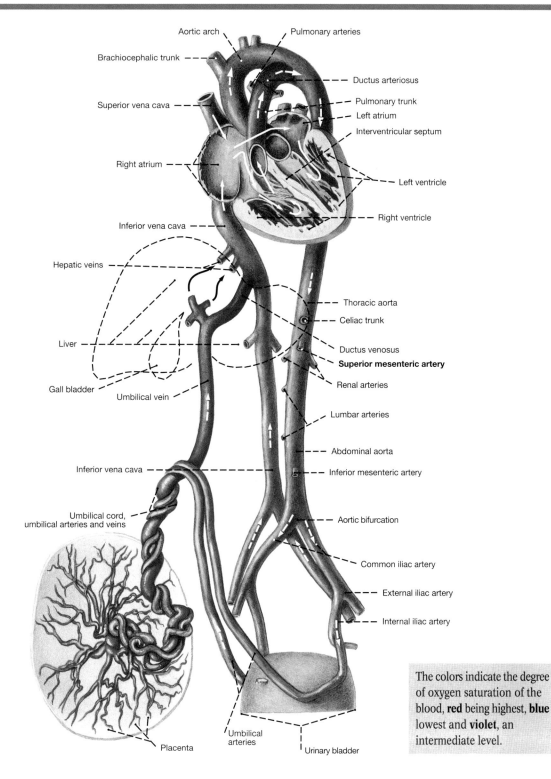

Aortic arch

Pulmonary arteries

Brachiocephalic trunk

Ductus arteriosus

Superior vena cava

Pulmonary trunk

Left atrium

Interventricular septum

Right atrium

Left ventricle

Right ventricle

Inferior vena cava

Hepatic veins

Thoracic aorta

Celiac trunk

Liver

Ductus venosus

Superior mesenteric artery

Renal arteries

Gall bladder

Lumbar arteries

Umbilical vein

Inferior vena cava

Abdominal aorta

Inferior mesenteric artery

Umbilical cord,
umbilical arteries and veins

Aortic bifurcation

Common iliac artery

External iliac artery

Internal iliac artery

The colors indicate the degree
of oxygen saturation of the
blood, **red** being highest, **blue**
lowest and **violet**, an
intermediate level.

Umbilical
arteries

Placenta

Urinary bladder

Fig. 224: Diagrammatic Representation of the Circulation in the Fetus

NOTE: Changes in the vascular system after birth; because the newborn infant becomes dependent on the lungs for oxygen,

1) breathing commences and the lungs begin to function thereby oxygenating the blood and removing carbon dioxide,

2) the **foramen ovale** decreases in size and blood ceases to cross from the right atrium to the left atrium,

3) the **ductus arteriosus** that interconnected the pulmonary artery and aorta constricts and gradually closes to become a fibrous cord called the **ligamentum arteriosum,**

4) the **umbilical arteries** cease to carry blood to the placenta, and they become fibrosed to form the **medial umbilical ligaments,**

5) the **umbilical vein** becomes fibrosed and forms the **ligamentum teres** (of the liver), while the **ductus venosus** is no longer functional and forms the **ligamentum venosum.**

Fig. 224   **II**

PLATE 142   Systemic Arteries in the Adult

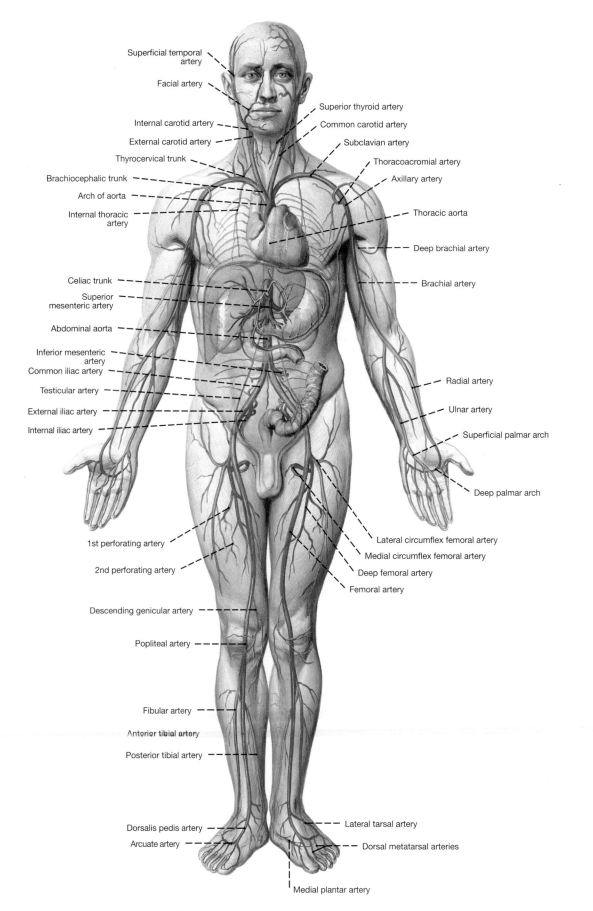

Superficial temporal artery
Facial artery
Superior thyroid artery
Internal carotid artery
Common carotid artery
External carotid artery
Subclavian artery
Thyrocervical trunk
Thoracoacromial artery
Brachiocephalic trunk
Axillary artery
Arch of aorta
Internal thoracic artery
Thoracic aorta
Deep brachial artery
Celiac trunk
Brachial artery
Superior mesenteric artery
Abdominal aorta
Inferior mesenteric artery
Common iliac artery
Radial artery
Testicular artery
Ulnar artery
External iliac artery
Internal iliac artery
Superficial palmar arch
Deep palmar arch
1st perforating artery
Lateral circumflex femoral artery
2nd perforating artery
Medial circumflex femoral artery
Deep femoral artery
Femoral artery
Descending genicular artery
Popliteal artery
Fibular artery
Anterior tibial artery
Posterior tibial artery
Lateral tarsal artery
Dorsalis pedis artery
Arcuate artery
Dorsal metatarsal arteries
Medial plantar artery

Fig. 225: Adult Systemic Arterial System (Male)
NOTE: most, but not all, of the named arteries in the systemic circulation are shown in this figure. Additionally, the pulmonary arteries coursing to the lungs from the right ventricle are not included.

Fig. 225

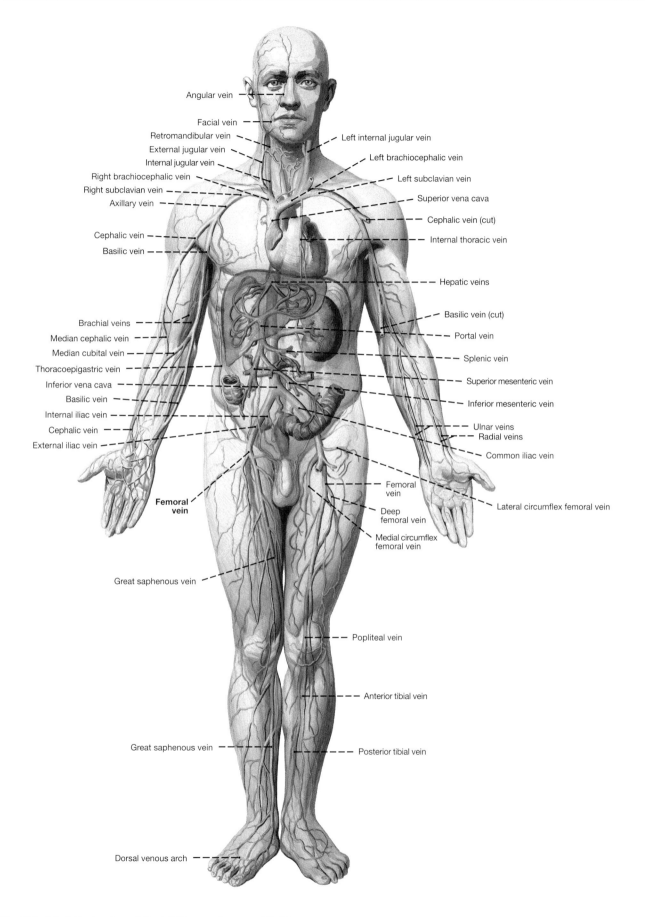

Fig. 226: Adult Systemic and Portal Venous Systems (Male)
NOTE: many, but not all, of the named veins are shown in this figure. The pulmonary veins that return blood to the left atrium from the lungs are not included. The portal system is shown in purple while the other veins are blue.

Fig. 226   ▌▌

PLATE 144   Mediastinum: Midsagittal Section

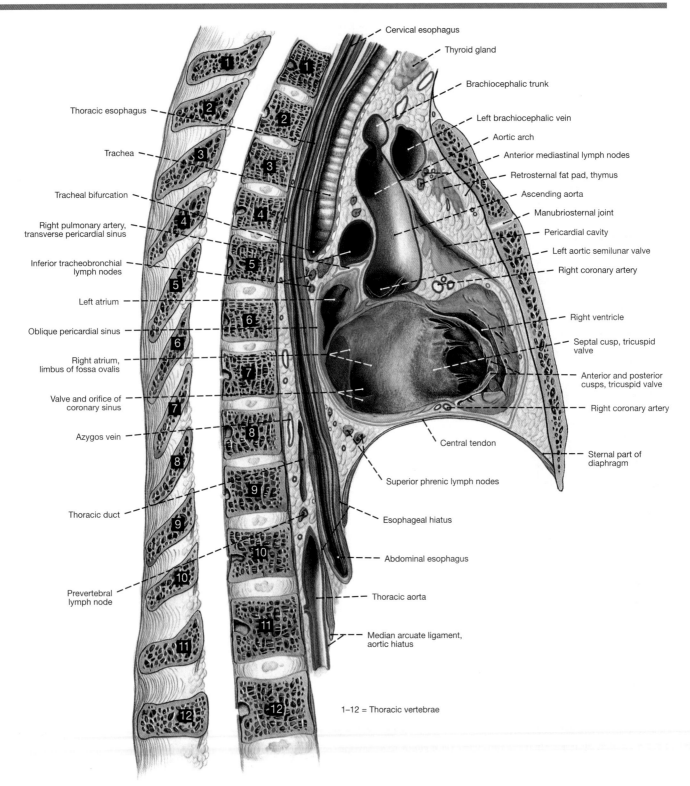

Cervical esophagus
Thyroid gland
Brachiocephalic trunk
Left brachiocephalic vein
Aortic arch
Anterior mediastinal lymph nodes
Retrosternal fat pad, thymus
Ascending aorta
Manubriosternal joint
Pericardial cavity
Left aortic semilunar valve
Right coronary artery
Right ventricle
Septal cusp, tricuspid valve
Anterior and posterior cusps, tricuspid valve
Right coronary artery
Sternal part of diaphragm
Central tendon
Superior phrenic lymph nodes
Esophageal hiatus
Abdominal esophagus
Thoracic aorta
Median arcuate ligament, aortic hiatus

Thoracic esophagus
Trachea
Tracheal bifurcation
Right pulmonary artery, transverse pericardial sinus
Inferior tracheobronchial lymph nodes
Left atrium
Oblique pericardial sinus
Right atrium, limbus of fossa ovalis
Valve and orifice of coronary sinus
Azygos vein
Thoracic duct
Prevertebral lymph node

1–12 = Thoracic vertebrae

Fig. 227: Median Sagittal Section of the Thorax and Vertebral Column Viewed from the Right Side

NOTE: 1) **vertebral levels** of important anatomical landmarks:

a) superior border of the sternum: T2
b) manubriosternal junction: T4
c) tracheal bifurcation: T4–T5
d) lower level of xiphoid process: T9
e) esophageal hiatus: T10
f) aortic hiatus: T11–12

2) a median sagittal section of the thorax goes through the right atrium and right ventricle, since $^1/_3$rd of the normal heart lies to the right of the midsternal line, and $^2/_3$rds lies to the left of the midline.

3) the **transverse pericardial sinus** located posterior to the aorta. The sinus also crosses the midline behind the pulmonary trunk, but in this figure the pulmonary trunk has already bifurcated and, thus, the sinus is shown below the right pulmonary artery.

4) in its course to the right atrium, the **left brachiocephalic vein** crosses the midline anterior to the arch of the aorta at the site where the brachiocephalic trunk arises from the aorta (see also Figs. 190, 193).

Fig. 227

LEFT

RIGHT

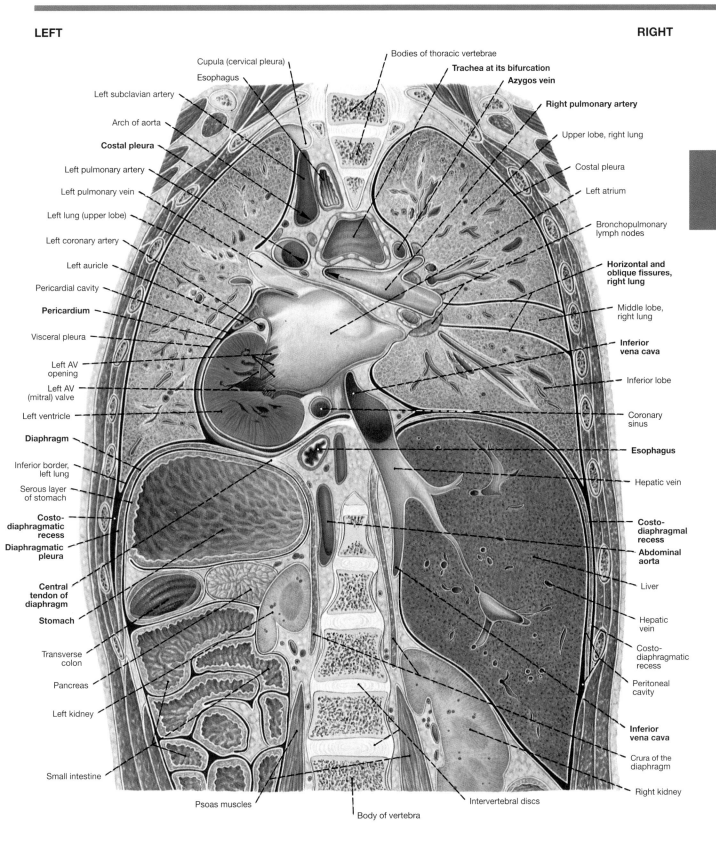

Cupula (cervical pleura)

Esophagus

Left subclavian artery

Arch of aorta

Costal pleura

Left pulmonary artery

Left pulmonary vein

Left lung (upper lobe)

Left coronary artery

Left auricle

Pericardial cavity

Pericardium

Visceral pleura

Left AV opening

Left AV (mitral) valve

Left ventricle

Diaphragm

Inferior border, left lung

Serous layer of stomach

Costo-diaphragmatic recess

Diaphragmatic pleura

Central tendon of diaphragm

Stomach

Transverse colon

Pancreas

Left kidney

Small intestine

Psoas muscles

Body of vertebra

Bodies of thoracic vertebrae

Trachea at its bifurcation

Azygos vein

Right pulmonary artery

Upper lobe, right lung

Costal pleura

Left atrium

Bronchopulmonary lymph nodes

Horizontal and oblique fissures, right lung

Middle lobe, right lung

Inferior vena cava

Inferior lobe

Coronary sinus

Esophagus

Hepatic vein

Costo-diaphragmal recess

Abdominal aorta

Liver

Hepatic vein

Costo-diaphragmatic recess

Peritoneal cavity

Inferior vena cava

Crura of the diaphragm

Right kidney

Intervertebral discs

Fig. 228: Frontal Section of the Thorax and Abdomen from Behind (Dorsal View)

NOTE: 1)   from this dorsal view, the right side of the specimen is on the reader's right. The pulmonary arteries and their branches are shown in blue, as are veins (such as the hepatic veins) that also carry blood with low levels of oxygen saturation.

2)   the AP plane of this frontal section in the thorax lies through the inferior vena cava and in front of the descending aorta. The esophagus is seen only in the superior mediastinum and at its entrance into the abdomen just below the diaphragm, while the trachea has been cut at its point of bifurcation.

Fig. 228   II

PLATE 146   Posterior Mediastinum: Esophagus, Aorta, and Trachea

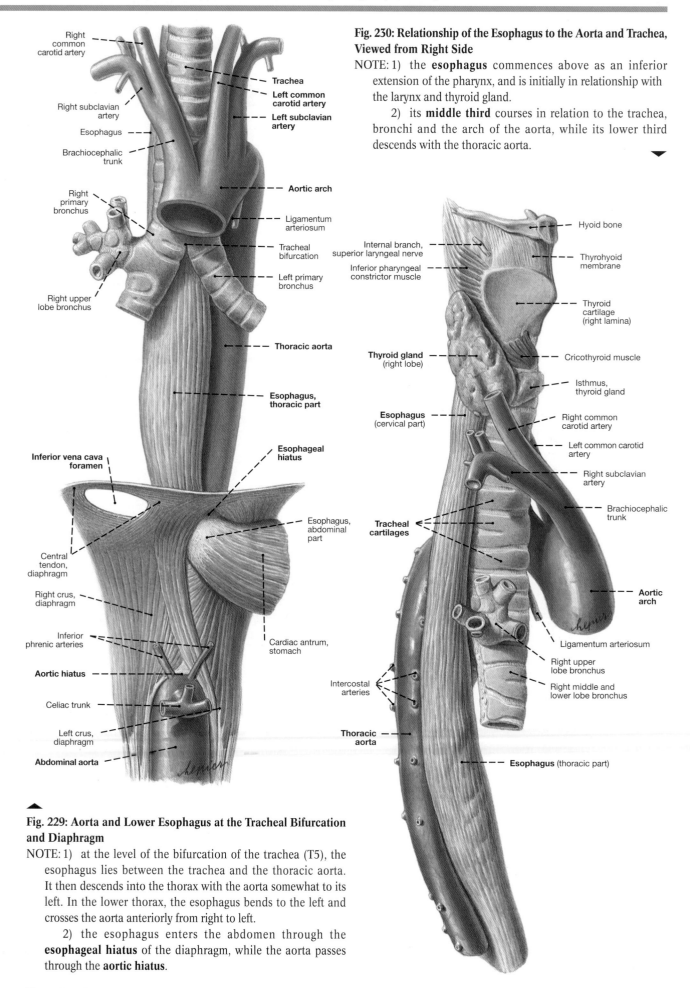

Fig. 230: Relationship of the Esophagus to the Aorta and Trachea, Viewed from Right Side

NOTE: 1) the **esophagus** commences above as an inferior extension of the pharynx, and is initially in relationship with the larynx and thyroid gland.

2) its **middle third** courses in relation to the trachea, bronchi and the arch of the aorta, while its lower third descends with the thoracic aorta.

Fig. 229: Aorta and Lower Esophagus at the Tracheal Bifurcation and Diaphragm

NOTE: 1) at the level of the bifurcation of the trachea (T5), the esophagus lies between the trachea and the thoracic aorta. It then descends into the thorax with the aorta somewhat to its left. In the lower thorax, the esophagus bends to the left and crosses the aorta anteriorly from right to left.

2) the esophagus enters the abdomen through the **esophageal hiatus** of the diaphragm, while the aorta passes through the **aortic hiatus**.

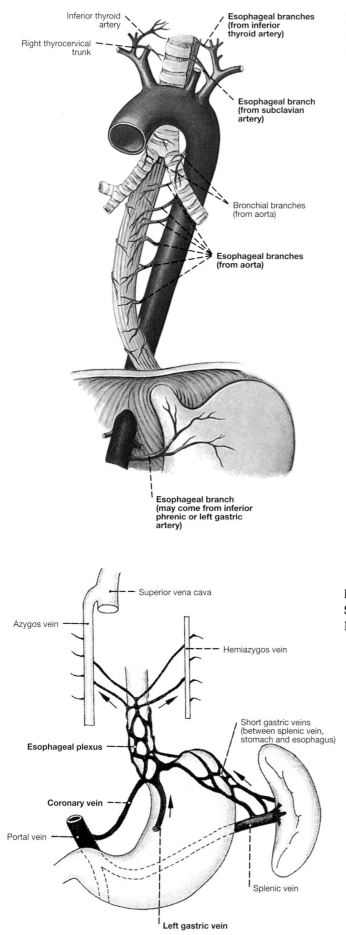

Fig. 231: Diagram of the Arterial Blood Supply of the Esophagus

NOTE: 1) because the esophagus is an elongated organ extending from the neck to the abdomen, it receives arterial blood from at least three sources:

a) **in the neck:** most frequently from the **inferior thyroid branch** of the **thyrocervical trunk,** but it may also come directly from the subclavian, or vertebral arteries or from the costocervical trunk,

b) **in the thorax:** multiple **esophageal branches** that come directly from the **aorta,**

c) **in the abdomen:** from the **inferior phrenic artery** or the **left gastric artery.**

2) these vessels anastomose with each other in the substance of the esophagus.

Fig. 232: Anastomosis Between the Portal Vein and the Superior Vena Cava Through the Esophageal Venous Plexus

NOTE: 1) veins from the **cervical part** of the esophagus drain into the inferior thyroid vein, while those from the **thoracic part** drain into the azygos, hemiazygos and accessory hemiazygos veins.

2) veins from the **abdominal part** drain partially into the left gastric vein and partially into the azygos vein.

3) **this figure shows** the anastomosis sometimes used to return blood from the portal vein to the inferior vena cava. Persons who have hypertension in the portal system may have blood diverted from the **portal vein** to the **coronary and left gastric veins,** then to the **hemiazygos and azygos veins,** and finally into the **superior vena cava.**

4) this shunt of venous blood from the liver results in enlargement or varicosities of the esophageal veins, a condition that could lead to serious esophageal hemorrhage.

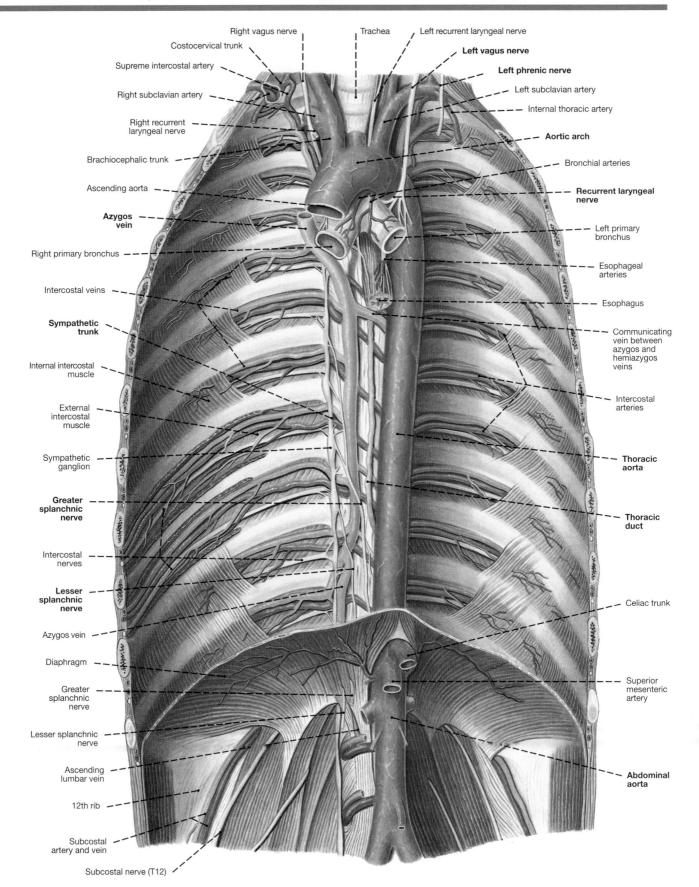

Fig. 233: Vessels and Nerves of the Dorsal Thoracic Wall

NOTE: 1) the aorta ascends from the left ventricle, arches behind the left pulmonary hilum, and descends through most of the thorax just to the left side of the vertebral column.

2) in its course through the posterior mediastinum, the aorta gradually shifts toward the midline which it has achieved when it traverses the diaphragm at the aortic hiatus to enter the abdomen.

Fig. 233

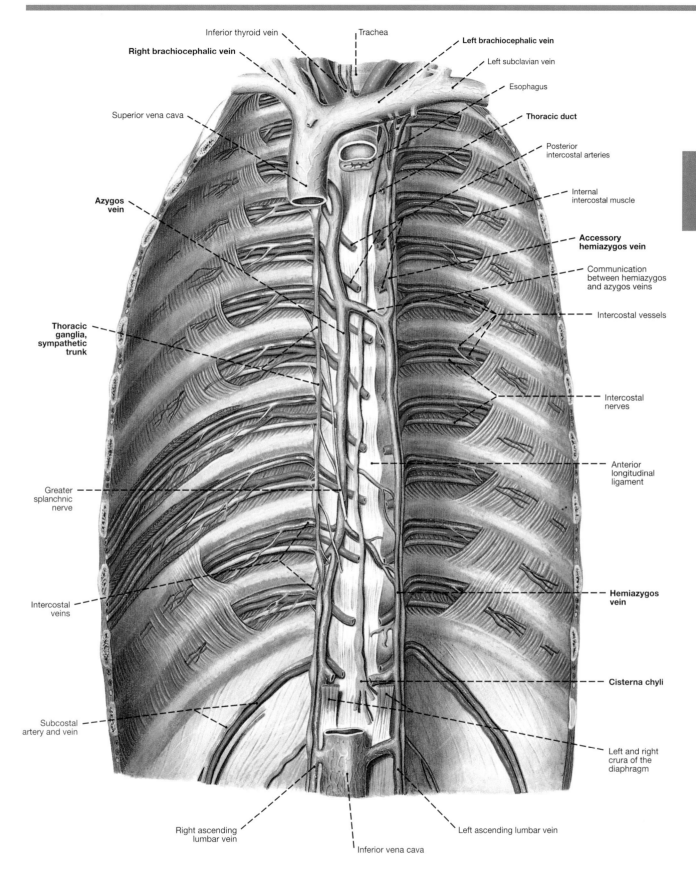

Fig. 234: Azygos System of Veins, the Thoracic Duct and Other Posterior Thoracic Wall Structures

NOTE: 1)   with most of the organs of the thorax and mediastinum removed or cut, the **hemiazygos and accessory hemiazygos veins** to the left of the vertebral column are seen communicating across the midline with the larger **azygos vein.**

2)   the azygos vein is seen ascending in the right thorax to open into the superior vena cava.

3)   the **thoracic duct.** It arises from the cysterna chyli at the 1st lumbar level and ascends in the thorax anterior to the vertebral column.

Fig. 234   II

PLATE 150   Superior and Posterior Mediastina: Posterior View

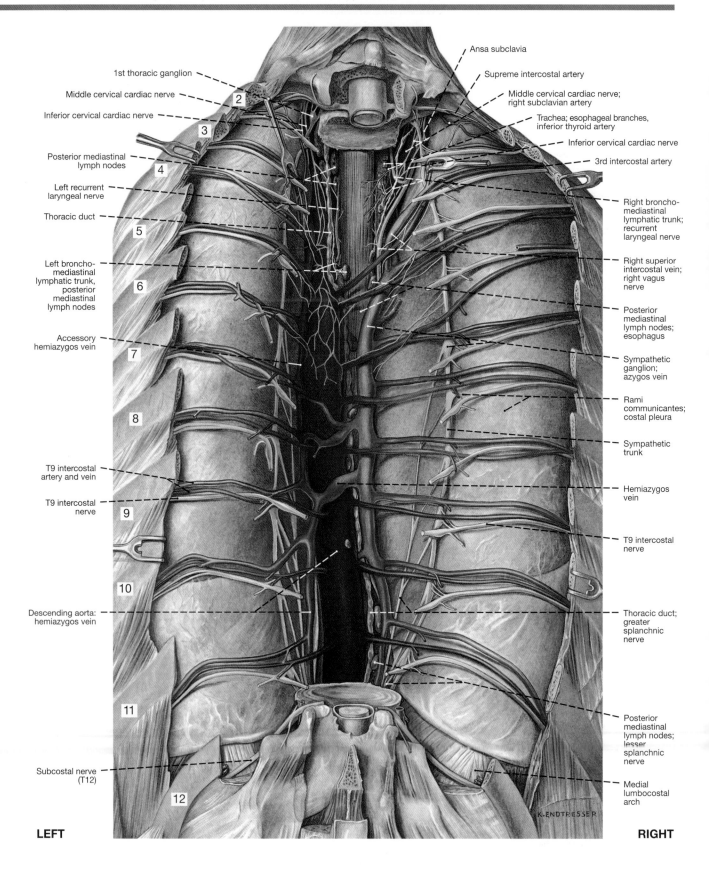

Ansa subclavia

1st thoracic ganglion

Middle cervical cardiac nerve

Inferior cervical cardiac nerve

Supreme intercostal artery

Middle cervical cardiac nerve; right subclavian artery

Trachea; esophageal branches, inferior thyroid artery

Inferior cervical cardiac nerve

Posterior mediastinal lymph nodes

3rd intercostal artery

Left recurrent laryngeal nerve

Thoracic duct

Right broncho-mediastinal lymphatic trunk; recurrent laryngeal nerve

Left broncho-mediastinal lymphatic trunk, posterior mediastinal lymph nodes

Right superior intercostal vein; right vagus nerve

Posterior mediastinal lymph nodes; esophagus

Accessory hemiazygos vein

Sympathetic ganglion; azygos vein

Rami communicantes; costal pleura

Sympathetic trunk

T9 intercostal artery and vein

Hemiazygos vein

T9 intercostal nerve

T9 intercostal nerve

Descending aorta: hemiazygos vein

Thoracic duct; greater splanchnic nerve

Posterior mediastinal lymph nodes; lesser splanchnic nerve

Subcostal nerve (T12)

Medial lumbocostal arch

K.ENDTRESSER

LEFT   RIGHT

Fig. 235: Dorsal View of the Mediastinum and Lungs with the Thoracic Vertebral Column Removed
NOTE: 1)   the **azygos, hemiazygos, and accessory azygos venous pattern** drains the intercostal spaces and flows superiorly in the mediastinum behind the esophagus.

2)   the relationship of the thoracic sympathetic chain and its ganglia to the intercostal nerves, and the formation of the **greater and lesser splanchnic nerves.**

3)   the **right and left bronchomediastinal lymphatic trunks** and the **thoracic duct.**

Fig. 235

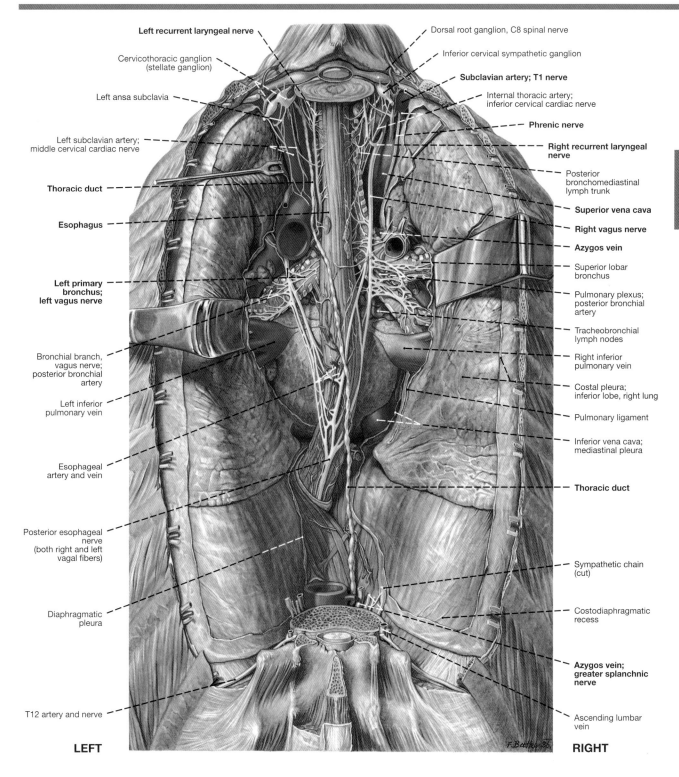

Left recurrent laryngeal nerve

Cervicothoracic ganglion
(stellate ganglion)

Left ansa subclavia

Left subclavian artery;
middle cervical cardiac nerve

Thoracic duct

Esophagus

**Left primary
bronchus;
left vagus nerve**

Bronchial branch,
vagus nerve;
posterior bronchial
artery

Left inferior
pulmonary vein

Esophageal
artery and vein

Posterior esophageal
nerve
(both right and left
vagal fibers)

Diaphragmatic
pleura

T12 artery and nerve

Dorsal root ganglion, C8 spinal nerve

Inferior cervical sympathetic ganglion

Subclavian artery; T1 nerve

Internal thoracic artery;
inferior cervical cardiac nerve

Phrenic nerve

**Right recurrent laryngeal
nerve**

Posterior
bronchomediastinal
lymph trunk

Superior vena cava

Right vagus nerve

Azygos vein

Superior lobar
bronchus

Pulmonary plexus;
posterior bronchial
artery

Tracheobronchial
lymph nodes

Right inferior
pulmonary vein

Costal pleura;
inferior lobe, right lung

Pulmonary ligament

Inferior vena cava;
mediastinal pleura

Thoracic duct

Sympathetic chain
(cut)

Costodiaphragmatic
recess

**Azygos vein;
greater splanchnic
nerve**

Ascending lumbar
vein

LEFT

RIGHT

F. Batke 35

Fig. 236: Dorsal View of the Mediastinum after Removal of the Vertebral Column and Retraction of the Lungs

NOTE: 1) the vertebral column and the thoracic aorta have been removed to reveal the mediastinal course of the **thoracic duct** and **esophagus.** Observe the gradual right to left course of the thoracic duct as it ascends in the mediastinum.

2) the esophagus descends behind the trachea in the superior mediastinum and lies directly behind the pericardium below the bifurcation of the trachea.

3) the autonomic plexus of nerves, lymph nodes, and bronchial vessels, which are found on the posterior surface of the primary bronchi at the hilum of each lung.

4) the course of the **right vagus nerve,** and observe that the **right recurrent laryngeal nerve** arches behind the subclavian artery to achieve the neck and ascend to the larynx.

Fig. 236

II

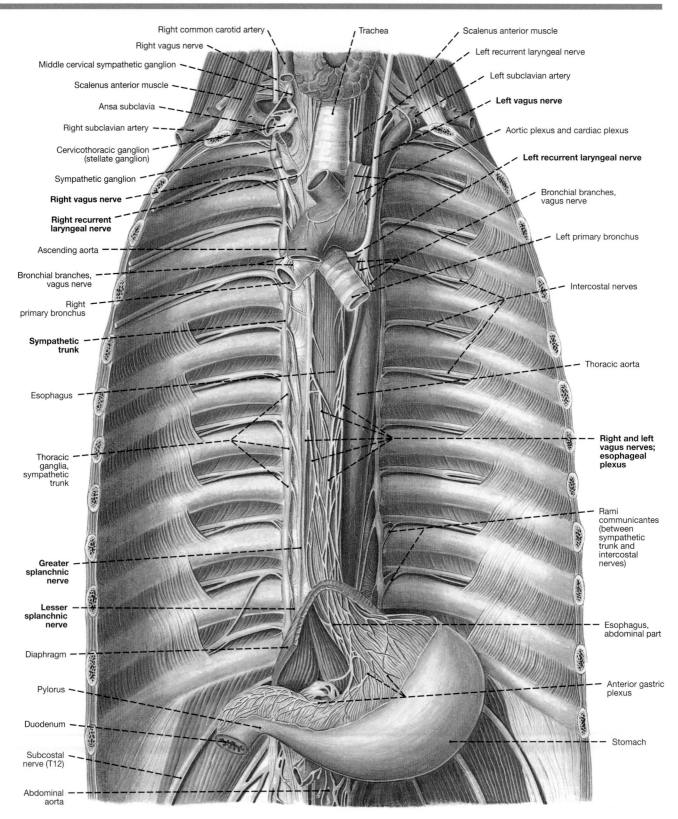

Right common carotid artery

Right vagus nerve

Middle cervical sympathetic ganglion

Scalenus anterior muscle

Ansa subclavia

Right subclavian artery

Cervicothoracic ganglion
(stellate ganglion)

Sympathetic ganglion

Right vagus nerve

**Right recurrent
laryngeal nerve**

Ascending aorta

Bronchial branches,
vagus nerve

Right
primary bronchus

**Sympathetic
trunk**

Esophagus

Thoracic
ganglia,
sympathetic
trunk

**Greater
splanchnic
nerve**

**Lesser
splanchnic
nerve**

Diaphragm

Pylorus

Duodenum

Subcostal
nerve (T12)

Abdominal
aorta

Trachea

Scalenus anterior muscle

Left recurrent laryngeal nerve

Left subclavian artery

Left vagus nerve

Aortic plexus and cardiac plexus

Left recurrent laryngeal nerve

Bronchial branches,
vagus nerve

Left primary bronchus

Intercostal nerves

Thoracic aorta

**Right and left
vagus nerves;
esophageal
plexus**

Rami
communicantes
(between
sympathetic
trunk and
intercostal
nerves)

Esophagus,
abdominal part

Anterior gastric
plexus

Stomach

Fig. 237: Sympathetic Trunks and Vagus Nerves in the Thorax and Upper Abdomen

NOTE: 1)   the ganglionated sympathetic trunks lie lateral to the bodies of the thoracic vertebrae on each side and are continued into the neck superiorly and the abdomen inferiorly.

2)   each ganglion is connected to an intercostal nerve by means of **rami communicantes. White rami** consist principally of preganglionic sympathetic fibers coursing to the ganglia, while the **gray rami** carry postganglionic fibers back to the spinal nerves.

3)   the course of the vagus nerves in the thorax. Below the aortic arch they send branches to the bronchi and then descend to form much of the esophageal plexus.

4)   below the diaphragm most of the fibers of the **left vagus** form the **anterior gastric nerve,** while most of the fibers of the **right vagus** form the **posterior gastric nerve.**

Fig. 237

PLATE 158   Diaphragm and Its Openings: Superior (Thoracic) Aspect

Fig. 245

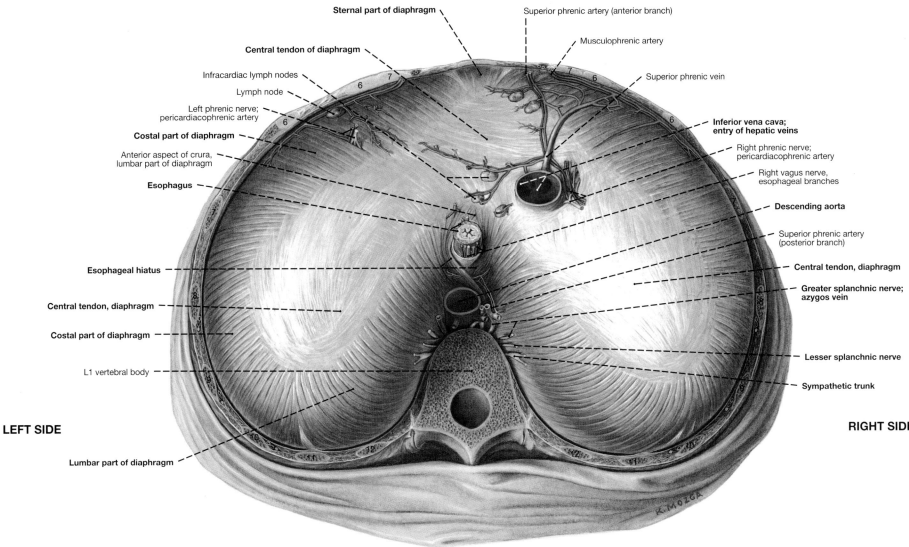

Sternal part of diaphragm

Central tendon of diaphragm

Infracardiac lymph nodes

Lymph node

Left phrenic nerve;
pericardiacophrenic artery

Costal part of diaphragm

Anterior aspect of crura,
lumbar part of diaphragm

Esophagus

Esophageal hiatus

Central tendon, diaphragm

Costal part of diaphragm

L1 vertebral body

Lumbar part of diaphragm

Superior phrenic artery (anterior branch)

Musculophrenic artery

Superior phrenic vein

Inferior vena cava;
entry of hepatic veins

Right phrenic nerve;
pericardiacophrenic artery

Right vagus nerve,
esophageal branches

Descending aorta

Superior phrenic artery
(posterior branch)

Central tendon, diaphragm

Greater splanchnic nerve;
azygos vein

Lesser splanchnic nerve

Sympathetic trunk

LEFT SIDE

RIGHT SIDE

Fig. 245: Diaphragm: Its Openings, Blood Vessels, and Nerves Viewed From Above

NOTE: 1) the thoracic cage has been severed transversely in a plane extending from the lower end of the sternum anteriorly to the body of the first lumbar vertebra posteriorly. The diaphragmatic pleurae and the pericardium have been stripped from the superior (thoracic) surface of the diaphragm.

2) the relative location of the vena cava orifice, and the esophageal and aortic hiatuses:

a) the **vena caval opening** lies to the right of the midline and is more anterior and higher (T8 to T9) than the other two,

b) the **aortic hiatus** lies in the midline and is the most posterior and inferior (L1) of the large apertures,

c) the **esophageal hiatus,** also in the midline, lies anterior to the aortic hiatus at about the level of T10.

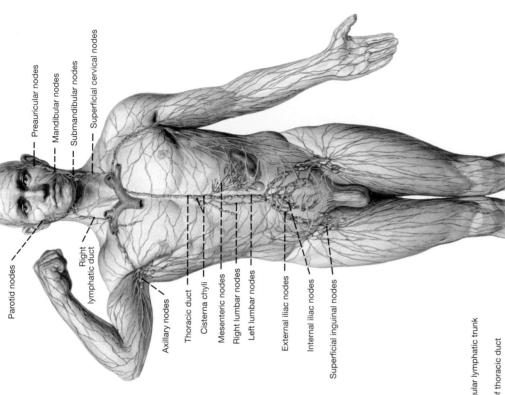

Fig. 243: Certain Lymphatics of the Head, Abdomen, Pelvis, and Limbs

NOTE: 1) in addition to its physiologic importance in returning tissue fluids and cells to the blood vascular system, the lymphatic system may serve as pathways for the spread of disease.

2) lymph channels may be used as preformed tubes for the spread of infectious diseases as well as metastatic cells from established tumors.

3) enlarged or painful lymph nodes are often clinical signs of disease processes elsewhere in the body or of the lymphoid organs themselves.

4) this figure shows the lymphatic channels that drain the upper limb into axillary nodes and those of the lower limb into the inguinal nodes. Also seen are the iliac and lumbar nodes as well as the mesenteric nodes. **Not shown** are the deep nodes of the head, neck, and thorax nor many of the visceral nodes of the thorax, abdomen, and pelvis.

Parotid nodes
Preauricular nodes
Mandibular nodes
Submandibular nodes
Superficial cervical nodes
Right lymphatic duct
Axillary nodes
Thoracic duct
Cisterna chyli
Mesenteric nodes
Right lumbar nodes
Left lumbar nodes
External iliac nodes
Internal iliac nodes
Superficial inguinal nodes

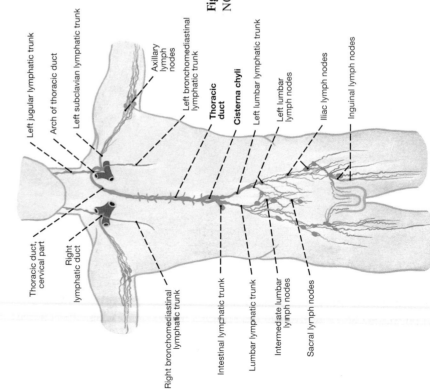

Left jugular lymphatic trunk
Arch of thoracic duct
Left subclavian lymphatic trunk
Axillary lymph nodes
Left bronchomediastinal lymphatic trunk
Thoracic duct
Cisterna chyli
Left lumbar lymphatic trunk
Left lumbar lymph nodes
Iliac lymph nodes
Inguinal lymph nodes
Thoracic duct, cervical part
Right lymphatic duct
Right bronchomediastinal lymphatic trunk
Intestinal lymphatic trunk
Lumbar lymphatic trunk
Intermediate lumbar lymph nodes
Sacral lymph nodes

Fig. 244: Large Lymphatic Vessels

NOTE: 1) the **inguinal lymph nodes** drain the lower limb. The **inguinal nodes** drain into the **iliac nodes** which also receive lymph from the pelvic organs.

2) the iliac nodes drain into the **right and left lumbar nodes**. The lumbar lymphatic trunks join the **intestinal trunk(s)** to form the **cisterna chyli** which opens into the **thoracic duct.**

3) the thoracic duct receives the **left jugular** and **left subclavian trunks** as well as the **left bronchomediastinal trunk** before it opens into the **left subclavian vein.**

4) the **right lymphatic duct** drains the **right jugular trunk** and the **right subclavian trunk** (shown but not labelled), as well as the **right bronchomediastinal trunk** before opening into the **right subclavian vein.**

Figs. 243, 244

PLATE 156 **Thoracic Duct and Lymphatic Drainage**

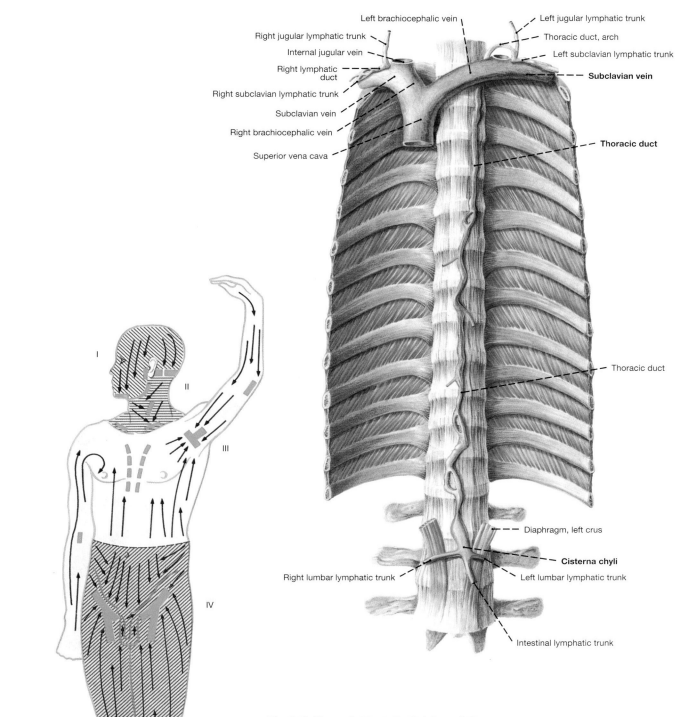

Left brachiocephalic vein
Right jugular lymphatic trunk
Internal jugular vein
Right lymphatic duct
Right subclavian lymphatic trunk
Subclavian vein
Right brachiocephalic vein
Superior vena cava

Left jugular lymphatic trunk
Thoracic duct, arch
Left subclavian lymphatic trunk
Subclavian vein
Thoracic duct

Thoracic duct

Diaphragm, left crus
Cisterna chyli
Right lumbar lymphatic trunk
Left lumbar lymphatic trunk
Intestinal lymphatic trunk

→ = Direction of flow of lymph in the following large areas of the body:
I = Head
II = Neck
III = Upper extremity and thorax
IV = Lower trunk and lower extremity
▪ = Sites of lymphatic channel convergence

Fig. 241: Diagram of Lymphatic Channel Flow

Fig. 242: Thoracic Duct: Its Origin and Course

1) the **thoracic duct** collects lymph from most of the body regions and conveys it back into the blood stream. The duct originates in the abdomen anterior to the 2nd lumbar vertebra at the **cisterna chyli.**

2) the thoracic duct enters the thorax through the **aortic hiatus** of the diaphragm, slightly to the right of the midline. Within the posterior mediastinum of the thorax, still coursing just ventral to the vertebral column, it gradually crosses the midline from right to left.

3) the duct then ascends into the root of the neck on the left side and opens into the **left subclavian vein** near the junction of the **left internal jugular vein.**

4) the **right lymphatic duct** receives lymph from the right side of the head, neck and trunk and from the right upper extremity. It empties into the **right subclavian vein.**

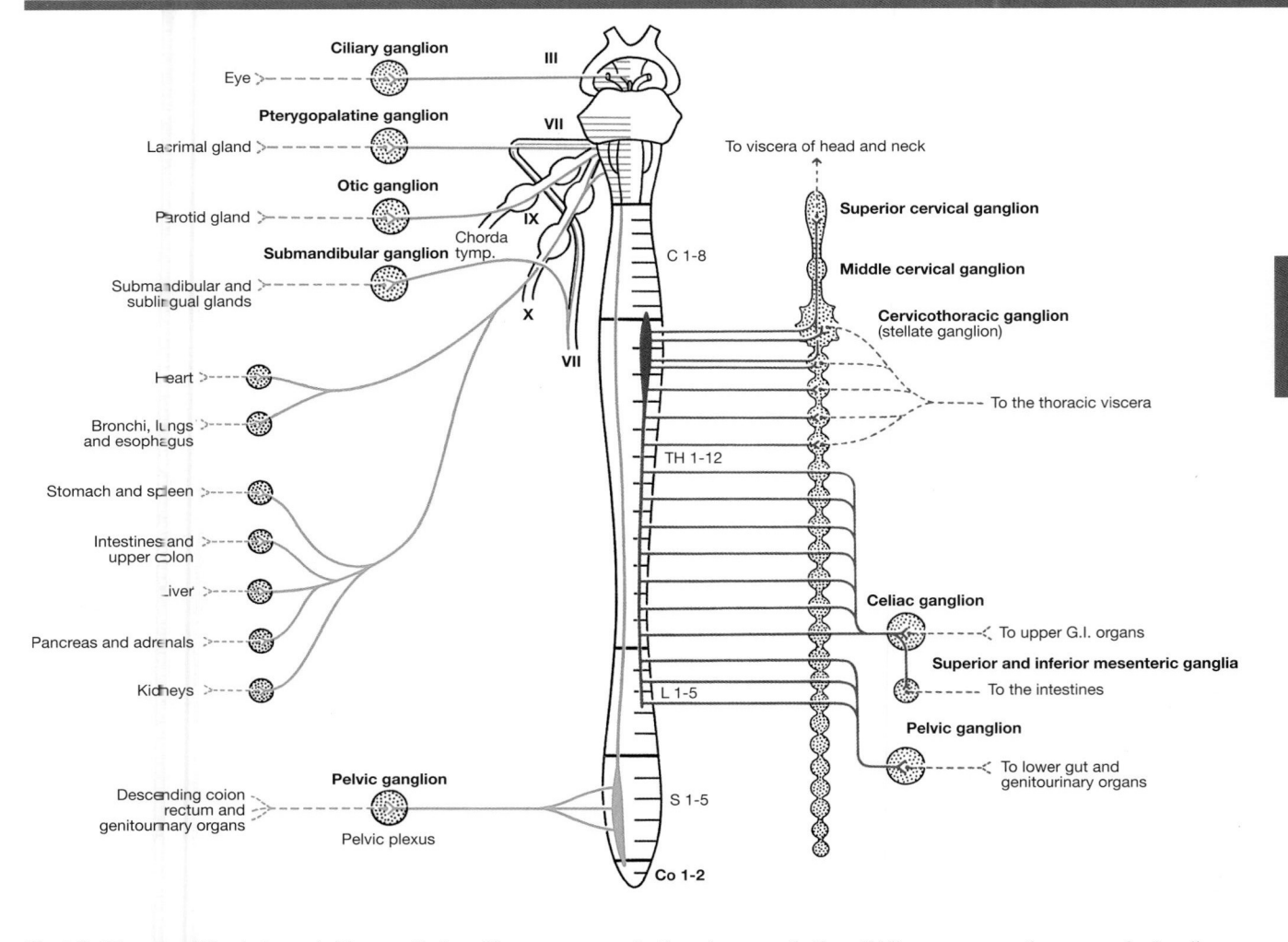

Fig. 240: Diagram of the Autonomic Nervous System. Blue = parasympathetic; red = sympathetic; solid lines = presynaptic neurons; broken lines = postsynaptic neurons.

NOTE: 1)   the autonomic nervous system, by definition, is a two-motor neuron system with the neuron cell bodies of the *presynaptic neurons* (solid lines) somewhere within the central nervous system, and the cell bodies of the *postsynaptic neurons* (broken lines) located in ganglia distributed peripherally in the body.

2)   the autonomic nervous system is comprised of the nerve fibers, which supply all the glands and blood vessels of the body including the heart. In so doing, all the smooth and cardiac muscle tissues (sometimes called involuntary muscles) are thereby innervated.

3)   the autonomic nervous system is composed of two major divisions called the parasympathetic (in blue) and sympathetic (in red) divisions. The autonomic regulation of visceral function is, therefore, a dualistic control, i.e., most organs receive postganglionic fibers of both parasympathetic and sympathetic source.

4)   the *parasympathetic division* is sometimes called a craniosacral outflow because the preganglionic cell bodies of this division lie in the brainstem and in the sacral segments of the spinal cord. Parasympathetic preganglionic fibers are found in four cranial nerves, III (oculomotor), VII (facial), IX (glossopharyngeal) and X (vagus) and in the 2nd, 3rd and 4th sacral nerves.

5)   these *pre*ganglionic parasympathetic fibers then synapse with *post*ganglionic parasympathetic cell bodies in peripheral ganglia. From these ganglia the *post*ganglionic nerve fibers innervate the various organs.

6)   the *sympathetic division* is sometimes called the thoracolumbar outflow because the *pre*ganglionic sympathetic neuron cell bodies are located in the lateral horn of the spinal cord between the 1st thoracic spinal segment and the 2nd or 3rd lumbar spinal segment, (i.e., from T1 to L3).

7)   these *pre*ganglionic fibers emerge from the cord with their corresponding spinal roots and communicate with the sympathetic trunk and its ganglia where some *pre*synaptic sympathetic fibers synapse with *post*ganglionic sympathetic neurons. Other presynaptic fibers (especially those of the upper thoracic segments) ascend in the sympathetic chain and synapse with *post*ganglionic neurons in the cervicothoracic, middle and superior cervical ganglia. *Post*ganglionic fibers from these latter ganglia are then distributed to the viscera of the head and neck. Still other *pre*synaptic sympathetic fibers do not synapse in the sympathetic chain of ganglia at all, but collect to form the splanchnic nerves. These nerves course to the collateral sympathetic ganglia (celiac, superior and inferior mesenteric and pelvic ganglia) where synapse with the *post*ganglionic neuron occurs. The *post*ganglionic neurons of the sympathetic division then course to the viscera to supply sympathetic innervation.

8)   the functions of the parasympathetic and sympathetic divisions of the autonomic nervous system are antagonistic to each other. The parasympathetic division constricts the pupil, decelerates the heart, lowers blood pressure, relaxes the sphincters of the gut and contracts the longitudinal musculature of the hollow organs. It is the division which is active during periods of calm and tranquility and aids in digestion and absorption. In contrast, the *sympathetic division* dilates the pupil, accelerates the heart, increases blood pressure, contracts the sphincters of the gut and relaxes the longitudinal musculature of hollow organs. It is active when the organism is challenged. It prepares for fight and flight and generally comes to the individual's defense during periods of stress and adversity.

Fig. 240   **II**

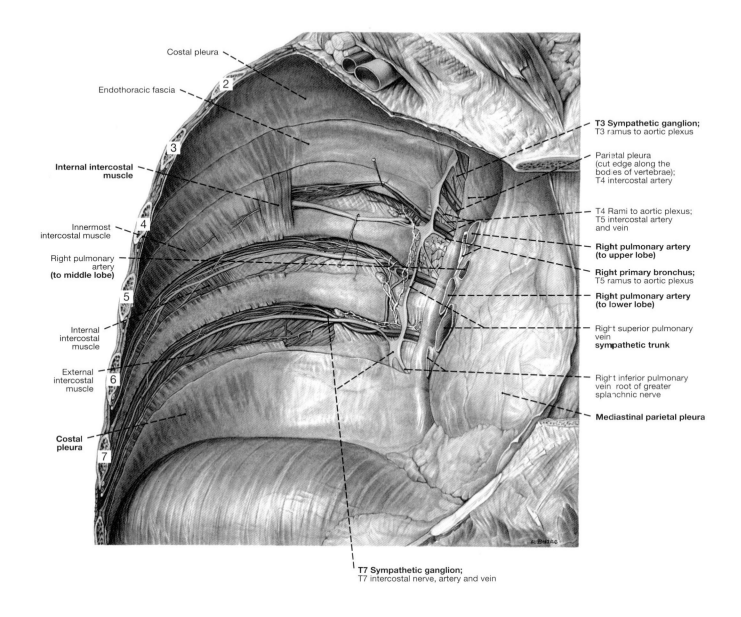

Costal pleura

Endothoracic fascia

Internal intercostal muscle

Innermost intercostal muscle

Right pulmonary artery **(to middle lobe)**

Internal intercostal muscle

External intercostal muscle

Costal pleura

T3 Sympathetic ganglion; T3 ramus to aortic plexus

Parietal pleura (cut edge along the bodies of vertebrae); T4 intercostal artery

T4 Rami to aortic plexus; T5 intercostal artery and vein

Right pulmonary artery (to upper lobe)

Right primary bronchus; T5 ramus to aortic plexus

Right pulmonary artery (to lower lobe)

Right superior pulmonary vein **sympathetic trunk**

Right inferior pulmonary vein root of greater splanchnic nerve

Mediastinal parietal pleura

T7 Sympathetic ganglion; T7 intercostal nerve, artery and vein

Fig. 239: Right Posterior Thoracic Wall, Sympathetic Trunk, and Intercostal Nerves and Vessels, Anterior View

NOTE: 1) the right lung has been removed from the thoracic cavity. Observe the cut structures at the pulmonary hilum: the **right primary bronchus,** the **right pulmonary artery** (severed distally enough to show its 3 lobar branches), and the **pulmonary veins.**

2) the costal and mediastinal reflections of parietal pleura have been stripped away to reveal the 5th, 6th, and 7th intercostal spaces and the intercostal vessels and nerves that course within them around the thoracic wall.

3) the intercostal vessels and nerves lie just below the ribs, the nerve being slightly more inferior to the vessels. This close relationship of the vessels and nerve to the lower border of the ribs explains why it is safer to guide a needle through the intercostal space along the **superior border** of the rib when access to the thoracic cavity is necessary.

4) the sympathetic trunk and the 3rd to 7th sympathetic ganglia. Observe that, in addition to the rami communicantes, the sympathetic trunk contributes sympathetic fibers to the aortic plexus (seen coursing toward the left from this right sympathetic trunk), as well as to the splanchnic nerves.

Fig. 239

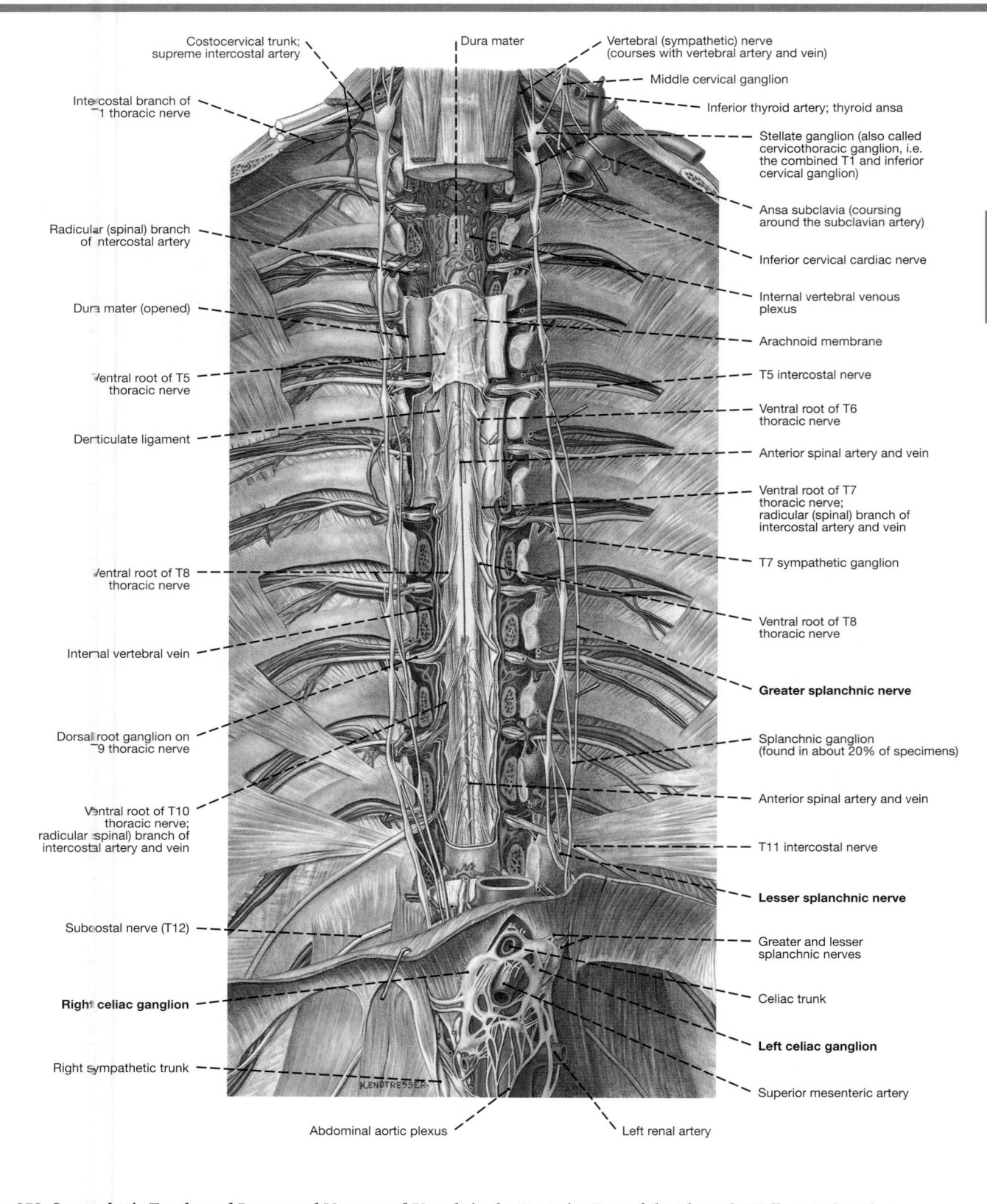

Costocervical trunk;
supreme intercostal artery

Intercostal branch of
T1 thoracic nerve

Radicular (spinal) branch
of intercostal artery

Dura mater (opened)

Ventral root of T5
thoracic nerve

Denticulate ligament

Ventral root of T8
thoracic nerve

Internal vertebral vein

Dorsal root ganglion on
T9 thoracic nerve

Ventral root of T10
thoracic nerve;
radicular (spinal) branch of
intercostal artery and vein

Subcostal nerve (T12)

Right celiac ganglion

Right sympathetic trunk

Abdominal aortic plexus

Dura mater

Vertebral (sympathetic) nerve
(courses with vertebral artery and vein)

Middle cervical ganglion

Inferior thyroid artery; thyroid ansa

Stellate ganglion (also called
cervicothoracic ganglion, i.e.
the combined T1 and inferior
cervical ganglion)

Ansa subclavia (coursing
around the subclavian artery)

Inferior cervical cardiac nerve

Internal vertebral venous
plexus

Arachnoid membrane

T5 intercostal nerve

Ventral root of T6
thoracic nerve

Anterior spinal artery and vein

Ventral root of T7
thoracic nerve;
radicular (spinal) branch of
intercostal artery and vein

T7 sympathetic ganglion

Ventral root of T8
thoracic nerve

Greater splanchnic nerve

Splanchnic ganglion
(found in about 20% of specimens)

Anterior spinal artery and vein

T11 intercostal nerve

Lesser splanchnic nerve

Greater and lesser
splanchnic nerves

Celiac trunk

Left celiac ganglion

Superior mesenteric artery

Left renal artery

K. ENDTRESSER

Fig. 238: Sympathetic Trunks and Intercostal Nerves and Vessels in the Posterior Part of the Thoracic Wall, Anterior View

NOTE: 1) the sympathetic trunks, their ganglia and the rami communicantes that interconnect the ganglia with the intercostal nerves.

2) the bodies of the lower seven or eight thoracic vertebrae have been removed to show the ventral surface of the spinal cord and its anterior roots.

3) the **greater splanchnic nerve** formed by sympathetic fibers through ganglia T5 to T9 and the **lesser splanchnic nerve** formed by fibers through ganglia T10 and T11. These nerves descend parallel to the sympathetic trunks, perforate the crura of the diaphragm and terminate on postganglionic neurons in the **celiac ganglia,** the **superior mesenteric ganglia,** and the **aorticorenal ganglia** (shown near the renal arteries, but not labelled).

Fig. 238   **II**

PART III
THE ABDOMEN

(PLATES 159–248 – FIGURES 246–375)

PART III   THE ABDOMEN

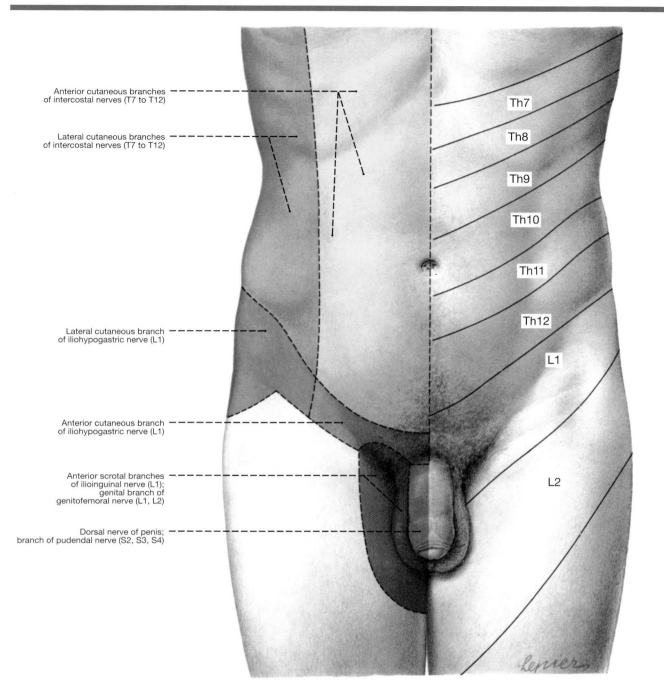

Anterior cutaneous branches
of intercostal nerves (T7 to T12)

Lateral cutaneous branches
of intercostal nerves (T7 to T12)

Lateral cutaneous branch
of iliohypogastric nerve (L1)

Anterior cutaneous branch
of iliohypogastric nerve (L1)

Anterior scrotal branches
of ilioinguinal nerve (L1);
genital branch of
genitofemoral nerve (L1, L2)

Dorsal nerve of penis;
branch of pudendal nerve (S2, S3, S4)

Th7
Th8
Th9
Th10
Th11
Th12
L1
L2

Fig. 246: Cutaneous Innervation and Dermatomes of the Anterior Abdominal Wall
NOTE: 1) the anterior abdominal wall is innervated by the ventral primary rami (anterior and lateral cutaneous branches) of the **lower six thoracic** (intercostal) **nerves** and by the **iliohypogastric** and **ilioinguinal** branches of the **first lumbar nerve.**

2) the tenth thoracic (T10) nerve supplies the dermatome that includes the umbilicus.

3) the upper medial thigh and the anterior and lateral part of the scrotum receive sensory fibers from the anterior scrotal branches of the **ilioinguinal nerve** (L1) and the genital branch of the **genitofemoral nerve** (L1, L2).

4) the dorsum of the penis is NOT supplied by lumbar segments. It receives its sensory innervation from the **dorsal nerve of the penis,** a branch of the **pudendal nerve** (S2, S3, S4).

Fig. 246   **III**

PLATE 160   Anterior Abdominal Wall: Fascia and Superficial Vessels

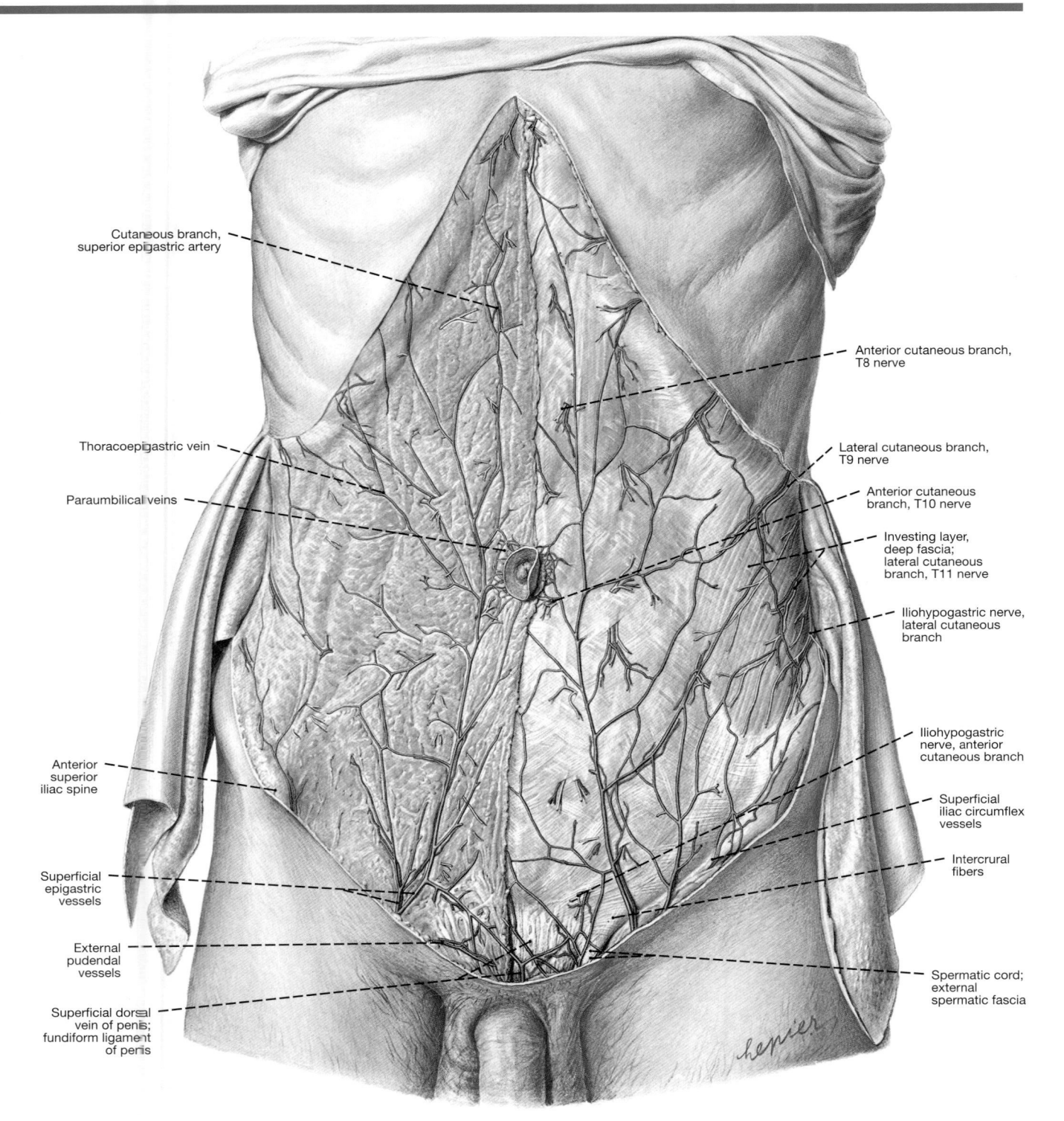

Cutaneous branch,
superior epigastric artery

Thoracoepigastric vein

Paraumbilical veins

Anterior
superior
iliac spine

Superficial
epigastric
vessels

External
pudendal
vessels

Superficial dorsal
vein of penis;
fundiform ligament
of penis

Anterior cutaneous branch,
T8 nerve

Lateral cutaneous branch,
T9 nerve

Anterior cutaneous
branch, T10 nerve

Investing layer,
deep fascia;
lateral cutaneous
branch, T11 nerve

Iliohypogastric nerve,
lateral cutaneous
branch

Iliohypogastric
nerve, anterior
cutaneous branch

Superficial
iliac circumflex
vessels

Intercrural
fibers

Spermatic cord;
external
spermatic fascia

Fig. 247: Superficial and Deep Fascial Layers Over the Anterior Abdominal Wall

NOTE: 1) on the right side (reader's left), the skin has been removed to expose the superficial fatty layer of superficial fascia, often called **Camper's fascia.** On the inner surface of this fatty layer is a fibrous deep layer of superficial fascia (not exposed in this figure) called **Scarpa's fascia.**

2) the superficial fatty layer (Camper's) is continuous over the inguinal ligament with the superficial fascia of the thigh.

3) the fibrous layer (Scarpa's) of superficial fascia, however, **in the lateral inguinal region** fuses with the fascia lata of the thigh below the inguinal ligament. In the **medial inguinal region,** the two layers of superficial fascia blend to form the **dartos layer** of the scrotum and continue in the perineum as Colles' fascia.

4) on the left side (reader's right), both layers of the superficial fascia have been removed exposing the superficial vessels and nerves and the deep fascial layer that invests the abdominal muscles.

Fig. 247

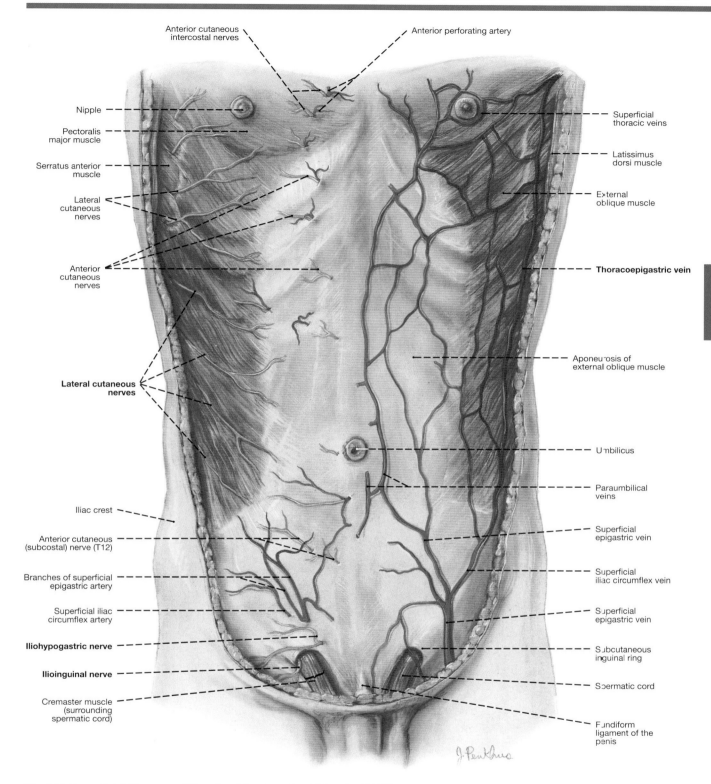

Anterior cutaneous
intercostal nerves

Anterior perforating artery

Nipple

Pectoralis
major muscle

Serratus anterior
muscle

Lateral
cutaneous
nerves

Anterior
cutaneous
nerves

**Lateral cutaneous
nerves**

Iliac crest

Anterior cutaneous
(subcostal) nerve (T12)

Branches of superficial
epigastric artery

Superficial iliac
circumflex artery

Iliohypogastric nerve

Ilioinguinal nerve

Cremaster muscle
(surrounding
spermatic cord)

Superficial
thoracic veins

Latissimus
dorsi muscle

External
oblique muscle

Thoracoepigastric vein

Aponeurosis of
external oblique muscle

Umbilicus

Paraumbilical
veins

Superficial
epigastric vein

Superficial
iliac circumflex vein

Superficial
epigastric vein

Subcutaneous
inguinal ring

Spermatic cord

Fundiform
ligament of the
penis

Fig. 248: Superficial Nerves and Vessels of the Anterior Abdominal Wall

NOTE: 1) the distribution of the superficial vessels and cutaneous nerves upon the removal of the skin and fascia from the lower thoracic and anterior abdominal wall.

2) the intercostal nerves supply the abdominal surface with lateral and anterior cutaneous branches.

3) the ilioinguinal and iliohypogastric branches of the 1st lumbar nerve become superficial in the region of the **superficial inguinal ring.**

4) the branches of the **superficial epigastric artery** (which arises from the femoral artery) ascending toward the umbilicus from the inguinal region.

5) the **thoracoepigastric vein** serves as a means of communication between the femoral vein and the axillary vein. In cases of portal vein obstruction, these superficial veins become greatly enlarged (varicosed), a condition called **caput medusae.**

Fig. 248   III

PLATE 62 Anterior Abdominal Wall: External Oblique Muscle

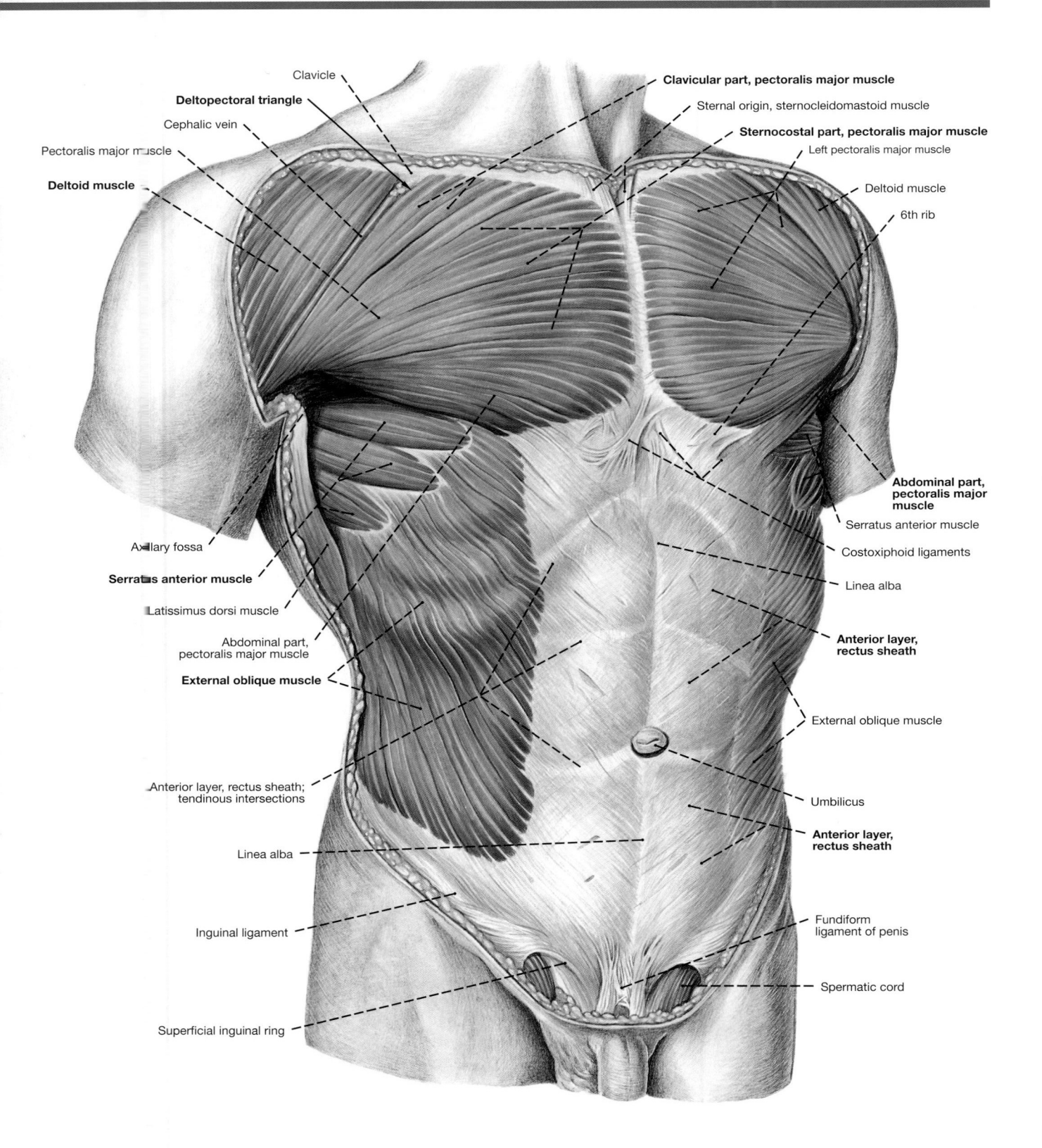

Clavicle

Clavicular part, pectoralis major muscle

Deltopectoral triangle

Sternal origin, sternocleidomastoid muscle

Cephalic vein

Sternocostal part, pectoralis major muscle

Pectoralis major muscle

Left pectoralis major muscle

Deltoid muscle

Deltoid muscle

6th rib

Abdominal part, pectoralis major muscle

Serratus anterior muscle

Costoxiphoid ligaments

Axillary fossa

Linea alba

Serratus anterior muscle

Latissimus dorsi muscle

Anterior layer, rectus sheath

Abdominal part, pectoralis major muscle

External oblique muscle

External oblique muscle

Anterior layer, rectus sheath; tendinous intersections

Umbilicus

Anterior layer, rectus sheath

Linea alba

Inguinal ligament

Fundiform ligament of penis

Spermatic cord

Superficial inguinal ring

Fig. 249: Superficial Musculature of the Anterior Abdominal and Thoracic Wall

NOTE: 1) the first layer of muscles on the anterior abdominal wall consists of the **external oblique muscle** and its broad flat aponeurosis. Medially, this aponeurosis helps form the sheath of the rectus abdominis muscle and inferiorly, it becomes the **inguinal ligament.**

2) the external oblique arises by means of seven or eight fleshy slips from the outer surfaces of the lower seven ribs, thereby interdigitating with the fleshy origin of the **serratus anterior muscle.**

Fig. 249

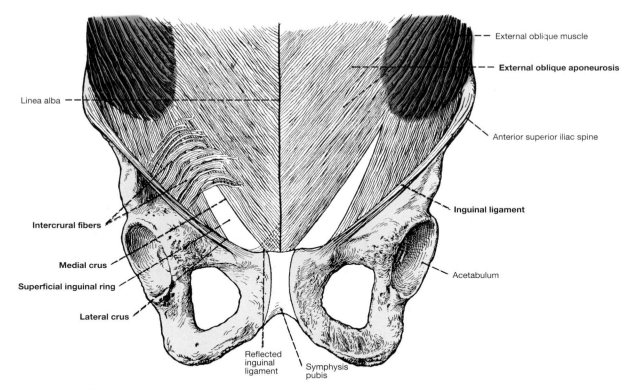

Fig. 250: Aponeurosis of the External Oblique Muscle

NOTE: 1) the **superficial inguinal ring** is a triangular slit-like opening in the aponeurosis of the external oblique muscle. Observe how the **intercrural fibers** strengthen the lateral aspect of the superficial ring by extending between the **medial** and **lateral crura.**

2) the **inguinal ligament** extends between the anterior superior iliac spine and the pubic tubercle. This ligament is formed by the lowermost fibers of the external oblique aponeurosis and lends support to the inferior portion of the anterior abdominal wall.

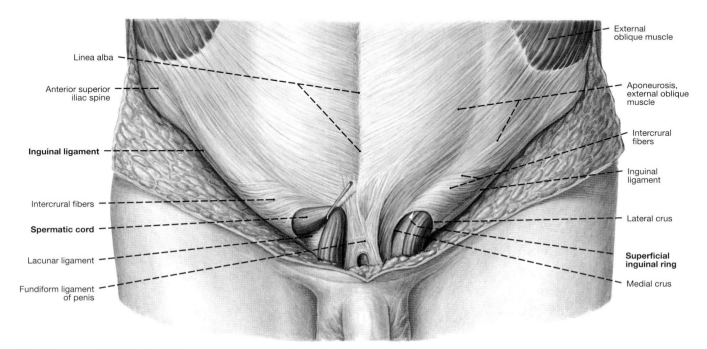

Fig. 251: Superficial Inguinal Ring and Spermatic Cord

NOTE: 1) the superficial inguinal ring transmits the **spermatic cord** in the male and the **round ligament of the uterus** in the female. In this dissection, the right spermatic cord has been lifted to show the lateral crus of the ring as well as the **lacunar ligament.**

2) the tendinous fibers of the aponeurosis are continuous with the fleshy fibers of the external oblique. They are directed inferomedially and decussate across the linea alba.

PLATE 164   Anterior Abdominal Wall: Internal Oblique Muscle

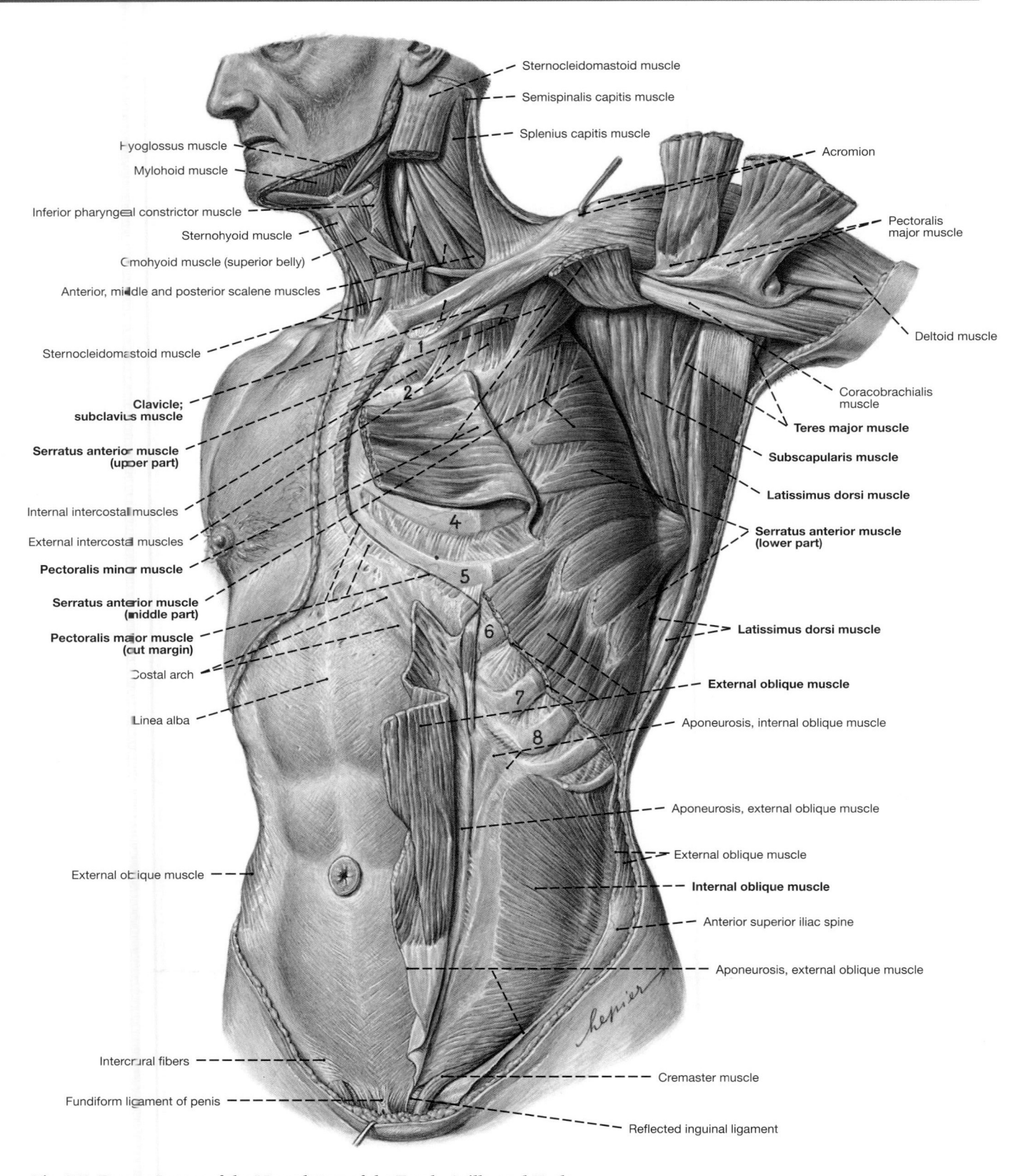

Sternocleidomastoid muscle

Semispinalis capitis muscle

Splenius capitis muscle

Acromion

Hyoglossus muscle

Mylohoid muscle

Inferior pharyngeal constrictor muscle

Sternohyoid muscle

Omohyoid muscle (superior belly)

Anterior, middle and posterior scalene muscles

Sternocleidomastoid muscle

Clavicle; subclavius muscle

Serratus anterior muscle (upper part)

Internal intercostal muscles

External intercostal muscles

Pectoralis minor muscle

Serratus anterior muscle (middle part)

Pectoralis major muscle (cut margin)

Costal arch

Linea alba

External oblique muscle

Intercrural fibers

Fundiform ligament of penis

Pectoralis major muscle

Deltoid muscle

Coracobrachialis muscle

Teres major muscle

Subscapularis muscle

Latissimus dorsi muscle

Serratus anterior muscle (lower part)

Latissimus dorsi muscle

External oblique muscle

Aponeurosis, internal oblique muscle

Aponeurosis, external oblique muscle

External oblique muscle

Internal oblique muscle

Anterior superior iliac spine

Aponeurosis, external oblique muscle

Cremaster muscle

Reflected inguinal ligament

Fig. 252: Deeper Layers of the Musculature of the Trunk, Axilla, and Neck

NOTE: 1)   the pectoralis major and minor muscles have been reflected to expose the underlying digitations of the serratus anterior muscle, which attach to the upper nine ribs.

2)   the external oblique muscle and the lower lateral part of its aponeurosis have been severed in a semicircular manner near their origin to reveal the underlying internal oblique muscle which comprises the 2nd layer of anterior abdominal wall muscles.

3)   the muscle fibers of the external oblique course inferomedially (or in the same direction as you would put your hands in your side pockets), whereas **most** of the fibers of the internal oblique course in the opposite direction at a 90 degree angle.

Fig. 252

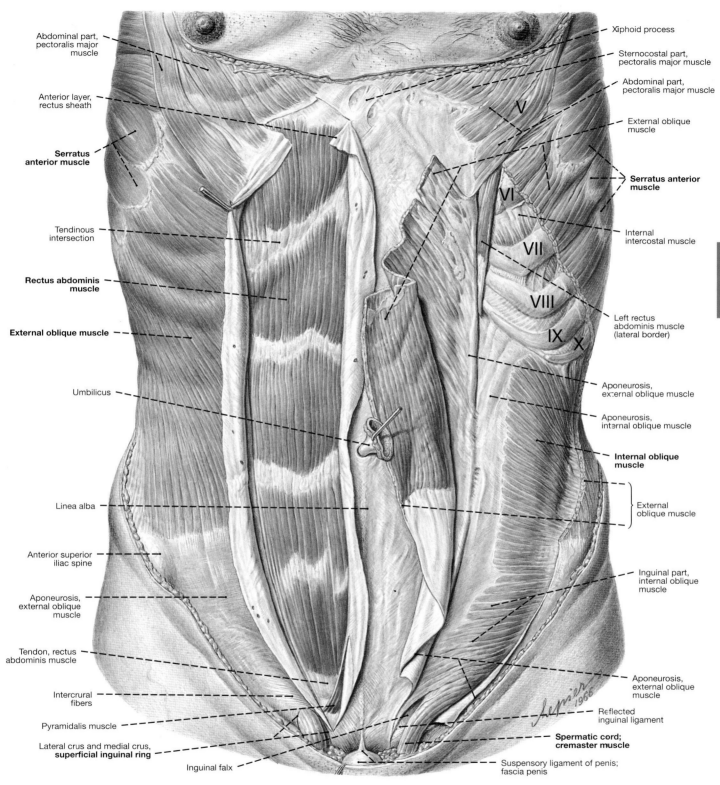

Fig. 253: Anterior Abdominal Wall: Rectus Abdominis and Internal Oblique Muscles

Muscle	Origin	Insertion	Innervation	Action
External Oblique	Fleshy slips from the outer surface of the lower 8 ribs (ribs 5 to 12)	Outer lip of the iliac crest; aponeurosis of external oblique which ends in a midline raphe, the **linea alba**	Lower 6 thoracic nerves (T7–T12)	Compresses the abdominal viscera; **both muscles**: flex the trunk forward; **each muscle**: bends the trunk to that side and rotates the front of the abdomen to the **opposite** side

Fig. 253   III

PLATE 166   Anterior Abdominal Wall: Rectus Sheath; Second Muscle Layer

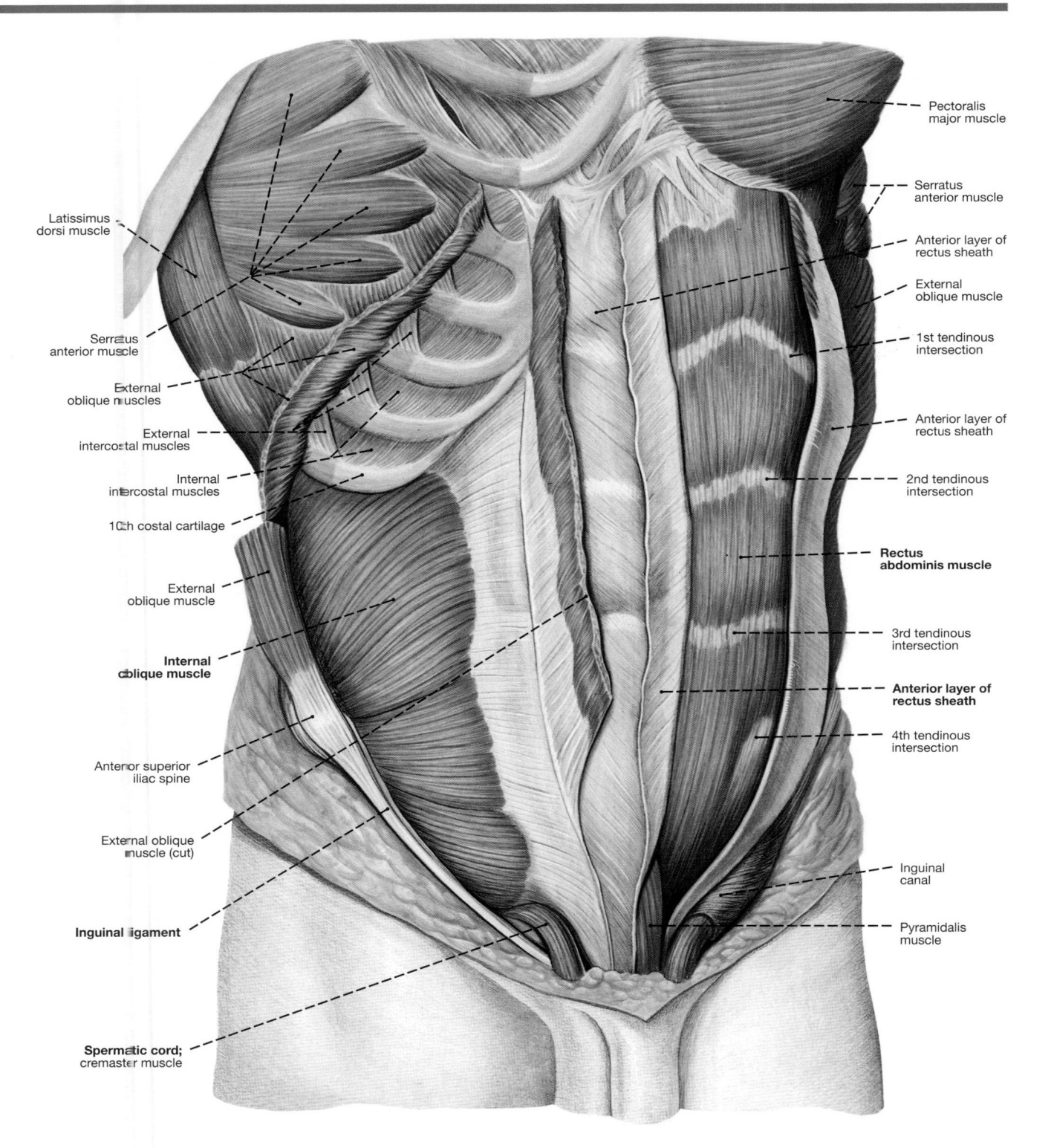

Pectoralis major muscle

Serratus anterior muscle

Anterior layer of rectus sheath

External oblique muscle

1st tendinous intersection

Anterior layer of rectus sheath

2nd tendinous intersection

Rectus abdominis muscle

3rd tendinous intersection

Anterior layer of rectus sheath

4th tendinous intersection

Inguinal canal

Pyramidalis muscle

Latissimus dorsi muscle

Serratus anterior muscle

External oblique muscles

External intercostal muscles

Internal intercostal muscles

10th costal cartilage

External oblique muscle

Internal oblique muscle

Anterior superior iliac spine

External oblique muscle (cut)

Inguinal ligament

Spermatic cord; cremaster muscle

Fig. 254: Middle Layer of Abdominal Musculature: Internal Oblique Muscle

Muscle	Origin	Insertion	Innervation	Action
Internal Oblique	Lateral ⅔ rds of inguinal ligament; the middle lip of the iliac crest; the thoracolumbar fascia	Inferior border of the lower 3 or 4 ribs; the **linea alba**; aponeurosis fuses with that of the external oblique to help form the rectus sheath	Lower 5 thoracic nerves and the 1st lumbar nerve (T8–L1)	Compresses the abdominal viscera; **both muscles:** flex the trunk forward; **each muscle:** bends the trunk to that side but rotates the front of the abdomen toward the **same** side

Fig. 254

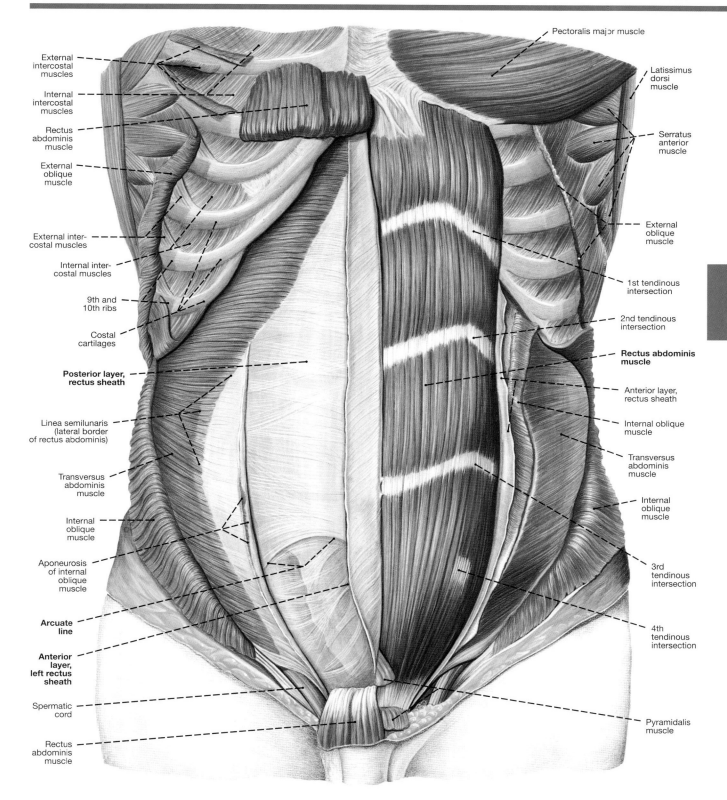

External intercostal muscles

Internal intercostal muscles

Rectus abdominis muscle

External oblique muscle

External inter-costal muscles

Internal inter-costal muscles

9th and 10th ribs

Costal cartilages

Posterior layer, rectus sheath

Linea semilunaris (lateral border of rectus abdominis)

Transversus abdominis muscle

Internal oblique muscle

Aponeurosis of internal oblique muscle

Arcuate line

Anterior layer, left rectus sheath

Spermatic cord

Rectus abdominis muscle

Pectoralis major muscle

Latissimus dorsi muscle

Serratus anterior muscle

External oblique muscle

1st tendinous intersection

2nd tendinous intersection

Rectus abdominis muscle

Anterior layer, rectus sheath

Internal oblique muscle

Transversus abdominis muscle

Internal oblique muscle

3rd tendinous intersection

4th tendinous intersection

Pyramidalis muscle

Fig. 255: Deep Layer of Abdominal Musculature: The Transversus Abdominis Muscle

Muscle	Origin	Insertion	Innervation	Action
Transversus Abdominis	Lateral $\frac{1}{3}$rd of inguinal ligament and inner lip of iliac crest; thoracolumbar fascia; inner surface of lower 6 ribs	Ends in an aponeurosis; **upper fibers**: to linea alba, help form posterior layer of rectus sheath; **lower fibers**: attach to pubis to form **conjoined tendon**	Lower 6 thoracic and 1st lumbar nerves (T7–L1)	Tenses abdominal wall; compresses abdominal contents

Fig. 255   III

PLATE 168   Anterior Abdominal Wall: Rectus Sheath

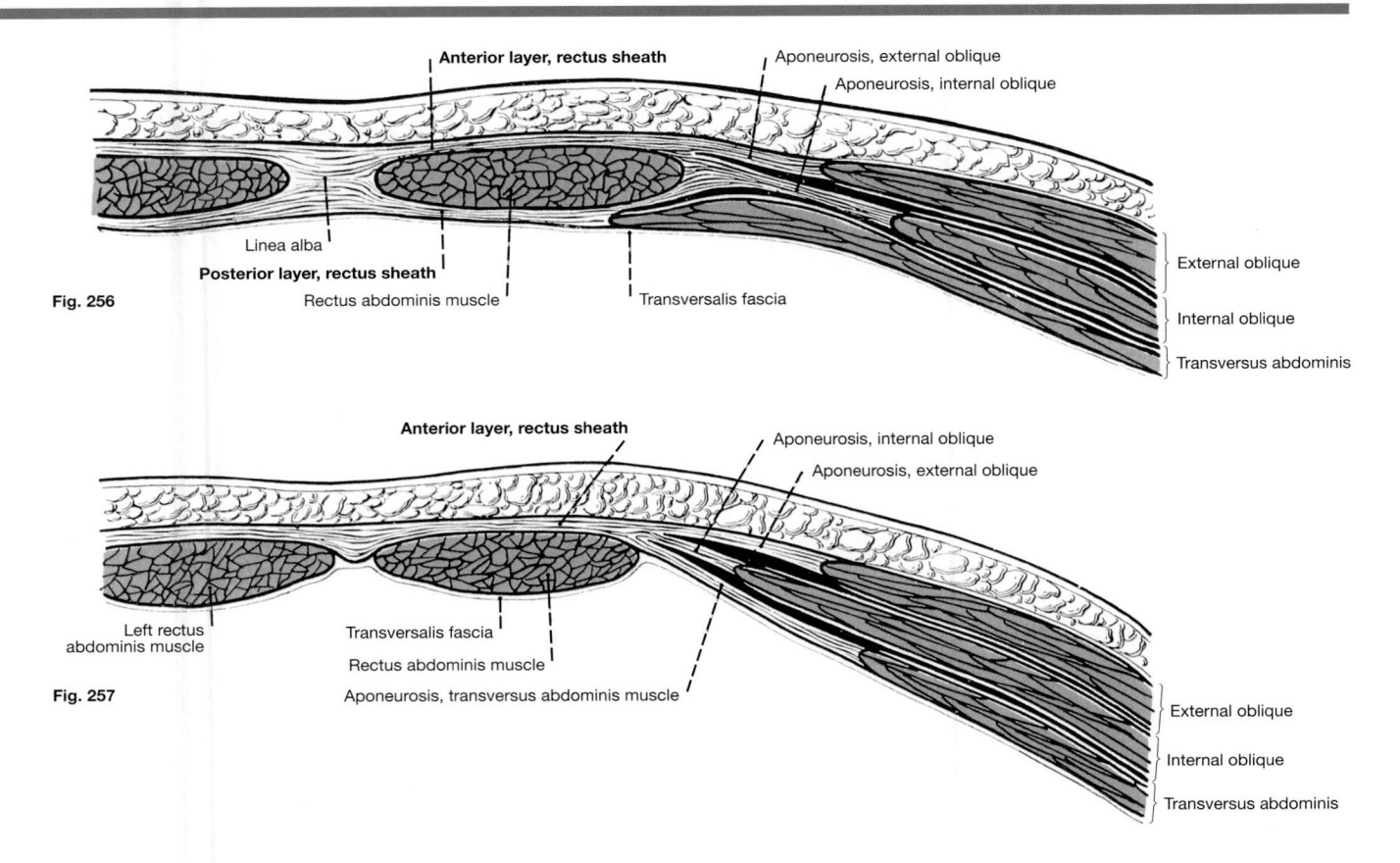

Fig. 256

Fig. 257

Figs. 256, 257: Transverse Sections of the Anterior Abdominal Wall: Above the Umbilicus and Below the Arcuate Line

NOTE: 1) the sheath of the rectus abdominis is formed by the aponeurosis of the external oblique, internal oblique, and transversus abdominis muscles.

2) the upper two-thirds of the sheath encloses the rectus muscle both anteriorly and posteriorly. To accomplish this, the internal oblique aponeurosis splits. Part of the internal oblique aponeurosis joins the aponeurosis of the external oblique to form the **anterior layer,** while the other portion joins the aponeurosis of the transversus abdominis to form the **posterior layer** (Fig. 256).

3) the lower one-third of the sheath, located below the arcuate line, is deficient posteriorly, since the aponeuroses of all three muscles pass anterior to the rectus abdominis muscle (Fig. 257).

4) deep to the sheath and transversus muscle is located the **transversalis fascia,** interposed between the peritoneum and the anterior wall structures.

Muscle	Origin	Insertion	Innervation	Action
Rectus Abdominis	5th, 6th and 7th costal cartilages; costoxiphoid ligaments and xiphoid process	Crest of pubis and pubic tubercle; front of symphysis pubis	Lower 7 thoracic nerves (T6–T12)	Flexes vertebral column; tenses anterior abdominal wall; compresses abdominal contents
Cremaster	Midway along the inguinal ligament as a continuation of internal oblique muscle	Onto tubercles and crest of pubis and sheath of rectus abdominis muscle (forms loops over spermatic cord that reach as far as testis)	Genital branch of genitofemoral nerve (L1, L2)	Pulls the testis upward toward the superficial inguinal ring
Pyramidalis	Anterior surface of pubis and anterior pubic ligament	Into **linea alba** between umbilicus and symphysis pubis (muscle variable in size, average 6 to 7 cm in length)	12th thoracic nerve (T12)	Tenses **linea alba**

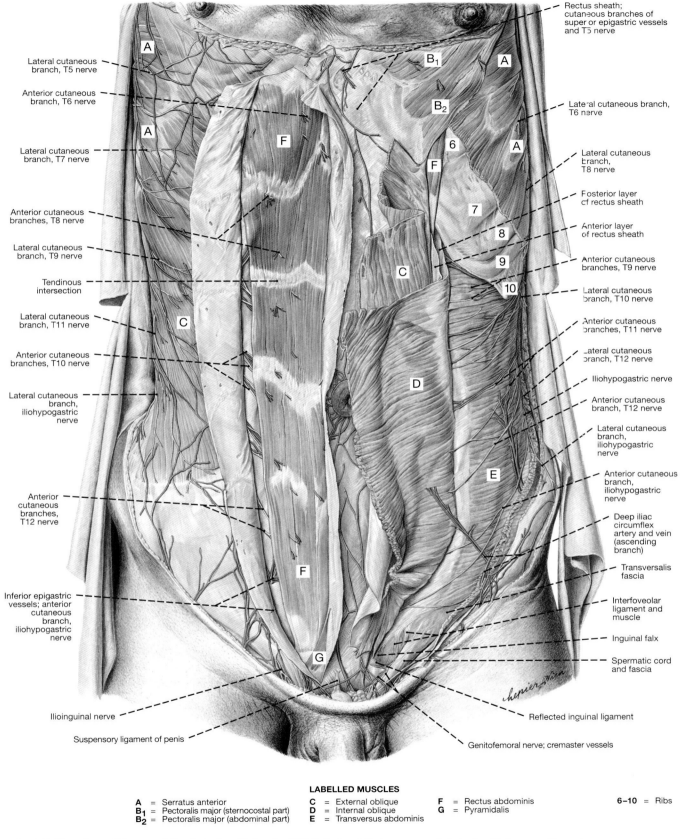

Rectus sheath; cutaneous branches of superior epigastric vessels and T5 nerve

Lateral cutaneous branch, T5 nerve

Anterior cutaneous branch, T6 nerve

Lateral cutaneous branch, T7 nerve

Anterior cutaneous branches, T8 nerve

Lateral cutaneous branch, T9 nerve

Tendinous intersection

Lateral cutaneous branch, T11 nerve

Anterior cutaneous branches, T10 nerve

Lateral cutaneous branch, iliohypogastric nerve

Anterior cutaneous branches, T12 nerve

Inferior epigastric vessels; anterior cutaneous branch, iliohypogastric nerve

Ilioinguinal nerve

Suspensory ligament of penis

Lateral cutaneous branch, T6 nerve

Lateral cutaneous branch, T8 nerve

Posterior layer of rectus sheath

Anterior layer of rectus sheath

Anterior cutaneous branches, T9 nerve

Lateral cutaneous branch, T10 nerve

Anterior cutaneous branches, T11 nerve

Lateral cutaneous branch, T12 nerve

Iliohypogastric nerve

Anterior cutaneous branch, T12 nerve

Lateral cutaneous branch, iliohypogastric nerve

Anterior cutaneous branch, iliohypogastric nerve

Deep iliac circumflex artery and vein (ascending branch)

Transversalis fascia

Interfoveolar ligament and muscle

Inguinal falx

Spermatic cord and fascia

Reflected inguinal ligament

Genitofemoral nerve; cremaster vessels

LABELLED MUSCLES

A = Serratus anterior	**C** = External oblique	**F** = Rectus abdominis	**6–10** = Ribs
B₁ = Pectoralis major (sternocostal part)	**D** = Internal oblique	**G** = Pyramidalis	
B₂ = Pectoralis major (abdominal part)	**E** = Transversus abdominis		

Fig. 258: Vessels and Nerves of the Anterior Abdominal Wall: Lateral Cutaneous and Anterior Cutaneous Branches
NOTE: this figure shows the **lateral** and **anterior cutaneous branches** of the lower six thoracic and 1st lumbar nerves. The lateral branches emerge between the ribs in the mid-axillary line, while the anterior branches course around the body between the internal oblique and transversus abdominis muscles. They are accompanied by similarly named branches of the intercostal vessels. Note also the **ascending branch** of the **deep circumflex iliac artery and vein.**

Fig 258   III

PLATE 170 **Anterior Abdominal Wall: Rectus Sheath, Deep Dissection**

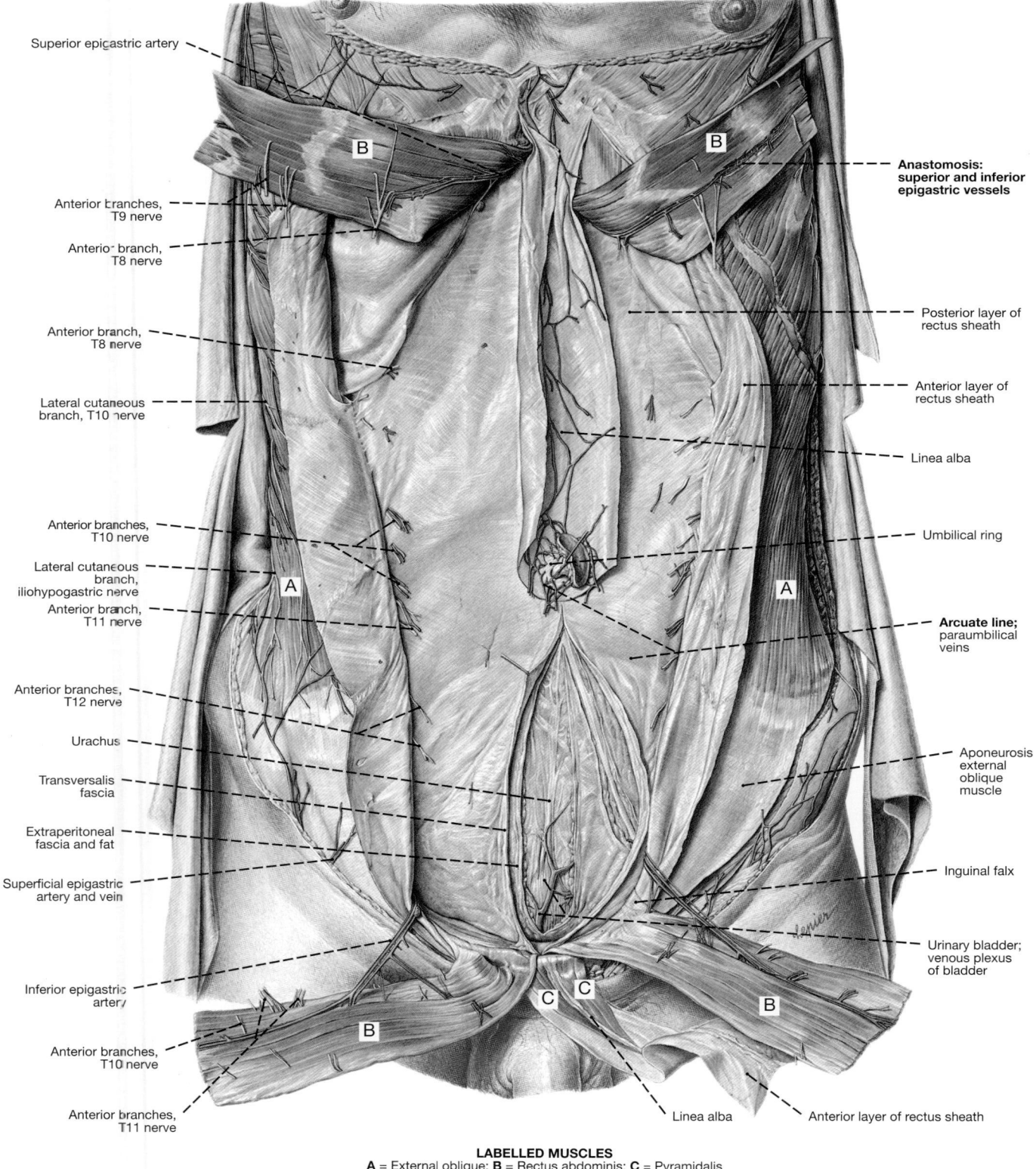

Superior epigastric artery

Anterior branches, T9 nerve

Anterior branch, T8 nerve

Anterior branch, T8 nerve

Lateral cutaneous branch, T10 nerve

Anterior branches, T10 nerve

Lateral cutaneous branch, iliohypogastric nerve

Anterior branch, T11 nerve

Anterior branches, T12 nerve

Urachus

Transversalis fascia

Extraperitoneal fascia and fat

Superficial epigastric artery and vein

Inferior epigastric artery

Anterior branches, T10 nerve

Anterior branches, T11 nerve

Anastomosis: superior and inferior epigastric vessels

Posterior layer of rectus sheath

Anterior layer of rectus sheath

Linea alba

Umbilical ring

Arcuate line; paraumbilical veins

Aponeurosis external oblique muscle

Inguinal falx

Urinary bladder; venous plexus of bladder

Linea alba

Anterior layer of rectus sheath

LABELLED MUSCLES
A = External oblique; **B** = Rectus abdominis; **C** = Pyramidalis

Fig. 259: Vessels and Nerves of the Anterior Abdominal Wall: Epigastric Vessels
NOTE: 1) the anterior layer of the rectus sheath has been opened on both sides and the two rectus abdominis muscles have been cut.

2) the descending course of the **superior epigastric vessels** and the ascending course of the **inferior epigastric vessels** found between the posterior layer of the rectus sheath and the rectus abdominis muscle on each side.

3) the superior and inferior epigastric vessels anastomose within the substance of the rectus abdominis muscle.

Fig. 259

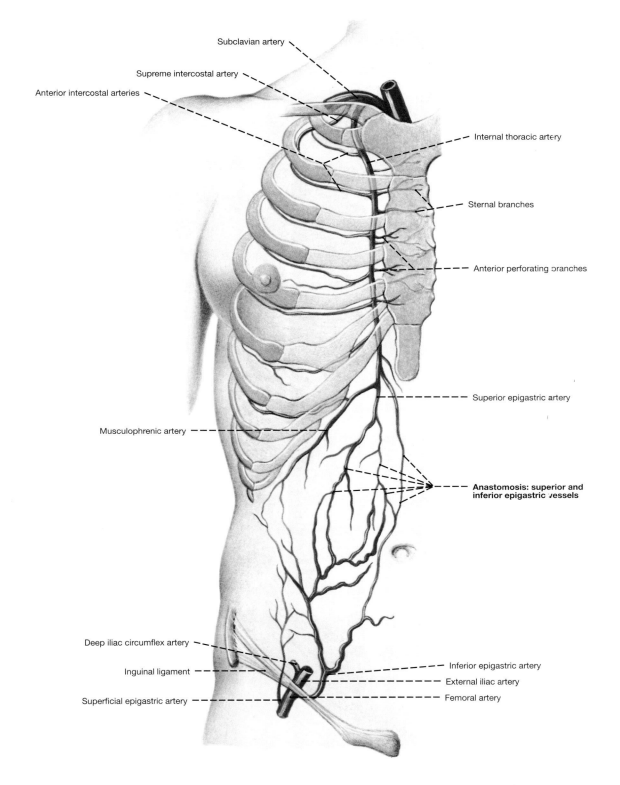

Subclavian artery

Supreme intercostal artery

Anterior intercostal arteries

Internal thoracic artery

Sternal branches

Anterior perforating branches

Superior epigastric artery

Musculophrenic artery

Anastomosis: superior and inferior epigastric vessels

Deep iliac circumflex artery

Inguinal ligament

Superficial epigastric artery

Inferior epigastric artery

External iliac artery

Femoral artery

Fig. 260: Schematic Diagram of the Epigastric Anastomosis

NOTE: 1) the **internal thoracic artery** arises from the subclavian artery and descends behind the ribs parallel to the sternum.

2) below the sternum the internal thoracic artery terminates by dividing into the **musculophrenic** and **superior epigastric arteries.**

3) the musculophrenic artery courses laterally adjacent to the costal margin and helps supply the diaphragm, while the superior epigastric artery descends within the rectus sheath where it enters the substance of the rectus abdominis muscle.

4) the inferior epigastric artery is a branch of the external iliac artery. It ascends and enters the rectus sheath at the arcuate line and also ramifies within the rectus abdominis muscle where it anastomoses with the superior epigastric. This anastomosis forms a functional interconnection between arteries that serve the upper and lower limbs.

Fig. 260   **III**

PLATE 172   **Anterior Abdominal and Thoracic Wall: Inner Surface, Muscles**

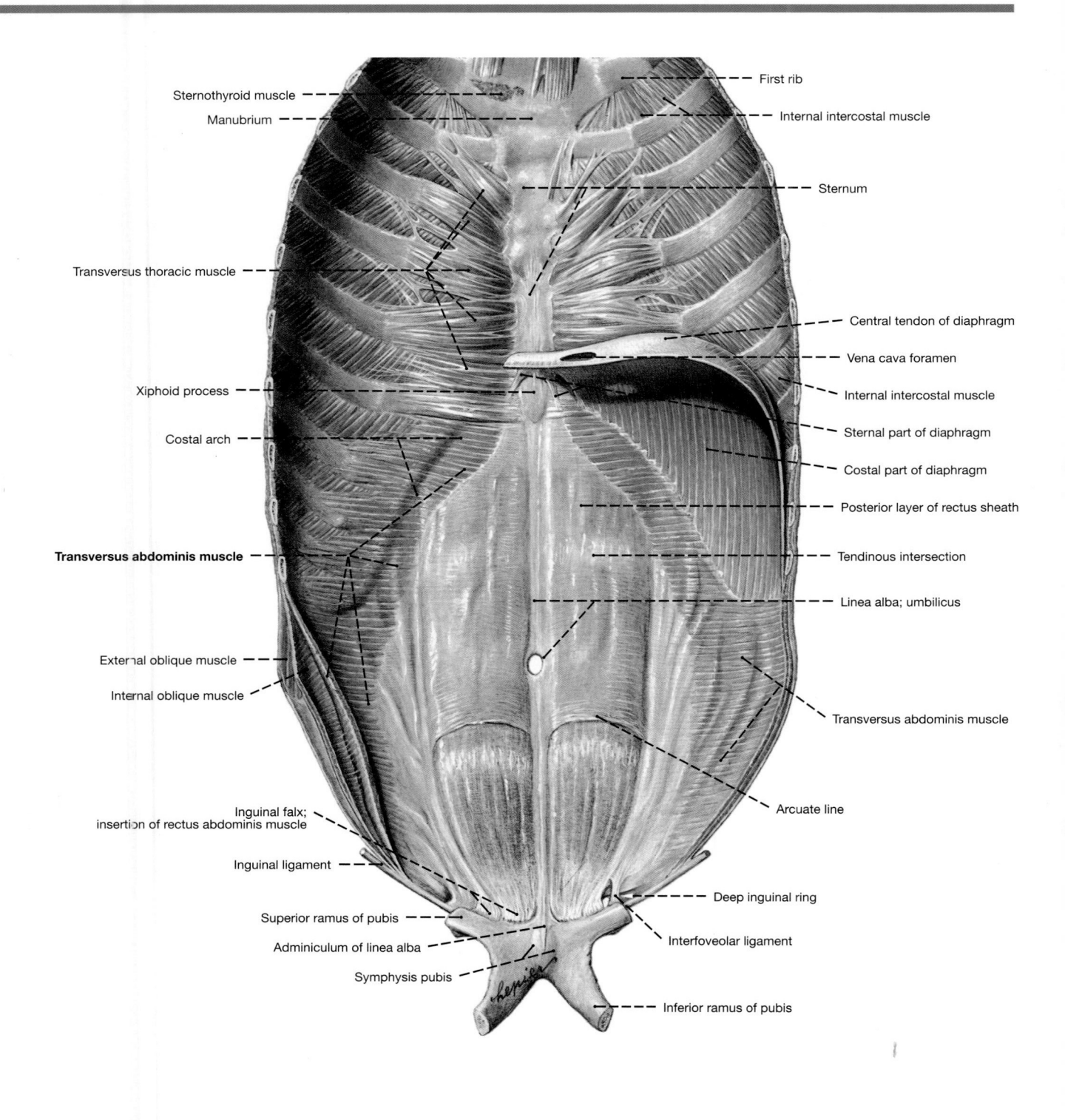

Sternothyroid muscle

Manubrium

Transversus thoracic muscle

Xiphoid process

Costal arch

Transversus abdominis muscle

External oblique muscle

Internal oblique muscle

Inguinal falx;
insertion of rectus abdominis muscle

Inguinal ligament

Superior ramus of pubis

Adminiculum of linea alba

Symphysis pubis

First rib

Internal intercostal muscle

Sternum

Central tendon of diaphragm

Vena cava foramen

Internal intercostal muscle

Sternal part of diaphragm

Costal part of diaphragm

Posterior layer of rectus sheath

Tendinous intersection

Linea alba; umbilicus

Transversus abdominis muscle

Arcuate line

Deep inguinal ring

Interfoveolar ligament

Inferior ramus of pubis

Fig. 261: Inner Aspect of the Anterior Thoracic and Abdominal Wall

NOTE: 1) this posterior view of the anterior abdominal and thoracic wall shows to good advantage inferiorly the posterior layer of the rectus sheath and the relationship of the **arcuate line** to the umbilicus. Also note the transverse thoracis muscle on the inner surface of the rib cage.

2) the opening of the **deep inguinal** (abdominal) **ring** and the **interfoveolar ligament,** a fibrous band that forms the medial edge of the deep inguinal ring and then courses superiorly and medially.

3) the breadth of the transversus abdominis muscle which lies adjacent to the next inner layer, the transversalis fascia (not shown).

4) the transversus thoracis lies in the same plane as the transversus abdominis below. It **arises** on the inner surface of the sternum and the 3rd to 6th costal cartilages. Its fibers course laterally and upward and **insert** on the costal cartilages of the 2nd to 6th ribs, acting as **depressors** of the ribs.

Fig. 261

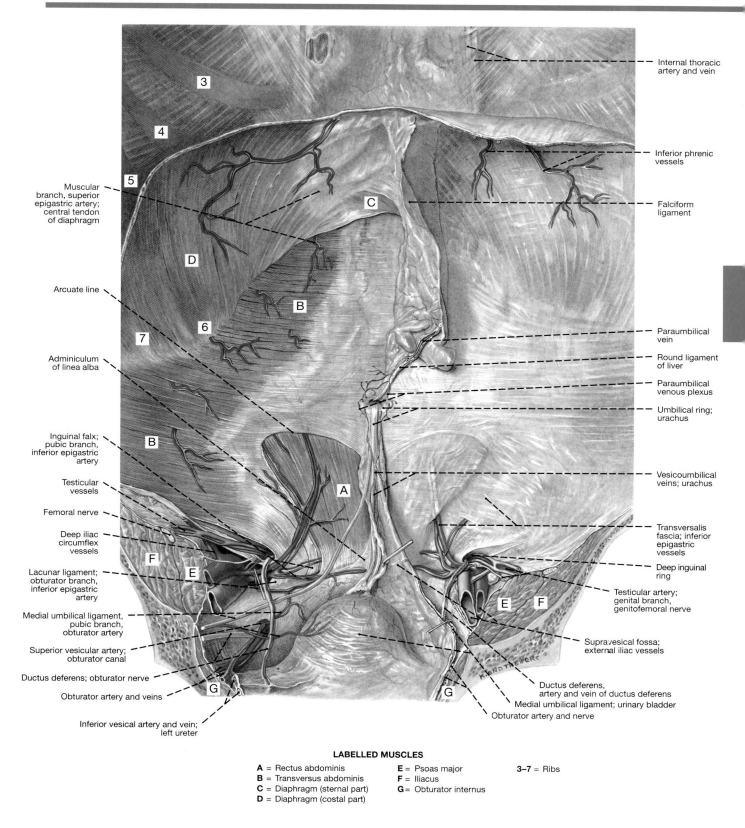

Internal thoracic artery and vein

Inferior phrenic vessels

Falciform ligament

Muscular branch, superior epigastric artery; central tendon of diaphragm

Arcuate line

Adminiculum of linea alba

Paraumbilical vein

Round ligament of liver

Paraumbilical venous plexus

Umbilical ring; urachus

Inguinal falx; pubic branch, inferior epigastric artery

Testicular vessels

Femoral nerve

Deep iliac circumflex vessels

Lacunar ligament; obturator branch, inferior epigastric artery

Medial umbilical ligament, pubic branch, obturator artery

Superior vesicular artery; obturator canal

Ductus deferens; obturator nerve

Obturator artery and veins

Inferior vesical artery and vein; left ureter

Vesicoumbilical veins; urachus

Transversalis fascia; inferior epigastric vessels

Deep inguinal ring

Testicular artery; genital branch, genitofemoral nerve

Supravesical fossa; external iliac vessels

Ductus deferens, artery and vein of ductus deferens

Medial umbilical ligament; urinary bladder

Obturator artery and nerve

LABELLED MUSCLES

A = Rectus abdominis	**E** = Psoas major	**3–7** = Ribs
B = Transversus abdominis	**F** = Iliacus	
C = Diaphragm (sternal part)	**G** = Obturator internus	
D = Diaphragm (costal part)		

Fig. 262: Vessels on the Inner Surface of the Anterior Abdominal Wall

NOTE: 1)   the **inferior epigastric** and **deep iliac circumflex** branches of the external iliac artery. Observe the anastomosis between the inferior epigastric and **obturator** arteries by means of their **pubic** branches.

2)   the **abdominal inguinal** ring through which courses the ductus deferens, the testicular vessels and the genital branch of the genitofemoral nerve (to the cremaster muscle).

3)   the **arcuate line,** clearly seen on the left. On the right side this line is somewhat obscured by the transversalis fascia which lines the deep surface of the transversus abdominis muscle.

Fig. 262   III

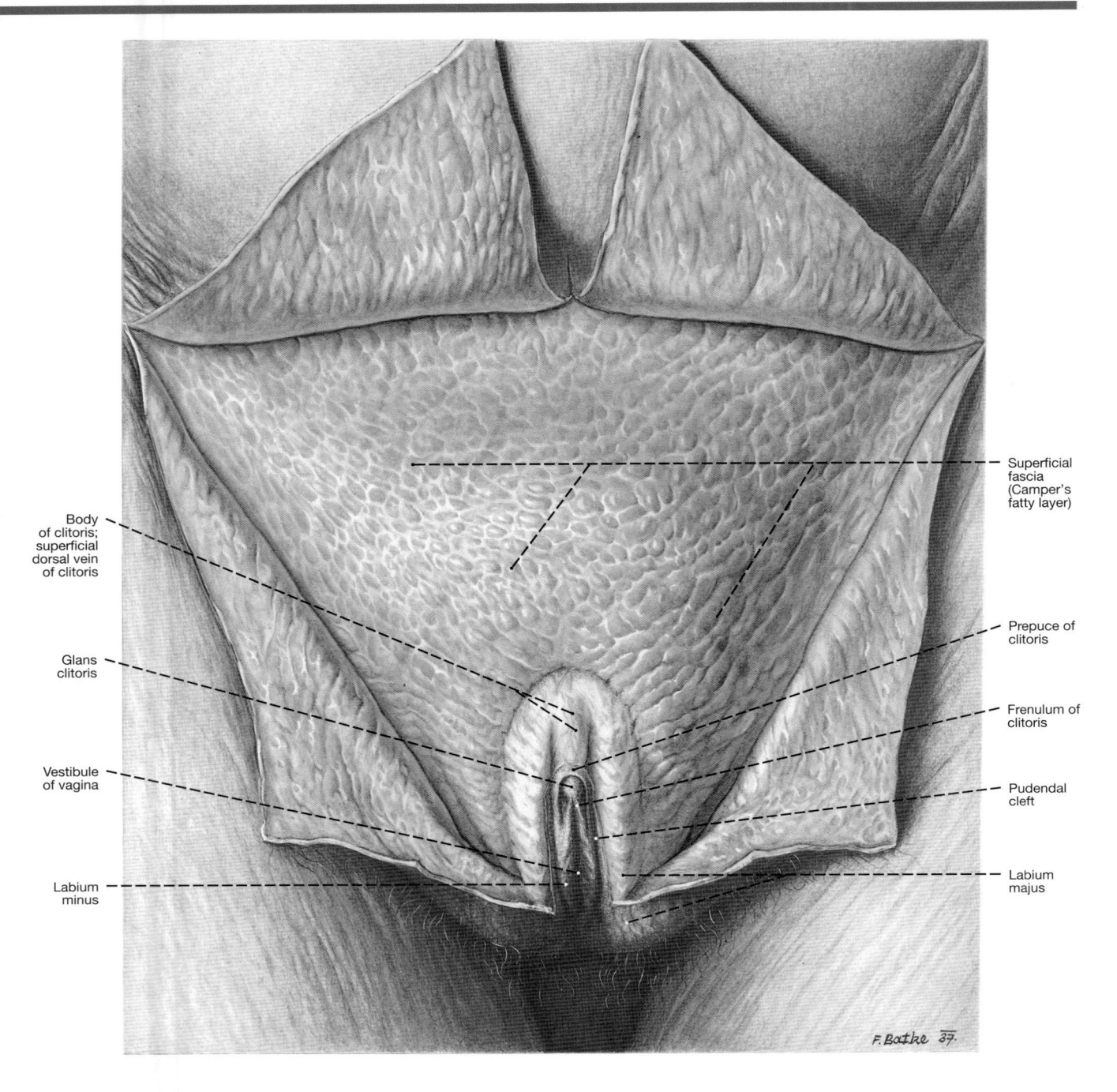

Superficial
fascia
(Camper's
fatty layer)

Body
of clitoris;
superficial
dorsal vein
of clitoris

Prepuce of
clitoris

Glans
clitoris

Frenulum of
clitoris

Vestibule
of vagina

Pudendal
cleft

Labium
minus

Labium
majus

F. Batke 37.

Fig. 263: Inguinal Region of the Anterior Abdominal Wall in the Female (1): Superficial Fascia (Fatty Layer)

NOTE: 1)   the superficial fascia of the lower anterior abdominal wall is usually described as consisting of a superficial fatty layer, often called **Camper's fascia,** and a deeper fibrous layer of superficial fascia which condenses into a strong membrane called **Scarpa's fascia** (see Fig. 264).

2)   this figure shows the skin reflected from the lower anterior abdominal wall and inguinal region exposing the superficial fatty layer of Camper that overlies these sites.

3)   this superficial fatty layer can be followed downward over the inguinal ligaments where it becomes continuous with the superficial fascia of the thigh.

4)   the skin has been removed from the body of the clitoris and from the labium majus on both sides. Essentially, the labia majora are composed of skin and superficial fascial structures and consist principally of fatty tissue.

Fig. 263

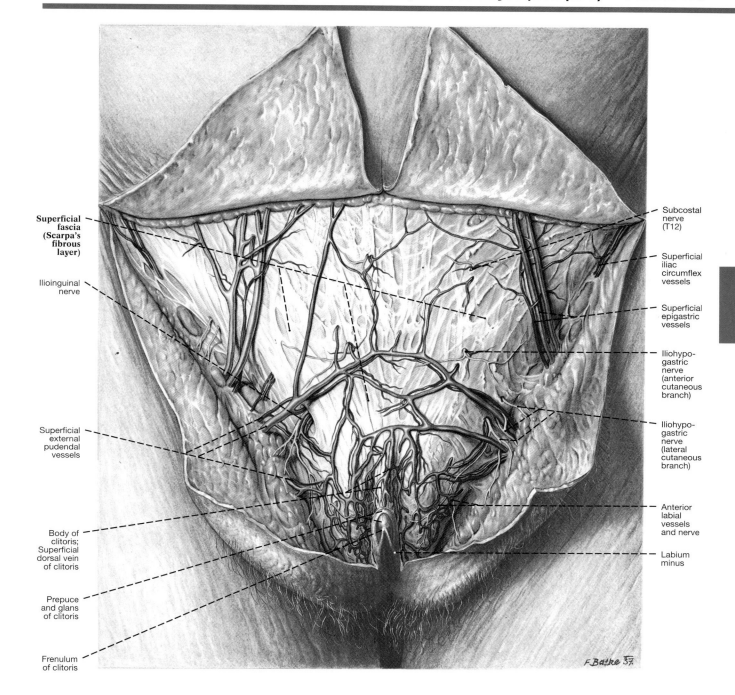

Superficial
fascia
(Scarpa's
fibrous
layer)

Ilioinguinal
nerve

Superficial
external
pudendal
vessels

Body of
clitoris;
Superficial
dorsal vein
of clitoris

Prepuce
and glans
of clitoris

Frenulum
of clitoris

Subcostal
nerve
(T12)

Superficial
iliac
circumflex
vessels

Superficial
epigastric
vessels

Iliohypo-
gastric
nerve
(anterior
cutaneous
branch)

Iliohypo-
gastric
nerve
(lateral
cutaneous
branch)

Anterior
labial
vessels
and nerve

Labium
minus

F.Batke 57

Fig. 264: Inguinal Region of the Anterior Abdominal Wall in the Female (2): Superficial Fascia (Fibrous Layer of Scarpa).

NOTE: 1) the superficial fatty layer of superficial fascia (Camper's) has been removed, thereby exposing the condensed fibrous deep layer of superficial fascia, often called **Scarpa's fascia.**

    2) as Scarpa's fascia descends in the inguinal region, on each side **laterally** its deep surface fuses with the fascia lata of the thigh just below the inguinal ligament, unlike Camper's fascia which is continuous with the fatty layer in the thigh. Medially, however, there is no deep fusion and Scarpa's fascia continues into the perineum as a membranous layer called **Colles' fascia.**

    3) vessels supplying and draining this region include the **superficial external pudendal, superficial iliac circumflex,** and **superficial epigastric arteries** and **veins.** All three of the arteries arise from the femoral artery, while the veins all drain into the great saphenous vein in the upper medial thigh.

    4) the anterior cutaneous branches of the T12 nerve (subcostal nerve) and the anterior and lateral cutaneous branches of the L1 nerve (branches of the ilioinguinal and iliohypogastric nerves) are seen to penetrate through Scarpa's fascia to become cutaneous in their distribution.

Fig. 264   III

PLATE 176   Female Inguinal Region III: Superficial Inguinal Ring

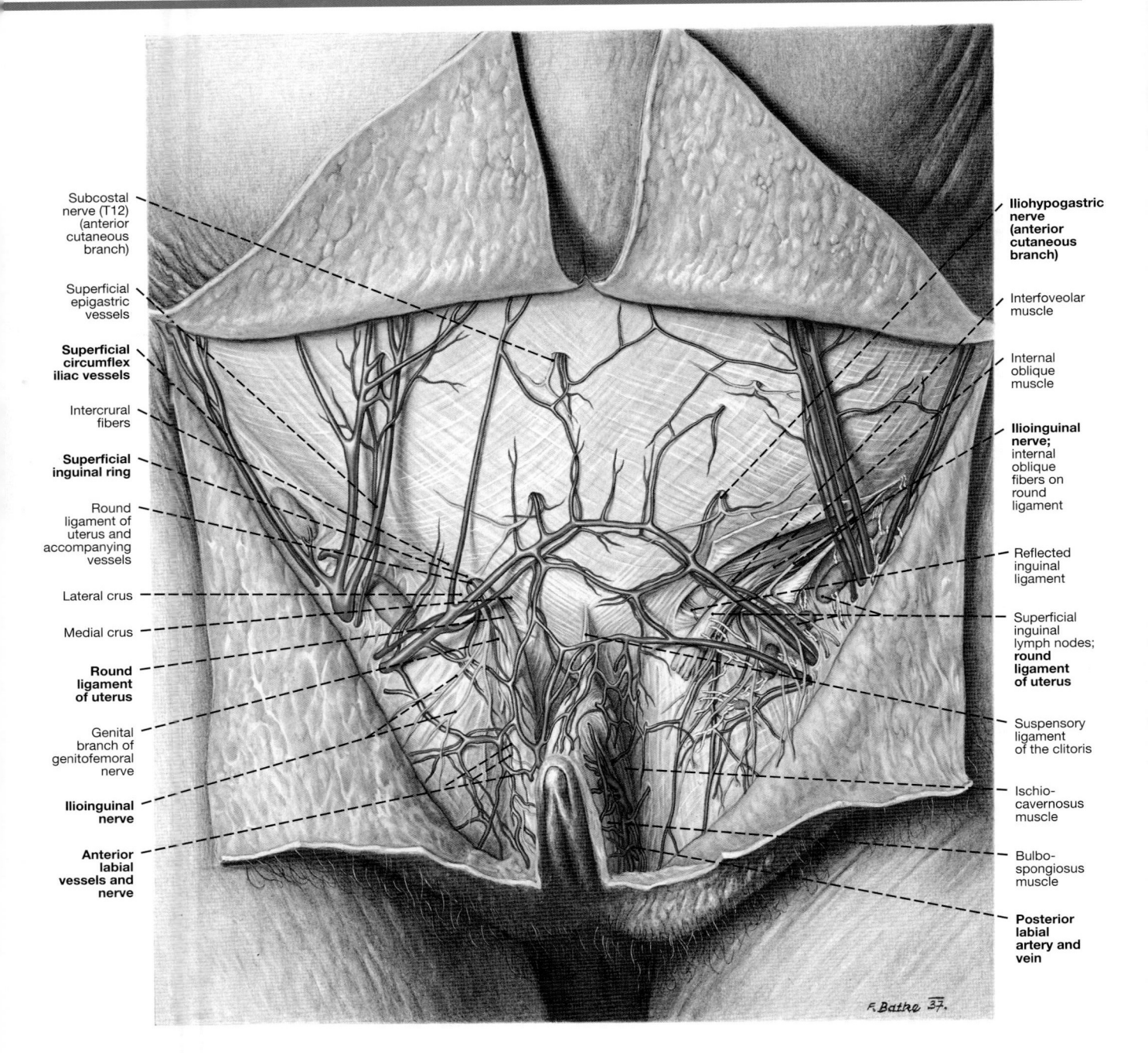

Subcostal nerve (T12) (anterior cutaneous branch)

Superficial epigastric vessels

Superficial circumflex iliac vessels

Intercrural fibers

Superficial inguinal ring

Round ligament of uterus and accompanying vessels

Lateral crus

Medial crus

Round ligament of uterus

Genital branch of genitofemoral nerve

Ilioinguinal nerve

Anterior labial vessels and nerve

Iliohypogastric nerve (anterior cutaneous branch)

Interfoveolar muscle

Internal oblique muscle

Ilioinguinal nerve; internal oblique fibers on round ligament

Reflected inguinal ligament

Superficial inguinal lymph nodes; **round ligament of uterus**

Suspensory ligament of the clitoris

Ischio-cavernosus muscle

Bulbo-spongiosus muscle

Posterior labial artery and vein

F.Bathe 37.

Fig. 265: Inguinal Region of the Anterior Abdominal Wall in the Female (3): Aponeurosis of the External Oblique

NOTE: 1) the skin and superficial fascia have been reflected from the inguinal region exposing the aponeurosis of the external oblique muscle, the superficial inguinal ring, the superficial vessels and nerves of the lower abdominal wall and the muscles and nerves of the clitoris.

2) the **superficial inguinal ring** is an opening in the aponeurosis of the external oblique muscle. On the specimen's left (reader's right) the ring has been opened to reveal the lower course of the round ligament and the ilioinguinal nerve.

3) the iliohypogastric nerve (branch of L1) as it penetrates the aponeurosis to become a sensory nerve after supplying motor fibers to the underlying musculature.

4) of the superficial vessels, observe the **superficial external pudendal** (labelled in Fig. 264), the **superficial iliac circumflex** and **superficial epigastric.** The latter vessels ascend within the superficial fascia between its superficial fatty (Camper's) and deep (Scarpa's) layers.

5) the **superficial dorsal vein of the clitoris**, which may drain into either the left or right superficial external pudendal vein.

Fig. 265

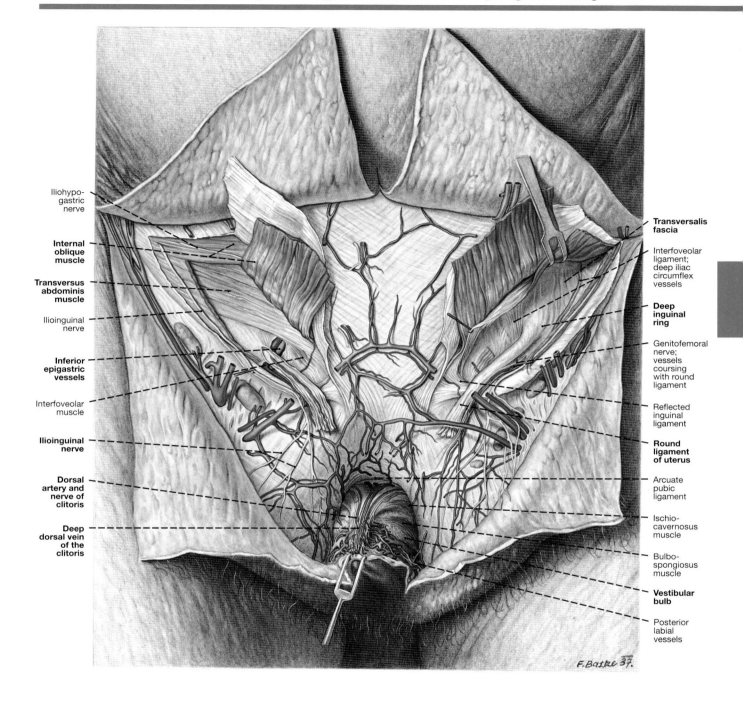

Iliohypo-
gastric
nerve

Internal
oblique
muscle

Transversus
abdominis
muscle

Ilioinguinal
nerve

Inferior
epigastric
vessels

Interfoveolar
muscle

Ilioinguinal
nerve

Dorsal
artery and
nerve of
clitoris

Deep
dorsal vein
of the
clitoris

Transversalis
fascia

Interfoveolar
ligament;
deep iliac
circumflex
vessels

Deep
inguinal
ring

Genitofemoral
nerve;
vessels
coursing
with round
ligament

Reflected
inguinal
ligament

Round
ligament
of uterus

Arcuate
pubic
ligament

Ischio-
cavernosus
muscle

Bulbo-
spongiosus
muscle

Vestibular
bulb

Posterior
labial
vessels

F. Batke 37.

Fig. 266: Inguinal Region of the Anterior Abdominal Wall in the Female (4): Opened Inguinal Canal
NOTE: 1)   the **left** (reader's right) **inguinal canal** has been completely opened by severing the overlying transversus abdominis and internal oblique muscles as well as the lower lateral part of the aponeurosis of the external oblique muscle.

2)   the female inguinal canal contains the **round ligament of the uterus** and its accompanying vessels. The **ilioinguinal branch of the L1 nerve** and the **genital branch of the genitofemoral nerve** (L1 and L2) both emerge with the round ligament through the superficial inguinal ring.

3)   the genital branch of the genitofemoral nerve enters the inguinal canal with the round ligament from within the pelvis. The ilioinguinal nerve does not enter the canal from within the pelvis, but it joins the canal just deep to the aponeurosis of the external oblique.

4)   the ilioinguinal nerve and the genital branch of the genitofemoral nerve in females are both sensory to the inguinal region and to the labia majora.

5)   after leaving the superficial inguinal ring, the round ligament splits into fibrous strands that blend with the subcutaneous tissue of the labium majus on each side. The labia majora are the homologues of the scrotal sac in the male.

Fig 266   **III**

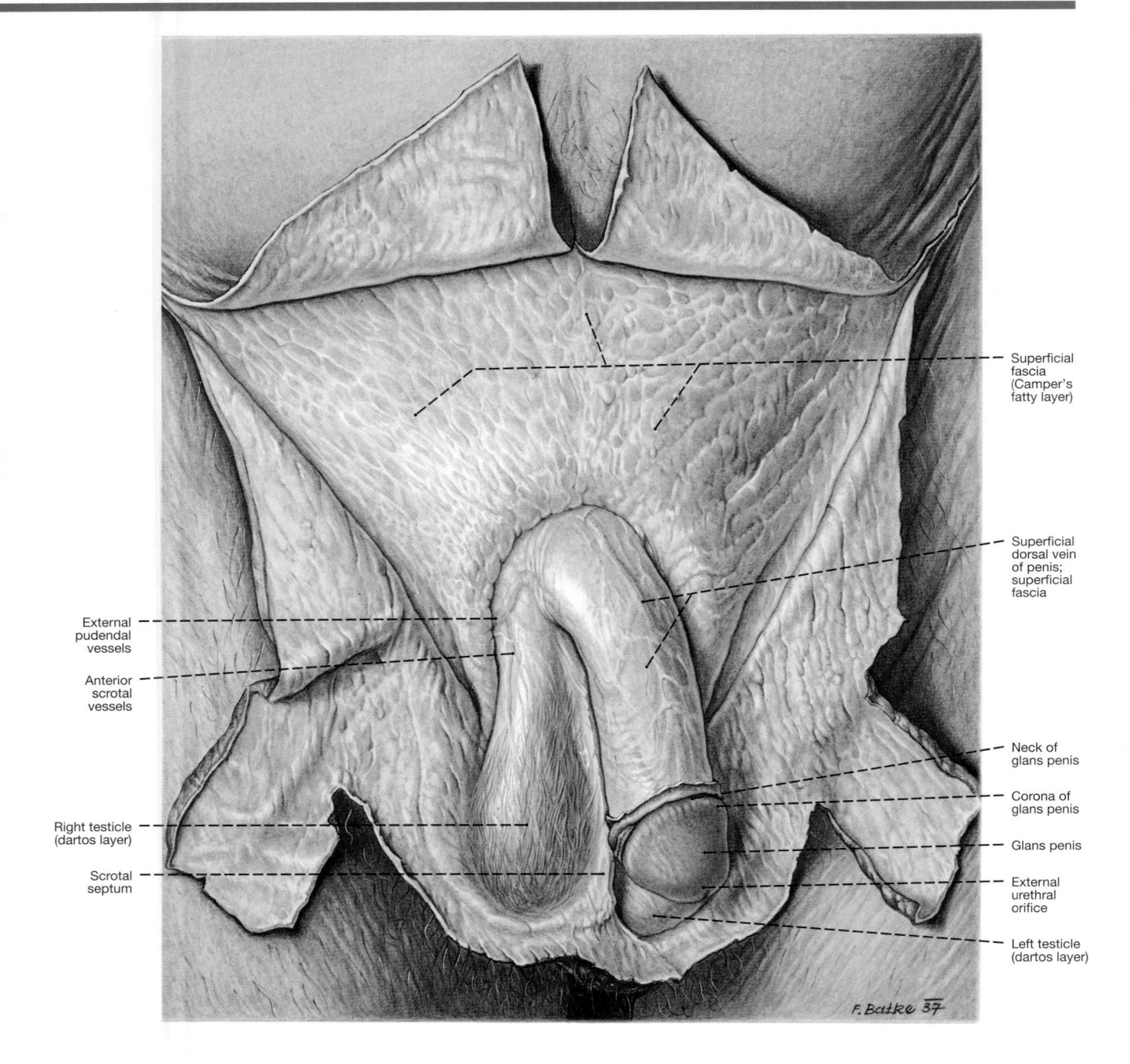

Superficial fascia (Camper's fatty layer)

Superficial dorsal vein of penis; superficial fascia

External pudendal vessels

Anterior scrotal vessels

Neck of glans penis

Corona of glans penis

Right testicle (dartos layer)

Glans penis

Scrotal septum

External urethral orifice

Left testicle (dartos layer)

F. Batke 37

Fig. 267: Inguinal Region of the Anterior Abdominal Wall in the Male (1): Superficial Fascia (Fatty Layer)

NOTE: 1)   the skin has been reflected from the lower anterior abdominal wall, inguinal region, scrotum, and penis.

     2)   removal of the skin exposes the superficial layer of superficial fascia, often called Camper's fascia, over the anterior abdominal wall, the dartos layer of the scrotal wall and the superficial fascia just deep to the skin of the scrotum.

     3)   the superficial fatty layer in males (as in females) extends downward over the inguinal ligament to be continuous with the fatty layer of superficial fascia covering the thigh.

     4)   the subcutaneous layer of the scrotum contains no fat but has a thin layer of smooth muscle, called the **dartos muscle,** contraction of which results in the formation of rugae or wrinkles on the scrotal skin surface.

Fig. 267

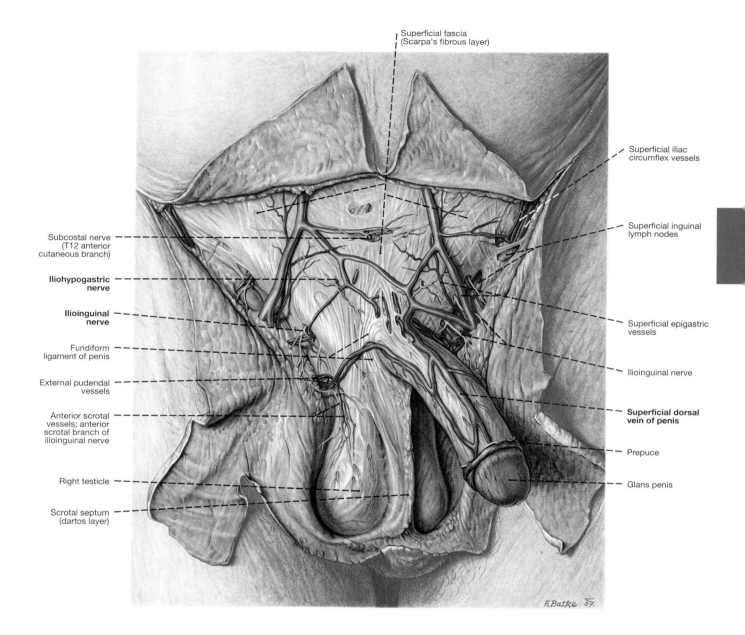

Superficial fascia
(Scarpa's fibrous layer)

Superficial iliac
circumflex vessels

Superficial inguinal
lymph nodes

Subcostal nerve
(T12 anterior
cutaneous branch)

Iliohypogastric
nerve

Ilioinguinal
nerve

Superficial epigastric
vessels

Fundiform
ligament of penis

Ilioinguinal nerve

External pudendal
vessels

Anterior scrotal
vessels; anterior
scrotal branch of
ilioinguinal nerve

Superficial dorsal
vein of penis

Prepuce

Right testicle

Glans penis

Scrotal septum
(dartos layer)

F.Batke 37.

Fig. 268: Inguinal Region of the Anterior Abdominal Wall in the Male (2): Superficial Fascia (Fibrous Layer of Scarpa)

NOTE: 1) the fibrous layer of superficial fascia (Scarpa's fascia) is exposed after removal of the superficial fatty layer (Camper's fascia).

2) Scarpa's fascia fuses to the **fascia lata** of the thigh laterally just below the inguinal ligaments, but it continues into the perineum as a dissectable sheet along the penis and as a distinct layer on the inner surface of the scrotal skin to help form the dartos layer of the scrotal wall.

3) in the perineum, this layer is called **Colles' fascia** and, as it becomes prolonged along the penile shaft it blends with the **fascia penis** (Buck's deep fascia) overlying the deep dorsal vein and the two dorsal arteries and two dorsal nerves of the penis.

4) the superficial dorsal vein of the penis drains into the superficial external pudendal vein or into a network that includes the superficial epigastric vein.

5) the cutaneous nerves include branches from T12 (subcostal) and L1 (ilioinguinal and iliohypogastric).

Fig. 268   III

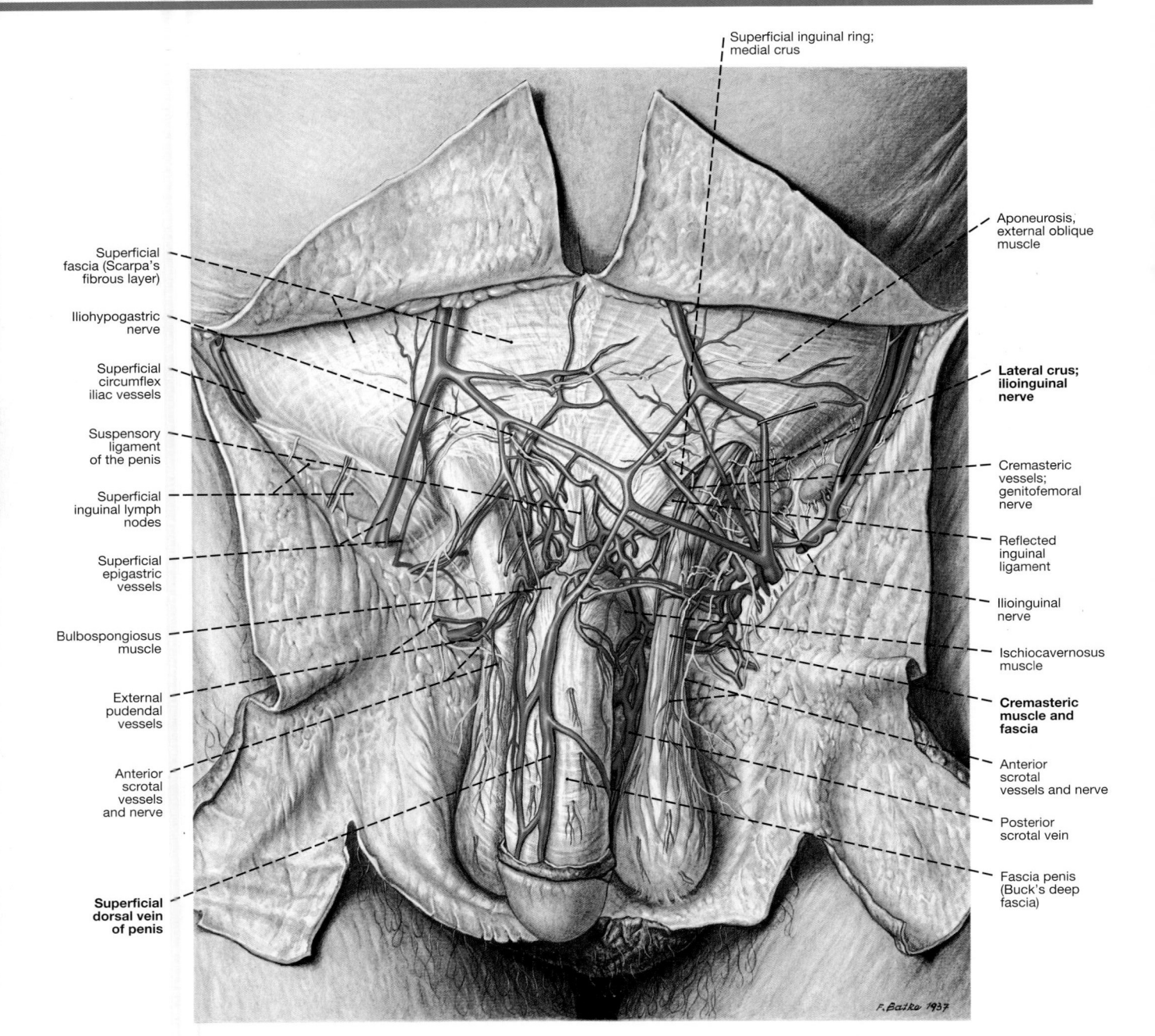

Superficial inguinal ring;
medial crus

Aponeurosis;
external oblique
muscle

Superficial
fascia (Scarpa's
fibrous layer)

Iliohypogastric
nerve

Superficial
circumflex
iliac vessels

Suspensory
ligament
of the penis

Superficial
inguinal lymph
nodes

Superficial
epigastric
vessels

Bulbospongiosus
muscle

External
pudendal
vessels

Anterior
scrotal
vessels
and nerve

**Superficial
dorsal vein
of penis**

**Lateral crus;
ilioinguinal
nerve**

Cremasteric
vessels;
genitofemoral
nerve

Reflected
inguinal
ligament

Ilioinguinal
nerve

Ischiocavernosus
muscle

**Cremasteric
muscle and
fascia**

Anterior
scrotal
vessels and nerve

Posterior
scrotal vein

Fascia penis
(Buck's deep
fascia)

F. Batke 1937

**Fig. 269: Inguinal Region of the Anterior Abdominal Wall in the Male (3): Superficial Inguinal Rings and
the Cremaster Muscle**

NOTE: 1) on the specimen's right (reader's left), the skin and superficial fatty layer (Camper's) has been removed, while
on the left side the skin, fatty layer and superficial fibrous layer (Scarpa's) have been resected revealing the aponeurosis of the
external oblique muscle.

2) the superficial inguinal rings have been exposed and the scrotal sacs opened. Observe the course of the **spermatic cord**
from the scrotum to the superficial inguinal ring and the cremaster muscle and fascia surrounding the spermatic cord on the left.

3) the **iliohypogastric nerve** penetrating the aponeurosis of the external oblique just above the superficial inguinal ring, and
the **ilioinguinal nerve** emerging from the ring to supply the inguinal region and then continuing as the **anterior scrotal nerve.**

4) the external spermatic fascia (not labelled) covering the spermatic cord is seen on the right while the cremasteric fascia
and cremaster muscle is seen on the left after removal of the external spermatic fascia.

Fig. 269

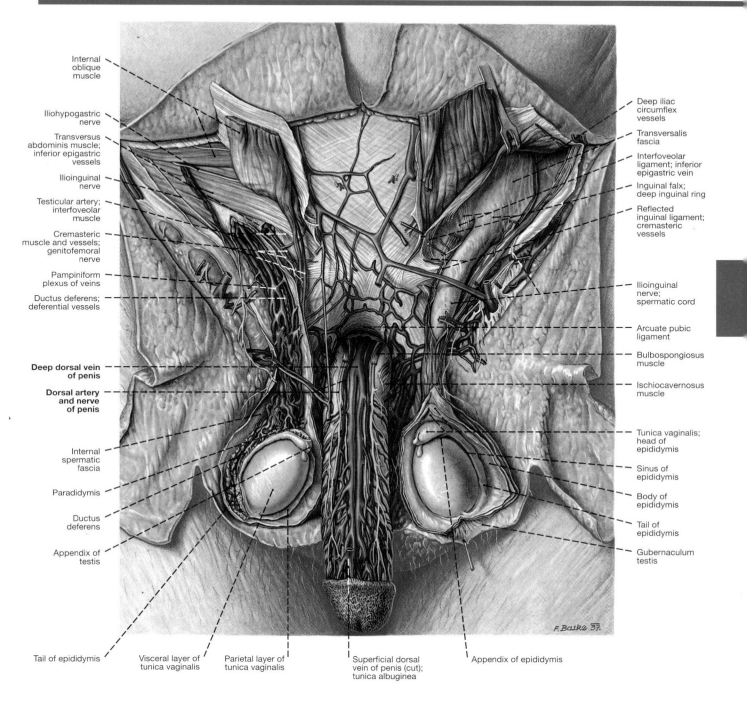

Internal oblique muscle

Iliohypogastric nerve

Transversus abdominis muscle; inferior epigastric vessels

Ilioinguinal nerve

Testicular artery; interfoveolar muscle

Cremasteric muscle and vessels; genitofemoral nerve

Pampiniform plexus of veins

Ductus deferens; deferential vessels

Deep dorsal vein of penis

Dorsal artery and nerve of penis

Internal spermatic fascia

Paradidymis

Ductus deferens

Appendix of testis

Deep iliac circumflex vessels

Transversalis fascia

Interfoveolar ligament; inferior epigastric vein

Inguinal falx; deep inguinal ring

Reflected inguinal ligament; cremasteric vessels

Ilioinguinal nerve; spermatic cord

Arcuate pubic ligament

Bulbospongiosus muscle

Ischiocavernosus muscle

Tunica vaginalis; head of epididymis

Sinus of epididymis

Body of epididymis

Tail of epididymis

Gubernaculum testis

F. Batke 37.

Tail of epididymis

Visceral layer of tunica vaginalis

Parietal layer of tunica vaginalis

Superficial dorsal vein of penis (cut); tunica albuginea

Appendix of epididymis

Fig. 270: Inguinal Region of the Anterior Abdominal Wall in the Male (4): Opened Inguinal Canal and Spermatic Cord.

NOTE: 1) the entire extent of the inguinal canal has been opened on the left side (reader's right) by severing the anterior abdominal muscles. The cremaster muscle and fascia have also been opened as have the other coverings of the testis.

    2) on the right side, the internal spermatic fascia has been opened to reveal the contents of the spermatic cord. These include:
      a) the ductus deferens,
      b) the testicular, cremasteric, and deferential arteries,
      c) the testicular veins which form a venous network called the **pampiniform plexus,**
      d) the cremaster muscle and its nerve (genital branch of the genitofemoral nerve),
      e) lymphatic vessels and sympathetic nerve fibers.

    3) the ilioinguinal nerve courses within the canal for a distance along the surface of the spermatic cord and emerges with the cord through the superficial inguinal ring.

Fig. 270   **III**

PLATE 132   Spermatic Cord and Testis

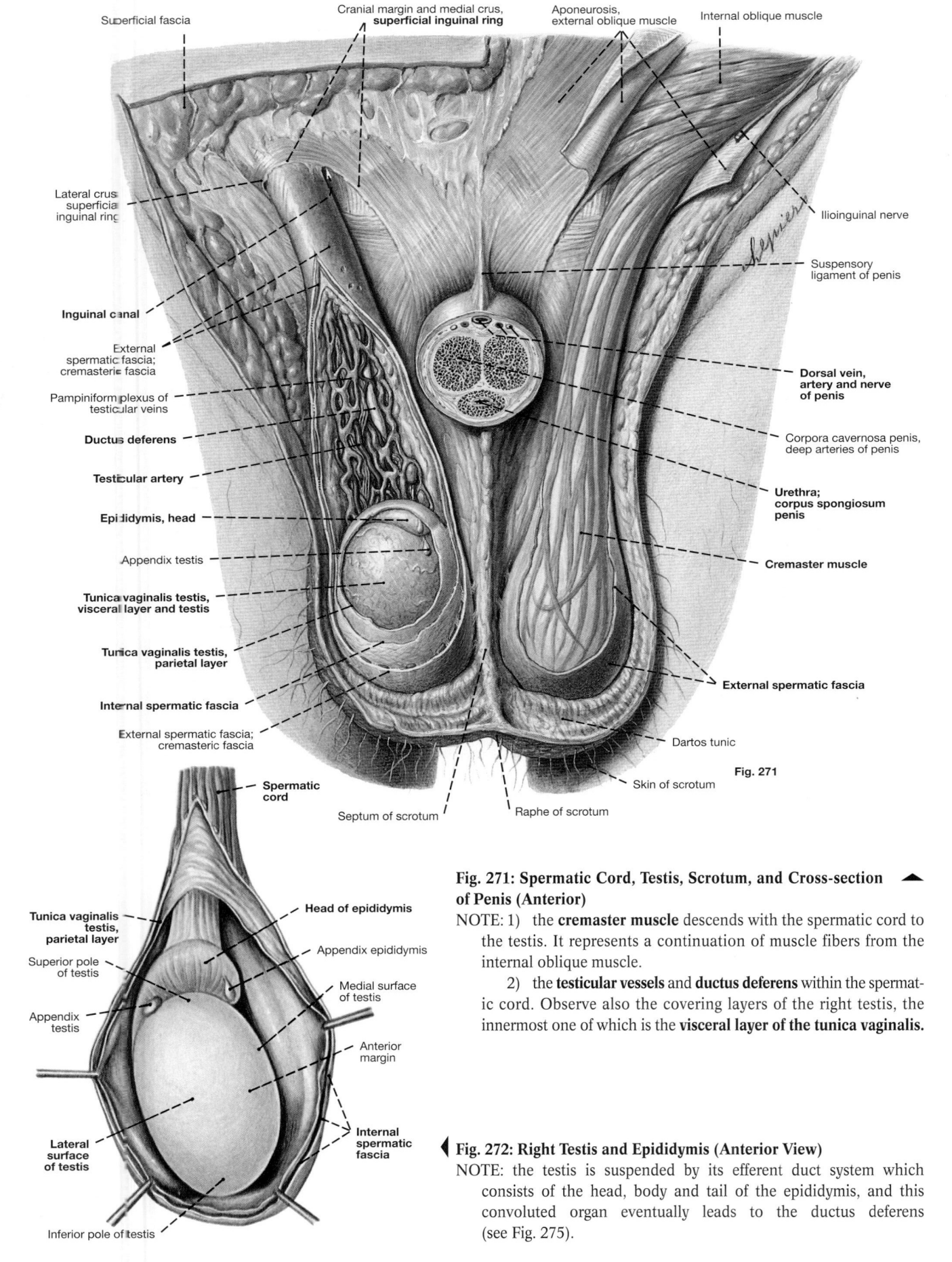

Superficial fascia

Cranial margin and medial crus, **superficial inguinal ring**

Aponeurosis, external oblique muscle

Internal oblique muscle

Lateral crus superficial inguinal ring

Ilioinguinal nerve

Suspensory ligament of penis

Inguinal canal

External spermatic fascia; cremasteric fascia

Dorsal vein, artery and nerve of penis

Pampiniform plexus of testicular veins

Corpora cavernosa penis, deep arteries of penis

Ductus deferens

Urethra; corpus spongiosum penis

Testicular artery

Epididymis, head

Appendix testis

Cremaster muscle

Tunica vaginalis testis, visceral layer and testis

Tunica vaginalis testis, parietal layer

External spermatic fascia

Internal spermatic fascia

Dartos tunic

External spermatic fascia; cremasteric fascia

Fig. 271

Spermatic cord

Skin of scrotum

Septum of scrotum

Raphe of scrotum

Fig. 271: Spermatic Cord, Testis, Scrotum, and Cross-section of Penis (Anterior)

NOTE: 1) the **cremaster muscle** descends with the spermatic cord to the testis. It represents a continuation of muscle fibers from the internal oblique muscle.

   2) the **testicular vessels** and **ductus deferens** within the spermatic cord. Observe also the covering layers of the right testis, the innermost one of which is the **visceral layer of the tunica vaginalis.**

Tunica vaginalis testis, parietal layer

Head of epididymis

Appendix epididymis

Superior pole of testis

Medial surface of testis

Appendix testis

Anterior margin

Lateral surface of testis

Internal spermatic fascia

Inferior pole of testis

Fig. 272: Right Testis and Epididymis (Anterior View)

NOTE: the testis is suspended by its efferent duct system which consists of the head, body and tail of the epididymis, and this convoluted organ eventually leads to the ductus deferens (see Fig. 275).

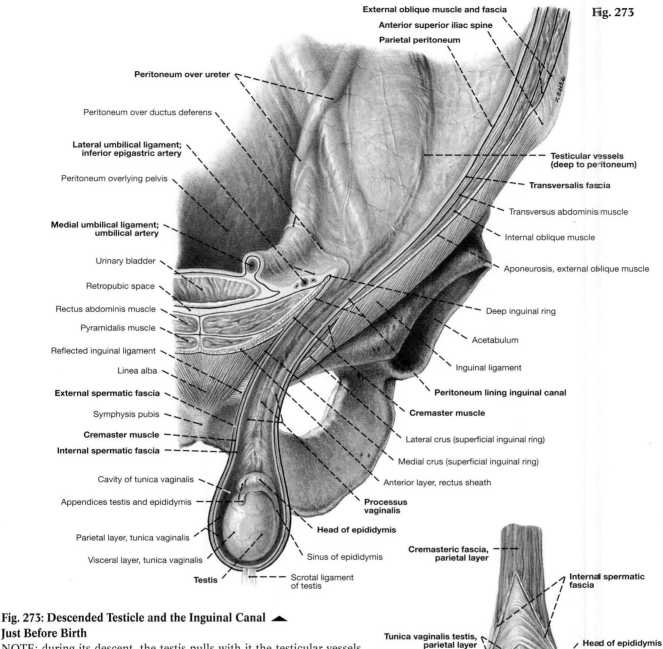

Fig. 273

External oblique muscle and fascia
Anterior superior iliac spine
Parietal peritoneum

Peritoneum over ureter

Peritoneum over ductus deferens

Lateral umbilical ligament; inferior epigastric artery

Peritoneum overlying pelvis

Medial umbilical ligament; umbilical artery

Urinary bladder

Retropubic space

Rectus abdominis muscle

Pyramidalis muscle

Reflected inguinal ligament

Linea alba

External spermatic fascia

Symphysis pubis

Cremaster muscle

Internal spermatic fascia

Cavity of tunica vaginalis

Appendices testis and epididymis

Parietal layer, tunica vaginalis

Visceral layer, tunica vaginalis

Testis

Testicular vessels (deep to peritoneum)

Transversalis fascia

Transversus abdominis muscle

Internal oblique muscle

Aponeurosis, external oblique muscle

Deep inguinal ring

Acetabulum

Inguinal ligament

Peritoneum lining inguinal canal

Cremaster muscle

Lateral crus (superficial inguinal ring)

Medial crus (superficial inguinal ring)

Anterior layer, rectus sheath

Processus vaginalis

Head of epididymis

Sinus of epididymis

Scrotal ligament of testis

Cremasteric fascia, parietal layer

Internal spermatic fascia

Tunica vaginalis testis, parietal layer

Head of epididymis

Superior ligament of epididymis

Appendix testis

Appendix epididymis

Sinus of epididymis

Testis, posterior margin

Testis, lateral surface

Inferior ligament of epididymis

Tail of epididymis

Testis, anterior margin

Fig. 274

Fig. 273: Descended Testicle and the Inguinal Canal ▲
Just Before Birth

NOTE: during its descent, the testis pulls with it the testicular vessels and a peritoneal covering called the **processus vaginalis.** This figure shows the formed inguinal canal at the time of birth, with the testis already in the scrotum.

Fig. 274: Right Testis and Epididymis (Lateral View) ▶

NOTE: the coverings of the testis represent evaginations of the layers forming the anterior abdominal wall. These evaginations precede the testis during its descent in the latter half of gestation. The comparable layers are as follows:

Anterior Abdominal Wall
1. Skin
2. Superficial fascia
3. External oblique
4. Internal oblique
5. Transversus abdominis
6. Transversalis fascia
7. Extraperitoneal fat
8. Peritoneum

Coverings of Testis
1. Skin
2. Dartos tunic } Scrotum
3. External spermatic fascia
4. Cremaster muscle and
5. Cremasteric fascia
6. Internal spermatic fascia
7. Fatty layer
8. Processus vaginalis

PLATE 184   Testis and Epididymis

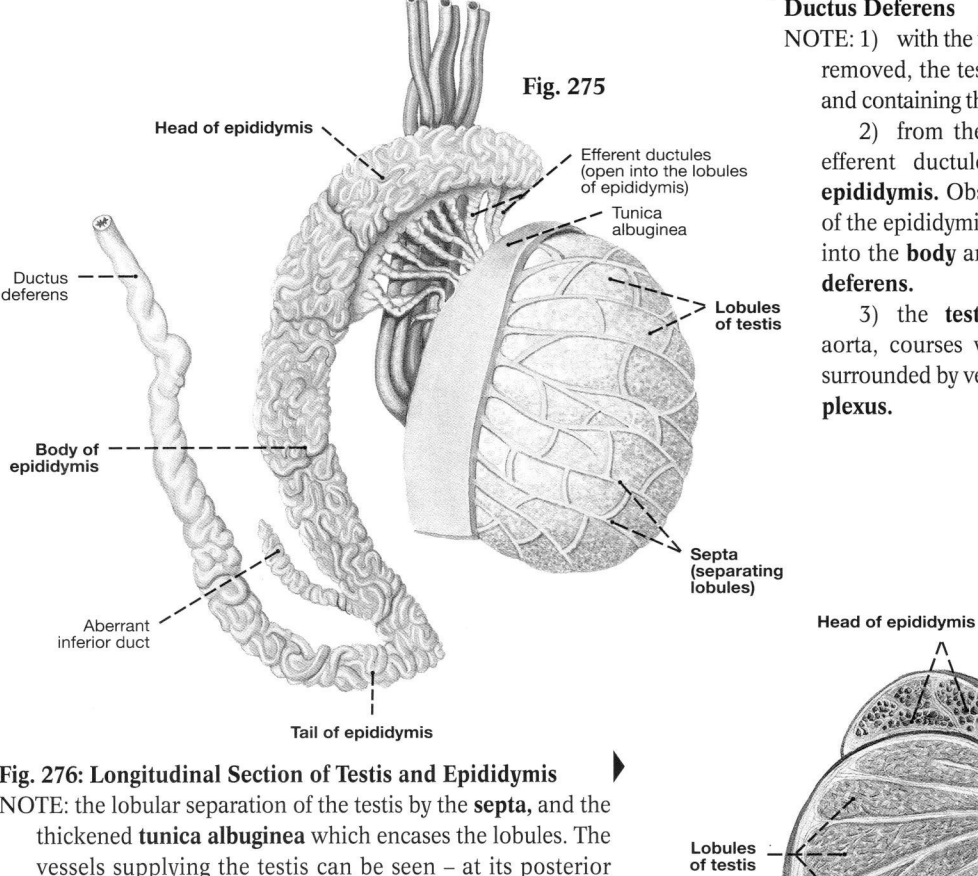

Testicular vessels

Fig. 275

Head of epididymis

Efferent ductules
(open into the lobules
of epididymis)

Tunica
albuginea

Ductus
deferens

Lobules
of testis

Body of
epididymis

Septa
(separating
lobules)

Aberrant
inferior duct

Tail of epididymis

Fig. 275: Testis, Epididymis, and the Beginning of the Ductus Deferens

NOTE: 1) with the tunica vaginalis and tunica albuginea removed, the testicular lobules, separated by septa and containing the **seminiferous tubules** are exposed.

2) from the lobules a group of 8 to 12 fine efferent ductules open into the **head of the epididymis.** Observe the highly convoluted nature of the epididymis. The head of the epididymis leads into the **body** and **tail,** which becomes the **ductus deferens.**

3) the **testicular artery,** derived from the aorta, courses with the spermatic cord and it is surrounded by venous plexus, called the **paminiform plexus.**

Fig. 276: Longitudinal Section of Testis and Epididymis

NOTE: the lobular separation of the testis by the **septa,** and the thickened **tunica albuginea** which encases the lobules. The vessels supplying the testis can be seen – at its posterior border (mediastinum).

Head of epididymis

Spermatic cord

Mediastinum testis
(posterior border)

Lobules
of testis

Septa

Fig. 276

Tunica albuginea

Tail of epididymis

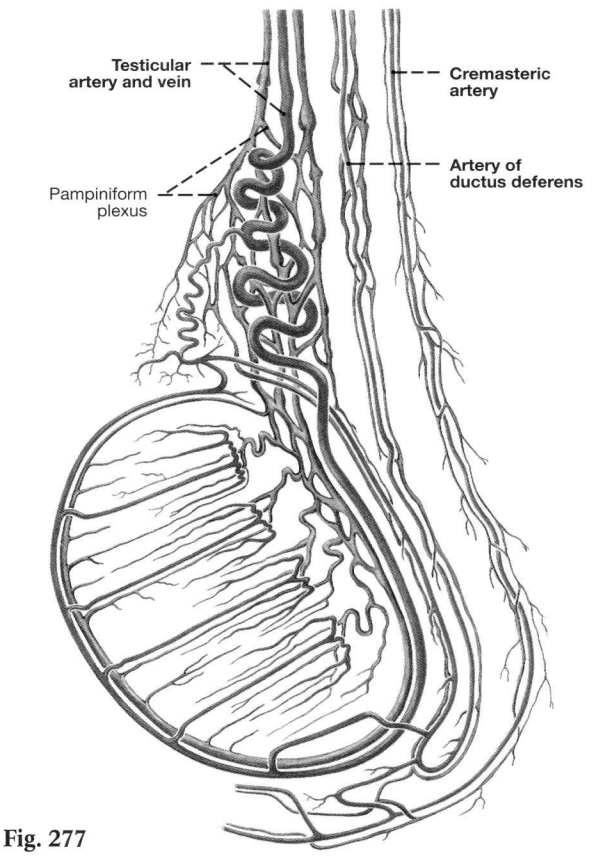

Testicular
artery and vein

Cremasteric
artery

Artery of
ductus deferens

Pampiniform
plexus

Fig. 277

Fig. 277: Schematic Representation of the Blood Supply of the Testis and Epididymis

1) the testis and epididymis are served by the **testicular artery** (from the aorta), the **artery of the ductus deferens** (usually from the superior vesical artery) and the **cremasteric artery** (from the inferior epigastric artery).

2) the **pampiniform plexus** of veins drains into the testicular vein, which on the left side flows into the left renal vein, and on the right side opens into the inferior vena cava.

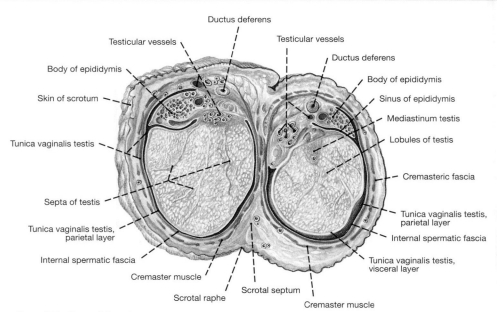

Fig. 278: Cross-section of Testis and Scrotum

NOTE: 1) the scrotum is divided by the median raphe and septum into two lateral compartments, each surrounding an ovoid-shaped testis. The two scrotal compartments normally do not communicate.

2) the **tunica vaginalis testis** consists of a **visceral layer** closely adherent to the testis and a **parietal layer**, which lines the inner surface of the internal spermatic fascia in the scrotum. A serous cavity or potential space between these two layers is a site where fluid might collect to form a **hydrocele.** These may be acquired or congenital.

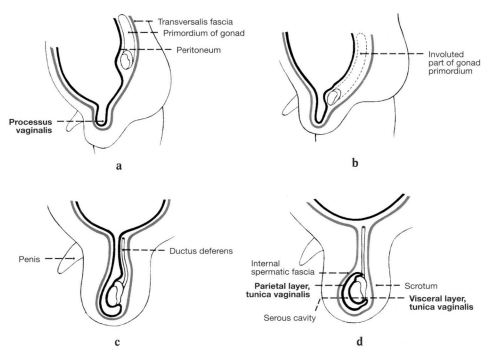

Fig. 279: Diagrammatic Representation of Four Stages in the Descent of the Testis

NOTE: 1) the testes commence development on the posterior wall of the fetus (a), during the 2nd trimester they attach to the posterior wall of the lower trunk at the boundary between the abdomen and pelvis in what is often called the "false pelvis" (b),

2) during the latter half of the 7th month, the testes begin their descent into the scrotum (b and c); this is normally completed by the 9th month (d),

3) attached to the peritoneum, each testis carries with it a peritoneal sac which surrounds the organ in the scrotum as the **parietal and visceral layers of the tunica vaginalis.** The peritoneum lining the inguinal canal then fuses, closing off its communication with the abdominal cavity.

4) when this fusion does not occur, the pathway may be used by a loop of intestine to enter the scrotum forming an **indirect or congenital hernia.**

PLATE 186   **Newborn Child: Anterior Abdominal Wall and Scrotum**

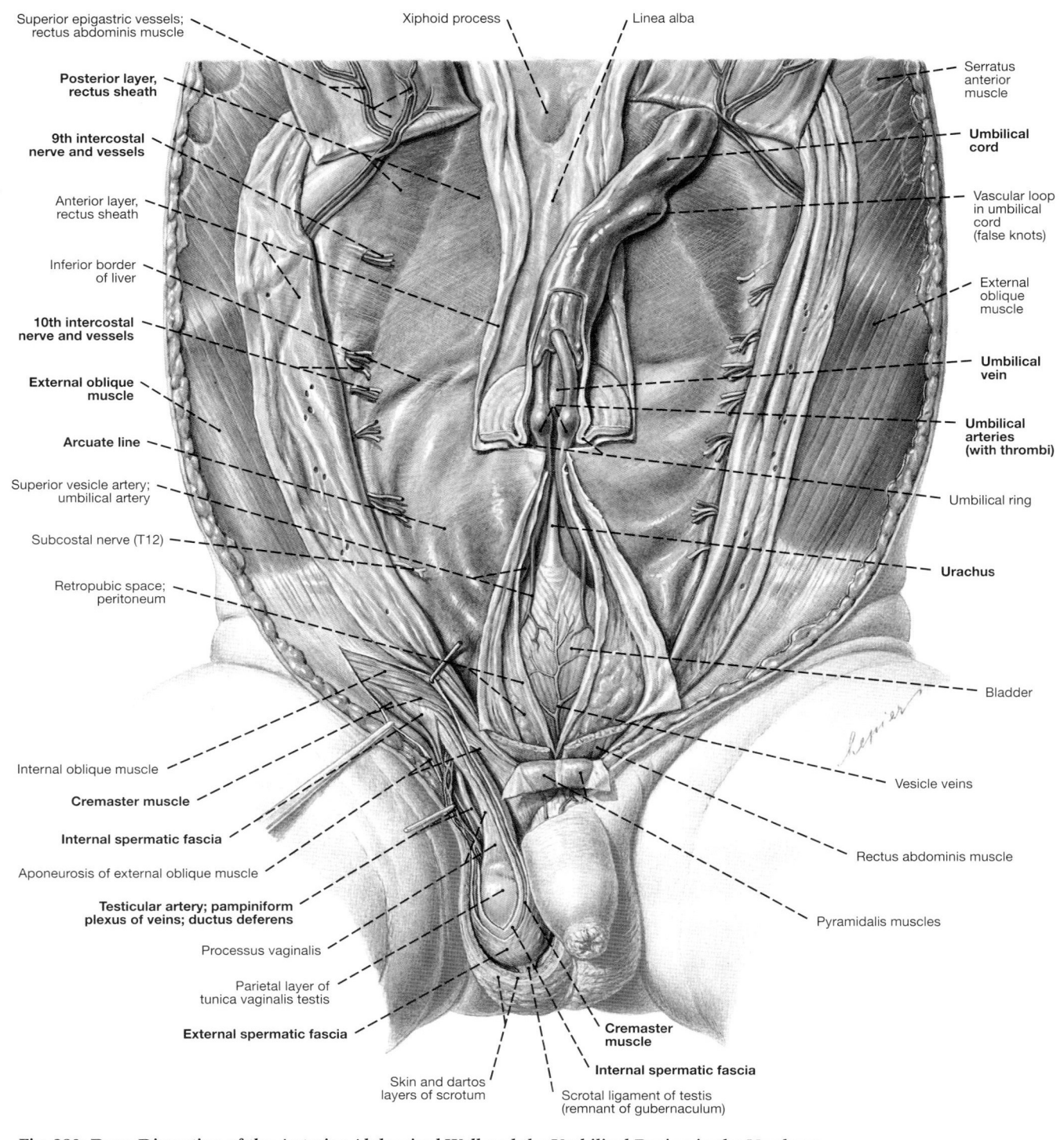

Superior epigastric vessels; rectus abdominis muscle

Posterior layer, rectus sheath

9th intercostal nerve and vessels

Anterior layer, rectus sheath

Inferior border of liver

10th intercostal nerve and vessels

External oblique muscle

Arcuate line

Superior vesicle artery; umbilical artery

Subcostal nerve (T12)

Retropubic space; peritoneum

Internal oblique muscle

Cremaster muscle

Internal spermatic fascia

Aponeurosis of external oblique muscle

Testicular artery; pampiniform plexus of veins; ductus deferens

Processus vaginalis

Parietal layer of tunica vaginalis testis

External spermatic fascia

Xiphoid process

Linea alba

Serratus anterior muscle

Umbilical cord

Vascular loop in umbilical cord (false knots)

External oblique muscle

Umbilical vein

Umbilical arteries (with thrombi)

Umbilical ring

Urachus

Bladder

Vesicle veins

Rectus abdominis muscle

Pyramidalis muscles

Cremaster muscle

Internal spermatic fascia

Skin and dartos layers of scrotum

Scrotal ligament of testis (remnant of gubernaculum)

Fig. 280: Deep Dissection of the Anterior Abdominal Wall and the Umbilical Region in the Newborn

NOTE: 1) the anterior layer of the rectus sheath is reflected laterally, and the two rectus abdominis muscles have been cut near the symphysis pubis and turned upward (almost out of view). This exposes the posterior layer of the rectus sheath and the **arcuate line.**

2) an incision has been made in the midline between the umbilicus and the pubic symphysis exposing the **bladder, urachus, the umbilical arteries** and the **umbilical vein.**

3) the anterior aspect of the right spermatic cord and scrotal sac have been opened to show the ductus deferens and the **tunica vaginalis testis** surrounding the testis.

4) the severed umbilical cord, usually 1 to 2 cm in diameter and about 50 cm or 20 inches long. It contains the two umbilical arteries and the umbilical vein surrounded by a mucoid form of connective tissue called Wharton's jelly.

5) at times, the umbilical vessels form harmless loops in the umbilical cord called "false knots." More rarely looping of the cord may be of functional significance and such "true knots" may alter the circulation to and from the fetus.

6) the bulges in the umbilical arteries. These are **in situ** blood clots that occlude the arteries, but which are probably postmortem phenomena in this dissection.

Fig. 280

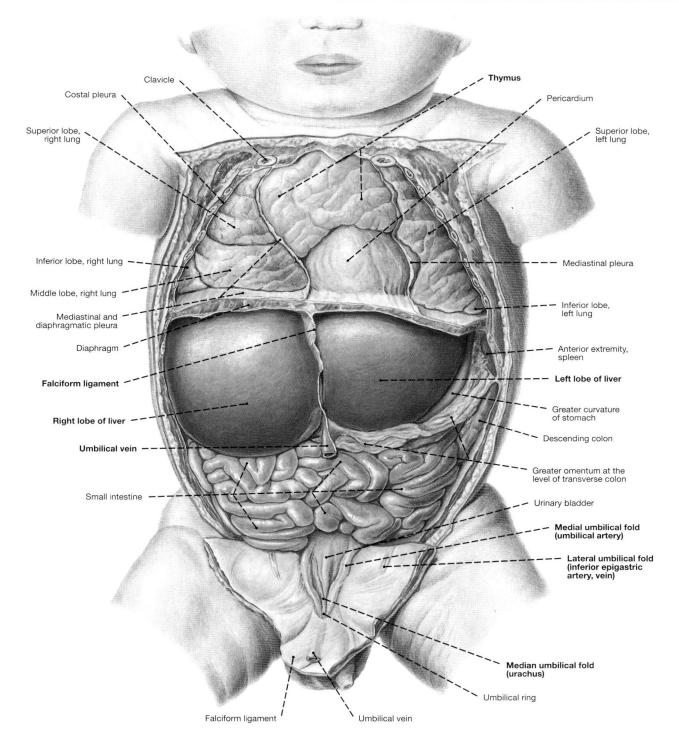

Clavicle

Costal pleura

Superior lobe,
right lung

Inferior lobe, right lung

Middle lobe, right lung

Mediastinal and
diaphragmatic pleura

Diaphragm

Falciform ligament

Right lobe of liver

Umbilical vein

Small intestine

Thymus

Pericardium

Superior lobe,
left lung

Mediastinal pleura

Inferior lobe,
left lung

Anterior extremity,
spleen

Left lobe of liver

Greater curvature
of stomach

Descending colon

Greater omentum at the
level of transverse colon

Urinary bladder

**Medial umbilical fold
(umbilical artery)**

**Lateral umbilical fold
(inferior epigastric
artery, vein)**

**Median umbilical fold
(urachus)**

Umbilical ring

Falciform ligament

Umbilical vein

Fig. 281: Abdominal and Thoracic Viscera Observed In Situ in the Newborn Child

NOTE: 1)   the anterior body wall has been removed in this newborn child, uncovering the viscera. Observe the umbilical ligaments on the inner surface of the lower wall.

2)   the average newborn child weighs about 3300 g (7 lb) and measures about 50 cm (20 in) from the top of the head to the sole of the foot. The umbilicus is located about 1.5 cm below the mid-point of this crown-heel length.

3)   the transverse diameter of the abdomen in the newborn is greatest above the umbilicus, due to the inordinate proportion of the abdomen occupied by the liver. The average weight of the liver in the neonate is about 120 g (4% of the body weight). In the adult the liver weighs 12 to 13 times that at birth (but only 2.5 to 3.5% of the body weight).

4)   the truncated shape of the thorax and the large thymus, weighing about 10 g at birth (0.42% of body weight at birth compared with 0.03 to 0.05% in the adult).

5)   the facts above taken from: Crelin ES. Functional Anatomy of the Newborn, New Haven, Yale Univ. Press, 1973, an excellent and short monograph (87 pages).

Fig. 281   III

PLATE 188   Projections of Viscera I: Anterior View of Male

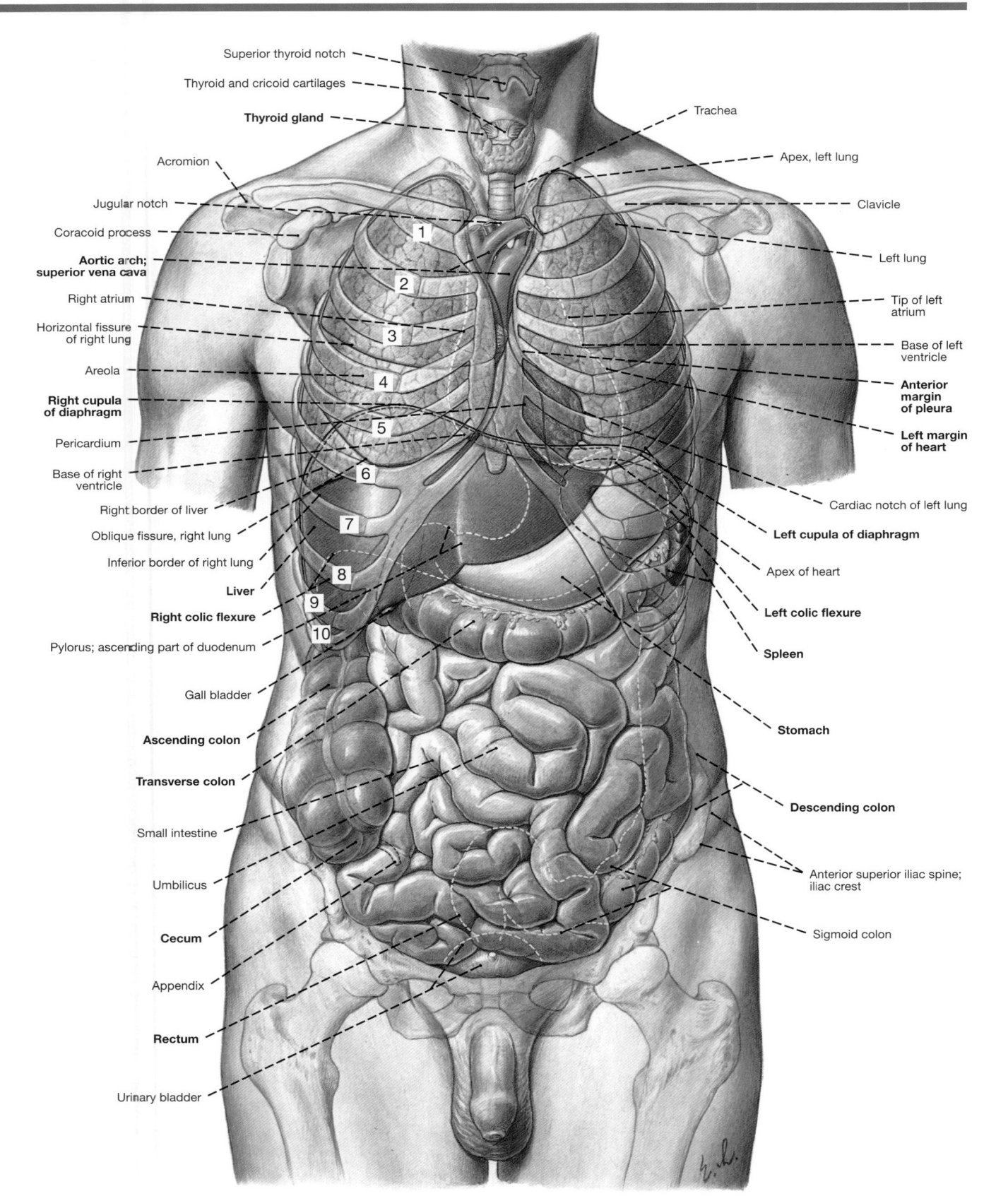

Superior thyroid notch
Thyroid and cricoid cartilages
Thyroid gland
Acromion
Jugular notch
Coracoid process
Aortic arch; superior vena cava
Right atrium
Horizontal fissure of right lung
Areola
Right cupula of diaphragm
Pericardium
Base of right ventricle
Right border of liver
Oblique fissure, right lung
Inferior border of right lung
Liver
Right colic flexure
Pylorus; ascending part of duodenum
Gall bladder
Ascending colon
Transverse colon
Small intestine
Umbilicus
Cecum
Appendix
Rectum
Urinary bladder

Trachea
Apex, left lung
Clavicle
Left lung
Tip of left atrium
Base of left ventricle
Anterior margin of pleura
Left margin of heart
Cardiac notch of left lung
Left cupula of diaphragm
Apex of heart
Left colic flexure
Spleen
Stomach
Descending colon
Anterior superior iliac spine; iliac crest
Sigmoid colon

Fig. 282: Frontal View of Thoracic and Abdominal Viscera
NOTE: the surface projections of the heart, stomach, gall bladder, transverse colon, descending and sigmoid colon, rectum, and urinary bladder are indicated by **white broken outlines.** The limits of the pleura are shown as **solid blue lines** and the spleen as a **purple broken line.** The gall bladder is shown as a **broken blue line.**

Fig. 282

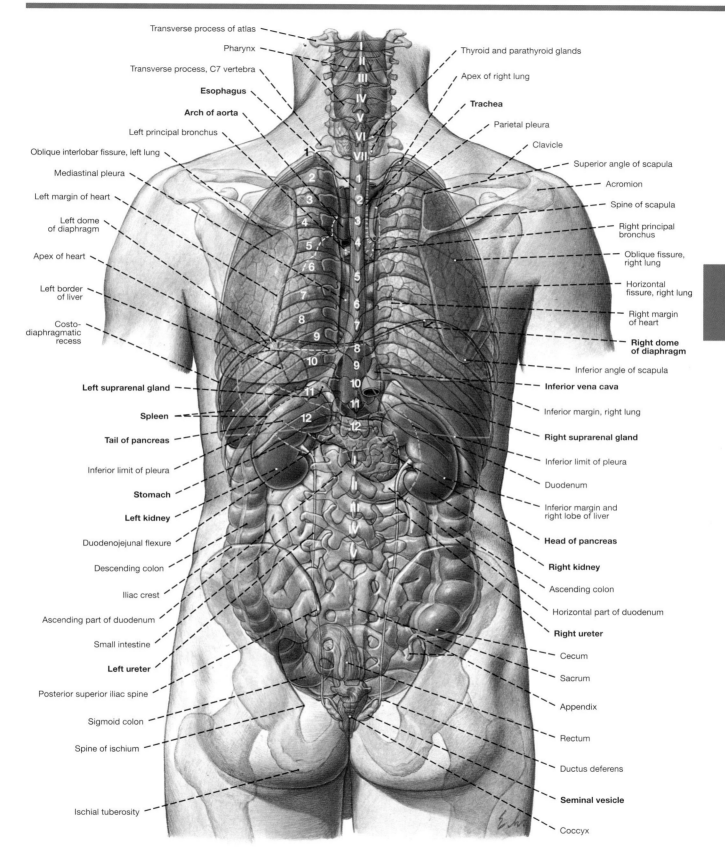

Transverse process of atlas
Pharynx
Transverse process, C7 vertebra
Esophagus
Arch of aorta
Left principal bronchus
Oblique interlobar fissure, left lung
Mediastinal pleura
Left margin of heart
Left dome of diaphragm
Apex of heart
Left border of liver
Costo-diaphragmatic recess
Left suprarenal gland
Spleen
Tail of pancreas
Inferior limit of pleura
Stomach
Left kidney
Duodenojejunal flexure
Descending colon
Iliac crest
Ascending part of duodenum
Small intestine
Left ureter
Posterior superior iliac spine
Sigmoid colon
Spine of ischium
Ischial tuberosity

Thyroid and parathyroid glands
Apex of right lung
Trachea
Parietal pleura
Clavicle
Superior angle of scapula
Acromion
Spine of scapula
Right principal bronchus
Oblique fissure, right lung
Horizontal fissure, right lung
Right margin of heart
Right dome of diaphragm
Inferior angle of scapula
Inferior vena cava
Inferior margin, right lung
Right suprarenal gland
Inferior limit of pleura
Duodenum
Inferior margin and right lobe of liver
Head of pancreas
Right kidney
Ascending colon
Horizontal part of duodenum
Right ureter
Cecum
Sacrum
Appendix
Rectum
Ductus deferens
Seminal vesicle
Coccyx

Fig. 283: Posterior View of Thoracic and Abdominal Viscera
NOTE: surface projections of the heart, stomach, and duodenum are shown as **white broken lines,** the body and tail of the pancreas as **yellow broken lines,** the superior pole of the spleen as a **purple broken line,** and the limits of the pleura as **solid blue lines.**

Fig. 283   **III**

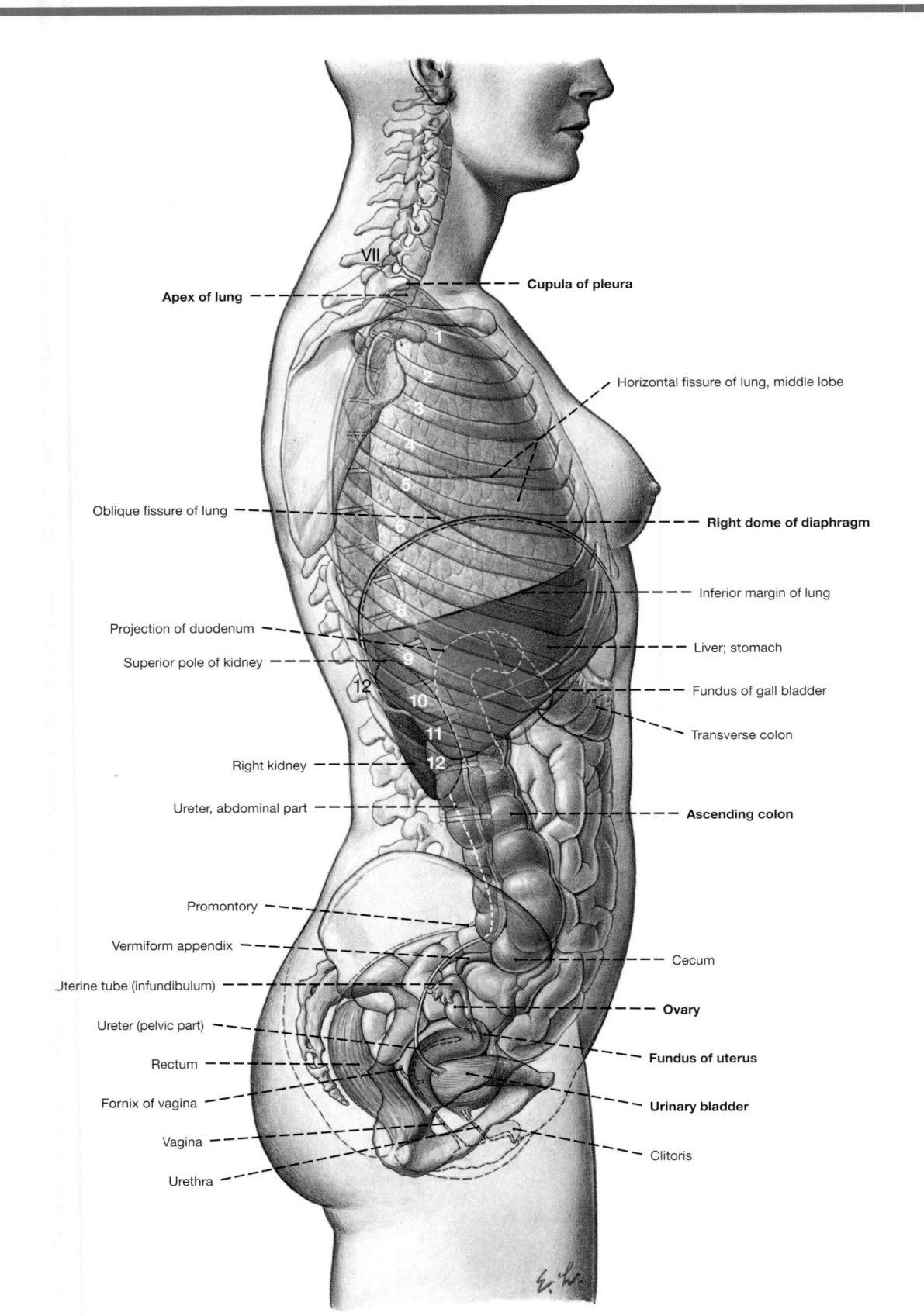

VII

Apex of lung ---- — — — — — — — — — — **Cupula of pleura**

— — Horizontal fissure of lung, middle lobe

Oblique fissure of lung — — — — — — — — — — **Right dome of diaphragm**

— — Inferior margin of lung

Projection of duodenum — — — —

Superior pole of kidney — — — — — — — — — — Liver; stomach

12 — — Fundus of gall bladder

— — Transverse colon

Right kidney — — — 12

Ureter, abdominal part — — — — — — — — — **Ascending colon**

Promontory — — — —

Vermiform appendix — — — —

— — Cecum

Uterine tube (infundibulum) — — — —

— — **Ovary**

Ureter (pelvic part) — — — —

Rectum — — — — — — **Fundus of uterus**

Fornix of vagina — — — — — — **Urinary bladder**

Vagina — — — — — — Clitoris

Urethra — — — —

Fig. 284: Right Lateral View of the Thoracic, Abdominal and Pelvic Viscera in the Female
NOTE: the projection of the duodenum and the course of the right ureter are indicated as **broken white lines.** The pleura is outlined
by a **solid blue line** while the gall bladder is shown by a **broken green line.** Within the pelvis and perineum the cavities of the vagina
and uterus are shown in **broken red lines.** The 12 ribs are numbered.

Fig. 284

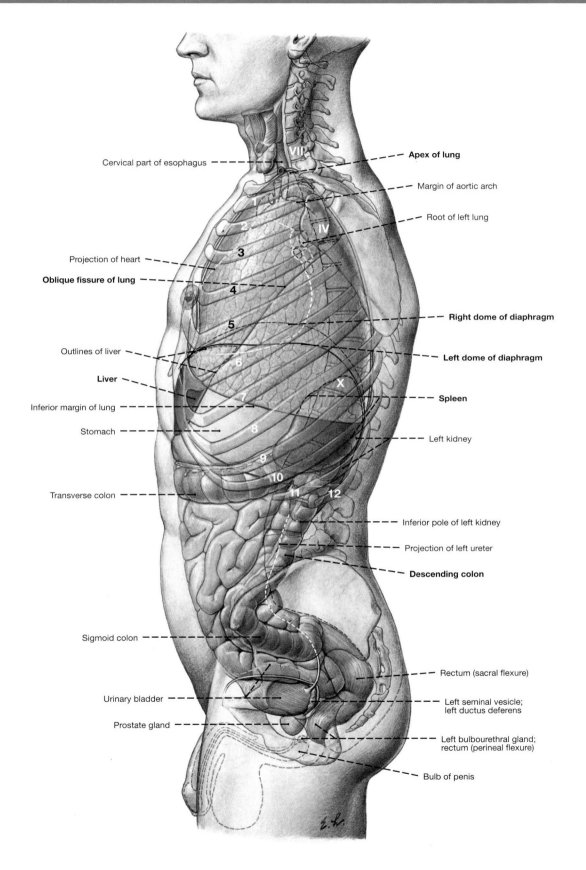

Cervical part of esophagus

Apex of lung

Margin of aortic arch

Root of left lung

Projection of heart

Oblique fissure of lung

Right dome of diaphragm

Outlines of liver

Left dome of diaphragm

Liver

Inferior margin of lung

Spleen

Stomach

Left kidney

Transverse colon

Inferior pole of left kidney

Projection of left ureter

Descending colon

Sigmoid colon

Rectum (sacral flexure)

Urinary bladder

Left seminal vesicle;
left ductus deferens

Prostate gland

Left bulbourethral gland;
rectum (perineal flexure)

Bulb of penis

Fig. 285: Left Lateral View of the Thoracic, Abdominal and Pelvic Viscera in the Male
NOTE: the projection of the heart and the course of the left ureter are shown in **broken white lines.** The pleura is shown in **solid blue lines,** whereas the urethra and corpora cavernosum and spongiosum are shown in **broken blue lines.** The aortic arch, the left kidney and the bulbourethral gland are all shown in **broken red lines.**

Fig. 285   **III**

PLATE 192   Abdominal Cavity I: Greater Omentum

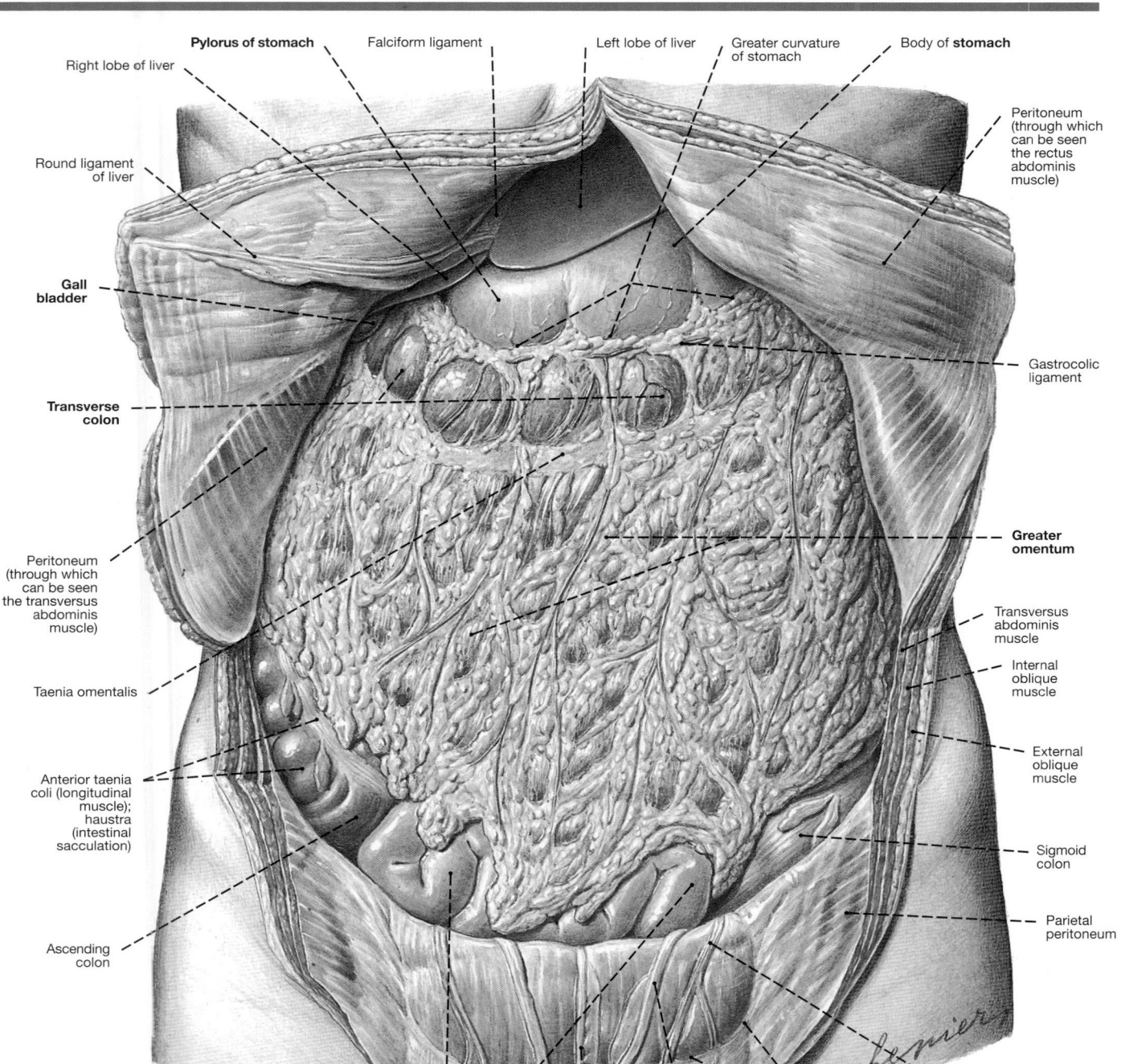

Right lobe of liver

Round ligament of liver

Gall bladder

Transverse colon

Peritoneum (through which can be seen the transversus abdominis muscle)

Taenia omentalis

Anterior taenia coli (longitudinal muscle); haustra (intestinal sacculation)

Ascending colon

Pylorus of stomach

Falciform ligament

Left lobe of liver

Greater curvature of stomach

Body of **stomach**

Peritoneum (through which can be seen the rectus abdominis muscle)

Gastrocolic ligament

Greater omentum

Transversus abdominis muscle

Internal oblique muscle

External oblique muscle

Sigmoid colon

Parietal peritoneum

Lateral umbilical fold

Arcuate line

Small intestine (ileum)

Medial umbilical fold (umbilical artery)

Median umbilical fold (urachus)

Fig. 286: Abdominal Cavity (1), Viscera Left Intact

NOTE: 1) the **greater omentum**. It attaches along the greater curvature of the stomach, covers the intestines like an apron and extends inferiorly almost to the pelvis.

2) the falciform ligament, a remnant of the ventral mesogastrium, extends between the liver and the anterior body wall and separates the left and right lobes of the liver. The **round ligament** is the remnant of the obliterated umbilical vein.

3) on the inner surface of the anterior abdominal wall identify the following folds:

a) **median umbilical fold:** remnant of the urachus, which extended between the bladder and the umbilicus in the fetus.

b) **medial umbilical folds:** the obliterated umbilical arteries, which were the continuation of the superior vesical arteries to the umbilicus in the fetus.

c) **lateral umbilical folds:** a fold of peritoneum over the inferior epigastric vessels.

Fig. 286

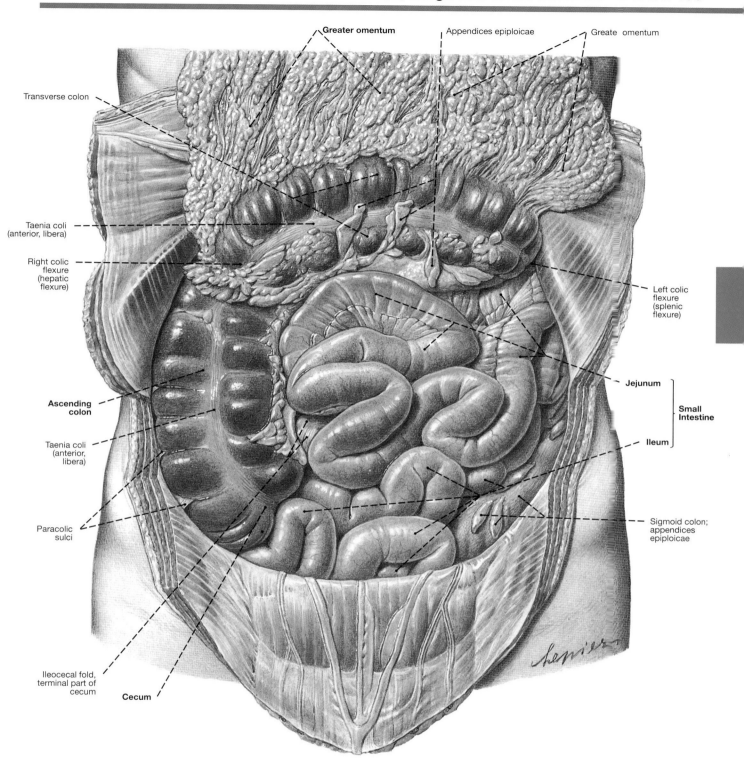

Greater omentum
Appendices epiploicae
Greate omentum
Transverse colon
Taenia coli (anterior, libera)
Right colic flexure (hepatic flexure)
Left colic flexure (splenic flexure)
Jejunum
Small Intestine
Ascending colon
Ileum
Taenia coli (anterior, libera)
Sigmoid colon; appendices epiploicae
Paracolic sulci
Ileocecal fold, terminal part of cecum
Cecum

Fig. 287: Abdominal Cavity (2), Ascending Colon, Transverse Colon and Its Mesocolon

NOTE: 1) with the greater omentum reflected upward, the **transverse colon** is crossing the abdominal cavity from right to left in continuity with the ascending colon on the right and the descending colon on the left.

2) longitudinal muscles called **taeniae,** along the outer surface of the colon. These muscles are shorter than the other coats of the large intestine causing sacculations, which are called **haustrae.**

3) smooth irregular fatty masses called **appendices epiploicae** are suspended from the large intestine. These assist in the identification of the large gut.

4) below the mesocolon (inframesocolic) can be seen the small intestine, which consists of 3 portions: the **duodenum, jejunum,** and **ileum.** The outer wall of the small intestine is smooth and glistening and is not sacculated.

Fig. 287   III

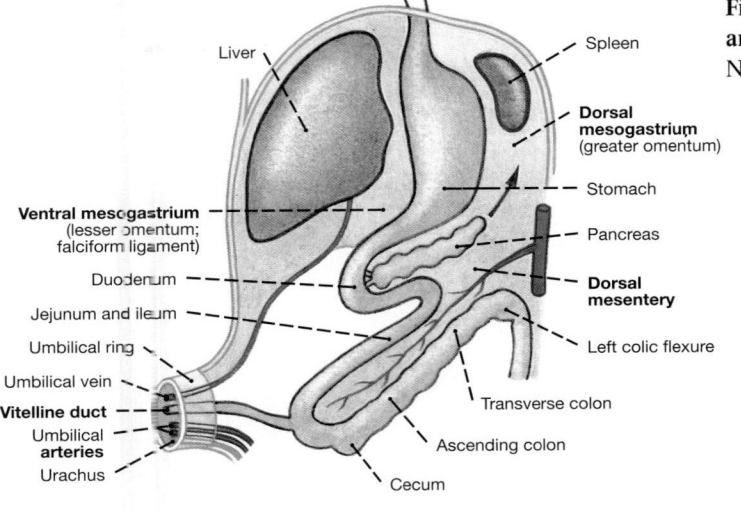

Fig. 288: Developing Gastrointestinal Organs and Their Mesenteries

NOTE: 1) as the primitive gastrointestinal tube develops within the abdominal celom, it is suspended to the body wall by primitive peritoneal reflections, both ventrally and dorsally. The early peritoneal attachments to the expanding stomach are called the ventral mesogastrium and dorsal mesogastrium, whereas the dorsal mesentery develops on the posterior aspect of the primitive small and large intestine.

2) the embryonic liver develops into the ventral mesogastrium, thereby dividing this ventral peritoneal attachment into:

   a) a portion between the anterior body wall and the liver, which eventually becomes the falciform ligament, and

   b) a portion between the liver and the stomach, which becomes the lesser omentum.

3) on the dorsal aspect:

   a) the pancreas develops in relation to the primitive duodenum, both of which lose their mesenteries during gut rotation to become retroperitoneal;

   b) the dorsal mesogastrium, attaching along the greater curvature of the stomach and rotating with the stomach, becomes the greater omentum. This eventually encases the transverse colon;

   c) the dorsal mesentery remains attached to the small intestine, while the ascending and descending colon become displaced to the right and left side, respectively, becoming adherent to the posterior body wall;

   d) the sigmoid colon usually retains its mesentery while that of the rectum becomes obliterated.

4) near the cecal end of the small intestine, the developing G.I. canal communicates with the vitelline duct. Before birth, this duct usually becomes resorbed; when it persists (3% of cases), it results in a diverticulum of the ileum called Meckel's diverticulum.

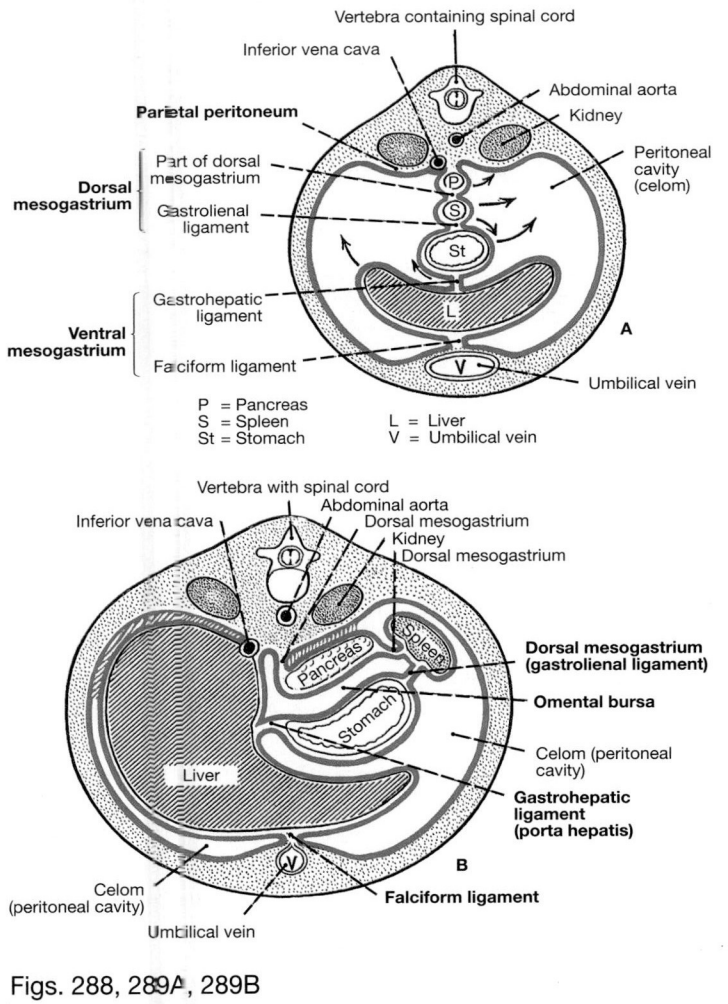

P = Pancreas
S = Spleen
St = Stomach
L = Liver
V = Umbilical vein

Fig. 289A: Cross-sectional Diagram of Development of Mesogastria: Early Stage (about 6 weeks)

NOTE: 1) the primitive peritoneal reflections are indicated in red. The arrows show the direction of growth and movement by the various organs shown in Fig. 289B.

2) at this early stage, the peritoneum completely surrounds the organs in the upper abdominal region (visceral peritoneum) and attaches peripherally to the body wall (parietal peritoneum). Attaching along the posterior border of the stomach, the dorsal mesogastrium then surrounds the spleen and pancreas. Anterior to the stomach, the liver becomes interposed between the stomach and the anterior body wall. This forms the gastrohepatic ligament (also called lesser omentum) between the lesser curvature of the stomach and the liver, and the falciform ligament between the liver and the anterior body wall.

Fig. 289B: Cross-sectional Diagram of Development of Mesogastria: Late Fetal Stage

NOTE: 1) with the rotation of the organs (in the direction of the arrows in Fig. 289A), the liver grows into the celomic cavity toward the right and contacts the inferior vena cava, while the stomach rotates such that its dorsal mesogastrium (greater curvature) is shifted to the left.

2) the reflection of dorsal mesogastrium between the stomach and spleen becomes established as the gastrolienal ligament, while one layer of mesogastrium surrounding the pancreas and duodenum fuses to the posterior body wall. This fixates these two organs with a layer of peritoneum on their anterior surface, causing them to become retroperitoneal. The omental bursa also develops posterior to the stomach and anterior to the pancreas.

Figs. 288, 289A, 289B

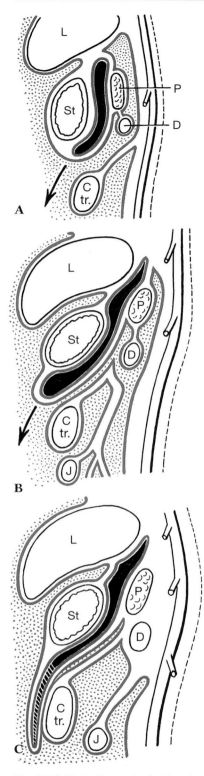

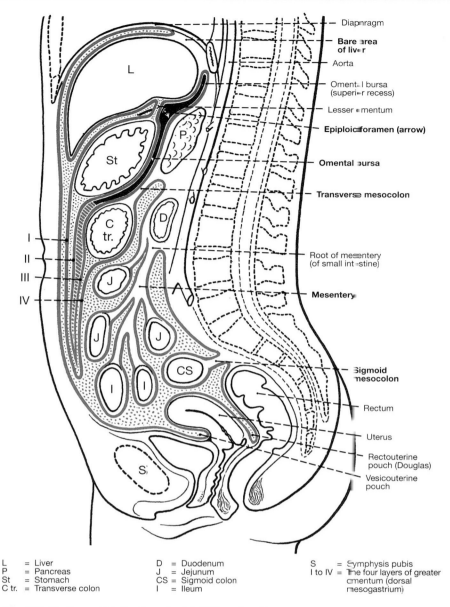

L = Liver	D = Duodenum
P = Pancreas	J = Jejunum
St = Stomach	CS = Sigmoid colon
C tr. = Transverse colon	I = Ileum

S = Symphysis pubis
I to IV = The four layers of greater omentum (dorsal mesogastrium)

Fig. 291: Peritoneal Reflections in Adult Female ▲

NOTE: 1) the greater peritoneal sac (red stippled) lies between the layers of visceral and parietal peritoneum. The greater peritoneal sac communicates with the lesser peritoneal sac (omental bursa; black) through the epiploic foramen (of Winslow).

2) dorsally, the roots of three distinct peritoneal mesenteries can be observed: a) the transverse mesocolon, b) the mesentery surrounding the small intestine, and c) the sigmoid mesocolon.

3) behind the stomach and transverse colon, observe the retroperitoneal pancreas and duodenum. A portion of the liver is not surrounded by peritoneum (bare area of the liver) and lies adjacent to the diaphragm.

Fig. 290A, B, C: Stages in the Development of the Omental Bursa (Sagittal Diagrams)

NOTE: 1) at 4 weeks, the dorsal border of the stomach grows faster than the ventral border assisting in rotation of the stomach on its long axis. The greater curvature and its dorsal mesogastrium becomes directed to the left, whereas the lesser curvature and the ventral mesogastrium is directed to the right.

2) by 8 weeks (Fig. 290A) the omental bursa (black) forms behind the stomach between the two leaves of dorsal mesogastrium. The pancreas and duodenum are still surrounded by dorsal mesentery. As gut rotation continues the dorsal mesogastrium extends inferiorly (Fig. 290B, arrow) to form the greater omentum, which becomes a double reflection (4 leaves) of the dorsal mesogastrium "trapping" the cavity of the omental bursa between the 2nd and 3rd leaves.

3) continued development (Fig. 290C) results in a further descent of the greater omentum over the abdominal viscera and a fusion (cross-hatched) of the 2nd and 3rd leaves inferiorly.

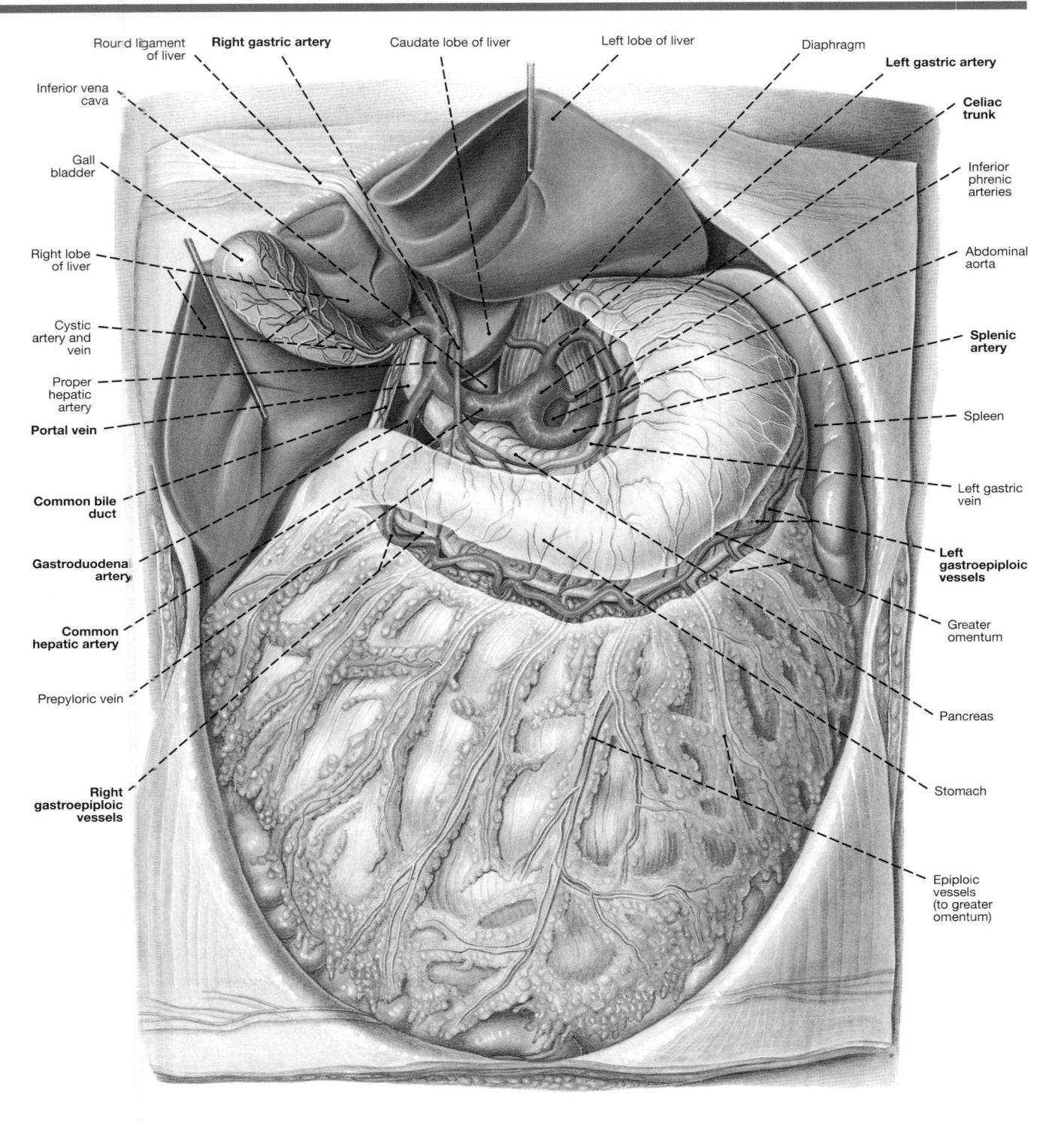

Round ligament of liver

Right gastric artery

Caudate lobe of liver

Left lobe of liver

Diaphragm

Left gastric artery

Celiac trunk

Inferior vena cava

Gall bladder

Right lobe of liver

Cystic artery and vein

Proper hepatic artery

Portal vein

Common bile duct

Gastroduodenal artery

Common hepatic artery

Prepyloric vein

Right gastroepiploic vessels

Inferior phrenic arteries

Abdominal aorta

Splenic artery

Spleen

Left gastric vein

Left gastroepiploic vessels

Greater omentum

Pancreas

Stomach

Epiploic vessels (to greater omentum)

Fig. 292: Abdominal Cavity (3): Celiac Trunk and Its Branches

NOTE: 1)   the lobes of the liver have been elevated and the lesser omentum has been removed between the lesser curvature of the stomach and the liver to reveal the **celiac trunk** (located anterior to the T12 vertebra) and its branches. These are:

    a) the **left gastric artery**, which courses along the lesser curvature of the stomach and anastomoses with the right gastric artery, a branch of the hepatic artery.

    b) the **splenic artery**, which courses to the left toward the hilum of the spleen, and

    c) the **hepatic artery**, which courses to the right and gives off the gastroduodenal artery before dividing to enter the lobes of the liver.

    2) the **gastroduodenal artery** gives rise to the **right gastroepiploic artery**, which follows along the greater curvature of the stomach to anastomose with the **left gastroepiploic branch** of the splenic artery.

Fig. 292

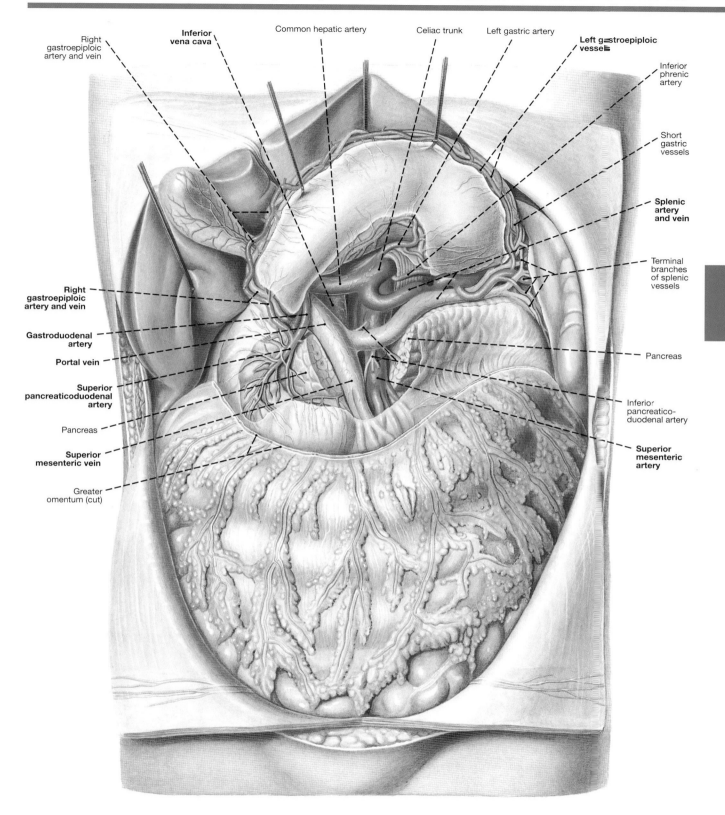

Right gastroepiploic artery and vein

Inferior vena cava

Common hepatic artery

Celiac trunk

Left gastric artery

Left gastroepiploic vessels

Inferior phrenic artery

Short gastric vessels

Splenic artery and vein

Terminal branches of splenic vessels

Right gastroepiploic artery and vein

Gastroduodenal artery

Portal vein

Superior pancreaticoduodenal artery

Pancreas

Superior mesenteric vein

Greater omentum (cut)

Pancreas

Inferior pancreatico-duodenal artery

Superior mesenteric artery

Fig. 293: Abdominal Cavity (4): Splenic Vessels and Formation of the Portal Vein

NOTE: 1) the greater omentum has been cut along the greater curvature of the stomach. The stomach is lifted to xpose its posterior surface and the underlying pancreas, duodenum, and blood vessels. A part of the pancreas has been removed o reveal the **portal vein** formed by the junction of the **splenic and superior mesenteric veins.**

    2) the tortuous **splenic artery** in its course to the splenic hilum, and the **gastroduodenal artery,** behind th pyloric end of the stomach dividing into **right gastroepiploic** and **superior pancreaticoduodenal arteries.**

Fig 293   III

PLATE 193   Stomach: Arteries and Veins

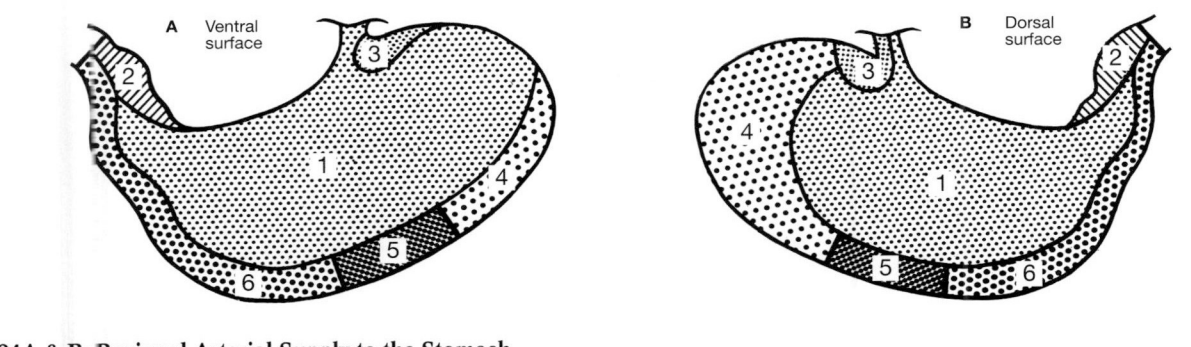

Fig. 294A & B: Regional Arterial Supply to the Stomach

1. Left gastric artery
2. Right gastric artery
3. Left inferior phrenic artery

4. Short gastric artery
5. Left gastroepiploic artery
6. Right gastroepiploic artery

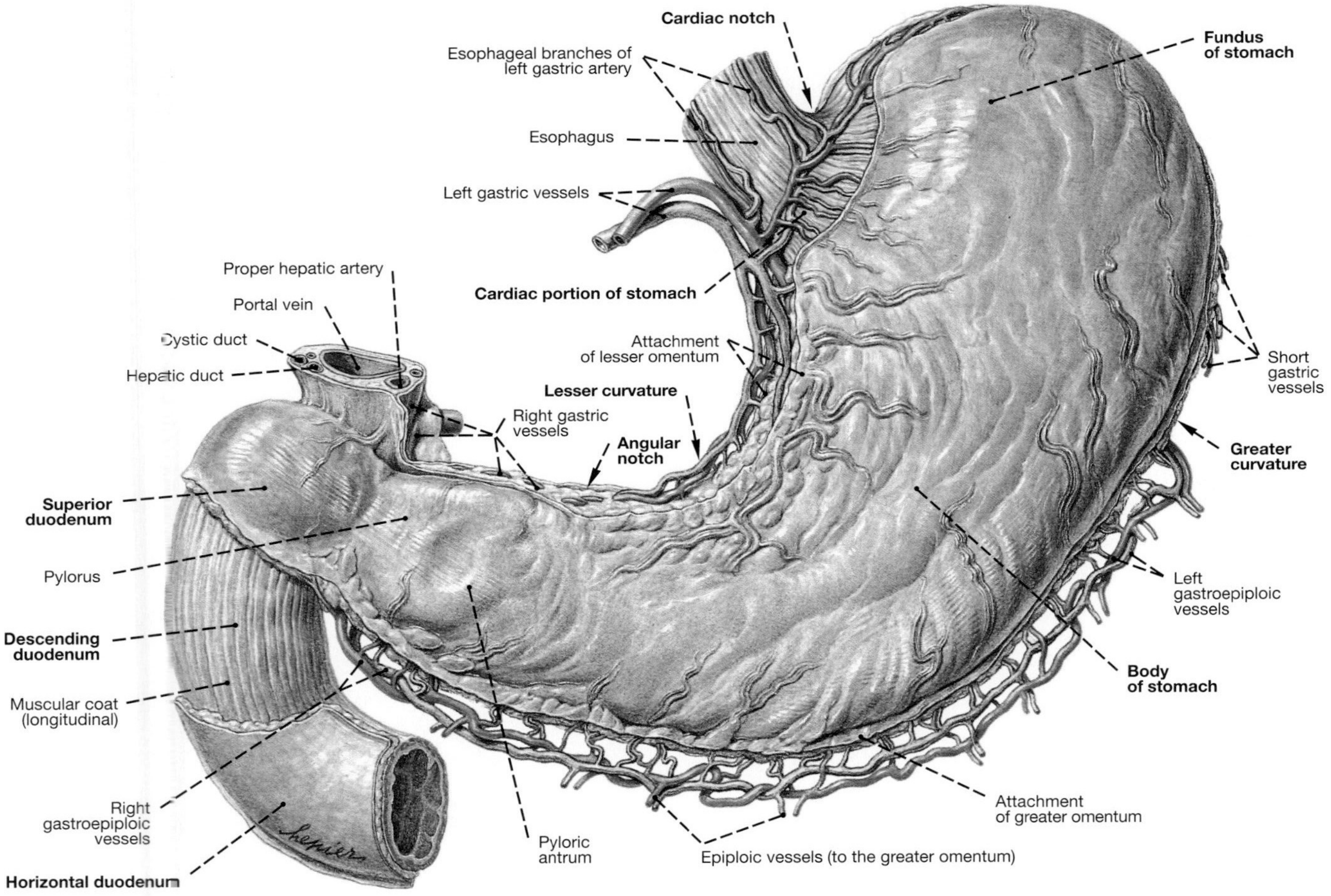

Fig. 295: Anterior View of Stomach

NOTE: 1) the stomach is a dilated muscular sac situated in the gastrointestinal tract between the esophagus (cardiac end) and duodenum (pyloric end). It consists of an upper portion called the **fundus,** a middle portion, the **body,** and a tapering lower part, the **pyloric region.**

2) although the shape of the stomach varies, it presents two curvatures as borders. The **greater curvature** is directed toward the left and to it is attached the **greater omentum.** This border forms an acute angle with the esophagus called the **cardiac notch.**

3) the **lesser curvature** constitutes the right border of the stomach and along this edge the **lesser omentum** is attached.

4) the blood vessels supplying the stomach include a) the **left and right gastric arteries** along the lesser curvature, b) the **left and right gastroepiploic arteries** along the greater curvature, and c) the **short gastric branches** of the **splenic artery.** Observe that the **esophageal branches** of the **left gastric artery** supply the cardiac end of the stomach.

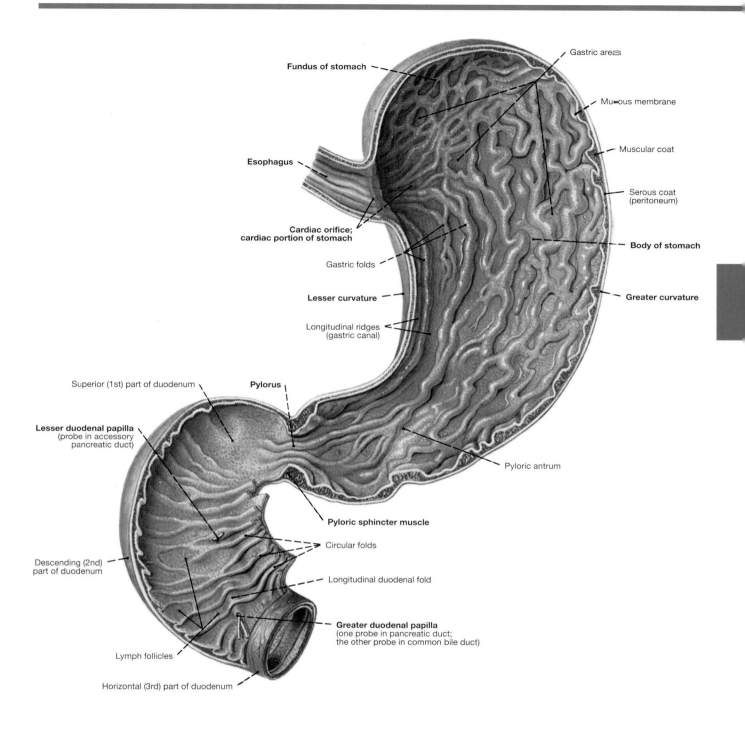

Fundus of stomach

Gastric areas

Esophagus

Mucous membrane

Muscular coat

Serous coat
(peritoneum)

Cardiac orifice;
cardiac portion of stomach

Body of stomach

Gastric folds

Lesser curvature

Greater curvature

Longitudinal ridges
(gastric canal)

Superior (1st) part of duodenum

Pylorus

Lesser duodenal papilla
(probe in accessory
pancreatic duct)

Pyloric antrum

Pyloric sphincter muscle

Circular folds

Descending (2nd)
part of duodenum

Longitudinal duodenal fold

Greater duodenal papilla
(one probe in pancreatic duct;
the other probe in common bile duct)

Lymph follicles

Horizontal (3rd) part of duodenum

Fig. 296: Interior of the Stomach and Upper Duodenum

NOTE: 1)   the mucosal lining of the stomach shows a series of longitudinally oriented gastric folds or empty rugae, which tend to disappear when the stomach is full and distended. These folds are more regular along the lesser curvature and form the grooved gastric canal. The concept that food travels along this canal (magenstrasse) is not correct.

2)   the surface of the first part of the duodenum is smooth, but the circular ridges characteristic of the small intestine commence in the 2nd or descending portion of the duodenum.

3)   a circular muscle, the **pyloric sphincter,** guards the pyloric junction of the stomach with the duodenum. It diminishes the lumen of the gastrointestinal tract at this point. The pylorus is to the right of midline at the level of the 1st lumbar vertebra.

4)   the openings in the wall of the duodenum. The **greater duodenal papilla** serves as the site of the openings of both the common bile duct and the main pancreatic duct. The accessory pancreatic duct opens 2 cm more proximally through the lesser duodenal papilla.

Fig 296   III

PLATE 200   Celiac Trunk and Its Branches

Fig. 297: Celiac Trunk Arteriogram

NOTE: 1)   this figure is a negative print from an x-ray of the upper abdomen after injection of a contrast medium through a catheter (21, arrow) in the abdominal aorta directed upward to the point where the **celiac trunk** (5) branches from the aorta.

2)   the three primary vessels arising from the celiac trunk (5) are the **left gastric artery** (2), the **splenic artery** (4), directed toward the spleen (1), and the **common hepatic artery** (5), which courses directly to the right.

3)   the **left gastroepiploic artery** arises from one of the lower hilar branches of the splenic artery. As it courses along the greater curvature to anastomose with the **right gastroepiploic**, the **left gastroepiploic** gives rise to **epiploic arteries** (7, arrows) which descend to supply the greater omentum. The right gastroepiploic (9) arises from the **gastroduodenal artery** (8) which courses downward from the **common hepatic artery** (5).

4)   beyond the origin of the gastroduodenal artery (8) the **common hepatic artery** (5) is called the **proper hepatic artery** (10).

5)   the proper hepatic artery (10) divides into the **right hepatic artery** (11), from which branches the **cystic artery** (12) to the gall bladder, t:1e **middle hepatic artery** (13), and the **left hepatic artery** (14, arrow). The hepatic vessels supply the liver.

6)   from the right hepatic artery (14) in this individual branches the **right gastric artery** (15, arrow). Just as frequently the right gastr:c a:tery arises from the common hepatic (5). The right gastric artery courses along the lesser curvature of the stomach to anastomose with the **left gastric** (2).

7)   the right renal pelvis (17) and the right ureter (18, arrow) can be seen inferiorly. Because of the liver, these structures on the right side a:e significantly lower than the left renal pelvis (19) and the origin of the left ureter (20, arrow).

(From Wicke L.: Atlas of Radiologic Anatomy, 4th Ed. Baltimore, Urban & Schwarzenberg, 1985).

Fig. 297

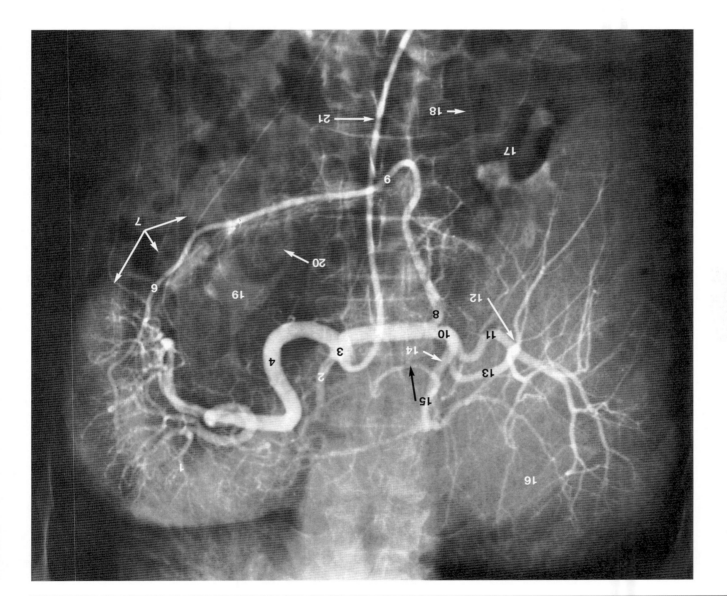

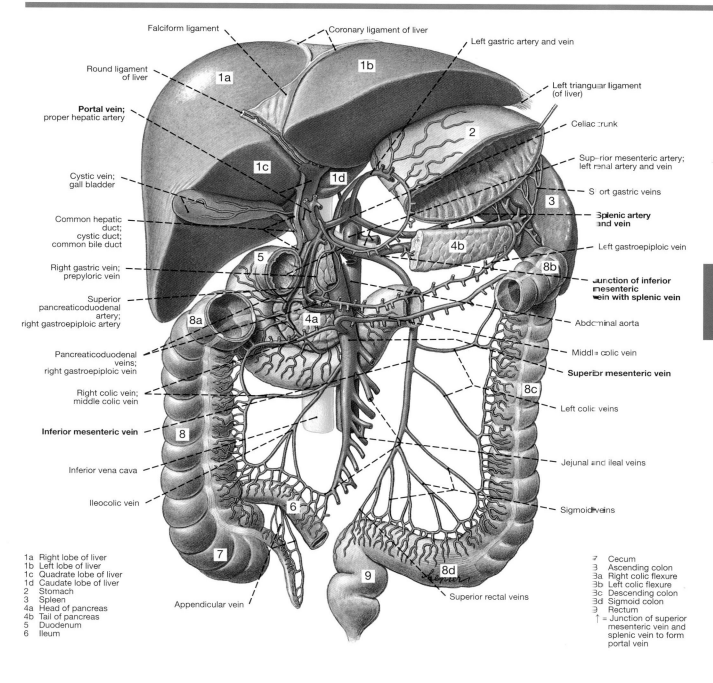

Falciform ligament

Coronary ligament of liver

Left gastric artery and vein

Round ligament of liver

1a

1b

2

Left triangular ligament (of liver)

Celiac trunk

Portal vein; proper hepatic artery

1c

1d

Superior mesenteric artery; left renal artery and vein

Cystic vein; gall bladder

Short gastric veins

3

Splenic artery and vein

Common hepatic duct; cystic duct; common bile duct

4b

Left gastroepiploic vein

Right gastric vein; prepyloric vein

5

8b

Junction of inferior mesenteric vein with splenic vein

Superior pancreaticoduodenal artery; right gastroepiploic artery

8a

4a

Abdominal aorta

Middle colic vein

Pancreaticoduodenal veins; right gastroepiploic vein

Superior mesenteric vein

Right colic vein; middle colic vein

8c

Left colic veins

Inferior mesenteric vein

8

Jejunal and ileal veins

Inferior vena cava

Ileocolic vein

6

Sigmoid veins

7

9

8d

Appendicular vein

Superior rectal veins

1a Right lobe of liver
1b Left lobe of liver
1c Quadrate lobe of liver
1d Caudate lobe of liver
2   Stomach
3   Spleen
4a Head of pancreas
4b Tail of pancreas
5   Duodenum
6   Ileum

7   Cecum
8   Ascending colon
8a Right colic flexure
8b Left colic flexure
8c Descending colon
8d Sigmoid colon
9   Rectum
↑ = Junction of superior mesenteric vein and splenic vein to form portal vein

Fig. 298: Abdominal Portal System of Veins

NOTE: 1)   the abdominal portal system of veins drains venous blood from the gastrointestinal tract, the gall bladder, pancreas, and spleen through the liver via the large **portal vein.** This is done to expose venous blood to various functions of the liver before it is returned to the general systemic circulation by way of the **hepatic veins** into the **inferior vena cava.**

2)   the portal vein is formed by the union of the **superior mesenteric** and **splenic veins.** The **inferior mesenteric vein** drains into the splenic vein. At the esophageal end of the stomach (esophageal veins) and at the distal end of the rectum (inferior rectal veins), the portal system of veins anastomoses with the systemic veins. Disease states that cause a reduction of blood flow through the liver result in use of these anastomotic channels in the return of blood to the heart from the portal system.

3)   the functions of the liver are numerous and vital to life. It secretes bile, which is stored in the gall bladder and released when food appears in the duodenum. Bile aids in the digestion of fats. The liver converts glucose to glycogen and then reconverts it to glucose when needed. The liver is involved in the synthesis of vitamin A, heparin, prothrombin, and fibrinogen. It also detoxifies substances in the blood and is involved in the breakdown of hemoglobin and the storing of both iron and copper.

Fig 298   III

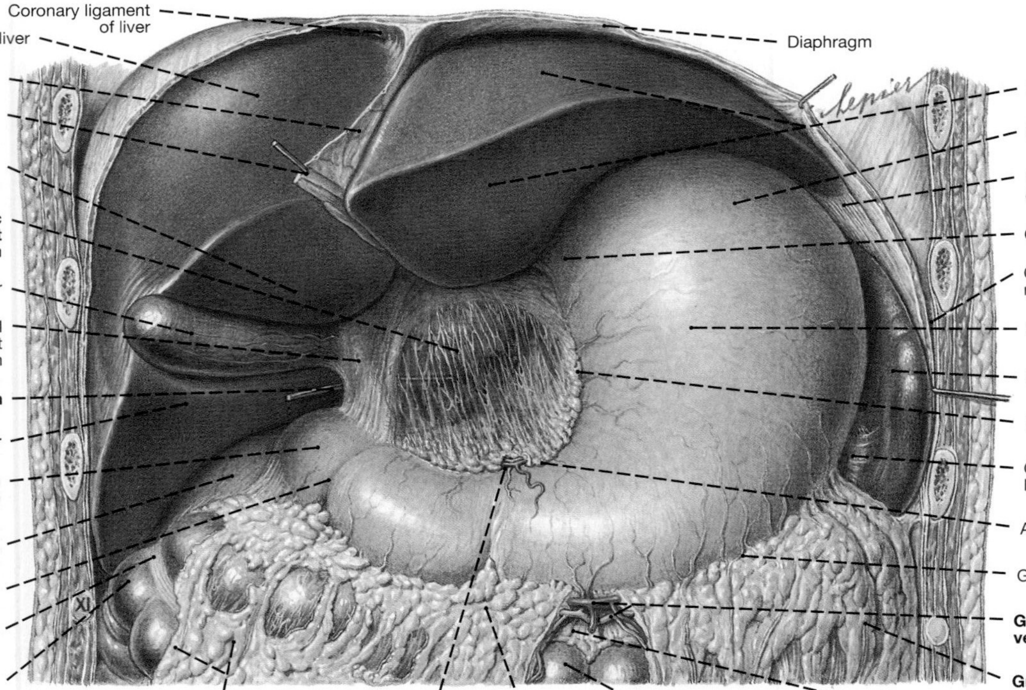

PLATE 202   Stomach, In Situ; Spleen (Visceral Surface)

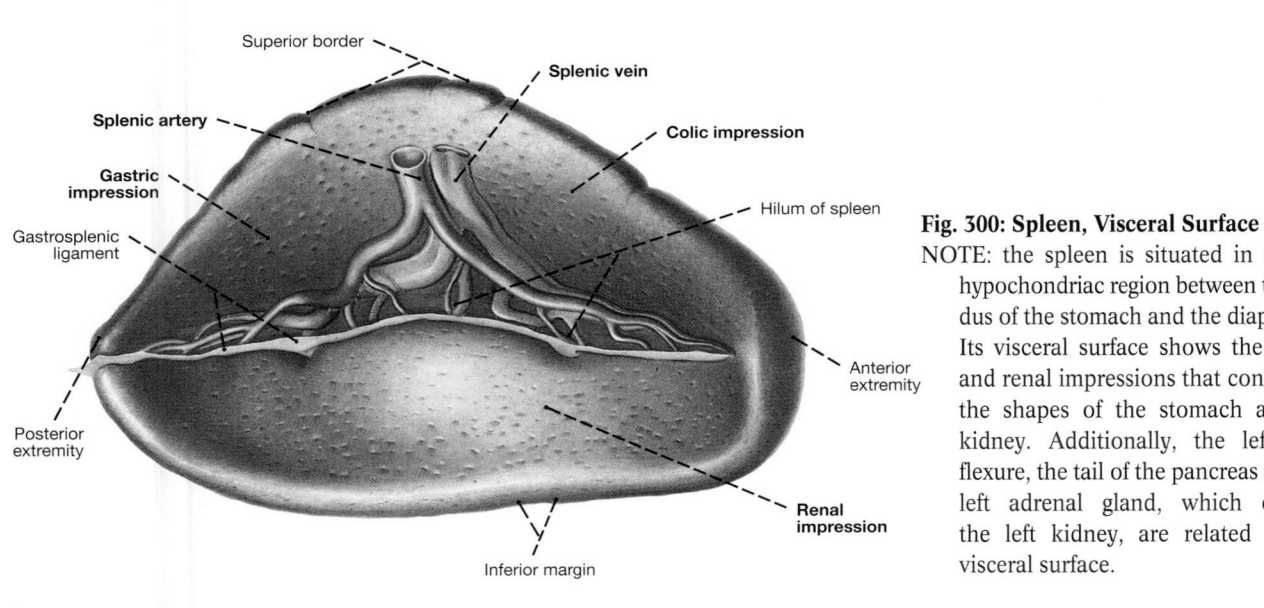

Coronary ligament of liver
Right lobe of liver
Falciform ligament
Round ligament of liver
Quadrate lobe of liver
Hepatogastric ligament of lesser omentum
Gall bladder
Hepatoduodenal ligament of lesser omentum
Epiploic foramen
Right lobe of liver
Duodenum (superior, or 1st part)
Right kidney
Pylorus
Taenia coli (omentalis)
Hepatic flexure
Greater omentum
Left gastric vessels
Gastrocolic ligament

Diaphragm
Left lobe of liver
Fundus of stomach
Fibrous appendix of liver
Cardia of stomach
Costodiaphragmatic recess
Body of stomach
Spleen
Lesser curvature
Gastrosplenic ligament
Angular notch
Greater curvature
Gastroepiploic vessels
Greater omentum
Transverse colon
Transverse mesocolon

Fig. 299: Lesser Omentum, Stomach, Liver, and Spleen

NOTE: 1) the liver is elevated and a probe inserted through the **epiploic foramen** into the vestibule of the **omental bursa.** By way of this opening, the greater peritoneal sac communicates with the lesser peritoneal sac (omental bursa). The **lesser omentum** consists of the **hepatogastric** and **hepatoduodenal ligaments.**

2) the epiploic foramen is situated just below the liver and readily admits two fingers. It is bound **superiorly** by the caudate lobe of the liver, **inferiorly** by the superior part of the duodenum, **posteriorly** by the inferior vena cava, and **anteriorly** by the lesser omentum which ensheathes the hepatic artery, portal vein, and bile ducts at the **porta hepatis.**

3) the greater omentum extends along the greater curvature from spleen to duodenum.

4) the gall bladder is situated between the right and quadrate lobes of the liver and projects just beyond the inferior border of the liver, thereby coming into contact directly with the anterior abdominal wall at this site.

Superior border
Splenic vein
Splenic artery
Colic impression
Gastric impression
Gastrosplenic ligament
Hilum of spleen
Posterior extremity
Anterior extremity
Renal impression
Inferior margin

Fig. 300: Spleen, Visceral Surface

NOTE: the spleen is situated in the left hypochondriac region between the fundus of the stomach and the diaphragm. Its visceral surface shows the gastric and renal impressions that conform to the shapes of the stomach and left kidney. Additionally, the left colic flexure, the tail of the pancreas and the left adrenal gland, which overlies the left kidney, are related to this visceral surface.

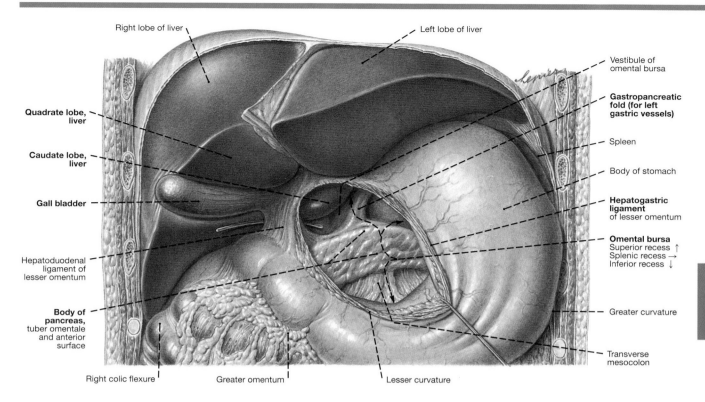

Right lobe of liver

Left lobe of liver

Vestibule of omental bursa

Gastropancreatic fold (for left gastric vessels)

Quadrate lobe, liver

Spleen

Body of stomach

Caudate lobe, liver

Hepatogastric ligament of lesser omentum

Gall bladder

Omental bursa
Superior recess ↑
Splenic recess →
Inferior recess ↓

Hepatoduodenal ligament of lesser omentum

Greater curvature

Body of pancreas,
tuber omentale and anterior surface

Transverse mesocolon

Right colic flexure

Greater omentum

Lesser curvature

Fig. 301: The Omental Bursa, Caudate Lobe of Liver and Body of Pancreas

NOTE: 1) with the liver elevated and the lesser curvature of the stomach pulled to the left, the exposure obtained by opening the omental bursa through the hepatogastric part of the lesser omentum has been enlarged. The superior, splenic, and inferior recesses of this bursa are indicated by arrows.

2) the portion of the omental bursa adjacent to the epiploic foramen is called the **vestibule.** Observe the **gastropancreatic fold** which crosses the dorsal wall of the bursa. This fold is a reflection of peritoneum covering the left gastric artery coursing from the celiac trunk to its destination, the lesser curvature of the stomach.

3) exposure of the omental bursa reveals the **caudate lobe** of the liver situated on the dorsal surface of the **right lobe.** Also seen is the anterior surface of the body of the pancreas coursing transversely behind the stomach.

4) the **left lobe** of the liver overlies the lesser curvature, the fundus, and part of the body of the stomach. The **caudate lobe** behind the porta hepatis and the **quadrate lobe,** located between the fossa of the gall bladder and the round ligament, come into contact with the pylorus and the first part of the duodenum.

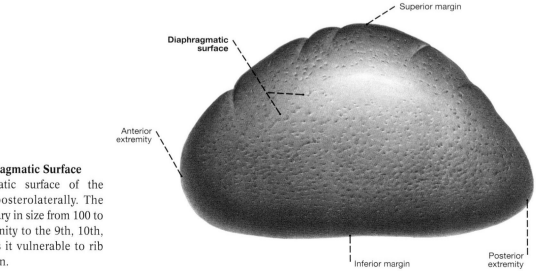

Superior margin

Diaphragmatic surface

Anterior extremity

Fig. 302: Spleen, Diaphragmatic Surface

NOTE: the diaphragmatic surface of the spleen is directed posterolaterally. The normal spleen may vary in size from 100 to 400 grams. Its proximity to the 9th, 10th, and 11th ribs makes it vulnerable to rib fractures in this region.

Inferior margin

Posterior extremity

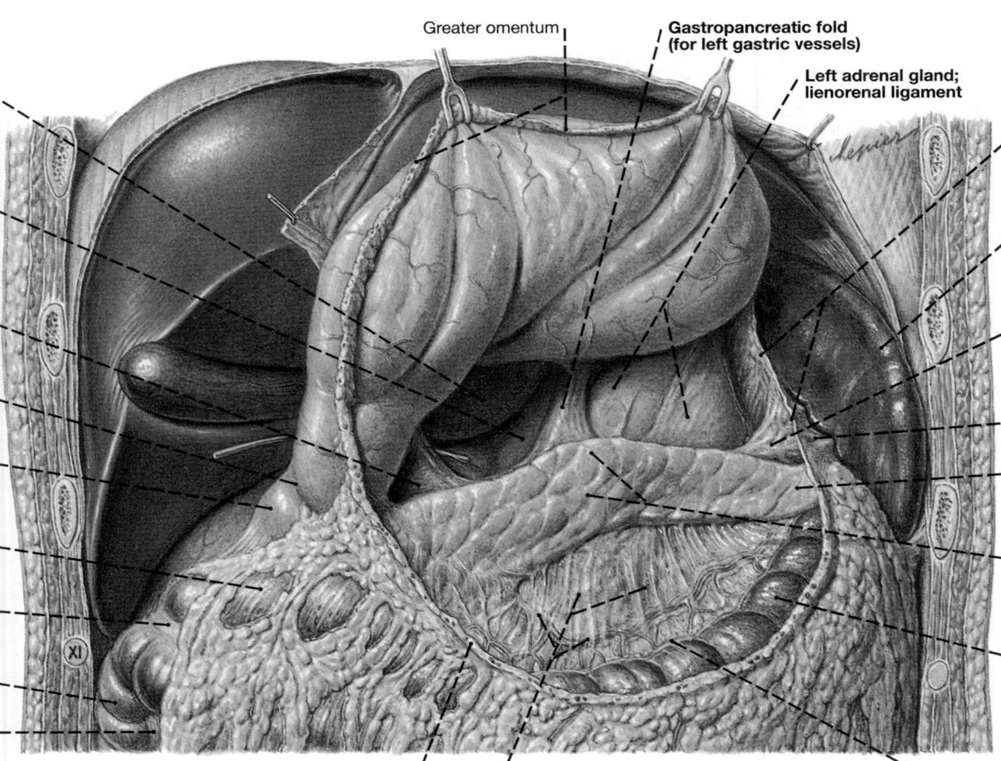

PLATE 204   **Omental Bursa, Stomach Reflected; Radiograph of Stomach**

Caudate lobe of liver

Vestibule of
omental bursa

Hepatoduodenal
ligament

Pylorus

Duodenum
(superior,
or 1st part)

**Transverse
colon**

**Taenia coli
(omentalis)**

Ascending colon

Taenia coli (libera)

Greater omentum

Gastropancreatic fold
(for left gastric vessels)

Left adrenal gland;
lienorenal ligament

**Gastrosplenic
ligament**

Spleen

Splenic vessels

Hilum of spleen

Tail of pancreas

**Tuber omentale
and body
of pancreas**

Transverse colon

Greater omentum

Transverse mesocolon;
middle colic artery and vein

Taenia coli (mesocolic)

Fig. 303: Omental Bursa and Structures of the Stomach Bed

NOTE: 1)   the attachment of the greater omentum has been cut along the entire greater curvature of the stomach, and the stomach has been elevated to expose the omental bursa.

2)   the transverse course of the pancreas across the posterior abdomen and the pointed direction of the tail of the pancreas toward the hilum of the spleen.

3)   the severed peritoneal reflection between the stomach and the spleen, the **gastrosplenic ligament,** and its continuation from the spleen to the kidney, the **lienorenal ligament.**

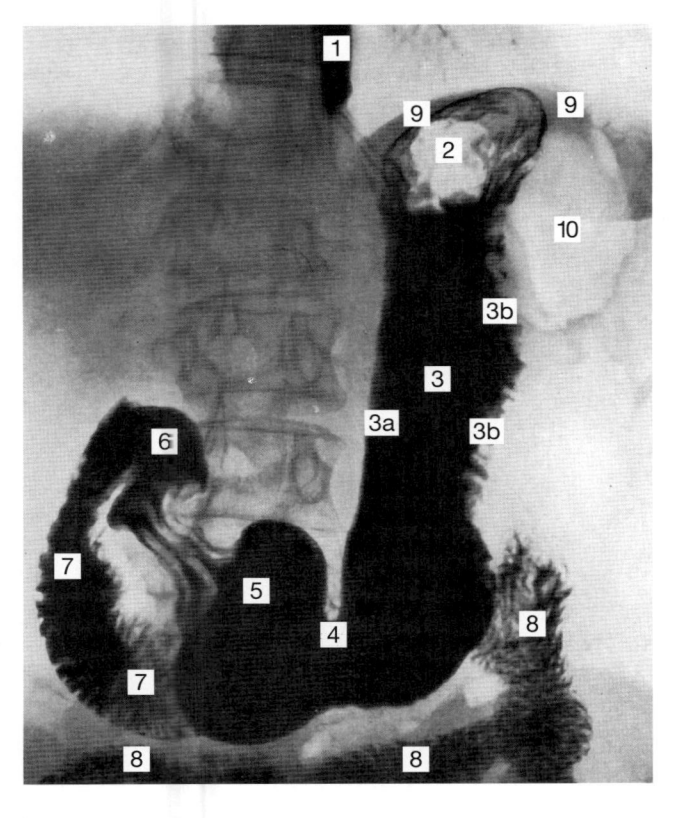

Fig. 304: Radiograph of the Lower Esophagus, Stomach, Duodenum, and Proximal Jejunum

NOTE: this is a normal "J-shaped" or "fishhook" stomach. The cardiac and pyloric ends of the stomach are more securely attached to the posterior body wall, whereas the body and pyloric parts are more mobile. Frequently in the upright position, the greater curvature hangs as low as the brim of the pelvis.

1. Esophagus
2. Stomach fundus (air bubble)
3. Body of stomach
   3a Lesser curvature
   3b Greater curvature
4. Peristaltic constriction
   at angular notch
5. Pyloric antrum (expanded)
6. Bulb of superior duodenum (1st part)
7. Descending duodenum (2nd part)
8. Jejunum
9. Left dome of diaphragm
10. Gas in left colic flexure

Figs. 303, 304

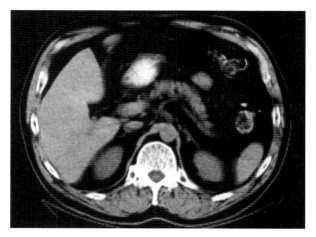

Fig. 305A: CT Scan, Abdomen (about L1)
Computerized tomographic scan of the upper abdominal
organs at the level of the **superior pole of the kidney.**

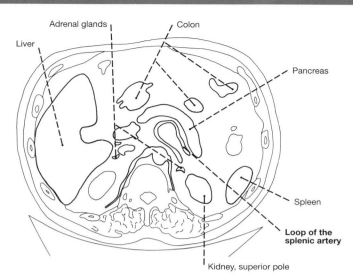

Fig. 305B: Outline Diagram for Fig. 305A

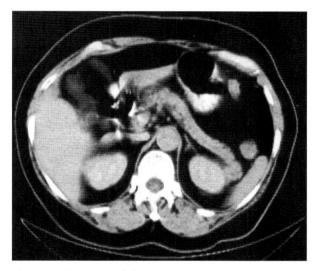

Fig. 306A: CT Scan, Abdomen (L1 to L2)
Computerized tomographic scan of the upper abdominal
organs at the level of the **body of the pancreas.**

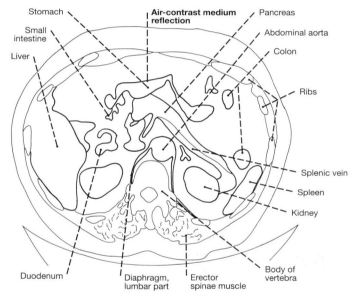

Fig. 306B: Outline Diagram for Fig. 306A

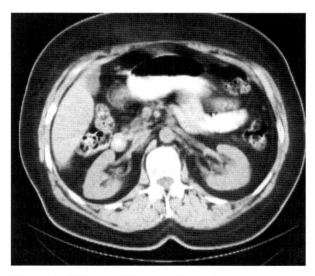

Fig. 307A: CT Scan, Abdomen (about L2)
Computerized tomographic scan of the upper abdominal
organs at the level of the **renal vessels.**

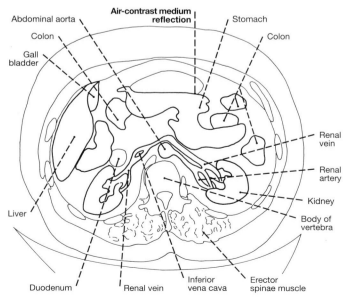

Fig. 307B: Outline Diagram for Fig. 307A

Figs. 305 A–307 B   **III**

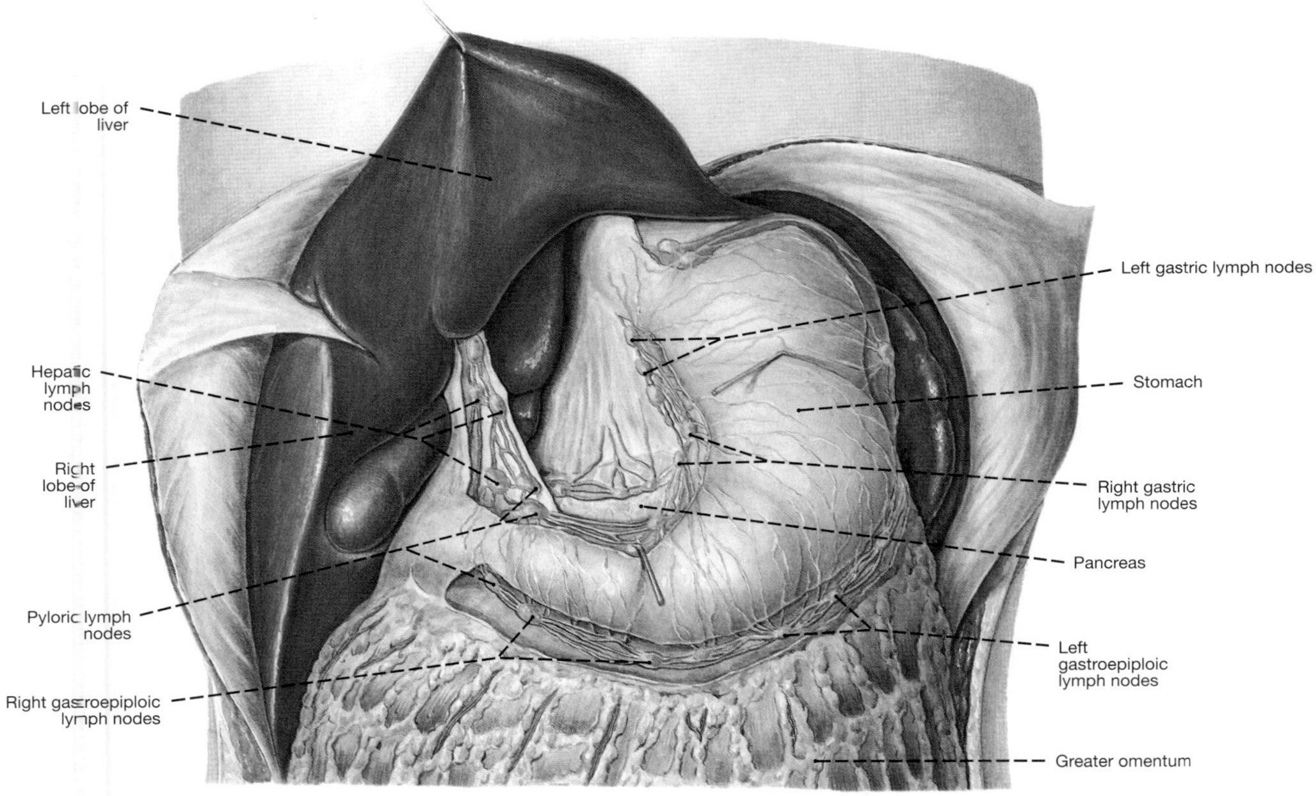

PLATE 206   Upper Abdominal Lymphatics; Liver; Diaphragmatic Surface

Left lobe of liver

Left gastric lymph nodes

Hepatic lymph nodes

Stomach

Right lobe of liver

Right gastric lymph nodes

Pancreas

Pyloric lymph nodes

Left gastroepiploic lymph nodes

Right gastroepiploic lymph nodes

Greater omentum

Fig. 308: Lymphatic Vessels and Nodes of the Stomach, the Porta Hepatis, and Pancreas

NOTE: lymph nodes for the stomach are found with the gastroepiploic arteries and veins along the greater curvature and with the right and left gastric vessels along the lesser curvature. Those in the porta hepatis follow the branches of the hepatic artery and, behind the stomach, pancreatic nodes are located along the splenic vessels. Most of these nodes drain toward the **preaortic nodes** around the celiac trunk.

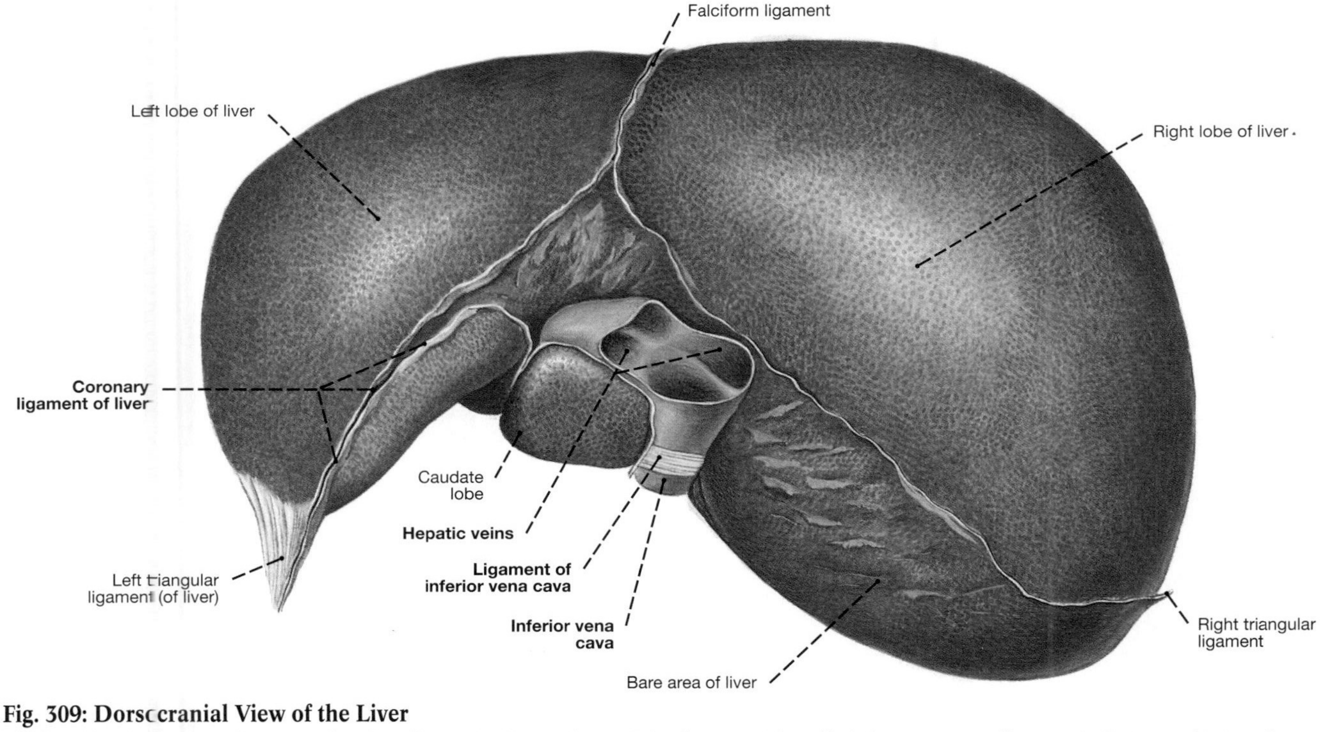

Falciform ligament

Left lobe of liver

Right lobe of liver

Coronary ligament of liver

Caudate lobe

Hepatic veins

Ligament of inferior vena cava

Left triangular ligament (of liver)

Inferior vena cava

Right triangular ligament

Bare area of liver

Fig. 309: Dorsocranial View of the Liver

NOTE: 1) visceral peritoneum closely adheres to the surface of the liver and is called the **coronary ligament.** Between its two leaves a portion of the liver, called the **bare area,** is devoid of peritoneum and is in contact with the abdominal surface of the diaphragm.

2) the **hepatic veins** converge superiorly to empty into the superior vena cava.

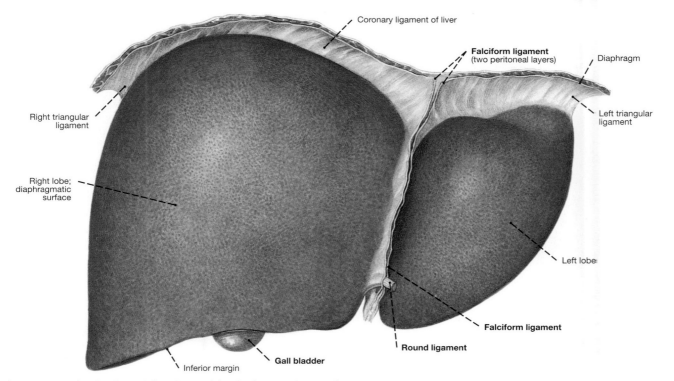

Fig. 310: Anterior Surface of the Liver (with Diaphragmatic Attachment)
NOTE: the **falciform ligament** separates the right and left lobes of the liver. It contains a fibrous cord, the **round ligament of the liver,** which was the **umbilical vein** during fetal life. Observe also the fundus of the gall bladder below the inferior margin of the liver.

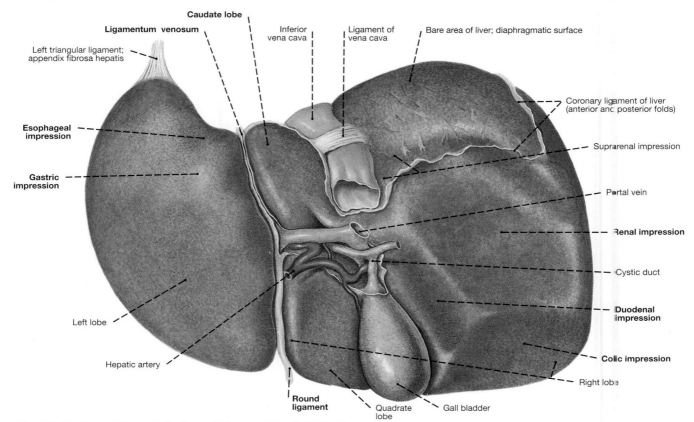

Fig. 311: Posterior (Visceral) Surface of Liver and the Gall Bladder
NOTE: the impressions made by the abdominal organs on the ventral surface of the liver, and the inferior vena cava which separates the **caudate** and **right lobes.** The gall bladder, portal vein, hepatic artery, and common bile duct bound the **quadrate lobe,** and the **ligamentum venosus** (ductus venosus) extends from the **round ligament** (umbilical vein).

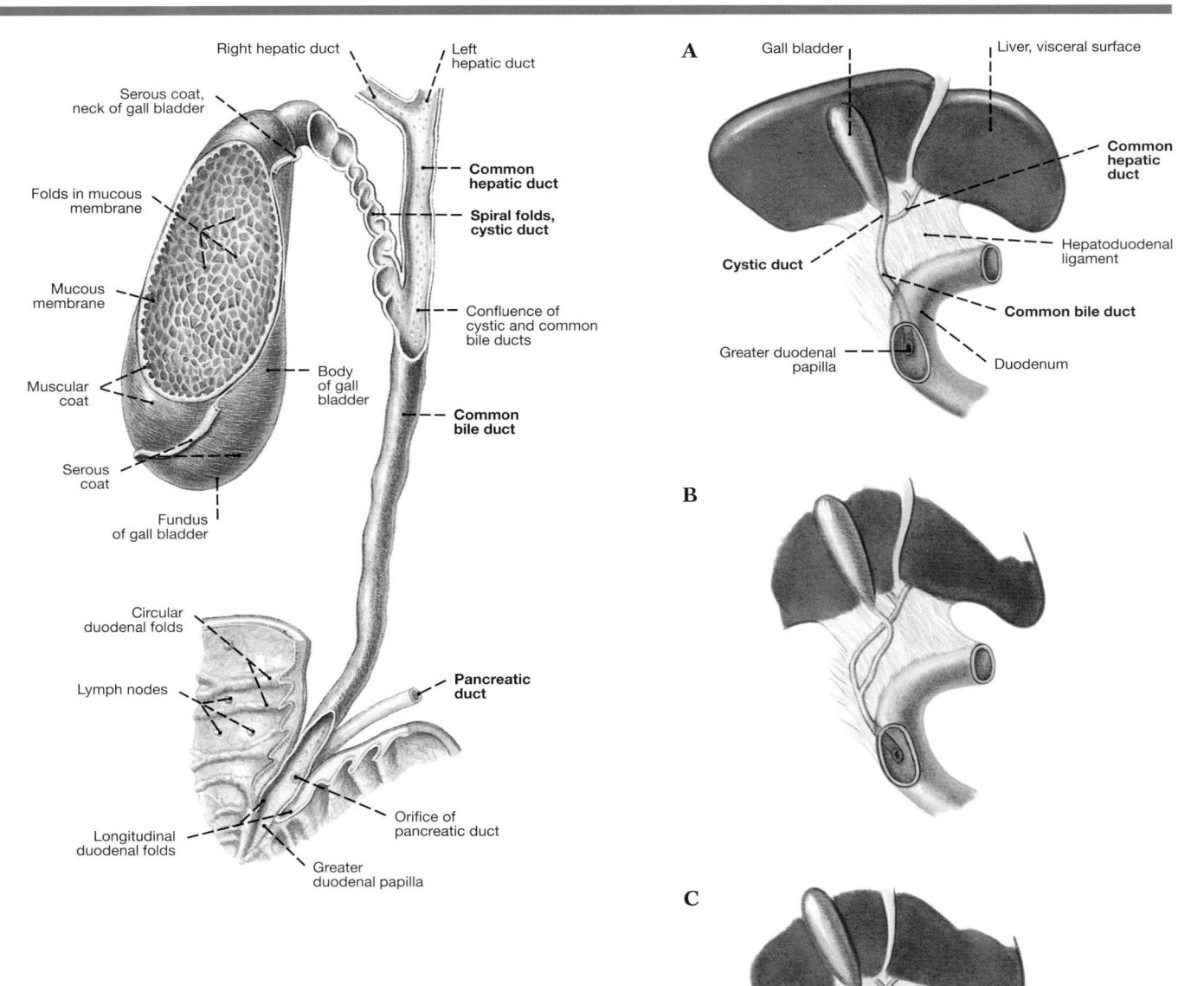

Fig. 312: Gall Bladder and Biliary Duct System

NOTE: 1)   the wall of the gall bladder has been opened to reveal the meshwork characteristic of the surface of the mucosal layer. The pear-shaped gall bladder stores bile, which reaches it from the liver. Its capacity is about 35 cc.

2)   the spiral nature of the **cystic duct,** which emerges from the neck of the gall bladder. Normally, the cystic duct measures about 1½ inches in length and joins the **common hepatic duct** (which also is about 1½ inches long) to form the **common bile duct.**

3)   the common bile duct descends about 3 inches to open into the 2nd or descending portion of the duodenum.

4)   at its point of entrance into the duodenum (greater duodenal papilla), the common bile duct is joined by the **main pancreatic duct** (duct of Wirsung).

Fig. 313A, B, C: Variations in the Union of the Cystic and Common Hepatic Ducts

NOTE: usually the cystic duct lies to the right of the common hepatic duct at a point just superior to the level of the 1st part of the duodenum. Variations in this schema occur as is indicated in the following three examples:

A. the union of the cystic and common hepatic ducts occurs close to the liver, resulting in short cystic and common hepatic ducts and a long common bile duct.

B. the cystic duct crosses to the left of the common hepatic duct and joins the hepatic duct low, resulting in a short common bile duct.

C. the cystic duct remains to the right of the common hepatic duct but still joins it close to the site of penetration of the duodenum, again resulting in a short common bile duct.

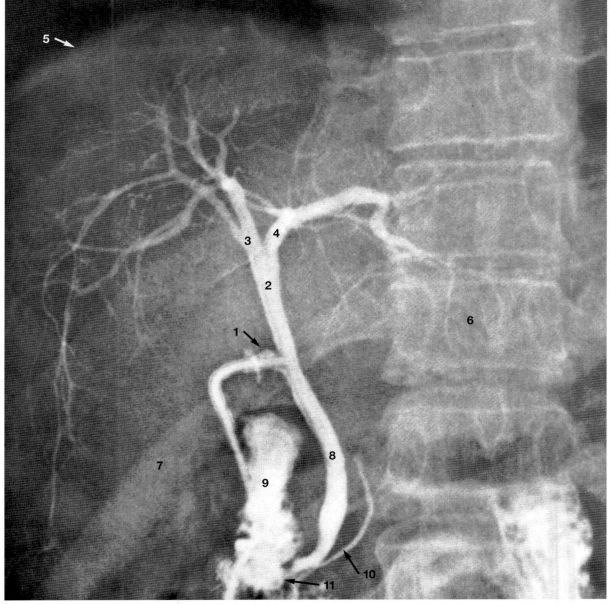

Fig. 314: Intraoperative Cholangiogram: Radiograph of Biliary Duct System

NOTE: the gall bladder has been removed and a catheter and tube has been inserted through the stump of the cystic duct (1) into the common hepatic duct (2) and contrast medium injected into the biliary system. Other structures are numbered as follows:

(3) Right hepatic duct
(4) Left hepatic duct
(5) Diaphragm
(6) 11th thoracic vertebra
(7) 11th rib
(8) Common bile duct
(9) Duodenum (2nd, desc. part)
(10) Main pancreatic duct
(11) Greater duodenal papilla

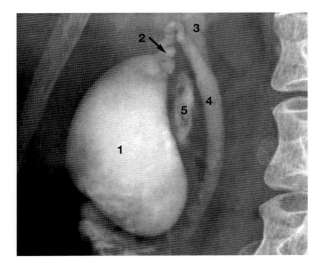

◀ **Fig. 315: Radiograph of Gall Bladder and Biliary Ducts**

(1) Body of the gall bladder
(2) Cystic duct with spiral valves
(3) Common hepatic duct
(4) Union of common hepatic and cystic ducts to form common bile duct
(5) Contrast medium in duodenum

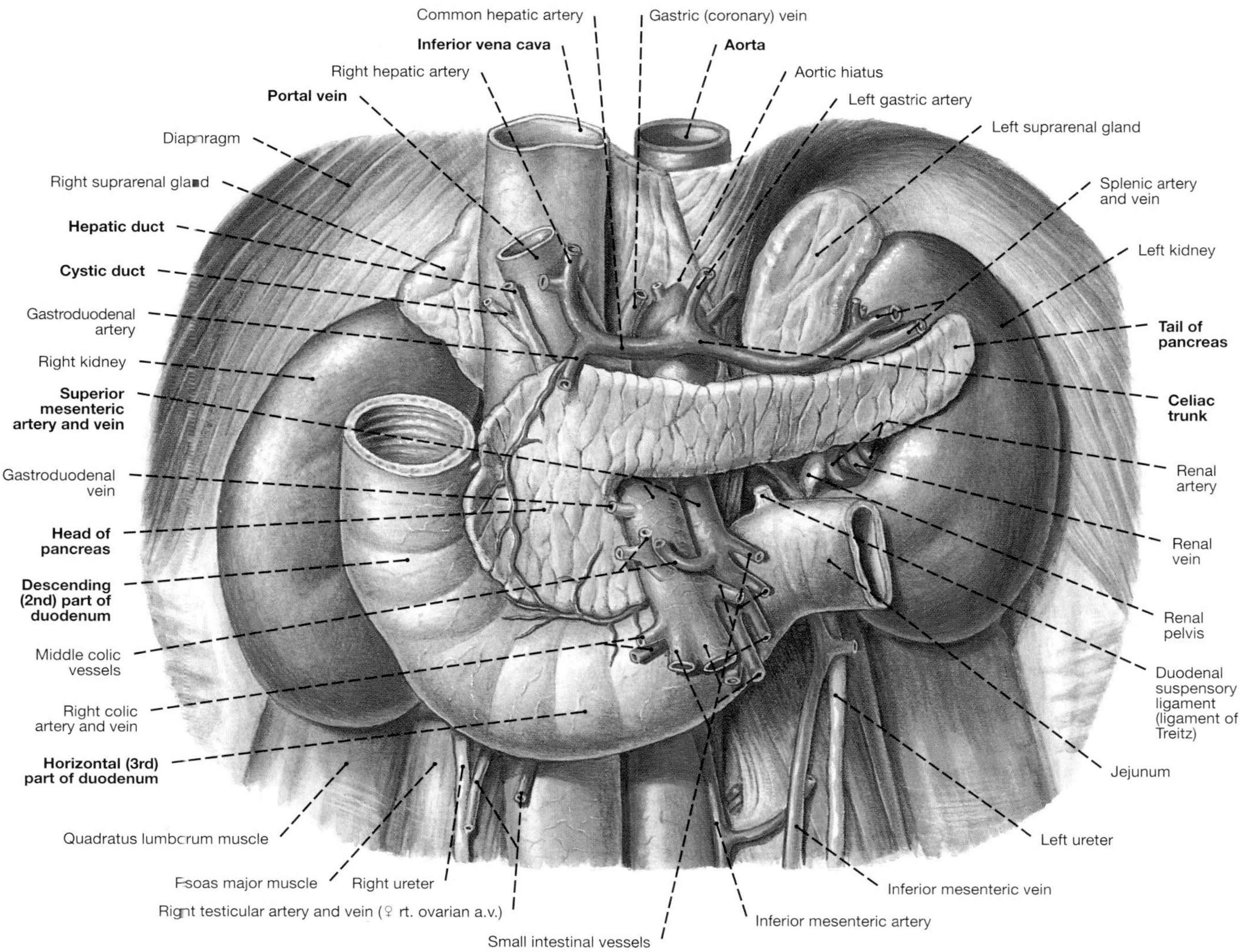

PLATE 210   Pancreas and Duodenum

Common hepatic artery

Gastric (coronary) vein

Inferior vena cava

Aorta

Right hepatic artery

Aortic hiatus

Portal vein

Left gastric artery

Left suprarenal gland

Diaphragm

Splenic artery and vein

Right suprarenal gland

Left kidney

Hepatic duct

Cystic duct

Tail of pancreas

Gastroduodenal artery

Celiac trunk

Right kidney

Superior mesenteric artery and vein

Renal artery

Gastroduodenal vein

Renal vein

Head of pancreas

Renal pelvis

Descending (2nd) part of duodenum

Duodenal suspensory ligament (ligament of Treitz)

Middle colic vessels

Right colic artery and vein

Jejunum

Horizontal (3rd) part of duodenum

Quadratus lumborum muscle

Left ureter

Psoas major muscle

Right ureter

Inferior mesenteric vein

Right testicular artery and vein (♀ rt. ovarian a.v.)

Inferior mesenteric artery

Small intestinal vessels

Fig. 316: Pancreas and Duodenum

NOTE: 1) the **head** of the pancreas lies to the right of midline and in contact with the inferior vena cava and common bile duct dorsally and transverse colon (not shown) ventrally.

2) the **body** of the pancreas crosses the midline at the L1 level, and it is in contact posteriorly with the aorta, superior mesenteric vessels, and left kidney and adrenal gland.

3) the **tail** of the pancreas is in contact with the spleen laterally, the left kidney behind and the splenic flexure of the colon anteriorly.

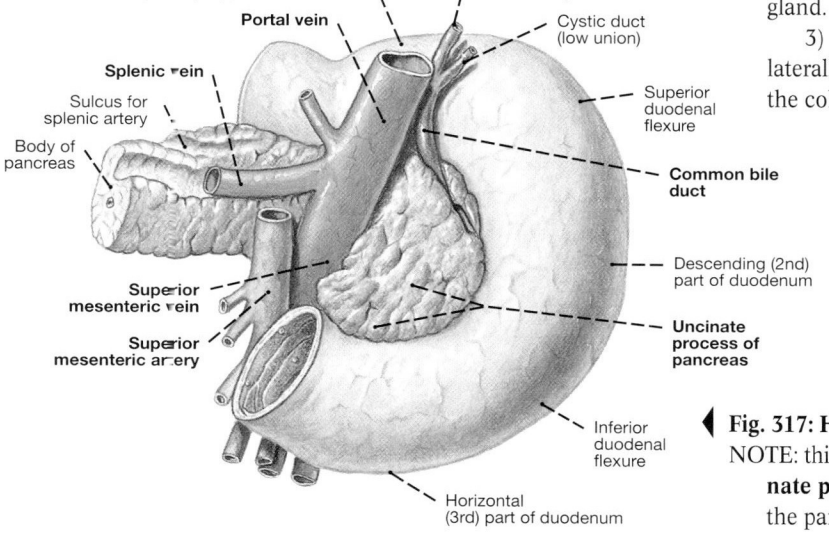

Superior (1st) part of duodenum

Common hepatic duct

Portal vein

Cystic duct (low union)

Splenic vein

Superior duodenal flexure

Sulcus for splenic artery

Body of pancreas

Common bile duct

Descending (2nd) part of duodenum

Superior mesenteric vein

Uncinate process of pancreas

Superior mesenteric artery

Inferior duodenal flexure

Fig. 317: Head of Pancreas and Duodenum (Dorsal View)

NOTE: this posterior view of the pancreatic head and its **uncinate process** shows the common bile duct embedded in the pancreas as it descends adjacent to the duodenum.

Horizontal (3rd) part of duodenum

Figs. 316, 317

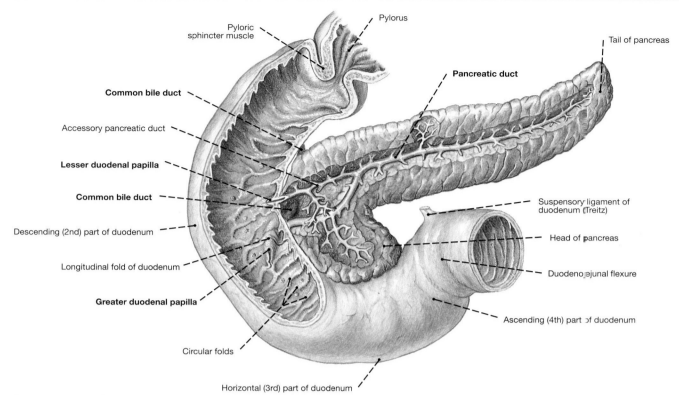

Fig. 318: Pancreatic Duct System

NOTE: 1) the main pancreatic duct system has been dissected in this specimen. Observe how the accessory pancreatic duct extends straight into the duodenum through the lesser duodenal papilla. The main pancreatic duct, however, bends caudally to drain most of the head of the pancreas and then opens into the greater duodenal papilla with the common bile duct.

    2) from the pylorus to the duodenojejunal flexure, the duodenum measures about 10 inches. At its termination, a suspensory ligament (of Treitz) marks the commencement of the jejunum. Here the small intestine becomes surrounded by peritoneum and is suspended from the posterior abdominal wall by the mesentery of the small intestine.

    3) the duodenum and pancreas are both retroperitoneal structures.

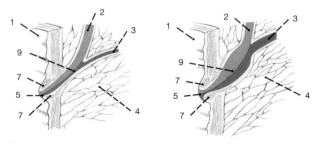

| **Fig. 319** | **Fig. 320** | **Fig. 321** | **Fig. 322** |

Figs. 319–324: Variations in Union of Common Bile Duct and Pancreatic Duct

Fig. 319: Pancreatic and common bile ducts join early, resulting in a long hepatopancreatic duct.

Fig. 320: A long hepatopancreatic duct is modified by an expanded ampulla.

Fig. 321: Pancreatic and common bile ducts join very close to the greater duodenal papilla, resulting in a short hepatopancreatic duct.

Fig. 322: Both pancreatic and common bile ducts open separately on a somewhat larger duodenal papilla.

Fig. 323: Pancreatic and common bile ducts drain through a single opening, but the ducts are separated by a septum.

Fig. 324: Long hepatopancreatic duct along with a well-developed accessory pancreatic duct, which opens through the lesser duodenal papilla.

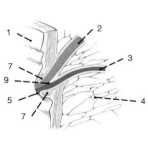

Fig. 323

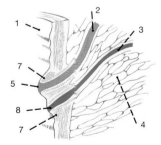

Fig. 324

1 Duodenum
2 Common bile duct
3 Pancreatic duct (Wirsung)
4 Pancreas
5 Greater duodenal papilla

6 Accessory pancreatic duct (Santorini)
7 Sphincter (Oddi) at duodenal papilla
8 Pancreatic duct separate opening
9 Hepatopancreatic duct

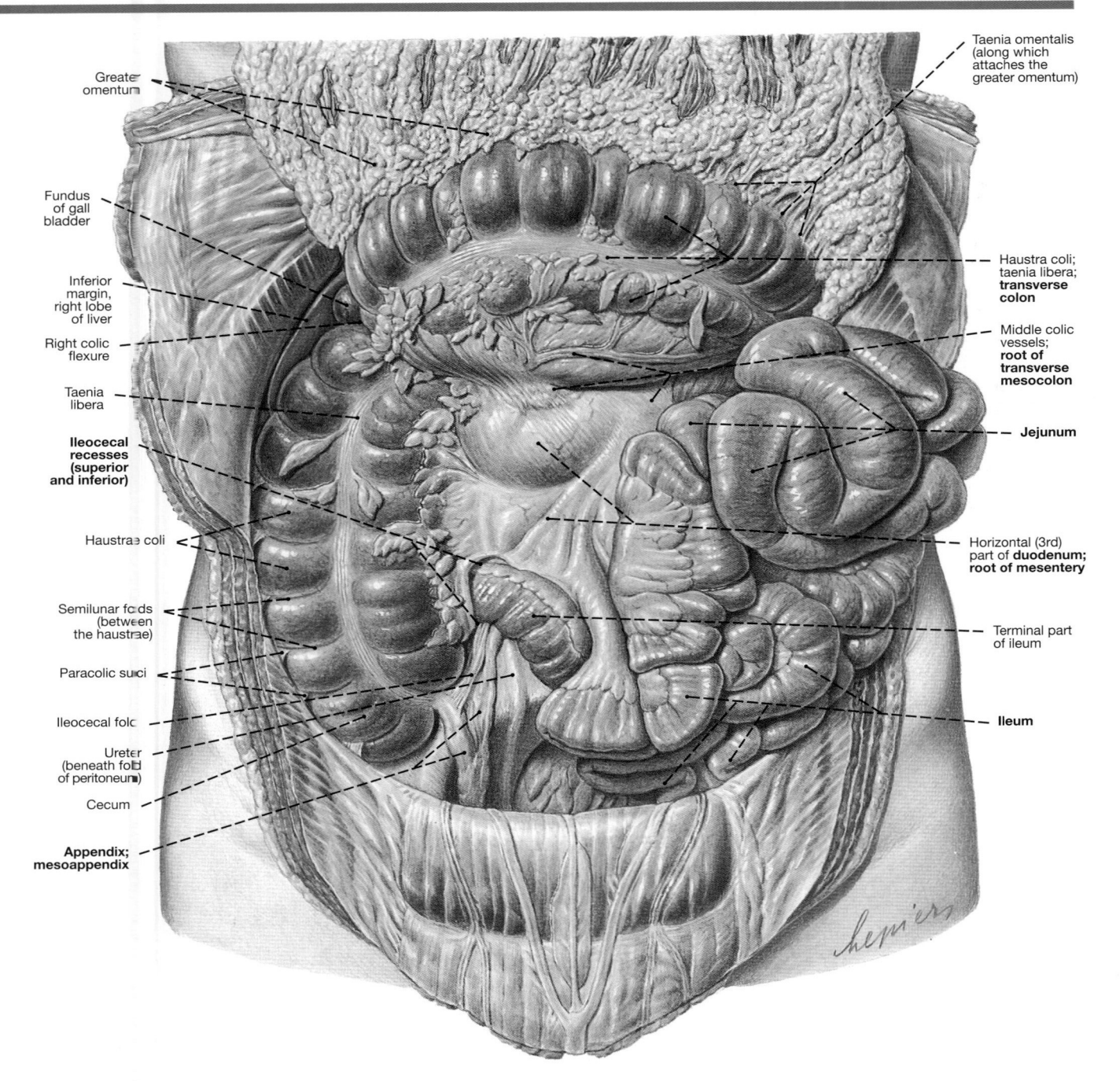

Greater omentum

Taenia omentalis (along which attaches the greater omentum)

Fundus of gall bladder

Haustra coli; taenia libera; **transverse colon**

Inferior margin, right lobe of liver

Middle colic vessels; **root of transverse mesocolon**

Right colic flexure

Taenia libera

Jejunum

Ileocecal recesses (superior and inferior)

Haustrae coli

Horizontal (3rd) part of **duodenum; root of mesentery**

Semilunar folds (between the haustrae)

Terminal part of ileum

Paracolic sulci

Ileocecal fold

Ileum

Ureter (beneath fold of peritoneum)

Cecum

Appendix; mesoappendix

Fig. 325: Abdominal Cavity (5): Jejunum, Ileum, Ascending and Transverse Colon

NOTE: 1) the greater omentum has been reflected superiorly and the jejunum and ileum have been pulled to the left to expose the **root of the mesentery of the small intestine.**

2) the horizontal (3rd) part of the duodenum which is retroperitoneal and which is covered by the smooth and glistening peritoneum.

3) the junction of the distal portion of the ileum with the cecum. At this **ileocecal junction** identify the **ileocecal fold,** the **appendix** and the **mesoappendix.** The appendix may extend cranially behind the cecum, toward the left and behind the ileum, or as demonstrated here, inferiorly over the pelvic brim.

4) the transverse colon and the small intestine beyond the duodenal junction are more mobile than most other organs because they are attached to the transverse mesocolon and the mesentery.

5) the retroperitoneal position of the **right ureter** as it descends over the pelvic brim on its course toward the urinary bladder in the pelvis.

Fig. 325

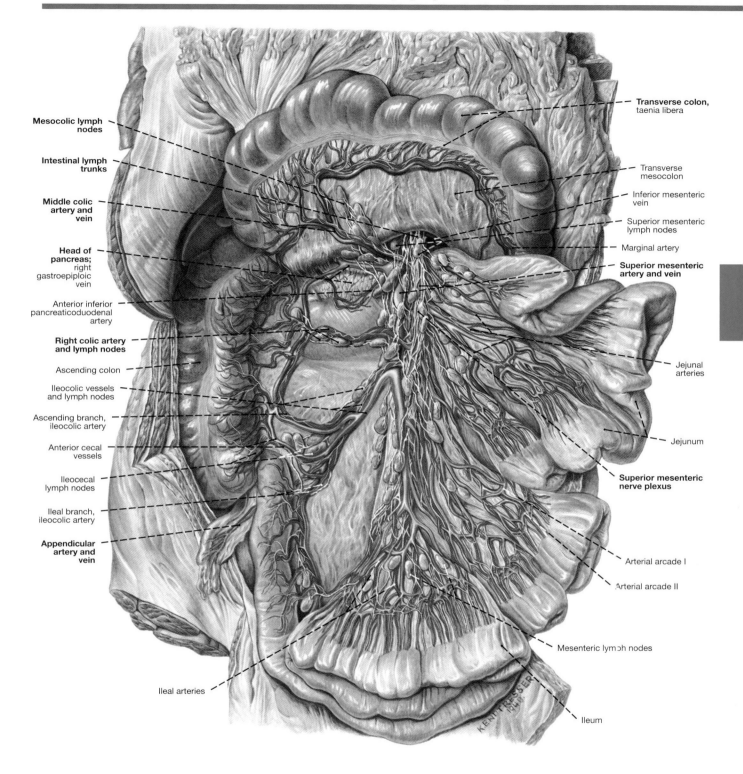

Mesocolic lymph nodes

Intestinal lymph trunks

Middle colic artery and vein

Head of pancreas; right gastroepiploic vein

Anterior inferior pancreaticoduodenal artery

Right colic artery and lymph nodes

Ascending colon

Ileocolic vessels and lymph nodes

Ascending branch, ileocolic artery

Anterior cecal vessels

Ileocecal lymph nodes

Ileal branch, ileocolic artery

Appendicular artery and vein

Ileal arteries

Transverse colon, taenia libera

Transverse mesocolon

Inferior mesenteric vein

Superior mesenteric lymph nodes

Marginal artery

Superior mesenteric artery and vein

Jejunal arteries

Jejunum

Superior mesenteric nerve plexus

Arterial arcade I

Arterial arcade II

Mesenteric lymph nodes

Ileum

Fig. 326: Abdominal Cavity (6); Lymph Nodes, Vessels, and Nerves Serving the Jejunum, Ileum, Ascending, and Transverse Colon
NOTE: 1)   the transverse colon has been lifted to reveal its mesocolon along with the retroperitoneal head of the pancreas and the horizontal part of the duodenum.

2)   the loops of the jejunum and ileum have been reflected to the left to show the root of the mesentery with its network of lymphatics, blood vessels, and autonomic nerves.

3)   chains of mesenteric lymph nodes follow the branches of the superior mesenteric vessels as well as the iliocolic, right colic, and middle colic branches of the same vessels.

4)   the lymphatics from both the small and large intestine drain centrally and superiorly, and eventually interconnect with preaortic chains of nodes.

Fig. 326   **III**

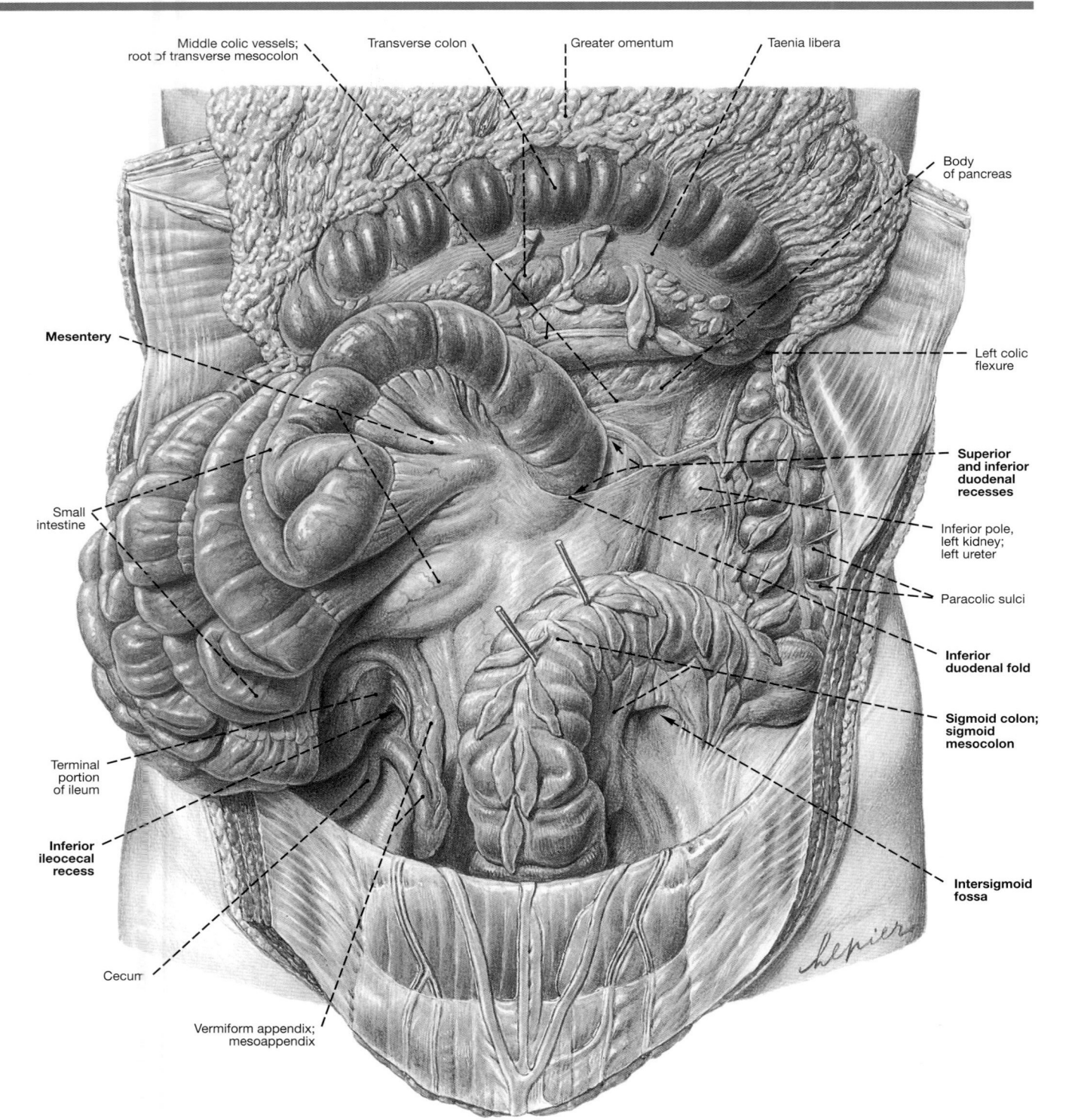

Middle colic vessels;
root of transverse mesocolon

Transverse colon

Greater omentum

Taenia libera

Body
of pancreas

Mesentery

Left colic
flexure

Superior
and inferior
duodenal
recesses

Small
intestine

Inferior pole,
left kidney;
left ureter

Paracolic sulci

Inferior
duodenal fold

Sigmoid colon;
sigmoid
mesocolon

Terminal
portion
of ileum

Inferior
ileocecal
recess

Intersigmoid
fossa

Cecum

Vermiform appendix;
mesoappendix

Fig. 327: Abdominal Cavity (7): Descending and Sigmoid Colon and the Duodenojejunal Junction
NOTE: 1) the transverse colon and greater omentum have been reflected upward and the jejunum and ileum have been pulled to the right to reveal the **duodenojejunal junction** and the **descending** and **sigmoid colon.**

2) at the duodenojejunal junction the small intestine acquires a mesentery. At this site, there are frequently found duodenal fossae or recesses located in relationship to the junction. Among these, the **superior** and **inferior duodenal recesses** are found in more than 50% of cases. These are of importance because they represent possible sites of herniation.

3) the mobility of the sigmoid colon (because of its mesocolic attachment), whereas the descending colon is fixed to the posterior wall of the abdomen.

4) the **intersigmoid fossa** located behind the sigmoid mesocolon, and between that mesocolon and the peritoneum reflected over the external iliac vessels.

Fig. 327

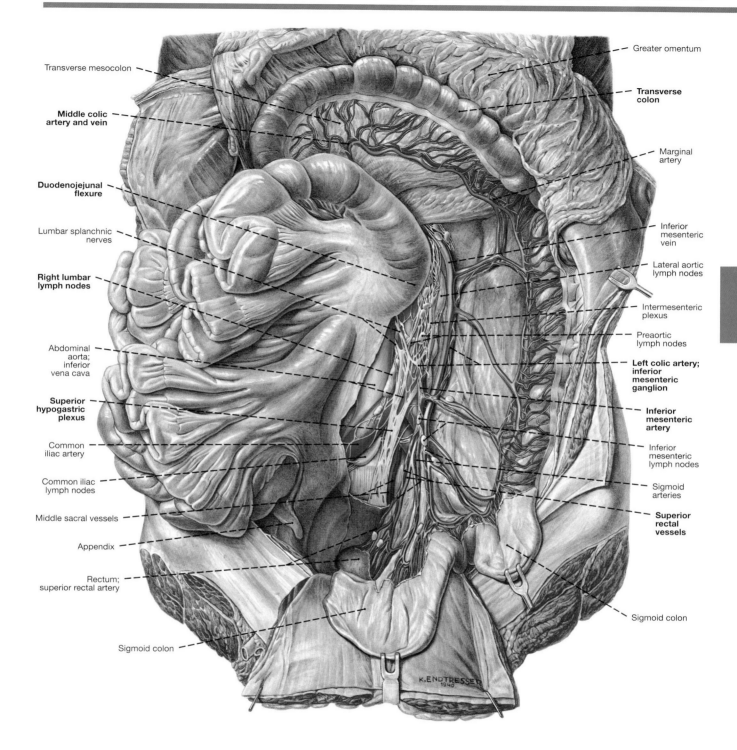

Transverse mesocolon

Middle colic
artery and vein

Duodenojejunal
flexure

Lumbar splanchnic
nerves

Right lumbar
lymph nodes

Abdominal
aorta;
inferior
vena cava

Superior
hypogastric
plexus

Common
iliac artery

Common iliac
lymph nodes

Middle sacral vessels

Appendix

Rectum;
superior rectal artery

Sigmoid colon

Greater omentum

Transverse
colon

Marginal
artery

Inferior
mesenteric
vein

Lateral aortic
lymph nodes

Intermesenteric
plexus

Preaortic
lymph nodes

Left colic artery;
inferior
mesenteric
ganglion

Inferior
mesenteric
artery

Inferior
mesenteric
lymph nodes

Sigmoid
arteries

Superior
rectal
vessels

Sigmoid colon

K.ENDTRESSER
1940

**Fig. 328: Abdominal Cavity (8): Blood Vessels, Lymph Nodes, and Autonomic Nerves in the Region
of the Descending Colon and Sigmoid Colon**

NOTE: 1) the small intestine has been deflected to the right and the peritoneum has been dissected over the abdominal aorta and inferior
vena cava.

2) the **left colic artery** is derived from the inferior mesenteric artery and it supplies much of the descending colon.

3) the anastomoses made above by the left colic artery with branches of the middle colic artery, and below with the sigmoid arteries.

4) the **superior hypogastric plexus** in front of the aortic bifurcation. It contains:

a) **postganglionic sympathetic fibers descending** to supply organs in the pelvis,

b) **preganglionic parasympathetic** fibers from S2, S3, and S4 **ascending** to supply part of the transverse colon and the
descending and sigmoid colon, and the rectum.

c) **visceral afferent** fibers that carry sensory information from lower abdominal and pelvic organs.

Fig. 328   III

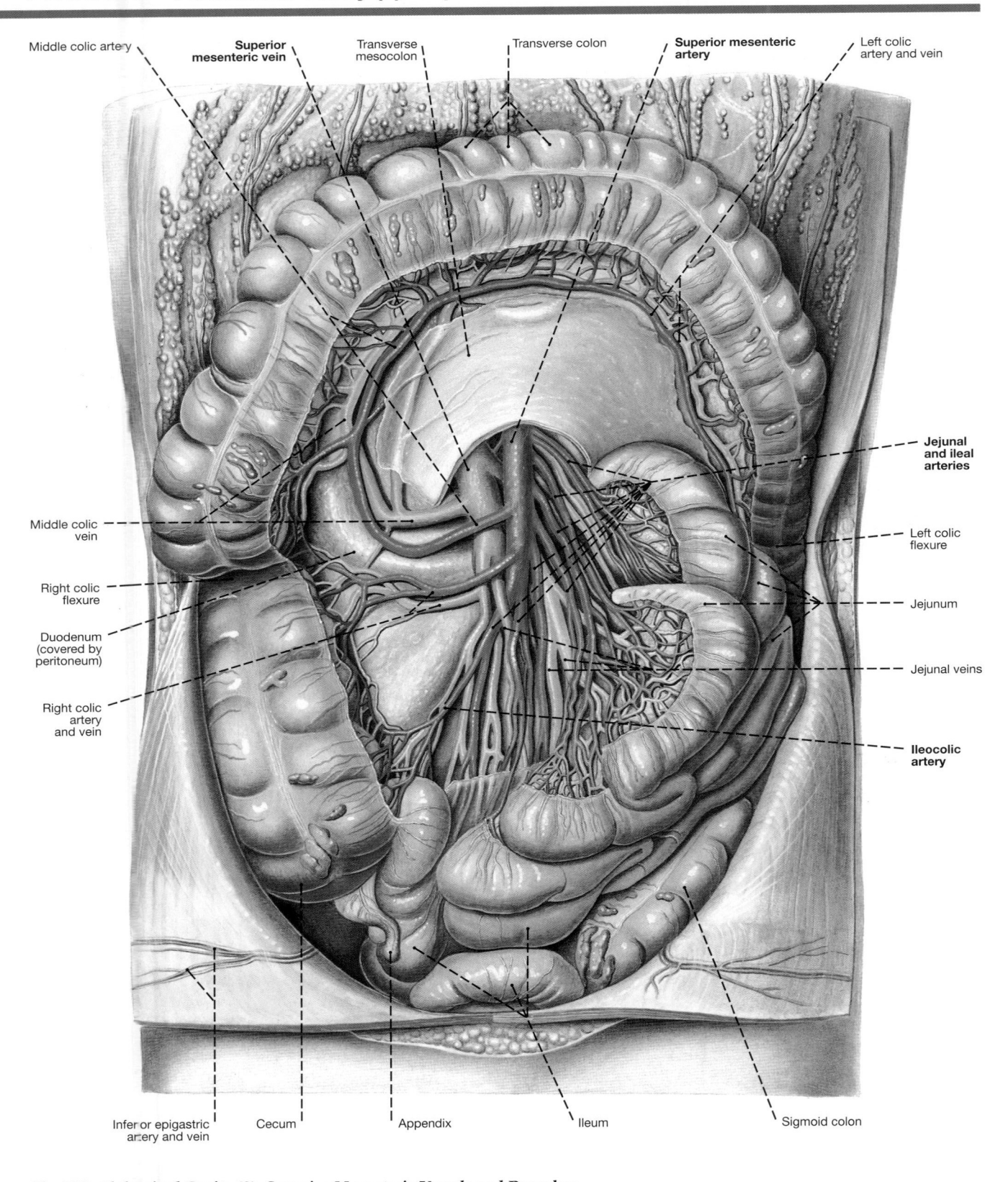

Middle colic artery · Superior mesenteric vein · Transverse mesocolon · Transverse colon · Superior mesenteric artery · Left colic artery and vein

Jejunal and ileal arteries

Middle colic vein

Right colic flexure

Duodenum (covered by peritoneum)

Right colic artery and vein

Left colic flexure

Jejunum

Jejunal veins

Ileocolic artery

Inferior epigastric artery and vein · Cecum · Appendix · Ileum · Sigmoid colon

Fig. 329: Abdominal Cavity (9): Superior Mesenteric Vessels and Branches
NOTE: 1) the small intestine is pushed to the left and the loops of bowel have been dissected to expose the branches of the superior mesenteric vessels.

2) the **jejunal and ileal arteries** branch from the left side of the mesenteric artery. There are about 15 of these vessels.

3) branching from the right side of the superior mesenteric artery are the **ileocolic, right colic,** and **middle colic arteries.** These vessels form rich anatomoses.

4) the small intestine measures about 22 feet in length, commencing at the pyloric end of the stomach and extending to the ileocecal junction where the large intestine starts.

Fig. 329

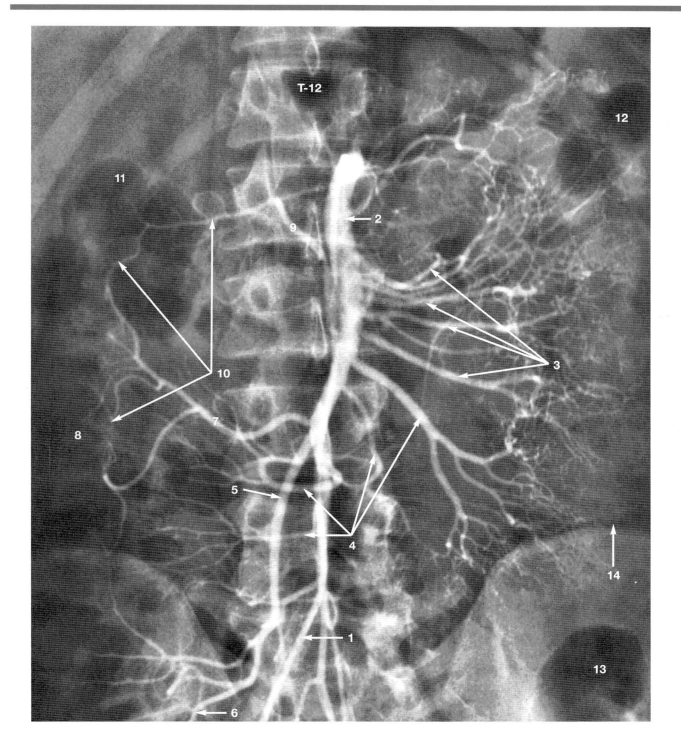

Fig. 330: Superior Mesenteric Arteriogram

NOTE: 1) a catheter (1) has been inserted into the common iliac artery and through the abdominal aorta to the point of branching of the superior mesenteric artery (2). Contrast medium was injected to visualize the principal branches of that vessel. The original radiograph is shown as a negative print.

2) the jejunal (3) and ileal (4) arteries branching as a sequence of vessels (about 15 in number), which supply all of the small intestine beyond the duodenum.

3) the ileocolic artery (5) and its appendicular branch (6), the right colic (7) and middle colic (9) arteries, which supply the cecum, ascending colon (8) and transverse colon. Anastomoses among these vessels along the margin of the colon contribute to the formation of the marginal artery (10).

4) other structures can be identified. These include the right colic flexure (11), the left colic flexure (12), the sigmoid colon (13), the body of the T12 vertebra, and the iliac crest (14). (From Wicke L. Atlas of Radiologic Anatomy, 3rd Edition. Baltimore, Urban & Schwarzenberg, 1982).

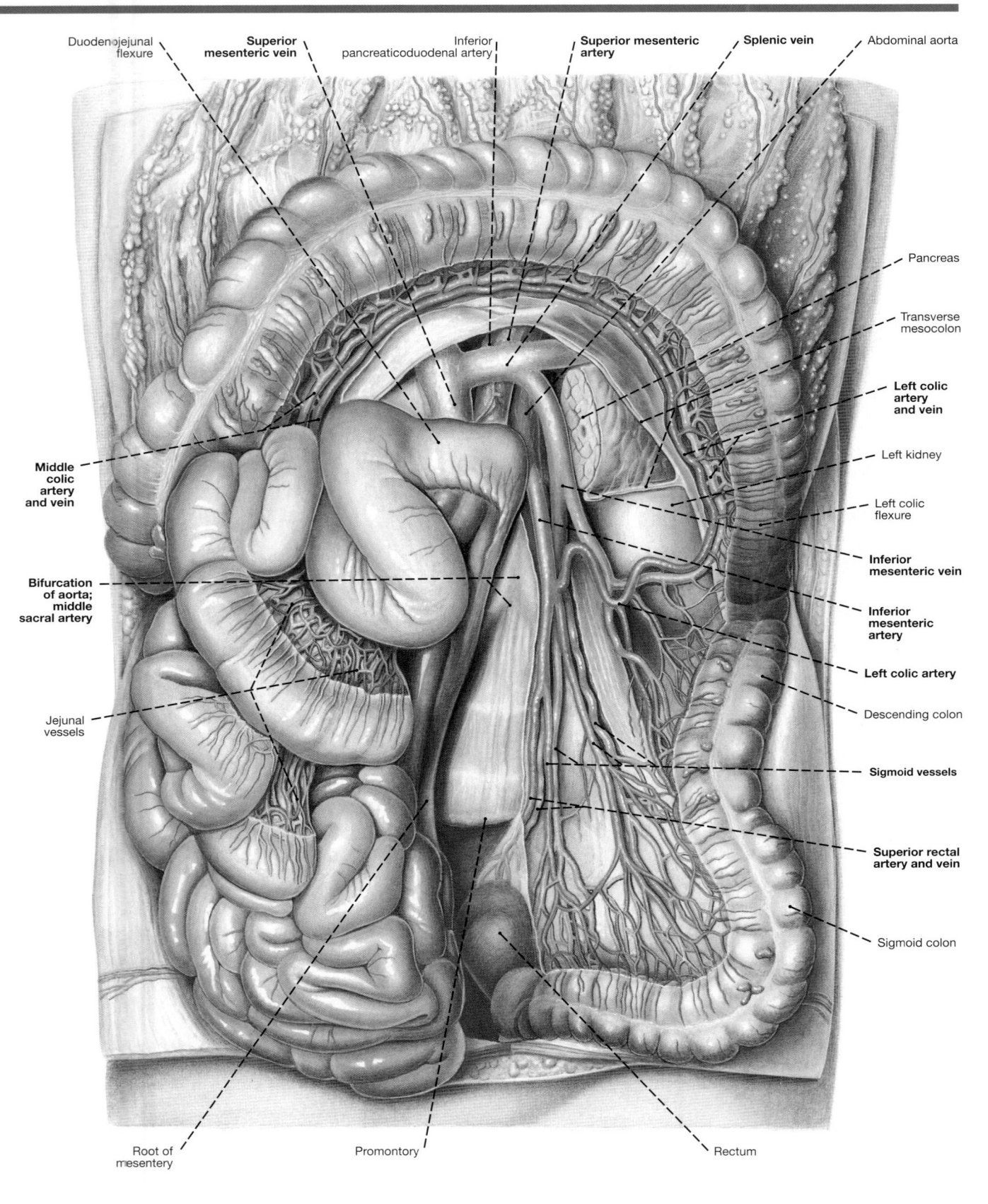

Fig. 331: Abdominal Cavity (10): Inferior Mesenteric Vessels and Branches

NOTE: 1) the small intestine has been pushed to the right and parts of the pancreas and transverse mesocolon removed to expose the origin of the superior mesenteric artery from the aorta and the drainage of the superior mesenteric vein into the splenic vein.

2) the inferior mesenteric artery supplies the descending colon via the **left colic artery** and the sigmoid colon and rectum via the **sigmoid** and **superior rectal arteries.**

Fig. 331

1. Catheter
2. Inferior mesenteric artery
3. Left colic artery
4. Ascending branch of left colic artery
5. Descending branch of left colic artery
6. Sigmoid arteries
7. Superior rectal artery
8. Left common iliac artery
9. Barium in appendix
10. Ascending colon
11. Left colic flexure
12. Descending colon
13. Sigmoid colon
14. Right renal pelvis
15. Right ureter

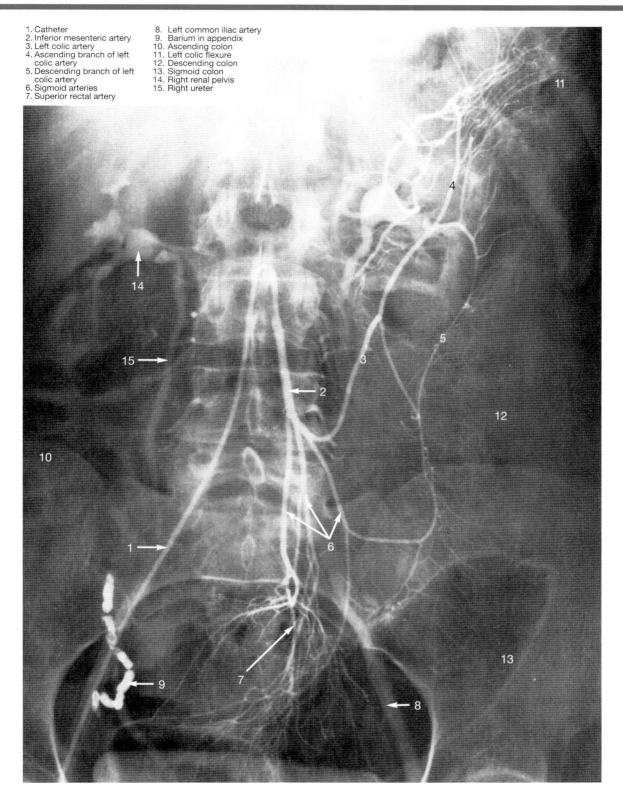

Fig. 332: Inferior Mesenteric Arteriogram

NOTE: 1) a catheter (1) was inserted through the right internal iliac artery and directed upward into the abdominal aorta to the origin of the **inferior mesenteric artery.** Contrast medium was injected into that artery to demonstrate its field of distribution.

2) the branches of the inferior mesenteric artery shown above are normal. The **left colic artery** (3) shows both an ascending (4) and a descending branch (5).

3) several **sigmoid arteries** (6) supply the sigmoid colon (13) and these anastomose above with branches of the left colic artery (3) and below with the **superior rectal artery** (7). (From Wicke L. Atlas of Radiologic Anatomy, 3rd Ed. Baltimore, Urban & Schwarzenberg, 1982).

Fig. 332   III

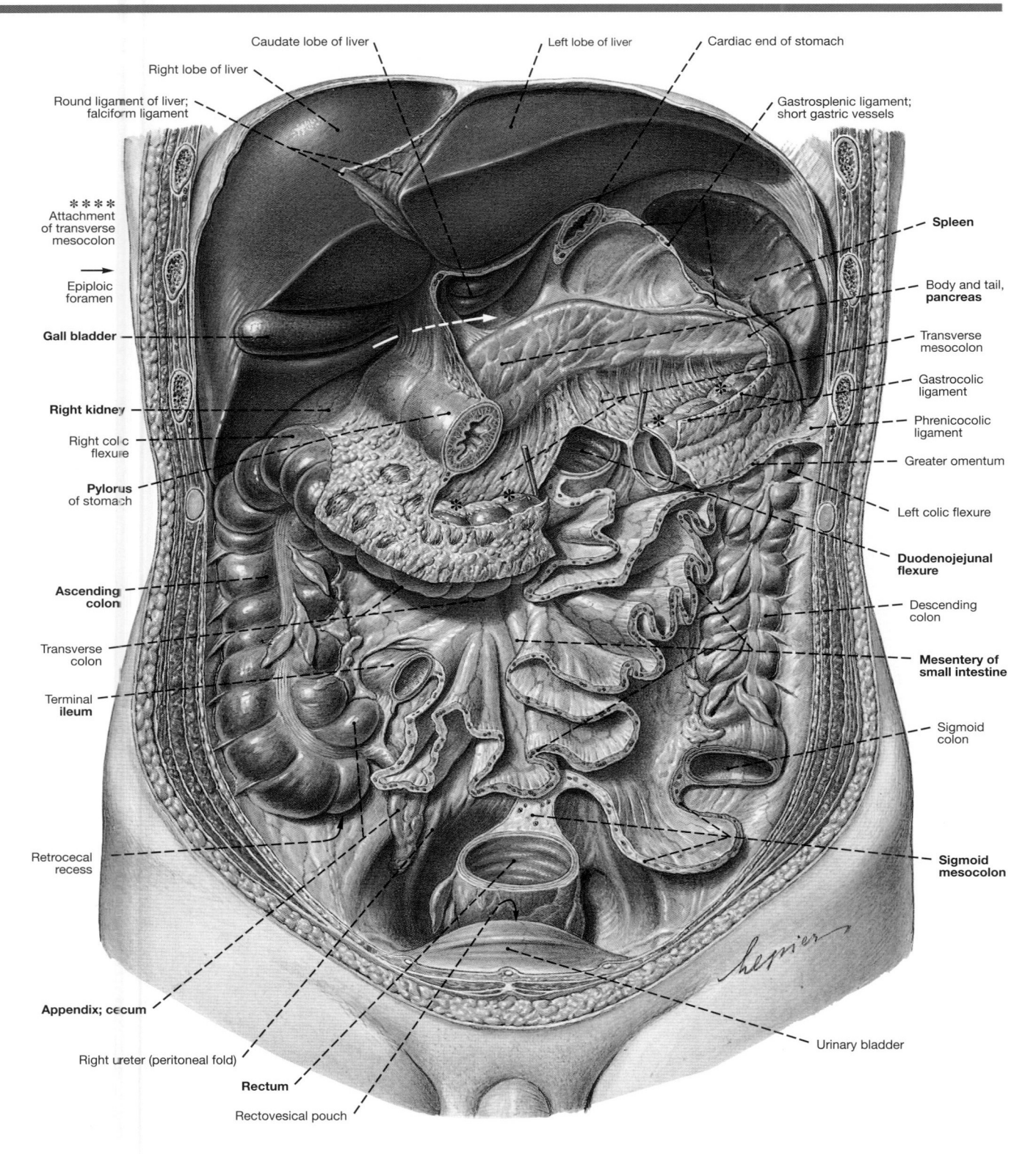

Caudate lobe of liver

Left lobe of liver

Cardiac end of stomach

Right lobe of liver

Round ligament of liver;
falciform ligament

Gastrosplenic ligament;
short gastric vessels

✳✳✳✳
Attachment
of transverse
mesocolon

Spleen

→
Epiploic
foramen

Body and tail,
pancreas

Gall bladder

Transverse
mesocolon

Gastrocolic
ligament

Right kidney

Phrenicocolic
ligament

Right colic
flexure

Greater omentum

Pylorus
of stomach

Left colic flexure

**Duodenojejunal
flexure**

**Ascending
colon**

Descending
colon

Transverse
colon

**Mesentery of
small intestine**

Terminal
ileum

Sigmoid
colon

Retrocecal
recess

**Sigmoid
mesocolon**

Appendix; cecum

Urinary bladder

Right ureter (peritoneal fold)

Rectum

Rectovesical pouch

Fig. 333: Abdominal Cavity (11): Large Intestine and Mesenteries

NOTE: 1) the stomach was cut just proximal to the pylorus and removed, the small intestine was severed at the duodenojejunal junction and at the distal ileum and also removed (by cutting the mesentery). A part of the transverse colon was resected along the greater omentum, and the sigmoid colon was removed to reveal its mesocolon.

2) the **mesentery of the small intestine** extends obliquely across the posterior abdominal wall from the **duodenojejunal junction** to the **ileocecal junction.** In this distance of 6 or 7 inches, the mesenteric folds accommodate all of the loops of jejunum and ileum.

3) the **ascending colon** and **descending colon** are fused to the posterior abdominal wall, whereas the **transverse colon** and **sigmoid colon** are suspended by their respective mesocolons.

4) the vessels and nerves supplying the small intestine course **between** the layers of the mesentery to achieve the organ.

Fig. 333

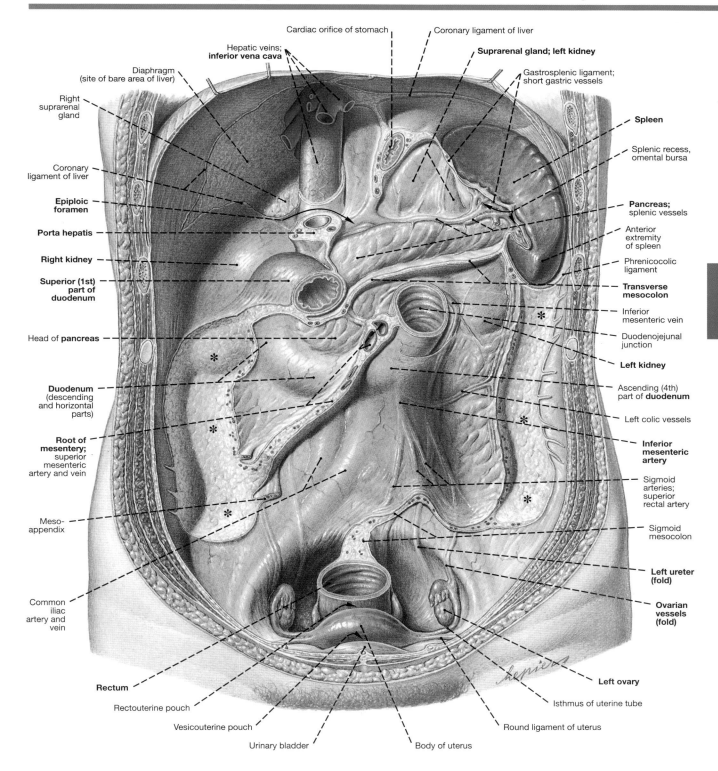

Cardiac orifice of stomach

Coronary ligament of liver

Hepatic veins;
inferior vena cava

Suprarenal gland; left kidney

Diaphragm
(site of bare area of liver)

Gastrosplenic ligament;
short gastric vessels

Right
suprarenal
gland

Spleen

Splenic recess,
omental bursa

Coronary
ligament of liver

Pancreas;
splenic vessels

**Epiploic
foramen**

Anterior
extremity
of spleen

Porta hepatis

Phrenicocolic
ligament

Right kidney

**Transverse
mesocolon**

**Superior (1st)
part of
duodenum**

Inferior
mesenteric vein

Duodenojejunal
junction

Head of **pancreas**

Left kidney

Ascending (4th)
part of **duodenum**

Duodenum
(descending
and horizontal
parts)

Left colic vessels

**Inferior
mesenteric
artery**

**Root of
mesentery;**
superior
mesenteric
artery and vein

Sigmoid
arteries;
superior
rectal artery

Sigmoid
mesocolon

Meso-
appendix

**Left ureter
(fold)**

**Ovarian
vessels
(fold)**

Common
iliac
artery and
vein

Left ovary

Rectum

Isthmus of uterine tube

Rectouterine pouch

Round ligament of uterus

Vesicouterine pouch

Urinary bladder

Body of uterus

Fig. 334: Abdominal Cavity (12): Posterior Abdominal Peritoneum (Female)

NOTE: 1) the stomach and the intestines (except for the duodenum and rectum) have been removed and their mesenteries cut close to their roots on the posterior abdominal wall. The liver and gall bladder were also removed, but the spleen and the retroperitoneal organs (duodenum, pancreas, adrenal glands, kidneys and ureters, aorta and inferior vena cava) are intact.

2) the ascending and descending portions of the large intestine are fused to the posterior abdominal wall (sites marked by *) with peritoneum covering their anterior surfaces.

3) the course of the ureters and ovarian vessels descending over the pelvic brim. Observe the ovaries, uterine tubes and uterus located in the pelvis, and their relationship to the rectum and bladder.

Fig. 334   **III**

PLATE 222   Ileocecal Junction and Cecum

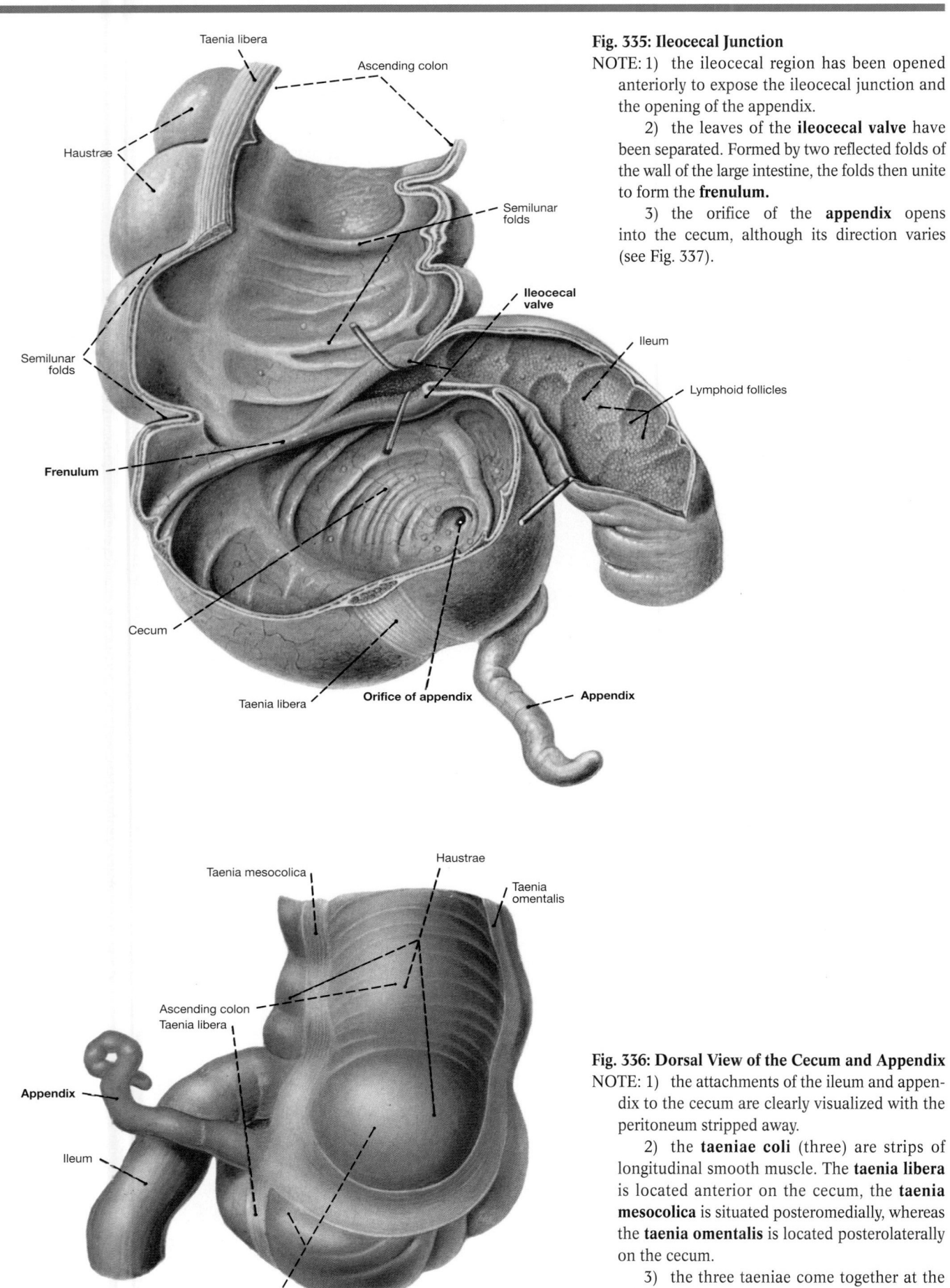

Taenia libera

Ascending colon

Haustrae

Semilunar folds

Semilunar folds

Ileocecal valve

Ileum

Lymphoid follicles

Frenulum

Cecum

Taenia libera

Orifice of appendix

Appendix

Fig. 335: Ileocecal Junction

NOTE: 1) the ileocecal region has been opened anteriorly to expose the ileocecal junction and the opening of the appendix.

2) the leaves of the **ileocecal valve** have been separated. Formed by two reflected folds of the wall of the large intestine, the folds then unite to form the **frenulum.**

3) the orifice of the **appendix** opens into the cecum, although its direction varies (see Fig. 337).

Taenia mesocolica

Haustrae

Taenia omentalis

Ascending colon
Taenia libera

Appendix

Ileum

Cecum

Fig. 336: Dorsal View of the Cecum and Appendix

NOTE: 1) the attachments of the ileum and appendix to the cecum are clearly visualized with the peritoneum stripped away.

2) the **taeniae coli** (three) are strips of longitudinal smooth muscle. The **taenia libera** is located anterior on the cecum, the **taenia mesocolica** is situated posteromedially, whereas the **taenia omentalis** is located posterolaterally on the cecum.

3) the three taeniae come together at the origin of the appendix on the cecum.

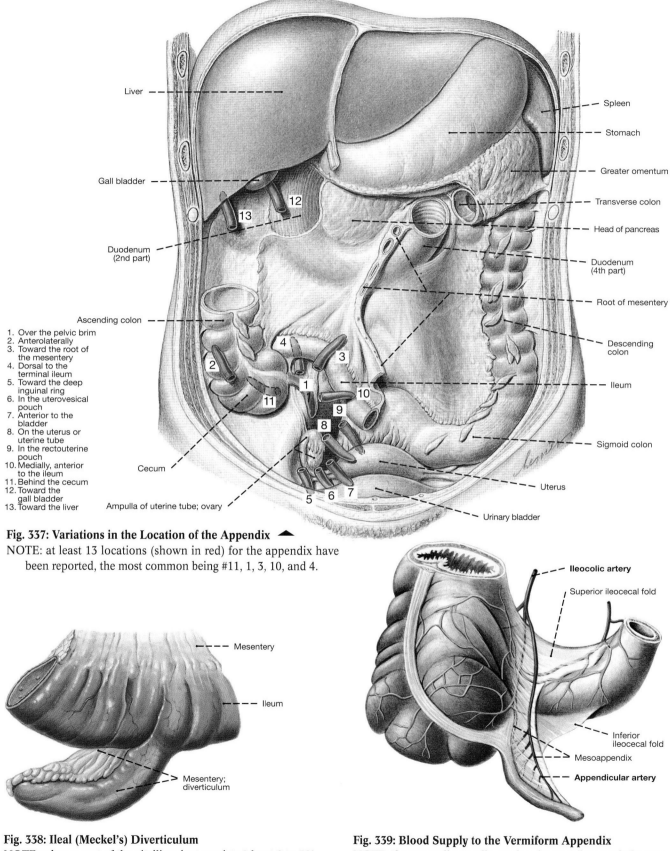

Liver

Spleen

Stomach

Greater omentum

Gall bladder

Transverse colon

Head of pancreas

Duodenum
(2nd part)

Duodenum
(4th part)

Root of mesentery

Ascending colon

Descending
colon

1. Over the pelvic brim
2. Anterolaterally
3. Toward the root of
   the mesentery
4. Dorsal to the
   terminal ileum
5. Toward the deep
   inguinal ring
6. In the uterovesical
   pouch
7. Anterior to the
   bladder
8. On the uterus or
   uterine tube
9. In the rectouterine
   pouch
10. Medially, anterior
    to the ileum
11. Behind the cecum
12. Toward the
    gall bladder
13. Toward the liver

Ileum

Sigmoid colon

Cecum

Uterus

Ampulla of uterine tube; ovary

Urinary bladder

Fig. 337: Variations in the Location of the Appendix ▲
NOTE: at least 13 locations (shown in red) for the appendix have
    been reported, the most common being #11, 1, 3, 10, and 4.

Mesentery

Ileocolic artery

Superior ileocecal fold

Ileum

Mesentery;
diverticulum

Inferior
ileocecal fold

Mesoappendix

Appendicular artery

Fig. 338: Ileal (Meckel's) Diverticulum
NOTE: when a part of the vitelline duct persists (about 2 to 3%
    of cases), it is found as a diverticulum (2 to 15 cm in
    length) of the ileum and is located about 2 to 3 feet proximal
    to the cecum.

Fig. 339: Blood Supply to the Vermiform Appendix
NOTE: the appendix usually receives its vascular supply by way
    of the **appendicular artery,** a branch of the ileocolic, and it
    descends either anterior to the ileocecal junction (as shown)
    or behind it.

PLATE 224   Large Intestine

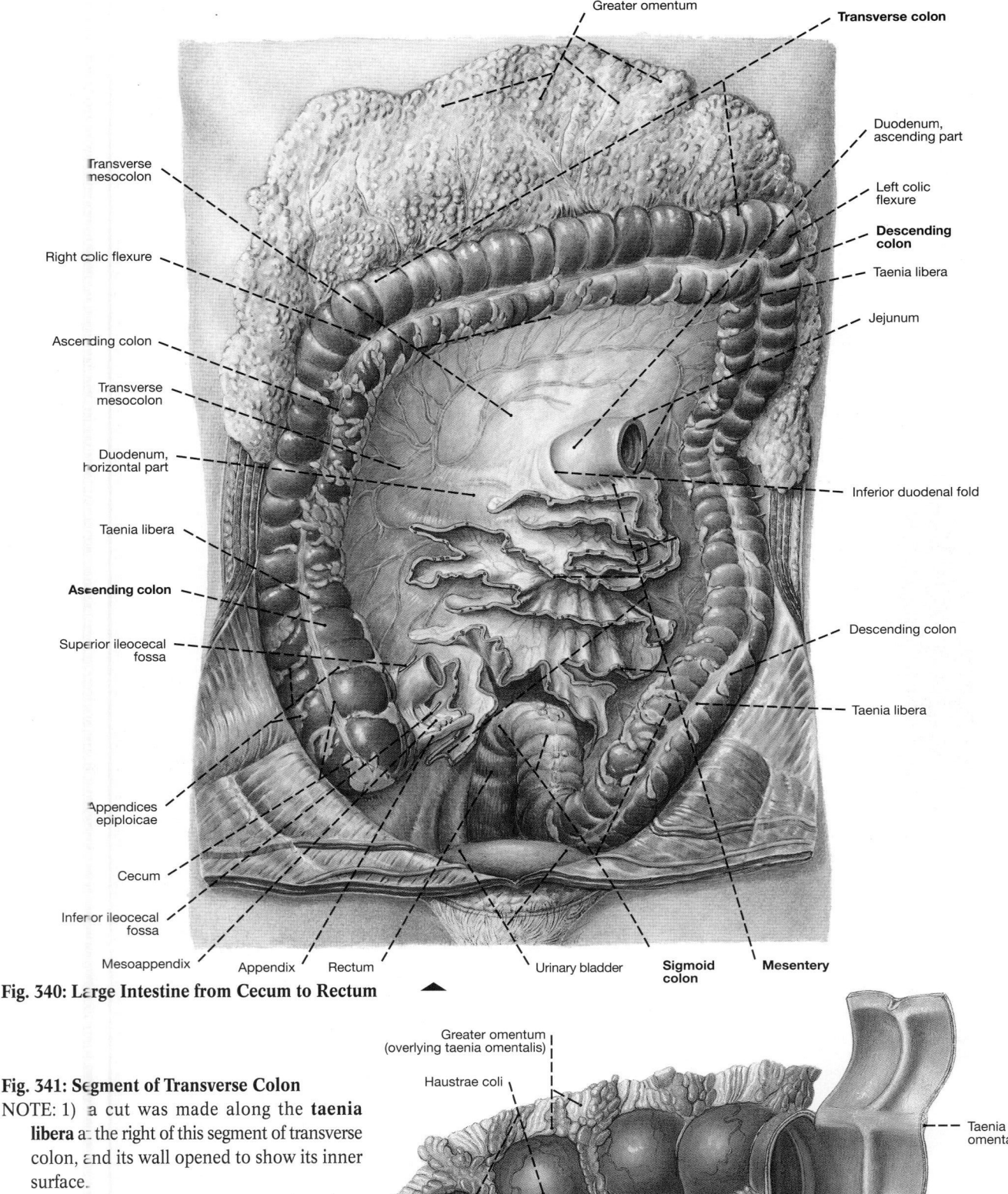

Fig. 340: Large Intestine from Cecum to Rectum

Fig. 341: Segment of Transverse Colon

NOTE: 1) a cut was made along the **taenia libera** at the right of this segment of transverse colon, and its wall opened to show its inner surface.

2) the greater omentum attaches along the **taenia omentalis,** the transverse mesocolon attaches along the **taenia mesocolica,** whereas the **taenia libera** is free from such attachments.

3) the large intestine is about 5 feet long and its diameter (1.5 to 3 inches) varies, being widest at the cecum, then narrowing, and dilating again at the rectal ampulla.

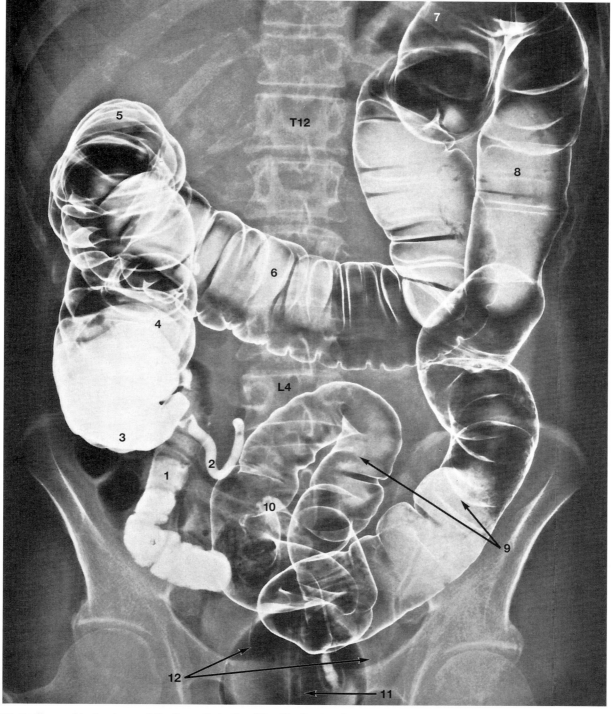

Fig. 342: Radiographic Anatomy of the Large Intestine (Double Contrast)

NOTE: 1) in this patient barium sulfate was administered as an enema and the mixture was then expelled and the colon insufflated with air (barium-air double contrast method).

2) the cecum (3) is usually located in the iliac fossa of the lower right quadrant, and it forms a cul-de-sac that opens into the ascending colon (4). The terminal ileum (1) most often joins the cecum on its medial or posterior surface. The appendix (2) extends from the cecum about 2 cm below the ileocecal opening. The right colic flexure (5) continues to the left to become the transverse colon (6).

3) the transverse colon, suspended by its mesentery, crosses the abdomen. It turns inferiorly at the left colic flexure (7) as the descending colon (8).

4) the descending colon becomes the sigmoid colon (9) at the inlet to the lesser pelvis. With its mesentery, the sigmoid colon leads into the rectum (10), within the true pelvis.

5) the locations of the T12 and L4 vertebrae, the symphysis pubis (11), and an air-filled balloon (12). (From Wicke L. Atlas of Radiologic Anatomy, 3rd Edition. Baltimore, Urban & Schwarzenberg, 1982).

Fig. 342   III

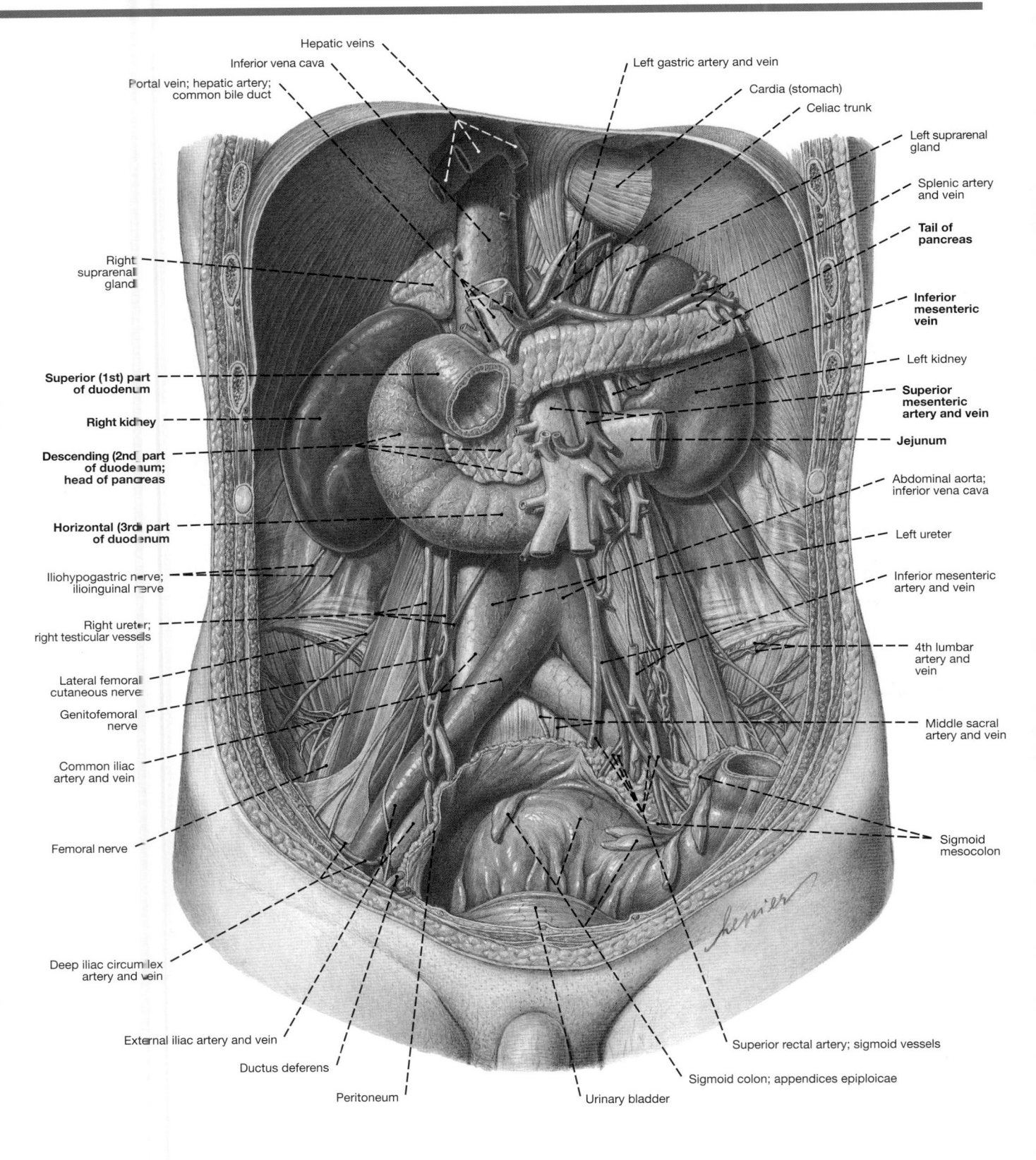

Hepatic veins

Inferior vena cava

Portal vein; hepatic artery; common bile duct

Left gastric artery and vein

Cardia (stomach)

Celiac trunk

Left suprarenal gland

Splenic artery and vein

Tail of pancreas

Inferior mesenteric vein

Left kidney

Superior mesenteric artery and vein

Jejunum

Abdominal aorta; inferior vena cava

Left ureter

Inferior mesenteric artery and vein

4th lumbar artery and vein

Middle sacral artery and vein

Sigmoid mesocolon

Superior rectal artery; sigmoid vessels

Sigmoid colon; appendices epiploicae

Right suprarenal gland

Superior (1st) part of duodenum

Right kidney

Descending (2nd part of duodenum; head of pancreas

Horizontal (3rd) part of duodenum

Iliohypogastric nerve; ilioinguinal nerve

Right ureter; right testicular vessels

Lateral femoral cutaneous nerve

Genitofemoral nerve

Common iliac artery and vein

Femoral nerve

Deep iliac circumflex artery and vein

External iliac artery and vein

Ductus deferens

Peritoneum

Urinary bladder

Fig. 343: Abdominal Cavity (13): Retroperitoneal Organs (Male)

NOTE: 1) the curvature of the duodenum lies ventral to the hilum of the right kidney, and the duodenojejunal junction is ventral to the lower medial border of the left kidney. The right kidney is slightly lower than the left.

2) the head of the pancreas lies anterior to the inferior vena cava and within the curve of the duodenum. An extension of the pancreatic head, the uncinate process (see Fig. 317) lies behind the root of the superior mesenteric vessels.

3) upon crossing the midline at the L1 level, the posterior surface of the body and tail of the pancreas is in contact with the middle third of the left kidney.

Fig. 343

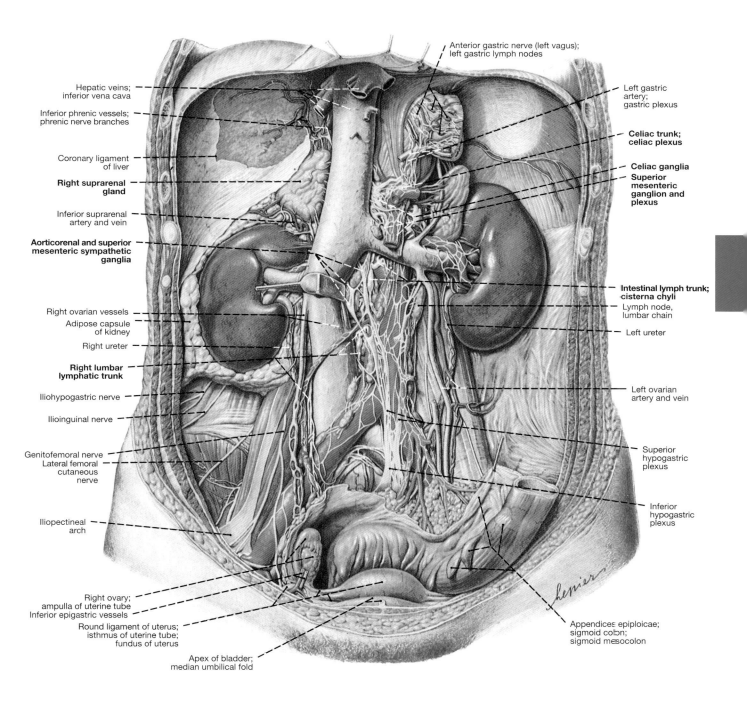

Anterior gastric nerve (left vagus); left gastric lymph nodes

Hepatic veins; inferior vena cava

Inferior phrenic vessels; phrenic nerve branches

Coronary ligament of liver

Right suprarenal gland

Inferior suprarenal artery and vein

Aorticorenal and superior mesenteric sympathetic ganglia

Right ovarian vessels

Adipose capsule of kidney

Right ureter

Right lumbar lymphatic trunk

Iliohypogastric nerve

Ilioinguinal nerve

Genitofemoral nerve
Lateral femoral cutaneous nerve

Iliopectineal arch

Right ovary; ampulla of uterine tube
Inferior epigastric vessels

Round ligament of uterus; isthmus of uterine tube; fundus of uterus

Apex of bladder; median umbilical fold

Left gastric artery; gastric plexus

Celiac trunk; celiac plexus

Celiac ganglia
Superior mesenteric ganglion and plexus

Intestinal lymph trunk; cisterna chyli

Lymph node, lumbar chain

Left ureter

Left ovarian artery and vein

Superior hypogastric plexus

Inferior hypogastric plexus

Appendices epiploicae; sigmoid colon; sigmoid mesocolon

Fig. 344: Abdominal Cavity (14): Lymphatics and Nerves of the Posterior Abdominal Wall

NOTE: 1) lymphatic channels draining the pelvic organs and the structures of the posterior abdominal wall course along iliac nodes to the right and left chains of lumbar nodes, which parallel the aorta.

2) the lumbar lymphatic trunks are joined by intestinal trunks draining the gastrointestinal organs to form the cisterna chyli.

3) the complexity of the sympathetic ganglia and autonomic plexuses found in relationship to the abdominal aorta and its branches.

4) the **superior hypogastric plexus** contains autonomic nerve fibers along with visceral afferent fibers. The autonomic fibers include **postganglionic sympathetic fibers descending** from ganglia in the abdomen to supply pelvic organs and **preganglionic parasympathetic fibers** from S2, S3, and S4 **ascending** to the abdomen to supply innervation of the large intestine beyond the transverse colon where the vagal fibers cease.

Fig. 344   III

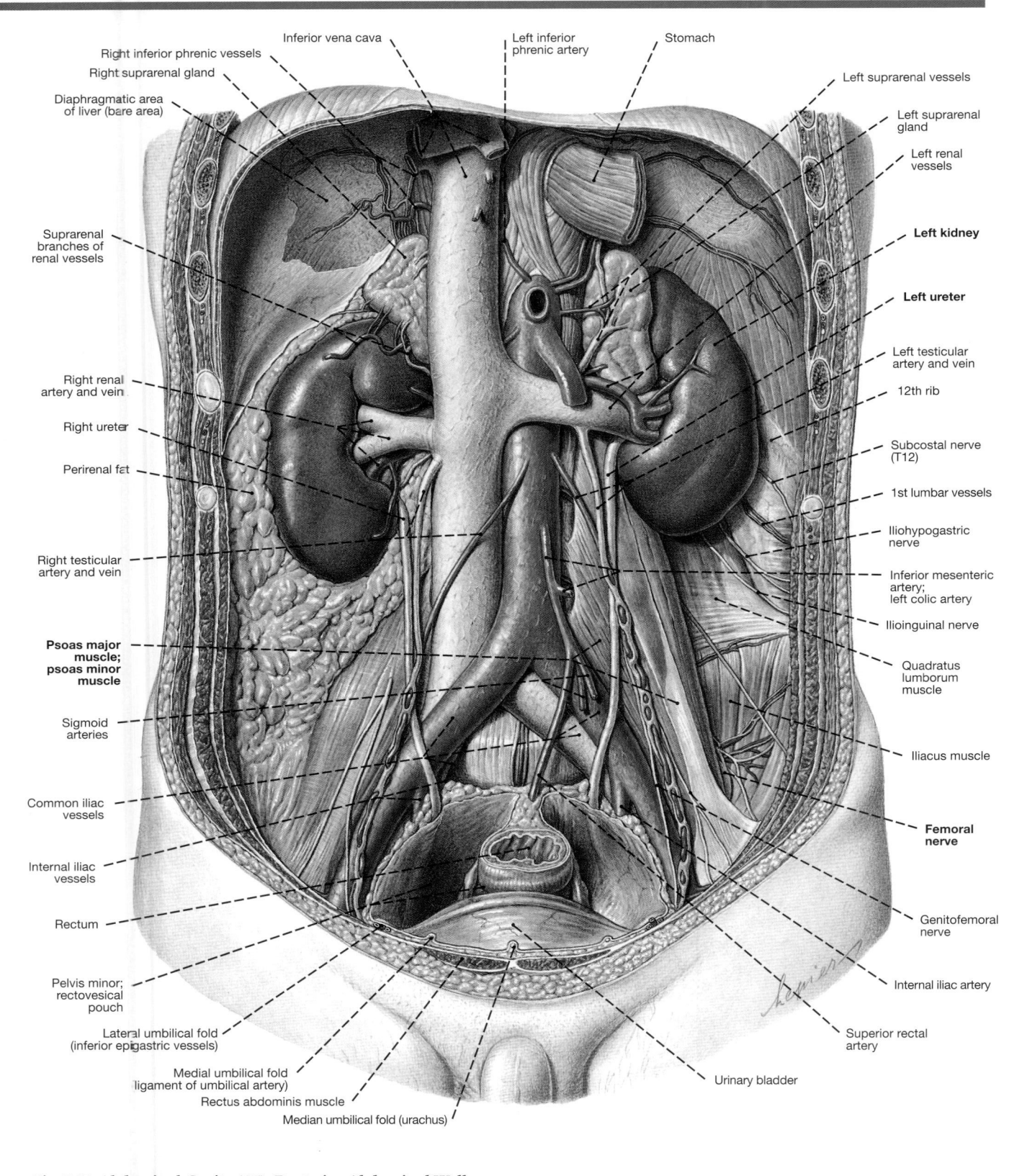

Fig. 345: Abdominal Cavity (15): Posterior Abdominal Wall

NOTE: 1) the kidneys, ureters, suprarenal glands, and the great vessels and their branches in the posterior abdominal wall.

2) the kidneys extend between T12 and L3 and the ureters course inferiorly over the pelvic brim near the iliac bifurcation to terminate in the bladder.

3) the suprarenal glands capping the upper pole of each kidney. These are highly vascular and vital organs of internal secretion (endocrine).

4) the aorta enters the abdomen through the aortic hiatus (T12) and the inferior vena cava lies to the right of the vertebral column.

Fig. 345

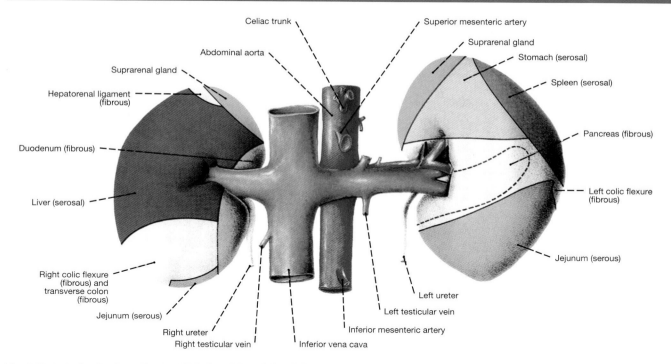

Celiac trunk

Superior mesenteric artery

Suprarenal gland

Abdominal aorta

Stomach (serosal)

Suprarenal gland

Hepatorenal ligament (fibrous)

Spleen (serosal)

Duodenum (fibrous)

Pancreas (fibrous)

Liver (serosal)

Left colic flexure (fibrous)

Jejunum (serous)

Right colic flexure (fibrous) and transverse colon (fibrous)

Jejunum (serous)

Left ureter

Right ureter

Left testicular vein

Right testicular vein

Inferior mesenteric artery

Inferior vena cava

Fig. 346: Anterior Surface Contact Relationships of the Kidneys

NOTE: 1)   the relationships of abdominal organs to the anterior surface of the kidneys are characterized either by a peritoneal reflection **(serosal)** intervening between the overlying organ and the kidney or a direct contact between the kidney and the overlying organ **(fibrous).**

2)   the structures in contact with the anterior surface of the **right kidney** are the right suprarenal gland, the hepatorenal ligament, the duodenum (2nd part), the liver, the right colic flexure and transverse colon and a small area of the jejunum.

3)   the structures in contact with the anterior surface of the **left kidney** are the left suprarenal gland, the stomach, the spleen, pancreas, jejunum, and left colic flexure.

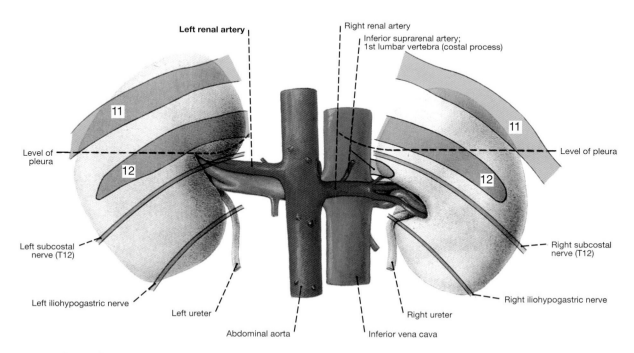

Left renal artery

Right renal artery

Inferior suprarenal artery; 1st lumbar vertebra (costal process)

11

11

Level of pleura

Level of pleura

12

12

Left subcostal nerve (T12)

Right subcostal nerve (T12)

Left iliohypogastric nerve

Right iliohypogastric nerve

Left ureter

Right ureter

Abdominal aorta

Inferior vena cava

Fig. 347: Posterior Surface Contact Relationships of the Kidneys

NOTE: 1)   the 11th and 12th ribs along with the T12 (subcostal) nerve and iliohypogastric nerve course behind the kidneys on both sides.

2)   not shown in this figure are the following muscles that help form the posterior abdominal wall and are directly behind the kidneys: the diaphragm, psoas major, quadratus lumborum, and the tendon of the transversus abdominis (see Fig. 369).

3)   the dashed lines indicate the inferior extent of the pleura on the posterior aspect of the body.

PLATE 230   Suprarenal Glands and Kidneys

Superior suprarenal arteries
(from inferior phrenic)

Superior border

Suprarenal gland

Anterior surface

Middle suprarenal arteries
(from aorta)

Fatty renal capsule

Right suprarenal veins

Fibrous renal capsule

Medial border

Inferior suprarenal artery
(from renal artery)

Right renal artery

Right renal vein

Right ureter

◀ **Fig. 348: Right Kidney and Suprarenal Gland**

NOTE: 1)   the suprarenal or adrenal gland is an endocrine gland whose secretions are vital of life. The glands are located in the posterior abdominal region and situated adjacent to the superior poles of the kidneys.

2)   the **right suprarenal gland** is pyramidal in shape and its anterior surface lies behind the inferior vena cava and adjacent to the right lobe of the liver. Its posterior surface is in contact with the diaphragm and the right kidney.

3)   the suprarenal glands are highly vascular and receive arterial blood from branches directly of the aorta and others from the inferior phrenic and renal arteries. Venous blood is drained by a single or by a pair of veins which, on the right side, flow directly into the inferior vena cava and on the left into the renal vein.

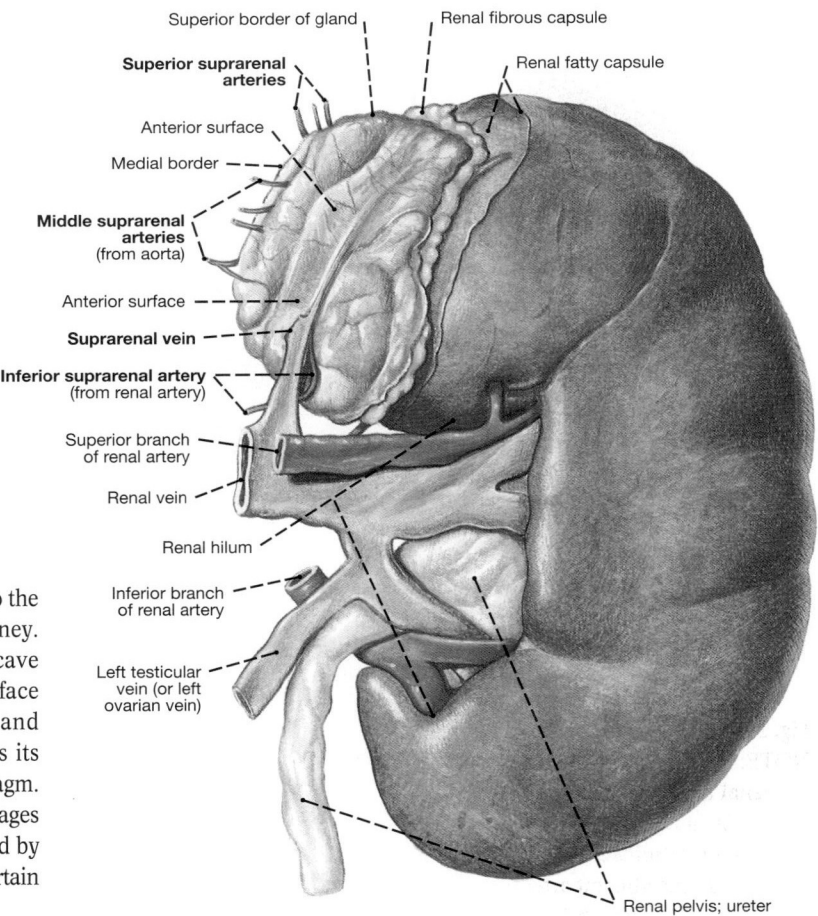

Superior border of gland

Renal fibrous capsule

Superior suprarenal arteries

Renal fatty capsule

Anterior surface

Medial border

Middle suprarenal arteries
(from aorta)

Anterior surface

Suprarenal vein

Inferior suprarenal artery
(from renal artery)

Superior branch of renal artery

Renal vein

Renal hilum

Inferior branch of renal artery

Left testicular vein (or left ovarian vein)

Renal pelvis; ureter

Fig. 349: Left Kidney and Suprarenal Gland ▶

NOTE: 1)   the **left suprarenal gland** is oriented onto the medial surface of the upper pole of the left kidney. It presents a crescenteric shape with its concave surface adjacent to the kidney. Its anterior surface lies behind the cardiac end of the stomach and pancreas (behind the omental bursa), whereas its posterior surface rests on the crus of the diaphragm.

2)   the combined weight of both glands averages about 10 grams. The glands are each surrounded by an investing fibrous capsule, around which is a certain amount of areolar tissue.

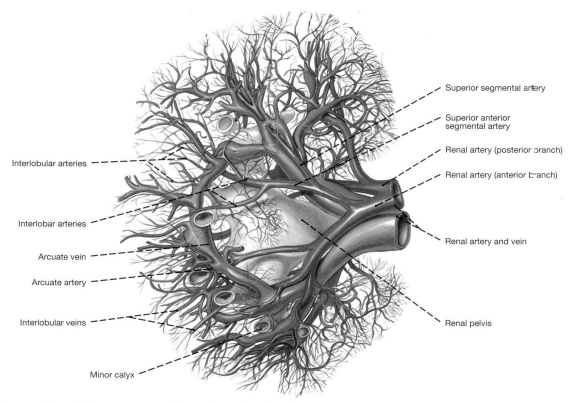

Fig. 350: Vessels of Right Kidney, Anterior View (a Corrosion Preparation)

NOTE: the main renal artery divides into **anterior** and **posterior branches** and these divide to form a variable number of **segmental arteries.** While still in the renal sinus, the segmental arteries branch into **interlobar arteries** that send **arcuate arteries** across the medullary pyramids. The arcuate arteries give rise to the **interlobular arteries** that course in the renal cortex between the renal lobules.

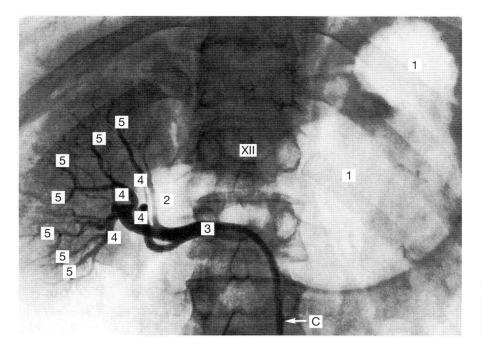

1 – Stomach
2 – Superior (1st) part of
        duodenum
3 – Right renal artery
4 – Interlobar arteries
5 – Interlobular arteries
C – Catheter
XII – 12th thoracic vertebra

Fig. 351: Arteriogram of Right Renal Artery and Its Branches

NOTE: 1) an arterial catheter (C) has been inserted into the femoral artery, passed through the abdominal aorta and then the **right renal artery.** Observe the division of the renal artery successively into **interlobar arteries.**

  2) as the interlobar arteries reach the junction of the renal cortex and medulla, they arch over the bases of the pyramids forming **arcuate arteries** (not numbered in this figure). From the arcuate arteries branch a series of **interlobular arteries** (5), which extend through the afferent arterioles entering the renal glomeruli.

  3) the stomach (1) and superior part of the duodenum (2), which are filled with air.

PLATE 232   Kidneys: Hilar Structures

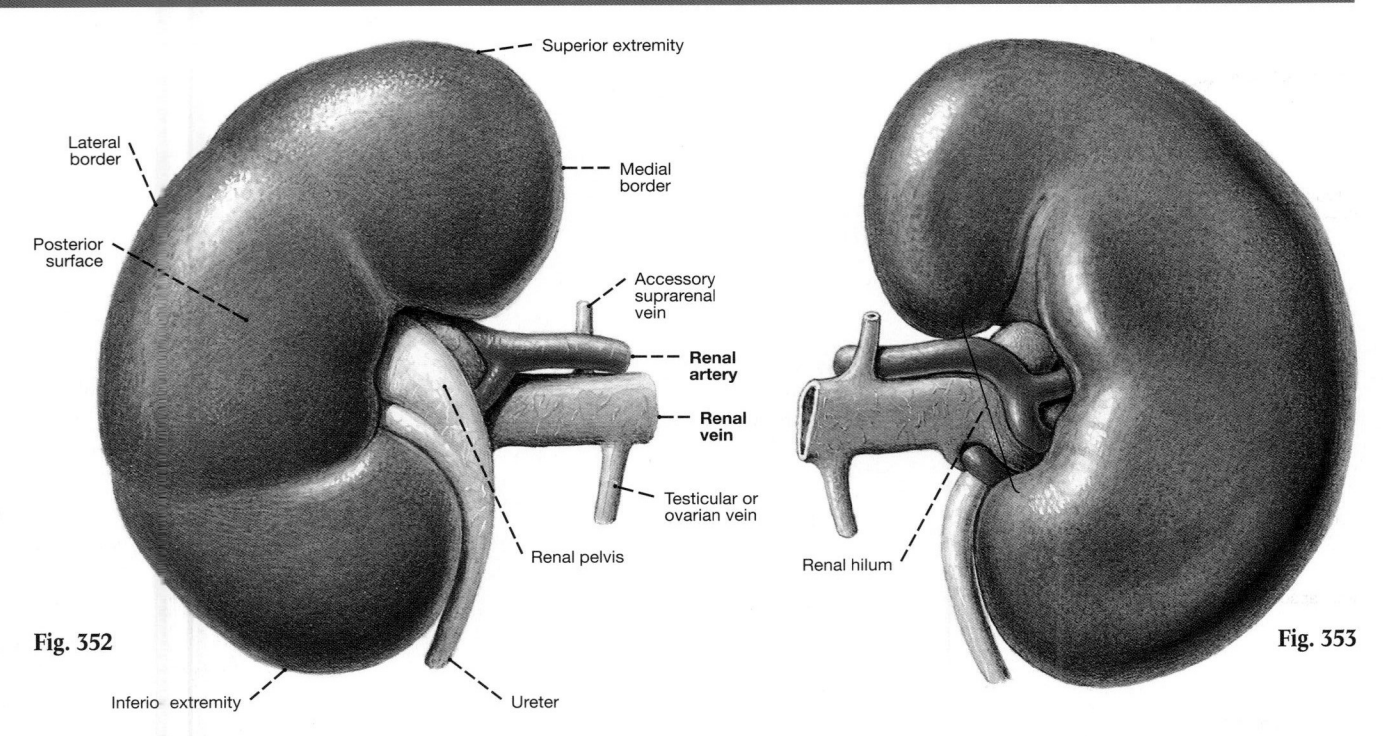

Superior extremity

Lateral border

Medial border

Posterior surface

Accessory suprarenal vein

Renal artery

Renal vein

Testicular or ovarian vein

Renal pelvis

Renal hilum

Fig. 352

Fig. 353

Inferior extremity

Ureter

Figs. 352 and 353: Left Kidney, Dorsal View (Fig. 352) and Ventral View (Fig. 353)

NOTE: 1) the kidneys are paired, bean-shaped organs and normally weigh about 125 to 150 grams each. Their lateral borders are convex and their medial borders concave, the latter being interrupted by the renal vessels and the ureter.

2) the **ureter** is the most posterior structure at the hilum (see Fig. 352). The **renal vein** is the most anterior structure at the hilum, but the **renal artery** frequently divides into anterior and posterior branches (or divisions), and the anterior branch often enters the kidney ventral to the renal vein as shown in Fig. 353.

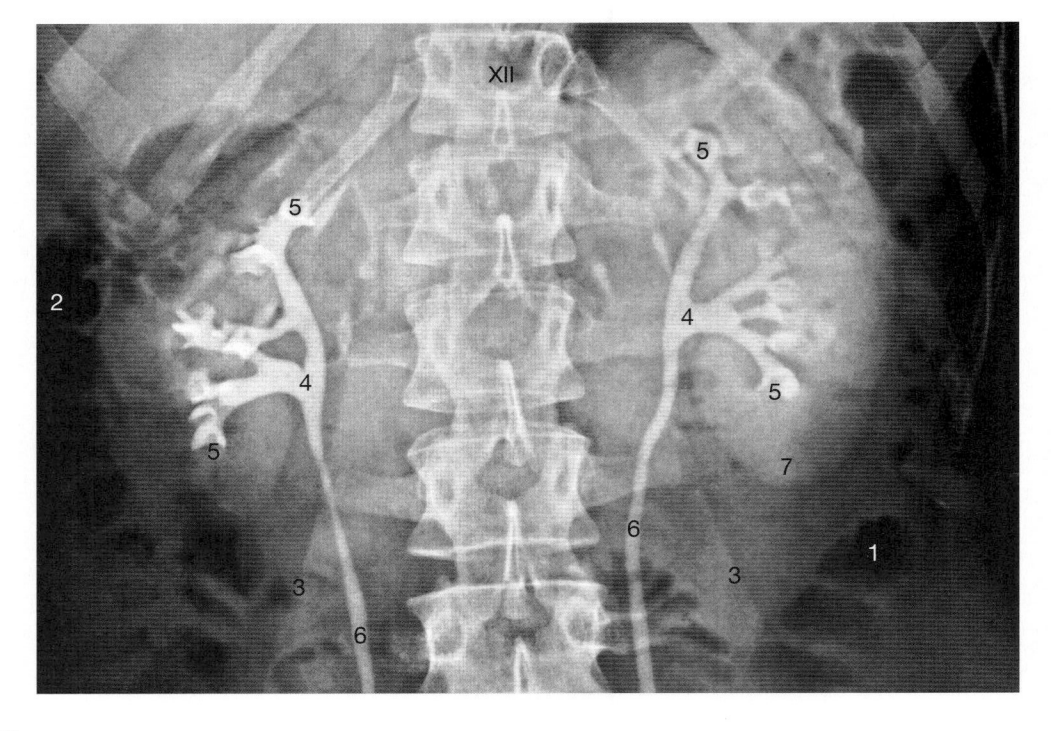

1 – Descending colon
2 – Ascending colon
3 – Psoas major muscle (lateral border)
4 – Renal pelvis
5 – Renal papilla
6 – Ureter
7 – Inferior pole of left kidney
XII – 12th thoracic vertebra

Fig. 354: Retrograde Pyelogram

NOTE: 1) a radio-opaque substance has been introduced into each ureter and forced into the renal pelvis, major calyces and minor calyces of each side. Observe that into the minor calyces project the renal papillae (5), resulting in radiolucent invaginations into the radio-opaque minor calyces.

2) the shadow of the superior extremity of the left kidney extending to top of the body of the T12 vertebra, while the right kidney is somewhat more inferior.

3) the lateral margins of the psoas major muscles (3). The ureters course toward the pelvis along their anterior surfaces.

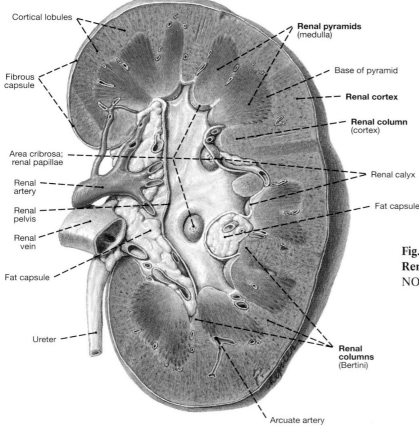

Cortical lobules

Fibrous capsule

Area cribrosa; renal papillae

Renal artery

Renal pelvis

Renal vein

Fat capsule

Ureter

Renal pyramids (medulla)

Base of pyramid

Renal cortex

Renal column (cortex)

Renal calyx

Fat capsule

Renal columns (Bertini)

Arcuate artery

Fig. 355: Left Kidney: Frontal Section Through Renal Vessels

NOTE: 1) the **cortex** of the kidney consists of an outer layer of somewhat lighter and granular-looking tissue which is also seen to dip as **renal columns** (of Bertini) toward the pelvis of the kidney, thereby separating the conical **renal pyramids** of the **medulla.**

2) within the cortex are found the tufted glomeruli and convoluted tubules, whereas the renal pyramids principally contain the loops of Henle and the collecting tubes.

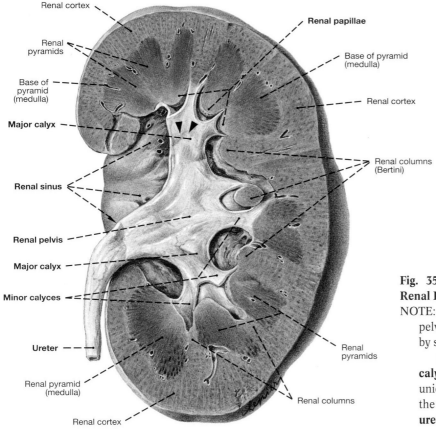

Renal cortex

Renal pyramids

Base of pyramid (medulla)

Major calyx

Renal sinus

Renal pelvis

Major calyx

Minor calyces

Ureter

Renal pyramid (medulla)

Renal cortex

Renal papillae

Base of pyramid (medulla)

Renal cortex

Renal columns (Bertini)

Renal pyramids

Renal columns

Fig. 356: Left Kidney: Frontal Section Through Renal Pelvis

NOTE: 1) this frontal section cuts through the renal pelvis and ureter. The **renal papillae** are cupped by small collecting tubes, the **minor calyces.**

2) several minor calyces unite to form a **major calyx,** whereas the **renal pelvis** is formed by the union of two or three major calyces. Leading from the renal pelvis is the somewhat more narrowed **ureter.**

PLATE 234   Fetal Kidney; Lobulation and Horseshoe Kidney

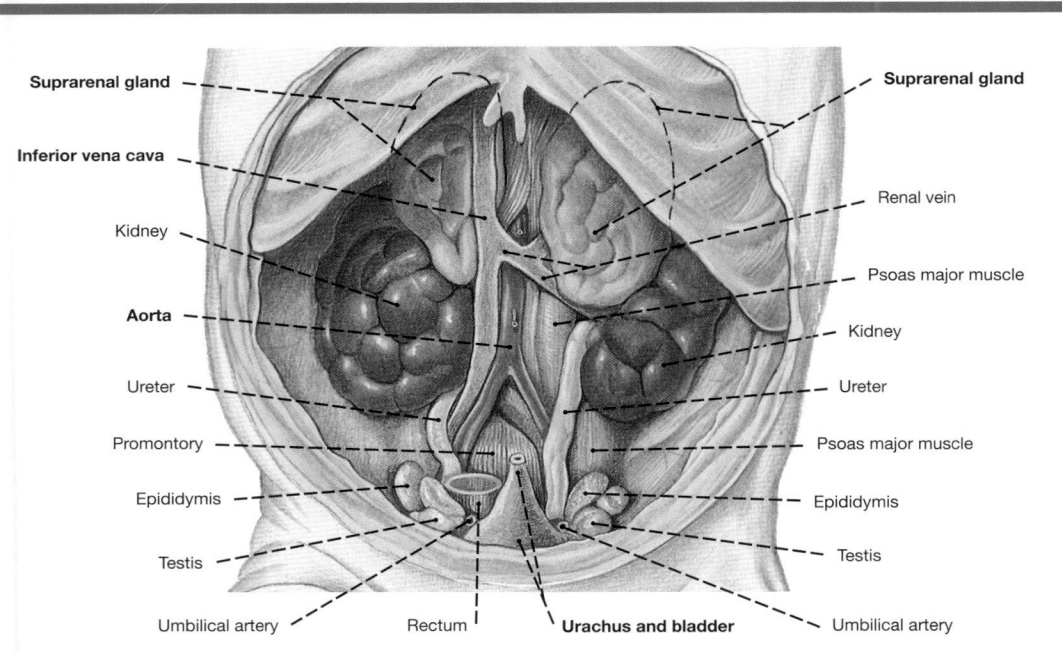

Fig. 357: Posterior Abdominal Wall in 5-Month Fetus

NOTE: 1) the kidneys and adrenal glands in this 5-month fetus. The upper abdominal organs and the intestines have been removed. The part of the adrenal glands lying behind the costal margin is indicated by dashed lines.

2) the **lobulated** appearance of the **fetal kidneys.** Even at birth this lobulation is obvious, but as maturation proceeds the surface slowly becomes smooth.

3) the large **suprarenal glands** and the enlarged and tortuous **ureters.** The testes and epididymis are still located in the lesser pelvis adjacent to the point where the abdominal inguinal ring will form the entrance to the inguinal canal.

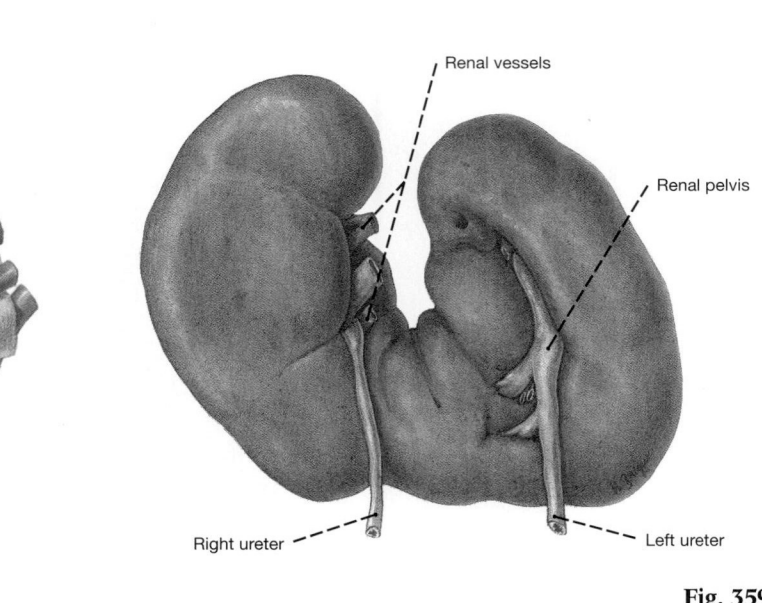

Fig. 358   **Fig. 359**

Fig. 358: Fetal Lobulation May Persist in the Adult Kidney

NOTE: the kidney of the fetus is divided into small lobules that are separated by interlacing grooves on the renal surface. This lobulation usually disappears during the 1st postnatal year but may persist in the adult but with **no functional impairment.**

Fig. 359: Horseshoe Kidney, Anterior View

NOTE: 1) **horseshoe kidney** is a common anomaly (1 in 500 persons) in which the lower poles of the kidneys are fused.

2) the fusion crosses the midline and is often found at the level of the aortic bifurcation. The ureters in the horseshoe kidney lie ventral to the renal vessels.

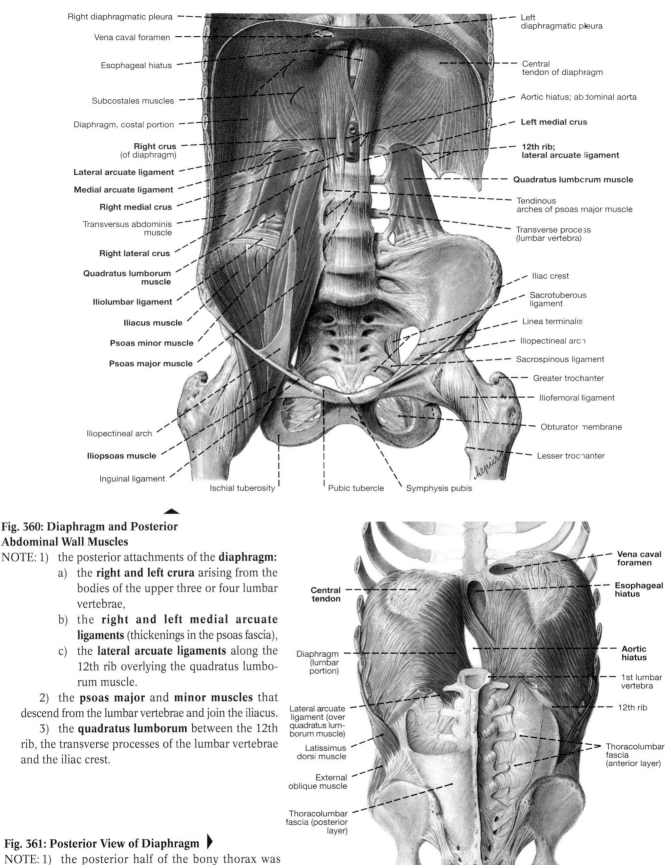

Fig. 360: Diaphragm and Posterior Abdominal Wall Muscles

NOTE: 1) the posterior attachments of the **diaphragm:**

    a) the **right and left crura** arising from the bodies of the upper three or four lumbar vertebrae,

    b) the **right and left medial arcuate ligaments** (thickenings in the psoas fascia),

    c) the **lateral arcuate ligaments** along the 12th rib overlying the quadratus lumborum muscle.

    2) the **psoas major** and **minor muscles** that descend from the lumbar vertebrae and join the iliacus.

    3) the **quadratus lumborum** between the 12th rib, the transverse processes of the lumbar vertebrae and the iliac crest.

Fig. 361: Posterior View of Diaphragm ▶

NOTE: 1) the posterior half of the bony thorax was removed to show the diaphragm from behind.

    2) the muscle fibers of the diaphragm converge to insert into a central tendon. The right dome of the diaphragm is higher than the left.

PLATE 236   Posterior Abdominal Wall Muscles Including the Diaphragm

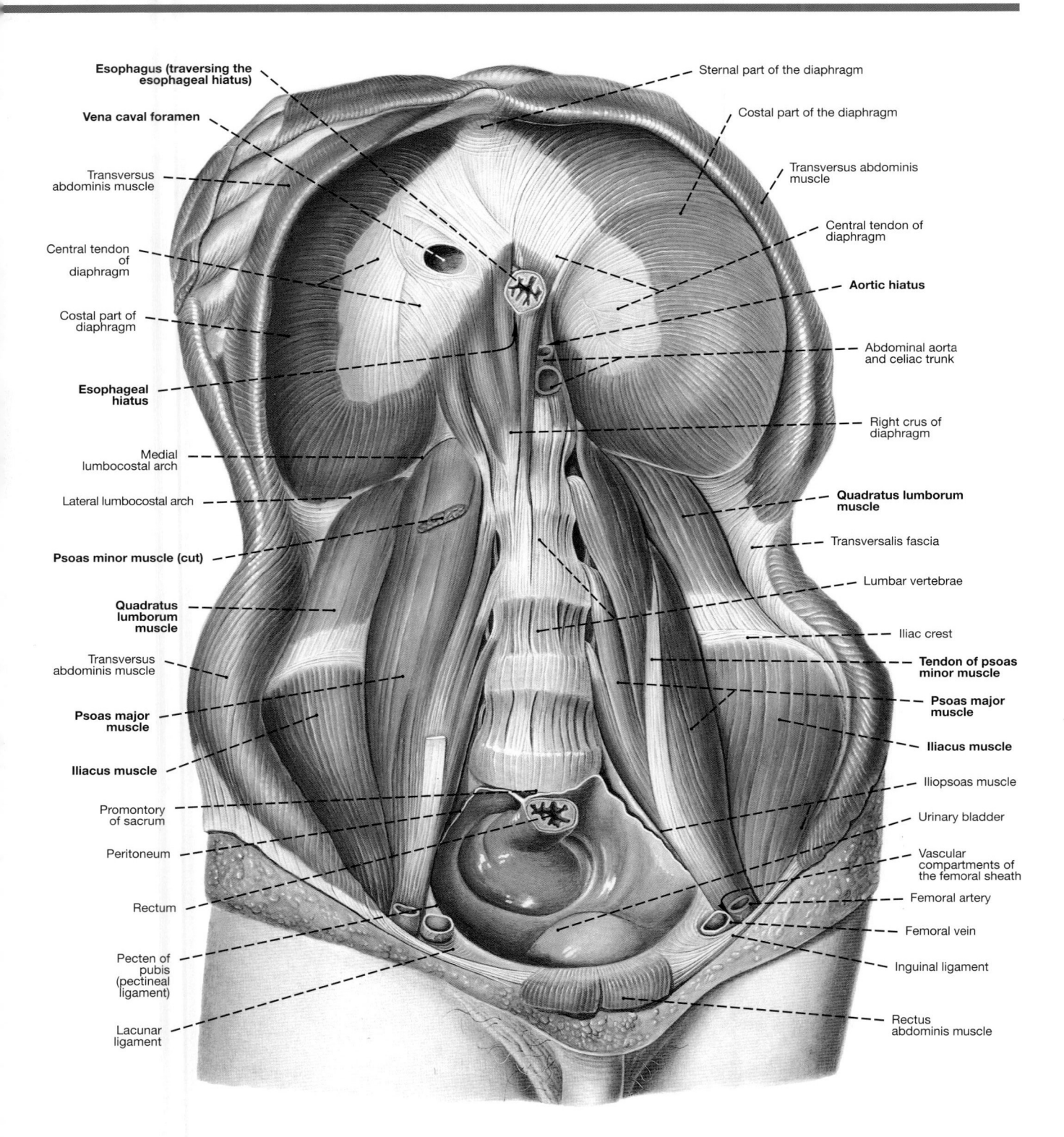

Esophagus (traversing the esophageal hiatus)

Vena caval foramen

Transversus abdominis muscle

Central tendon of diaphragm

Costal part of diaphragm

Esophageal hiatus

Medial lumbocostal arch

Lateral lumbocostal arch

Psoas minor muscle (cut)

Quadratus lumborum muscle

Transversus abdominis muscle

Psoas major muscle

Iliacus muscle

Promontory of sacrum

Peritoneum

Rectum

Pecten of pubis (pectineal ligament)

Lacunar ligament

Sternal part of the diaphragm

Costal part of the diaphragm

Transversus abdominis muscle

Central tendon of diaphragm

Aortic hiatus

Abdominal aorta and celiac trunk

Right crus of diaphragm

Quadratus lumborum muscle

Transversalis fascia

Lumbar vertebrae

Iliac crest

Tendon of psoas minor muscle

Psoas major muscle

Iliacus muscle

Iliopsoas muscle

Urinary bladder

Vascular compartments of the femoral sheath

Femoral artery

Femoral vein

Inguinal ligament

Rectus abdominis muscle

Fig. 362: Psoas Minor, Psoas Major, Iliacus, and Quadratus Lumborum Muscles and Diaphragm

NOTE: 1) the **psoas minor muscle** lies anterior to the psoas major and it merges with the lower part of the psoas major above the inguinal ligament.

2) the **psoas major muscle** descends deep to the inguinal ligament and is joined by the iliacus muscle.

3) the **iliacus muscle** arises from the iliac fossa, converges with the psoas major, and their joint tendon inserts onto the lesser trochanter of the femur.

4) the **quadratus lumborum muscle** is a four-sided muscle on the dorsal wall of the abdomen, and it is located between the 12th rib, the iliac crest, and the transverse processes of the upper four lumbar vertebrae.

Fig. 362

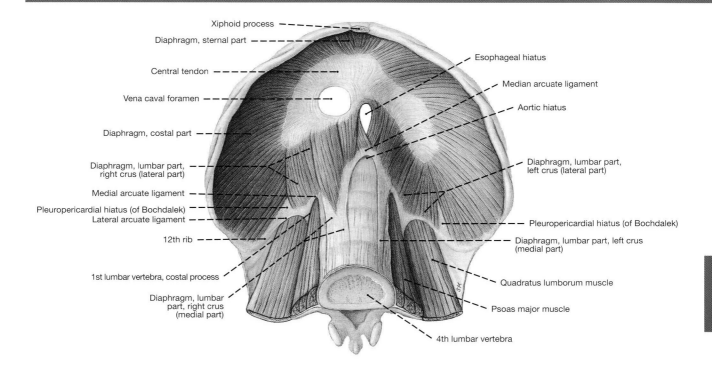

Fig. 363: Diaphragm (from below) and Arcuate Ligaments ▲

Muscle	Origin	Insertion	Innervation	Action
Diaphragm	STERNAL PART Dorsum of xiphoid process COSTAL PART Inner surfaces of cartilages and adjacent parts of lower six ribs LUMBAR PART Medial and lateral arcuate ligaments; crura from bodies of upper two or three lumbar vertebrae	Central tendon of diaphragm	Phrenic nerve C3, C4, C5	Active during inspiration; assists in increasing intraabdominal pressure
Quadratus Lumborum	Iliolumbar ligament and the adjacent iliac crest	Medial half of the 12th rib and into the transverse processes of upper four lumbar vertebrae	Branches from T12, L1, L2, L3 (L4) nerves	Flexes vertebral column to the same side; fixes 12th rib in breathing; both muscles together extend lumbar vertebrae
Psoas Major	Transverse process and body of T12 and upper four lumbar vertebrae; intervertebral discs between T12 and L5	Lesser trochanter of femur (receives also the fibers of iliacus muscle)	Branches from upper four lumbar nerves	Powerful flexor of thigh at hip; when femurs are fixed, they flex the trunk, as in sitting up from a supine position
Psoas Minor (muscle present in about 40% of cadavers)	Lateral surface of bodies of T12 and L1 vertebrae	Pectineal line and iliopectineal eminence and the iliac fascia (often merges with psoas major tendon)	Branch from L1 nerve	Weak flexor of the thigh at the hip joint
Iliacus	Iliac fossa; anterior inferior iliac spine	Lesser trochanter of femur in common with tendon of psoas major muscle	Femoral nerve (L2, L3)	Powerful flexor of thigh at the hip joint

Fig. 363   **III**

PLATE 238   **Posterior Abdominal Wall: Vessels and Nerves**

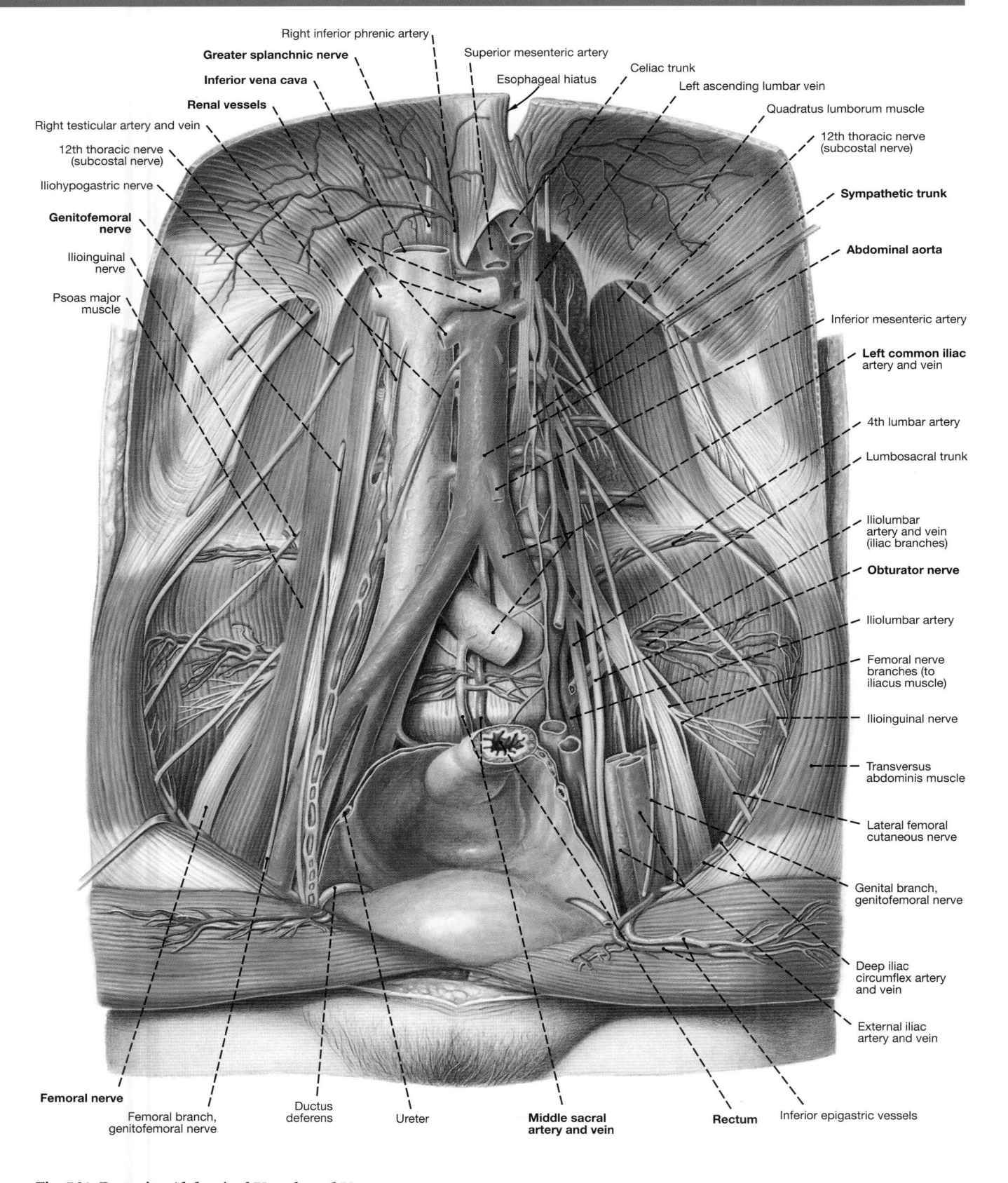

Right inferior phrenic artery

Greater splanchnic nerve

Inferior vena cava

Superior mesenteric artery

Esophageal hiatus

Celiac trunk

Left ascending lumbar vein

Renal vessels

Quadratus lumborum muscle

Right testicular artery and vein

12th thoracic nerve
(subcostal nerve)

12th thoracic nerve
(subcostal nerve)

Iliohypogastric nerve

Sympathetic trunk

**Genitofemoral
nerve**

Abdominal aorta

Ilioinguinal
nerve

Inferior mesenteric artery

Psoas major
muscle

Left common iliac
artery and vein

4th lumbar artery

Lumbosacral trunk

Iliolumbar
artery and vein
(iliac branches)

Obturator nerve

Iliolumbar artery

Femoral nerve
branches (to
iliacus muscle)

Ilioinguinal nerve

Transversus
abdominis muscle

Lateral femoral
cutaneous nerve

Genital branch,
genitofemoral nerve

Deep iliac
circumflex artery
and vein

External iliac
artery and vein

Femoral nerve

Femoral branch,
genitofemoral nerve

Ductus
deferens

Ureter

**Middle sacral
artery and vein**

Rectum

Inferior epigastric vessels

Fig. 364: Posterior Abdominal Vessels and Nerves

NOTE: 1)   the abdominal organs and the left psoas muscle have been removed. See the **greater splanchnic nerves** enter the abdomen
through the diaphragmatic crura. Identify the **inferior phrenic arteries** and the **abdominal sympathetic chain.**

2)   the **testicular arteries** arising from the aorta below the renal arteries. Inferiorly, the testicular artery and vein join the **ductus
deferens** to enter the inguinal canal through the abdominal inguinal ring just lateral to the inferior epigastric vessels. Observe the
middle sacral vessels descending into the pelvis in the midline.

Fig. 364

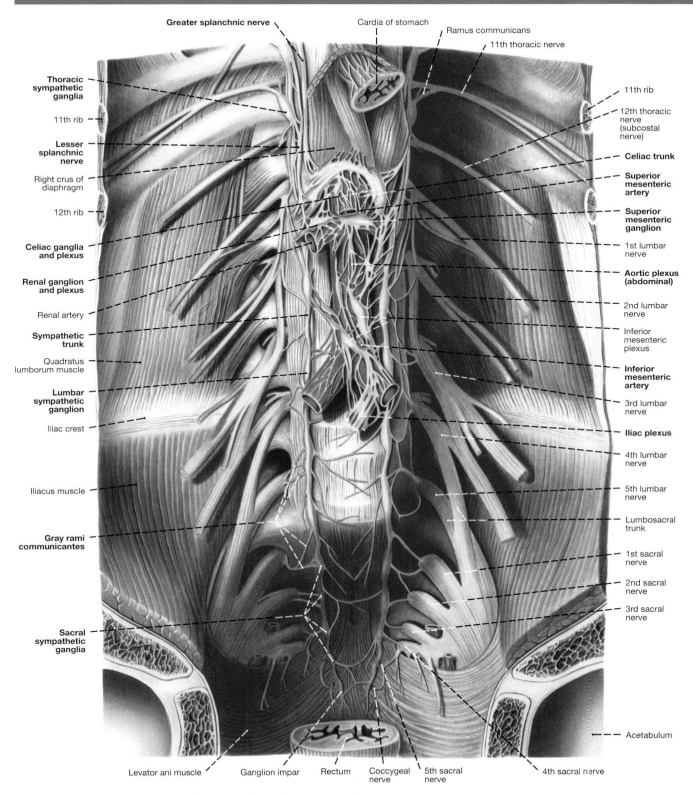

Greater splanchnic nerve

Cardia of stomach

Ramus communicans

11th thoracic nerve

Thoracic sympathetic ganglia

11th rib

Lesser splanchnic nerve

Right crus of diaphragm

12th rib

Celiac ganglia and plexus

Renal ganglion and plexus

Renal artery

Sympathetic trunk

Quadratus lumborum muscle

Lumbar sympathetic ganglion

Iliac crest

Iliacus muscle

Gray rami communicantes

Sacral sympathetic ganglia

11th rib

12th thoracic nerve (subcostal nerve)

Celiac trunk

Superior mesenteric artery

Superior mesenteric ganglion

1st lumbar nerve

Aortic plexus (abdominal)

2nd lumbar nerve

Inferior mesenteric plexus

Inferior mesenteric artery

3rd lumbar nerve

Iliac plexus

4th lumbar nerve

5th lumbar nerve

Lumbosacral trunk

1st sacral nerve

2nd sacral nerve

3rd sacral nerve

Acetabulum

Levator ani muscle   Ganglion impar   Rectum   Coccygeal nerve   5th sacral nerve   4th sacral nerve

Fig. 365: Lumbar Sympathetic Trunk and Abdominal Autonomic Ganglia

NOTE: 1) the two sympathetic chains of ganglia descending from the thorax through the abdomen and into the pelvis, and observe the plexuses and their associated ganglia, which overlie the major arteries branching from the aorta.

2) the **celiac plexuses** and the **superior mesenteric, inferior mesenteric, renal, aortic,** and **iliac plexuses** form dense networks of autonomic fibers from which many of the abdominal and pelvic viscera receive sympathetic innervation.

3) the **splanchnic nerves** (containing preganglionic sympathetic fibers) join the upper abdominal ganglia where their fibers synapse with postganglionic neurons.

4) below L2 only **gray rami** connect the ganglia of the sympathetic chain with the segmental nerves, since preganglionic fibers do not emerge from the spinal cord below L2.

Fig. 365   **III**

PLATE 240   Lumbar, Sacral, and Coccygeal Plexuses: Diagram

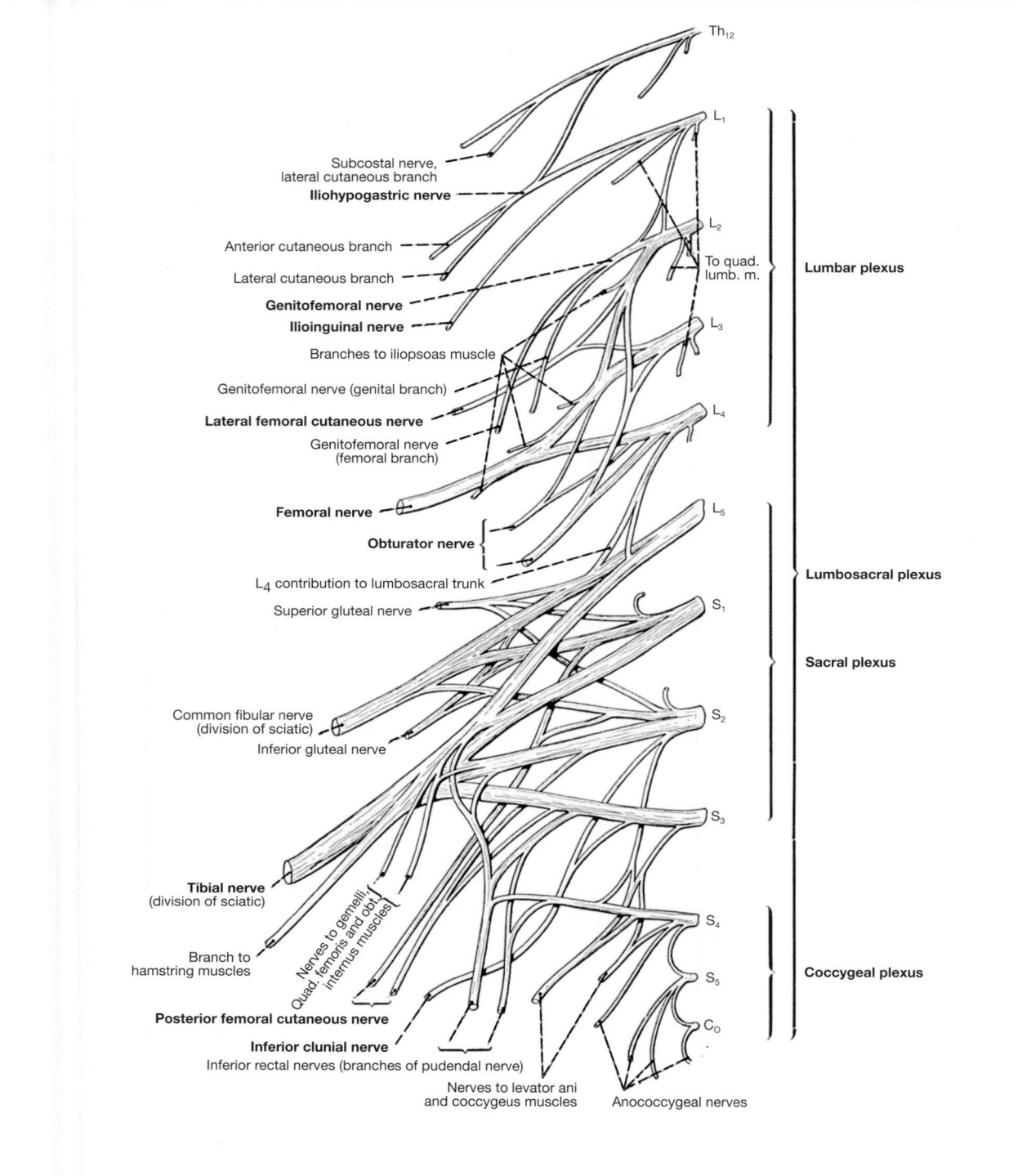

Fig. 366: Diagram of the Lumbar, Sacral, Pudendal, and Coccygeal Nerve Plexuses

NOTE: 1) the **subcostal (T12)** and **L1 nerves** are mainly distributed to the lower abdominal wall, and L1 divides into the **ilioinguinal** and **iliohypogastric nerves.**

2) **L2, L3,** and **L4** are the principal segments forming the **lumbar plexus. L1** contributes some fibers to the **genitofemoral nerve.** From these segments are derived the:

a) **genitofemoral nerve**   (L1, L2)   c) **obturator nerve**   (L2, L3, L4)
b) **lateral femoral cutaneous nerve**   (L2, L3)   d) **femoral nerve**   (L2, L3, L4)

3) **L5, S1, S2,** and **S3** with some contribution from **L4** form the **sacral plexus.** From these segments are derived:

a) **superior gluteal nerve**   (L4, L5, S1)   d) **sciatic nerve:**
b) **inferior gluteal nerve**   (L5, S1, S2)   **common fibular nerve**   (L4, L5, S1, S2)
c) **posterior femoral cutaneous nerve** (S1, S2, S3)   **tibial nerve**   (L4, L5, S1, S2, S3)

4) **S2, S3,** and **S4** also contribute to the **pudendal nerve,** which is the main sensory and motor nerve of the perineum.

Fig. 366

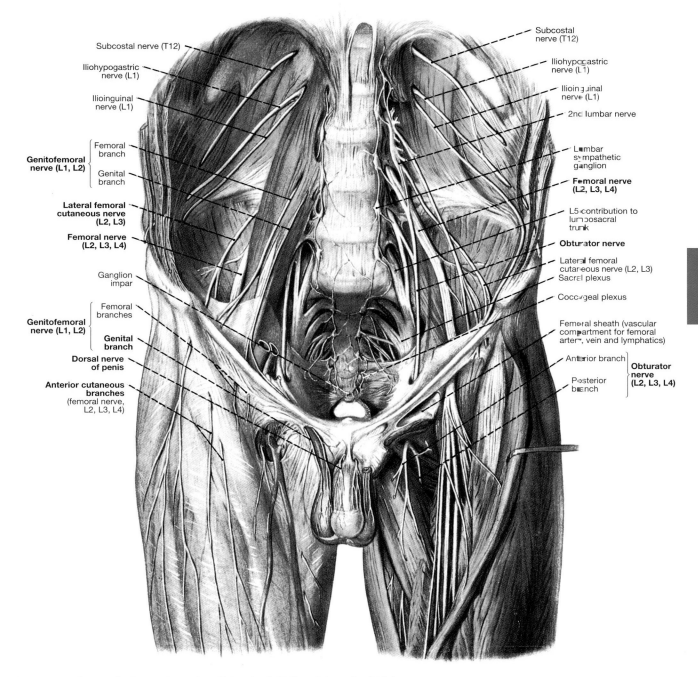

Subcostal nerve (T12)

Iliohypogastric nerve (L1)

Ilioinguinal nerve (L1)

Genitofemoral nerve (L1, L2) { Femoral branch / Genital branch

Lateral femoral cutaneous nerve (L2, L3)

Femoral nerve (L2, L3, L4)

Ganglion impar

Genitofemoral nerve (L1, L2) { Femoral branches / **Genital branch**

Dorsal nerve of penis

Anterior cutaneous branches (femoral nerve, L2, L3, L4)

Subcostal nerve (T12)

Iliohypogastric nerve (L1)

Ilioinguinal nerve (L1)

2nd lumbar nerve

Lumbar sympathetic ganglion

Femoral nerve (L2, L3, L4)

L5 contribution to lumbosacral trunk

Obturator nerve

Lateral femoral cutaneous nerve (L2, L3)
Sacral plexus

Coccygeal plexus

Femoral sheath (vascular compartment for femoral artery, vein and lymphatics)

Anterior branch } **Obturator nerve (L2, L3, L4)**
Posterior branch

Fig. 367: Lumbosacral Plexus: Posterior Abdominal Wall and Anterior Thigh

NOTE: 1)   on the left side the psoas muscles have been removed to reveal the **lumbar plexus** more completely. The lumbar nerves emerge from the spinal cord and descend along the posterior abdominal wall within the substance of the psoas muscles. The **12th thoracic** (subcostal) **nerve** courses around the abdominal wall below the 12th rib.

   2)   the **1st lumbar nerve** divides into **iliohypogastric** and **ilioinguinal branches.** The ilioinguinal nerve descends obliquely toward the iliac crest, penetrates the transversus and internal oblique muscles to join the spermatic cord, becoming cutaneous at the superficial inguinal ring.

   3)   the **genitofemoral nerve** courses superficially on the surface of the psoas major muscle. It divides into a **genital branch** (which supplies the cremaster muscle and the skin of the scrotum) and a **femoral branch** (which is sensory to the upper anterior thigh).

   4)   the **femoral** and **obturator nerves** derived from the posterior and anterior divisions of **L2, L3,** and **L4,** respectively descend to innervate the anterior and medial groups of femoral muscles.

   5)   the femoral nerve enters the thigh beneath the inguinal ligament and divides into both sensory and motor branches, whereas the obturator nerve courses more medially through the obturator foramen to innervate the adductor muscle group.

   6)   **L4** and **L5** nerve roots **(lumbosacral trunk)** join with the upper three sacral nerves to form the **sacral plexus,** from which is derived, among other nerves, the large **sciatic nerve,** which reaches the gluteal region through the greater sciatic foramen.

Fig 367   **III**

PLATE 242   Posterior Abdominal Wall and Pelvis: Vessels and Nerves

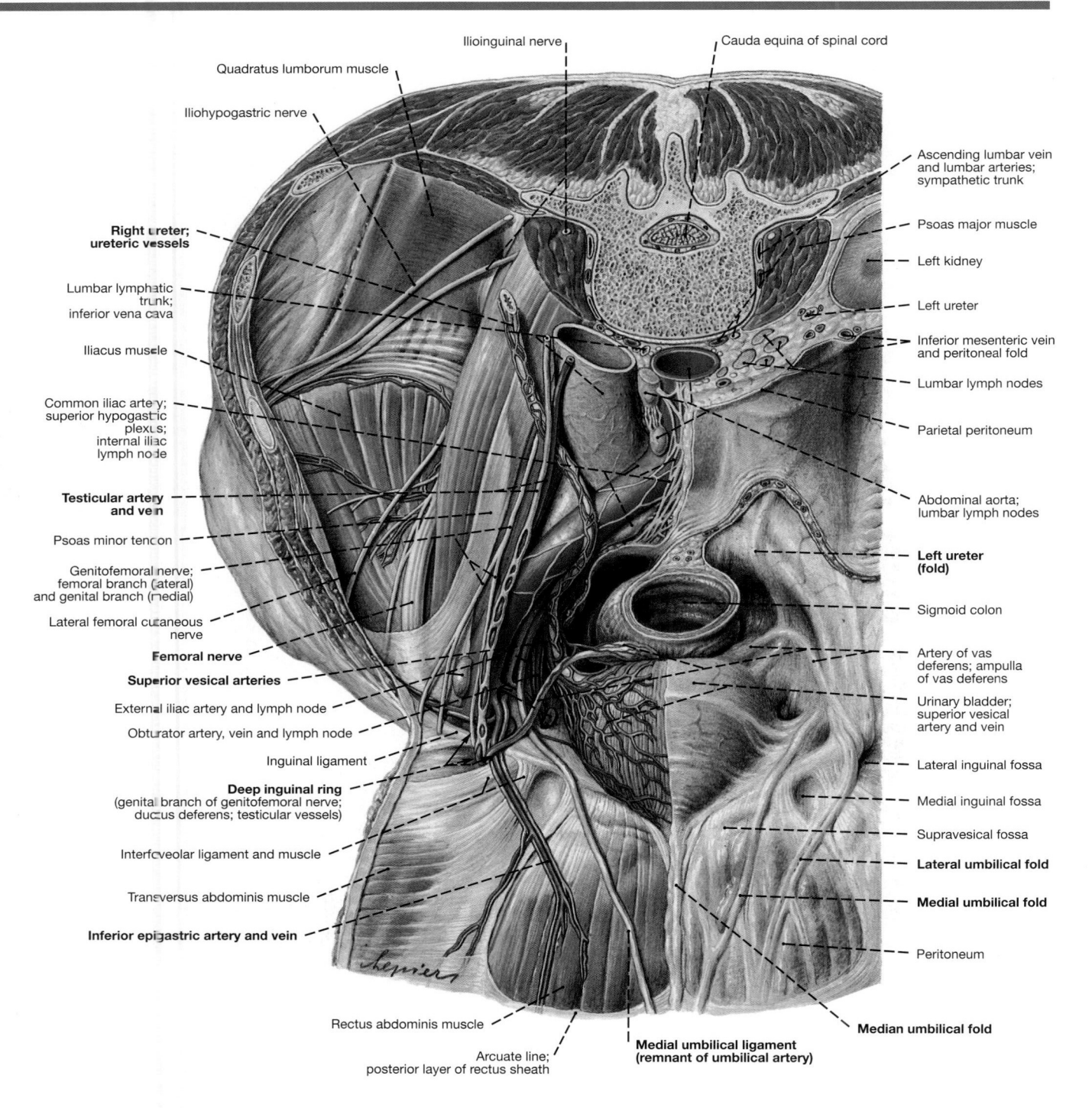

Fig. 368: Vessels and Nerves of the Inferior Abdomen and Pelvis

NOTE: 1) the entire anterior abdominal wall has been opened and reflected downward, thereby exposing its inner (posterior) surface. The body has been transected through the lumbar region just below the 3rd lumbar vertebra and the peritoneum has been stripped away on the right side but, left intact on the left.

2) this dissection shows the intact male pelvic viscera viewed from above. Observe the course of the **ureters** as they cross the pelvic brim anterior to the **common iliac arteries.** The ureter surrounded by blood vessels is seen to course medially toward the bladder, whereas the **ductus deferens** (on its path to the seminal vesicle) courses ventral to the ureter.

3) the convergence of the **testicular vessels, ductus deferens,** and **genital branch** of the **genitofemoral nerve** at the abdominal inguinal ring to help form the **spermatic cord.**

4) the origins within the pelvis of the umbilical ligaments and folds:

a) the **median umbilical fold** extending from the bladder to the umbilicus **(urachus).**

b) the **medial umbilical fold** formed by a peritoneal reflection over the obliterated umbilical artery, and

c) the **lateral umbilical fold** formed by peritoneum covering the inferior epigastric vessels.

Fig. 368

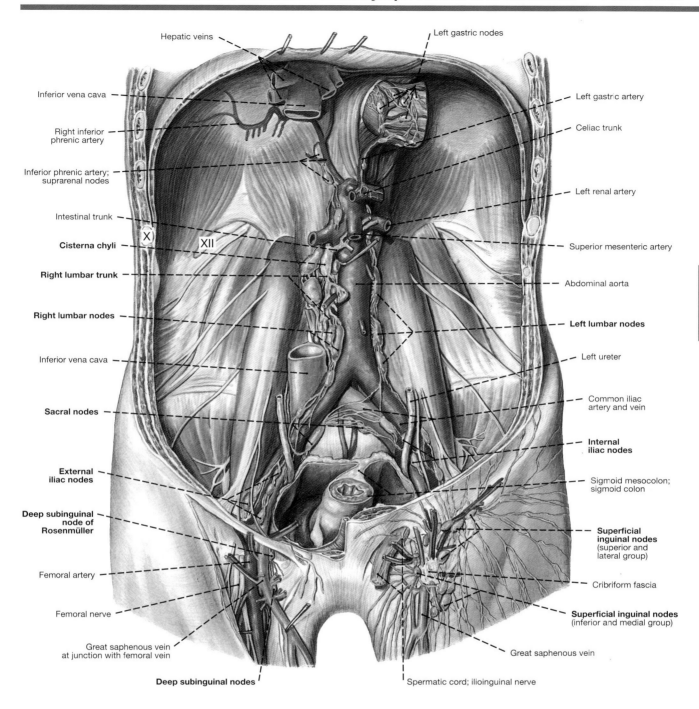

Hepatic veins

Left gastric nodes

Inferior vena cava

Left gastric artery

Right inferior phrenic artery

Celiac trunk

Inferior phrenic artery; suprarenal nodes

Left renal artery

Intestinal trunk

Cisterna chyli

Superior mesenteric artery

Right lumbar trunk

Abdominal aorta

Right lumbar nodes

Left lumbar nodes

Inferior vena cava

Left ureter

Sacral nodes

Common iliac artery and vein

Internal iliac nodes

External iliac nodes

Sigmoid mesocolon; sigmoid colon

Deep subinguinal node of Rosenmüller

Superficial inguinal nodes (superior and lateral group)

Femoral artery

Cribriform fascia

Femoral nerve

Superficial inguinal nodes (inferior and medial group)

Great saphenous vein at junction with femoral vein

Great saphenous vein

Deep subinguinal nodes

Spermatic cord; ilioinguinal nerve

Fig. 369: Inguinal, Pelvic, and Lumbar (Aortic) Lymph Nodes

NOTE: 1)   chains of lymph nodes and lymphatic vessels lie along the paths of major blood vessels from the inguinal region to the diaphragm. The **superficial inguinal nodes** lie just distal to the inguinal ligament within the superficial fascia.

2)   there are 10 to 20 superficial inguinal nodes and they receive drainage from the genitalia, perineum, gluteal region, and the anterior abdominal wall. More deeply, **subinguinal nodes** drain the lower extremity, one of which lies in the femoral ring (Rosenmüller's or Cloquet's node).

3)   within the pelvis, visceral lymph nodes lie close to the organs that they drain and they channel lymph along the paths of major blood vessels such as the **external, internal,** and **common iliac nodes** located along these vessels in the pelvis.

4)   on the posterior abdominal wall are located the **right** and **left lumbar** chains coursing along the abdominal aorta, while **preaortic nodes** are arranged around the roots of the major unpaired aortic branches, forming the **celiac** and **superior** and **inferior mesenteric nodes.**

5)   at the level of the L2 vertebra, there is a confluence of lymph channels that forms a dilated sac, the **cisterna chyli.** This is located somewhat posterior and to the right of the aorta, and it marks the commencement of the **thoracic duct.**

Fig. 369   **III**

Fig. 370

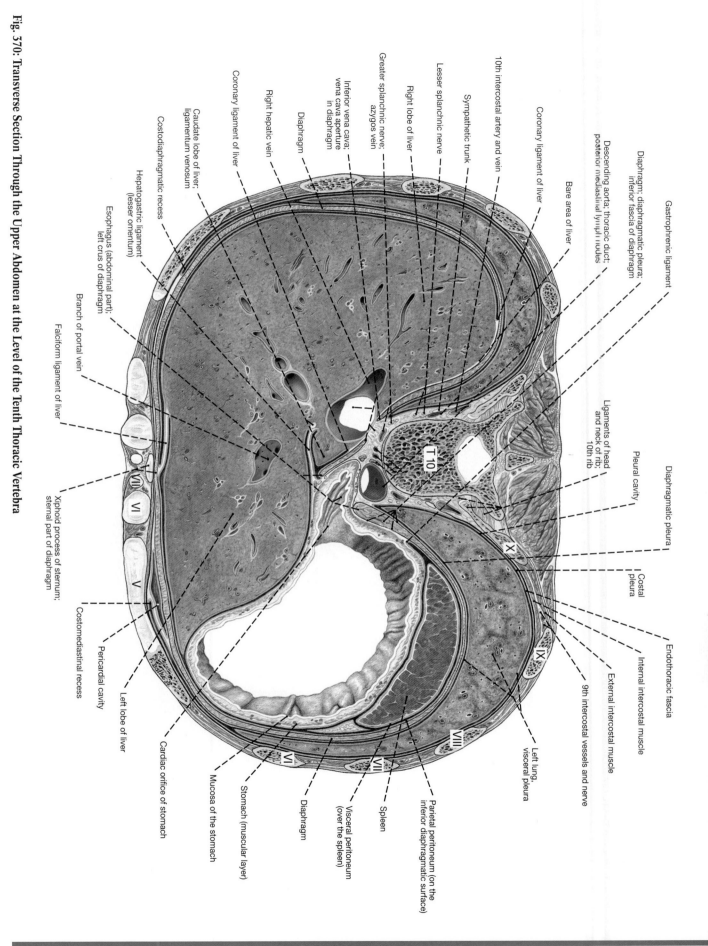

Fig. 370: Transverse Section Through the Upper Abdomen at the Level of the Tenth Thoracic Vertebra

Gastrophrenic ligament

Diaphragm; diaphragmatic pleura; inferior fascia of diaphragm

Descending aorta; thoracic duct; posterior mediastinal lymph nodes

10th intercostal artery and vein

Coronary ligament of liver

Bare area of liver

Lesser splanchnic nerve

Sympathetic trunk

Right lobe of liver

Greater splanchnic nerve

Inferior vena cava; vena cava aperture in diaphragm

Diaphragm

Right hepatic vein

Coronary ligament of liver

Costodiaphragmatic recess

Hepatogastric ligament (lesser omentum)

Caudate lobe of liver; ligamentum venosum

Esophagus (abdominal part); left crus of diaphragm

Branch of portal vein

Falciform ligament of liver

Xiphoid process of sternum; sternal part of diaphragm

Costomediastinal recess

Pericardial cavity

Left lobe of liver

Cardiac orifice of stomach

Mucosa of the stomach

Stomach (muscular layer)

Diaphragm

Spleen

Visceral peritoneum (over the spleen)

Parietal peritoneum (on the inferior diaphragmatic surface)

Left lung, visceral pleura

9th intercostal vessels and nerve

External intercostal muscle

Internal intercostal muscle

Endothoracic fascia

Costal pleura

Pleural cavity

Ligaments of head and neck of rib; 10th rib

Diaphragmatic pleura

Inferior splanchnic nerve; azygos vein

T 10

IX

X

VIII

VII

VI

V

VII

VI

PLATE 244   Cross-section of Abdomen: T10 Level

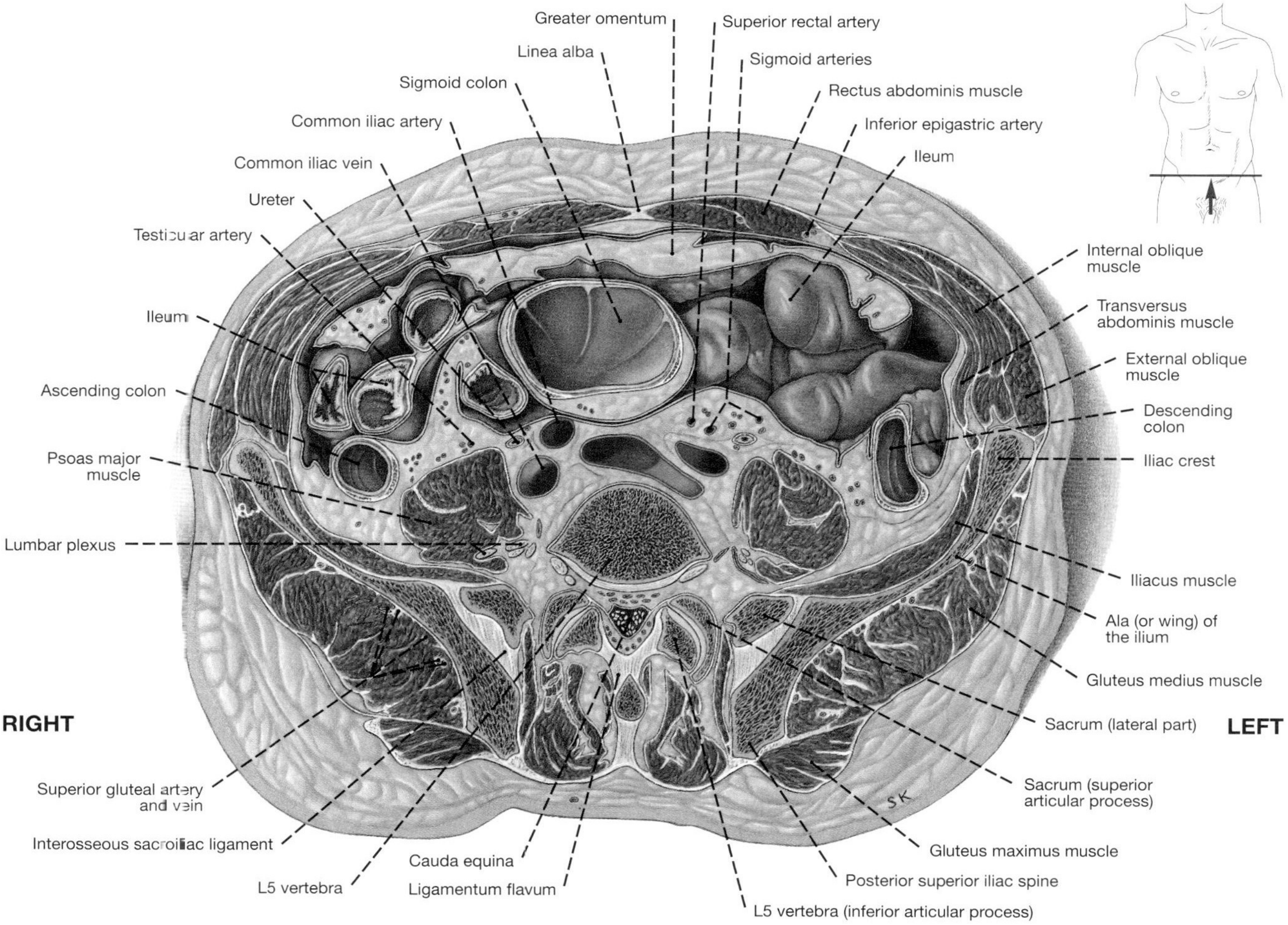

PLATE 248   **Cross-section and CT Scan of Abdomen at L5 Level**

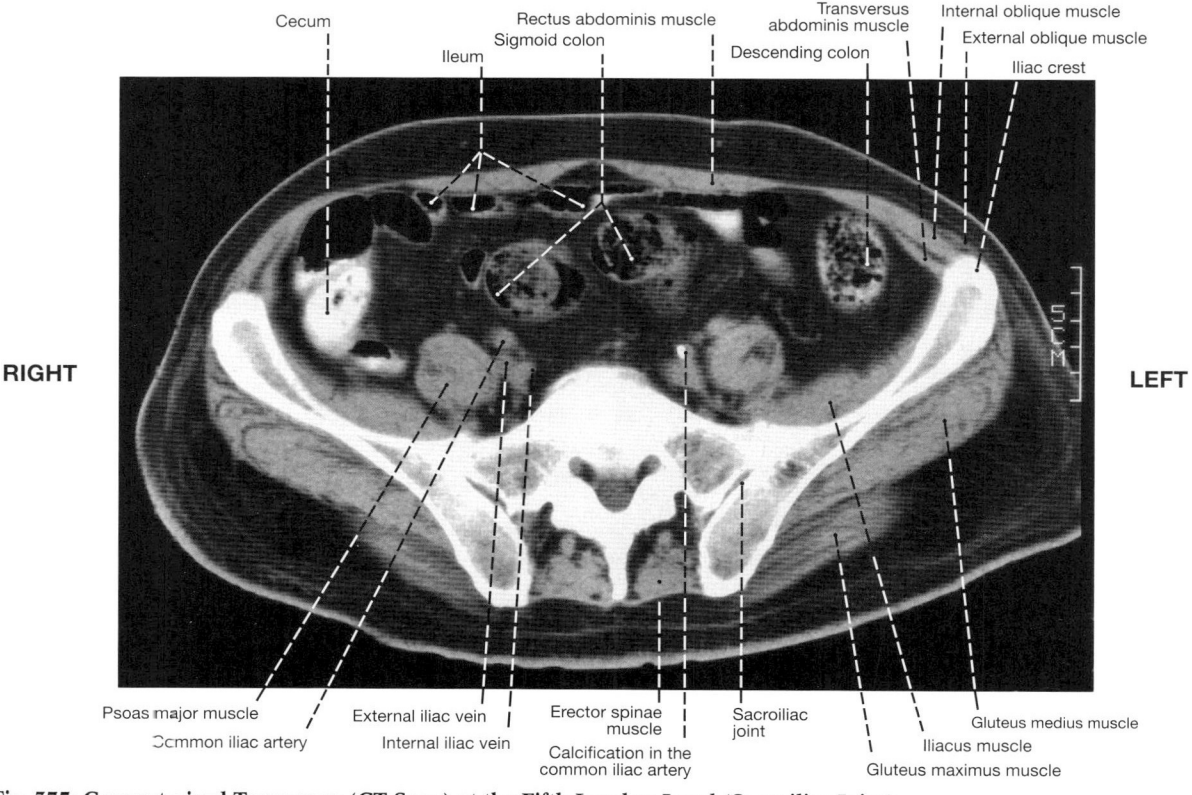

Fig. 374: Transverse Section Through the Abdomen at the Fifth Lumbar Level (Sacroiliac Joint)

Fig. 375: Computerized Tomogram (CT Scan) at the Fifth Lumbar Level (Sacroiliac Joint)

Figs. 374, 375

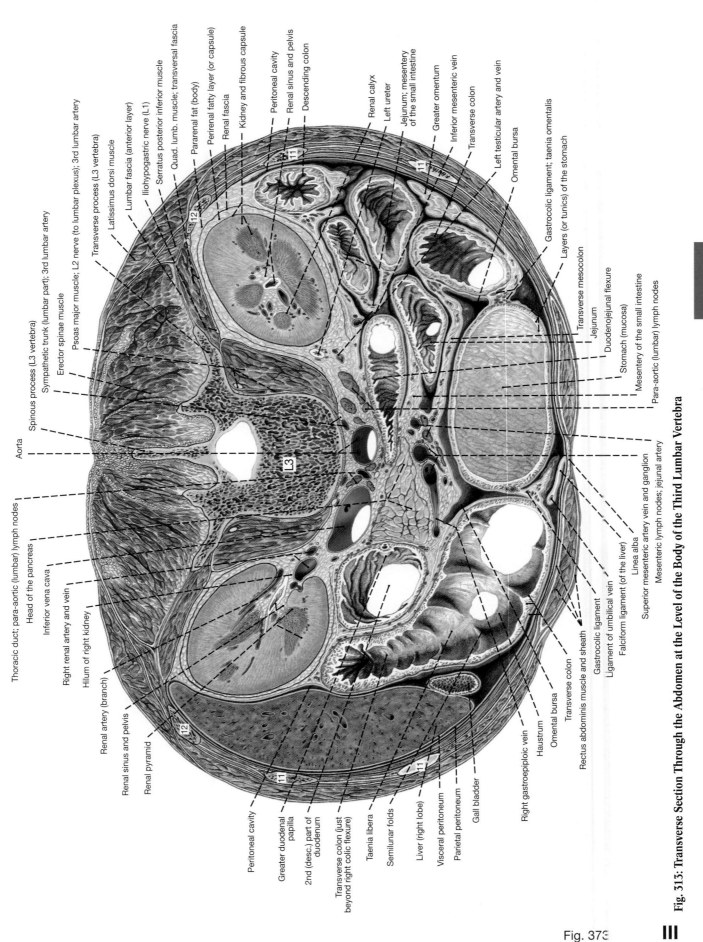

Fig. 315: Transverse Section Through the Abdomen at the Level of the Body of the Third Lumbar Vertebra

Thoracic duct; para-aortic (lumbar) lymph nodes
Head of the pancreas
Inferior vena cava
Right renal artery and vein
Hilum of right kidney

Renal artery (branch)
Renal sinus and pelvis
Renal pyramid

Peritoneal cavity
Greater duodenal papilla
2nd (desc.) part of duodenum
Transverse colon (just beyond right colic flexure)
Taenia libera
Semilunar folds
Liver (right lobe)
Visceral peritoneum
Parietal peritoneum
Gall bladder
Right gastroepiploic vein
Haustrum
Omental bursa
Transverse colon
Gastrocolic ligament
Ligament of umbilical vein
Falciform ligament (of the liver)
Linea alba
Superior mesenteric artery vein and ganglion
Mesenteric lymph nodes; jejunal artery
Rectus abdominis muscle and sheath
Para-aortic (lumbar) lymph nodes
Mesentery of the small intestine
Stomach (mucosa)
Duodenojejunal flexure
Jejunum
Transverse mesocolon
Layers (or tunics) of the stomach
Gastrocolic ligament; taenia omentalis
Left testicular artery and vein
Omental bursa
Transverse colon
Inferior mesenteric vein
Greater omentum
Jejunum; mesentery of the small intestine
Left ureter
Renal calyx
Descending colon
Renal sinus and pelvis
Peritoneal cavity
Kidney and fibrous capsule
Renal fascia
Perirenal fatty layer (or capsule)
Pararenal fat (body)
Quad. lumb. muscle; transversal fascia
Serratus posterior inferior muscle
Iliohypogastric nerve (L1)
Lumbar fascia (anterior layer)
Transverse process (L3 vertebra)
Latissimus dorsi muscle
Psoas major muscle; L2 nerve (to lumbar plexus); 3rd lumbar artery
Erector spinae muscle
Sympathetic trunk (lumbar part); 3rd lumbar artery
Spinous process (L3 vertebra)
Aorta

Fig. 373

III

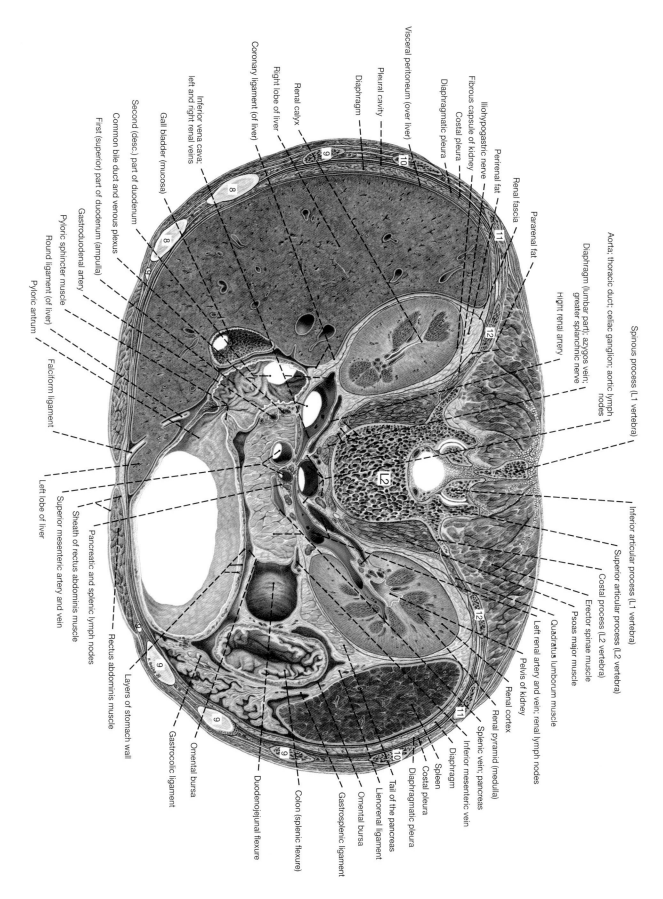

Fig. 372

Fig. 372: Transverse Section Through the Abdomen at the Level of the Body of the Second Lumbar Vertebra

Spinous process (L1 vertebra)

Aorta; thoracic duct; celiac ganglion; aortic lymph nodes

Diaphragm (lumbar part); azygos vein; greater splanchnic nerve

Right renal artery

Inferior articular process (L1 vertebra)

Superior articular process (L2 vertebra)

Costal process (L2 vertebra)

Erector spinae muscle

Psoas major muscle

Quadratus lumborum muscle

Left renal artery and vein; renal lymph nodes

Pelvis of kidney

Renal cortex

Renal pyramid (medulla)

Splenic vein; pancreas

Inferior mesenteric vein

Diaphragm

Costal pleura

Diaphragmatic pleura

Spleen

Tail of the pancreas

Omental bursa

Lienorenal ligament

Gastrosplenic ligament

Omental bursa

Gastrocolic ligament

Colon (splenic flexure)

Duodenojejunal flexure

Layers of stomach wall

Rectus abdominis muscle

Pancreatic and splenic lymph nodes

Superior mesenteric artery and vein

Sheath of rectus abdominis muscle

Left lobe of liver

Pyloric antrum

Falciform ligament

Round ligament (of liver)

Pyloric sphincter muscle

Gastroduodenal artery

First (superior) part of duodenum

Common bile duct and venous plexus

Second (desc.) part of duodenum

Gall bladder (mucosa)

Inferior vena cava; left and right renal veins

Coronary ligament (of liver)

Right lobe of liver

Renal calyx

Diaphragm

Pleural cavity

Diaphragmatic pleura

Costal pleura

Fibrous capsule of kidney

Iliohypogastric nerve

Visceral peritoneum (over liver)

Perirenal fat

Renal fascia

Pararenal fat

PLATE 246   Cross-section of Abdomen: L2 Level

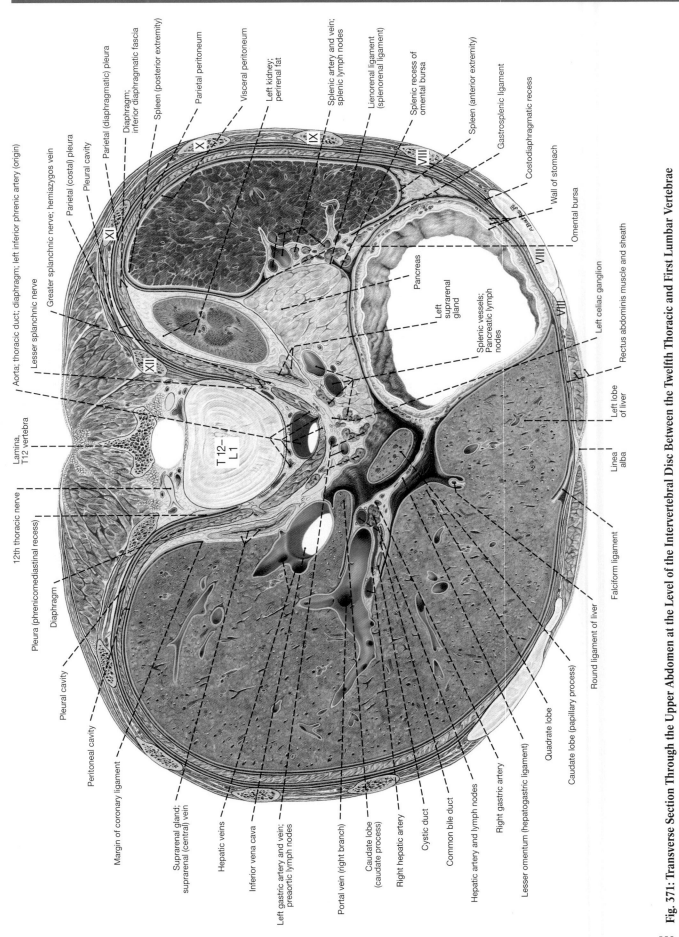

Fig. 371: Transverse Section Through the Upper Abdomen at the Level of the Intervertebral Disc Between the Twelfth Thoracic and First Lumbar Vertebrae

Fig. 371

PART IV
THE PELVIS AND PERINEUM

(PLATES 249–308 – FIGURES 376–478)

PART IV   The Pelvis and Perineum

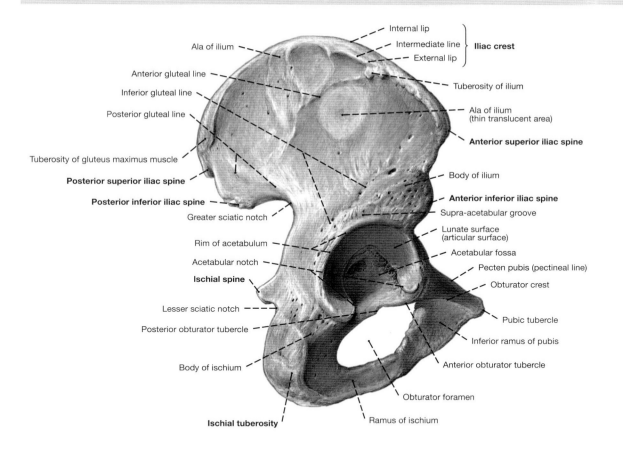

Internal lip
Intermediate line } Iliac crest
External lip

Ala of ilium

Anterior gluteal line

Inferior gluteal line

Posterior gluteal line

Tuberosity of gluteus maximus muscle

Posterior superior iliac spine

Posterior inferior iliac spine

Greater sciatic notch

Rim of acetabulum

Acetabular notch

Ischial spine

Lesser sciatic notch

Posterior obturator tubercle

Body of ischium

Ischial tuberosity

Ramus of ischium

Obturator foramen

Anterior obturator tubercle

Inferior ramus of pubis

Pubic tubercle

Obturator crest

Pecten pubis (pectineal line)

Acetabular fossa

Lunate surface (articular surface)

Supra-acetabular groove

Anterior inferior iliac spine

Body of ilium

Anterior superior iliac spine

Ala of ilium (thin translucent area)

Tuberosity of ilium

Fig. 376: Lateral View of the Adult Right Hip Bone

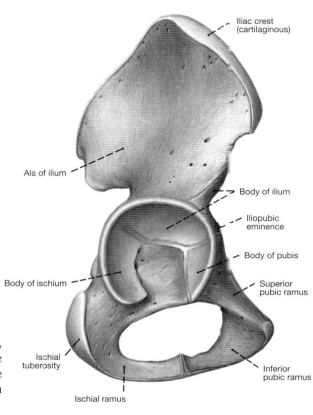

Iliac crest (cartilaginous)

Ala of ilium

Body of ilium

Iliopubic eminence

Body of pubis

Superior pubic ramus

Body of ischium

Ischial tuberosity

Inferior pubic ramus

Ischial ramus

Fig. 377: Hip Bone of 5-Year-Old Child: Lateral View
NOTE: the hip bone is formed by a fusion of the **ilium** (yellow),
ischium (green), and **pubis** (blue). Although ossification of the
inferior pubic ramus occurs during the 7th or 8th year, complete
fusion of the three bones at the **acetabulum** occurs sometime between
the 15th and 20th year.

PLATE 250   Bones of the Pelvis: Medial and Anterior Views

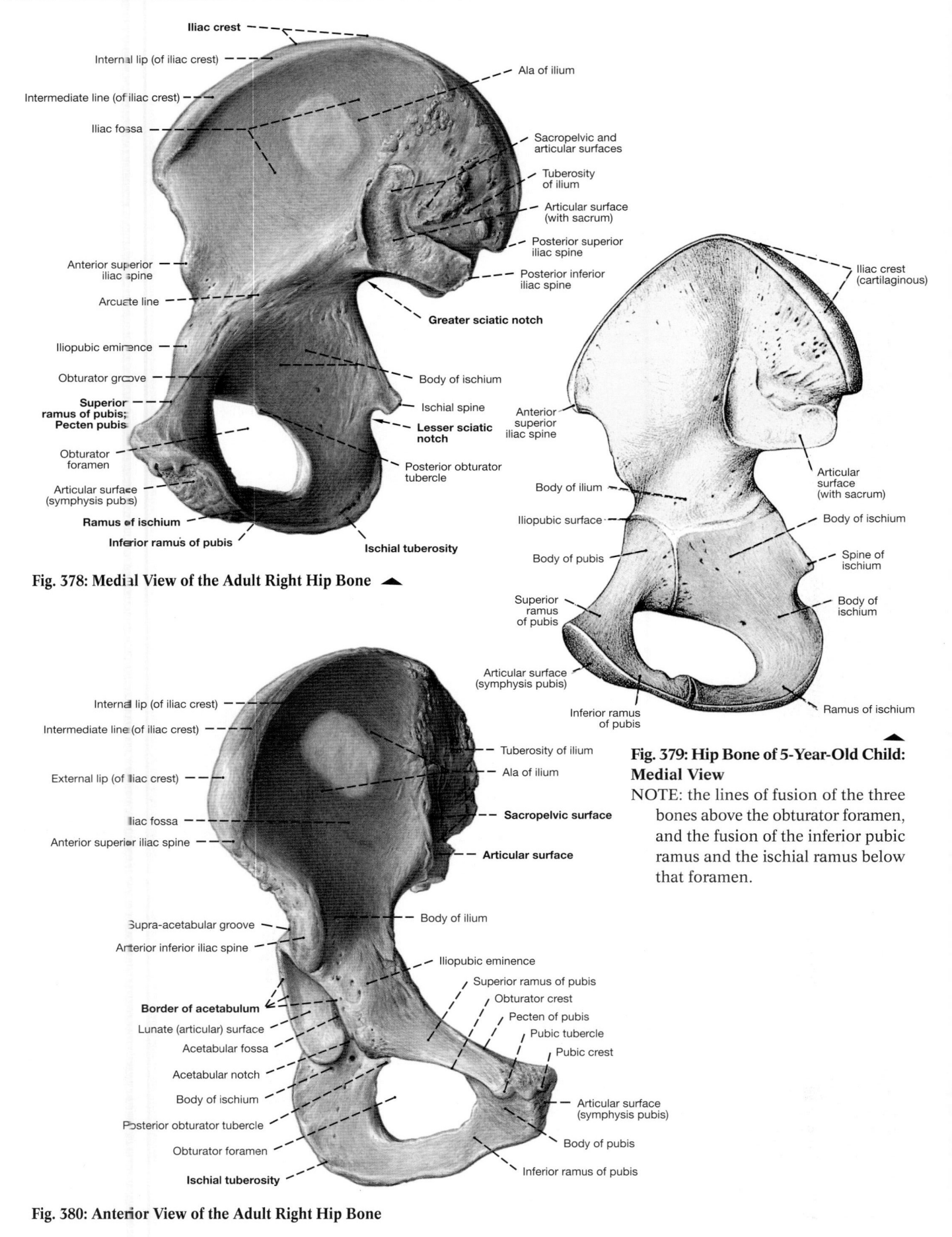

Iliac crest

Internal lip (of iliac crest)

Intermediate line (of iliac crest)

Iliac fossa

Ala of ilium

Sacropelvic and articular surfaces

Tuberosity of ilium

Articular surface (with sacrum)

Anterior superior iliac spine

Posterior superior iliac spine

Arcuate line

Posterior inferior iliac spine

Iliopubic eminence

Greater sciatic notch

Obturator groove

Body of ischium

Superior ramus of pubis; Pecten pubis

Ischial spine

Lesser sciatic notch

Obturator foramen

Articular surface (symphysis pubis)

Posterior obturator tubercle

Ramus of ischium

Inferior ramus of pubis

Ischial tuberosity

Fig. 378: Medial View of the Adult Right Hip Bone ▲

Iliac crest (cartilaginous)

Anterior superior iliac spine

Articular surface (with sacrum)

Body of ilium

Iliopubic surface

Body of ischium

Body of pubis

Spine of ischium

Superior ramus of pubis

Body of ischium

Articular surface (symphysis pubis)

Inferior ramus of pubis

Ramus of ischium

Fig. 379: Hip Bone of 5-Year-Old Child: Medial View

NOTE: the lines of fusion of the three bones above the obturator foramen, and the fusion of the inferior pubic ramus and the ischial ramus below that foramen.

Internal lip (of iliac crest)

Intermediate line (of iliac crest)

Tuberosity of ilium

Ala of ilium

External lip (of iliac crest)

Sacropelvic surface

Iliac fossa

Anterior superior iliac spine

Articular surface

Body of ilium

Supra-acetabular groove

Anterior inferior iliac spine

Iliopubic eminence

Superior ramus of pubis

Obturator crest

Border of acetabulum

Pecten of pubis

Lunate (articular) surface

Pubic tubercle

Acetabular fossa

Pubic crest

Acetabular notch

Body of ischium

Articular surface (symphysis pubis)

Posterior obturator tubercle

Body of pubis

Obturator foramen

Inferior ramus of pubis

Ischial tuberosity

Fig. 380: Anterior View of the Adult Right Hip Bone

Figs. 378, 379, 380

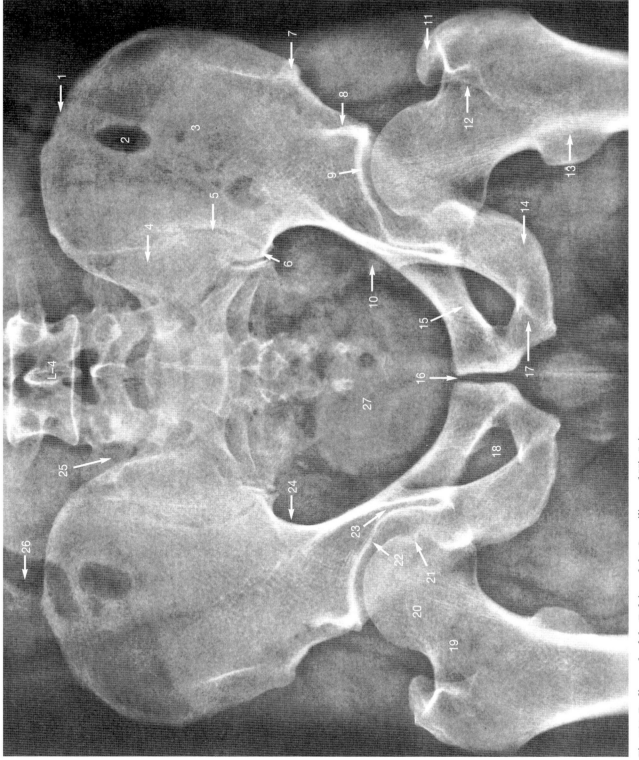

1. Iliac crest
2. Gas bubble in colon
3. Ala of ilium
4. Lateral part of sacrum
5. Sacroiliac joint
6. Posterior inferior iliac spine
7. Anterior superior iliac spine
8. Anterior inferior iliac spine
9. Lunate surface of acetabulum
10. Spine of ischium
11. Greater trochanter
12. Intertrochanteric crest
13. Lesser trochanter
14. Ischial tuberosity
15. Superior ramus of pubis
16. Symphysis pubis
17. Inferior ramus of pubis
18. Obturator foramen
19. Neck of femur
20. Head of femur
21. Fovea on head of femur
22. Acetabular fossa
23. Iliopubic eminence
24. Greater sciatic notch
25. Transverse process, L5 vertebra
26. Gas bubble in colon
27. Urinary bladder

Fig. 381: Radiograph of the Pelvis and the Sacroiliac and Hip Joints
(From Wicke L. Atlas of Radiographic Anatomy, 5th Edition. Philadelphia, Lea and Febiger, 1994).

Fig. 381   IV

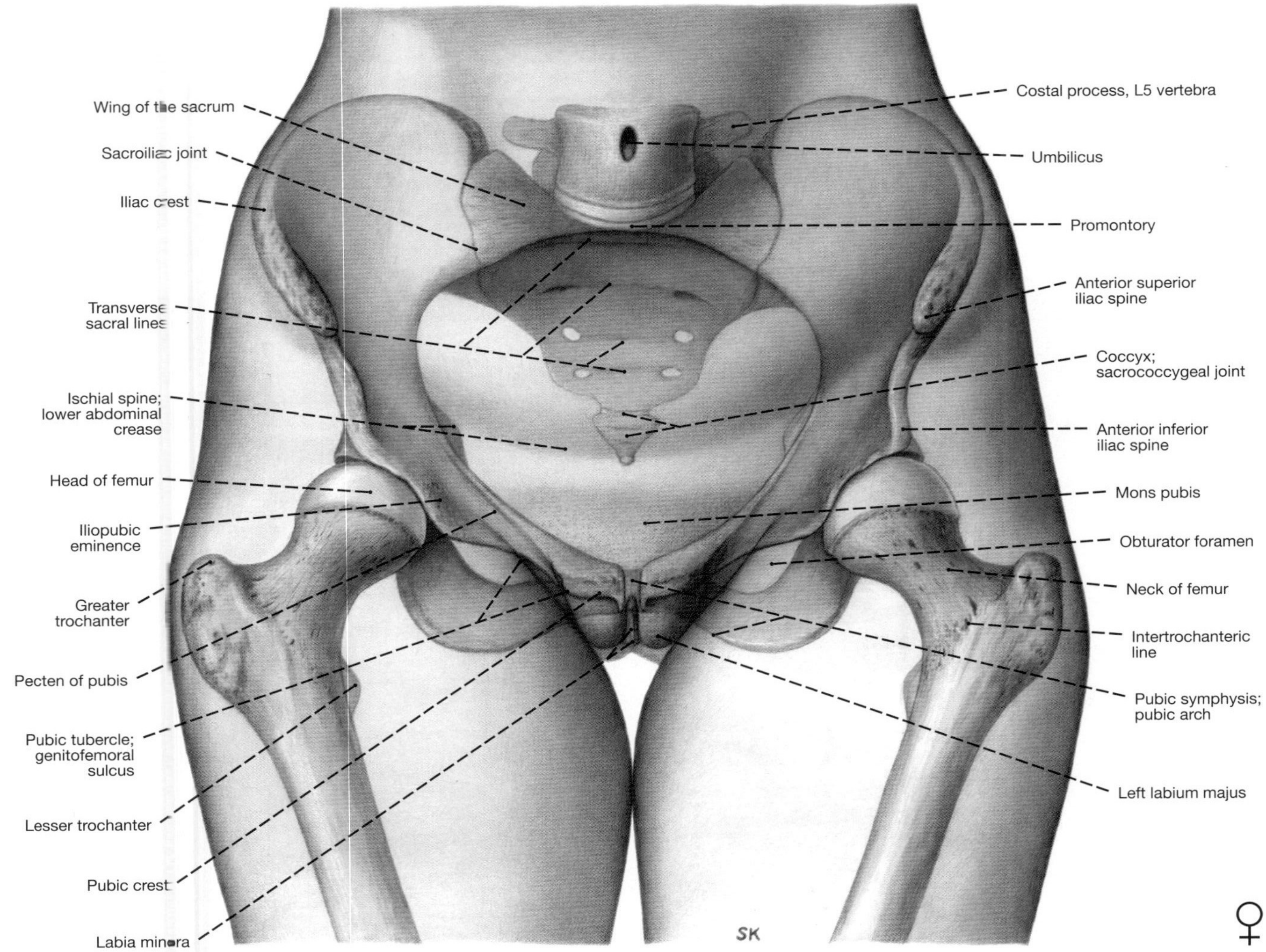

PLATE 252   Bones of the Female Pelvis: Sex Differences

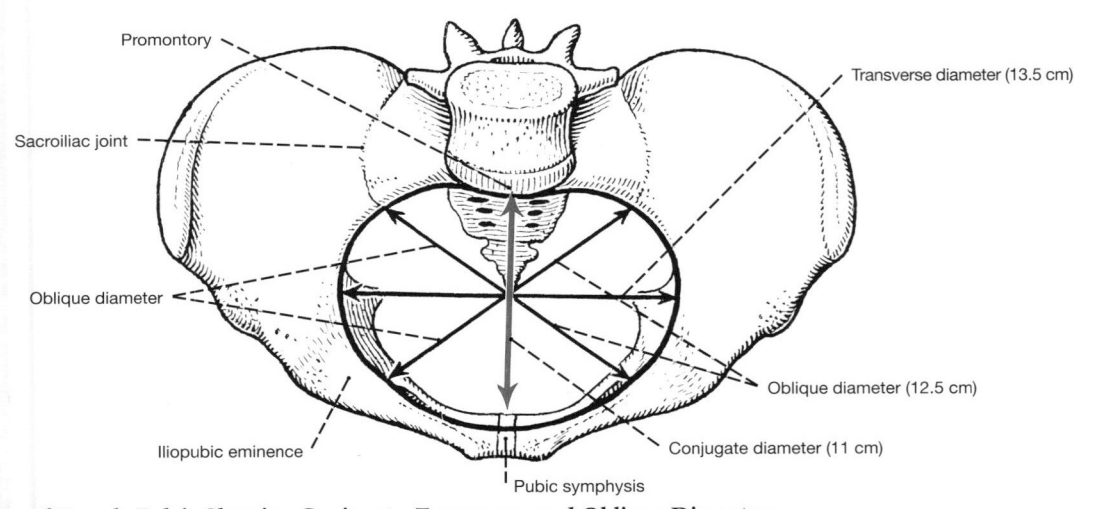

Wing of the sacrum

Sacroiliac joint

Iliac crest

Transverse sacral lines

Ischial spine; lower abdominal crease

Head of femur

Iliopubic eminence

Greater trochanter

Pecten of pubis

Pubic tubercle; genitofemoral sulcus

Lesser trochanter

Pubic crest

Labia minora

Costal process, L5 vertebra

Umbilicus

Promontory

Anterior superior iliac spine

Coccyx; sacrococcygeal joint

Anterior inferior iliac spine

Mons pubis

Obturator foramen

Neck of femur

Intertrochanteric line

Pubic symphysis; pubic arch

Left labium majus

Fig. 382: Female Pelvis: Anterosuperior View

NOTE: the enlarged portion of the pelvic cavity located above and anterior to the pelvic brim (or **linea terminalis**) is called the **false** or **greater pelvis,** whereas that part of the pelvic cavity situated below the pelvic brim is called the **true** or **lesser pelvis.**

Promontory

Sacroiliac joint

Oblique diameter

Iliopubic eminence

Pubic symphysis

Transverse diameter (13.5 cm)

Oblique diameter (12.5 cm)

Conjugate diameter (11 cm)

Fig. 383: Diagram of Female Pelvis Showing Conjugate, Transverse, and Oblique Diameters

NOTE: the following differences between the female and male pelvis;

1) the **cavity of the true pelvis** in women is more shallow and wider than in men.

2) the **superior aperture** is oval or rounded in females, but heart-shaped in males.

3) the **inferior aperture** is comparatively larger in females and the female coccyx is more movable than in males (cont. under Fig. 385).

Figs. 382, 383

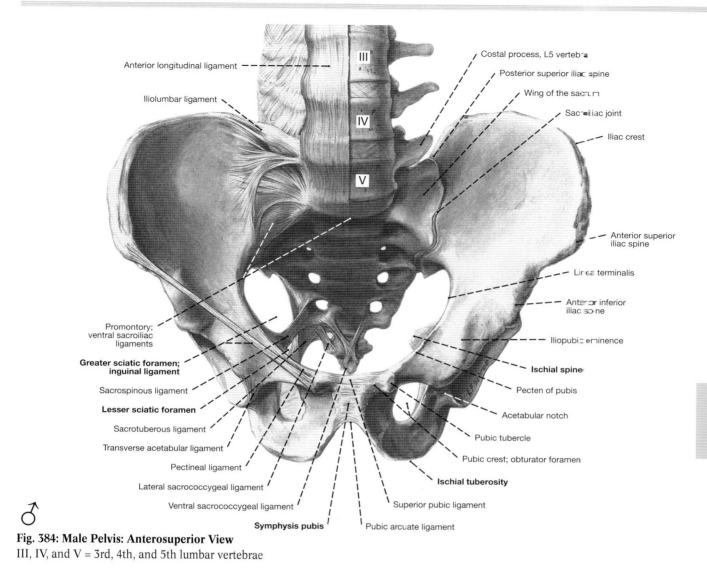

Anterior longitudinal ligament

Iliolumbar ligament

Costal process, L5 vertebra

Posterior superior iliac spine

Wing of the sacrum

Sacroiliac joint

Iliac crest

Anterior superior iliac spine

Linea terminalis

Anterior inferior iliac spine

Iliopubic eminence

Promontory; ventral sacroiliac ligaments

Greater sciatic foramen; inguinal ligament

Sacrospinous ligament

Lesser sciatic foramen

Sacrotuberous ligament

Transverse acetabular ligament

Pectineal ligament

Lateral sacrococcygeal ligament

Ventral sacrococcygeal ligament

Symphysis pubis

Superior pubic ligament

Pubic arcuate ligament

Ischial spine

Pecten of pubis

Acetabular notch

Pubic tubercle

Pubic crest; obturator foramen

Ischial tuberosity

Fig. 384: Male Pelvis: Anterosuperior View
III, IV, and V = 3rd, 4th, and 5th lumbar vertebrae

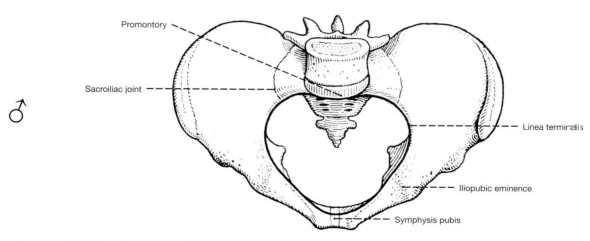

Promontory

Sacroiliac joint

Linea terminalis

Iliopubic eminence

Symphysis pubis

Fig. 385: Diagram of the Male Pelvis
Differences between the female and male pelvis (cont.):
4) the **pubic arch (subpubic angle)** is greater in females and, therefore, the **ischial tuberosities** are farther apart than in males.
5) the **obturator foramen** is usually oval in shape in women but more rounded in men.
6) the female **pelvic bones** are more delicate and lighter than the male pelvic bones.
7) the **sacrum** is shorter and wider in females and it is usually less curved than in males.
8) the **ischial spines** project less in females and the **sciatic notches** are usually wider and more shallow than in males.

PLATE 254   Bones and Ligaments of the Female Pelvis

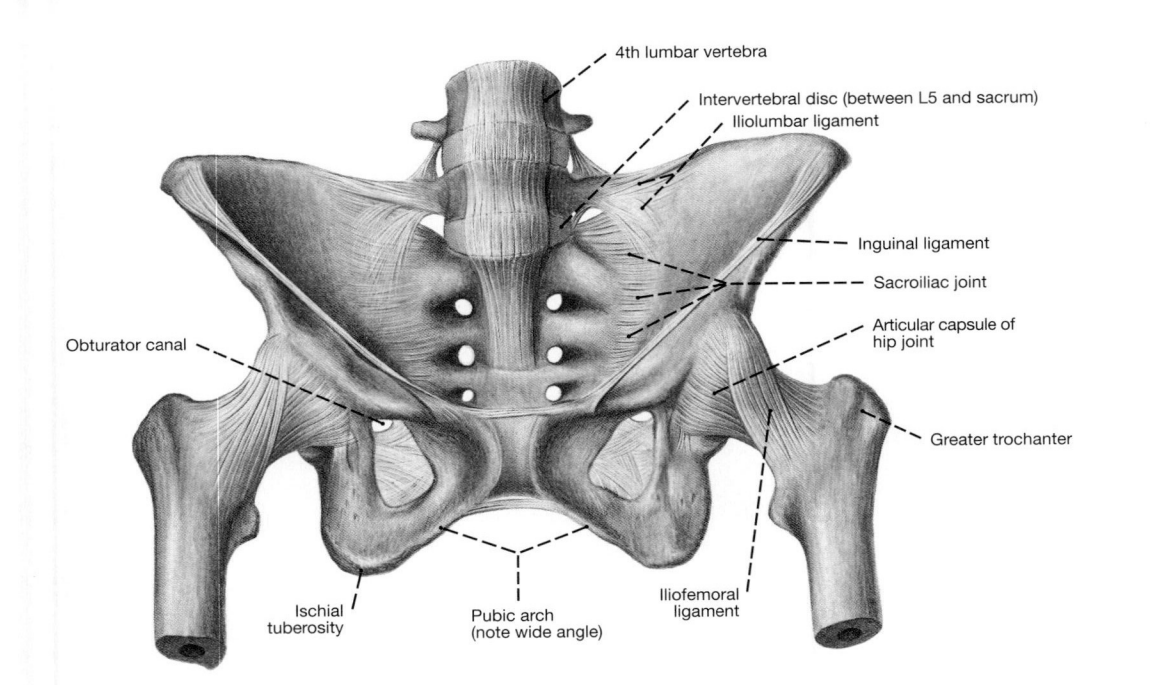

4th lumbar vertebra

Intervertebral disc (between L5 and sacrum)

Iliolumbar ligament

Inguinal ligament

Sacroiliac joint

Articular capsule of hip joint

Greater trochanter

Obturator canal

Iliofemoral ligament

Ischial tuberosity

Pubic arch (note wide angle)

Fig. 386: Female Pelvis and Ligaments: Articulations of the Pelvic Girdle and Hip Joints, Anteroinferior View

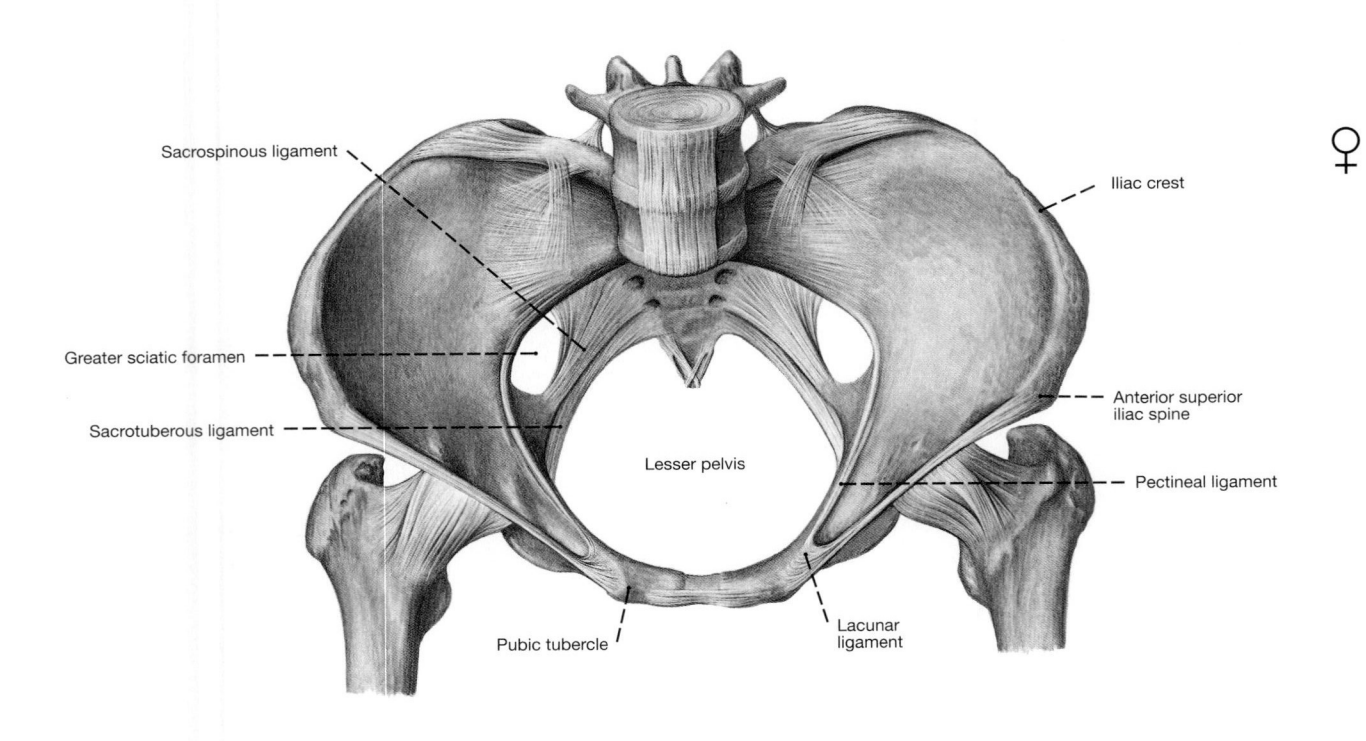

Sacrospinous ligament

Iliac crest

Greater sciatic foramen

Anterior superior iliac spine

Sacrotuberous ligament

Lesser pelvis

Pectineal ligament

Pubic tubercle

Lacunar ligament

Fig. 387: Female Pelvis and Ligaments Viewed from Above

NOTE: 1) the forward inclination of the pelvis shown here corresponds to the position of the pelvis while the person is standing upright.

2) in addition to having wider diameters, both at the pelvic inlet and outlet, the female lesser pelvis is more circular in shape than the male (compare with Fig. 389).

3) the larger capacity of the lesser or true pelvis in the female, and the fact that the female hormones of pregnancy tend to relax the pelvic ligaments, serve to facilitate the function of child bearing.

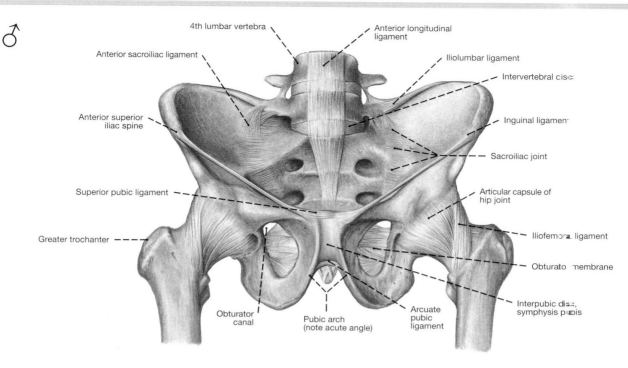

4th lumbar vertebra

Anterior longitudinal ligament

Iliolumbar ligament

Anterior sacroiliac ligament

Intervertebral disc

Anterior superior iliac spine

Inguinal ligament

Sacroiliac joint

Superior pubic ligament

Articular capsule of hip joint

Greater trochanter

Iliofemoral ligament

Obturator membrane

Interpubic disc, symphysis pubis

Obturator canal

Pubic arch (note acute angle)

Arcuate pubic ligament

Fig. 388: Male Pelvis and Associated Ligaments: Anterior Aspect

NOTE: 1)   the pelvis is formed by the articulations of the left and right hip bones anteriorly at the **symphysis pubis** and posteriorly with the sacrum, coccyx, and fifth lumbar vertebra of the vertebral column.

2)   the articulations inferiorly of the pelvis with the two femora allow the weight of the head, trunk, and upper extremities to be transmitted to the lower limbs, thereby maintaining the upright posture characteristic of the human.

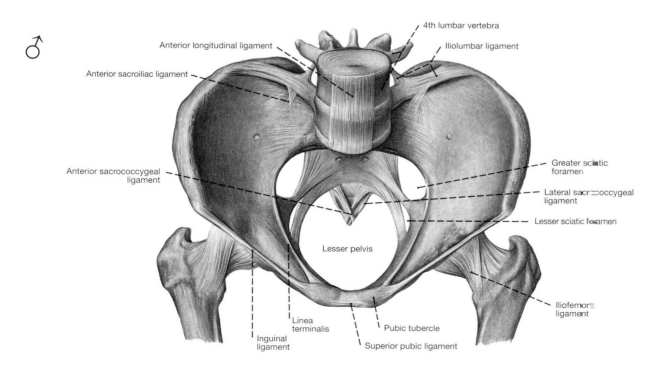

4th lumbar vertebra

Anterior longitudinal ligament

Iliolumbar ligament

Anterior sacroiliac ligament

Anterior sacrococcygeal ligament

Greater sciatic foramen

Lateral sacrococcygeal ligament

Lesser sciatic foramen

Lesser pelvis

Iliofemoral ligament

Linea terminalis

Pubic tubercle

Inguinal ligament

Superior pubic ligament

Fig. 389: Male Pelvis and Ligaments Viewed from Above

NOTE: the size of the **pelvic inlet** (superior aperture of the **lesser pelvis**) and **inferior outlet** of the male pelvis is smaller than that in the female (see Fig. 387). Thus, the **lesser pelvis** is deeper and more narrow in the male and its cavity has a smaller capacity than that seen in the female. In the male, the pelvic bones are thicker and heavier, and generally, the **major pelvis** (above the pelvic brim) is larger than in the female.

PLATE 256   Female Pelvis: Viewed from Below; Hemisected Pelvis

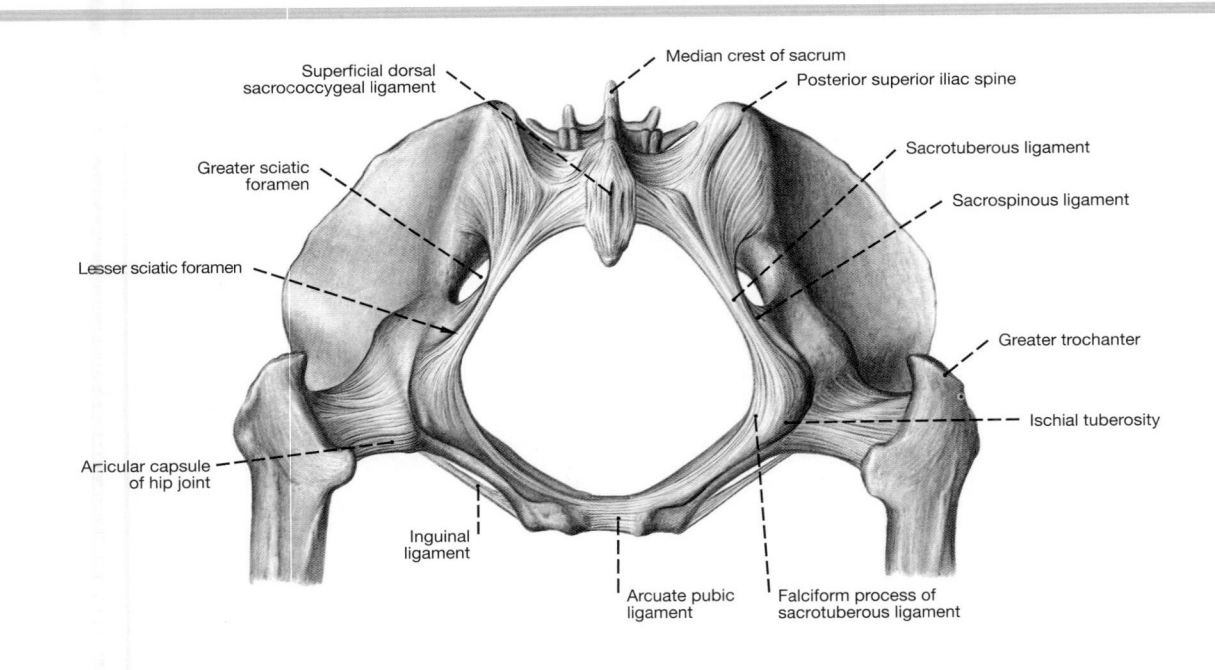

Fig. 390: Female Pelvic Outlet Showing the Pelvic Ligaments and Viewed from Below

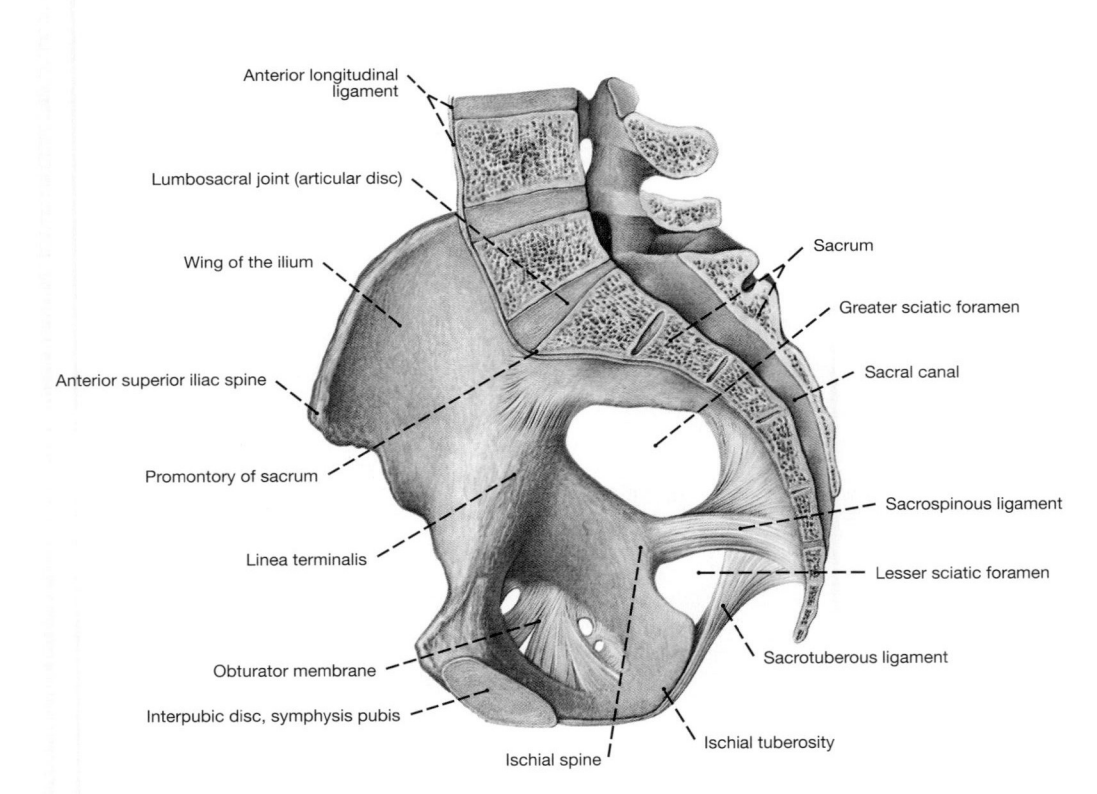

Fig. 391: Articulations and Ligaments of the Female Hemisected Pelvis

NOTE: 1)   the **sacrospinous ligament** courses between the **sacrum** and the **ischial spine** and forms the lower border of the **greater sciatic foramen.**

2)   the **lesser sciatic foramen** is bounded above by the **sacrospinous ligament** and below by the **sacrotuberous ligament.** The latter extends between the **sacrum** and the **ischial tuberosity.**

3)   these two foramina allow the emergence of muscles, nerves, and arteries from the pelvis to the gluteal region and the entrance of veins from the gluteal region to the pelvis.

4)   because the sacrum lies beneath the remainder of the vertebral column, considerable weight is transmitted to it from above. This tends to rotate the upper end of the sacrum forward and downward and its lower end and the coccyx backward and upward. The sacrotuberous and sacrospinous ligaments add stability to the sacroiliac joint by resisting these forces.

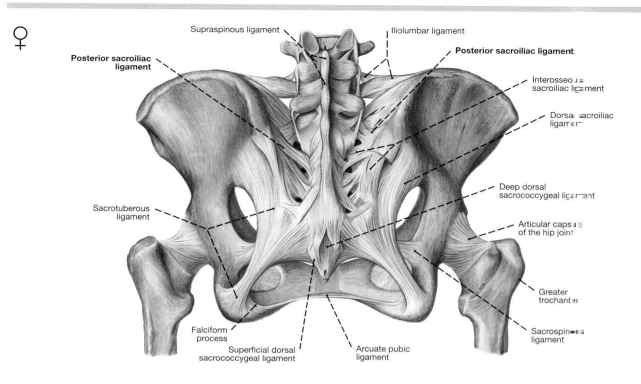

Fig. 392: Female Pelvis with Joints and Ligaments: Posterior Aspect

NOTE: 1)   broad ligamentous bands articulate the two hip bones posteriorly with the sacrum and coccyx. Observe the strong **posterior (dorsal) sacroiliac ligament.**

2)   the posterior sacroiliac ligament is composed of short **transverse fibers** that interconnect the ilium with the upper part of the lateral crest of the sacrum, whereas the longer **vertical fibers** attach the 3rd and 4th transverse tubercles of the sacrum to the superior and inferior posterior iliac spines, many blending with fibers of the sacrotuberous ligament.

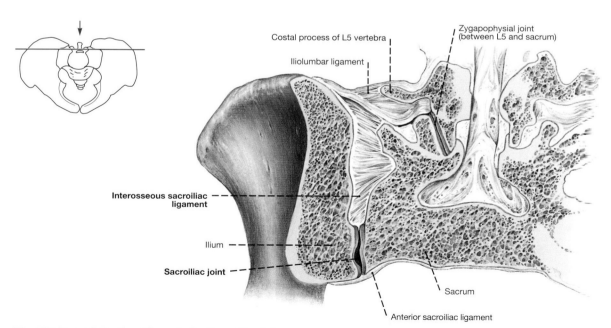

Fig. 393: Frontal Section Through the Sacroiliac Joint

NOTE: 1)   the **sacroiliac joint** is a synovial joint connecting the **auricular surface** of the sacrum with the reciprocally curved **auricular surface** of the ilium.

2)   this joint is bound by the **anterior** and **interosseous sacroiliac ligaments** (shown in this figure) as well as the **posterior** (dorsal) **sacroiliac ligament** shown in Figure 392.

3)   the interosseous sacroiliac ligament is the strongest ligament between the sacrum and ilium and it stretches above and behind the synovial joint.

PLATE 258   Female Pelvis: Midsagittal View

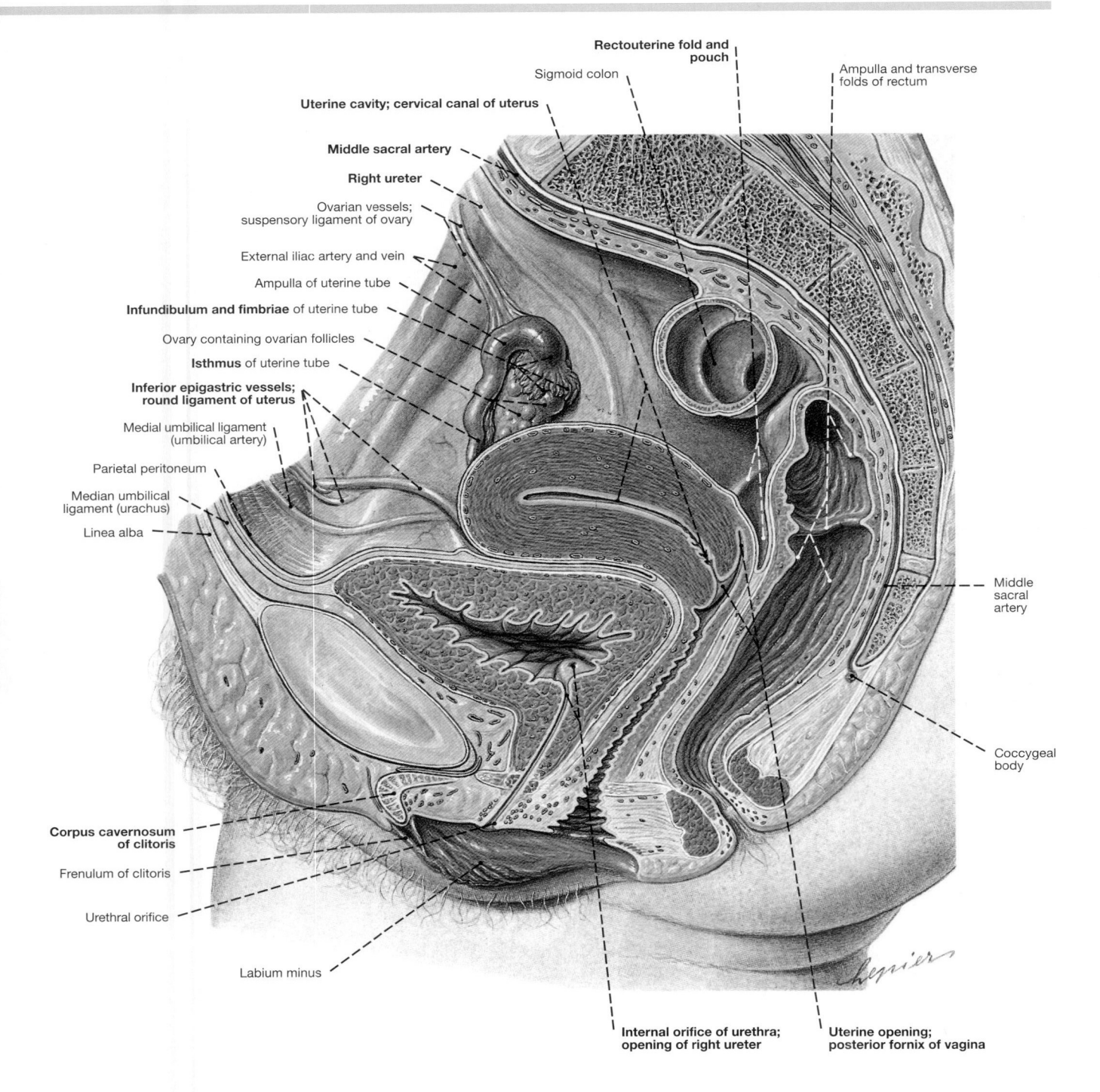

Rectouterine fold and pouch

Sigmoid colon

Ampulla and transverse folds of rectum

Uterine cavity; cervical canal of uterus

Middle sacral artery

Right ureter

Ovarian vessels; suspensory ligament of ovary

External iliac artery and vein

Ampulla of uterine tube

Infundibulum and fimbriae of uterine tube

Ovary containing ovarian follicles

Isthmus of uterine tube

Inferior epigastric vessels; round ligament of uterus

Medial umbilical ligament (umbilical artery)

Parietal peritoneum

Median umbilical ligament (urachus)

Linea alba

Middle sacral artery

Coccygeal body

Corpus cavernosum of clitoris

Frenulum of clitoris

Urethral orifice

Labium minus

Internal orifice of urethra; opening of right ureter

Uterine opening; posterior fornix of vagina

Fig. 394: Adult Female Pelvis, Median Sagittal Section

NOTE: 1) this medial view of the hemisected female pelvis shows the relationships of the **bladder, uterus, vagina, rectum, ovary,** and **uterine tube.** Observe the retropubic position of the empty bladder and the short course of the female **urethra,** leading from the bladder through the **urogenital diaphragm** to open in the midline, anterior to the vagina.

2) the **posterior fornix** of the vagina reaches superiorly to lie in front of the **rectouterine pouch (of Douglas),** being separated from it only by the vaginal wall. Observe that the vagina and uterus are interposed between the bladder and rectum.

3) the **round ligament of the uterus** is directed laterally and anteriorly to enter the abdominal inguinal ring, and note the course of the **inferior epigastric vessels** in relation to this ligament. Observe the **ovarian vessels** within the **suspensory ligament of the ovary,** and the **ureter** along the posterolateral wall of the pelvis.

4) the **large bowel** and the direct course of the **rectum** toward the **anal canal.** The peritoneum is reflected over the anterior surface of the rectum, thereby lining the rectouterine pouch.

Fig. 394

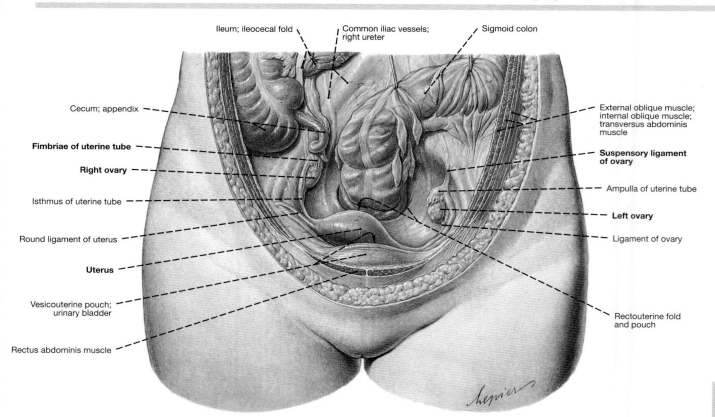

Ileum; ileocecal fold

Common iliac vessels;
right ureter

Sigmoid colon

Cecum; appendix

Fimbriae of uterine tube

Right ovary

Isthmus of uterine tube

Round ligament of uterus

Uterus

Vesicouterine pouch;
urinary bladder

Rectus abdominis muscle

External oblique muscle;
internal oblique muscle;
transversus abdominis
muscle

**Suspensory ligament
of ovary**

Ampulla of uterine tube

Left ovary

Ligament of ovary

Rectouterine fold
and pouch

Fig. 395: Pelvic Viscera of an Adult Female: Anterior View

NOTE: 1) the ovaries are situated on the posterolateral aspect of the true pelvis on each side. Having descended from the posterior abdominal wall to their location just below the pelvic brim, the ovaries are held in position by peritoneal ligamentous attachments. The suspensory ligament of the ovary transmits the ovarian vessels and ovarian autonomic nerves.

2) the position of the uterus between the bladder and rectum and frequently it is located somewhat to one or the other side of the midline.

3) the fimbriae of the uterine tubes as they extend from the ampullae of the tubes to encircle the upper medial surface of the ovaries. The uterine tubes vary from 3 to 6 inches in length and they convey the ova to the uterus. It is within the uterine tube that fertilization of the ovum usually occurs.

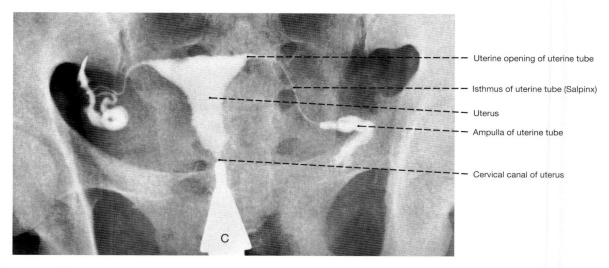

Uterine opening of uterine tube

Isthmus of uterine tube (Salpinx)

Uterus

Ampulla of uterine tube

Cervical canal of uterus

C

Fig. 396: Uterosalpingogram

NOTE: 1) a cannula (C) was placed in the vagina and radiopaque material was injected into the uterus and uterine tube. Observe the narrow lumen of the isthmus of the uterine tubes and how the tubes enlarge at the ampullae.

2) on the specimen's left side (reader's right), even the fimbriated end of the tube is discernible, whereas on the specimen's right side (reader's left) a small portion of the radiopaque material has been forced into the pelvis through the opening in the uterine tube.

PLATE 260 Female Genitourinary Organs (Diagrammatic)

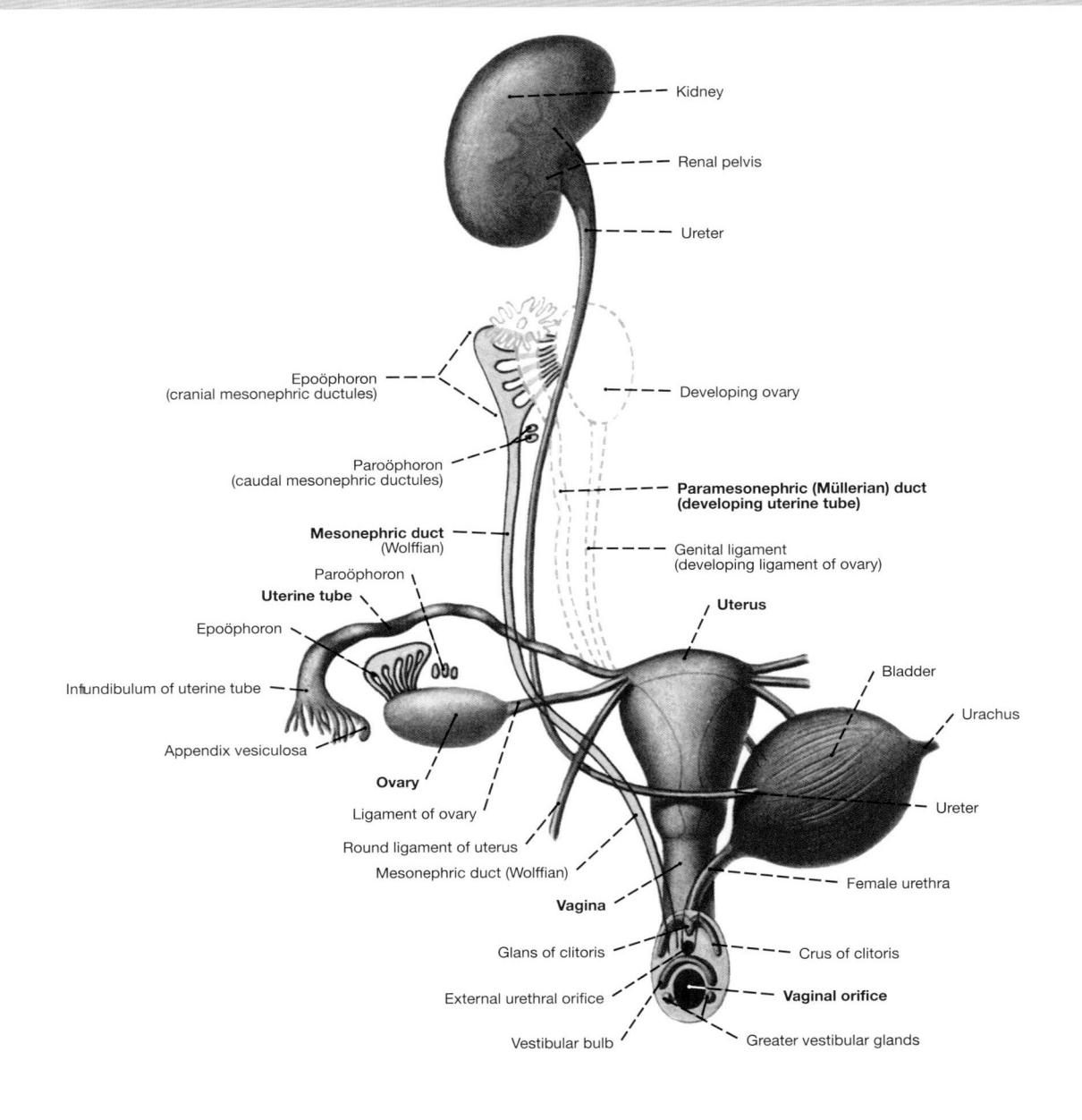

Kidney

Renal pelvis

Ureter

Epoöphoron
(cranial mesonephric ductules)

Developing ovary

Paroöphoron
(caudal mesonephric ductules)

**Paramesonephric (Müllerian) duct
(developing uterine tube)**

Mesonephric duct
(Wolffian)

Genital ligament
(developing ligament of ovary)

Paroöphoron

Uterine tube

Uterus

Epoöphoron

Bladder

Infundibulum of uterine tube

Urachus

Appendix vesiculosa

Ureter

Ovary

Ligament of ovary

Round ligament of uterus

Mesonephric duct (Wolffian)

Female urethra

Vagina

Glans of clitoris

Crus of clitoris

External urethral orifice

Vaginal orifice

Vestibular bulb

Greater vestibular glands

Fig. 397: Diagram of the Female Genitourinary Organs and Their Embryologic Precursors

NOTE: 1) this figure shows:

    a) all of the organs of the adult female genitourinary system (dark red-brown)

    b) the structures and relevant positions of the female genital organs (gonad and ligament of the ovary and uterine tube) prior to their descent into the pelvis (interrupted lines); and

    c) the structures that become atrophic during development (pink with red outline).

    2) the urinary system of females (as in males) includes the kidney, which produces urine from the blood, the ureter which conveys the urine to the bladder where it is stored. Leading from the bladder is the urethra through which urine passes to the external urethral orifice during micturition.

    3) the adult female genital system includes the **ovary, uterine tube, uterus,** and **vagina,** plus the associated glands and external genital organs.

    4) at one time during development, structures capable of developing into both male and female genital systems existed. In the female the Müllerian or paramesonephric duct becomes vestigial. Also the developing gonads become ovaries, while their attachments become the ligaments of the ovaries.

    5) the ovaries produce ova that are discharged periodically between adolescence and menopause. The ova are captured by the uterine tube where fertilization may occur. If this happens, the fertilized ovum is transported to the uterus, and about a week after fertilization, implantation occurs in the wall of the uterus.

Fig. 397

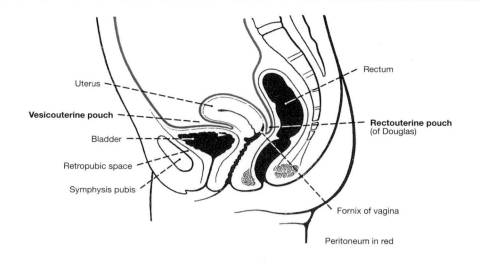

Fig. 398: Diagram of Peritoneal Reflections Over Female Pelvic Organs (Midsagittal Section)

NOTE: 1) the parietal peritoneum is reflected over the free abdominal surface of the pelvic organs. Observe that as the uterus and vagina are interposed between the bladder and rectum, peritoneal pouches are formed between the bladder and the uterus (vesicouterine) and between the rectum and the uterus (rectouterine pouch of Douglas).

2) the **vesicouterine pouch** is shallow. The forward tilt or inclination of the uterus (anteversion) toward the superior surface of the bladder reduces the potential size of the vesicouterine pouch.

3) the vesicouterine pouch does not extend as far inferiorly as the vagina, whereas the deeper **rectouterine pouch** dips to the level of the posterior fornix of the vagina. This important anatomical relationship stresses the fact that the posterior fornix is separated from the peritoneal cavity only by the thin vaginal wall and the peritoneum.

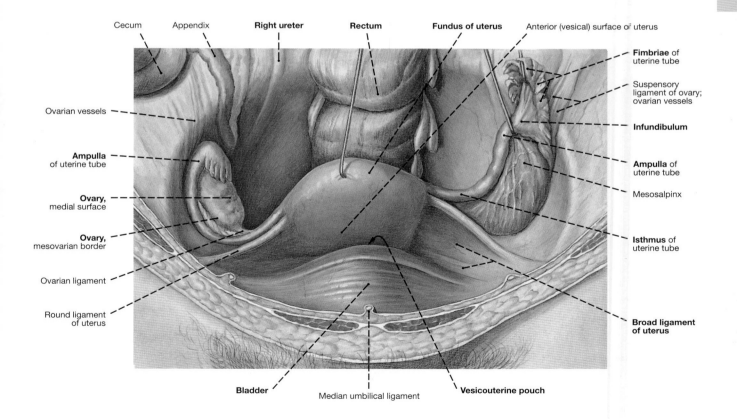

Fig. 399: Female Pelvic Organs: Anterosuperior View

NOTE: the body of the uterus has been elevated, thereby exposing the **vesicouterine pouch** and demonstrating the **broad ligaments.**

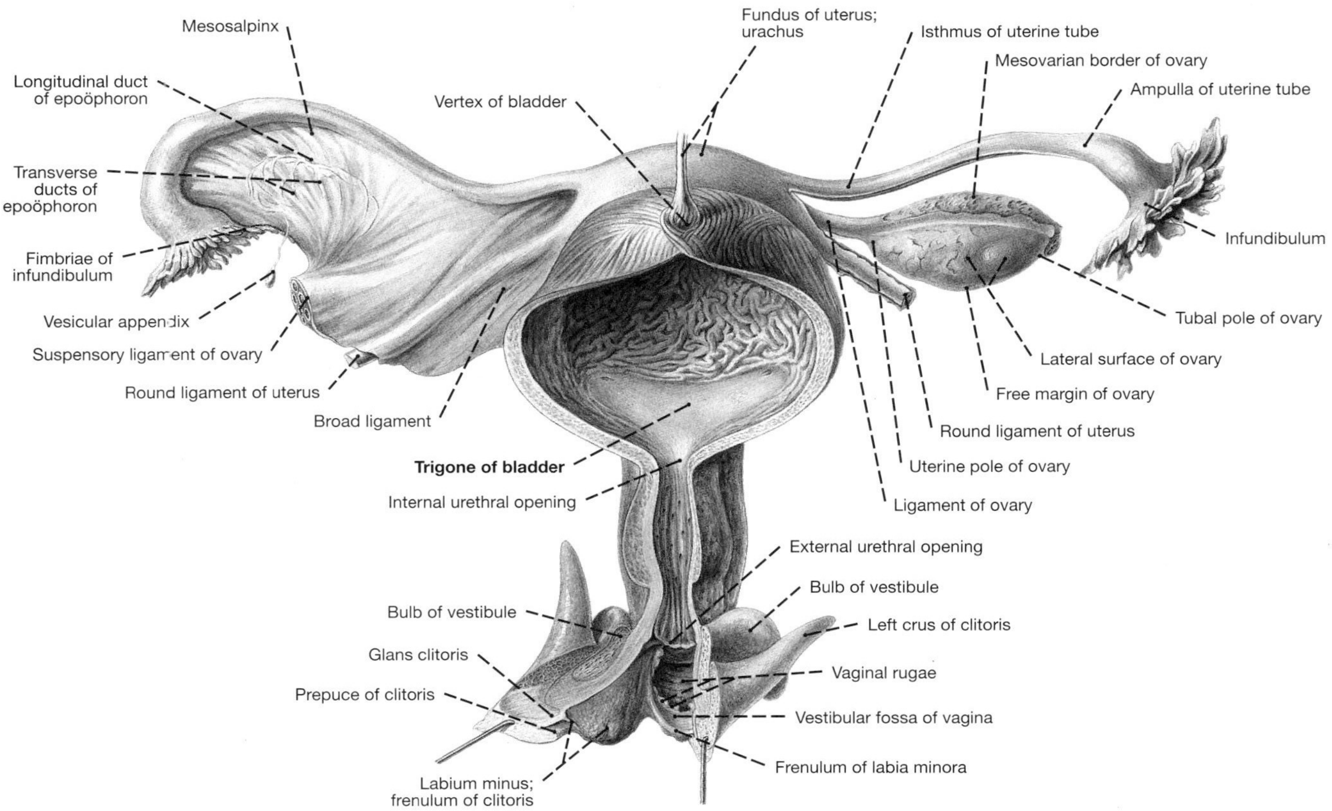

PLATE 262   Female Pelvis: Bladder and Urethra; Uterus and Adnexa

Mesosalpinx

Longitudinal duct
of epoöphoron

Transverse
ducts of
epoöphoron

Fimbriae of
infundibulum

Vesicular appendix

Suspensory ligament of ovary

Round ligament of uterus

Broad ligament

Trigone of bladder

Internal urethral opening

Fundus of uterus;
urachus

Vertex of bladder

Isthmus of uterine tube

Mesovarian border of ovary

Ampulla of uterine tube

Infundibulum

Tubal pole of ovary

Lateral surface of ovary

Free margin of ovary

Round ligament of uterus

Uterine pole of ovary

Ligament of ovary

Bulb of vestibule

Glans clitoris

Prepuce of clitoris

External urethral opening

Bulb of vestibule

Left crus of clitoris

Vaginal rugae

Vestibular fossa of vagina

Frenulum of labia minora

Labium minus;
frenulum of clitoris

Fig. 400: Opened Female Bladder and Urethra, Anterior View

NOTE: the position of the bladder and urethra in front of (anterior to) the uterus and vagina. Observe also the trigone of the bladder and the internal and external urethral openings.

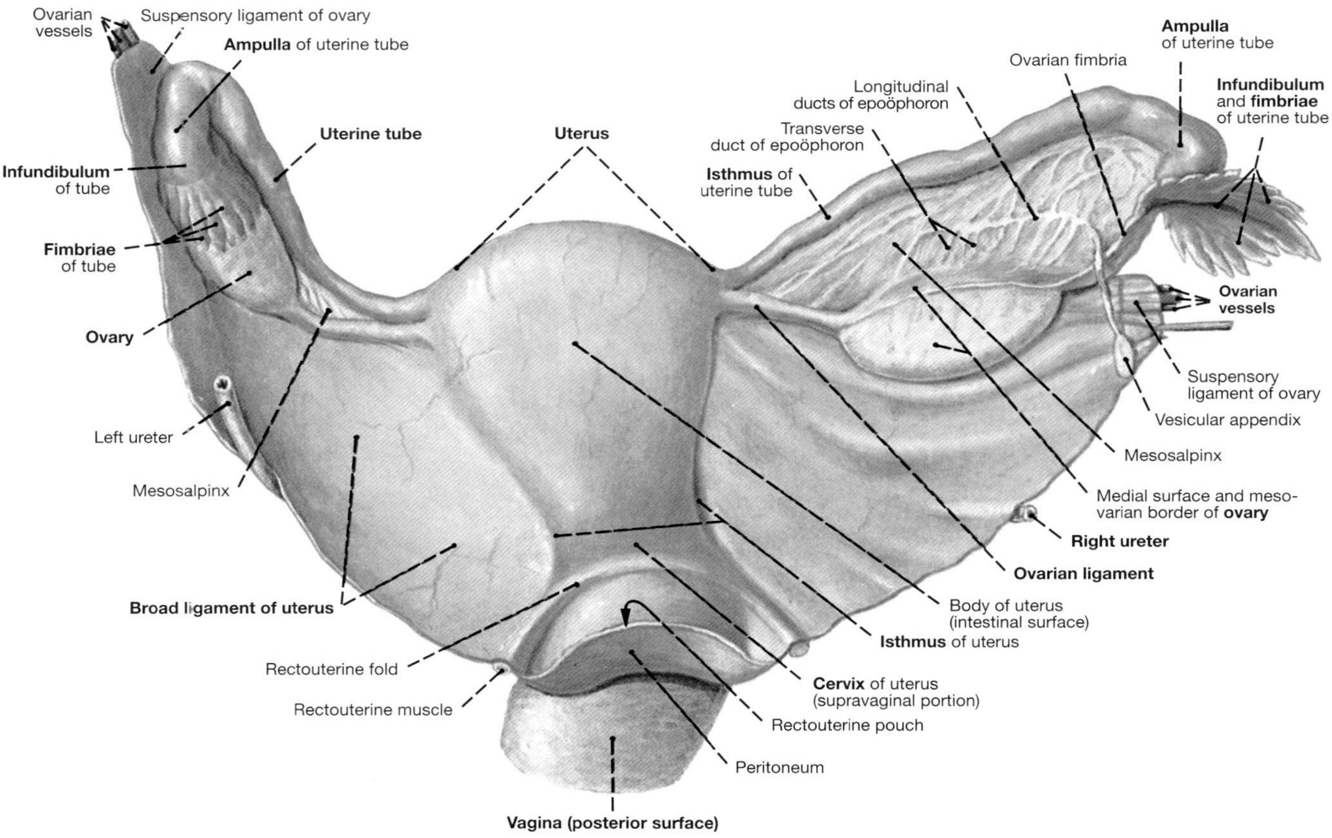

Ovarian
vessels

Suspensory ligament of ovary

Ampulla of uterine tube

Uterine tube

Uterus

Infundibulum
of tube

Fimbriae
of tube

Ovary

Left ureter

Mesosalpinx

Broad ligament of uterus

Rectouterine fold

Rectouterine muscle

Longitudinal
ducts of epoöphoron

Transverse
duct of epoöphoron

Isthmus of
uterine tube

Ovarian fimbria

Ampulla
of uterine tube

Infundibulum
and **fimbriae**
of uterine tube

**Ovarian
vessels**

Suspensory
ligament of ovary

Vesicular appendix

Mesosalpinx

Medial surface and meso-
varian border of **ovary**

Right ureter

Ovarian ligament

Body of uterus
(intestinal surface)

Isthmus of uterus

Cervix of uterus
(supravaginal portion)

Rectouterine pouch

Peritoneum

Vagina

Vagina (posterior surface)

Fig. 401: Pelvic Reproductive Organs of an Immature Girl, Posterior View

Fig. 400, 401

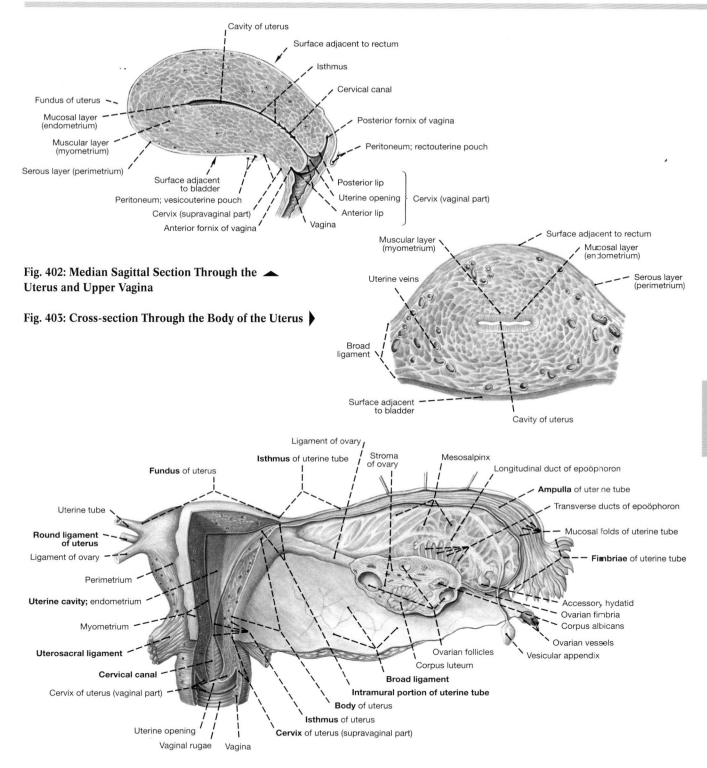

Cavity of uterus
Surface adjacent to rectum
Isthmus
Cervical canal
Posterior fornix of vagina
Peritoneum; rectouterine pouch
Fundus of uterus
Mucosal layer (endometrium)
Muscular layer (myometrium)
Serous layer (perimetrium)
Surface adjacent to bladder
Peritoneum; vesicouterine pouch
Cervix (supravaginal part)
Anterior fornix of vagina
Posterior lip
Uterine opening
Anterior lip
Cervix (vaginal part)
Vagina

**Fig. 402: Median Sagittal Section Through the ▲
Uterus and Upper Vagina**

Fig. 403: Cross-section Through the Body of the Uterus ▶

Muscular layer (myometrium)
Surface adjacent to rectum
Mucosal layer (endometrium)
Serous layer (perimetrium)
Uterine veins
Broad ligament
Surface adjacent to bladder
Cavity of uterus

Ligament of ovary
Isthmus of uterine tube
Stroma of ovary
Mesosalpinx
Longitudinal duct of epoöphoron
Fundus of uterus
Ampulla of uterine tube
Transverse ducts of epoöphoron
Uterine tube
Mucosal folds of uterine tube
Round ligament of uterus
Ligament of ovary
Fimbriae of uterine tube
Perimetrium
Uterine cavity; endometrium
Accessory hydatid
Ovarian fimbria
Corpus albicans
Myometrium
Ovarian vessels
Vesicular appendix
Uterosacral ligament
Cervical canal
Cervix of uterus (vaginal part)
Ovarian follicles
Corpus luteum
Broad ligament
Intramural portion of uterine tube
Body of uterus
Isthmus of uterus
Cervix of uterus (supravaginal part)
Uterine opening
Vaginal rugae   Vagina

Fig. 404: Frontal Section of Uterus, Uterine Tube, and Ovary

NOTE: 1) the vagina communicates with the pelvic cavity through the uterus and the uterine tube. The lumen of this pathway varies in diameter, and its most narrow sites are the isthmus of the uterus and the intrauterine (intramural) part of the uterine tube.

2) the uterus consists of the **cervix** (vaginal and supravaginal portions), the **body** and the **fundus**. The cervix and the body are interconnected by the **isthmus.**

3) the attachments of the uterus include:

a) the **broad ligaments** that attach to the lateral margins of the uterus

b) the fibrous **round ligaments** and the **ligaments of the ovaries** attached just below the uterine tubes

c) the **uterosacral ligaments,** and

d) the **cardinal ligaments (of Mackenrodt)** that attach along the lateral border of the uterus and vagina. With the pelvic diaphragm, the cardinal ligaments offer important support to the uterus and vagina.

PLATE 264   Female Pelvis: Blood Supply to Ovary, Uterus and Vagina

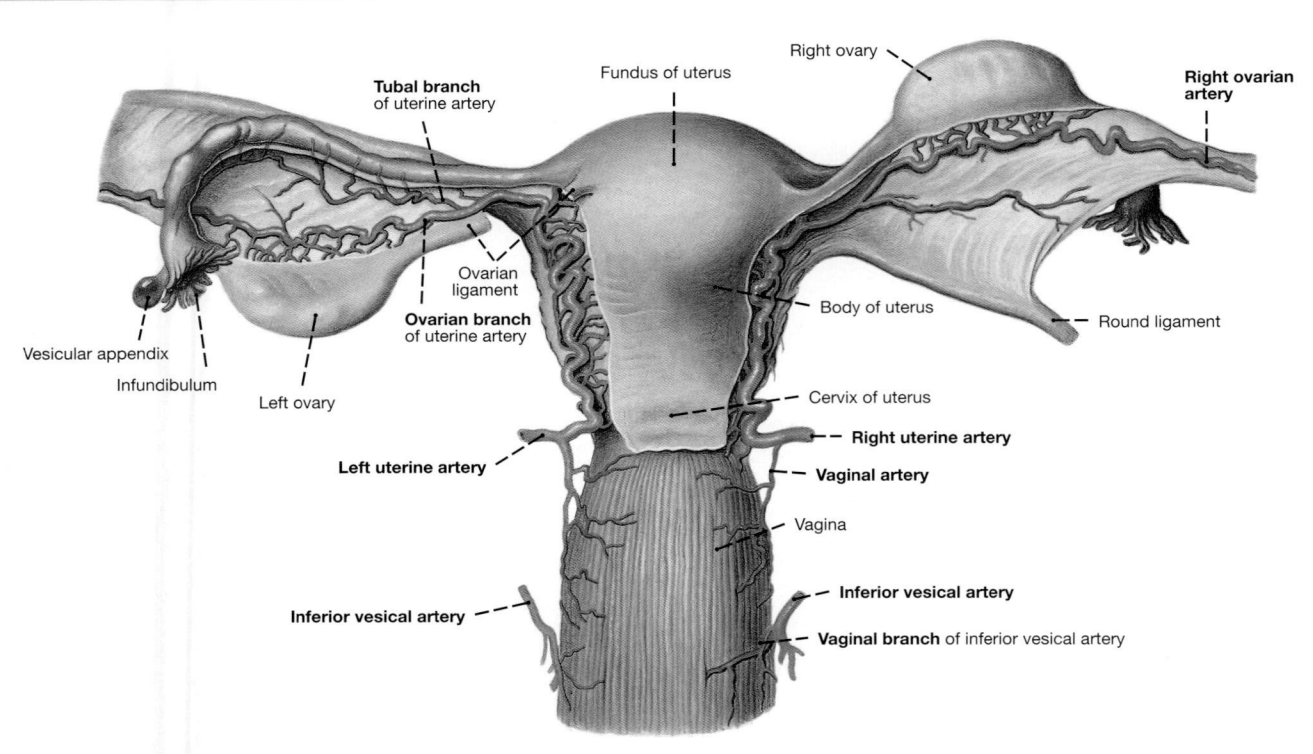

Fig. 405: Arterial Supply to Female Pelvic Genital Organs

NOTE: 1) the vessels supplying the female pelvic genital organs are the **uterine arteries** from the internal iliac and the **ovarian arteries** that stem from the aorta. They anastomose freely along both lateral borders of the uterus.

2) the uterine artery also anastomoses with the arterial supply to the vagina. Often the **vaginal arteries** arise from the uterine, but they may branch from the inferior vesical or even directly from the internal iliac.

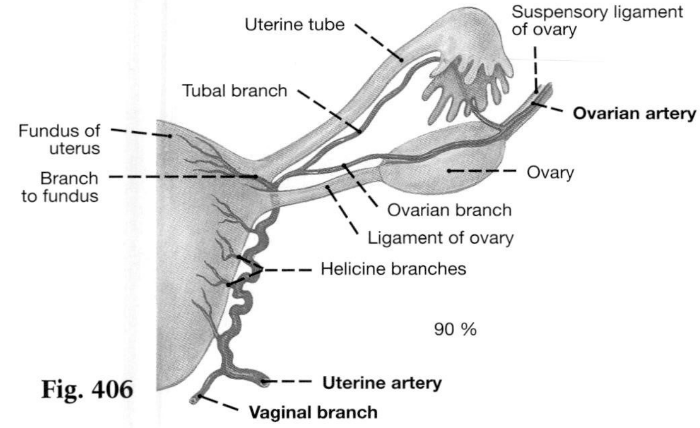

Fig. 406: Diagram of Uterine and Ovarian Arteries

◀ NOTE: this arterial pattern (similar to that shown in Fig. 405) is seen in about 90% of human cases.

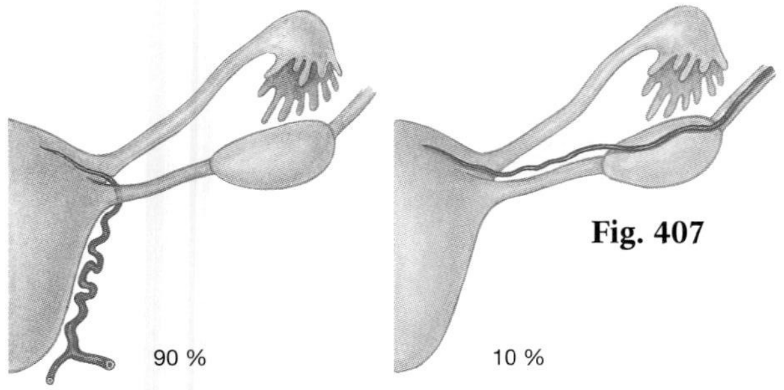

Fig. 407: Arterial Supply to the Fundus of the Uterus

NOTE: in 90% of cases the fundus gets blood from the uterine artery, whereas in 10% it comes from the ovarian artery.

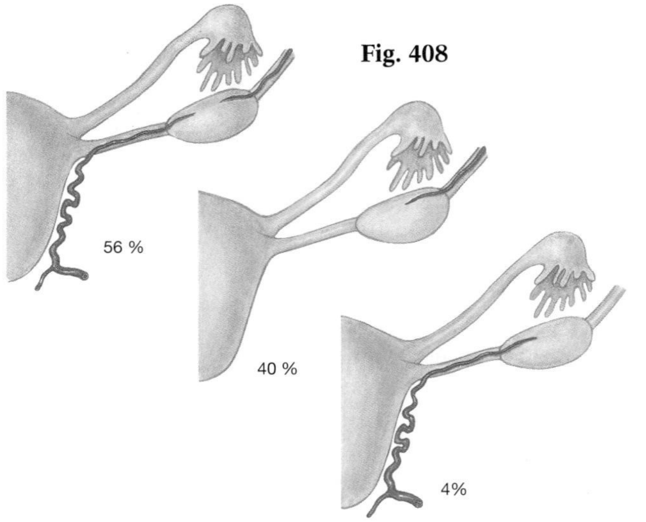

Fig. 408: Arterial Supply to the Ovary

NOTE: in 56% of cases blood to the ovary comes from both the ovarian and uterine arteries; in 40% from the ovarian artery only; in 4% from the uterine artery only.

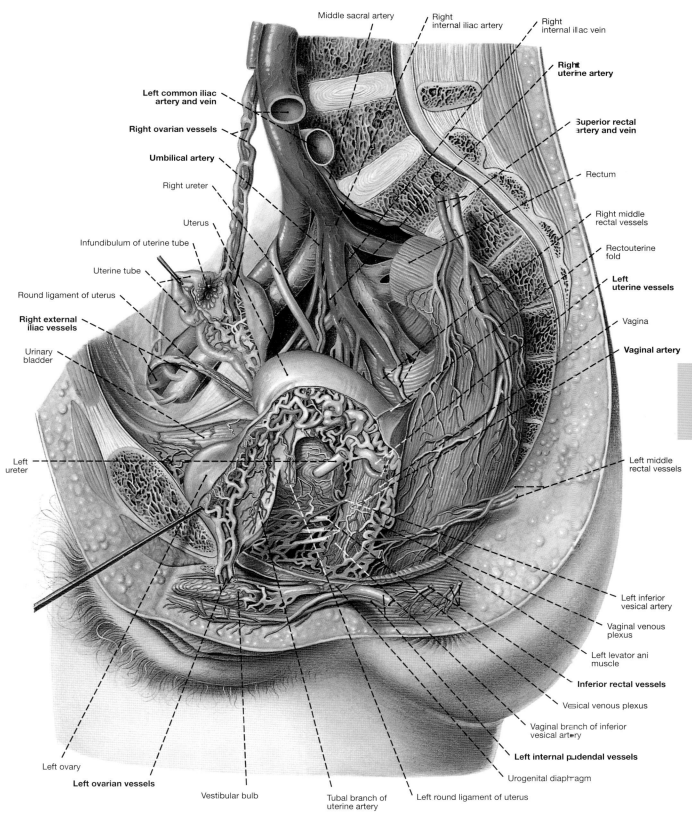

Middle sacral artery

Right internal iliac artery

Right internal iliac vein

Right uterine artery

Left common iliac artery and vein

Right ovarian vessels

Umbilical artery

Right ureter

Uterus

Infundibulum of uterine tube

Uterine tube

Round ligament of uterus

Right external iliac vessels

Urinary bladder

Left ureter

Left ovary

Left ovarian vessels

Vestibular bulb

Tubal branch of uterine tube

Left round ligament of uterus

Superior rectal artery and vein

Rectum

Right middle rectal vessels

Rectouterine fold

Left uterine vessels

Vagina

Vaginal artery

Left middle rectal vessels

Left inferior vesical artery

Vaginal venous plexus

Left levator ani muscle

Inferior rectal vessels

Vesical venous plexus

Vaginal branch of inferior vesical artery

Left internal pudendal vessels

Urogenital diaphragm

Fig. 409: Blood Vessels of the Female Pelvis and Genital System

NOTE: 1)   the left half of the pelvis has been removed to expose the pelvic organs and their dense plexuses of veins **(ovarian, vaginal, uterine** and **vesical)** which accompany their respective arteries.

2)   with the exception of the **ovarian artery** (from the aorta) and the **superior rectal artery** (from the inferior mesenteric) all other arteries to the pelvic organs, perineum, and genital tract are derived from the **internal iliac artery** or its branches.

3)   the descending course of the **ureter,** crossing the external iliac vessels over the pelvic brim. It then courses **under the uterine vessels** before entering the bladder.

Fig. 409   **IV**

PLATE 266   Female or Male Pelvis: Branches of Internal Iliac Artery

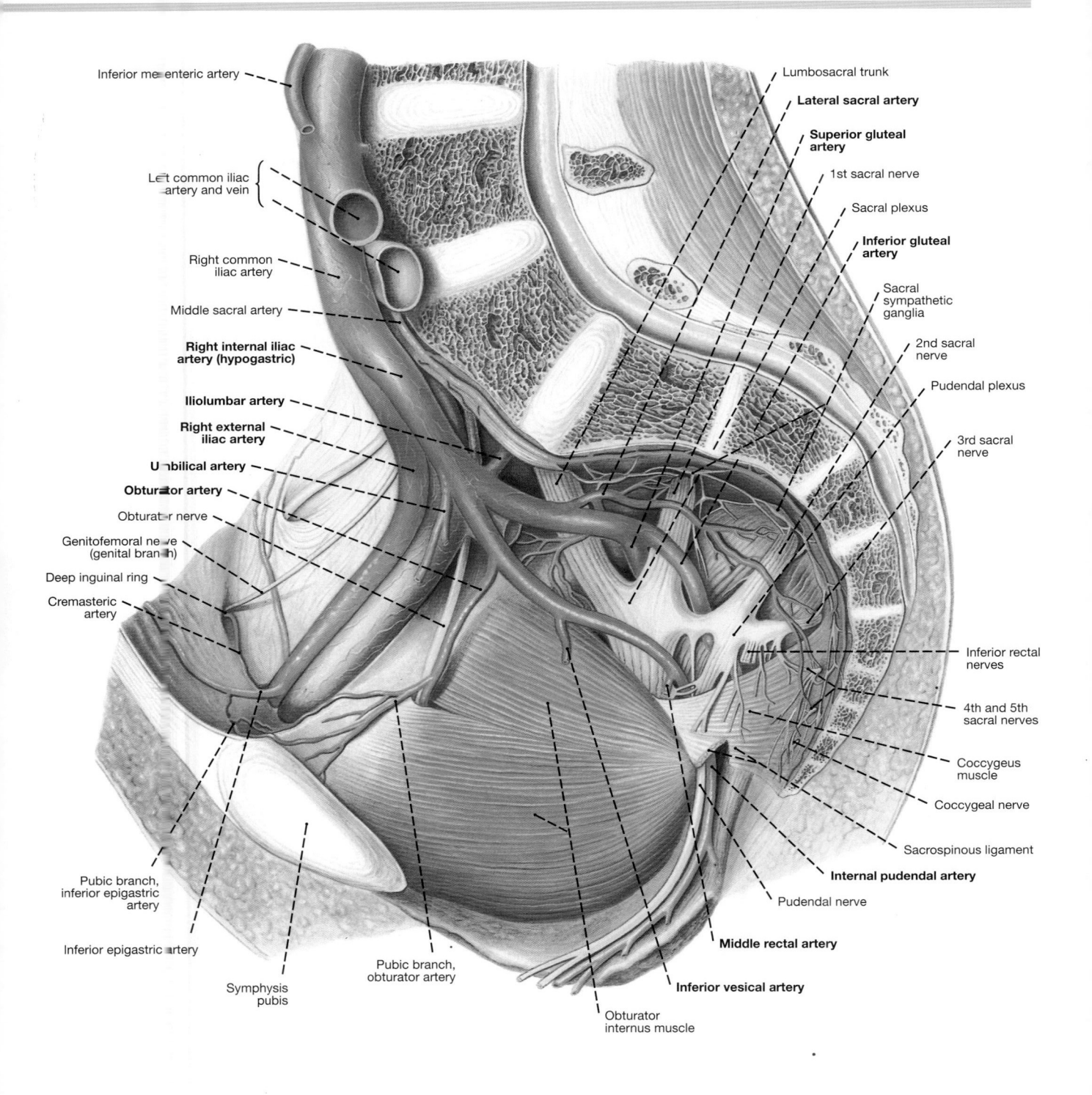

Inferior mesenteric artery
Left common iliac artery and vein
Right common iliac artery
Middle sacral artery
Right internal iliac artery (hypogastric)
Iliolumbar artery
Right external iliac artery
Umbilical artery
Obturator artery
Obturator nerve
Genitofemoral nerve (genital branch)
Deep inguinal ring
Cremasteric artery
Pubic branch, inferior epigastric artery
Inferior epigastric artery
Symphysis pubis
Pubic branch, obturator artery
Obturator internus muscle

Lumbosacral trunk
Lateral sacral artery
Superior gluteal artery
1st sacral nerve
Sacral plexus
Inferior gluteal artery
Sacral sympathetic ganglia
2nd sacral nerve
Pudendal plexus
3rd sacral nerve
Inferior rectal nerves
4th and 5th sacral nerves
Coccygeus muscle
Coccygeal nerve
Sacrospinous ligament
Internal pudendal artery
Pudendal nerve
Middle rectal artery
Inferior vesical artery

Fig. 410: Blood Vessels and Nerves of the Pelvic Wall

NOTE: 1)   this is a midsagittal view of the right pelvic wall seen from the left side with the pelvic viscera removed and the parietal blood vessels and nerves demonstrated.

2)   the principal arteries of the pelvic wall are derived from the internal iliac artery. Although the branches of this vessel are quite variable, it courses about 1½ inches toward the greater sciatic foramen before dividing, usually into **posterior** and **anterior divisions.**

3)   the posterior division vessels include (a) the **iliolumbar** (b) the **lateral sacral** c) the **superior gluteal,** which leaves the pelvis below the piriformis.

4)   the anterior division usually gives rise to four visceral arteries (**umbilical, inferior vesical, middle rectal** and **uterine** or **deferential,** see Fig. 409). Two parietal vessels from the anterior divisions are the **obturator,** which courses through the obturator canal to the medial thigh, and the **internal pudendal,** which leaves the pelvis through the greater sciatic foramen, crosses the ischial spine to enter the lesser sciatic foramen. It then courses toward the perineum by way of the **pudendal canal** to get to the perineum.

Fig. 410

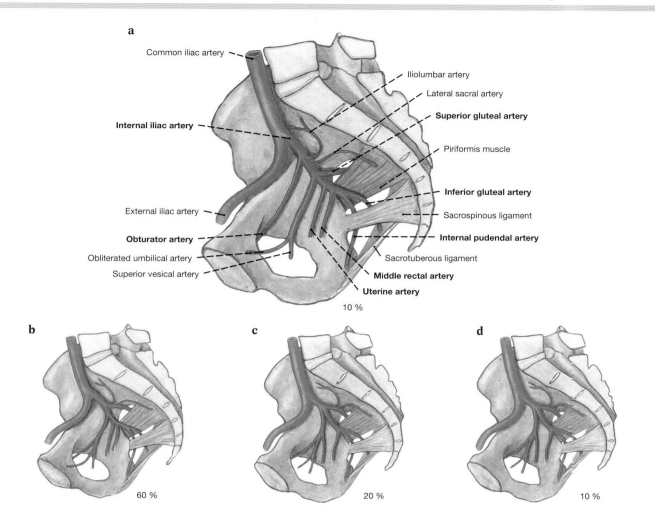

a

Common iliac artery

Internal iliac artery

External iliac artery

Obturator artery

Obliterated umbilical artery

Superior vesical artery

Iliolumbar artery

Lateral sacral artery

Superior gluteal artery

Piriformis muscle

Inferior gluteal artery

Sacrospinous ligament

Internal pudendal artery

Sacrotuberous ligament

Middle rectal artery

Uterine artery

10 %

b   60 %

c   20 %

d   10 %

Fig. 411: Variations in the Divisions of the Internal Iliac Artery

NOTE: 1) in 10% of specimens (shown in **a**) the internal iliac artery itself gives off all branches.

2) in 60% of specimens (shown in **b**) the internal iliac artery divides into two main branches, an anterior and a posterior trunk.

3) in 20% of specimens (shown in **c**) the internal iliac artery divides into three branches.

4) in 10% of specimens (shown in **d**) the internal iliac artery divides into more than three branches.

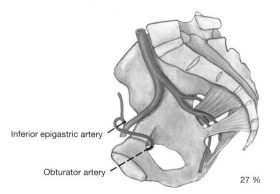

Inferior epigastric artery

Obturator artery

27 %

Fig. 412: Aberrant Origin of the Obturator Artery

NOTE: 1)   the obturator artery arises from the internal iliac artery or one of its branches in nearly 70% of bodies, but in 27% of cases the obturator artery arises from the **inferior epigastric artery** as shown in this figure.

2) if the course of the aberrant obturator artery is lateral to the lacunar ligament, then repair of a femoral hernia is relatively safe, but if it curves along the free margin of the lacunar ligament, the vessel could easily be injured during hernia repair. (From Pick, Anson, Ashley. Am J Anat 1942).

PLATE 268   Female Pelvis: Iliac Arteriogram

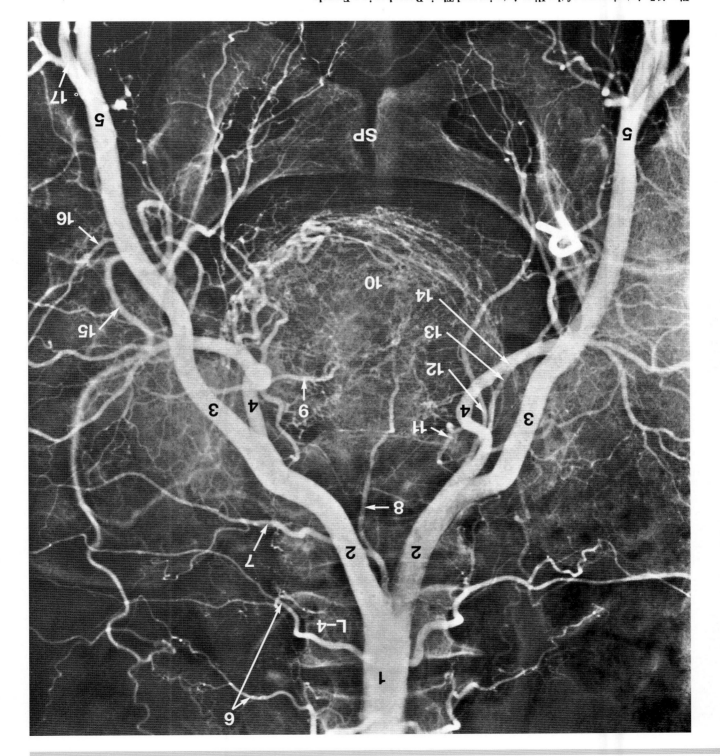

Fig. 413: Arteriogram of the Iliac Arteries and Their Branches in a Female

NOTE: the bifurcation of the aorta (1) into the two common iliac arteries (2) occurs at the lower border of the body of the L4 vertebra. The common iliac vessels branch into external (3) and internal iliac arteries (4) on each side serves a number of branches to the pelvis, perineum, and gluteal region, whereas the external iliac artery (3), after giving off the inferior epigastric (15) and deep circumflex iliac (16) arteries, becomes the femoral artery below the inguinal ligament. (From Wicke L. Atlas of Radiologic Anatomy, 4th Edition, Munich, Urban & Schwarzenberg, 1992).

1. Abdominal aorta	5. Femoral artery	9. Uterine artery	13. Internal pudendal artery
2. Common iliac artery	6. Lumbar arteries	10. Uterus	14. Superior gluteal artery
3. External iliac artery	7. Iliolumbar artery	11. Lateral sacral artery	15. Inferior epigastric artery
4. Internal iliac artery	8. Median sacral artery	12. Obturator artery	16. Deep circumflex iliac artery
			17. Deep femoral artery
			L4-4th lumbar vertebra
			SP-Symphysis pubis

Fig. 413

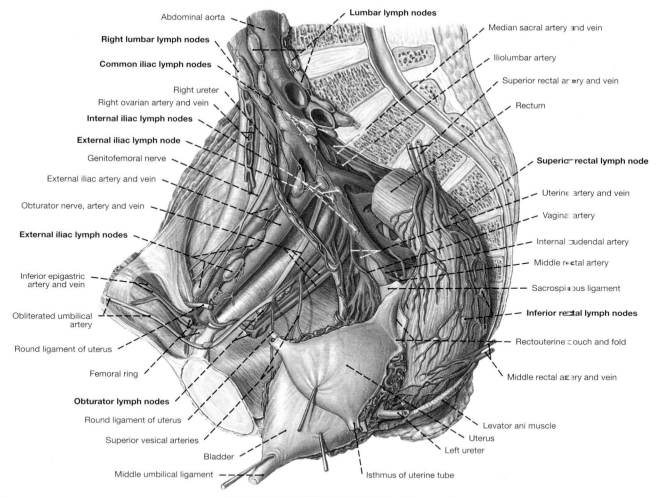

Abdominal aorta
Right lumbar lymph nodes
Common iliac lymph nodes
Right ureter
Right ovarian artery and vein
Internal iliac lymph nodes
External iliac lymph node
Genitofemoral nerve
External iliac artery and vein
Obturator nerve, artery and vein
External iliac lymph nodes
Inferior epigastric artery and vein
Obliterated umbilical artery
Round ligament of uterus
Femoral ring
Obturator lymph nodes
Round ligament of uterus
Superior vesical arteries
Bladder
Middle umbilical ligament

Lumbar lymph nodes
Median sacral artery and vein
Iliolumbar artery
Superior rectal artery and vein
Rectum
Superior rectal lymph node
Uterine artery and vein
Vaginal artery
Internal pudendal artery
Middle rectal artery
Sacrospinous ligament
Inferior rectal lymph nodes
Rectouterine couch and fold
Middle rectal artery and vein
Levator ani muscle
Uterus
Left ureter
Isthmus of uterine tube

Fig. 414: Lymph Vessels and Nodes ▲
of the Female Pelvis

NOTE: 1)   the lymph nodes in the pelvis lie along the course of the major vessels. Lymphatic channels drain superiorly and posteriorly to right and left **lumbar nodes,** which lie bilaterally along the psoas major muscles on both sides of the aorta.

2)   lymph from the bladder drains laterally to **external iliac** and **internal iliac nodes.** These nodes also receive lymph from the fundus, body and cervix of the uterus and the vagina in women, and the prostate and seminal vesicles in men.

Fig. 415: Lymphograph of Pelvis and ▶
Lumbar Region

NOTE: this lymphograph shows lymphatic channels along the femoral vessels (below) and their connections with iliac and lumbar lymph nodes (above).

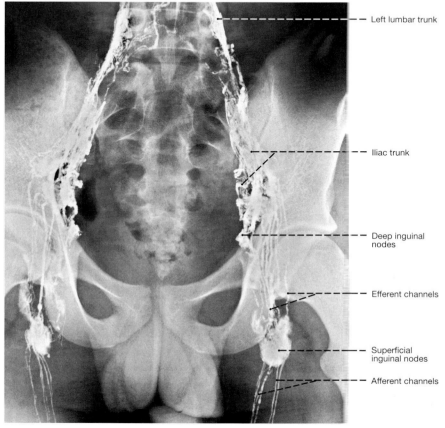

Left lumbar trunk

Iliac trunk

Deep inguinal nodes

Efferent channels

Superficial inguinal nodes

Afferent channels

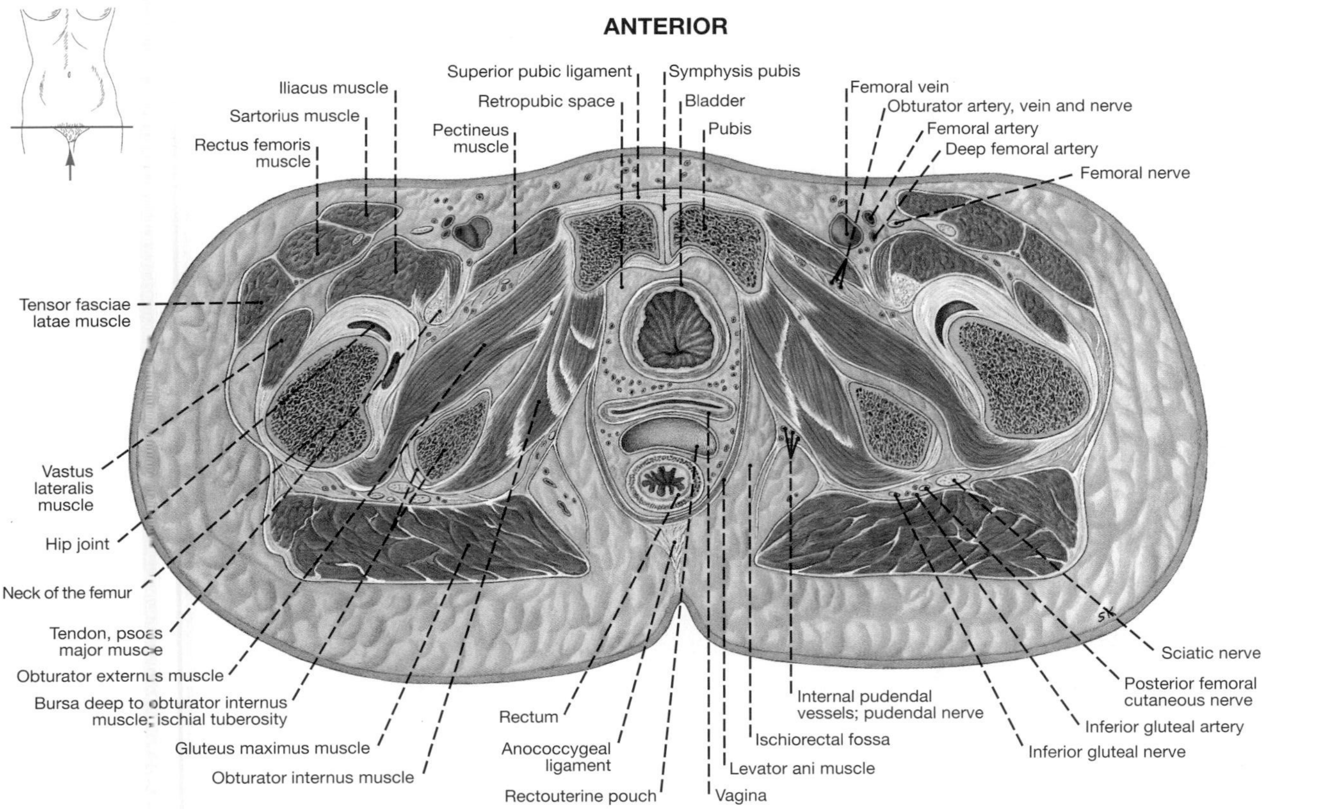

PLATE 270   Female Pelvis: Cross-section and CT Image

ANTERIOR

Iliacus muscle
Sartorius muscle
Rectus femoris muscle
Superior pubic ligament
Retropubic space
Pectineus muscle
Symphysis pubis
Bladder
Pubis
Femoral vein
Obturator artery, vein and nerve
Femoral artery
Deep femoral artery
Femoral nerve

Tensor fasciae latae muscle

Vastus lateralis muscle
Hip joint
Neck of the femur
Tendon, psoas major muscle
Obturator externus muscle
Bursa deep to obturator internus muscle; ischial tuberosity
Gluteus maximus muscle
Obturator internus muscle

Rectum
Anococcygeal ligament
Rectouterine pouch

Internal pudendal vessels; pudendal nerve
Ischiorectal fossa
Levator ani muscle
Vagina

Sciatic nerve
Posterior femoral cutaneous nerve
Inferior gluteal artery
Inferior gluteal nerve

Fig. 416: Cross-section of the Female Pelvis at the Level of the Symphysis Pubis
NOTE: the viscera medially and the **obturator internus muscle** laterally in the pelvis. Observe also the attachment of the **levator ani muscle** from the fascia overlying the obturator internus muscle and how the levator separates the pelvis from the perineum below. Compare this figure with Figures 417 and 418.

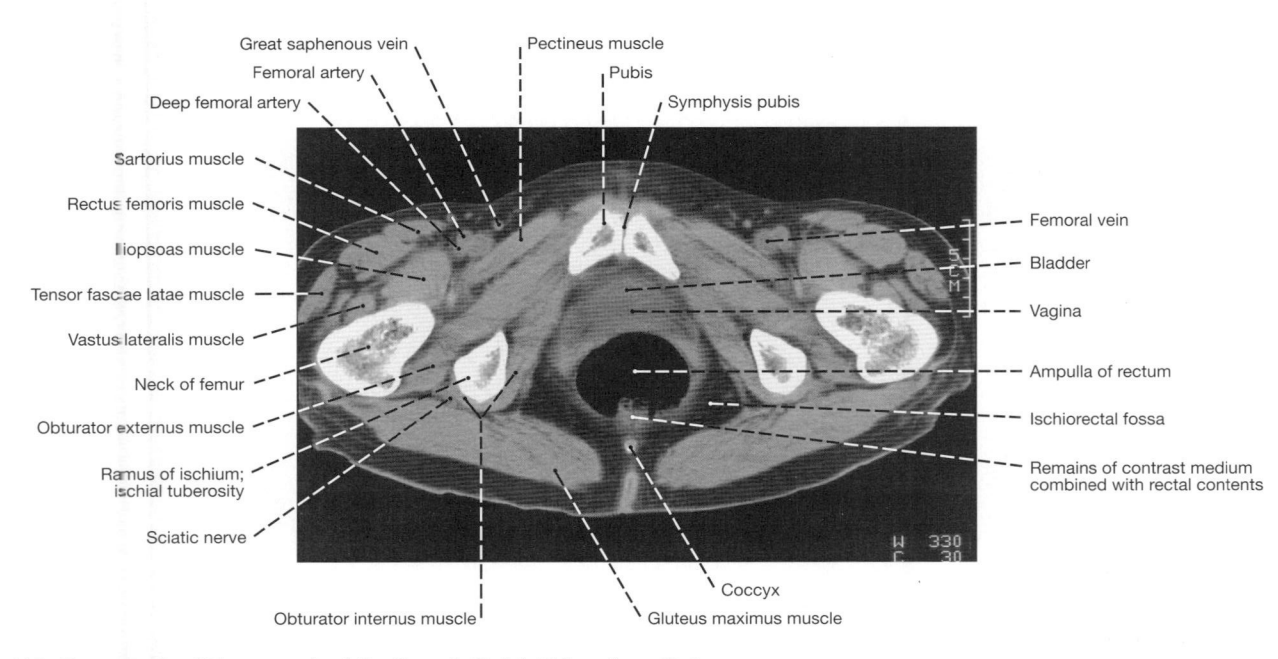

Great saphenous vein
Femoral artery
Deep femoral artery
Pectineus muscle
Pubis
Symphysis pubis

Sartorius muscle
Rectus femoris muscle
Iliopsoas muscle
Tensor fasciae latae muscle
Vastus lateralis muscle
Neck of femur
Obturator externus muscle
Ramus of ischium; ischial tuberosity
Sciatic nerve

Femoral vein
Bladder
Vagina
Ampulla of rectum
Ischiorectal fossa
Remains of contrast medium combined with rectal contents

Obturator internus muscle
Gluteus maximus muscle
Coccyx

Fig. 417: Computerized Tomograph of the Female Pelvis Taken from Below

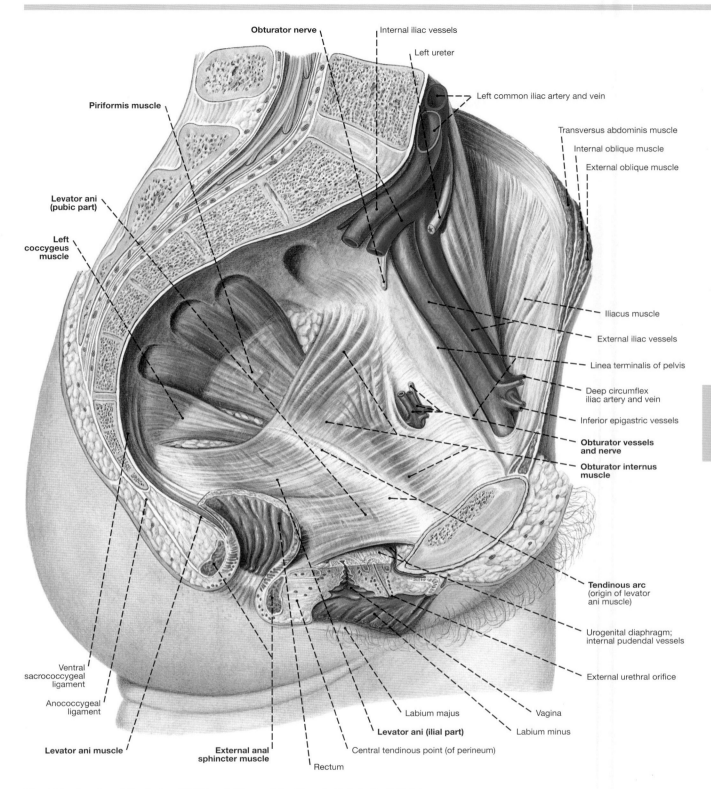

Obturator nerve

Internal iliac vessels

Left ureter

Piriformis muscle

Left common iliac artery and vein

Transversus abdominis muscle

Internal oblique muscle

External oblique muscle

Levator ani
(pubic part)

Left
coccygeus
muscle

Iliacus muscle

External iliac vessels

Linea terminalis of pelvis

Deep circumflex
iliac artery and vein

Inferior epigastric vessels

Obturator vessels
and nerve

Obturator internus
muscle

Tendinous arc
(origin of levator
ani muscle)

Urogenital diaphragm;
internal pudendal vessels

External urethral orifice

Ventral
sacrococcygeal
ligament

Anococcygeal
ligament

Labium majus

Vagina

Levator ani (ilial part)

Labium minus

Levator ani muscle

External anal
sphincter muscle

Central tendinous point (of perineum)

Rectum

Fig. 418: Muscles of the Lateral Wall and Floor of the Female Pelvis (Left Side)

NOTE: 1) the lateral wall of the true pelvis is covered by the piriformis and obturator internus muscles, whereas the floor is formed by the pubic and ischial parts of the levator ani muscle, and more posteriorly, by the coccygeus muscle.

2) the **piriformis muscle** arises from the ventral surface of the 2nd, 3rd, and 4th sacral vertebrae, but is studied with the gluteal muscles, because its fibers converge and leave the pelvis through the greater sciatic foramen.

3) the **obturator internus muscle** arises from the lateral and anterior wall of the true bony pelvis and it surrounds the obturator foramen (note obturator vessels and nerve). Its tendon passes out of the pelvis to the gluteal region through the lesser sciatic foramen.

4) both the **pubic** and **ischial** parts of the **levator ani muscle** arise from the tendinous arc of the obturator internus fascia.

Fig. 418   **IV**

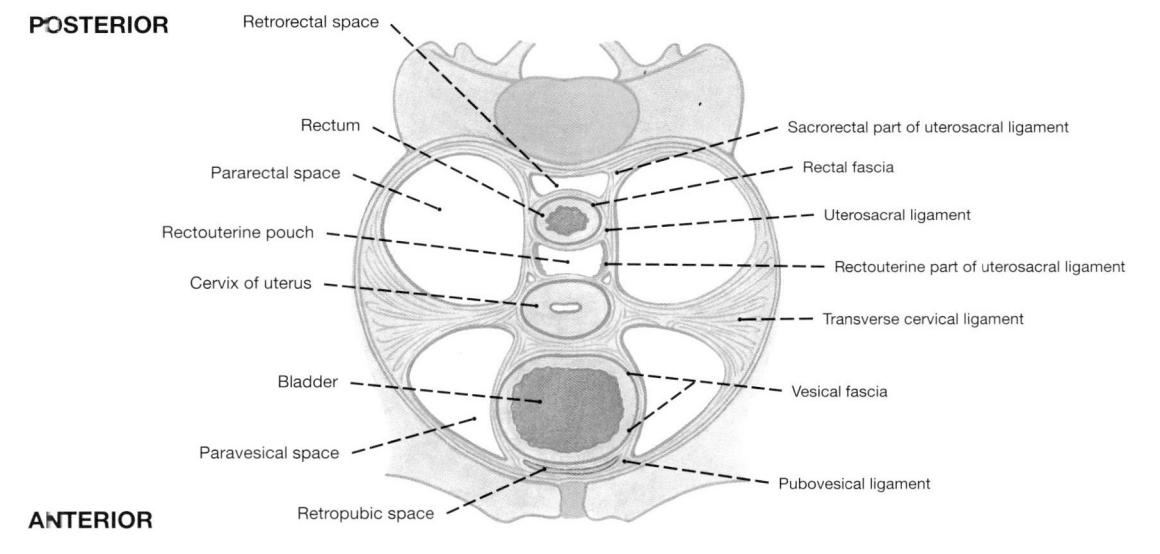

POSTERIOR

Retrorectal space

Rectum

Pararectal space

Rectouterine pouch

Cervix of uterus

Bladder

Paravesical space

Retropubic space

ANTERIOR

Sacrorectal part of uterosacral ligament

Rectal fascia

Uterosacral ligament

Rectouterine part of uterosacral ligament

Transverse cervical ligament

Vesical fascia

Pubovesical ligament

Fig. 419: Uterine Ligaments at the Cervix Just Above the Pelvic Floor (Diagram)

NOTE: 1) just above the floor of the pelvis (formed by the levator ani and coccygeus muscles), is located the cervix of the uterus in women. Extending laterally from the uterine cervix and from the upper vagina to the fascia covering the levator ani muscles are the **transverse cervical ligaments** (also called **lateral cervical, cardinal** or **Mackenrodt's ligaments**).

2) the transverse cervical ligaments are located at the base of the broad ligaments and below the uterine vessels. Observe that the **uterosacral ligaments** also attach to the cervix and upper vagina, but course backward around the rectum to the front of the sacrum.

3) the uterus is supported in position by a) its attachment to the bladder and rectum, b) the transverse cervical and uterosacral ligaments, and c) by the musculature that forms the pelvic floor and urogenital diaphragm.

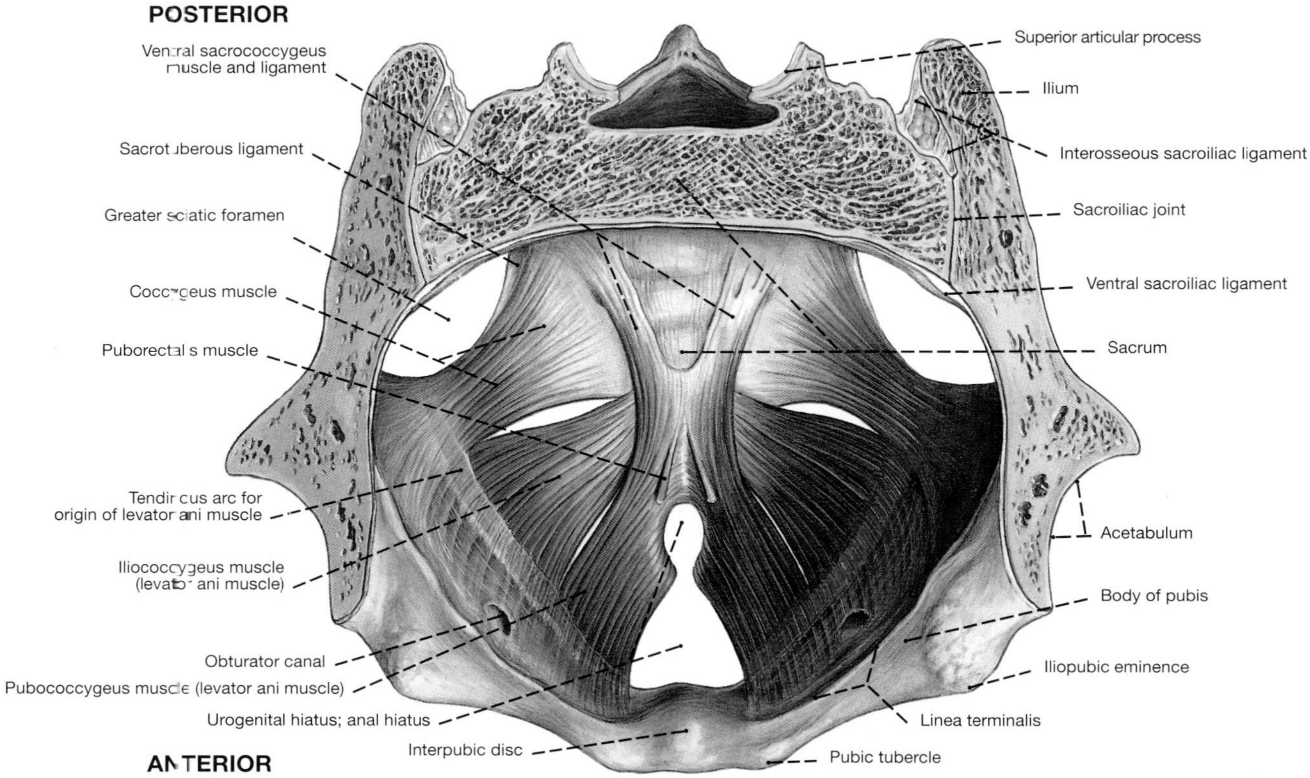

POSTERIOR

Ventral sacrococcygeus muscle and ligament

Sacrotuberous ligament

Greater sciatic foramen

Coccygeus muscle

Puborectalis muscle

Tendinous arc for origin of levator ani muscle

Iliococcygeus muscle (levator ani muscle)

Obturator canal

Pubococcygeus muscle (levator ani muscle)

Urogenital hiatus; anal hiatus

Interpubic disc

ANTERIOR

Superior articular process

Ilium

Interosseous sacroiliac ligament

Sacroiliac joint

Ventral sacroiliac ligament

Sacrum

Acetabulum

Body of pubis

Iliopubic eminence

Linea terminalis

Pubic tubercle

Fig. 420: Muscular Floor of the Female Pelvis, Viewed from Above

NOTE: 1) the muscular floor of the pelvis is formed anteriorly by the **pubococcygeus** and anterolaterally by the **iliococcygeus** portions of the **levator ani muscle** and posterolaterally the **coccygeus muscle,** which lies above the sacrotuberous ligament.

2) the **urogenital hiatus.** At this site is located the **urogenital (UG) diaphragm,** which is formed by the deep transverse perineal muscles and the membranous sphincter of the urethra, which lie between two layers of fascia (see Fig. 429). The urethra and vagina penetrate through the UG diaphragm in the female.

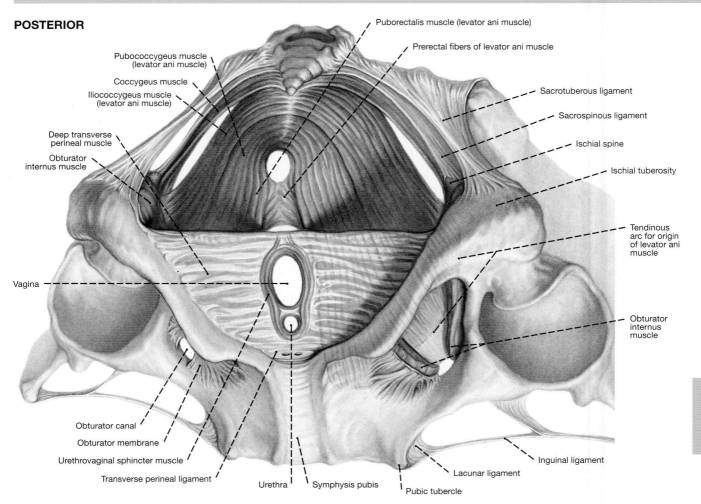

POSTERIOR

Puborectalis muscle (levator ani muscle)

Prerectal fibers of levator ani muscle

Pubococcygeus muscle (levator ani muscle)

Coccygeus muscle

Iliococcygeus muscle (levator ani muscle)

Deep transverse perineal muscle

Obturator internus muscle

Sacrotuberous ligament

Sacrospinous ligament

Ischial spine

Ischial tuberosity

Tendinous arc for origin of levator ani muscle

Vagina

Obturator internus muscle

Obturator canal

Obturator membrane

Urethrovaginal sphincter muscle

Transverse perineal ligament

Urethra

Symphysis pubis

Pubic tubercle

Lacunar ligament

Inguinal ligament

ANTERIOR

Fig. 421: Muscular Floor of the Female Pelvis Viewed from Below

NOTE: 1)   from this inferior view can be seen the parts of the **levator ani muscle** and **coccygeus muscle** (shown from above in Fig. 420) that form the floor of the pelvis (and the roof of the perineum).

2)   the **deep transverse perineal muscles** form the bulk of the urogenital diaphragm and with the **transverse perineal ligament** seal the borders of the urogenital hiatus. The vagina and urethra, however, still course through this site, penetrating the urogenital diaphragm.

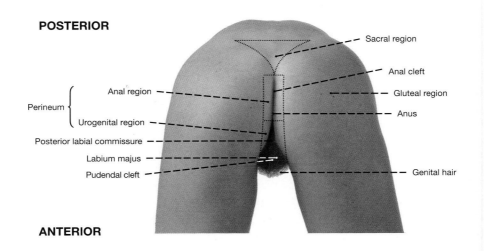

POSTERIOR

Sacral region

Anal cleft

Gluteal region

Anus

Anal region

Perineum

Urogenital region

Posterior labial commissure

Labium majus

Pudendal cleft

Genital hair

ANTERIOR

Fig. 422: Surface Anatomy of the Female Sacral, Gluteal and Perineal Regions, Posteroinferior View

PLATE 274   Female Perineum: External Genitalia

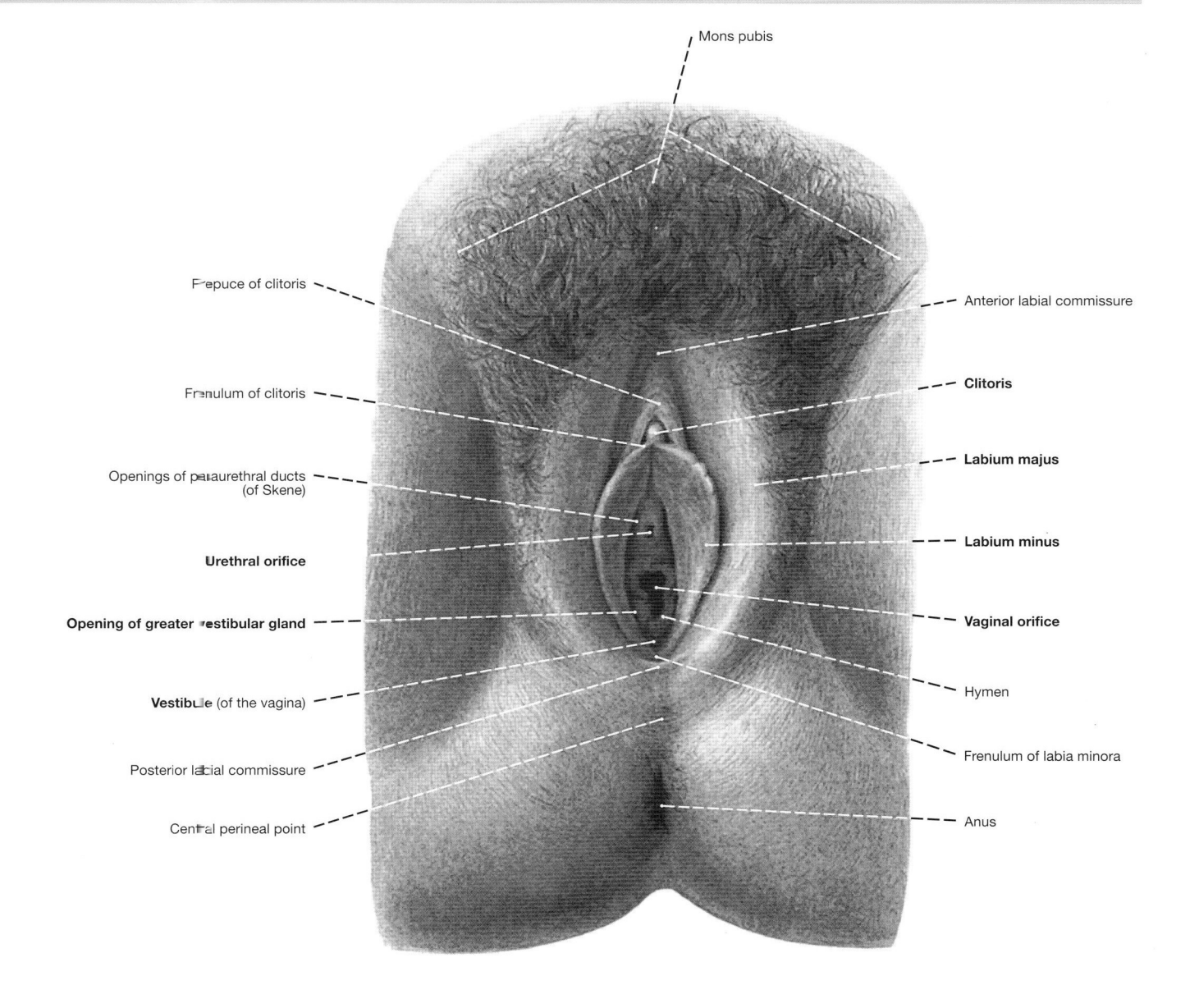

Mons pubis

Prepuce of clitoris

Frenulum of clitoris

Openings of paraurethral ducts
(of Skene)

Urethral orifice

Opening of greater vestibular gland

Vestibule (of the vagina)

Posterior labial commissure

Central perineal point

Anterior labial commissure

Clitoris

Labium majus

Labium minus

Vaginal orifice

Hymen

Frenulum of labia minora

Anus

Fig. 423: External Genitalia of an 18-Year-Old Virgin

NOTE: 1) the female **external genitalia** are a) the mons pubis, b) the labia majora, c) the labia minora, d) the clitoris, and e) the vestibule of the vagina. The **orifices** of the female perineum include the openings of the a) urethra, b) vagina, c) ducts of the two greater vestibular glands, d) small paraurethral ducts (of Skene), and e) anus.

2) the **mons pubis** is a rounded mound of skin and adipose tissue anterior to the symphysis pubis, and it is covered with genital hair in the adult.

3) the **labia majora** are two elongated folds of skin and fat extending from the mons pubis toward the anus. They vary in size and thickness dependent on age and obesity and their anterior ends receive the fibrous round ligaments of the uterus. The labia majora are the female homologous structures to the male scrotum.

4) the **labia minora** are two thin folds of skin situated between the labia majora. They commence at the glans clitoris and small extensions pass over the dorsum of the clitoris to form the **prepuce.** Posteriorly, they meet in the midline to form the **frenulum.**

5) the **clitoris** is the homologue of the male penis. It is an erectile organ that measures one inch or less in length and consists of two corpora cavernosa attached by crura to the pubic rami. It is suspended by a fibrous ligament and capped by the **glans.**

6) the **vestibule** of the vagina is the region between the two labia minora. Into it open the **urethra,** the **ducts of the greater vestibular glands,** and the **vagina.** In the virgin the vaginal orifice is partially closed by a thin membrane, the **hymen,** which usually is ruptured at first copulation. Since its form and extent are quite variable, establishment of virginity by its absence cannot be absolutely determined.

Fig. 423

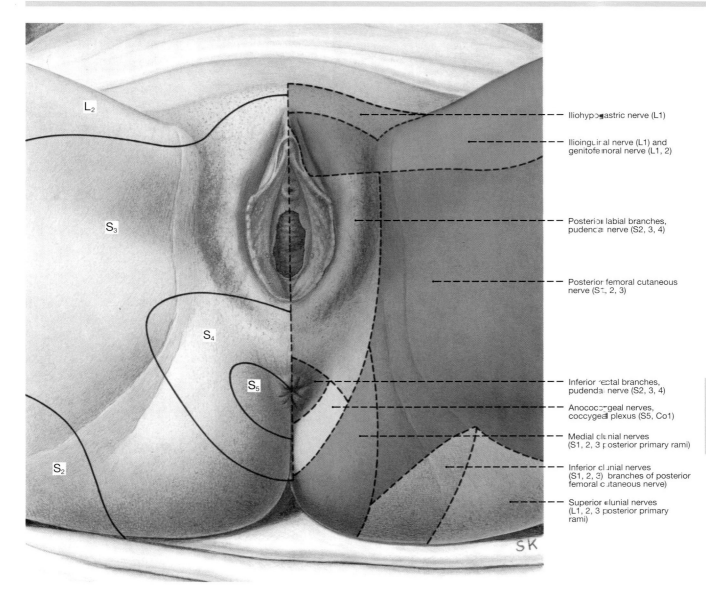

Fig. 424: Cutaneous Fields of Peripheral Nerves and Dermatomes: Female Urogenital Region

Labels on Fig. 424:

- Iliohypogastric nerve (L1)
- Ilioinguinal nerve (L1) and genitofemoral nerve (L1, 2)
- Posterior labial branches, pudendal nerve (S2, 3, 4)
- Posterior femoral cutaneous nerve (S1, 2, 3)
- Inferior rectal branches, pudendal nerve (S2, 3, 4)
- Anococcygeal nerves, coccygeal plexus (S5, Co1)
- Medial clunial nerves (S1, 2, 3 posterior primary rami)
- Inferior clunial nerves (S1, 2, 3 branches of posterior femoral cutaneous nerve)
- Superior clunial nerves (L1, 2, 3 posterior primary rami)

L₂   S₃   S₄   S₅   S₂

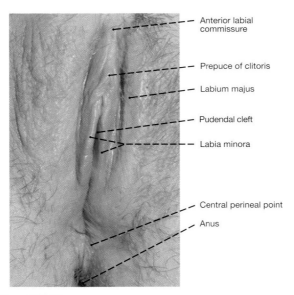

Labels on Fig. 425:

- Anterior labial commissure
- Prepuce of clitoris
- Labium majus
- Pudendal cleft
- Labia minora
- Central perineal point
- Anus

Fig. 425: Perineal Structures in a 26-Year-Old Woman
NOTE: in this photograph the labia minora are approximated so that the vaginal and urethral orifices are not visible.

PLATE 276   Female Perineum: Muscles

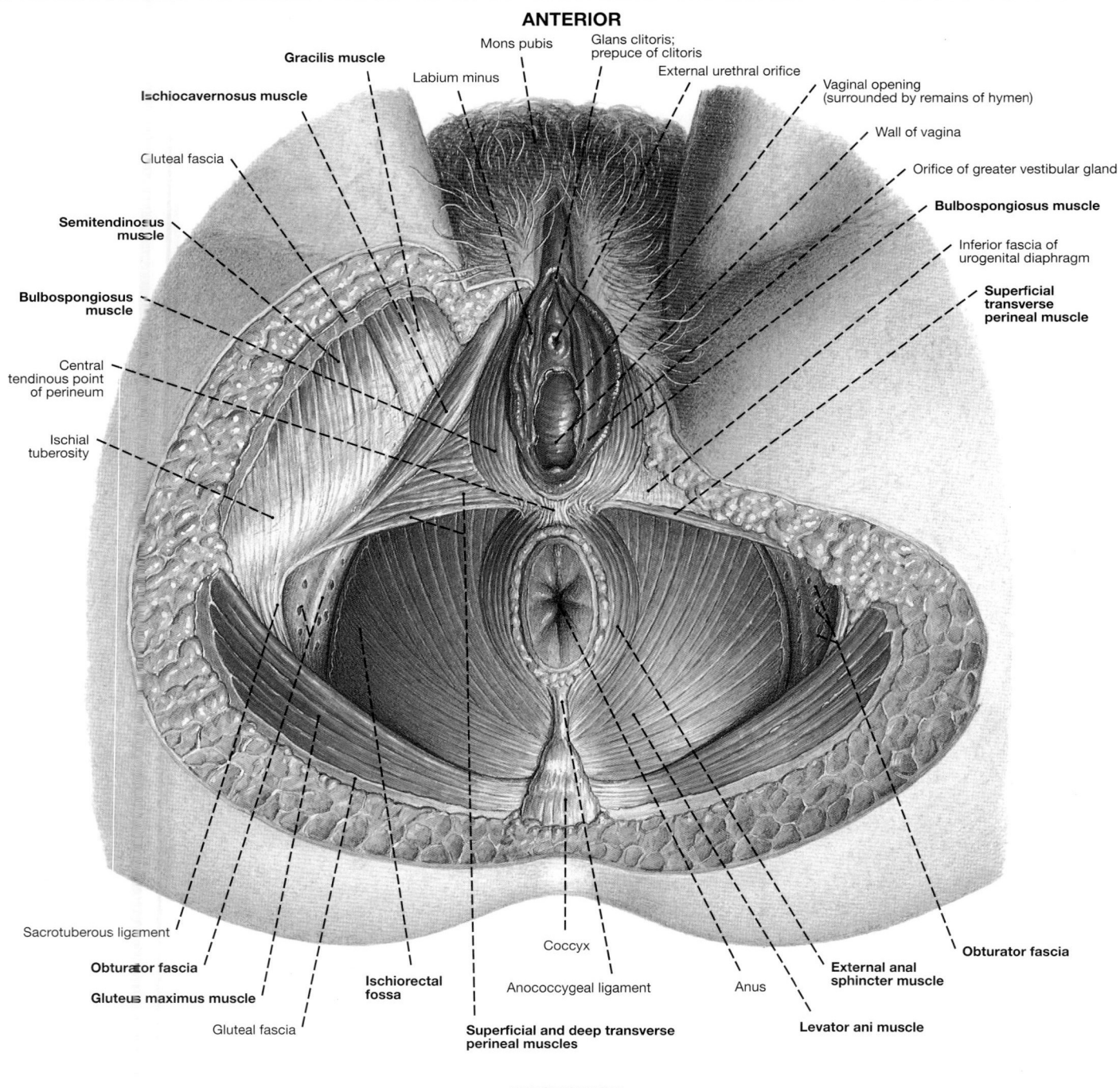

ANTERIOR

Gracilis muscle

Ischiocavernosus muscle

Gluteal fascia

Semitendinosus
muscle

Bulbospongiosus
muscle

Central
tendinous point
of perineum

Ischial
tuberosity

Mons pubis

Labium minus

Glans clitoris;
prepuce of clitoris

External urethral orifice

Vaginal opening
(surrounded by remains of hymen)

Wall of vagina

Orifice of greater vestibular gland

Bulbospongiosus muscle

Inferior fascia of
urogenital diaphragm

**Superficial
transverse
perineal muscle**

Sacrotuberous ligament

Obturator fascia

Gluteus maximus muscle

Gluteal fascia

**Ischiorectal
fossa**

Coccyx

Anococcygeal ligament

**Superficial and deep transverse
perineal muscles**

Anus

**External anal
sphincter muscle**

Levator ani muscle

Obturator fascia

POSTERIOR

Fig. 426: Muscles of the Female Perineum

NOTE: 1) the perineum is a diamond-shaped region located below the pelvis and separated from it by the muscular pelvic diaphragm. The perineum is bounded by the **symphysis pubis** anteriorly, the **coccyx** posteriorly and the two **ischial tuberosities** laterally. A line drawn across the perineum anterior to the anus between the two ischial tuberosities divides the perineum into an anterior **urogenital region** and a posterior **anal region.**

2) the *urogenital region* contains the external genitalia and the associated muscles and glands. Often books refer to *superficial and deep perineal compartments* (spaces or pouches). The **superficial perineal compartment** lies superficial to the inferior layer of fascia of the urogenital diaphragm and it contains the ischiocavernosus, bulbocavernosus, and superficial transverse perineal muscles and the perineal vessels and nerves. It is limited superficially by a layer of deep fascia (the external perineal fascia) just deep to **Colles' fascia.**

3) the **deep perineal compartment** is the space enclosed between the two layers of the urogenital diaphragm. It contains the deep transverse perineal and urethral sphincter muscles and is traversed by the urethra and vagina in the female.

4) the *anal region* is situated posterior to the urogenital region, and it contains the anus surrounded by the external anal sphincter muscle. A large portion of the anal region is occupied on by the two fat-filled **ischiorectal fossae.**

Fig. 426

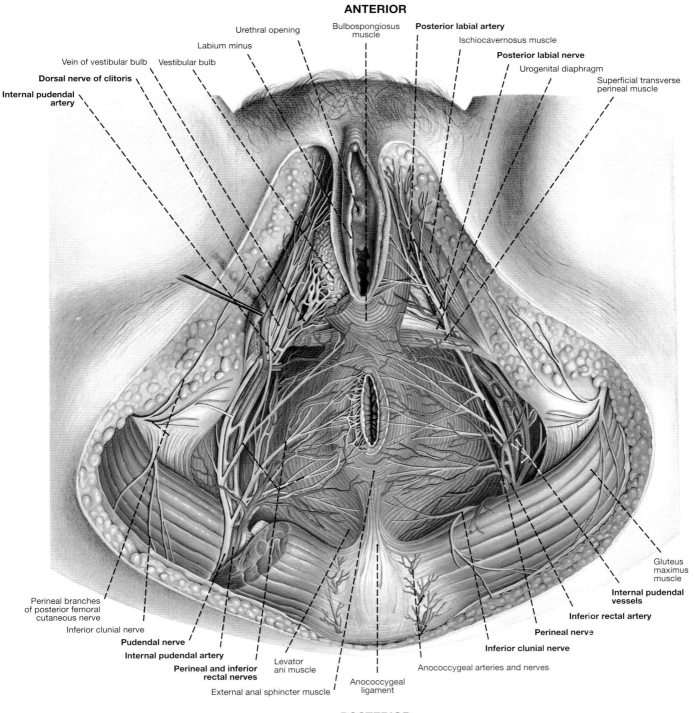

ANTERIOR

Urethral opening

Labium minus

Bulbospongiosus muscle

Posterior labial artery

Ischiocavernosus muscle

Vein of vestibular bulb   Vestibular bulb

Posterior labial nerve

Urogenital diaphragm

Superficial transverse perineal muscle

Dorsal nerve of clitoris

Internal pudendal artery

Perineal branches of posterior femoral cutaneous nerve

Inferior clunial nerve

Pudendal nerve

Internal pudendal artery

Perineal and inferior rectal nerves

External anal sphincter muscle

Levator ani muscle

Anococcygeal ligament

Anococcygeal arteries and nerves

Gluteus maximus muscle

Internal pudendal vessels

Inferior rectal artery

Perineal nerve

Inferior clunial nerve

POSTERIOR

Fig. 427: Nerves and Blood Vessels of the Female Perineum

NOTE: 1)   the branches of the **pudendal nerve** supply most of the perineal structures. This nerve arises from the 2nd, 3rd, and 4th sacral segments of the spinal cord. Within the pelvis it is joined by the **internal pudendal artery and vein.** The vessels and nerve leave the pelvis through the greater sciatic foramen along the lower border of the piriformis muscle, cross the ischial spine to reenter the pelvis through the lesser sciatic foramen.

2)   the pudendal structures reach the perineum by way of the **pudendal canal** (of Alcock) deep to the fascia of the obturator internus muscle. Their branches, the **inferior rectal vessels** and **nerves** cross the ischiorectal fossa toward the midline to supply the levator ani and external anal sphincter muscles as well as other structures in the anal region.

3)   the pudendal vessels and nerve then continue anteriorly as the **perineal vessels** and **nerve** and enter the urogenital region by penetrating the urogenital diaphragm. They branch again into superficial and deep branches to supply structures in the superficial and deep compartments. The superficial branches supply the labia majora and the external genital structures, whereas the deep branches supply the muscles, vestibular bulb, and clitoris.

Fig. 427   **IV**

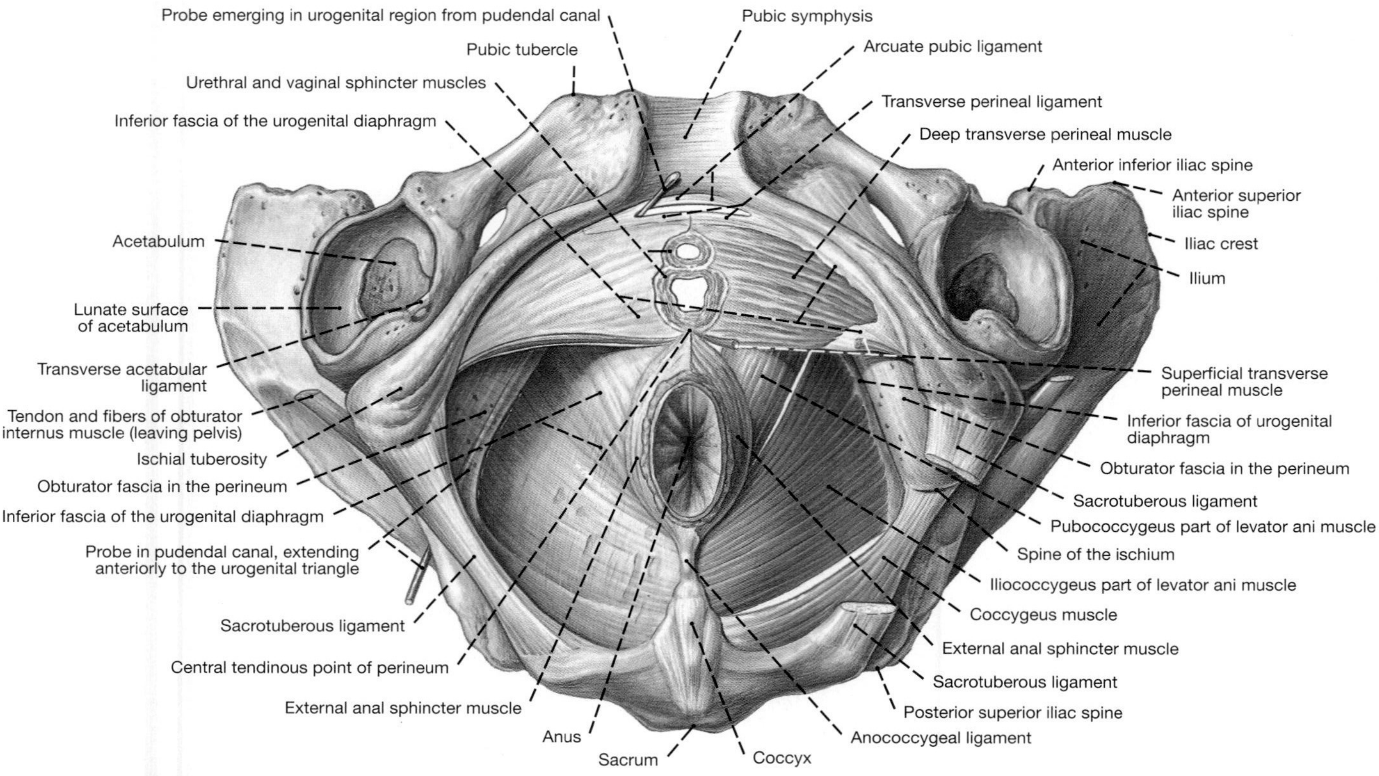

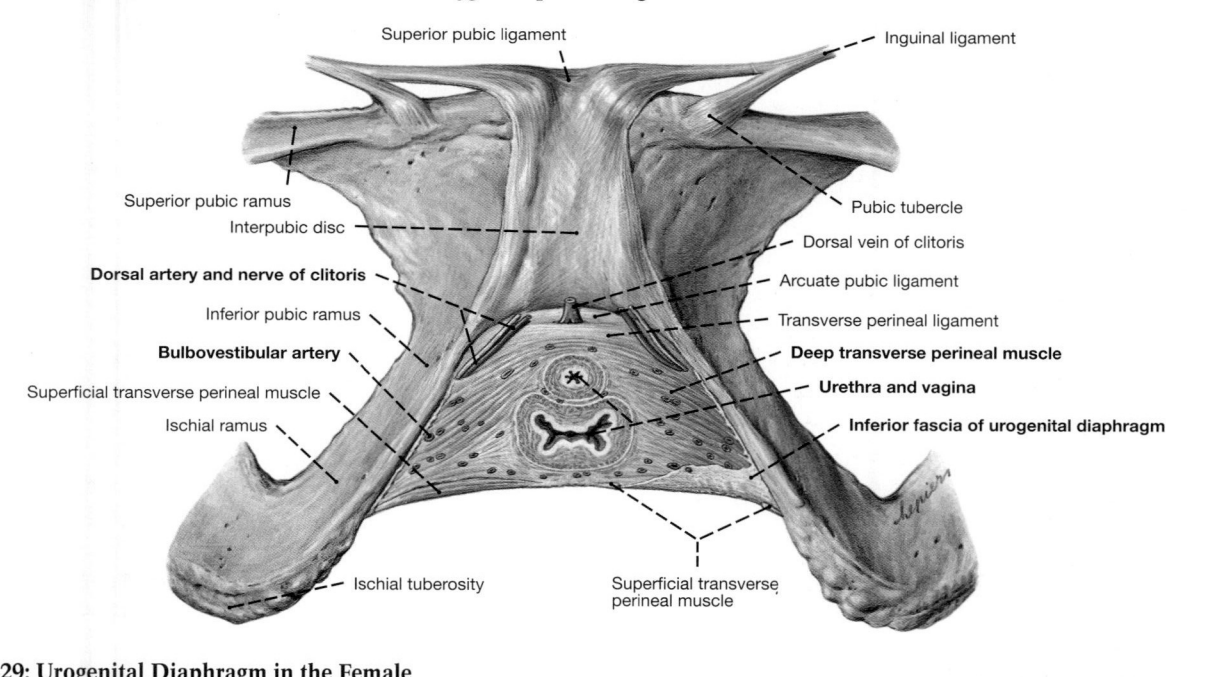

Probe emerging in urogenital region from pudendal canal
Pubic symphysis
Pubic tubercle
Arcuate pubic ligament
Urethral and vaginal sphincter muscles
Transverse perineal ligament
Inferior fascia of the urogenital diaphragm
Deep transverse perineal muscle
Anterior inferior iliac spine
Anterior superior iliac spine
Acetabulum
Iliac crest
Ilium
Lunate surface of acetabulum
Superficial transverse perineal muscle
Transverse acetabular ligament
Inferior fascia of urogenital diaphragm
Tendon and fibers of obturator internus muscle (leaving pelvis)
Obturator fascia in the perineum
Ischial tuberosity
Sacrotuberous ligament
Obturator fascia in the perineum
Pubococcygeus part of levator ani muscle
Inferior fascia of the urogenital diaphragm
Spine of the ischium
Probe in pudendal canal, extending anteriorly to the urogenital triangle
Iliococcygeus part of levator ani muscle
Coccygeus muscle
Sacrotuberous ligament
External anal sphincter muscle
Central tendinous point of perineum
Sacrotuberous ligament
External anal sphincter muscle
Posterior superior iliac spine
Anus
Anococcygeal ligament
Sacrum
Coccyx

Fig. 428: Musculature of the Floor of the Female Pelvis, Viewed from the Inferior or Perineal Aspect

NOTE: 1)   on the left side (reader's right) the inferior fascias of the pelvic and urogenital diaphragms have been removed.

2)   the musculature of the urogenital diaphragm completes the anterior part of the female pelvic floor but allows the urethra and vagina to traverse the urogenital hiatus.

3)   the **central point of the perineum** interposed in the midline between the urogenital diaphragm and the anterior end of the raphé formed by the two external anal sphincters.

4)   the anal hiatus is surrounded by the **pubococcygeus** parts of the levator ani muscles. These are reinforced above by the puborectalis muscle and below by the external sphincter. Observe that the **iliococcygeus** sweeps medially to the coccyx, but some fibers also insert into the short midline **anococcygeal raphé** and **ligament.**

Superior pubic ligament
Inguinal ligament
Superior pubic ramus
Interpubic disc
Pubic tubercle
Dorsal vein of clitoris
Dorsal artery and nerve of clitoris
Arcuate pubic ligament
Inferior pubic ramus
Transverse perineal ligament
Bulbovestibular artery
Deep transverse perineal muscle
Superficial transverse perineal muscle
Urethra and vagina
Ischial ramus
Inferior fascia of urogenital diaphragm
Ischial tuberosity
Superficial transverse perineal muscle

Fig. 429: Urogenital Diaphragm in the Female

NOTE: the female **urethra** and **vagina** both pass through the **urogenital diaphragm.** Observe the circular **sphincter** surrounding the membranous urethra and the **deep transverse perineal muscles** that are covered by deep fascia on both their superior and inferior surfaces.

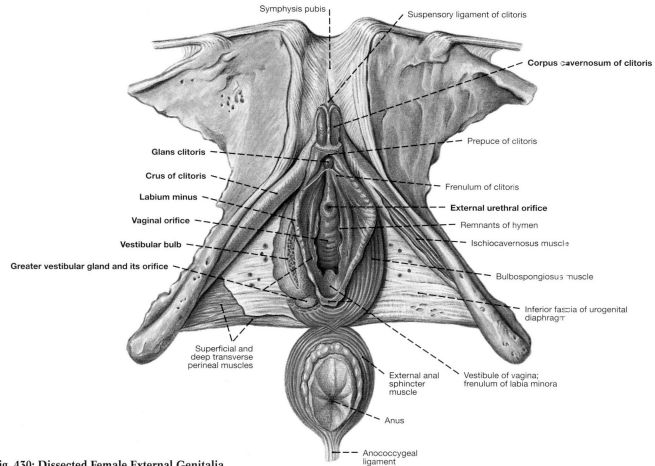

Fig. 430: Dissected Female External Genitalia

NOTE: 1) the skin and fascia of the labia majora have been removed. Observe the **crura, body** and **glans clitoris, the vestibular bulbs** and the location of the **greater vestibular glands.**

2) each crus of the clitoris is covered by an **ischiocavernosus muscle** and the vestibular bulbs are surrounded by the **bulbospongiosus muscles.**

3) the **greater vestibular glands** (of Bartholin) are found just behind the vestibular bulbs. During sexual stimulation, they secrete a viscous fluid that lubricates the vagina.

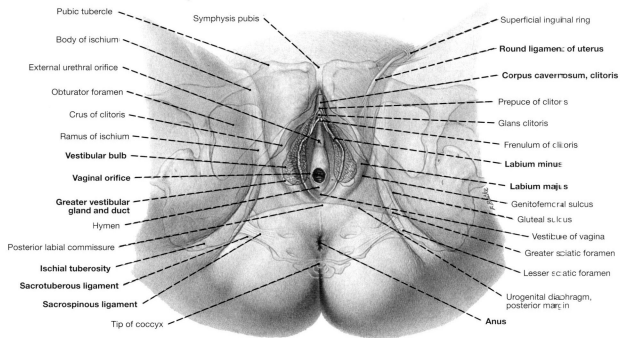

Fig. 431: Projection of External Female Genitalia on Bony Structures of the Pelvis

PLATE 280   Muscles of the Anal and Urogenital Regions; Chart

Muscles Related to the Pelvic Diaphragm

Muscle	Origin	Insertion	Innervation	Action
Levator ani consisting of: PUBOCOCCYGEUS ILIOCOCCYGEUS PUBOVAGINALIS LEVATOR of PROSTATE PUBORECTALIS	From a tendinous arch (along the fascia of the obturator internus muscle). The arch extends from the symphysis pubis to the ischial spine.	Into the coccyx; the anococcygeal raphe and ligament; the external anal sphincter; central tendinous point of the perineum.	Pudendal nerve (S3, 4 and 5)	Supports and slightly raises the floor of the pelvis; it resists intraabdominal pressure, as in forced expiration.
Coccygeus	Spine of the ischium; sacrospinous ligament	Lateral margin of coccyx and sacrum.	Pudendal plexus (S4, S5 nerves)	Draws coccyx forward during parturition or defecation. Supports pelvic floor.
External Anal Sphincter SUBCUTANEOUS PART A band of fibers just deep to the skin	Attached anteriorly to the perineal body and posteriorly to the anococcygeal ligament		Pudendal nerve, inferior rectal branch (S4)	Anal sphincter is in a state of tonic contraction; upon defecation the muscle relaxes.
SUPERFICIAL PART Lies deep to the subcutaneous part; main part of muscle	From the anococcygeal ligament	Into the perineal body		
DEEP PART Forms a complete sphincter of the anal canal	Fibers surround the anal canal and are applied closely to the internal anal sphincter.			

Deep Muscles of the Urogenital Region

Muscle	Origin	Insertion	Innervation	Action
Deep Transverse Perineal Muscle (FEMALE)	Inferior ramus of the ischium	To the side of the vagina, meeting fibers of the muscle from the other side.	Perineal branch of the pudendal nerve (S2, 3, 4)	Helps to fix the perineal body and assists the urethrovaginal sphincter.
Deep Transverse Perineal Muscle (MALE)	Inferior ramus of the ischium	Fibers course to the median line where they interlace in a tendinous raphe with fibers from the other side	Perineal branch of the pudendal nerve (S2, 3, 4)	Helps to fix the perineal body and assists the urethral sphincter
Urethrovaginal Sphincter (FEMALE)	*Inferior fibers:* from the transverse perineal ligament *Superior fibers:* from the inner surface of the pubic ramus	Course backward on both sides of the urethra Encircle the lower end of the urethra	Perineal branch of the pudendal nerve (S2, 3, 4)	Acts as a voluntary constrictor of the urethra and vagina.
Sphincter of the Urethra (MALE) Surrounds the membranous part of the urethra	*Superficial part:* from the transverse perineal ligament *Deep part:* from the ramus of the pubis	Most fibers form a circular sphincter that invests the membranous urethra; some fibers join the perineal body.	Perineal branch of the pudendal nerve (S2, 3, 4)	Acts as the voluntary constrictor of the membranous urethra.

Superficial Muscles of the Urogenital Region

Muscle	Origin	Insertion	Innervation	Action
Superficial Transverse Perineal Muscle (MALE and FEMALE)	Medial and anterior part of the ischial tuberosity	Into the perineal body in front of the anus	Perineal branch of the pudendal nerve (S2, 3, 4)	Simultaneous contraction of the two muscles helps to fix the central tendinous point of the perineum.
Ischiocavernosus Muscle (FEMALE)	Inner surface of the ischial tuberosity behind the crus clitoris and from the adjacent part of the ramus of the ischium.	Fibers end in an aponeurosis which inserts onto the sides and under surface of the crus clitoris.	Perineal branch of the pudendal nerve (S2, 3, 4)	Compresses the crus clitoris retarding the return of blood and thereby helping to maintain erection of the clitoris.
Ischiocavernosus Muscle (MALE)	Inner surface of the ischial tuberosity behind the crus penis and from the ramus of the ischium on each side of the crus.	Fibers end in an aponeurosis attached to the sides and under surface of the corpus cavernosum on each side as they join to form the body of the penis.	Perineal branch of the pudendal nerve (S2, 3, 4)	Compresses the crus penis and thereby helps to maintain erection.
Bulbospongiosus Muscle (FEMALE)	Fibers attached posteriorly to the perineal body	Fibers pass anteriorly around the vagina and are inserted into the corpora cavernosa clitoris.	Perineal branch of the pudendal nerve (S2, 3, 4)	Decreases the orifice of the vagina; anterior fibers assist erection of the clitoris by compressing the deep dorsal vein of the clitoris.
Bulbospongiosus Muscle (MALE)	From the perineal body and the ventral extension of the perineal body that forms a median raphe between the two bulbocavernosus muscles.	*Posterior fibers:* end in connective tissue of the fascia of UG diaphragm; *Middle fibers:* encircle the bulb of the penis and the corpus spongiosum; *Anterior fibers:* spread over the side of the corpus cavernosum and extend anteriorly as a tendinous expansion over the dorsal vessels	Perineal branch of the pudendal nerve (S2, 3, 4)	Aids in emptying the urethra at end of urination; by compressing the dorsal vein, it also helps maintain penile erection; contracts during ejaculation.

IV

PLATE 282   **Pregnant Uterus: Anterior View**

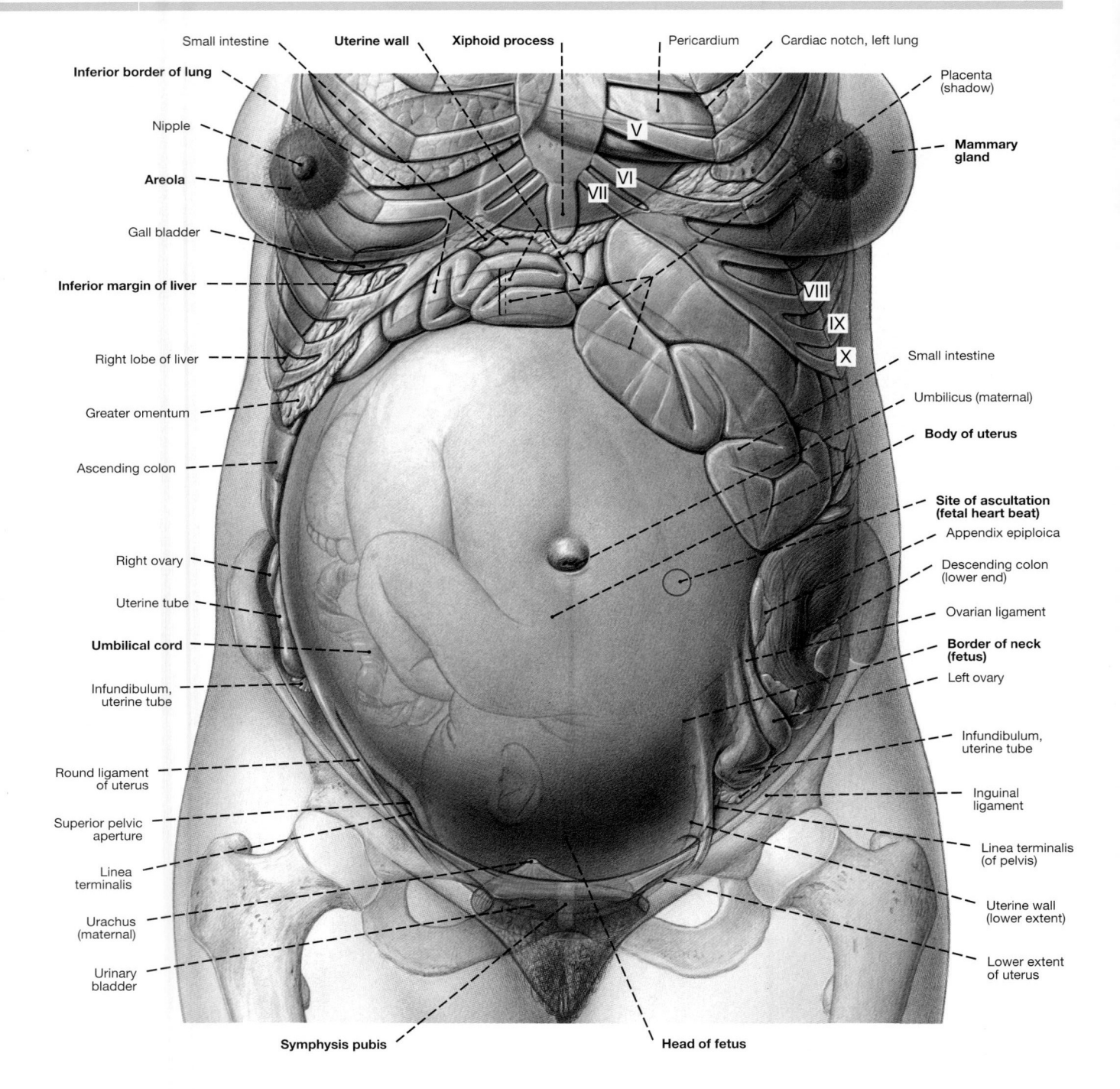

Fig. 432: Projection of Abdominal and Pelvic Organs in a Pregnant Woman Shortly Before Giving Birth: Anterior View
NOTE: 1)   in the maternal abdomen, the full-term fetus is characteristically in a longitudinal posture, with the dorsum of the head and back oriented toward the mother's anterior abdominal wall.

2)   the cephalic longitudinal presentation shown in this figure occurs in about 95% of births, whereas longitudinal pelvic presentation (breech) occurs in about 3% of births. In about 1% of births, a transverse presentation of the fetus occurs, with one of the fetal shoulders as the presenting part.

3)   near the end of pregnancy the maternal liver, stomach and intestines are displaced upward, while the diaphragm is elevated and the dimensions of the thoracic cavity are broadened. The breasts enlarge considerably through a proliferation of its glandular tissue in advance of lactation, and the areolar region around the nipple becomes more darkly pigmented.

Fig. 432

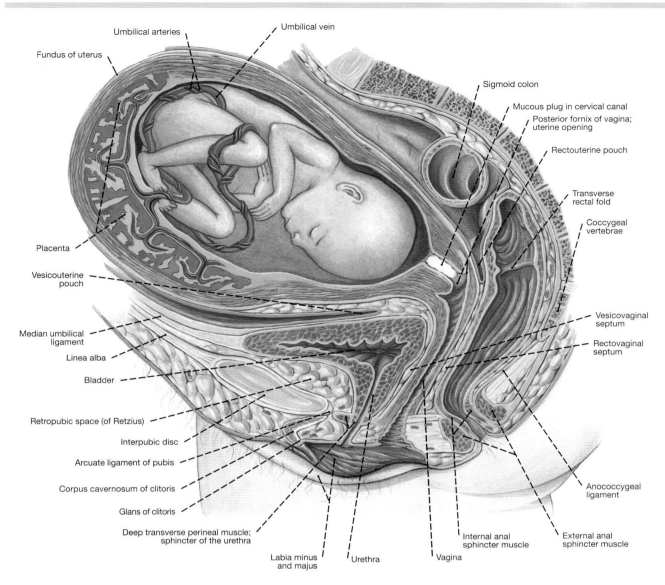

Umbilical arteries

Umbilical vein

Fundus of uterus

Sigmoid colon

Mucous plug in cervical canal

Posterior fornix of vagina; uterine opening

Rectouterine pouch

Transverse rectal fold

Coccygeal vertebrae

Placenta

Vesicouterine pouch

Vesicovaginal septum

Rectovaginal septum

Median umbilical ligament

Linea alba

Bladder

Retropubic space (of Retzius)

Interpubic disc

Arcuate ligament of pubis

Corpus cavernosum of clitoris

Glans of clitoris

Anococcygeal ligament

Deep transverse perineal muscle; sphincter of the urethra

Labia minus and majus

Urethra

Vagina

Internal anal sphincter muscle

External anal sphincter muscle

Fig. 433: Pregnant Uterus Shortly Before Birth, Right Half of Pelvis
NOTE: 1)   the pelvis, including the uterus, have been hemisected, while the new-born fetus is shown intact.

2)   in this cephalic longitudinal presentation of the fetus, the placenta is oriented toward the maternal anterior abdominal wall, in contrast to the longitudinal presentation shown in Figure 432, which shows the back of the fetus positioned anteriorly.

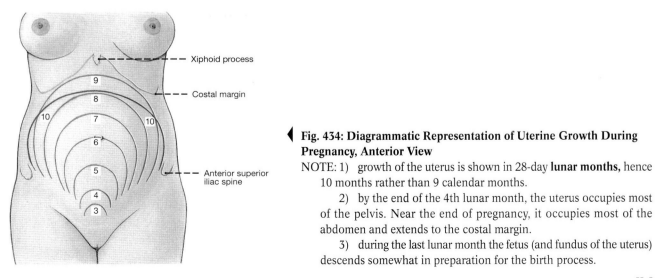

Xiphoid process

Costal margin

Anterior superior iliac spine

9

8

10

7

10

6

5

4

3

◀ **Fig. 434: Diagrammatic Representation of Uterine Growth During Pregnancy, Anterior View**
NOTE: 1)   growth of the uterus is shown in 28-day **lunar months,** hence 10 months rather than 9 calendar months.

2)   by the end of the 4th lunar month, the uterus occupies most of the pelvis. Near the end of pregnancy, it occupies most of the abdomen and extends to the costal margin.

3)   during the last lunar month the fetus (and fundus of the uterus) descends somewhat in preparation for the birth process.

PLATE 284   Pregnant Uterus: Fetal X-ray

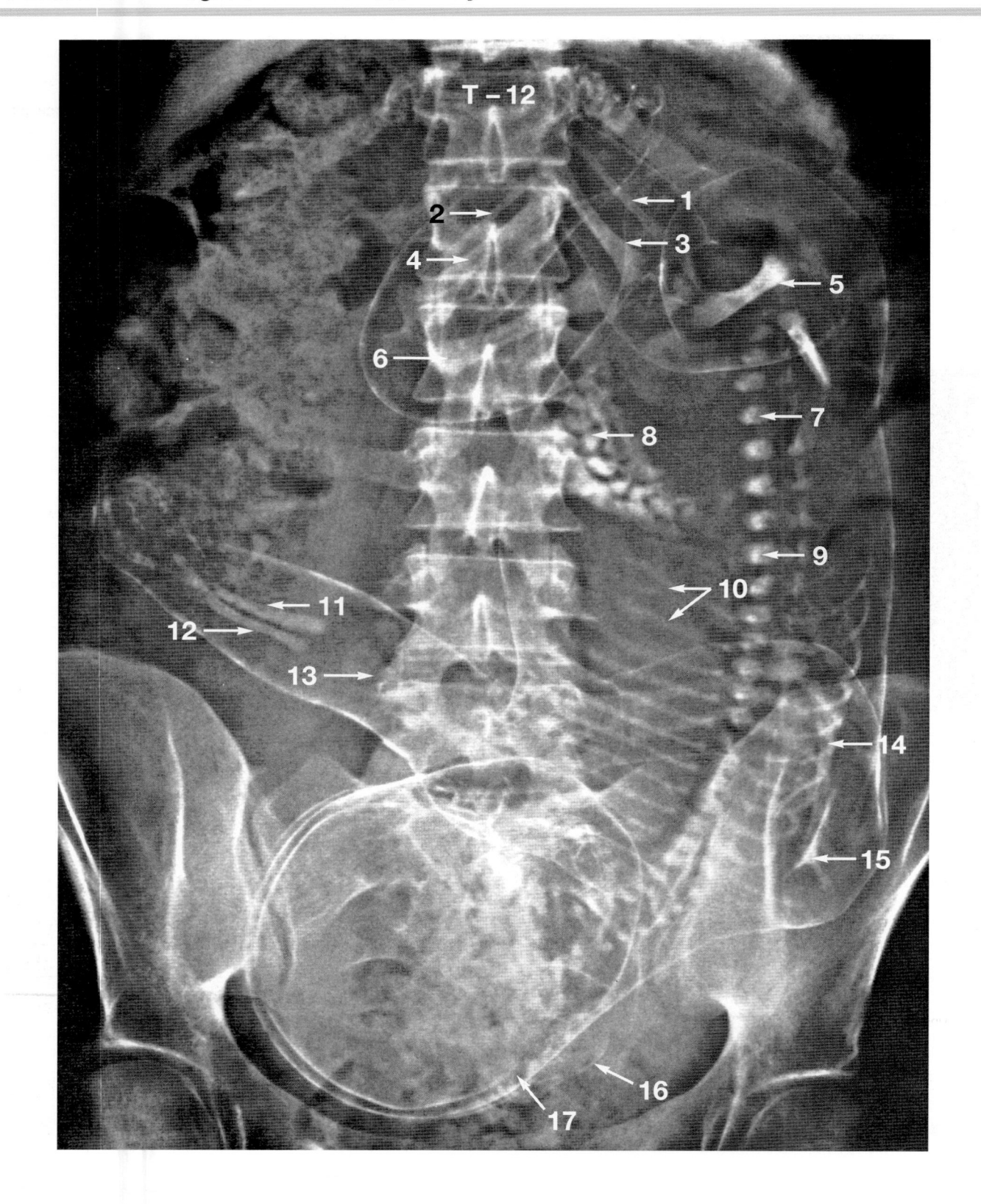

Fig. 435: Fetal Roentgenogram
NOTE: the body contours of the near-term fetus *in utero* and a number of the ossifying bones. Observe that the uterus extends to the maternal T12 vertebral body level. (From Wicke L. Atlas of Radiologic Anatomy. Philadelphia, Lea and Febiger, 1994).

1. Right fibula	6. Left femur	11. Left ulna	16. External ear
2. Left fibula	7. L5 vertebra (fetal)	12. Left radius	17. Fetal head
3. Right tibia	8. Small intestine (fetal)	13. Left humerus	
4. Left tibia	9. L1 vertebra (fetal)	14. Right humerus	
5. Right femur	10. Ribs	15. Right scapula	

Fig. 435

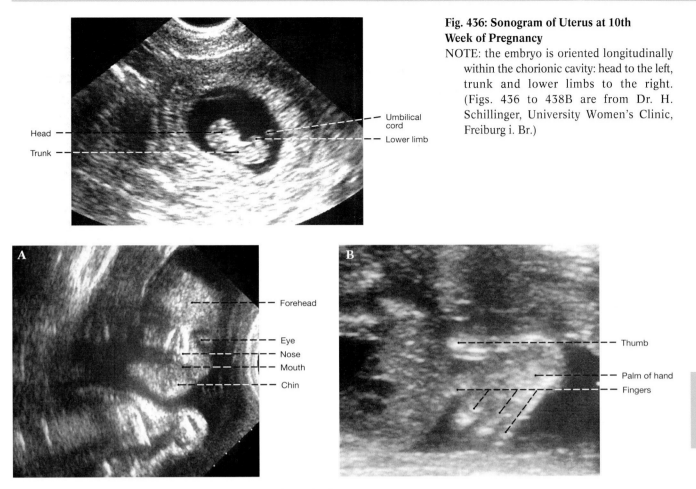

Head —

Trunk —

— — Umbilical cord

— — Lower limb

Fig. 436: Sonogram of Uterus at 10th Week of Pregnancy

NOTE: the embryo is oriented longitudinally within the chorionic cavity: head to the left, trunk and lower limbs to the right. (Figs. 436 to 438B are from Dr. H. Schillinger, University Women's Clinic, Freiburg i. Br.)

A

— Forehead

— Eye
— Nose
— Mouth

— Chin

B

— — Thumb

— — Palm of hand
— — Fingers

Fig. 437A and B: Sonogram of Uterus During the 24th Week of Pregnancy

NOTE: 1) in **A,** a frontal section through the face shows the facial features of the fetus, presenting the fetal "portrait".

2) in **B,** the sonogram shows the fetal hand, clearly demonstrating all of the fingers and the thumb.

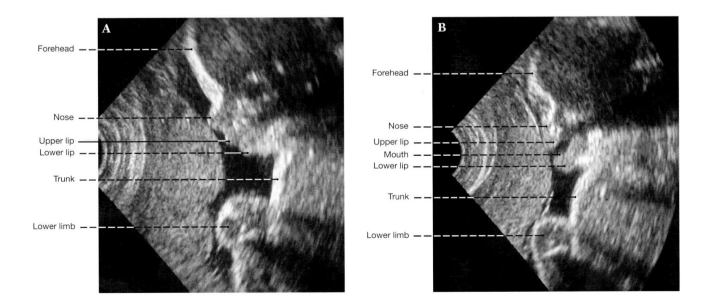

A

Forehead — —

Nose — —

Upper lip —
Lower lip — —

Trunk — —

Lower limb — —

B

Forehead — —

Nose — —
Upper lip — —
Mouth — —
Lower lip — —

Trunk — —

Lower limb — —

Fig. 438A and B: Sonogram of the Uterus During the 28th Week of Pregnancy

NOTE: 1) in **A,** the longitudinal section shows the fetal head and body in profile.

2) in **B,** the fetus has opened its mouth and expanded its trunk indicative of fete sporadic diaphragmatic and swallowing movements that occur during the latter part of fetal life when large amounts of amniotic fluid are ingested.

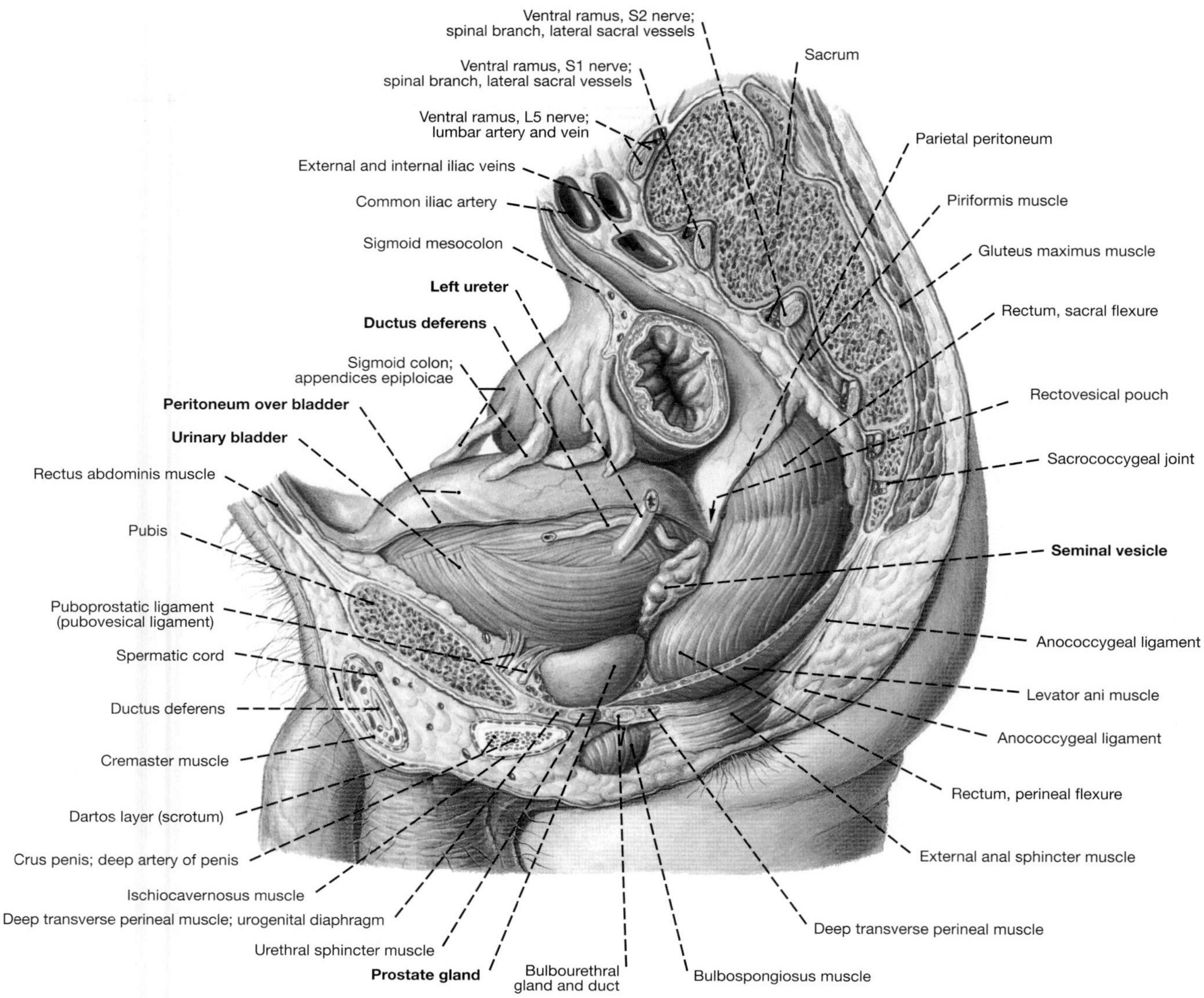

PLATE 286   Male Pelvic Organs and Peritoneal Reflections

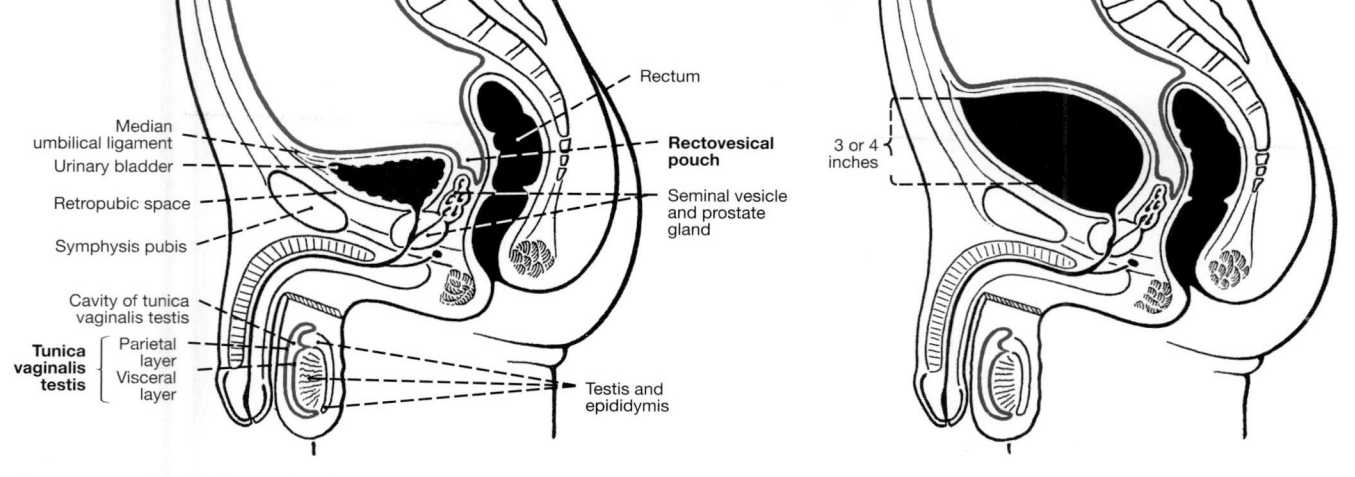

Ventral ramus, S2 nerve;
spinal branch, lateral sacral vessels

Sacrum

Ventral ramus, S1 nerve;
spinal branch, lateral sacral vessels

Ventral ramus, L5 nerve;
lumbar artery and vein

Parietal peritoneum

External and internal iliac veins

Piriformis muscle

Common iliac artery

Gluteus maximus muscle

Sigmoid mesocolon

Rectum, sacral flexure

Left ureter

Ductus deferens

Rectovesical pouch

Sigmoid colon;
appendices epiploicae

Peritoneum over bladder

Sacrococcygeal joint

Urinary bladder

Rectus abdominis muscle

Seminal vesicle

Pubis

Puboprostatic ligament
(pubovesical ligament)

Anococcygeal ligament

Spermatic cord

Levator ani muscle

Ductus deferens

Anococcygeal ligament

Cremaster muscle

Rectum, perineal flexure

Dartos layer (scrotum)

External anal sphincter muscle

Crus penis; deep artery of penis

Ischiocavernosus muscle

Deep transverse perineal muscle; urogenital diaphragm

Deep transverse perineal muscle

Urethral sphincter muscle

Prostate gland

Bulbourethral
gland and duct

Bulbospongiosus muscle

Fig. 439: Male Pelvic Organs Viewed from the Left Side

A

Rectum

Median
umbilical ligament

**Rectovesical
pouch**

Urinary bladder

Retropubic space

Seminal vesicle
and prostate
gland

Symphysis pubis

Cavity of tunica
vaginalis testis

**Tunica
vaginalis
testis** { Parietal
layer
Visceral
layer

Testis and
epididymis

B

3 or 4
inches

Fig. 440A and B: Peritoneal Reflection Over the Pelvic Organs: Empty and Full Bladder

NOTE: 1) when the bladder is empty **(A),** the peritoneum extends down to the level of the symphysis pubis, but when the bladder is full **(B),** the peritoneum is elevated 3 or 4 inches.

2) the prostate and bladder may be reached **without entering the peritoneal cavity** anteriorly above the pubis, and through the perineum by ascending in front of the rectum.

Figs. 439, 440A, B

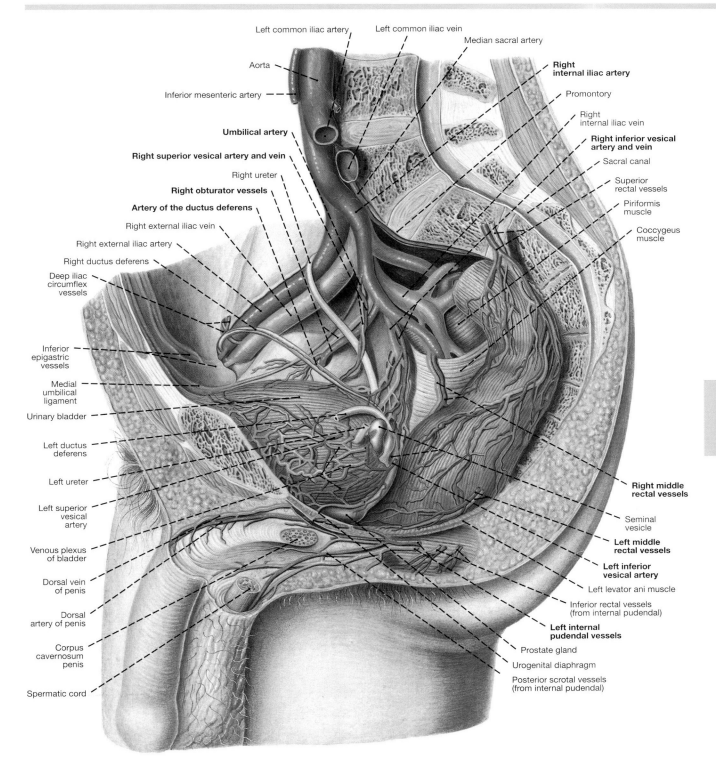

Left common iliac artery

Left common iliac vein

Median sacral artery

Aorta

Right internal iliac artery

Inferior mesenteric artery

Promontory

Right internal iliac vein

Umbilical artery

Right inferior vesical artery and vein

Right superior vesical artery and vein

Sacral canal

Right ureter

Superior rectal vessels

Right obturator vessels

Piriformis muscle

Artery of the ductus deferens

Coccygeus muscle

Right external iliac vein

Right external iliac artery

Right ductus deferens

Deep iliac circumflex vessels

Inferior epigastric vessels

Medial umbilical ligament

Urinary bladder

Left ductus deferens

Left ureter

Left superior vesical artery

Right middle rectal vessels

Seminal vesicle

Left middle rectal vessels

Left inferior vesical artery

Left levator ani muscle

Venous plexus of bladder

Dorsal vein of penis

Inferior rectal vessels (from internal pudendal)

Left internal pudendal vessels

Dorsal artery of penis

Corpus cavernosum penis

Prostate gland

Urogenital diaphragm

Posterior scrotal vessels (from internal pudendal)

Spermatic cord

Fig. 441: Blood Vessels of the Male Pelvis, Perineum, and External Genitalia

NOTE: 1) the aorta bifurcates into the **common iliac arteries,** which then divide into the **external** and **internal iliac arteries.** The external iliac becomes the principal arterial trunk of the lower extremity, whereas the internal iliac artery supplies the organs of the pelvis and perineum.

2) the **visceral branches** of the internal iliac are: (a) the umbilical (from which is derived the superior vesical artery), (b) the inferior vesical, (c) the artery of the vas deferens (uterine artery in females), and (d) the middle rectal, and

3) the **parietal branches** include: (a) the iliolumbar, (b) lateral sacral, (c) superior gluteal, (d) inferior gluteal, (e) obturator, and (f) internal pudendal.

Fig. 441   **IV**

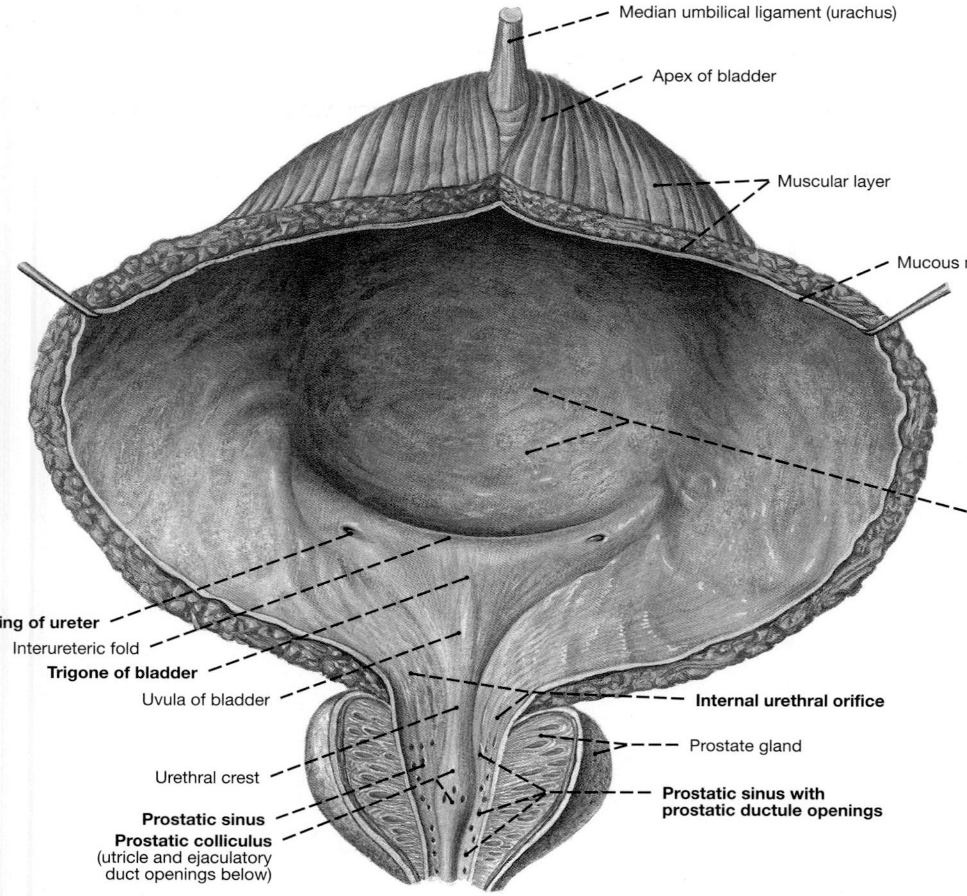

Median umbilical ligament (urachus)

Apex of bladder

Muscular layer

Mucous membrane

Mucosal folds

Opening of ureter

Interureteric fold

Trigone of bladder

Uvula of bladder

Internal urethral orifice

Prostate gland

Urethral crest

Prostatic sinus with prostatic ductule openings

Prostatic sinus

Prostatic colliculus
(utricle and ejaculatory duct openings below)

Fig. 442: Bladder and Prostatic Urethra Incised Anteriorly

NOTE: 1)   the smooth triangular area at the base of the bladder called the **trigone,** which is bounded by the two orifices of the ureters and the opening of the prostatic urethra.

   2)   the **colliculus** is a mound on the posterior wall of the prostatic urethra, on both sides of which lie the **prostatic sinuses.** Into these, open the ducts of the prostate gland. In the center of the colliculus is a small blind pouch, the **prostatic utricle,** on both sides of the utricle are the single orifices of the **ejaculatory ducts** (openings not labelled).

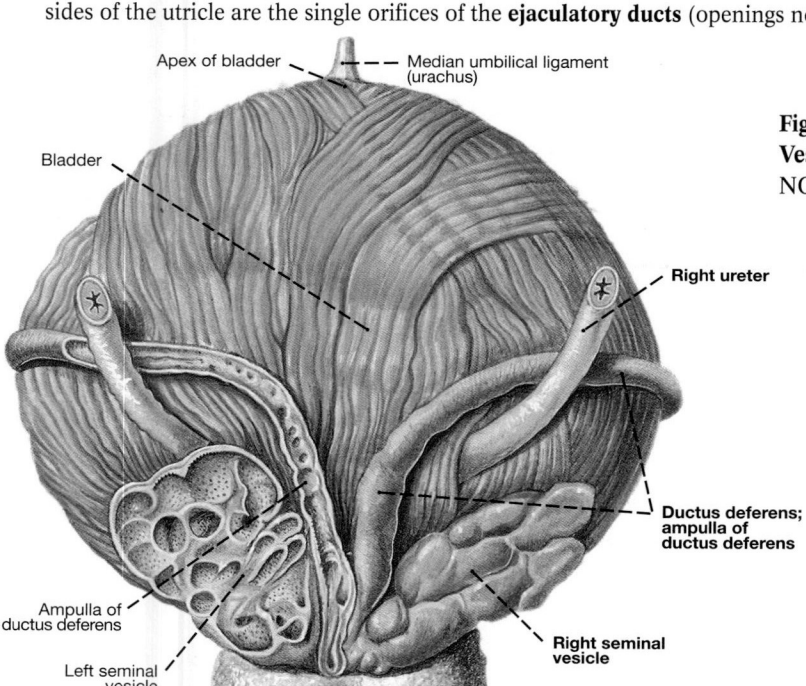

Apex of bladder

Median umbilical ligament (urachus)

Bladder

Right ureter

Ductus deferens; ampulla of ductus deferens

Ampulla of ductus deferens

Right seminal vesicle

Left seminal vesicle

Prostate gland

Fig. 443: Posterior Surface of the Bladder: the Seminal Vesicles, Ureters, and Deferent Ducts

NOTE: 1)   the ureters, deferent ducts, seminal vesicles, and prostate gland are all in contact with the inferior aspect of the posterior surface of the bladder.

   2)   the **ureters** penetrate the bladder diagonally at points about two inches apart. Upon entering the bladder, each ureter is crossed anteriorly by the ductus deferens.

   3)   the deferent ducts join the ducts of the lobulated seminal vesicles to form the two ejaculatory ducts.

   4)   the prostate hugs the bladder at its outlet, surrounding the prostatic urethra.

   5)   all of these organs lie directly in front of the rectum and can be palpated during a rectal examination.

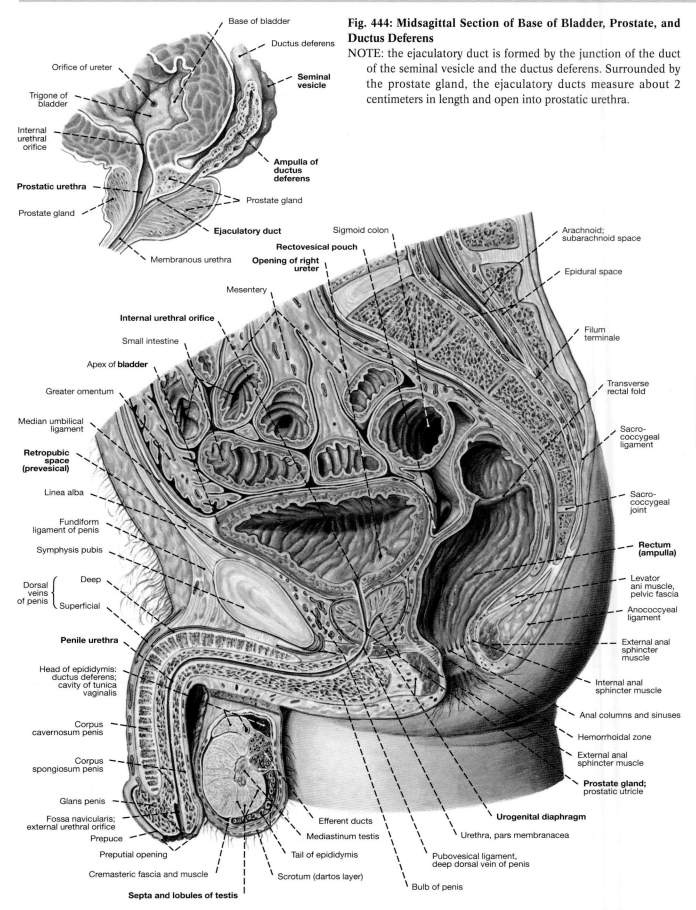

Base of bladder
Ductus deferens
Seminal vesicle
Orifice of ureter
Trigone of bladder
Internal urethral orifice
Ampulla of ductus deferens
Prostatic urethra
Prostate gland
Prostate gland
Ejaculatory duct
Membranous urethra
Opening of right ureter

Fig. 444: Midsagittal Section of Base of Bladder, Prostate, and Ductus Deferens
NOTE: the ejaculatory duct is formed by the junction of the duct of the seminal vesicle and the ductus deferens. Surrounded by the prostate gland, the ejaculatory ducts measure about 2 centimeters in length and open into prostatic urethra.

Sigmoid colon
Rectovesical pouch
Mesentery
Internal urethral orifice
Small intestine
Apex of **bladder**
Greater omentum
Median umbilical ligament
Retropubic space (prevesical)
Linea alba
Fundiform ligament of penis
Symphysis pubis
Dorsal veins of penis { Deep / Superficial }
Penile urethra
Head of epididymis; ductus deferens; cavity of tunica vaginalis
Corpus cavernosum penis
Corpus spongiosum penis
Glans penis
Fossa navicularis; external urethral orifice
Prepuce
Preputial opening
Cremasteric fascia and muscle
Septa and lobules of testis

Efferent ducts
Mediastinum testis
Tail of epididymis
Scrotum (dartos layer)

Arachnoid; subarachnoid space
Epidural space
Filum terminale
Transverse rectal fold
Sacro-coccygeal ligament
Sacro-coccygeal joint
Rectum (ampulla)
Levator ani muscle, pelvic fascia
Anococcygeal ligament
External anal sphincter muscle
Internal anal sphincter muscle
Anal columns and sinuses
Hemorrhoidal zone
External anal sphincter muscle
Prostate gland; prostatic utricle
Urogenital diaphragm
Urethra, pars membranacea
Pubovesical ligament, deep dorsal vein of penis
Bulb of penis

Fig. 445: Median Sagittal Section of the Male Pelvis and Perineum Showing the Pelvic Viscera and the External Genitalia

Figs. 444, 445   **IV**

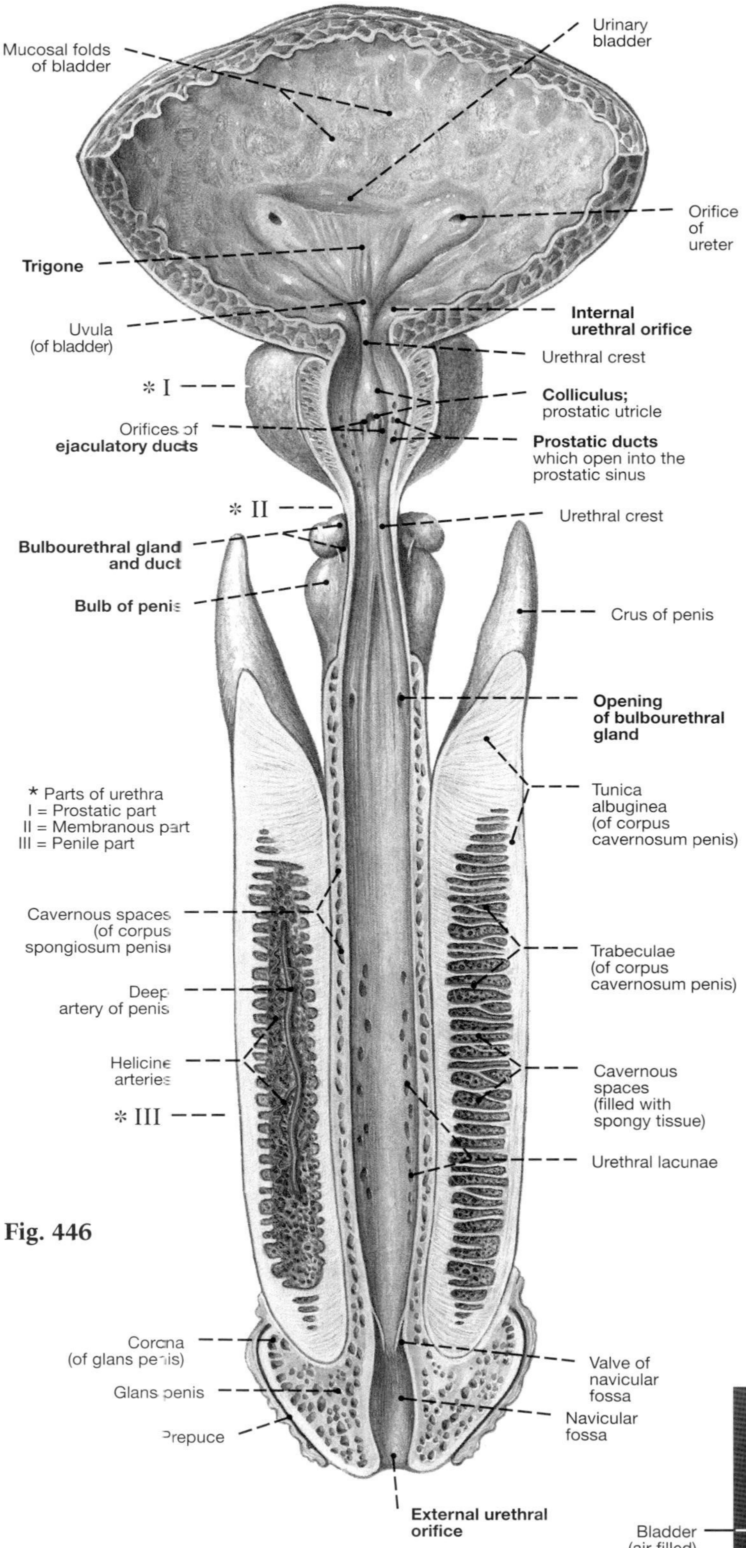

PLATE 290   Urethra, Seminal Vesicles, Deferent and Ejaculatory Ducts

Mucosal folds
of bladder

Urinary
bladder

Orifice
of
ureter

Trigone

Uvula
(of bladder)

**Internal
urethral orifice**

Urethral crest

✳ I

Colliculus;
prostatic utricle

Orifices of
ejaculatory ducts

Prostatic ducts
which open into the
prostatic sinus

✳ II

Urethral crest

**Bulbourethral gland
and duct**

Bulb of penis

Crus of penis

**Opening
of bulbourethral
gland**

Tunica
albuginea
(of corpus
cavernosum penis)

✳ Parts of urethra
I = Prostatic part
II = Membranous part
III = Penile part

Cavernous spaces
(of corpus
spongiosum penis)

Trabeculae
(of corpus
cavernosum penis)

Deep
artery of penis

Helicine
arteries

Cavernous
spaces
(filled with
spongy tissue)

✳ III

Urethral lacunae

Fig. 446

Corona
(of glans penis)

Glans penis

Valve of
navicular
fossa

Navicular
fossa

Prepuce

**External urethral
orifice**

Fig. 446: Male Urethra and its Associated Orifices

NOTE: 1)   the male urethra extends from the internal urethral orifice at the bladder to the external urethral orifice at the end of the glans penis. In males, it traverses the prostate gland, the urogenital diaphragm (membrane) and penis, and is, therefore, divided into **prostatic, membranous**, and **penile** parts.

2)   before ejaculation a viscous fluid from the **bulbourethral glands** (of Cowper) lubricates the urethra. These glands are located in the urogenital diaphragm, but their ducts open 1 inch distally in the penile urethra.

3)   the total urethra measures between 7 and 8 inches in length, the prostatic part about 1½ inches long, the membranous part about ½ inch and the penile part 5 to 6 inches. The **prostatic urethra** receives the secretions of the ejaculatory ducts along with those from the prostate. Enlargement of the prostate, often occuring in older men, tends to constrict the urethra at this site, resulting in difficulty in urination.

4)   the **membranous urethra** is short and narrow and it is completely surrounded by the circular fibers of the voluntary urethral sphincter muscle. Relaxation of this sphincter initiates urination while its tonic contraction constricts the urethra and maintains urinary continence.

5)   the **penile urethra** is surrounded initially by the bulb of the penis and the bulbospongiosus muscle. It traverses the penile shaft within the corpus spongiosum penis. The internal surface of the distal half is marked by small recesses called the urethral lacunae.

Fig. 447: Radiograph of Bladder, Seminal Vesicles, Deferent Ducts, and Ejaculatory Ducts ▶

NOTE: the bladder has been filled with air and appears light, while the seminal vesicles, deferent ducts and ejaculatory ducts stand out as dark because of an injected contrast medium.

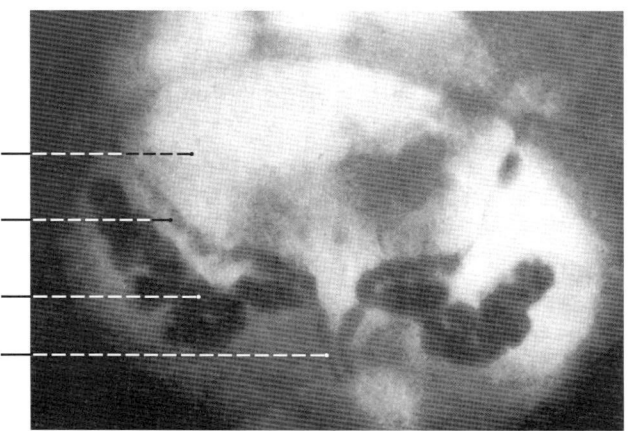

Bladder
(air filled)

Ductus
deferens

Seminal
vesicle

Ejaculatory
duct

Fig. 448: Diagram of the Male Genitourinary System

NOTE: 1)   this figure shows: (a) the organs of the adult male genitourinary system (dark red bown), (b) the structures of the genital system prior to the descent of the testis (interrupted blue lines), and (c) those structures that partially or entirely became atrophic and disappeared during development (pink structures with red outlines).

2)   the **urinary system** includes the *kidneys*, which produce urine by filtration of the blood, the *ureters*, which convey urine to the *bladder* where it is stored, and the *urethra* through which urine is discharged.

3)   the adult male genital system includes the *testis* where sperm are generated, the *epididymis* and *ductus deferens*, which transport sperm to the *ejaculatory duct* where the *seminal vesicle* joins the genital system. The *prostate* and *bulbourethral glands* along with the ejaculatory ducts join the *urethra* which then courses through the prostate and *penis*.

4)   embryologically, structures capable of developing into either sex exist in all individuals. In the male the **mesonephric duct** (Wolffian) becomes the epididymis, vas deferens, ejaculatory duct and seminal vesicle along with the penis, while the **paramesonephric duct** (Müllerian) is suppressed.

5)   the testes are developed on the posterior abdominal wall to which each is attached by a fibrous genital ligament called the **gubernaculum testis.** As development continues, each testis *migrates* from its site of formation, so that by the 5th month it lies adjacent to the abdominal inguinal ring. The gubernaculum is still attached to anterior abdominal wall tissue, which by this time has evaginated as the developing scrotum. The testes then commence their descent through the inguinal canal, so that by the 8th month they usually lie in the scrotum attached by a peritoneal reflection, the processus vaginalis testis, which becomes the **tunica vaginalis testis.**

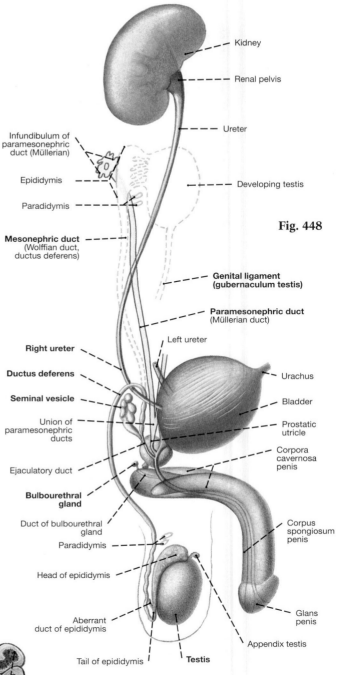

Fig. 448

Labels: Kidney; Renal pelvis; Ureter; Developing testis; Infundibulum of paramesonephric duct (Müllerian); Epididymis; Paradidymis; **Mesonephric duct** (Wolffian duct, ductus deferens); **Genital ligament (gubernaculum testis)**; **Paramesonephric duct** (Müllerian duct); Left ureter; **Right ureter**; **Ductus deferens**; **Seminal vesicle**; Union of paramesonephric ducts; Ejaculatory duct; **Bulbourethral gland**; Urachus; Bladder; Prostatic utricle; Corpora cavernosa penis; Duct of bulbourethral gland; Paradidymis; Head of epididymis; Corpus spongiosum penis; Aberrant duct of epididymis; Glans penis; Appendix testis; Tail of epididymis; **Testis**

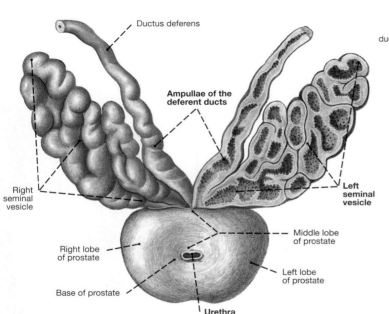

Labels: Ductus deferens; **Ampullae of the deferent ducts**; Right seminal vesicle; **Left seminal vesicle**; Middle lobe of prostate; Right lobe of prostate; Left lobe of prostate; Base of prostate; Urethra

Fig. 449: Prostate Gland, Seminal Vesicles, and Ampullae of the Deferent Ducts (Superior View)

NOTE: 1)   the left seminal vesicle and ductus deferens were cut longitudinally, while the urethra was cut transversely, distal to the bladder.

2)   the **prostate gland** is conical in shape and normally measures just over 1½ inches across, 1 inch in thickness and slightly longer than 1 inch vertically. In the young adult, it weighs about 25 grams and is formed by 2 lateral lobes surrounding a middle lobe.

PLATE 292   Rectum, Inner Surface (Male or Female)

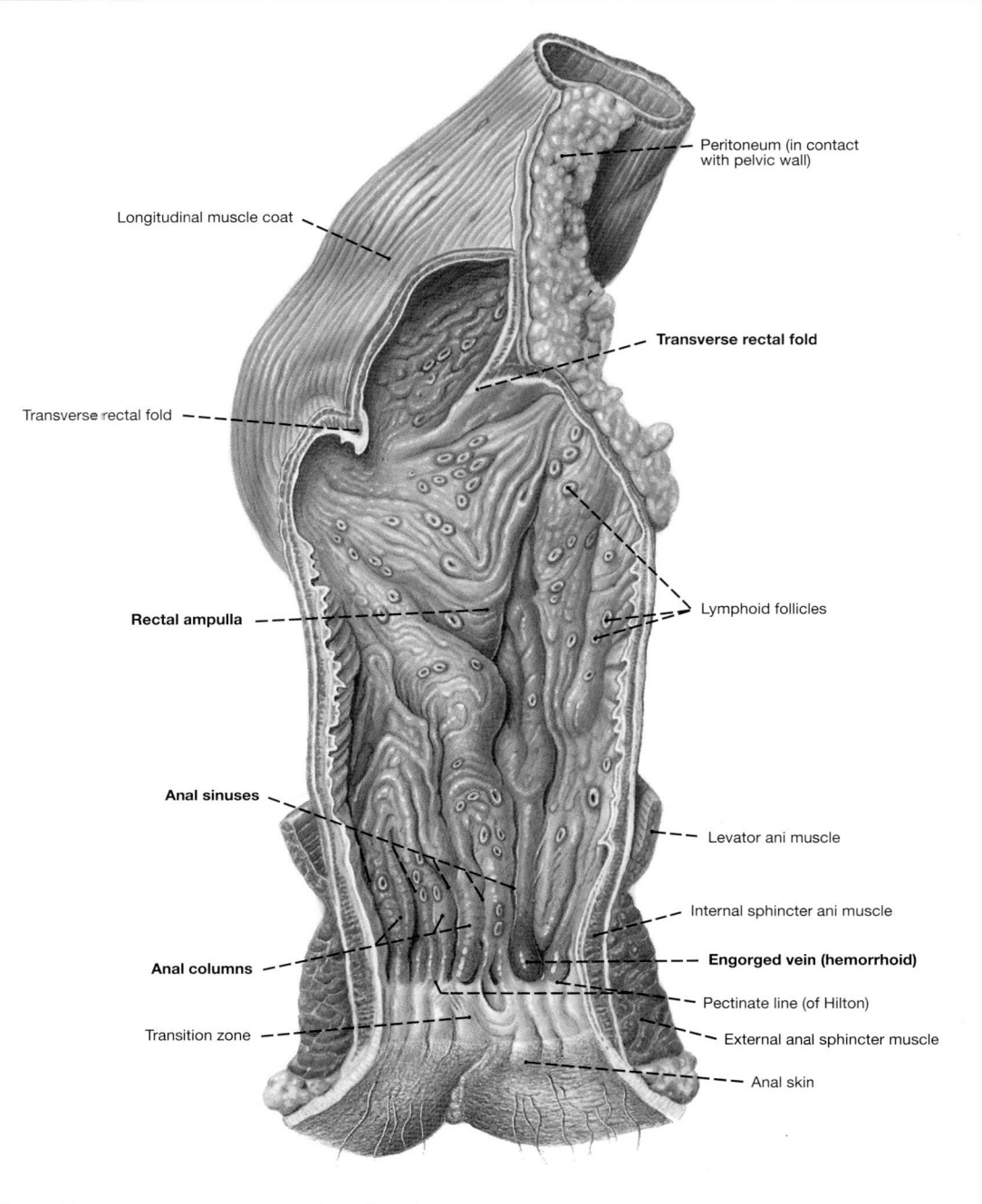

Peritoneum (in contact with pelvic wall)

Longitudinal muscle coat

Transverse rectal fold

Transverse rectal fold

Lymphoid follicles

Rectal ampulla

Levator ani muscle

Anal sinuses

Internal sphincter ani muscle

Engorged vein (hemorrhoid)

Anal columns

Pectinate line (of Hilton)

Transition zone

External anal sphincter muscle

Anal skin

Fig. 450: Inner Surface of the Rectum and Anal Canal

NOTE: 1) the sigmoid colon becomes the **rectum** at about the level of the middle of the sacrum. Measuring about 5 inches in length, the rectum then becomes the **anal canal,** which is the terminal 1½ inches of the intestinal tract. The rectum is dilated near its junction with the anal canal, giving rise to the **rectal ampulla.**

2) the internal mucosa of the rectum is thrown into transverse folds of which there are usually three in number. These are known as **horizontal folds** or **valves of Houston.**

3) below the rectal ampulla the mucosa of the anal canal presents a series of vertical folds called the **anal columns (columns of Morgagni),** each of which possesses an artery and vein. Between the anal columns are small fossae called the **anal sinuses.** The veins in this region are dilated and tortuous, and if they become varicosed, a condition results called hemorrhoids or piles.

4) distal to the anal columns is a zone where the epithelium abruptly changes. This zone is called **Hilton's line,** and the simple columnar epithelium of the rectum becomes the stratified squamous epithelium of the lower anal canal (slightly below the pectinate line).

Fig. 450

Fig. 451: External Surface of Rectum, Lateral View ▶

NOTE: 1) the rectum shows a dorsally directed **sacral flexure** proximally and a less pronounced **perineal flexure** distally. Peritoneum ensheathes the rectum ventrally almost as far as the ampulla (to the bladder in the male and the uterus in the female).

2) the fibers of the **levator ani muscle** (which form the floor of the pelvis) surround the rectum and are continued distally as the **external anal sphincter muscle.**

3) the **internal anal sphincter muscle** (seen in Figs. 450 and 452) is composed of smooth muscle and really represents a thickening of the muscular layer in the wall of the rectum.

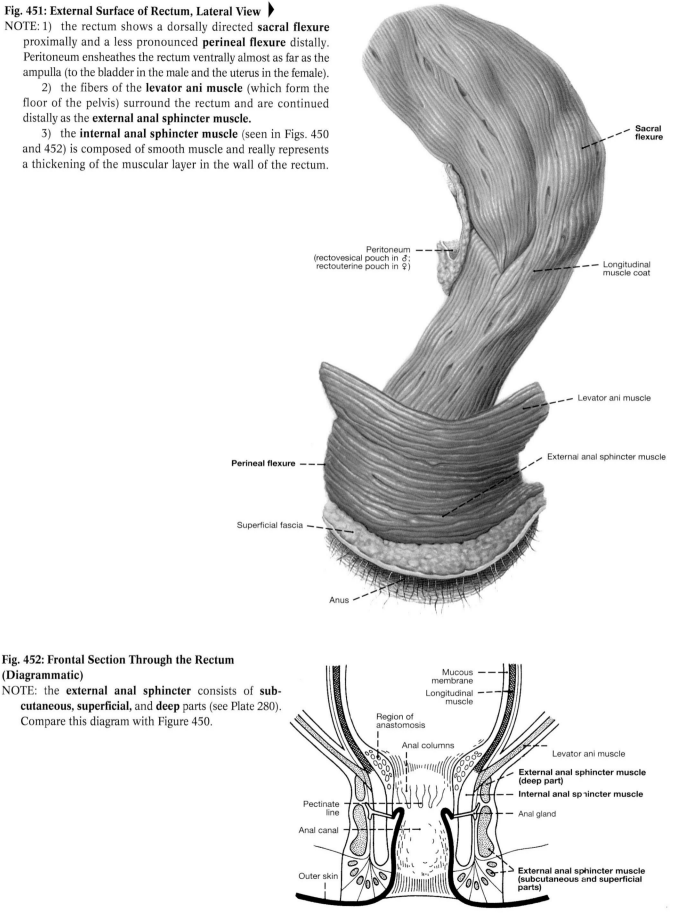

Fig. 452: Frontal Section Through the Rectum (Diagrammatic)

NOTE: the **external anal sphincter** consists of **subcutaneous, superficial,** and **deep** parts (see Plate 280). Compare this diagram with Figure 450.

PLATE 294   Rectum: Arterial Blood Supply (Male or Female)

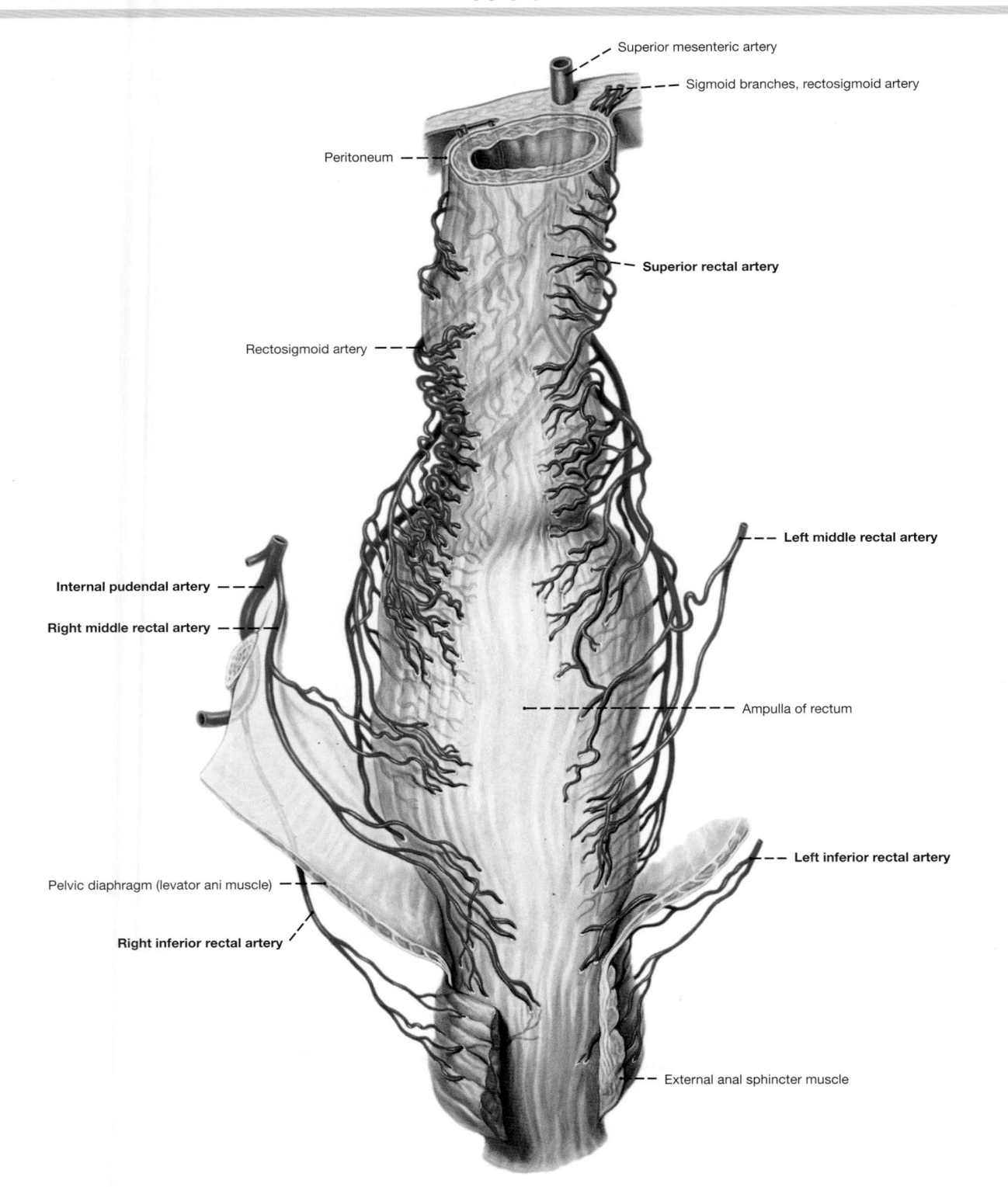

Superior mesenteric artery

Sigmoid branches, rectosigmoid artery

Peritoneum

Superior rectal artery

Rectosigmoid artery

Left middle rectal artery

Internal pudendal artery

Right middle rectal artery

Ampulla of rectum

Left inferior rectal artery

Pelvic diaphragm (levator ani muscle)

Right inferior rectal artery

External anal sphincter muscle

Fig. 453: Arterial Supply of the Rectum, Anterior View

NOTE: 1) this anterior view of the rectum shows its arterial supply coming by way of the superior, middle, and inferior rectal arteries which anastomose as they supply the organ.

2) the **superior rectal artery** is the vessel that continues distally from the inferior mesenteric artery after the sigmoid branches are given off and, thus, represents a source from within the **abdomen**. It distributes to the rectum as far as the ampulla.

3) the **middle rectal artery** at times arises with the inferior vesical artery from the internal iliac artery. More frequently, it arises from the internal pudendal artery (as shown here) or from the inferior gluteal artery, thus it has a source from the **pelvis.**

4) the **inferior rectal artery** arises from the internal pudendal artery. Its branches supply the lowermost part of the rectum and the muscles and skin of the anal region. Its source can be considered from the **perineum.**

Fig. 453

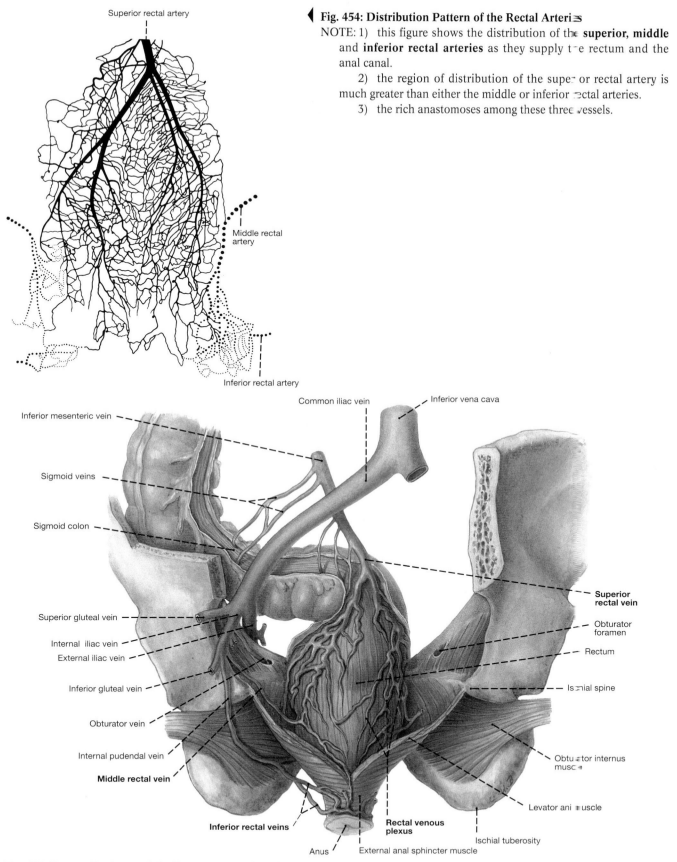

Superior rectal artery

Middle rectal artery

Inferior rectal artery

◀ **Fig. 454: Distribution Pattern of the Rectal Arteries**

NOTE: 1) this figure shows the distribution of the **superior, middle** and **inferior rectal arteries** as they supply the rectum and the anal canal.

2) the region of distribution of the superior rectal artery is much greater than either the middle or inferior rectal arteries.

3) the rich anastomoses among these three vessels.

Inferior mesenteric vein

Common iliac vein

Inferior vena cava

Sigmoid veins

Sigmoid colon

Superior rectal vein

Obturator foramen

Rectum

Superior gluteal vein

Internal iliac vein

External iliac vein

Inferior gluteal vein

Ischial spine

Obturator vein

Internal pudendal vein

Middle rectal vein

Obturator internus muscle

Levator ani muscle

Inferior rectal veins

Rectal venous plexus

Anus

External anal sphincter muscle

Ischial tuberosity

Fig. 455: Venous Drainage of the Rectum, Posterior View

NOTE: blood from the middle and inferior rectal veins eventually drains into the inferior vena cava, while blood returning from the superior rectal vein drains into the portal circulation by way of the inferior mesenteric vein. This allows a route of **collateral circulation** between these two venous systems.

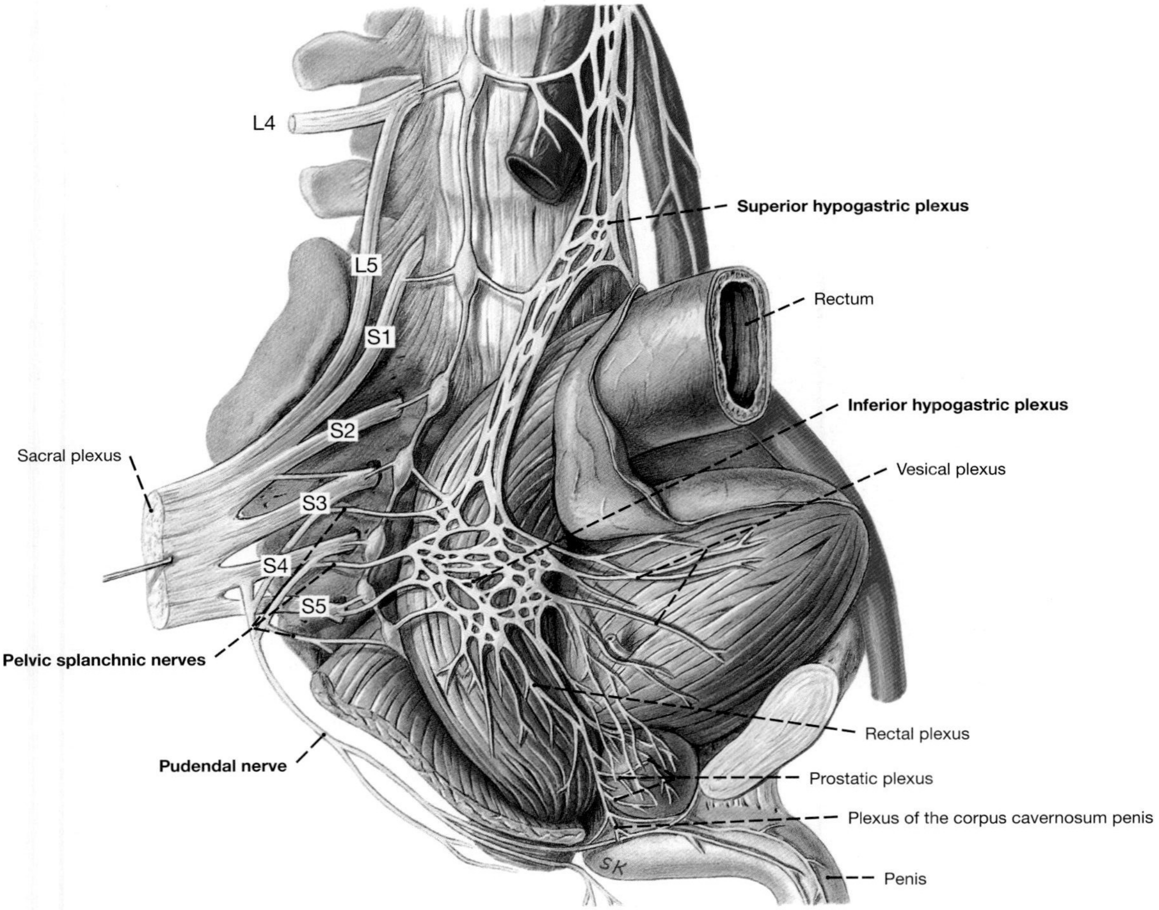

L4

Superior hypogastric plexus

L5

Rectum

S1

Inferior hypogastric plexus

S2

Vesical plexus

Sacral plexus

S3

S4

S5

Rectal plexus

Pelvic splanchnic nerves

Prostatic plexus

Plexus of the corpus cavernosum penis

Pudendal nerve

Penis

Fig. 456: Autonomic and Visceral Afferent Innervation of the Pelvic Organs

NOTE: 1) *post*gangionic *sympathetic fibers* course downward in the **superior hypogastric plexus** from lower lumbar ganglia and continue in the specific visceral plexuses (i.e., rectal, vesical, etc.) to supply pelvic organs with sympathetic innervation.

2) *pre*ganglionic *parasympathetic fibers* to the pelvic organs emerge from the S2, S3, and S4 spinal nerves to form the **pelvic splanchnic nerves.** They also course through the specific visceral plexuses and then synapse with postganglionic parasympathetic neurons within the walls of the viscera.

3) **visceral afferent fibers** from the pelvic organs course centrally along with these autonomic fibers. Their cell bodies lie in their respective dorsal root ganglia, and they enter the spinal cord by way of the dorsal roots from these ganglia.

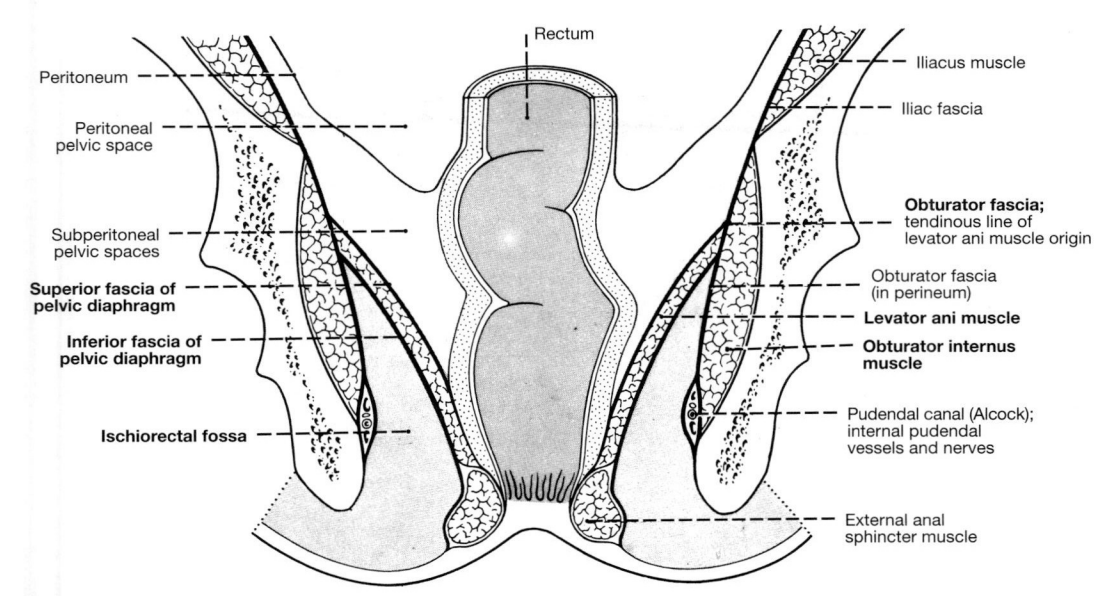

Rectum

Peritoneum

Iliacus muscle

Peritoneal pelvic space

Iliac fascia

Subperitoneal pelvic spaces

Obturator fascia; tendinous line of levator ani muscle origin

Obturator fascia (in perineum)

Superior fascia of pelvic diaphragm

Levator ani muscle

Inferior fascia of pelvic diaphragm

Obturator internus muscle

Pudendal canal (Alcock); internal pudendal vessels and nerves

Ischiorectal fossa

External anal sphincter muscle

Fig. 457: Diagram of Frontal Section Through Pelvis and Perineum

Figs. 456, 457

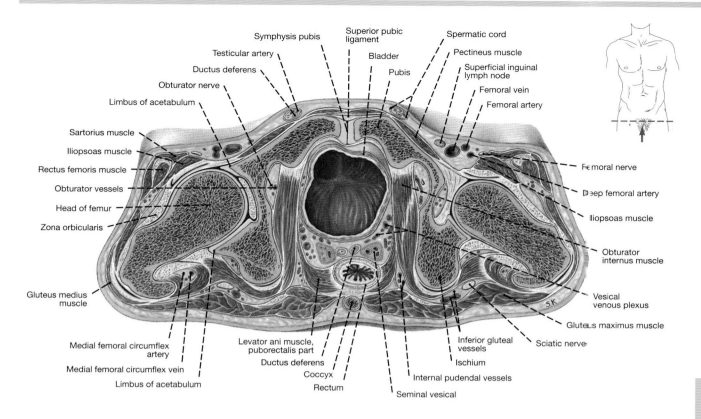

Fig. 458: Cross-section of the Male Pelvis at the Level of the Symphysis Pubis

NOTE: 1) the location of the **ductus deferens** and the **seminal vesical** behind the **bladder** on both sides, and behind these, observe the position of the **rectum.**

2) the **obturator internus muscle** forms the lateral wall of the true pelvis and the levator ani (in this figure, its puborectalis part) arises from the obturator fascia that covers its medial surface.

3) the **vesical plexus of veins** surrounding the bladder. This plexus anastomoses with the prostatic plexus below and both drain into the internal iliac vein. Thus, venous blood from the bladder and prostate usually enters the inferior vena cava and goes to the lungs, although anastomoses also exist with the rectal system of veins and with the vertebral system of veins.

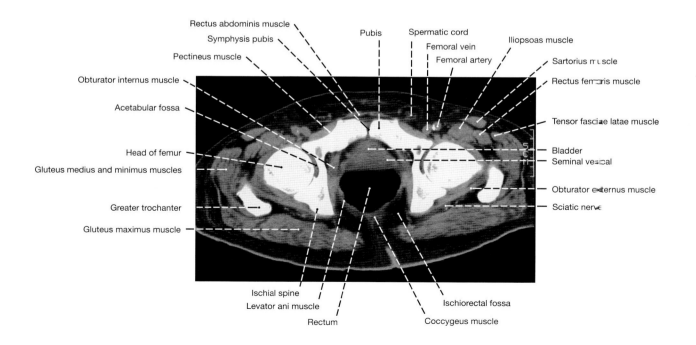

Fig. 459: Computerized Tomograph of the Male Pelvis Taken from Below

PLATE 298   Male Pelvis and Perineum: Frontal Section, Posterior View

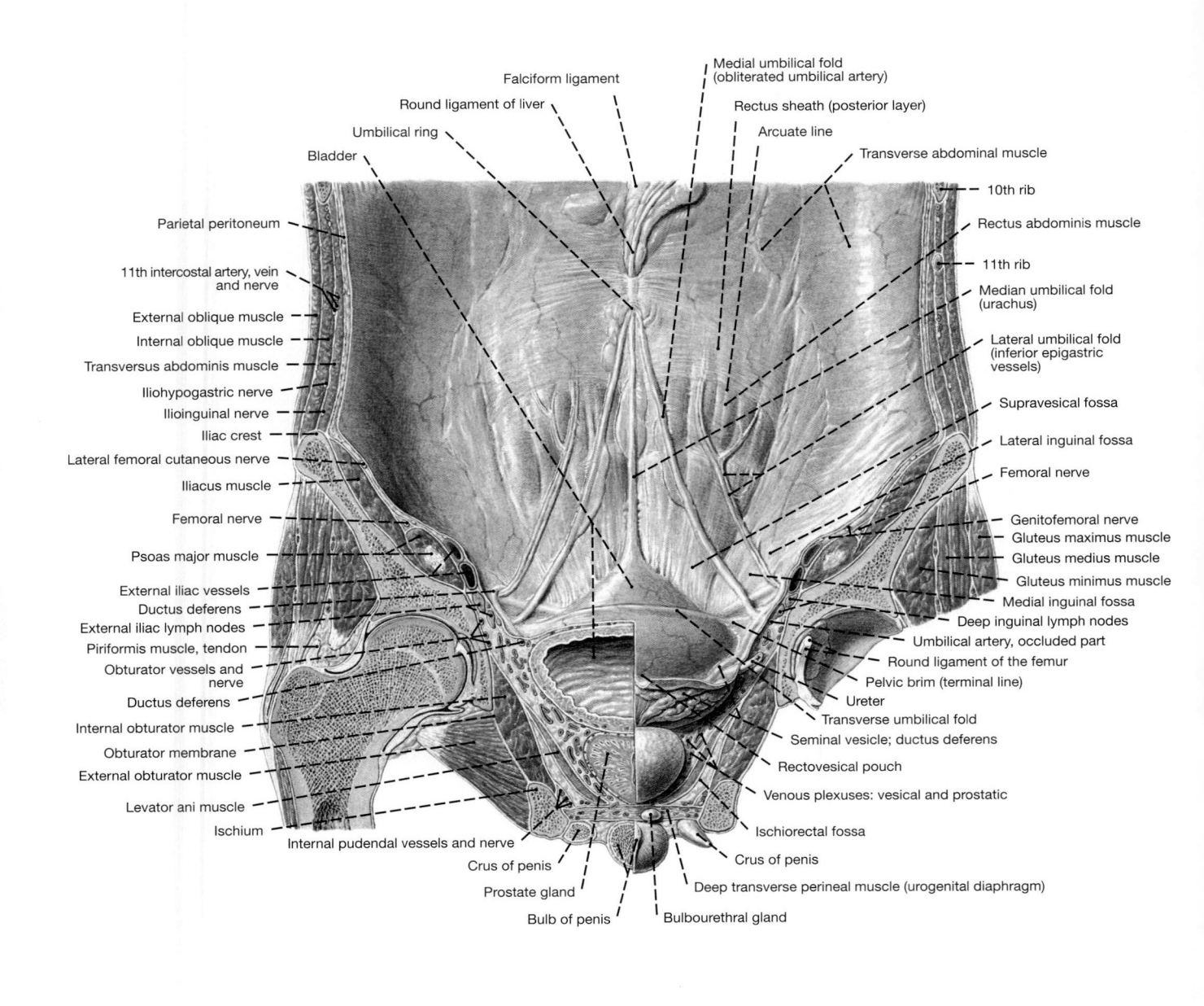

Falciform ligament

Round ligament of liver

Umbilical ring

Bladder

Parietal peritoneum

11th intercostal artery, vein and nerve

External oblique muscle

Internal oblique muscle

Transversus abdominis muscle

Iliohypogastric nerve

Ilioinguinal nerve

Iliac crest

Lateral femoral cutaneous nerve

Iliacus muscle

Femoral nerve

Psoas major muscle

External iliac vessels

Ductus deferens

External iliac lymph nodes

Piriformis muscle, tendon

Obturator vessels and nerve

Ductus deferens

Internal obturator muscle

Obturator membrane

External obturator muscle

Levator ani muscle

Ischium

Internal pudendal vessels and nerve

Crus of penis

Prostate gland

Bulb of penis

Medial umbilical fold (obliterated umbilical artery)

Rectus sheath (posterior layer)

Arcuate line

Transverse abdominal muscle

10th rib

Rectus abdominis muscle

11th rib

Median umbilical fold (urachus)

Lateral umbilical fold (inferior epigastric vessels)

Supravesical fossa

Lateral inguinal fossa

Femoral nerve

Genitofemoral nerve

Gluteus maximus muscle

Gluteus medius muscle

Gluteus minimus muscle

Medial inguinal fossa

Deep inguinal lymph nodes

Umbilical artery, occluded part

Round ligament of the femur

Pelvic brim (terminal line)

Ureter

Transverse umbilical fold

Seminal vesicle; ductus deferens

Rectovesical pouch

Venous plexuses: vesical and prostatic

Ischiorectal fossa

Crus of penis

Deep transverse perineal muscle (urogenital diaphragm)

Bulbourethral gland

Fig. 460: Posterior Aspect of the Male Pelvic Organs and of the Anterior Abdominal Wall

NOTE: 1) this is a frontal section through the bones of the pelvis. Observe the wings (alae) of each ilium, which extend laterally to reach the skin of the iliac crest and bound the greater (or false) pelvis. On their internal or pelvic surface lie the **iliacus** and **psoas muscles** along with the iliac vessels and nerves of the lumbar plexus.

2) the lesser (or true) pelvis lies below the pelvic brim. It is restricted by bone and bounds more snugly the pelvic organs: the **bladder, prostate, seminal vesicle, vas deferens,** and **rectum** (the latter not shown). Inferiorly, the pelvic organs are separated from the perineum by the **pelvic diaphragm** (levator ani muscles).

3) the reflection of peritoneum as it invests the inner surface of the anterior abdominal wall, curves over the superior surface of the bladder and dips somewhat posterior to bladder (rectovesical pouch) to come into contact with the seminal vesicles and deferent ducts.

4) the **obturator internus muscle,** which covers much of the inner surface of the lateral wall of the pelvis. Extending into the perineum, this muscle also forms the lateral boundary of the ischiorectal fossa.

5) the inner surface of the anterior abdominal wall shows the **umbilical ligaments** and the **round ligament of the liver,** as well as the smooth contour of the rectus abdominis muscle and the **arcuate line,** which marks the inferior limit of the rectus sheath.

Fig. 460

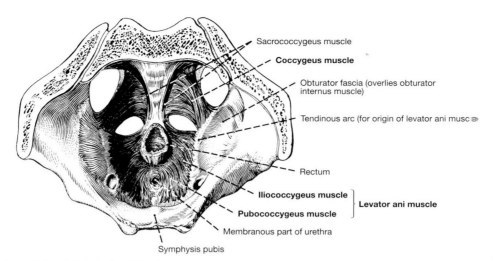

Sacrococcygeus muscle

Coccygeus muscle

Obturator fascia (overlies obturator internus muscle)

Tendinous arc (for origin of levator ani muscle)

Rectum

Iliococcygeus muscle
Pubococcygeus muscle
} **Levator ani muscle**

Membranous part of urethra

Symphysis pubis

Fig. 461: Muscular Floor of the Pelvis: Pelvic Diaphragm

NOTE: 1) the **pelvic diaphragm** consists of the **levator ani** (iliococcygeus and pubococcygeus parts) **muscle** and the **coccygeus muscle** along with two fascial layers, which cover the *pelvic* (supraanal fascia) and *perineal* (infraanal fascia) surfaces of these two muscles.

2) the muscles composing the pelvic diaphragm stretch across the pelvic floor in a concave sling-like manner and separate the structures of the pelvis from those in the perineum below. In males, the pelvic diaphragm is perforated by the anal canal and urethra.

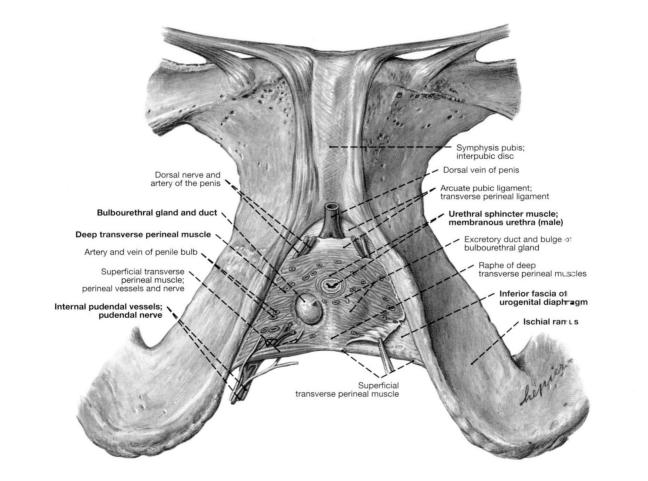

Symphysis pubis; interpubic disc

Dorsal vein of penis

Arcuate pubic ligament; transverse perineal ligament

Urethral sphincter muscle; membranous urethra (male)

Excretory duct and bulge of bulbourethral gland

Raphe of deep transverse perineal muscles

Inferior fascia of urogenital diaphragm

Ischial ramus

Dorsal nerve and artery of the penis

Bulbourethral gland and duct

Deep transverse perineal muscle

Artery and vein of penile bulb

Superficial transverse perineal muscle; perineal vessels and nerve

Internal pudendal vessels; pudendal nerve

Superficial transverse perineal muscle

Fig. 462: Urogenital Diaphragm; Deep Transverse Perineal Muscle (Male)

NOTE: 1) the **deep transverse perineal muscle** stretches between the ischial rami and is covered by fascia on both its internal (pelvic or superior) surface and its external (perineal or inferior) surface. These two fascias and the muscle form the **urogenital diaphragm.**

2) the region between the two fascias is often referred to as the **deep perineal compartment** (pouch, cleft or space). In the male it contains a) the deep transverse perineal muscle, b) the sphincter of the urethra, c) the bulbourethral glands, d) the membranous urethra, and e) branches of the internal pudendal vessels and nerve.

PLATE 300   **Male Perineum: Surface Anatomy; Muscles**

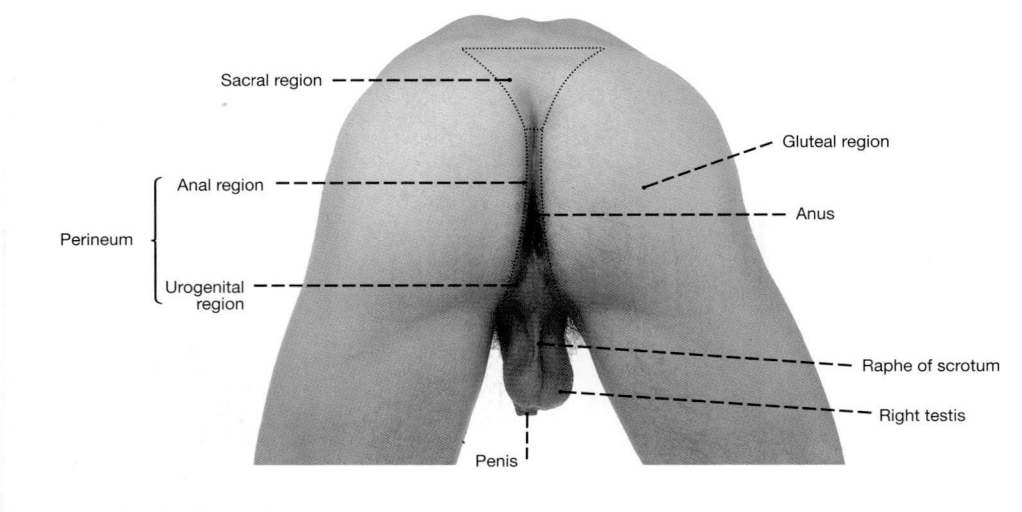

Sacral region

Gluteal region

Anal region

Anus

Perineum

Urogenital region

Raphe of scrotum

Right testis

Penis

Fig. 463: Surface Anatomy of the Male Perineum

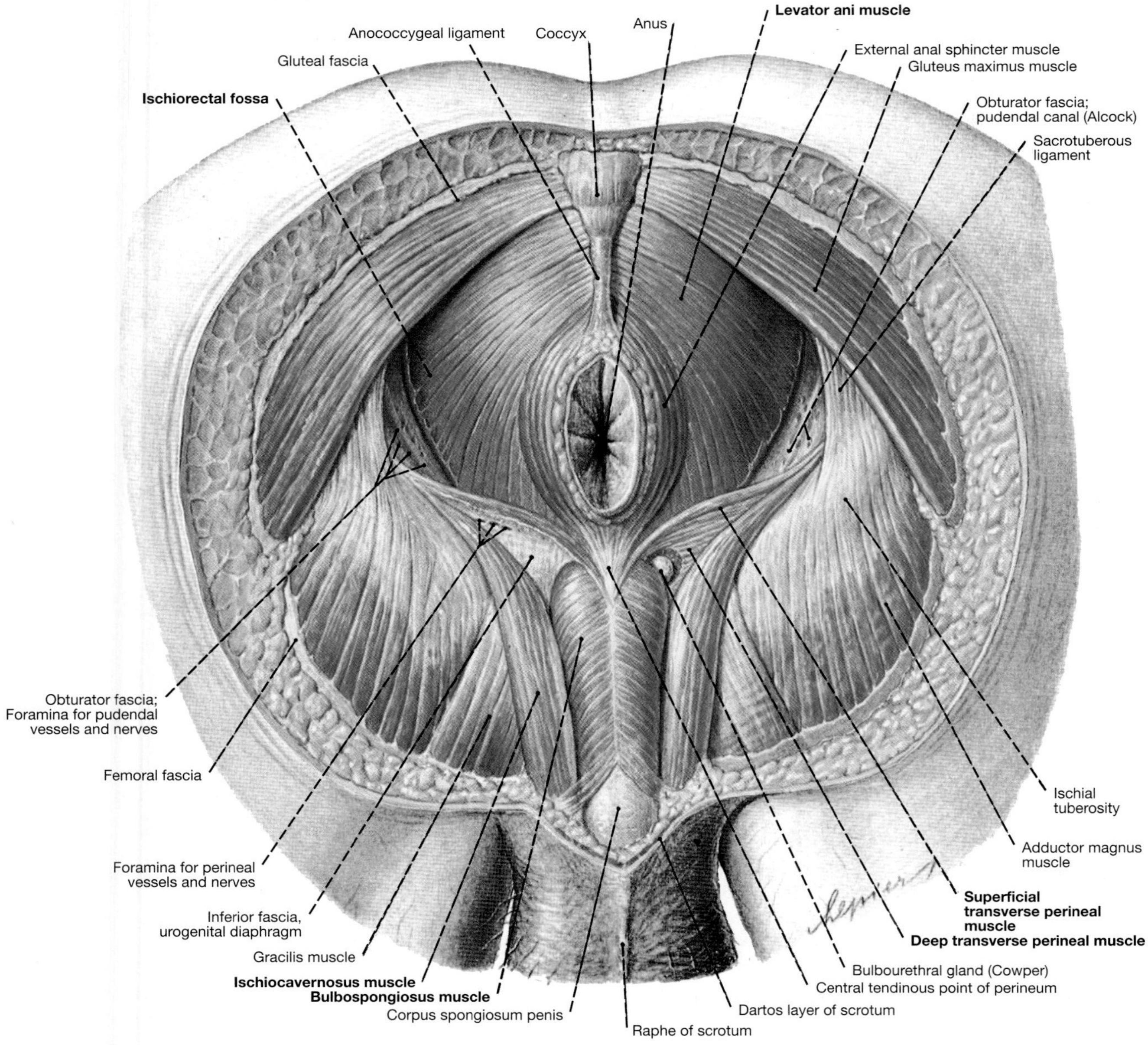

Anococcygeal ligament   Coccyx   Anus   **Levator ani muscle**

Gluteal fascia

External anal sphincter muscle
Gluteus maximus muscle

Ischiorectal fossa

Obturator fascia;
pudendal canal (Alcock)

Sacrotuberous
ligament

Ischial
tuberosity

Adductor magnus
muscle

Obturator fascia;
Foramina for pudendal
vessels and nerves

Femoral fascia

**Superficial
transverse perineal
muscle**
Deep transverse perineal muscle

Foramina for perineal
vessels and nerves

Bulbourethral gland (Cowper)
Central tendinous point of perineum

Inferior fascia,
urogenital diaphragm

Gracilis muscle

Dartos layer of scrotum

Ischiocavernosus muscle
Bulbospongiosus muscle

Corpus spongiosum penis

Raphe of scrotum

Fig. 464: Superficial Muscles of the Male Perineum

Figs. 463, 464

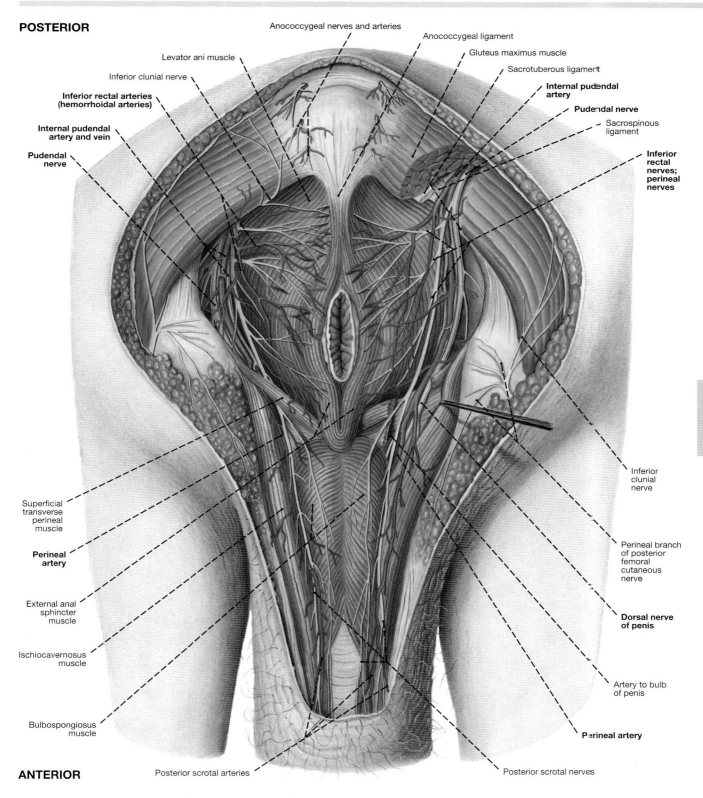

POSTERIOR

Anococcygeal nerves and arteries

Anococcygeal ligament

Levator ani muscle

Gluteus maximus muscle

Inferior clunial nerve

Sacrotuberous ligament

Inferior rectal arteries (hemorrhoidal arteries)

Internal pudendal artery

Pudendal nerve

Internal pudendal artery and vein

Sacrospinous ligament

Pudendal nerve

Inferior rectal nerves; perineal nerves

Inferior clunial nerve

Superficial transverse perineal muscle

Perineal branch of posterior femoral cutaneous nerve

Perineal artery

Dorsal nerve of penis

External anal sphincter muscle

Ischiocavernosus muscle

Artery to bulb of penis

Bulbospongiosus muscle

Perineal artery

ANTERIOR

Posterior scrotal arteries

Posterior scrotal nerves

Fig. 465: Nerves and Blood Vessels of the Male Perineum

NOTE: 1)   the skin of the perineum and the fat of the ischiorectal fossa have been removed to expose the muscles, vessels, and nerves of both the **anal** and **urogenital regions.**

2)   the **internal pudendal vessels** and **nerves** emerge from the pelvis to the gluteal region and then course to the perineum by way of the **pudendal canal** (of Alcock). At the lateral border of the **ischiorectal fossa** their branches, the **inferior rectal vessels** and **nerves,** cross the fossa transversely to supply the levator ani and external anal sphincter muscles.

3)   the main trunks of the vessels and nerve continue anteriorly, pierce the urogenital diaphragm and become the **perineal vessels** and **nerve** and the **dorsal vessels** and **nerve of the penis.** The muscles of the urogenital triangle are innervated by the perineal nerve, while the dorsal nerve of the penis is the main sensory nerve of that organ.

Fig. 465   **IV**

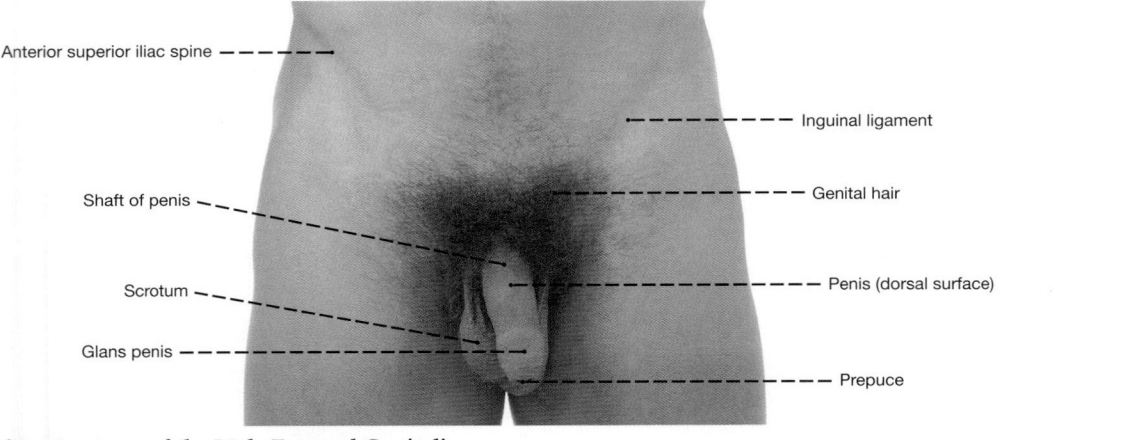

Anterior superior iliac spine

Inguinal ligament

Genital hair

Shaft of penis

Scrotum

Penis (dorsal surface)

Glans penis

Prepuce

Fig. 466: Surface Anatomy of the Male External Genitalia

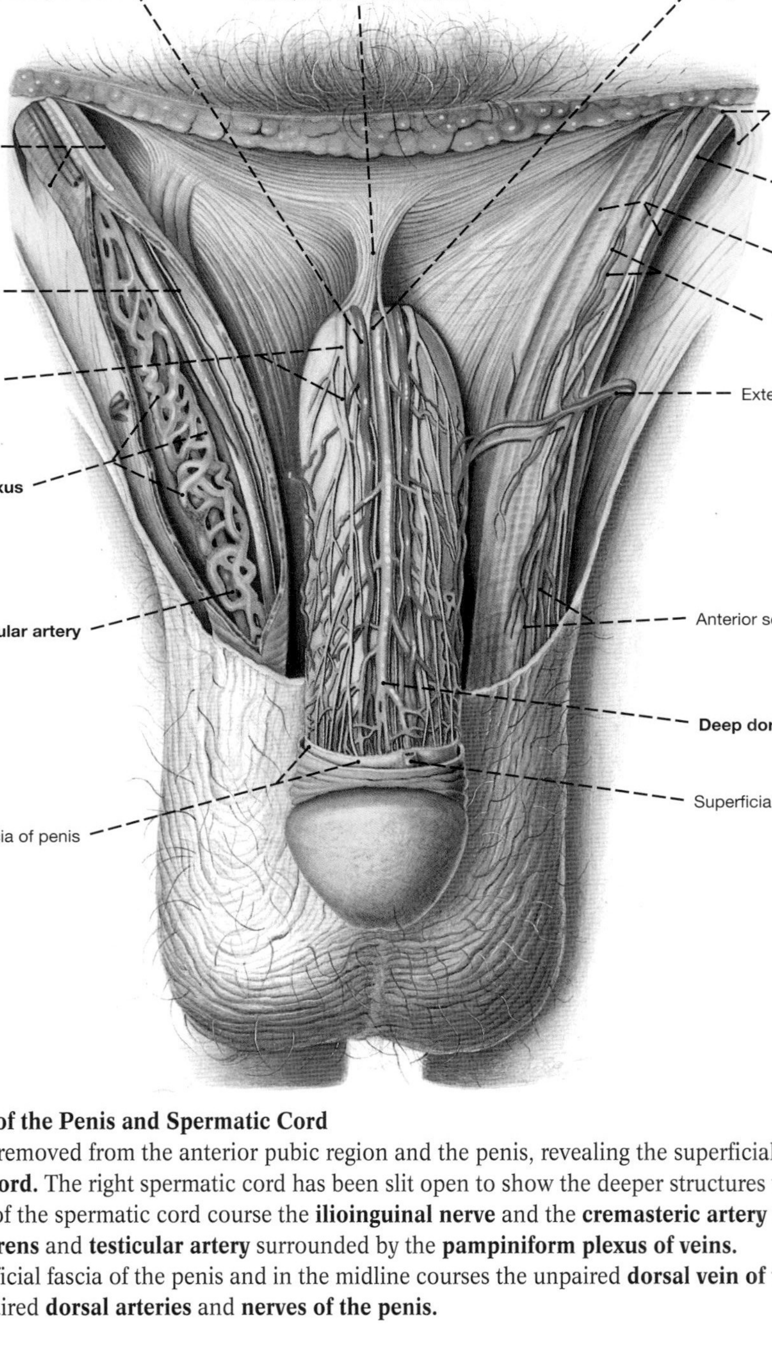

Dorsal artery of penis — Suspensory ligament of penis — **Deep dorsal vein of penis**

Spermatic cord

Superficial inguinal ring

Ilioinguinal nerve

Spermatic cord

Genital branch of genitofemoral nerve

Cremasteric artery and vein

Dorsal nerve of penis

External pudendal vessels

Pampiniform plexus

Testicular artery

Anterior scrotal vessels

Deep dorsal vein of penis

Superficial dorsal vein of penis

Superficial fascia of penis

Fig. 467: Vessels and Nerves of the Penis and Spermatic Cord

NOTE: 1)   the skin has been removed from the anterior pubic region and the penis, revealing the superficial vessels and nerves of the penis and left **spermatic cord.** The right spermatic cord has been slit open to show the deeper structures within (see Fig. 469).

  2)   along the surface of the spermatic cord course the **ilioinguinal nerve** and the **cremasteric artery** and **vein.** Within the cord are found the **ductus deferens** and **testicular artery** surrounded by the **pampiniform plexus of veins.**

  3)   beneath the superficial fascia of the penis and in the midline courses the unpaired **dorsal vein of the penis.** Along the sides of the vein, observe the paired **dorsal arteries** and **nerves of the penis.**

Fig. 466, 467

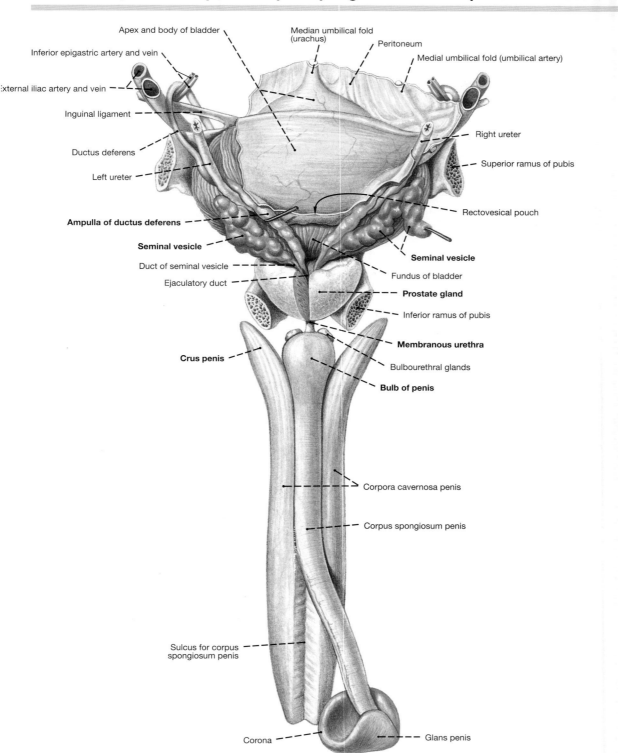

Apex and body of bladder

Inferior epigastric artery and vein

External iliac artery and vein

Inguinal ligament

Ductus deferens

Left ureter

Ampulla of ductus deferens

Seminal vesicle

Duct of seminal vesicle

Ejaculatory duct

Median umbilical fold
(urachus)

Peritoneum

Medial umbilical fold (umbilical artery)

Right ureter

Superior ramus of pubis

Rectovesical pouch

Seminal vesicle

Fundus of bladder

Prostate gland

Inferior ramus of pubis

Membranous urethra

Crus penis

Bulbourethral glands

Bulb of penis

Corpora cavernosa penis

Corpus spongiosum penis

Sulcus for corpus
spongiosum penis

Corona

Glans penis

Fig. 468: Erectile Bodies of the Penis Attached to the Bladder and Other Organs by the Membranous Urethra

NOTE: 1) the deep fascia, which closely invests the erectile bodies of the penis, has been removed, and the distal part of the **corpus spongiosum penis** (which contains the penile urethra), has been displaced from its position between the two **corpora cavernosa penis.**

2) the posterior surface of the **bladder** and **prostate** and the associated **seminal vesicles, ductus deferens,** and **bulbourethral glands** are also demonstrated. These structures all communicate with the **urethra,** the membranous part of which is in continuity with the **penile urethra.**

3) the tapered **crura** of the corpora cavernosa penis, which diverge laterally to become adherent to the ischial and pubic rami. They are surrounded by fibers of the ischiocavernosus muscles (see Fig. 465). The base of the corpus spongiosum penis is also expanded, and is called the **bulb of the penis.** It is surrounded by the bulbocavernosus muscle (see Fig. 464).

Fig. 468   **IV**

PLATE 304   Male Perineum: Superficial Dissection from Below

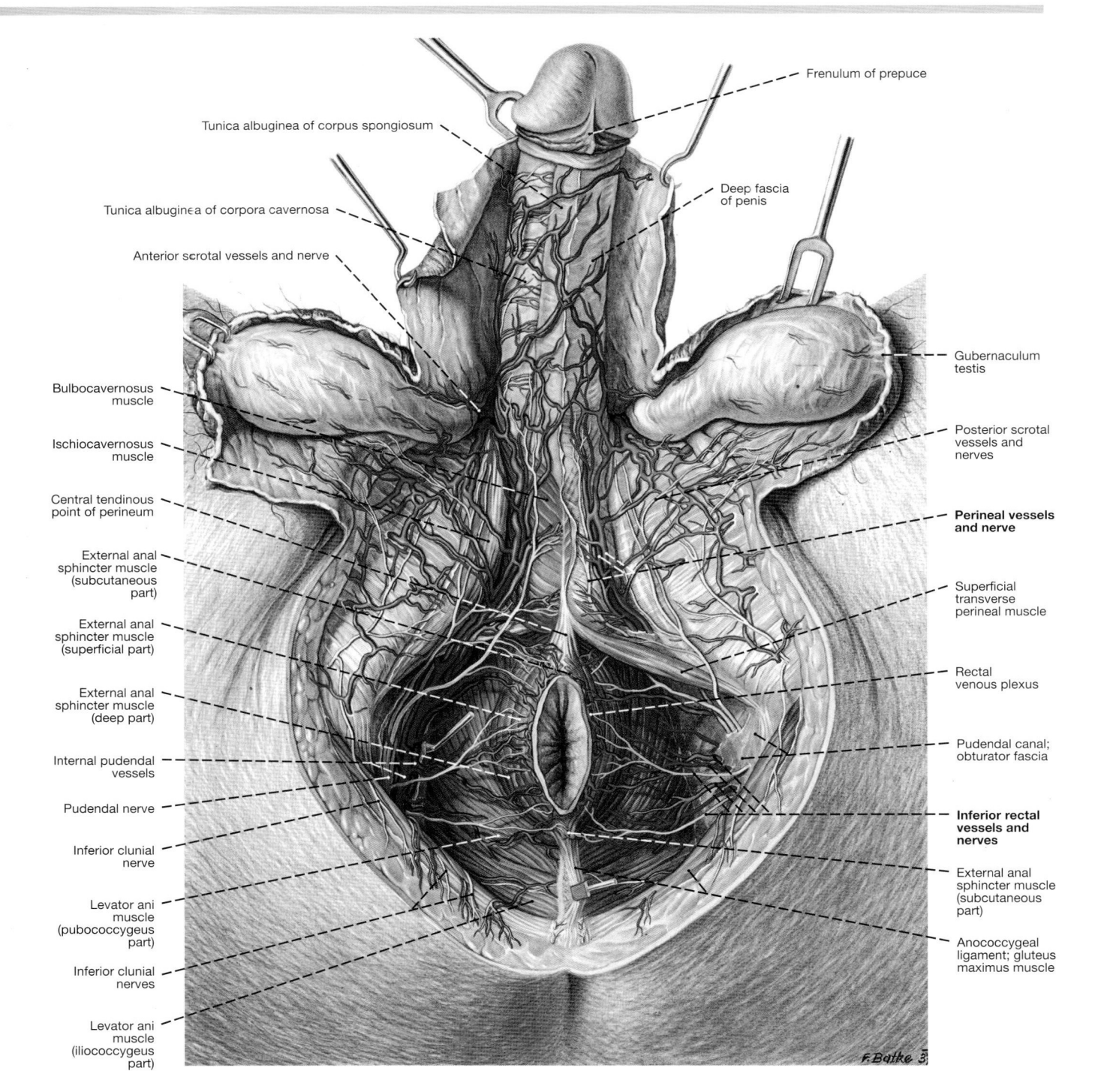

Frenulum of prepuce

Tunica albuginea of corpus spongiosum

Tunica albuginea of corpora cavernosa

Anterior scrotal vessels and nerve

Deep fascia of penis

Bulbocavernosus muscle

Ischiocavernosus muscle

Central tendinous point of perineum

External anal sphincter muscle (subcutaneous part)

External anal sphincter muscle (superficial part)

External anal sphincter muscle (deep part)

Internal pudendal vessels

Pudendal nerve

Inferior clunial nerve

Levator ani muscle (pubococcygeus part)

Inferior clunial nerves

Levator ani muscle (iliococcygeus part)

Gubernaculum testis

Posterior scrotal vessels and nerves

Perineal vessels and nerve

Superficial transverse perineal muscle

Rectal venous plexus

Pudendal canal; obturator fascia

Inferior rectal vessels and nerves

External anal sphincter muscle (subcutaneous part)

Anococcygeal ligament; gluteus maximus muscle

F. Batke 3

Fig. 469: Superficial Dissection of the Urogenital and Anal Regions of the Perineum

NOTE: 1)   this is a dissection of the perineum from below, and the superficial fascia and fat have been removed from the urogenital and anal regions.

2)   on the specimen's left (reader's right), the **deep fascia of the penis** and the **superficial** (or external) **perineal fascia** that covers the bulbocavernosus and ischiocavernosus muscles are left intact as are the **obturator fascia** and its underlying **pudendal canal.**

3)   on the specimen's right (reader's left), the external perineal fascia has been removed to expose the **ischiocavernosus** and **bulbocavernosus muscles,** as well as the **perineal vessels** and **nerves** that course forward as continuations of the internal pudendal vessels and the pudendal nerve.

4)   the **inferior rectal vessels** and **nerves** crossing the ischiorectal fossa to supply the **levator ani muscle** as well as the **subcutaneous, superficial** and **deep** parts of the **external anal sphincter muscle.**

Fig. 469

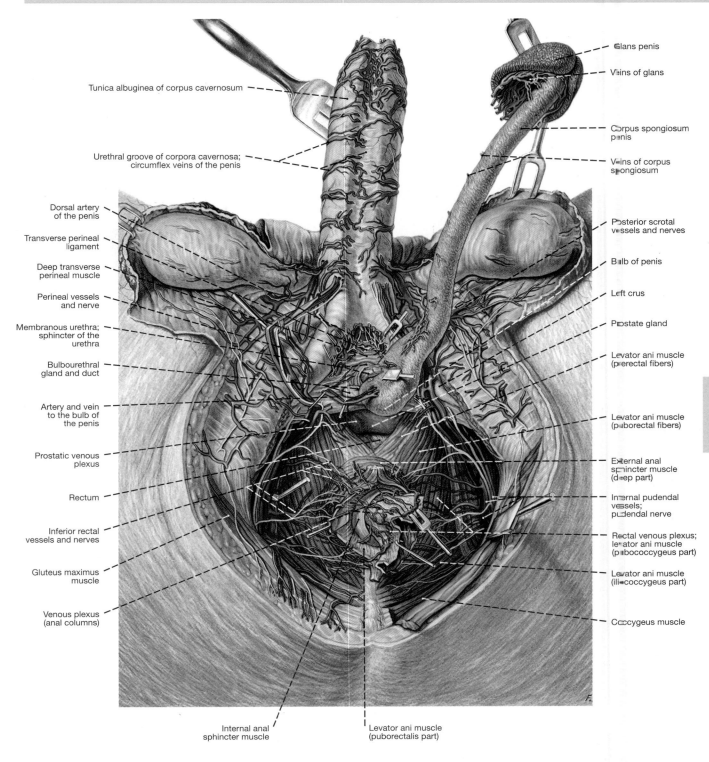

Tunica albuginea of corpus cavernosum

Urethral groove of corpora cavernosa; circumflex veins of the penis

Dorsal artery of the penis

Transverse perineal ligament

Deep transverse perineal muscle

Perineal vessels and nerve

Membranous urethra; sphincter of the urethra

Bulbourethral gland and duct

Artery and vein to the bulb of the penis

Prostatic venous plexus

Rectum

Inferior rectal vessels and nerves

Gluteus maximus muscle

Venous plexus (anal columns)

Glans penis

Veins of glans

Corpus spongiosum penis

Veins of corpus spongiosum

Posterior scrotal vessels and nerves

Bulb of penis

Left crus

Prostate gland

Levator ani muscle (prerectal fibers)

Levator ani muscle (puborectal fibers)

External anal sphincter muscle (deep part)

Internal pudendal vessels; pudendal nerve

Rectal venous plexus; levator ani muscle (pubococcygeus part)

Levator ani muscle (iliococcygeus part)

Coccygeus muscle

Internal anal sphincter muscle

Levator ani muscle (puborectalis part)

Fig. 470: Deep Dissection of the Urogenital and Anal Regions of the Perineum

NOTE: 1) this dissection is somewhat deeper than that shown in Figure 469. In the urogenital region, the **corpus spongiosum penis** has been detached from the **urethral groove** of the **corpora cavernosa penis.**

2) with the inferior fascia of the urogenital diaphragm removed, the **deep transverse perineal muscle,** the **bulbourethral gland,** the **membranous urethra** and its **sphincter** are exposed. Observe that the membranous urethra enters the **bulb of the penis** and thereby becomes the **penile urethra.**

3) with the ischiocavernosus muscles removed, the **crura of the corpora cavernosa penis** are exposed at their attachment to the rami of the ischium and pubis.

4) the lowermost part of the pelvis has been opened and the anterior surface of the rectum and the adjacent posterior surface of the prostate gland have been exposed. An important fascial layer (the **rectoprostatic** or **rectovesical fascia of Denonvillier**) separates these two organs. This allows the surgeon access to the prostate gland through a perineal approach.

Fig. 470   **IV**

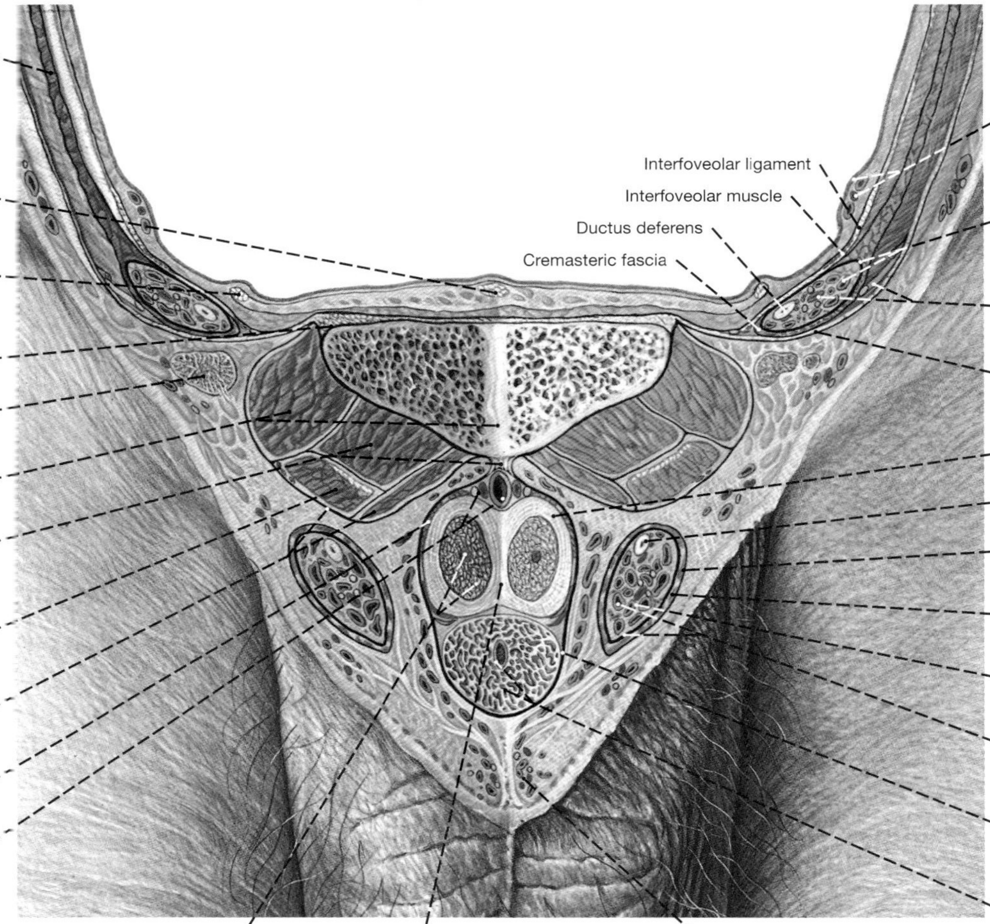

Internal oblique muscle

Urachus

Obliterated umbilical artery

Inguinal ligament

Superficial inguinal lymph node

Pectineus muscle; symphysis pubis

Adductor brevis muscle; suspensory ligament of penis

Adductor longus muscle

Gracilis muscle; adductor fascia

Ischiocavernosus muscle

Dorsal artery and nerve of penis; deep dorsal vein

Interfoveolar ligament

Interfoveolar muscle

Ductus deferens

Cremasteric fascia

Inferior epigastric vessels; lateral umbilical fold

Pampiniform plexus; internal spermatic fascia

Testicular artery; ilioinguinal nerve

External spermatic fascia

Tunica albuginea

Ductus deferens

External spermatic fascia

Cremasteric fascia and muscle

Testicular artery

Pampiniform plexus; internal spermatic fascia

Deep fascia of penis

Scrotal septum

Deep artery of penis; Corpus cavernosum penis

Septum of penis

Urethra; corpus spongiosum

Fig. 471: Transverse Section Through the Symphysis Pubis and the Erect Penis

NOTE: 1) the penis has been transected distal to its bulb. Observe the two corpora cavernosa with centrally located **deep arteries** and the corpus spongiosum containing the **penile urethra.**

    2) the **dorsal arteries** and **nerves of the penis** along with the **deep dorsal vein** course beneath the deep fascia of the penis.

    3) the two **spermatic cords** are both severed in the inguinal region and more distally in the scrotum.

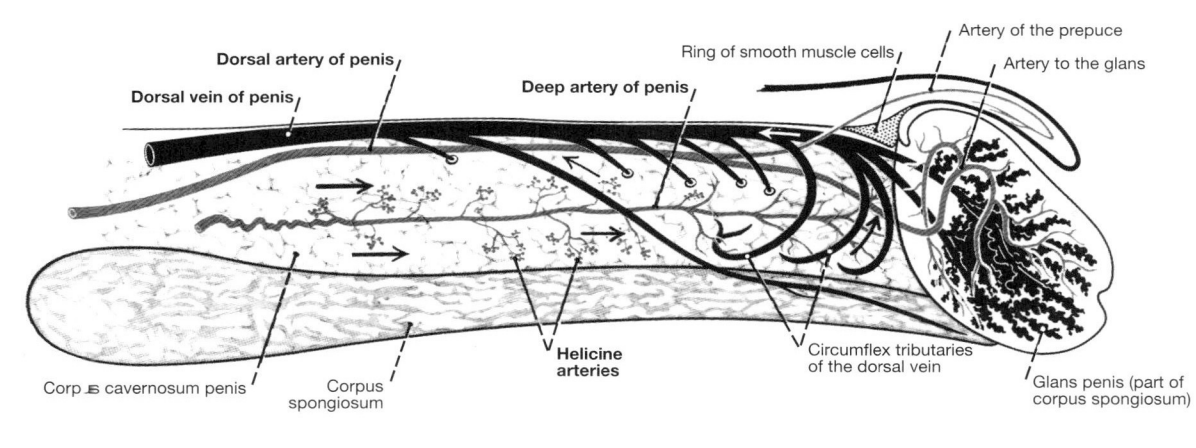

Dorsal artery of penis

Dorsal vein of penis

Deep artery of penis

Ring of smooth muscle cells

Artery of the prepuce

Artery to the glans

Helicine arteries

Circumflex tributaries of the dorsal vein

Glans penis (part of corpus spongiosum)

Corpus cavernosum penis

Corpus spongiosum

Fig. 472: Longitudinal Section Through the Penis Showing Its Vascular Circulation

NOTE: 1) the dorsal and deep arteries of the penis supply blood principally to the corpora cavernosa but also to the glans penis of the corpus spongiosum

    2) the **helicine branches** of the deep artery and the **circumflex tributaries** of the deep dorsal vein that return blood from the corpora and the glans.

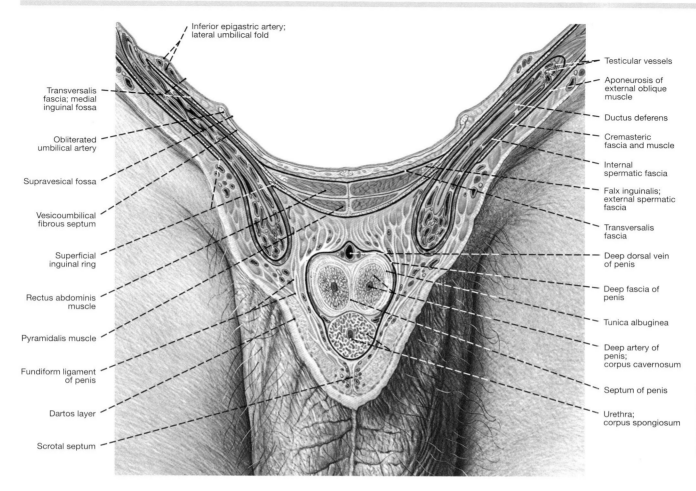

Inferior epigastric artery; lateral umbilical fold

Transversalis fascia; medial inguinal fossa

Obliterated umbilical artery

Supravesical fossa

Vesicoumbilical fibrous septum

Superficial inguinal ring

Rectus abdominis muscle

Pyramidalis muscle

Fundiform ligament of penis

Dartos layer

Scrotal septum

Testicular vessels

Aponeurosis of external oblique muscle

Ductus deferens

Cremasteric fascia and muscle

Internal spermatic fascia

Falx inguinalis; external spermatic fascia

Transversalis fascia

Deep dorsal vein of penis

Deep fascia of penis

Tunica albuginea

Deep artery of penis; corpus cavernosum

Septum of penis

Urethra; corpus spongiosum

Fig. 473: Oblique Section Through Both Inguinal Canals and Through the Penis

NOTE: the spermatic cord is demonstrated coursing through the inguinal canal from its entrance at the superficial inguinal ring nearly to the abdominal inguinal ring on both sides. The shaft of the penis has also seen sectioned.

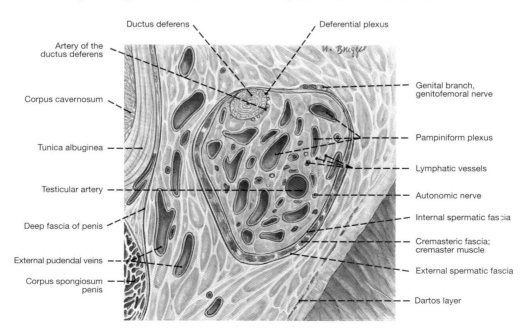

Ductus deferens

Artery of the ductus deferens

Corpus cavernosum

Tunica albuginea

Testicular artery

Deep fascia of penis

External pudendal veins

Corpus spongiosum penis

Deferential plexus

Genital branch, genitofemoral nerve

Pampiniform plexus

Lymphatic vessels

Autonomic nerve

Internal spermatic fascia

Cremasteric fascia; cremaster muscle

External spermatic fascia

Dartos layer

Fig. 474: Transverse Section of the Spermatic Cord Within the Scrotum

NOTE: the spermatic cord contains: 1) ductus deferens, 2) artery of the ductus deferens, 3) testicular artery, 4) cremasteric artery, 5) pampiniform plexus of veins, 6) lymphatic vessels, 7) sympathetic and sensory nerve fibers and some fat. These are surrounded by the internal and external spermatic fascial layers and the cremaster muscle.

PLATE 308   Male Perineum: Penis, Cross-sections Through the Shaft

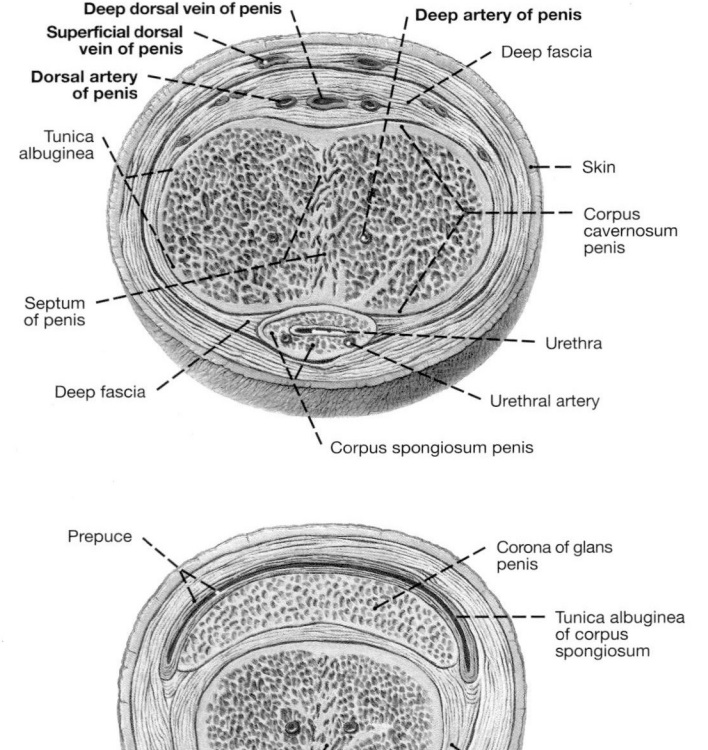

Fig. 475: Section Through Middle of Penis (see Fig. 478)

NOTE: 1) the penis is composed of two corpora cavernosa penis containing erectile tissue and one corpus spongiosum penis seen ventrally and in the midline that contains the penile portion of the urethra.

2) the three corpora are surrounded by a closely investing layer of deep fascia. In erection, blood fills the erectile tissue causing the corpora to become rigid. The thin-walled veins are compressed between the corpora and the deep fascia. Erection is maintained by the prevention of venous blood from draining back into the general circulation.

Deep dorsal vein of penis
Superficial dorsal vein of penis
Dorsal artery of penis
Deep artery of penis
Deep fascia
Tunica albuginea
Skin
Corpus cavernosum penis
Septum of penis
Urethra
Deep fascia
Urethral artery
Corpus spongiosum penis

Fig. 476: Section at Neck of the Glans Penis (see Fig. 478)

NOTE: this section is taken from the proximal part of the glans penis. The corpora cavernosa penis become smaller distally, while the corona of the glans penis is formed by the spongy tissue of the corpus spongiosum penis.

Prepuce
Corona of glans penis
Tunica albuginea of corpus spongiosum
Tunica albuginea of corpus cavernosum
Urethra
Septum of penis

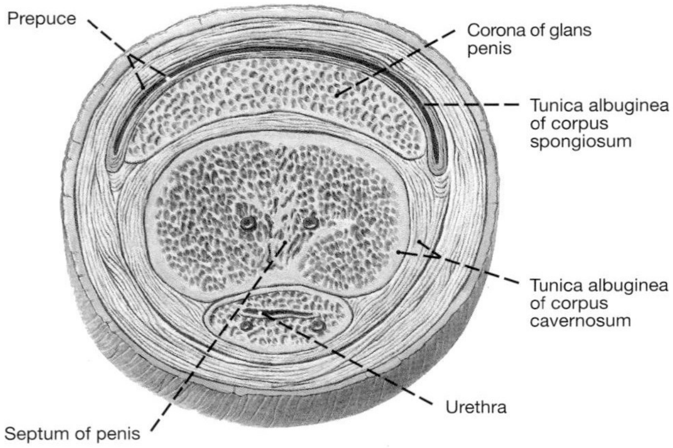

Fig. 477: Section Through Glans Penis (see Fig. 478)

NOTE: the glans penis is the expanded distal extremity of the corpus spongiosum penis. At its distal end is the opening of the urethra. In the uncircumcised male, the glans penis is covered by a duplication of thin skin, called the prepuce, which is attached to the glans penis ventrally by the frenulum.

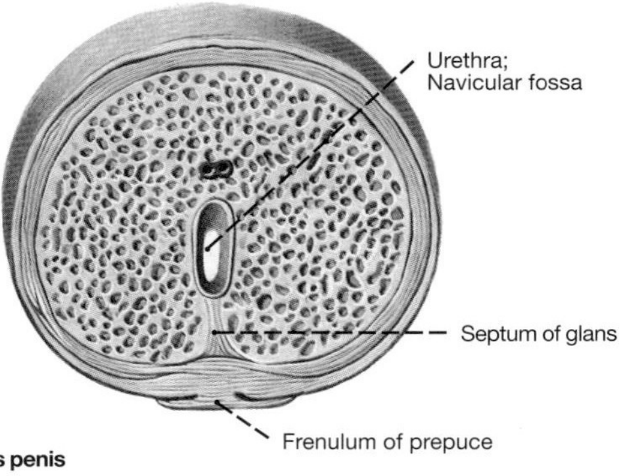

Urethra; Navicular fossa
Septum of glans
Frenulum of prepuce

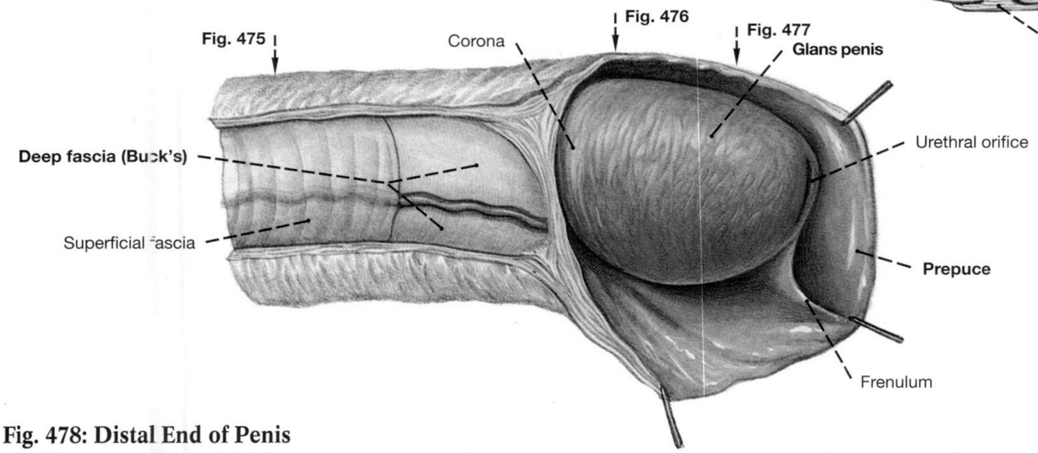

Fig. 475
Corona
Fig. 476
Fig. 477
Glans penis

Deep fascia (Buck's)
Urethral orifice
Superficial fascia
Prepuce
Frenulum

Fig. 478: Distal End of Penis

NOTE: the distal end of the penis consists of the glans penis which is attached by the frenulum to a duplicated fold of skin, the prepuce. Observe that the skin of the penis is thin and delicate and is loosely attached to the underlying deep fascia and corpora, accounting for its freely movable nature. (Arrows indicate cross-sections seen above).

Figs. 475–478

PART V
THE LOWER LIMB

(PLATES 309–402 – FIGURES 479–622)

PART V   The Lower Limb

PART V   The Lower Limb

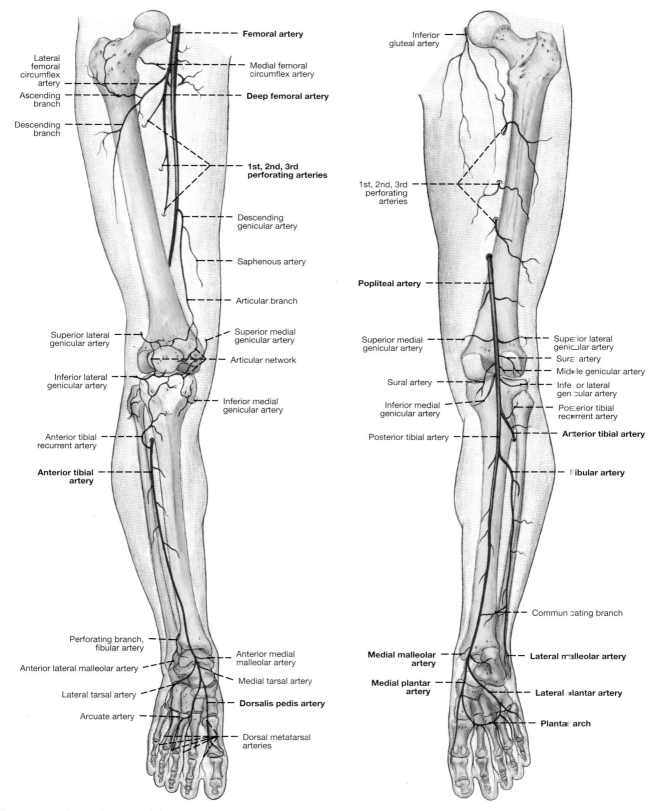

Fig. 479: **Arteries and Bones of the Lower Limb**
(Anterior View)
NOTE: the anastomoses in the hip and knee regions, and the
perforating branches of the **deep femoral artery.** In the
anterior leg, the **anterior tibial artery** descends between the
tibia and fibula to achieve the malleolar region and the foot
dorsum.

Fig. 480: **Arteries and Bones of the Lower Limb (Posterior View)**
NOTE: the branches of the **popliteal artery** at the knee, and its
continuation as the **posterior tibial artery.** In the foot this vessel
divides to form the **medial** and **lateral plantar arteries** which
then anastomose to form the **plantar arch.**

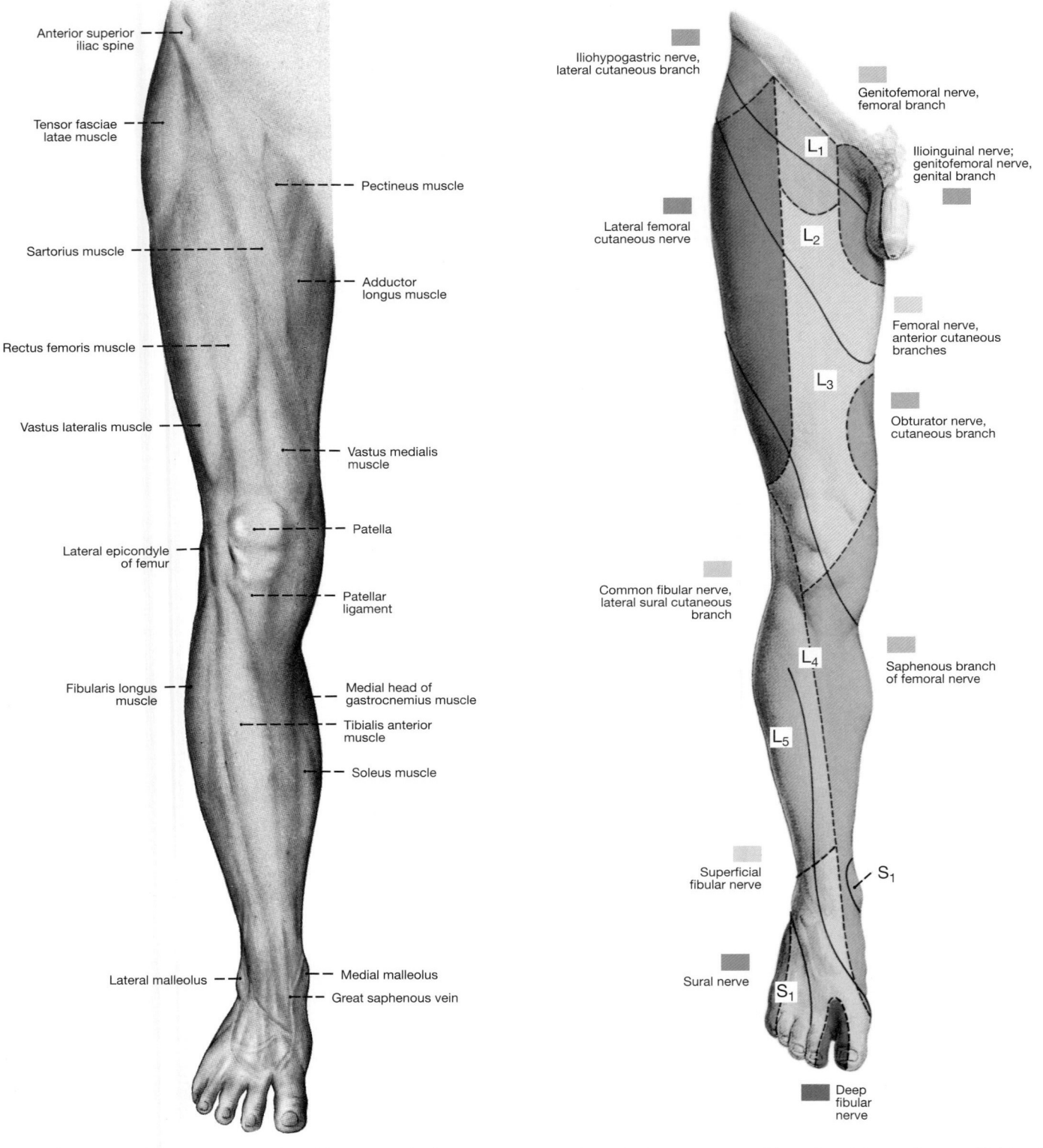

Fig. 481: Surface Anatomy of the Right Lower Limb, Anterior View

NOTE: 1) the pectineus and adductor longus muscles forming the floor of the femoral triangle. Observe also the sartorius muscle coursing inferomedially, and the tensor fasciae latae that shapes the rounded upper lateral contour of the thigh.

    2) the leg is shaped laterally by the fibularis muscles, anteriorly by the tibialis anterior, and medially by the gastrocnemius and soleus muscles.

Fig. 482: Dermatomes and Peripheral Nerve Sensory Fields of the Anterior Lower Limb

NOTE: 1) as a rule the lumbar segments of the spinal cord supply cutaneous innervation to the anterior aspect of the lower limb, and the dermatomes are segmentally arranged in order from L1 to L5.

    2) the 1st sacral segment supplies the skin over the medial malleolus and the dorsolateral aspect of the foot.

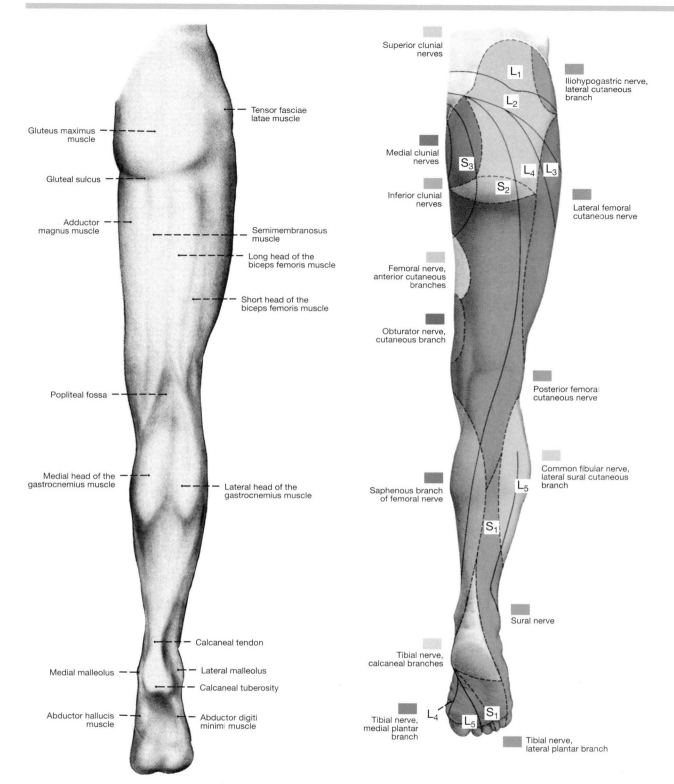

Tensor fasciae latae muscle

Gluteus maximus muscle

Gluteal sulcus

Adductor magnus muscle

Semimembranosus muscle

Long head of the biceps femoris muscle

Short head of the biceps femoris muscle

Popliteal fossa

Medial head of the gastrocnemius muscle

Lateral head of the gastrocnemius muscle

Calcaneal tendon

Medial malleolus

Lateral malleolus

Calcaneal tuberosity

Abductor hallucis muscle

Abductor digiti minimi muscle

Superior clunial nerves

Iliohypogastric nerve, lateral cutaneous branch

L_1

L_2

Medial clunial nerves

S_3 L_4 L_3

S_2

Inferior clunial nerves

Lateral femoral cutaneous nerve

Femoral nerve, anterior cutaneous branches

Obturator nerve, cutaneous branch

Posterior femoral cutaneous nerve

Common fibular nerve, lateral sural cutaneous branch

Saphenous branch of femoral nerve

L_5

S_1

Sural nerve

Tibial nerve, calcaneal branches

L_4 S_1

Tibial nerve, medial plantar branch

L_5

Tibial nerve, lateral plantar branch

Fig. 483: Surface Anatomy of the Right Lower Limb, Posterior View
NOTE: 1) the rounded contour of the buttock formed by the gluteus maximus muscle.

2) the outline of the hamstring muscles (semitendinosus, semimembranosus and biceps femoris) in the posterior thigh.

3) the popliteal fossa, below which are the heads of the gastrocnemius muscle. Note also the calcaneal tendon, which inserts between the two malleoli onto the calcaneus. On the plantar surface of the foot see the abductor hallucis medially and the abductor digiti minimi laterally.

Fig. 484: Dermatomes and Peripheral Nerve Sensory Fields of the Posterior Lower Limb
NOTE: 1) sensory innervation to a) the **posterior thigh** is by the posterior femoral cutaneous nerve (S1, S2, S3), b) the **medial calf** by the saphenous nerve (femoral: L2, L3, L4), and c) the **lateral calf** by the sural nerve (S1, S2).

2) the **heel** is supplied by the tibial nerve (S1, S2), and the **plantar foot** by the medial plantar nerve (L4, L5) and the lateral plantar nerve (S1, S2).

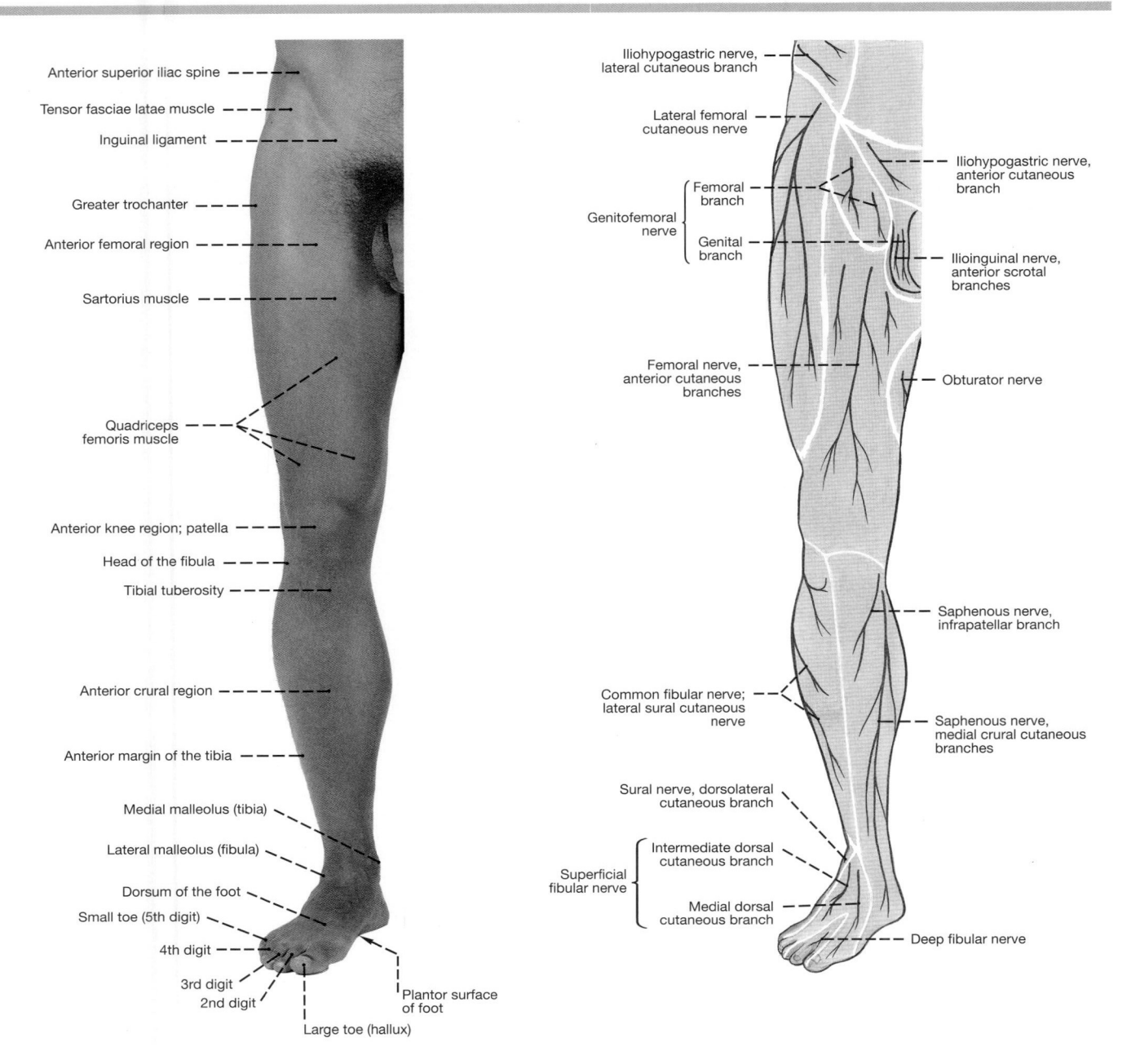

Fig. 485: Photograph of the Anterior Surface of the Lower Limb

NOTE: 1)   the following bony landmarks:
- a)   anterior superior iliac spine
- b)   greater trochanter
- c)   patella
- d)   head of the fibula
- e)   tibial tuberosity
- f)   anterior margin of the tibia
- g)   medial and lateral malleoli

2)   the inguinal ligament, which forms the lower anterior boundary of the abdominal wall, separating it from the anterior thigh, inferiorly.

3)   deep to the surface areas shown in this figure course branches of the cutaneous nerves that supply the anterior and lateral aspects of the thigh and leg and the dorsum of the foot. These branches are shown in Figure 486.

Fig. 486: Cutaneous Nerve Branches on the Anterior Surface of the Lower Limb

NOTE: 1)   compare the sites of emergence of sensory nerve branches with surface landmarks shown in Figure 485.

2)   cutaneous branches of the **femoral nerve** supply the anteromedial aspect of the thigh below the fields of the ilioinguinal and genitofemoral nerves, and the **saphenous nerve** is the largest cutaneous branch of the femoral nerve and it supplies the anteromedial and posteromedial aspects of the leg.

3)   the **lateral sural cutaneous branch** of the **common fibular nerve** which supplies the anteromedial and posteromedial surfaces of the leg.

4)   the large field supplied by the **superficial fibular nerve** on the anterior leg and foot dorsum, and the small field supplied by the **deep fibular nerve.**

5)   knowledge of the course of these branches is important in administering local anesthesia.

Figs. 485, 486

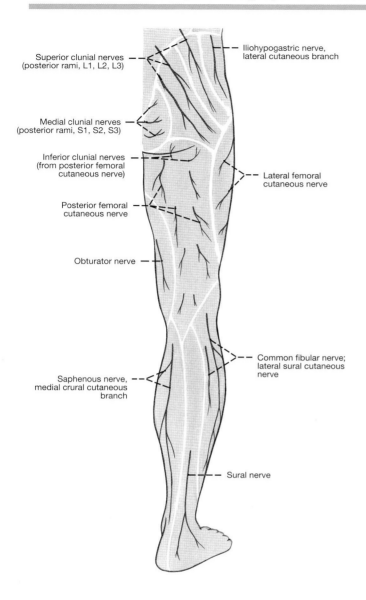

Superior clunial nerves (posterior rami, L1, L2, L3)

Iliohypogastric nerve, lateral cutaneous branch

Medial clunial nerves (posterior rami, S1, S2, S3)

Inferior clunial nerves (from posterior femoral cutaneous nerve)

Posterior femoral cutaneous nerve

Lateral femoral cutaneous nerve

Obturator nerve

Saphenous nerve, medial crural cutaneous branch

Common fibular nerve; lateral sural cutaneous nerve

Sural nerve

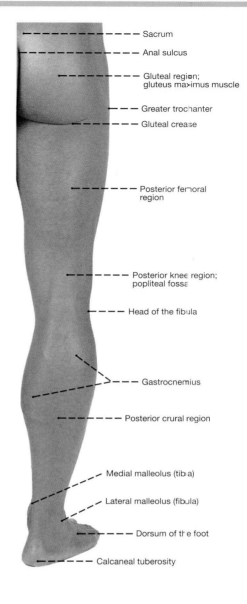

Sacrum

Anal sulcus

Gluteal region; gluteus maximus muscle

Greater trochanter

Gluteal crease

Posterior femoral region

Posterior knee region; popliteal fossa

Head of the fibula

Gastrocnemius

Posterior crural region

Medial malleolus (tibia)

Lateral malleolus (fibula)

Dorsum of the foot

Calcaneal tuberosity

Fig. 487: Cutaneous Nerve Branches on the Posterior Surface of the Lower Limb

NOTE: 1) cutaneous innervation of the **gluteal region** comes from four sources:

    a) lateral cutaneous branches of the **iliohypogastric nerve** (anterior ramus, L1)

    b) **superior clunial nerves** (posterior rami, L1, L2, L3)

    c) **medial clunial nerves** (posterior rami, S1, S2, S3)

    d) **inferior clunial nerves** (branches of the posterior femoral cutaneous nerve, anterior rami, S1, S2, S3)

2) the skin of the **posterior thigh** is supplied principally by the **posterior femoral cutaneous nerve** with small contributions from the **lateral femoral cutaneous nerve** and the **obturator nerve.**

3) the **posterior leg** receives cutaneous branches from:

    a) the **saphenous branch** of the femoral nerve

    b) the **sural nerve**

    c) the **lateral sural cutaneous branch** of the **common fibular nerve.**

Fig. 488: Photograph of the Posterior Surface of the Lower Limb

NOTE: 1) the following bony landmarks:

    a) sacrum

    b) greater trochanter

    c) head of the fibula

    d) medial and lateral malleoli

    e) calcaneal tuberosity

2) the **gluteal crease.** Midway between the greater trochanter laterally and the ischial tuberosity medially and deep to this crease is found the large **sciatic nerve** descending in the posterior thigh. The nerve is vulnerable at this site because only skin and superficial fascia overlie it.

3) the **popliteal fossa** located behind the knee joint. Deep to the skin at this site are found the tibial and fibular divisions of the sciatic nerve and the popliteal artery and vein.

4) the **calcaneal tuberosity** into which inserts the calcaneus tendon formed as the common tendon of the gastrocnemius, soleus and plantaris muscles.

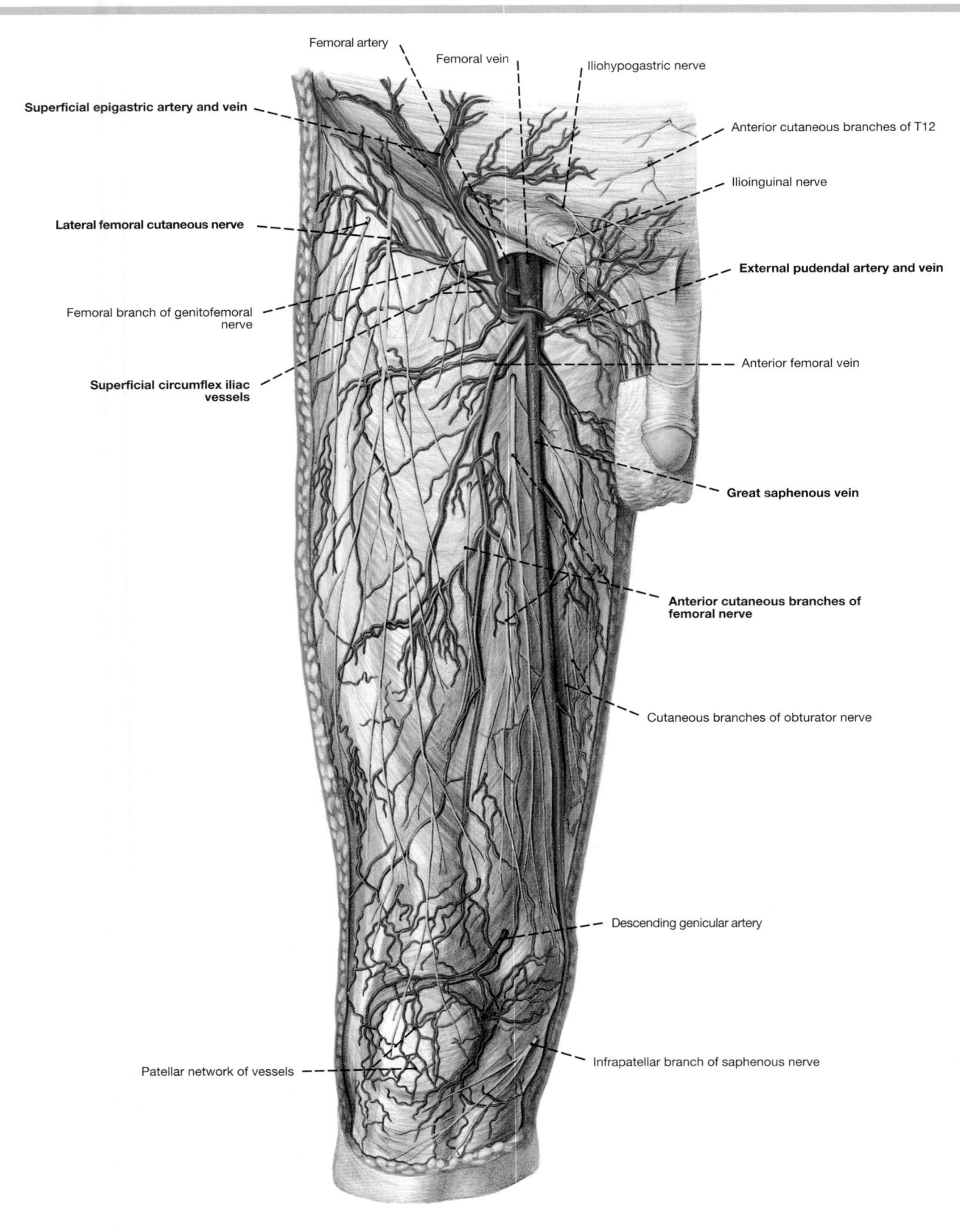

Femoral artery

Femoral vein

Iliohypogastric nerve

Superficial epigastric artery and vein

Anterior cutaneous branches of T12

Lateral femoral cutaneous nerve

Ilioinguinal nerve

External pudendal artery and vein

Femoral branch of genitofemoral nerve

Anterior femoral vein

Superficial circumflex iliac vessels

Great saphenous vein

Anterior cutaneous branches of femoral nerve

Cutaneous branches of obturator nerve

Descending genicular artery

Patellar network of vessels

Infrapatellar branch of saphenous nerve

Fig. 489: Superficial Nerves and Blood Vessels of the Anterior Thigh
NOTE: 1) the **great saphenous vein** as it ascends on the anterior and medial aspect of the thigh. Just below (1¹/₂ inches) the inguinal
ligament, it penetrates the deep fascia through the **saphenous opening** to enter the **femoral vein.**
2) the superficial branches of the **femoral artery** and the superficial vessels that drain into the **great saphenous vein.** These
include: 1) **the superficial epigastric,** 2) **the external pudendal,** and 3) **the superficial circumflex iliac** arteries and veins.
3) the principal cutaneous nerves of the anterior thigh. Compare these with those shown in Figure 486.

Fig. 489

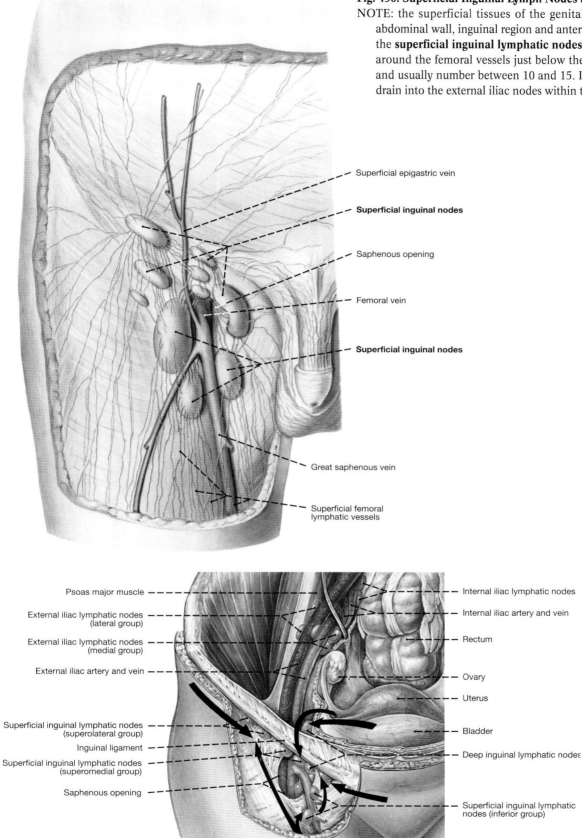

Fig. 490: Superficial Inguinal Lymph Nodes and Channels
NOTE: the superficial tissues of the genitalia, lower anterior abdominal wall, inguinal region and anterior thigh drain into the **superficial inguinal lymphatic nodes.** These are located around the femoral vessels just below the inguinal ligament and usually number between 10 and 15. In turn these nodes drain into the external iliac nodes within the pelvis.

Superficial epigastric vein

Superficial inguinal nodes

Saphenous opening

Femoral vein

Superficial inguinal nodes

Great saphenous vein

Superficial femoral lymphatic vessels

Psoas major muscle

External iliac lymphatic nodes (lateral group)

External iliac lymphatic nodes (medial group)

External iliac artery and vein

Superficial inguinal lymphatic nodes (superolateral group)

Inguinal ligament

Superficial inguinal lymphatic nodes (superomedial group)

Saphenous opening

Internal iliac lymphatic nodes

Internal iliac artery and vein

Rectum

Ovary

Uterus

Bladder

Deep inguinal lymphatic nodes

Superficial inguinal lymphatic nodes (inferior group)

Fig. 491: Superficial and Deep Inguinal Lymphatic Nodes
NOTE: the directions of flow (arrows) of lymph from adjacent tissues into deep superficial and deep inguinal nodes. The superficial nodes are divided into superolateral, superomedial and inferomedial groups, while the deep nodes are closest to the femoral vessels.

PLATE 316   Lower Extremity: Anterior Thigh, Fascia Lata

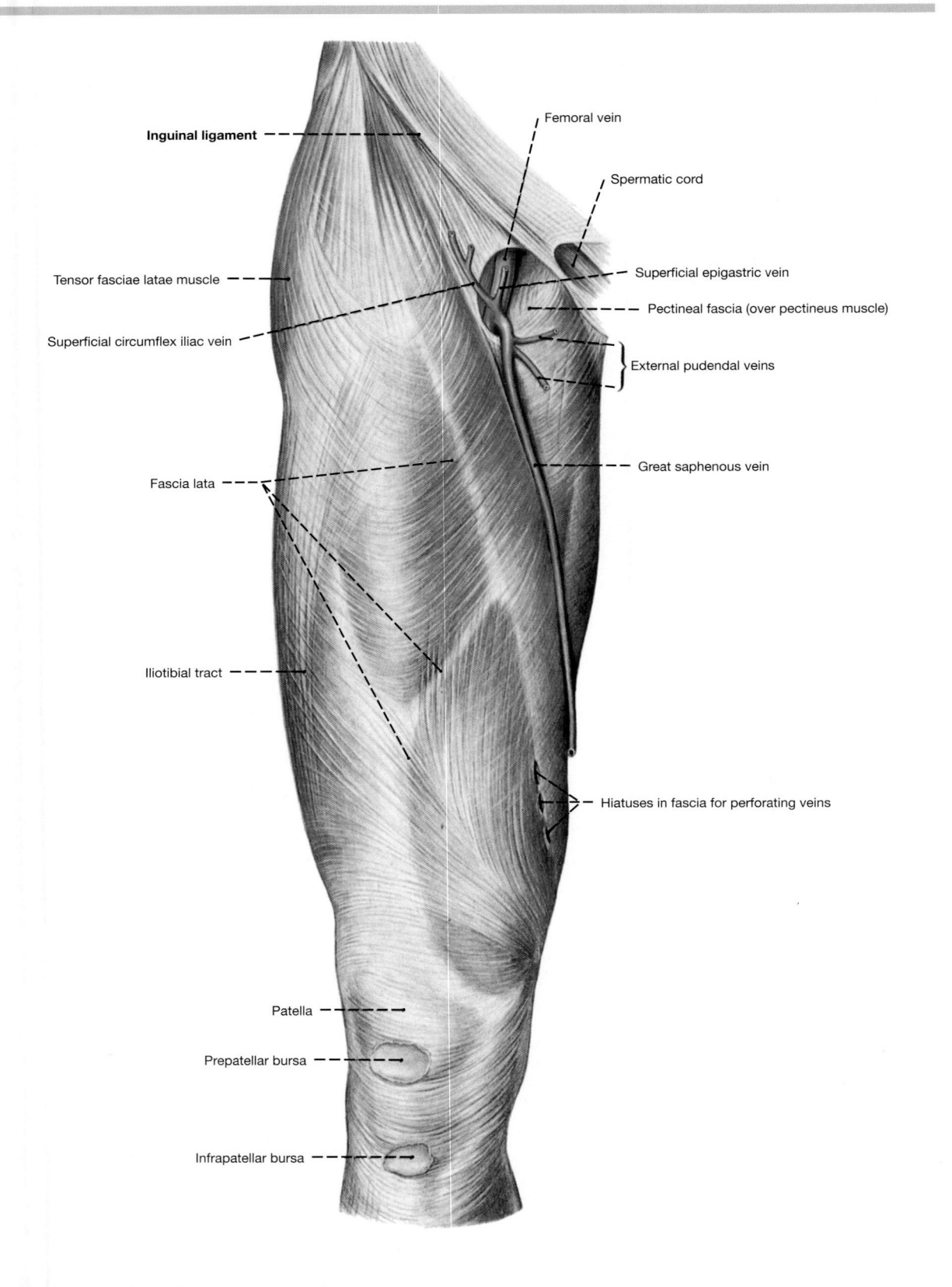

Inguinal ligament

Femoral vein

Spermatic cord

Tensor fasciae latae muscle

Superficial epigastric vein

Superficial circumflex iliac vein

Pectineal fascia (over pectineus muscle)

External pudendal veins

Great saphenous vein

Fascia lata

Iliotibial tract

Hiatuses in fascia for perforating veins

Patella

Prepatellar bursa

Infrapatellar bursa

Fig. 492: Fascia of the Anterior Thigh, Fascia Lata (right)

NOTE: 1)   the dense fascia, which closely invests the muscles of the hip and thigh, is called the **fascia lata.** It is attached above to the ischial and pubic rami and inguinal ligament anteriorly, the crest of the ilium laterally, and the ischial tuberosity, sacrotuberous ligament, sacrum and coccyx posteriorly.

2)   the fascia lata is most strong laterally where it forms the **iliotibial tract.** This thickened band descends to the lateral condyle of the tibia. Above, the fascia lata surrounds a muscle called the **tensor fascia latae** which, by pulling on the iliotibial tract can extend and laterally rotate the leg at the knee joint.

Fig. 492

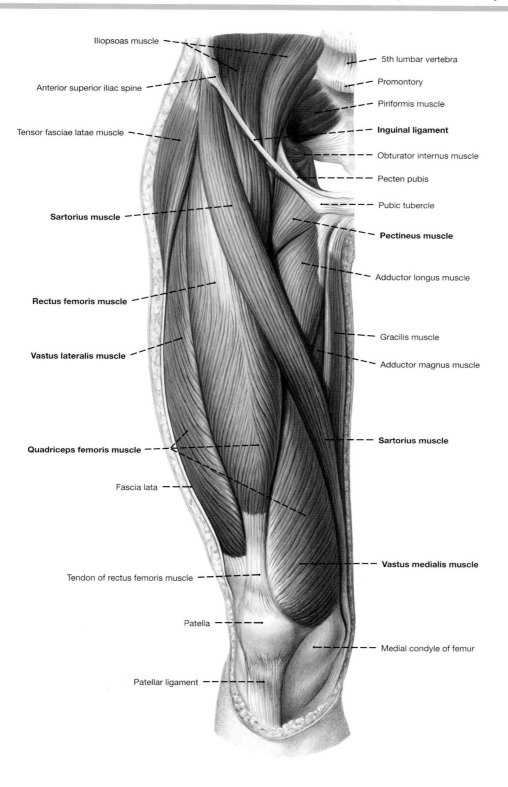

Iliopsoas muscle

Anterior superior iliac spine

Tensor fasciae latae muscle

Sartorius muscle

Rectus femoris muscle

Vastus lateralis muscle

Quadriceps femoris muscle

Fascia lata

Tendon of rectus femoris muscle

Patella

Patellar ligament

5th lumbar vertebra

Promontory

Piriformis muscle

Inguinal ligament

Obturator internus muscle

Pecten pubis

Pubic tubercle

Pectineus muscle

Adductor longus muscle

Gracilis muscle

Adductor magnus muscle

Sartorius muscle

Vastus medialis muscle

Medial condyle of femur

Fig. 493: Anterior Muscles of the Thigh: Superficial View (right)

NOTE: 1) the long narrow **sartorius muscle,** which arises on the anterior superior iliac spine and passes obliquely across the anterior femoral muscles to insert on the medial aspect of the body of the tibia. The sartorius flexes, abducts, and rotates the thigh laterally at the hip joint and it flexes and rotates the leg medially at the knee joint.

   2) the **quadriceps femoris muscle** forms the bulk of the anterior femoral muscles, and both the sartorius and quadriceps muscles are innervated by the femoral nerve.

   3) above and medial to the sartorius muscle are visible, in order, the iliopsoas, pectineus, adductor longus, adductor magnus and gracilis muscles.

Fig. 493   **V**

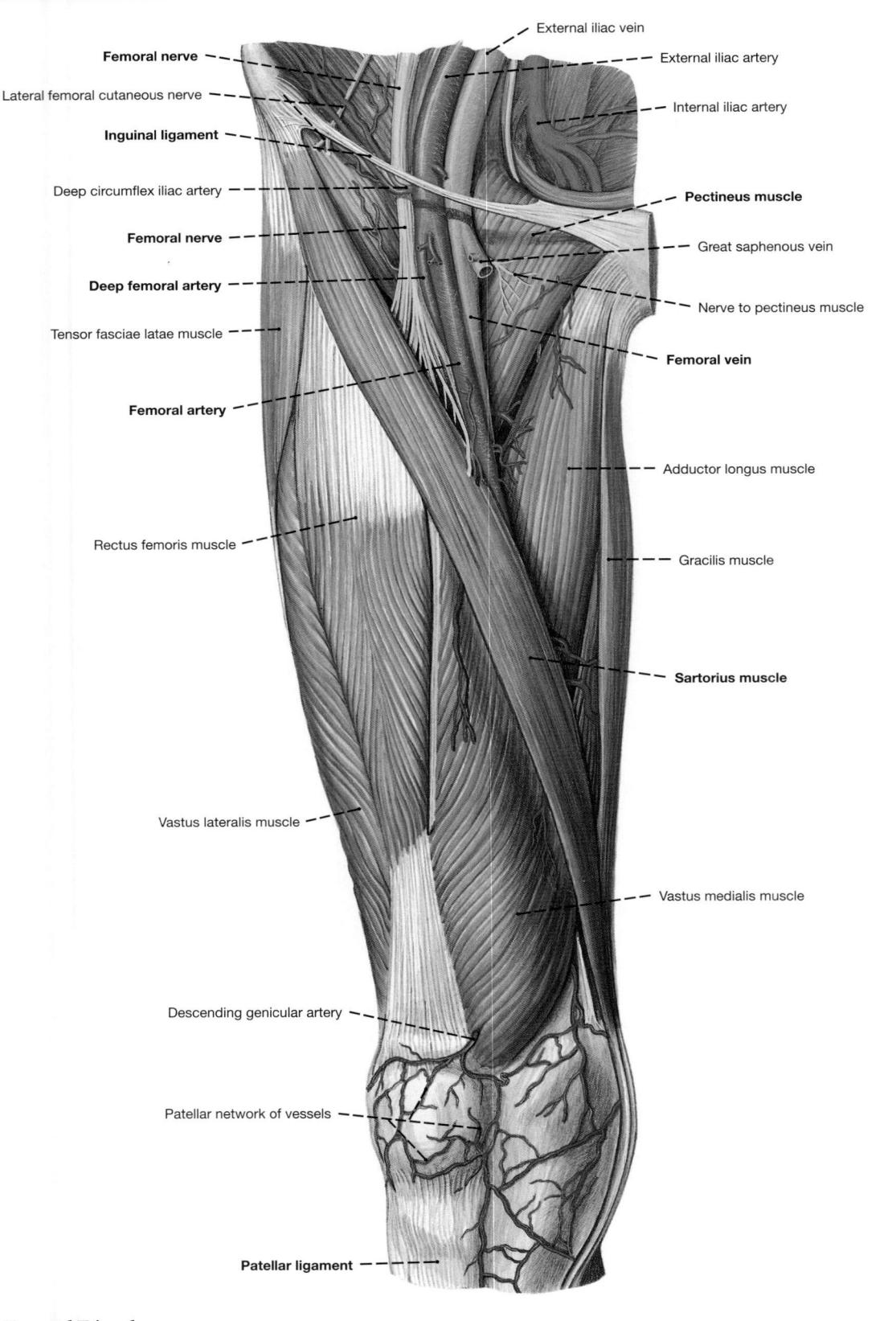

External iliac vein

Femoral nerve

External iliac artery

Lateral femoral cutaneous nerve

Internal iliac artery

Inguinal ligament

Deep circumflex iliac artery

Pectineus muscle

Femoral nerve

Great saphenous vein

Deep femoral artery

Nerve to pectineus muscle

Tensor fasciae latae muscle

Femoral vein

Femoral artery

Adductor longus muscle

Rectus femoris muscle

Gracilis muscle

Sartorius muscle

Vastus lateralis muscle

Vastus medialis muscle

Descending genicular artery

Patellar network of vessels

Patellar ligament

Fig. 494: Femoral Triangle

NOTE: 1) the boundaries of the **femoral triangle** are the inguinal ligament above, the medial border of the sartorius muscle laterally and the medial border of the adductor longus muscle medially. The floor is formed by the iliopsoas and pectineus muscles. The **femoral nerve, artery, and vein** traverse the triangle beneath the inguinal ligament.

2) of the neurovascular structures, the nerve is the most lateral within the triangle, then descend the artery and vein. The femoral artery can easily be located because it courses downward *midway* between the anterior superior iliac spine and the pubic tubercle, just below the inguinal ligament.

Fig. 494

Fig. 495: Saphenous Opening in the Fascia Lata

NOTE: 1)   the *femoral sheath* (dense connective tissue that surrounds the femoral artery and vein) has been removed in this dissection, revealing the sharply defined **falciform margin** of the **saphenous opening.**

2)   the great saphenous vein receives its superficial tributaries before it enters the saphenous opening.

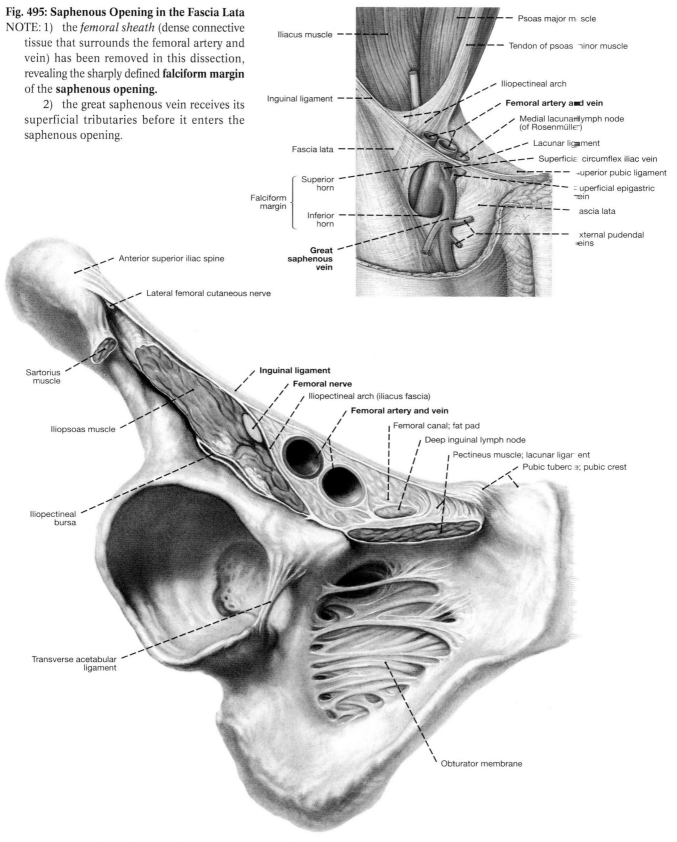

Psoas major muscle

Iliacus muscle

Tendon of psoas minor muscle

Iliopectineal arch

Inguinal ligament

Femoral artery and vein

Medial lacunar lymph node (of Rosenmüller)

Lacunar ligament

Fascia lata

Superficial circumflex iliac vein

Superior pubic ligament

Superficial epigastric vein

Superior horn

Fascia lata

Falciform margin

Inferior horn

External pudendal veins

Great saphenous vein

Anterior superior iliac spine

Lateral femoral cutaneous nerve

Sartorius muscle

Inguinal ligament

Femoral nerve

Iliopectineal arch (iliacus fascia)

Iliopsoas muscle

Femoral artery and vein

Femoral canal; fat pad

Deep inguinal lymph node

Pectineus muscle; lacunar ligament

Pubic tubercle; pubic crest

Iliopectineal bursa

Transverse acetabular ligament

Obturator membrane

Fig. 496: Section Through the Inguinal Ligament, Vascular Compartments, and Femoral Canal

NOTE: 1)   medial to the femoral vein is the **femoral canal,** a space containing lymph channels, an occasional lymph node and fat. The abdominal end of this canal is the **femoral ring,** through which a **femoral hernia** of a loop of intestine may occur. This is more frequent in women (especially during pregnancy) than men because the femoral ring is slightly larger.

2)   the **femoral nerve** enters the thigh on the surface of the **iliopsoas muscle** and deep to the iliopectineal arch (or iliac fascia).

PLATE 320 Lower Extremity: Anterior Thigh Muscles (Dissection 4)

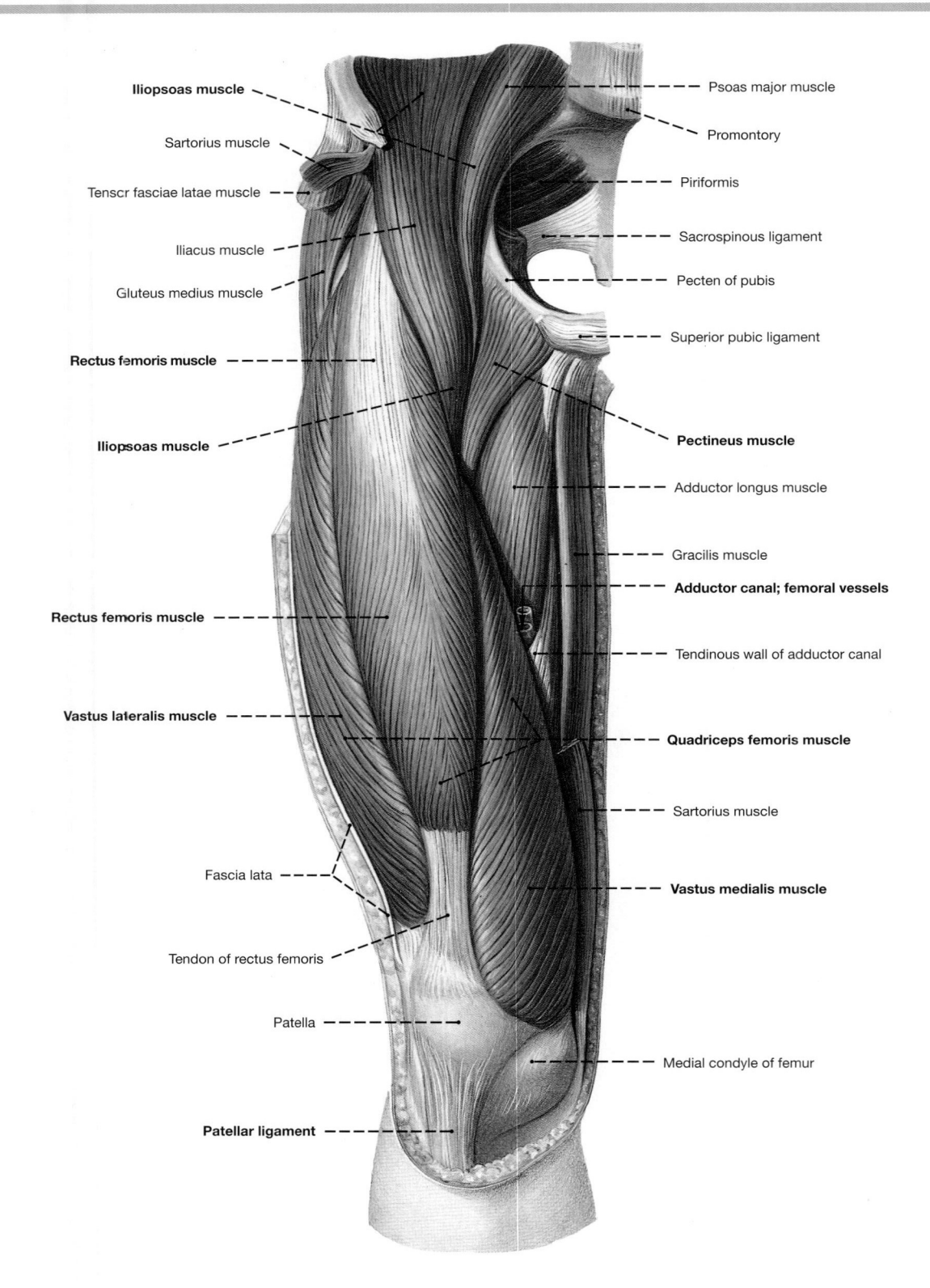

Iliopsoas muscle

Sartorius muscle

Tenscr fasciae latae muscle

Iliacus muscle

Gluteus medius muscle

Rectus femoris muscle

Iliopsoas muscle

Rectus femoris muscle

Vastus lateralis muscle

Fascia lata

Tendon of rectus femoris

Patella

Patellar ligament

Psoas major muscle

Promontory

Piriformis

Sacrospinous ligament

Pecten of pubis

Superior pubic ligament

Pectineus muscle

Adductor longus muscle

Gracilis muscle

Adductor canal; femoral vessels

Tendinous wall of adductor canal

Quadriceps femoris muscle

Sartorius muscle

Vastus medialis muscle

Medial condyle of femur

Fig. 497: Quadriceps Femoris, Iliopsoas, and Pectineus Muscles

NOTE: 1) the **quadriceps femoris muscle** consisting of the rectus femoris and the three vastus muscles (lateralis, intermedius and medialis) as it converges inferiorly to form a powerful tendon which encases the patella and inserts onto the **tuberosity of the tibia.** The entire quadriceps extends the leg at the knee, while the rectus femoris also flexes the thigh at the hip.

2) the **iliopsoas muscle** is the most powerful flexor of the thigh at the hip joint and it inserts on the **lesser trochanter.**

3) the quadrangular and flat **pectineus muscle** medial to the iliopsoas. Sometimes called the key to the femoral triangle, this muscle is normally supplied by the femoral nerve, but in slightly over 10% of cases it also receives a branch from one of the obturator nerves.

Fig. 497.

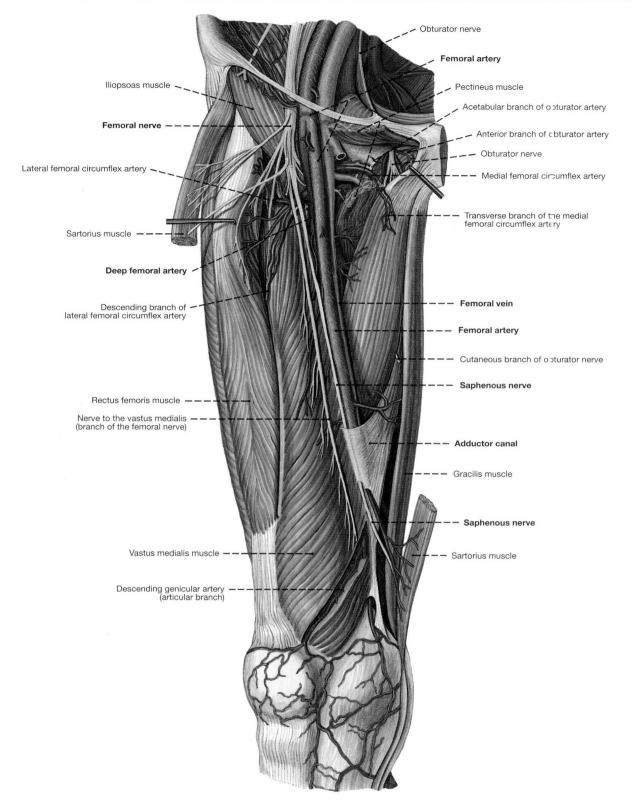

Obturator nerve

Femoral artery

Pectineus muscle

Acetabular branch of obturator artery

Anterior branch of obturator artery

Obturator nerve

Medial femoral circumflex artery

Transverse branch of the medial femoral circumflex artery

Femoral vein

Femoral artery

Cutaneous branch of obturator nerve

Saphenous nerve

Adductor canal

Gracilis muscle

Saphenous nerve

Sartorius muscle

Iliopsoas muscle

Femoral nerve

Lateral femoral circumflex artery

Sartorius muscle

Deep femoral artery

Descending branch of lateral femoral circumflex artery

Rectus femoris muscle

Nerve to the vastus medialis (branch of the femoral nerve)

Vastus medialis muscle

Descending genicular artery (articular branch)

Fig. 498: Femoral Vessels and Nerves

NOTE: 1)   the femoral vessels, the saphenous branch of the femoral nerve, and the nerve to the vastus medialis all enter the **adductor canal (of Hunter).**

2)   the **saphenous nerve,** after coursing some distance in the canal, penetrates the overlying fascia to reach the superficial leg region; the **nerve to the vastus medialis** traverses the more proximal part of the canal and then divides into muscular branches to supply the vastus medialis muscle.

3)   the **femoral artery and vein** course through the entire canal and then leave it by way of an opening in the adductor magnus muscle called the **adductor hiatus.** The vessels course to the back of the lower limb to become the **popliteal artery and vein.**

Fig. 498

V

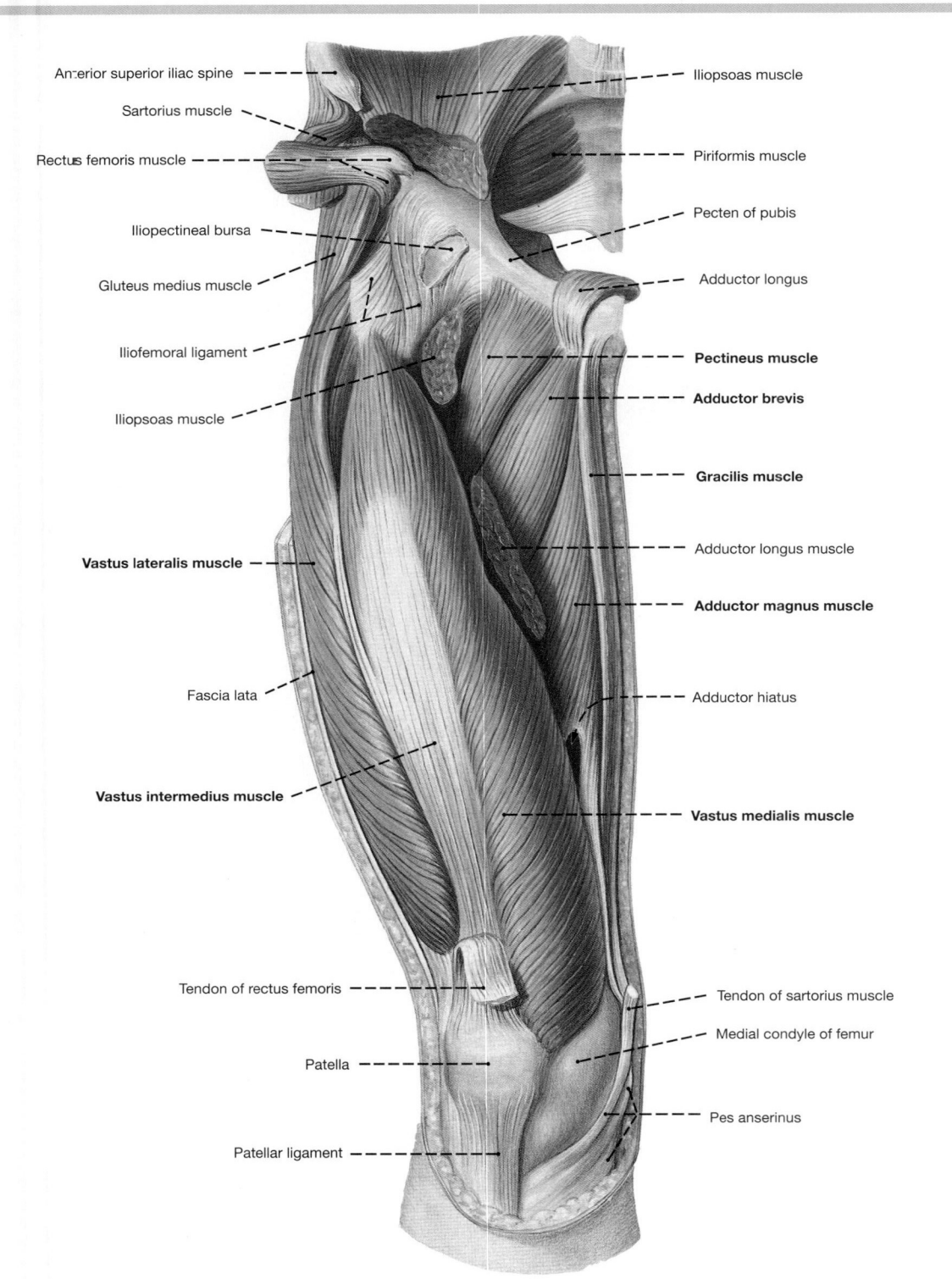

Anterior superior iliac spine

Sartorius muscle

Rectus femoris muscle

Iliopectineal bursa

Gluteus medius muscle

Iliofemoral ligament

Iliopsoas muscle

Vastus lateralis muscle

Fascia lata

Vastus intermedius muscle

Tendon of rectus femoris

Patella

Patellar ligament

Iliopsoas muscle

Piriformis muscle

Pecten of pubis

Adductor longus

Pectineus muscle

Adductor brevis

Gracilis muscle

Adductor longus muscle

Adductor magnus muscle

Adductor hiatus

Vastus medialis muscle

Tendon of sartorius muscle

Medial condyle of femur

Pes anserinus

Fig. 499: Intermediate Layer of Anterior and Medial Thigh Muscles

NOTE: 1)   the **rectus femoris** and **iliopsoas muscles** are cut to expose the underlying **vastus intermedius** situated between the **vastus lateralis** and **vastus medialis.**

2)   the **adductor longus** has also been reflected. This displays the **pectineus, adductor brevis and magnus muscles** and the long **gracilis muscle.**

3)   the quadriceps femoris is the most powerful extensor of the leg. During extension, however there is a natural tendency to displace the patella laterally out of its groove on the patellar surface of the femur because of the natural angulation of the femur with respect to the bones of the leg.

4)   the muscle fibers of the **vastus medialis** descend further inferiorly than those of the vastus lateralis and the lowest fibers insert directly along the medial border of the patella. The medial pull of these fibers are thought to be essential in maintaining the stability of the patella on the femur.

Fig. 499

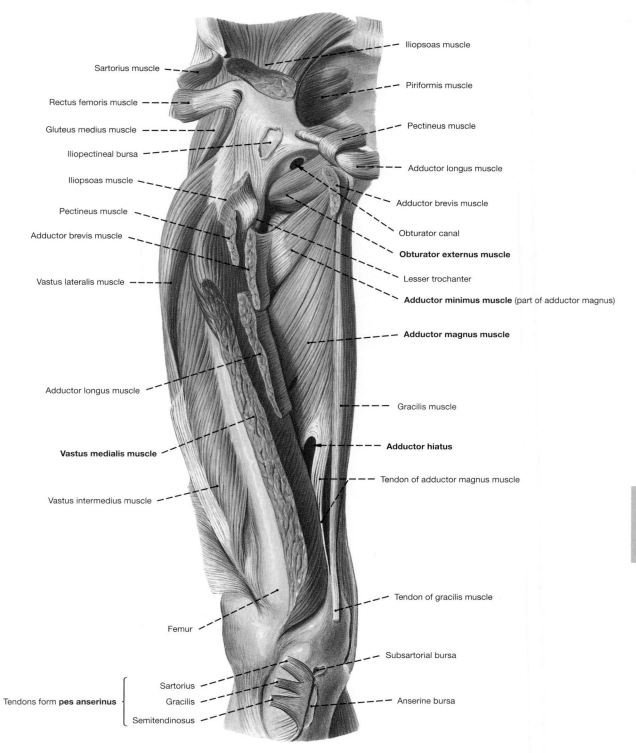

Iliopsoas muscle

Sartorius muscle

Piriformis muscle

Rectus femoris muscle

Pectineus muscle

Gluteus medius muscle

Iliopectineal bursa

Adductor longus muscle

Iliopsoas muscle

Adductor brevis muscle

Pectineus muscle

Obturator canal

Adductor brevis muscle

Obturator externus muscle

Lesser trochanter

Vastus lateralis muscle

Adductor minimus muscle (part of adductor magnus)

Adductor magnus muscle

Adductor longus muscle

Gracilis muscle

Vastus medialis muscle

Adductor hiatus

Tendon of adductor magnus muscle

Vastus intermedius muscle

Tendon of gracilis muscle

Femur

Subsartorial bursa

Tendons form **pes anserinus** { Sartorius
Gracilis
Semitendinosus

Anserine bursa

Fig. 500: Deep Layer of Anterior and Medial Thigh Muscles (Right)

NOTE: 1)   the rectus femoris and vastus medialis have been removed, thereby exposing the shaft of the femur. Likewise, the adductor longus and brevis and the pectineus muscles have been reflected, exposing the **obturator externus,** the **adductor magnus** and the adductor minimus (which usually is just the upper portion of the adductor magnus).

2)   the common insertion of the tendons of the **sartorius, gracilis,** and **semitendinosus muscles** on the medial aspect of the medial condyle of the tibia. The divergent nature of this insertion resembles a goose's foot (pes anserinus). This tendinous formation can be used by surgeons to strengthen the medial aspect of the capsule of the knee joint.

3)   the tendinous opening on the adductor magnus, called the **adductor hiatus,** through which the femoral vessels course to (or from) the popliteal fossa.

4)   the **obturator externus muscle** stretching across the inferior surface of the obturator membrane to insert laterally on the neck of the femur. This muscle laterally rotates the femur, and it is not part of the adductor group of muscles.

Fig. 500   **V**

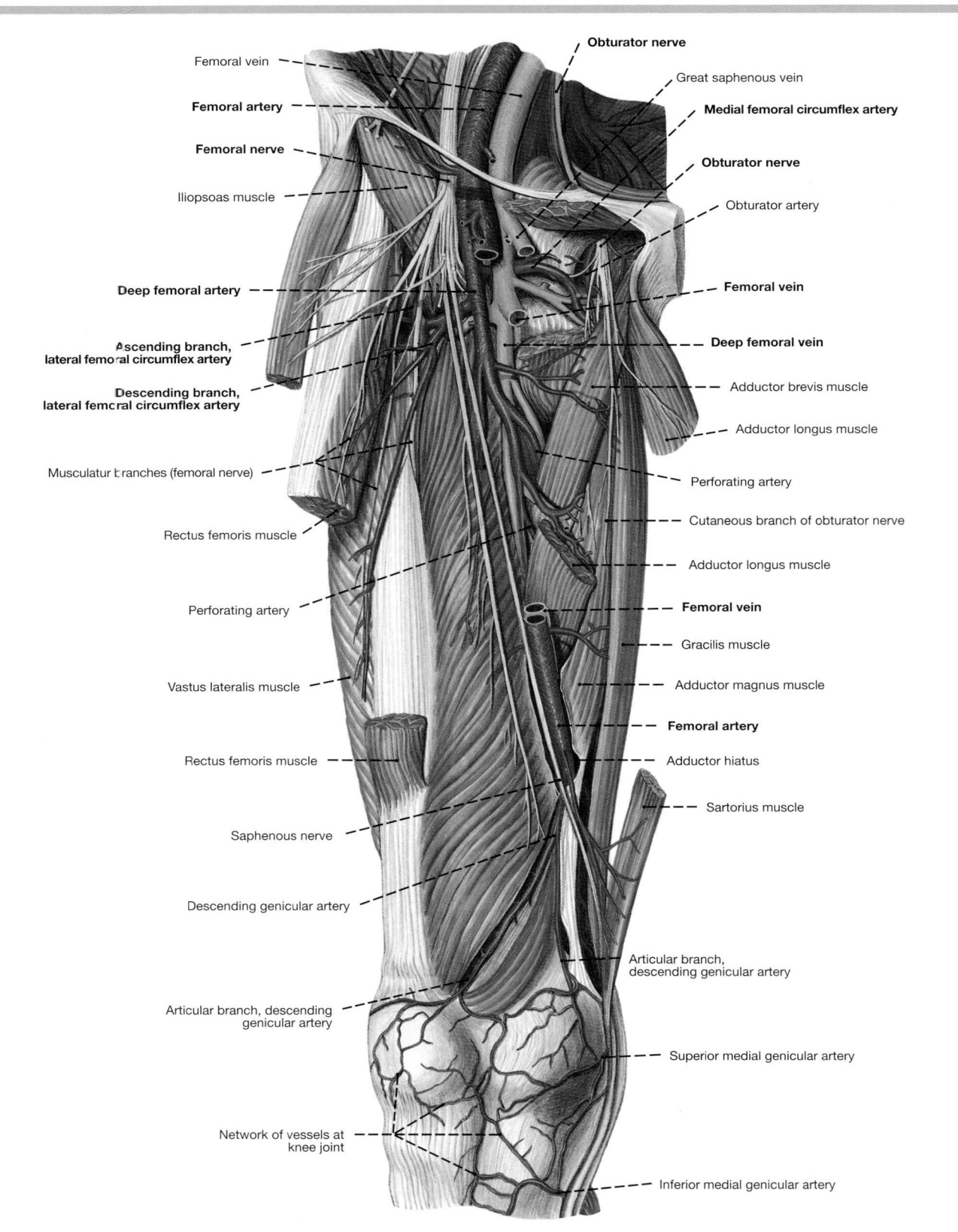

Femoral vein

Obturator nerve

Great saphenous vein

Femoral artery

Medial femoral circumflex artery

Femoral nerve

Obturator nerve

Iliopsoas muscle

Obturator artery

Deep femoral artery

Femoral vein

Ascending branch,
lateral femoral circumflex artery

Deep femoral vein

Descending branch,
lateral femoral circumflex artery

Adductor brevis muscle

Adductor longus muscle

Musculatur branches (femoral nerve)

Perforating artery

Cutaneous branch of obturator nerve

Rectus femoris muscle

Adductor longus muscle

Perforating artery

Femoral vein

Gracilis muscle

Vastus lateralis muscle

Adductor magnus muscle

Rectus femoris muscle

Femoral artery

Adductor hiatus

Saphenous nerve

Sartorius muscle

Descending genicular artery

Articular branch,
descending genicular artery

Articular branch, descending
genicular artery

Superior medial genicular artery

Network of vessels at
knee joint

Inferior medial genicular artery

Fig. 501: Femoral and Obturator Nerves and Deep Femoral Artery

NOTE: 1) the **obturator nerve** supplies the adductor muscles, the gracilis, and the obturator externus (not shown, see Fig. 500), while the femoral nerve innervates all the other anterior thigh muscles.

2) the **deep femoral artery** is the largest branch of the femoral artery and it gives off both the **medial** and **lateral femoral circumflex arteries.** Observe the femoral vessels disappearing in the femoral canal.

3) in about 50% of cases, the deep femoral artery branches from the lateral side of femoral artery; in 40%, it branches from the posterior aspect of the femoral and courses behind it; in 10%, the deep femoral arises from the medial side of the femoral.

Fig. 501

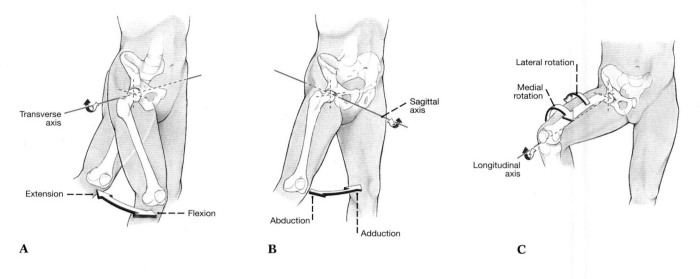

A   **B**   **C**

Fig. 502: Movements of the Thigh at the Hip Joint
In A: **Flexion** and **extension** occur through the transverse axis of the hip joint.
In B: **Abduction** and **adduction** occur through the sagittal axis of the hip joint.
In C: **Medial rotation** and **lateral rotation** occur around the longitudinal axis of the hip joint.

Anterior Thigh Muscles

Muscle	Origin	Insertion	Innervation	Action
Sartorius Muscle	Anterior superior iliac spine	Superior part of the medial surface of the tibia	Femoral nerve (L2, L3)	Flexes, abducts and laterally rotates the thigh at the hip joint; flexes and medially rotates the leg at the knee joint
Quadriceps Femoris Muscle **Rectus Femoris**	STRAIGHT HEAD Anterior inferior iliac spine REFLECTED HEAD the groove above the acetabulum	All four parts of the quadriceps femoris form a common tendon that encases the patella and finally inserts onto the tibial tuberosity	Femoral nerve (L2, L3, L4)	All four parts extend the leg at the knee joint; the rectus femoris also helps to flex the thigh at the hip joint
Vastus Medialis	Intertrochanteric line and the medial lip of the linea aspera on the femur			
Vastus Lateralis	Greater trochanter and the lateral lip of the linea aspera			
Vastus Intermedius	Anterior and lateral surface of the body of the femur			
Articularis Genu	Anterior surface of the lower part of the femur	Upper part of the synovial membrane of the knee joint	Femoral nerve (L2, L3, L4)	Draws the synovial membrane upward during extension of the leg to prevent its compression
The PSOAS MAJOR, PSOAS MINOR and ILIACUS MUSCLES are outlined on PLATE 237				

Fig. 502   **V**

PLATE 326 **Lower Extremity: Chart of Thigh Muscles**

Medial Thigh Muscles

Muscle	Origin	Insertion	Innervation	Action
Pectineus Muscle	Pectineal line of the pubis	Along the pectineal line of the femur, between the lesser trochanter and the linea aspera	Femoral nerve (L2, L3); may also receive a branch from the obturator or the accessory obturator nerve when present	Flexes, adducts and medially rotates the femur
Adductor Longus Muscle	From the anterior pubis, where the pubic crest joins the symphysis pubis	Middle one-third of the femur along the linea aspera	Obturator nerve (L2, L3, L4)	Adducts, flexes, and medially rotates the femur
Adductor Brevis Muscle	Outer surface of the inferior pubic ramus between the gracilis and the obturator externus	Along the pectineal line of the femur and the upper part of the linea aspera behind the pectineus	Obturator nerve (L2, L3, L4)	Adducts, flexes, and medially rotates the femur
Adductor Magnus Muscle	Inferior ramus of pubis; ramus of the ischium and the ischial tuberosity	Medial lip of the upper ²⁄₃rds of the linea aspera; the medial supracondylar line and the adductor tubercle	Obturator nerve (L2, L3, L4): sciatic nerve (tibial division) for the hamstring part of the muscle	Powerful adductor of the thigh; upper part flexes and medially rotates the thigh; lower part extends and laterally rotates the thigh
Adductor Minimus Muscle	The upper more horizontal part of the adductor magnus which receives the name adductor minimus when it forms a distinct muscle.			
Gracilis Muscle	From the body of the pubis and the adjacent inferior pubic ramus	Upper part of the medial surface of the tibia below the medial condyle	Obturator nerve (L2, L3)	Adducts the thigh; also flexes the leg at the knee and medially rotates the leg
Obturator Externus Muscle	Medial part of the outer surface of obturator membrane and medial margin of obturator foramen	Trochanteric fossa of the femur	Obturator nerve (L3, L4)	Laterally rotates the thigh

Lateral Thigh Muscle

Tensor Fasciae Latae Muscle	Outer lip of the iliac crest; also from the anterior superior iliac spine	Iliotibial tract which then descends to attach to the lateral condyle of the tibia	Superior gluteal nerve (L4, L5)	Abducts, flexes and medially rotates the thigh; tenses the iliotibial tract, thereby helping to extend the leg at the knee

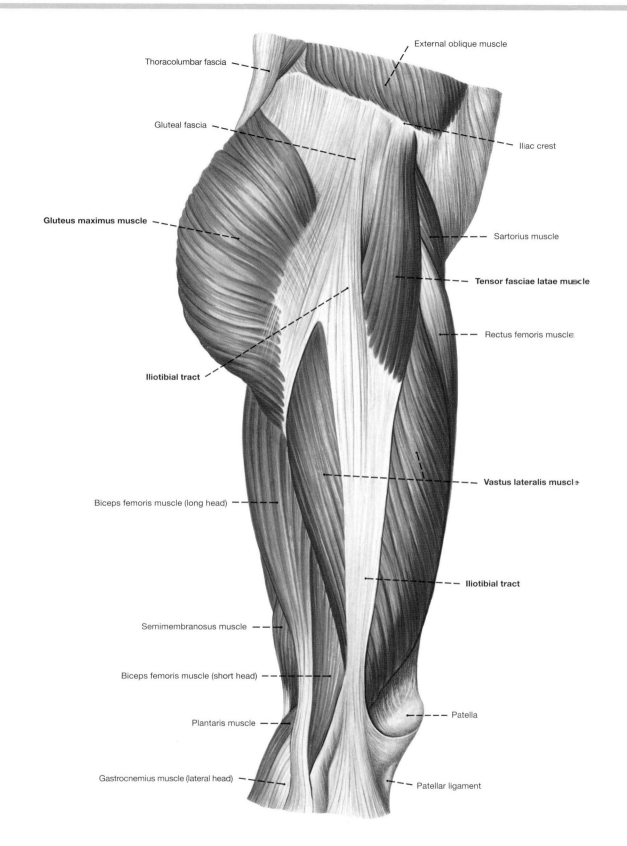

External oblique muscle

Thoracolumbar fascia

Gluteal fascia

Iliac crest

Gluteus maximus muscle

Sartorius muscle

Tensor fasciae latae muscle

Rectus femoris muscle

Iliotibial tract

Vastus lateralis muscle

Biceps femoris muscle (long head)

Iliotibial tract

Semimembranosus muscle

Biceps femoris muscle (short head)

Plantaris muscle

Patella

Gastrocnemius muscle (lateral head)

Patellar ligament

Fig. 503: Superficial Thigh and Gluteal Muscles (Lateral View)

NOTE: 1) the massive size of the **vastus lateralis, biceps femoris** and **gluteus maximus muscles** seen from this lateral side.

2) the **iliotibial tract** (or band) stretches, superficially, the length of the thigh. Its muscle, the **tensor fasciae latae,** helps to keep the dense fascia lata taut.

3) the fascia lata is a very tight layer of deep fascia that surrounds the thigh muscles (see Fig. 492). Because of this the tensor fasciae latae assists in extension of the leg at the knee joint and in helping to maintain an erect posture.

Fig. 503   **V**

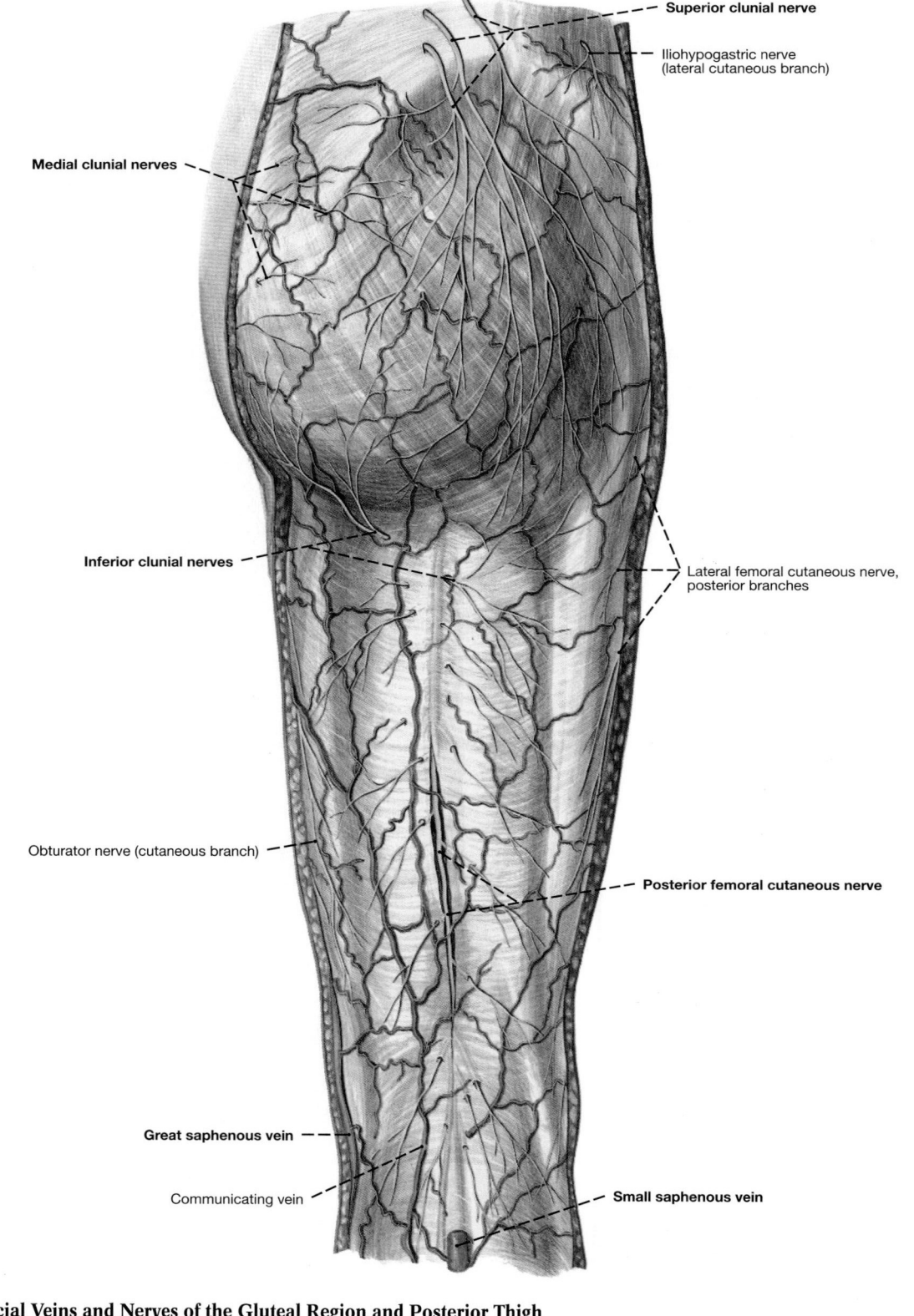

Superior clunial nerve

Iliohypogastric nerve
(lateral cutaneous branch)

Medial clunial nerves

Inferior clunial nerves

Lateral femoral cutaneous nerve,
posterior branches

Obturator nerve (cutaneous branch)

Posterior femoral cutaneous nerve

Great saphenous vein

Communicating vein

Small saphenous vein

Fig. 504: Superficial Veins and Nerves of the Gluteal Region and Posterior Thigh

NOTE: 1) the principal cutaneous nerves supplying the **gluteal region** are the:

    a) **superior clunial nerves** (from the posterior primary rami of **L1, L2, L3**),

    b) **medial clunial nerves** (from the posterior primary rami of **S1, S2, S3**), and

    c) **inferior clunial nerves** (from the posterior femoral cutaneous nerve: anterior primary rami of **S1, S2, S3**).

    2) the skin of the **posterior thigh** is supplied primarily by the **posterior femoral cutaneous nerve (S1, S2, S3),** but posterolaterally it also receives branches from the lateral femoral cutaneous nerve, and posteromedially, cutaneous branches from the obturator nerve.

Fig. 504

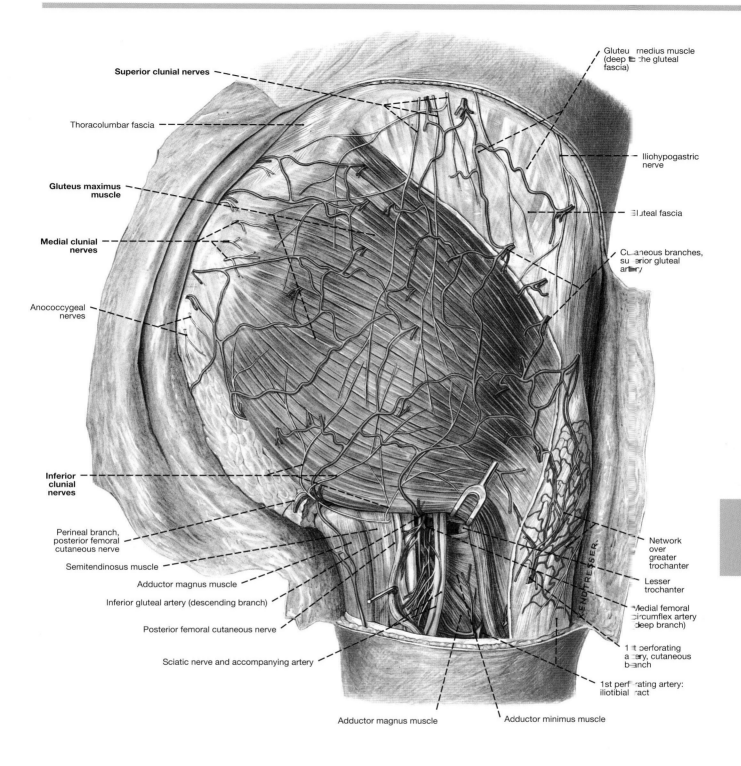

Superior clunial nerves

Thoracolumbar fascia

Gluteus maximus muscle

Medial clunial nerves

Anococcygeal nerves

Inferior clunial nerves

Perineal branch, posterior femoral cutaneous nerve

Semitendinosus muscle

Adductor magnus muscle

Inferior gluteal artery (descending branch)

Posterior femoral cutaneous nerve

Sciatic nerve and accompanying artery

Adductor magnus muscle

Adductor minimus muscle

Gluteus medius muscle (deep to the gluteal fascia)

Iliohypogastric nerve

Gluteal fascia

Cutaneous branches, superior gluteal artery

Network over greater trochanter

Lesser trochanter

Medial femoral circumflex artery (deep branch)

1st perforating artery, cutaneous branch

1st perforating artery: iliotibial tract

Fig. 505: Gluteus Maximus Muscle and Superficial Gluteal Vessels and Nerves

NOTE: 1)   the skin, superficial fascia and deep fascia overlying the **gluteus maximus muscle** have been removed exposing the entire mass of this quadrilateral muscle. Observe that its fibers course obliquely inferolaterally from their broad origin on the **ilium** (posterior gluteal line), the **sacrum** (posterior aspect), the **coccyx** (lateral border) and the **sacrotuberous ligament.**

2)   the gluteus maximus overlies the ischial tuberosity which can be felt deep to the lower part of the muscle. It inserts principally into the **iliotibial tract** of the fascia lata and onto the **gluteal tuberosity** of the femur, between the vastus lateralis and the adductor magnus.

3)   the gluteus maximus is the most powerful extensor and lateral rotator of the thigh at the hip joint and it is very active during running but is hardly used during ordinary walking. When its femoral attachment is fixed, it strongly extends the pelvis. This latter action occurs when we arise from a sitting position.

Fig. 505

V

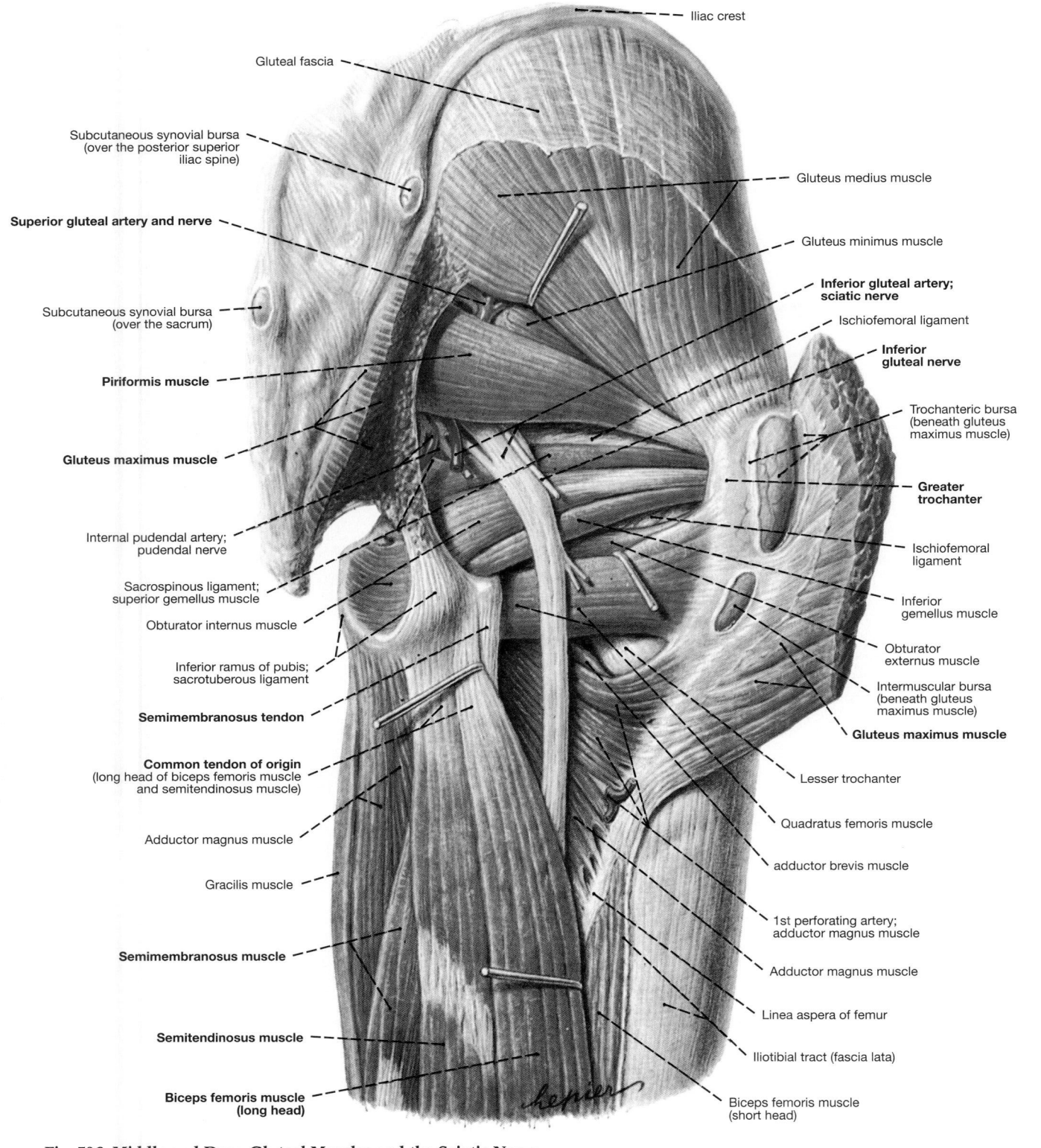

- Iliac crest
- Gluteal fascia
- Subcutaneous synovial bursa (over the posterior superior iliac spine)
- Gluteus medius muscle
- **Superior gluteal artery and nerve**
- Gluteus minimus muscle
- **Inferior gluteal artery; sciatic nerve**
- Ischiofemoral ligament
- Subcutaneous synovial bursa (over the sacrum)
- **Inferior gluteal nerve**
- **Piriformis muscle**
- Trochanteric bursa (beneath gluteus maximus muscle)
- **Gluteus maximus muscle**
- **Greater trochanter**
- Internal pudendal artery; pudendal nerve
- Ischiofemoral ligament
- Sacrospinous ligament; superior gemellus muscle
- Inferior gemellus muscle
- Obturator internus muscle
- Obturator externus muscle
- Inferior ramus of pubis; sacrotuberous ligament
- Intermuscular bursa (beneath gluteus maximus muscle)
- **Semimembranosus tendon**
- **Gluteus maximus muscle**
- **Common tendon of origin** (long head of biceps femoris muscle and semitendinosus muscle)
- Lesser trochanter
- Quadratus femoris muscle
- Adductor magnus muscle
- adductor brevis muscle
- Gracilis muscle
- 1st perforating artery; adductor magnus muscle
- **Semimembranosus muscle**
- Adductor magnus muscle
- Linea aspera of femur
- **Semitendinosus muscle**
- Iliotibial tract (fascia lata)
- **Biceps femoris muscle (long head)**
- Biceps femoris muscle (short head)

Fig. 506: Middle and Deep Gluteal Muscles and the Sciatic Nerve

NOTE: 1) the gluteus maximus has been reflected to show the centrally located **piriformis muscle,** which is the key structure in understanding the anatomy of this region.

2) the piriformis muscle, as do most other structures that leave the pelvis to enter the gluteal region, passes through the **greater sciatic foramen.** The nerves and vessels enter the gluteal region from the pelvis either above or below the piriformis muscle. The important **sciatic nerve** enters the gluteal region **below** the piriformis.

3) in addition to the piriformis, observe the **gluteus medius, the obturator internus** with two **gemelli** above and below it, and the **quadratus femoris** muscles. The gluteus medius and minimus muscles are abductors and medial rotators of the thigh and *all* the other muscles are lateral rotators.

Fig. 506

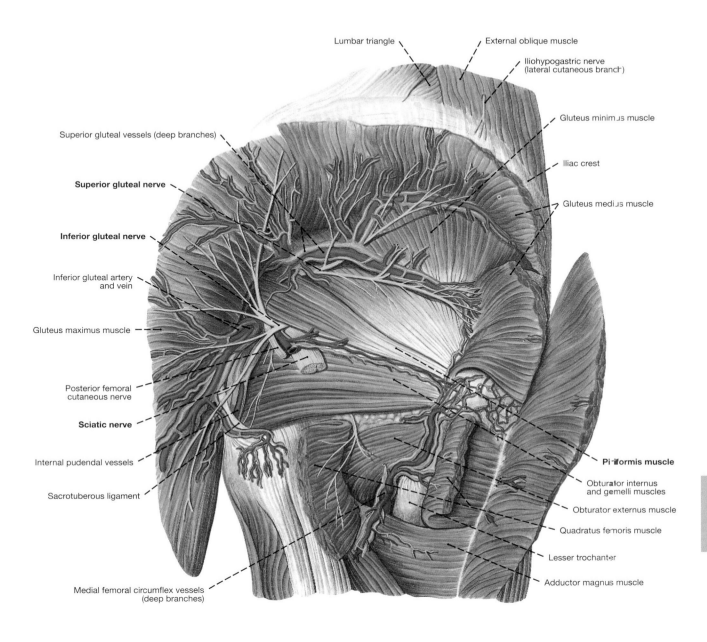

Lumbar triangle

External oblique muscle

Iliohypogastric nerve
(lateral cutaneous branch)

Gluteus minimus muscle

Iliac crest

Gluteus medius muscle

Superior gluteal vessels (deep branches)

Superior gluteal nerve

Inferior gluteal nerve

Inferior gluteal artery
and vein

Gluteus maximus muscle

Posterior femoral
cutaneous nerve

Sciatic nerve

Internal pudendal vessels

Sacrotuberous ligament

Medial femoral circumflex vessels
(deep branches)

Piriformis muscle

Obturator internus
and gemelli muscles

Obturator externus muscle

Quadratus femoris muscle

Lesser trochanter

Adductor magnus muscle

Fig. 507: Deep Vessels and Nerves of the Gluteal Region

NOTE: 1)   the gluteus maximus and gluteus medius muscles and the sciatic nerve have been cut to expose the short lateral rotators and the **gluteus minimus muscle.**

2)   **above the piriformis** the *superior gluteal artery, vein,* and *nerve* enter the gluteal region through the greater sciatic foramen; **below the piriformis** the following structures enter the gluteal region by way of the greater sciatic foramen: the *inferior gluteal vessels* and *nerve,* the *sciatic nerve,* the *nerve to the obturator internus muscle,* the *posterior femoral cutaneous nerve,* the *nerve to the quadratus femoris muscle* and the *internal pudendal vessels* and *pudendal nerve.*

3)   the internal pudendal artery and vein and the pudendal nerve, after entering the gluteal region through the greater sciatic foramen, cross the sacrospinous ligament and reenter the pelvis through the **lesser sciatic foramen** and course in the pudendal canal to get to the perineum. The other structure that passes through the lesser sciatic foramen is the *tendon of the obturator internus muscle.*

4)   to separate the gluteus medius muscle from the gluteus minimus muscle as shown in this figure, dissect along the course of the superior gluteal vessels and nerve, since these structures lie in the plane between the medius and minimus.

Fig. 507

V

PLATE 332   Muscles of the Gluteal Region and the Posterior Thigh (Chart)

Muscles of the Gluteal Region

Muscle	Origin	Insertion	Innervation	Action
Gluteus Maximus Muscle	Outer surface of the ilium and iliac crest; dorsal surface of the sacrum; lateral side of coccyx and the sacrotuberous ligament	Into the iliotibial band which then descends to attach to the lateral condyle of tibia, also onto the gluteal tuberosity of the femur	Inferior gluteal nerve (L5, S1, S2)	Powerful extensor of the thigh; lateral rotator of the thigh, helps steady the extended leg; extends the trunk when distal end is fixed
Gluteus Medius Muscle	External surface of the ilium between the anterior and posterior gluteal lines	Lateral surface of greater trochanter of the femur	Superior gluteal nerve (L4, L5, S1)	Abducts and medially rotates the thigh; helps steady the pelvis
Gluteus Minimus Muscle	Outer surface of ilium between the anterior and inferior gluteal lines	Anterior border of greater trochanter and on the fibrous capsule of the hip joint	Superior gluteal nerve (L4, L5, S1)	Abducts and medially rotates the thigh; helps steady the pelvis
Piriformis Muscle	Anterior (pelvic) surface of the sacrum and the inner surface of sacrotuberous ligament	Upper border of the greater trochanter of the femur	Muscular branches from the S1 and S2 nerves	Laterally rotates the extended thigh; when the thigh is flexed, it abducts the femur
Obturator Internus Muscle	Pelvic surface of obturator membrane and from the bone surrounding the obturator foramen	Medial surface of greater trochanter proximal to the trochanteric fossa	Nerve to the obturator internus (L5, S1)	Laterally rotates the extended thigh and abducts the flexed thigh
Superior Gemellus Muscle	Outer surface of the ischial spine	Medial surface of greater trochanter with tendon of the obturator internus	Nerve to the obturator internus (L5, S1)	Laterally rotates the extended thigh and abducts the flexed thigh
Inferior Gemellus Muscle	From the ischial tuberosity	Medial surface of greater trochanter with tendon of the obturator internus	Nerve to the quadratus femoris (L5, S1)	Laterally rotates the extended thigh and abducts the flexed thigh
Quadratus Femoris Muscle	Lateral border of the ischial tuberosity	Quadrate tubercle on the posterior surface of the femur; also onto the intertrochanteric crest of the femur	Nerve to the quadratus femoris (L5, S1)	Laterally rotates the thigh

Posterior Thigh Muscles

Muscle	Origin	Insertion	Innervation	Action
Biceps Femoris Muscle	LONG HEAD Ischial tuberosity in common with other hamstring muscles SHORT HEAD Lateral lip of the linea aspera of the femur	LONG HEAD Lateral surface of the head of the fibula and a small slip to lateral condyle of tibia SHORT HEAD	LONG HEAD Tibial part of sciatic nerve (S1, S2, S3) SHORT HEAD Peroneal part of the sciatic nerve (L5, S1, S2)	Flexes the leg and rotates the tibia laterally; long head also extends the thigh at the hip joint
Semitendinosus Muscle	Ischial tuberosity in common with other hamstring muscles	Medial surface of the upper part of the body of the tibia	Tibial part of the sciatic nerve (L5, S1, S2)	Flexes the leg and rotates the tibia medially; extends the thigh
Semimembranosus Muscle	Ischial tuberosity in common with other hamstring muscles	Posterior aspect of the medial condyle of the tibia	Tibial part of the sciatic nerve (L5, S1, S2)	Flexes the leg and rotates it medially; extends the thigh

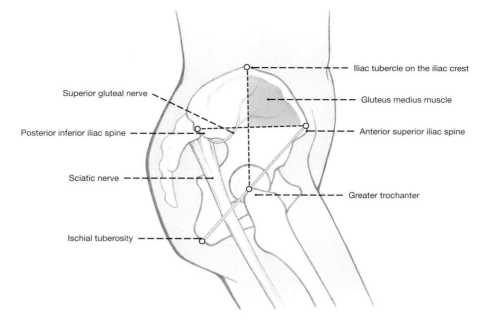

Fig. 508: Safe Quadrant for Injections Into the Gluteal Region

NOTE: in this figure the four quadrants of the gluteal region are determined by a **transverse line** between the *anterior superior iliac spine* anteriorly and the *posterior inferior iliac spine* posteriorly that intersects a **vertical line** between the *greater trochanter* inferiorly and the *iliac crest* superiorly. The colored upper lateral quadrant is the safe zone for intramuscular injection.

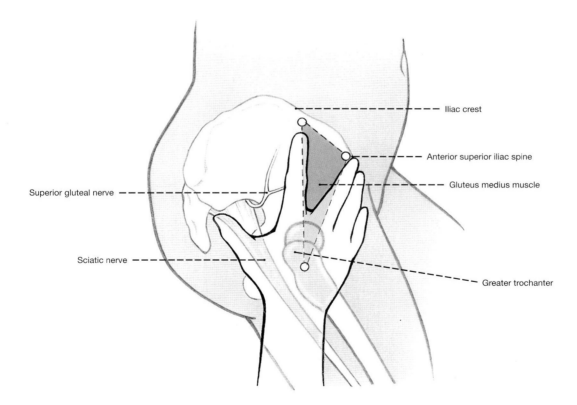

Fig. 509: Quick Method of Determining Safe Zone for Intramuscular Gluteal Injection

NOTE: the safe zone can be visualized quickly by

   1) placing the palm of the right hand over the right greater trochanter (or left hand over the left greater trochanter,

   2) directing the index finger vertically to the iliac crest and spreading the middle finger to the anterior superior iliac spine,

   3) the colored region shown in this diagram between the index and middle fingers is the safe zone and avoids the superior gluteal vessels and nerve as well as the sciatic nerve and other important gluteal structures.

PLATE 334   Lower Extremity: Posterior Thigh Muscles (Dissection 1)

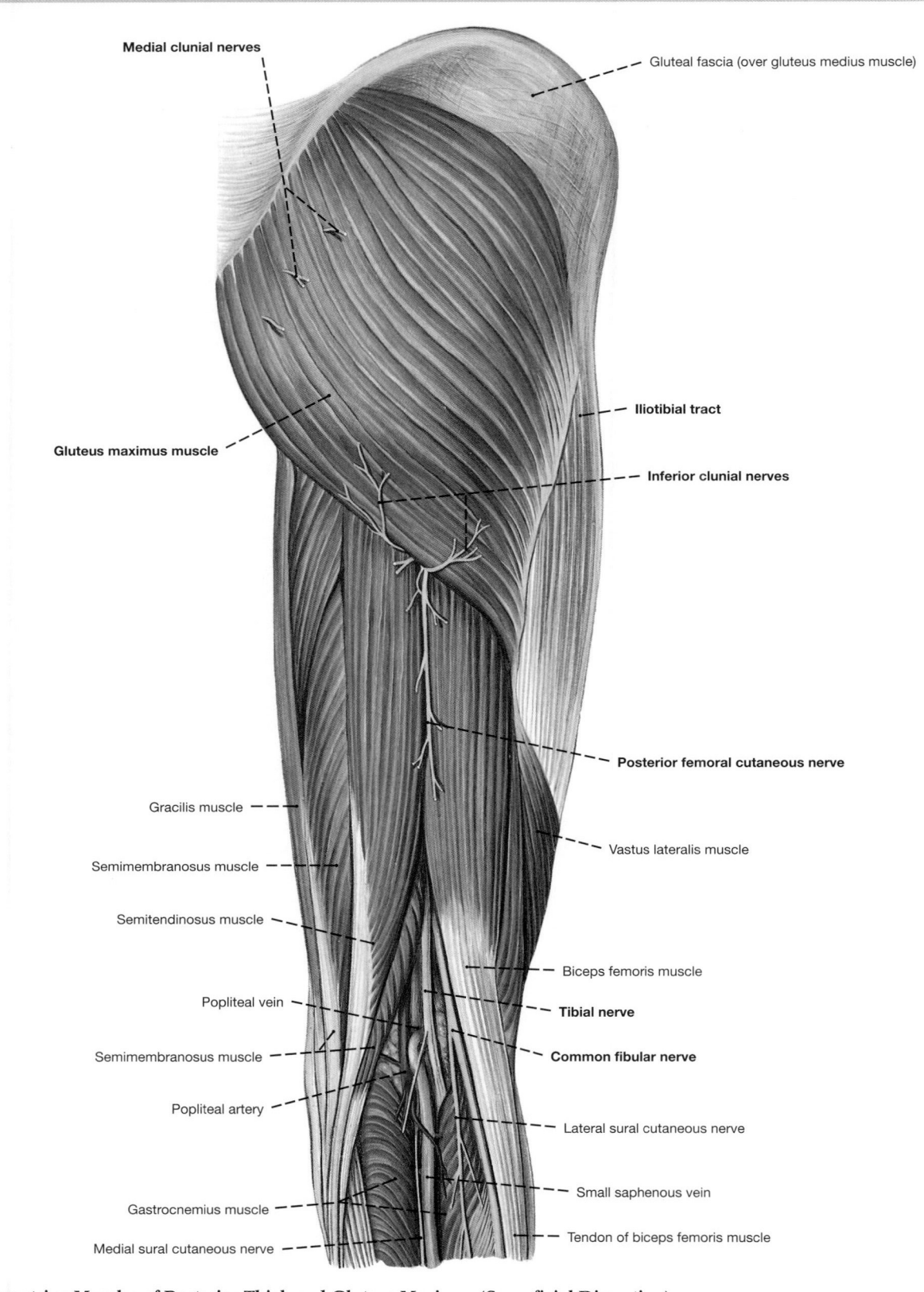

Medial clunial nerves

Gluteal fascia (over gluteus medius muscle)

Iliotibial tract

Gluteus maximus muscle

Inferior clunial nerves

Posterior femoral cutaneous nerve

Gracilis muscle

Semimembranosus muscle

Vastus lateralis muscle

Semitendinosus muscle

Biceps femoris muscle

Popliteal vein

Tibial nerve

Semimembranosus muscle

Common fibular nerve

Popliteal artery

Lateral sural cutaneous nerve

Small saphenous vein

Gastrocnemius muscle

Tendon of biceps femoris muscle

Medial sural cutaneous nerve

Fig. 510: Hamstring Muscles of Posterior Thigh and Gluteus Maximus (Superficial Dissection)
NOTE: 1)   the emergence of the posterior femoral cutaneous nerve below the inferior border of the gluteus maximus muscle, and its descent down the middle of the thigh.

2)   the appearance of the major vessels (popliteal artery and vein) and the sciatic nerve (tibial and common fibular nerves) in the popliteal fossa.

3)   the posterior thigh contains the **hamstring muscles.** These include four muscles, the **long head of the biceps femoris,** the **semitendinosus muscle,** the **semimembranosus muscle,** and the ischiocondylar part of the **adductor magnus muscle** (see Note 1 under Fig. 511).

Fig. 510

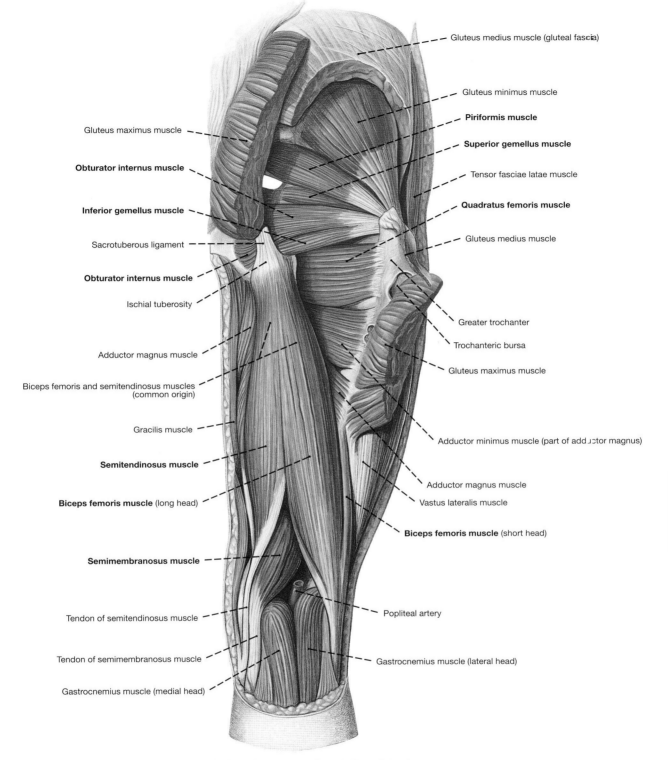

Gluteus medius muscle (gluteal fascia)

Gluteus minimus muscle

Piriformis muscle

Superior gemellus muscle

Tensor fasciae latae muscle

Quadratus femoris muscle

Gluteus medius muscle

Greater trochanter

Trochanteric bursa

Gluteus maximus muscle

Adductor minimus muscle (part of adductor magnus)

Adductor magnus muscle

Vastus lateralis muscle

Biceps femoris muscle (short head)

Popliteal artery

Gastrocnemius muscle (lateral head)

Gluteus maximus muscle

Obturator internus muscle

Inferior gemellus muscle

Sacrotuberous ligament

Obturator internus muscle

Ischial tuberosity

Adductor magnus muscle

Biceps femoris and semitendinosus muscles
(common origin)

Gracilis muscle

Semitendinosus muscle

Biceps femoris muscle (long head)

Semimembranosus muscle

Tendon of semitendinosus muscle

Tendon of semimembranosus muscle

Gastrocnemius muscle (medial head)

Fig. 511: Hamstring Muscles of Posterior Thigh and Deep Muscles of Gluteal Region

NOTE: 1) for a muscle to be considered a **hamstring muscle,** it must:
   a) arise from the **ischial tuberosity,**
   b) receive innervation from the **tibial division of the sciatic nerve,** and
   c) cross **both** the hip and knee joints.

   2) the long head of the biceps is a hamstring, but the short head **is not,** because it arises from the femur and is supplied by the fibular division of the sciatic nerve.

   3) the **ischiocondylar part** of the adductor magnus meets two criteria as a hamstring, but only crosses the hip joint. Its insertion, however, on the adductor tubercle is embryologically continuous with the tibial collateral ligament, which does attach below on the tibia.

Fig. 511   **V**

PLATE 336   Lower Extremity: Posterior Thigh, Deep Muscles (Dissection 3)

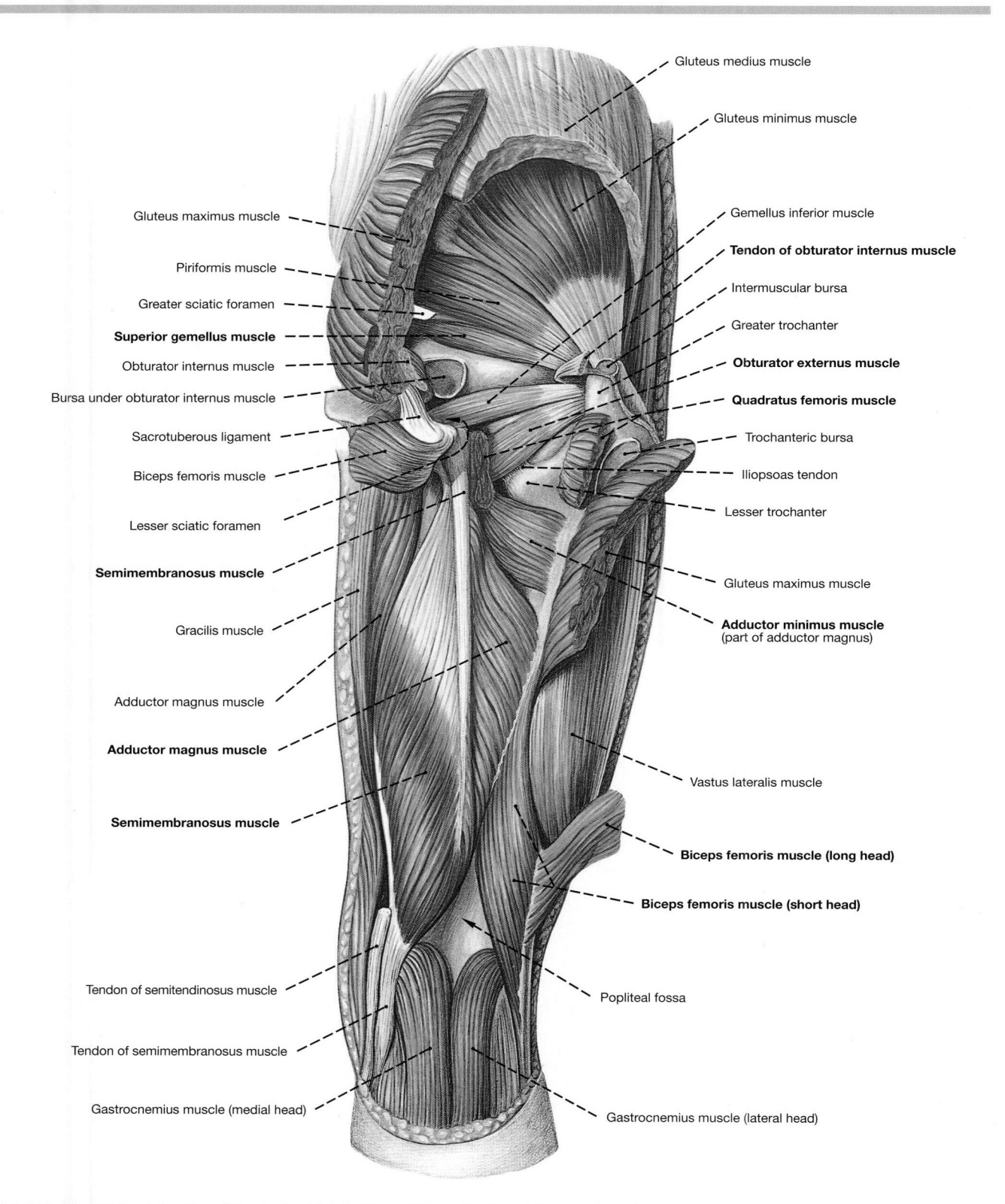

Gluteus medius muscle

Gluteus minimus muscle

Gemellus inferior muscle

Tendon of obturator internus muscle

Intermuscular bursa

Greater trochanter

Obturator externus muscle

Quadratus femoris muscle

Trochanteric bursa

Iliopsoas tendon

Lesser trochanter

Gluteus maximus muscle

Adductor minimus muscle
(part of adductor magnus)

Vastus lateralis muscle

Biceps femoris muscle (long head)

Biceps femoris muscle (short head)

Popliteal fossa

Gastrocnemius muscle (lateral head)

Gluteus maximus muscle

Piriformis muscle

Greater sciatic foramen

Superior gemellus muscle

Obturator internus muscle

Bursa under obturator internus muscle

Sacrotuberous ligament

Biceps femoris muscle

Lesser sciatic foramen

Semimembranosus muscle

Gracilis muscle

Adductor magnus muscle

Adductor magnus muscle

Semimembranosus muscle

Tendon of semitendinosus muscle

Tendon of semimembranosus muscle

Gastrocnemius muscle (medial head)

Fig. 512: Hamstring Muscles of Posterior Thigh (Deep Dissection) and Deep Gluteal Muscles

NOTE: 1) the common tendon of the long head of the biceps femoris and semitendinosus muscles has been cut in the thigh close to the ischial tuberosity. This exposes the origin of the **semimembranosus muscle,** the breadth of the **adductor magnus muscle,** and the **short head of the biceps femoris muscle.**

2) the **short head of the biceps femoris muscle** arising from the lateral lip of the linea aspera of the femur, between the attachments of the vastus lateralis and the adductor magnus muscles. It descends to join the tendon of the long head before insertion.

3) in the gluteal region, the quadratus femoris muscle has been severed and reflected, thereby revealing the **obturator externus muscle** beneath. Also the tendon of the obturator internus muscle has been cut (between the gemelli) exposing the bursa deep to that tendon.

Fig. 512

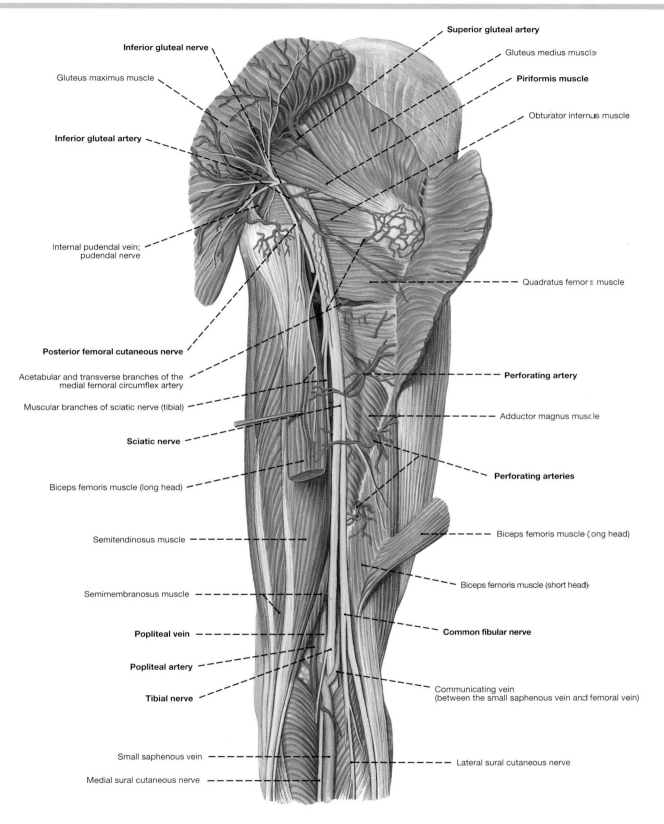

Superior gluteal artery

Inferior gluteal nerve

Gluteus medius muscle

Gluteus maximus muscle

Piriformis muscle

Obturator internus muscle

Inferior gluteal artery

Internal pudendal vein;
pudendal nerve

Quadratus femoris muscle

Posterior femoral cutaneous nerve

Perforating artery

Acetabular and transverse branches of the
medial femoral circumflex artery

Muscular branches of sciatic nerve (tibial)

Adductor magnus muscle

Sciatic nerve

Perforating arteries

Biceps femoris muscle (long head)

Biceps femoris muscle (long head)

Semitendinosus muscle

Biceps femoris muscle (short head)

Semimembranosus muscle

Popliteal vein

Common fibular nerve

Popliteal artery

Tibial nerve

Communicating vein
(between the small saphenous vein and femoral vein)

Small saphenous vein

Lateral sural cutaneous nerve

Medial sural cutaneous nerve

Fig. 513: Vessels and Nerves of the Posterior Thigh and Gluteal Region (Deep Dissection)

NOTE: 1) the course of **sciatic nerve** as it passes through the greater sciatic foramen in the gluteal region, inferior to the piriformis muscle, lateral to the ischial tuberosity and under cover of the gluteus maximus muscle. It enters the thigh nearly midway between the ischial tuberosity and the greater trochanter.

2) the **superior and inferior gluteal arteries** and the **posterior femoral cutaneous nerve** in the gluteal region. In the thigh observe the **perforating arteries,** branches of the **deep femoral artery,** and the fact that the sciatic nerve splits to become the **tibial and common fibular nerves.**

Fig. 513 **V**

PLATE 338   Popliteal Fossa, Vessels and Nerves (Dissections 1 and 2)

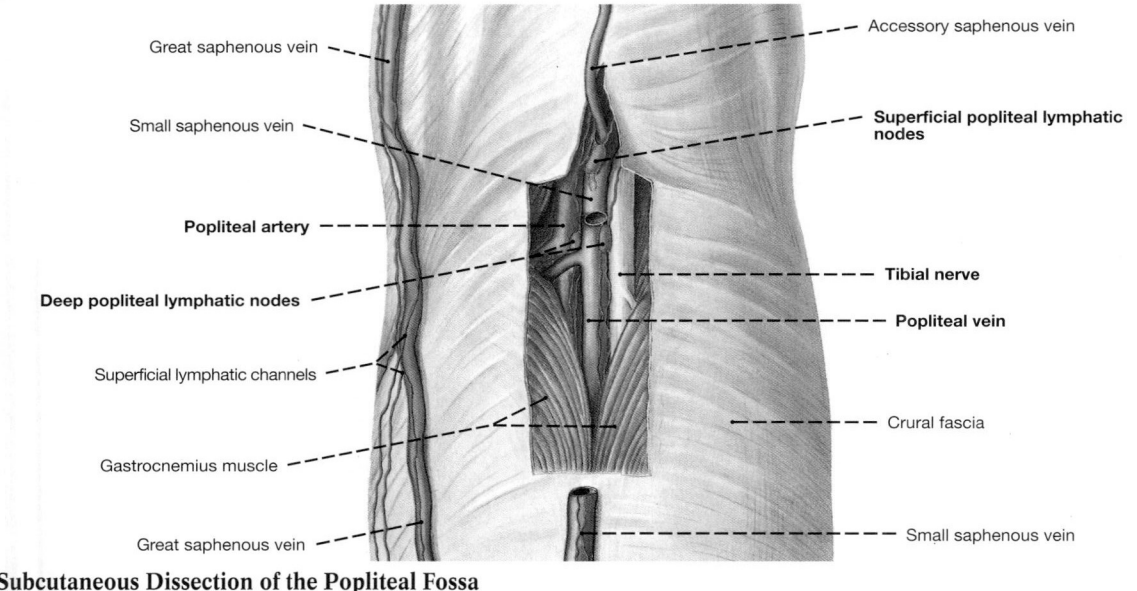

Great saphenous vein

Small saphenous vein

Popliteal artery

Deep popliteal lymphatic nodes

Superficial lymphatic channels

Gastrocnemius muscle

Great saphenous vein

Accessory saphenous vein

Superficial popliteal lymphatic nodes

Tibial nerve

Popliteal vein

Crural fascia

Small saphenous vein

Fig. 514: Subcutaneous Dissection of the Popliteal Fossa
NOTE: the skin and crural fascia have been removed over the popliteal fossa and a part of the small saphenous vein has been resected. Observe the popliteal vessels and nerves and the **popliteal lymphatic nodes** and **channels** deeper in the fossa.

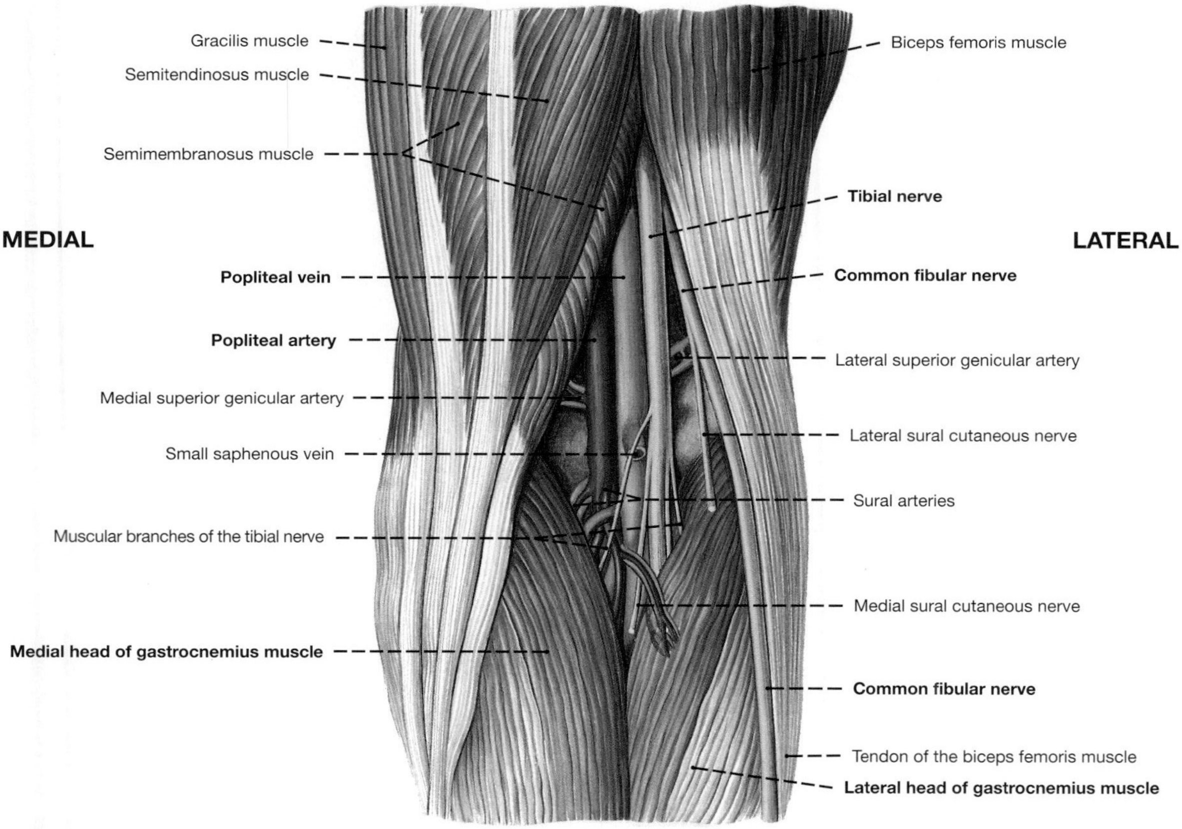

Gracilis muscle

Semitendinosus muscle

Semimembranosus muscle

MEDIAL

Popliteal vein

Popliteal artery

Medial superior genicular artery

Small saphenous vein

Muscular branches of the tibial nerve

Medial head of gastrocnemius muscle

Biceps femoris muscle

Tibial nerve

LATERAL

Common fibular nerve

Lateral superior genicular artery

Lateral sural cutaneous nerve

Sural arteries

Medial sural cutaneous nerve

Common fibular nerve

Tendon of the biceps femoris muscle

Lateral head of gastrocnemius muscle

Fig. 515: Nerves and Vessels of the Popliteal Fossa, Superficial View
NOTE: 1) the relationships of the **popliteal vessels** and **nerve** within the popliteal fossa. The **sciatic nerve** has already divided into the laterally directed **common fibular nerve** and the **tibial nerve** which continues directly into the calf. Both the common fibular and the tibial nerves lie superficial to the vessels in the popliteal fossa.

2) the popliteal vein is located between the tibial nerve and popliteal artery, while the artery is the deepest (most anterior) and most medial of three structures.

3) the two muscular branches of the tibial nerve innervating the two heads of the gastrocnemius muscle, and a descending sensory branch, the **medial sural cutaneous nerve,** to the calf. Also note the **lateral sural cutaneous nerve** from the common fibular nerve.

4) the popliteal fossa is about 2.5 cm (1 inch) wide at its maximum, and in the undissected specimen, the fossa is filled with fat, and the vessels and nerves are initially difficult to see.

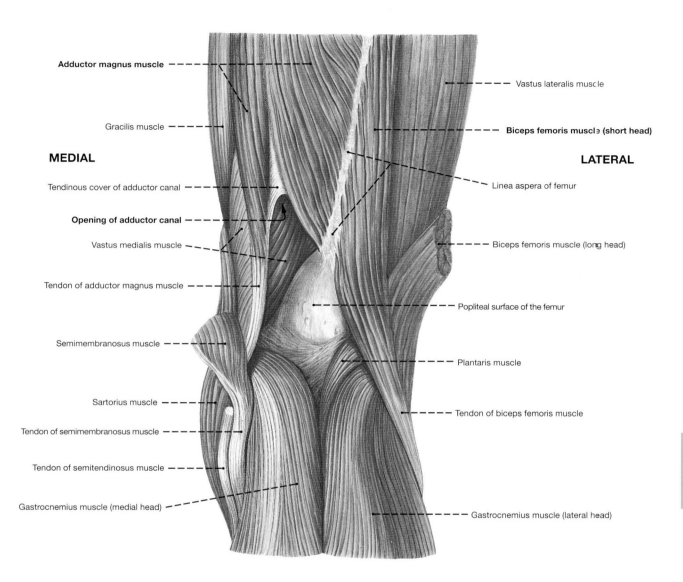

Adductor magnus muscle

Gracilis muscle

MEDIAL

Tendinous cover of adductor canal

Opening of adductor canal

Vastus medialis muscle

Tendon of adductor magnus muscle

Semimembranosus muscle

Sartorius muscle

Tendon of semimembranosus muscle

Tendon of semitendinosus muscle

Gastrocnemius muscle (medial head)

Vastus lateralis muscle

Biceps femoris muscle (short head)

LATERAL

Linea aspera of femur

Biceps femoris muscle (long head)

Popliteal surface of the femur

Plantaris muscle

Tendon of biceps femoris muscle

Gastrocnemius muscle (lateral head)

Fig. 516: Deep Muscles That Bound the Popliteal Fossa

NOTE: 1)   the **popliteal fossa** is a diamond-shaped space behind the knee joint. Its *superior boundaries* are the **long head of the biceps femoris muscle** laterally and the **semimembranosus** and **semitendinosus muscles** medially (see Fig. 515). All three of these muscles have been cut in this dissection, exposing the more deeply located **adductor magnus** and **vastus medialis** medially and the **short head of the biceps femoris** laterally.

2)   the *inferior boundaries* of the fossa are the **medial** and **lateral heads of the gastrocnemius muscle** which arise from the medial and lateral condyles of the femur.

3)   the inferior opening of the **adductor canal** which transmits the **femoral artery** and **vein** from and to the anterior aspect of the thigh.

4)   anterior to the upper part of the popliteal fossa is the **popliteal surface of the femur.** This flattened area of the femur is located just above the epicondyles.

Fig. 516   **V**

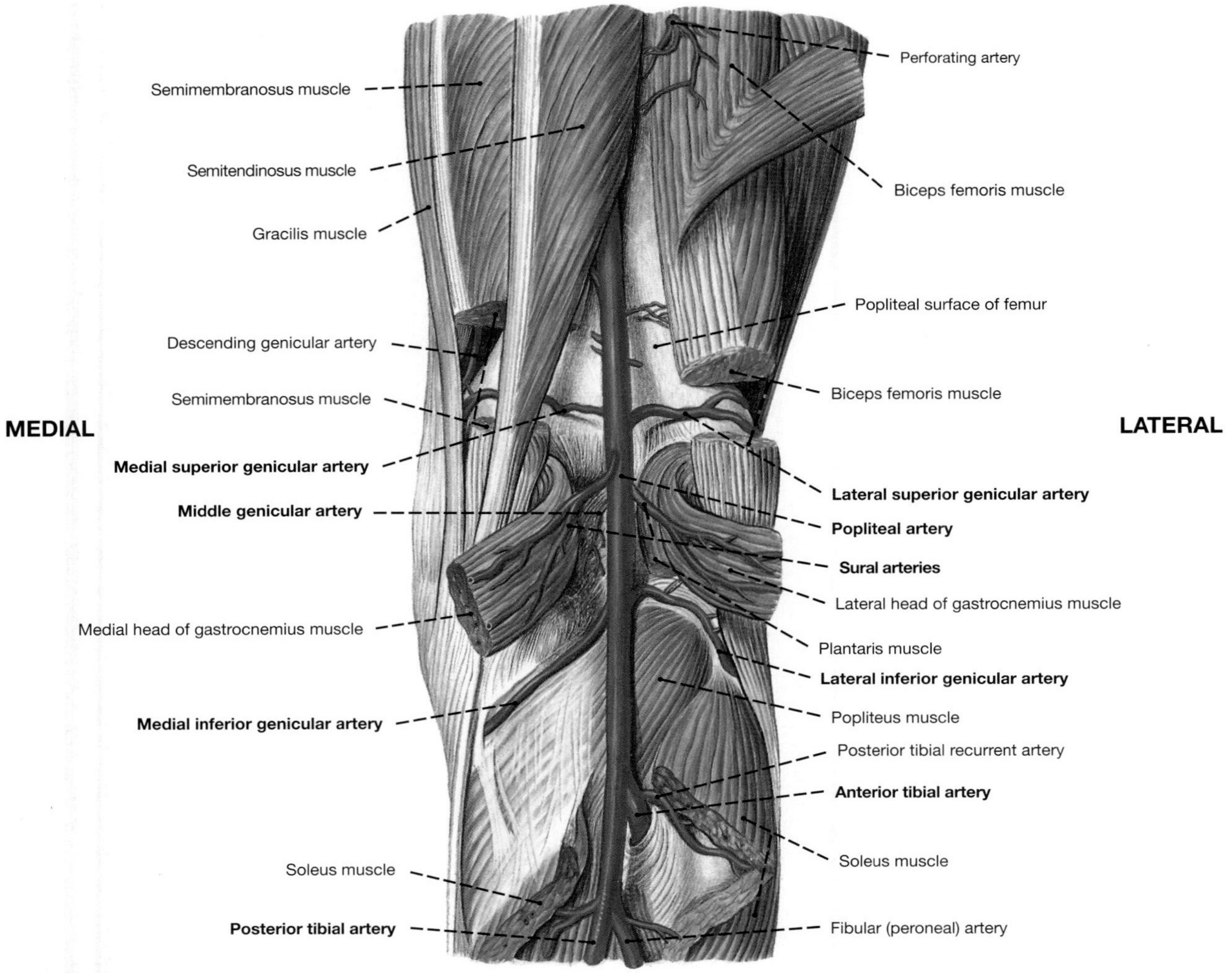

PLATE 340   Lower Extremity: Popliteal Fossa, Deep Arteries (Dissection 4)

Semimembranosus muscle

Semitendinosus muscle

Gracilis muscle

Descending genicular artery

Semimembranosus muscle

MEDIAL

Medial superior genicular artery

Middle genicular artery

Medial head of gastrocnemius muscle

Medial inferior genicular artery

Soleus muscle

Posterior tibial artery

Perforating artery

Biceps femoris muscle

Popliteal surface of femur

Biceps femoris muscle

LATERAL

Lateral superior genicular artery

Popliteal artery

Sural arteries

Lateral head of gastrocnemius muscle

Plantaris muscle

Lateral inferior genicular artery

Popliteus muscle

Posterior tibial recurrent artery

Anterior tibial artery

Soleus muscle

Fibular (peroneal) artery

Fig. 517: Branches of the Popliteal Artery

NOTE: 1)   within the popliteal fossa, the popliteal artery most frequently gives rise to two **superior (lateral** and **medial) genicular,** one **middle genicular** and two **inferior (lateral** and **medial) genicular arteries.**

2)   the **anterior tibial artery** branches from the **posterior tibial** and penetrates an aperture above the interosseous membrane to reach the anterior compartment. Somewhat lower, the **fibular artery** also branches from the posterior tibial. The pattern shown here occurs in about **90% of cases.** Variations in this pattern are shown in Figure 518.

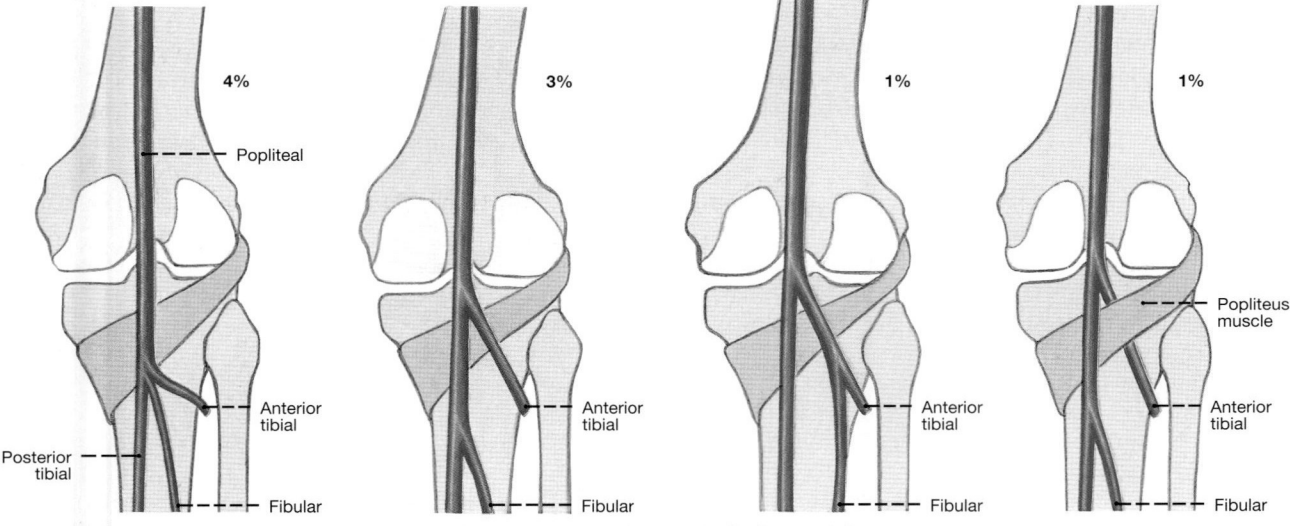

Fig. 518: Variations in the Branching Pattern of the Anterior Tibial and Fibular Arteries
See NOTE 2 under Figure 517.

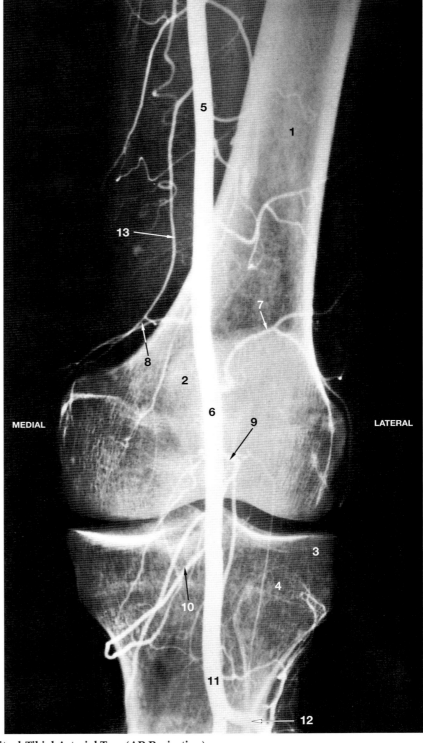

1. Femur
2. Patella
3. Tibia
4. Head of fibula
5. Femoral artery
6. Popliteal artery
7. Lateral superior genicular artery
8. Medial superior genicular artery
9. Middle genicular artery
10. Inferior genicular artery
11. Posterior tibial artery
12. Anterior tibial artery
13. Descending genicular artery

Fig. 519: Arteriogram of the Left Femoral-Popliteal-Tibial Arterial Tree (AP Projection)

NOTE: 1)   this arteriogram shows the branches from the femoral, popliteal and tibial arteries in the lower ⅓rd of the thigh and the upper part of the calf. Observe the following bony structures: **femur** (1), **patella** (2), **tibia** (3), and **fibula** (4).

2)   the course of the **femoral artery** (5) as it becomes the **popliteal artery** (6) just above the popliteal fossa. Observe the following branches from the popliteal artery: **superior genicular** (7, 8), **middle genicular** (9), and single **inferior genicular** (10) in this patient.

3)   below the popliteal fossa the **posterior tibial artery** (11) can be seen giving off the **anterior tibial artery** just above the lower edge of the angiogram.

4)   the **descending genicular artery** (13), a branch of the femoral above the popliteal fossa, as it courses downward to participate in the anastomosis around the knee joint. (From Wicke L. Atlas of Radiographic Anatomy, 5th Ed. Philadelphia, Lea & Febiger, 1994).

Fig. 519   **V**

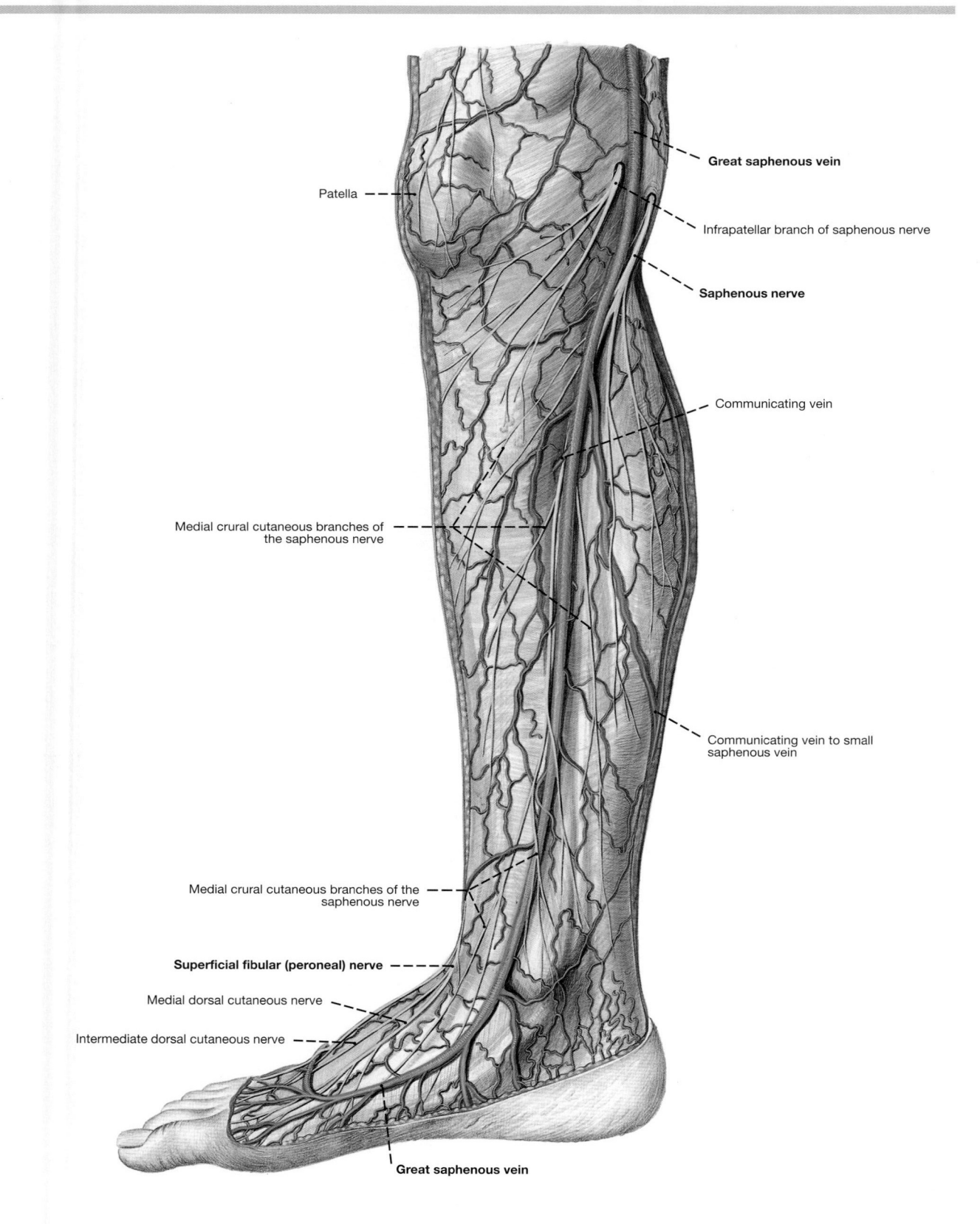

Patella

Great saphenous vein

Infrapatellar branch of saphenous nerve

Saphenous nerve

Communicating vein

Medial crural cutaneous branches of the saphenous nerve

Communicating vein to small saphenous vein

Medial crural cutaneous branches of the saphenous nerve

Superficial fibular (peroneal) nerve

Medial dorsal cutaneous nerve

Intermediate dorsal cutaneous nerve

Great saphenous vein

Fig. 520: Superficial Veins and Nerves on the Anterior and Medial Aspects of the Leg and Foot

NOTE: 1) the **great saphenous vein** is formed on the medial aspect of the foot, courses anterior to the medial malleolus, and ascends along the medial side of the leg.

    2) branches of the **saphenous nerve** accompany the great saphenous vein below the knee. This nerve becomes superficial medially just below the knee and is the largest branch of the femoral nerve. It functions as dsthe sensory nerve that supplies the skin over most of the medial half of the leg region (i.e., between the knee and ankle).

Fig. 520

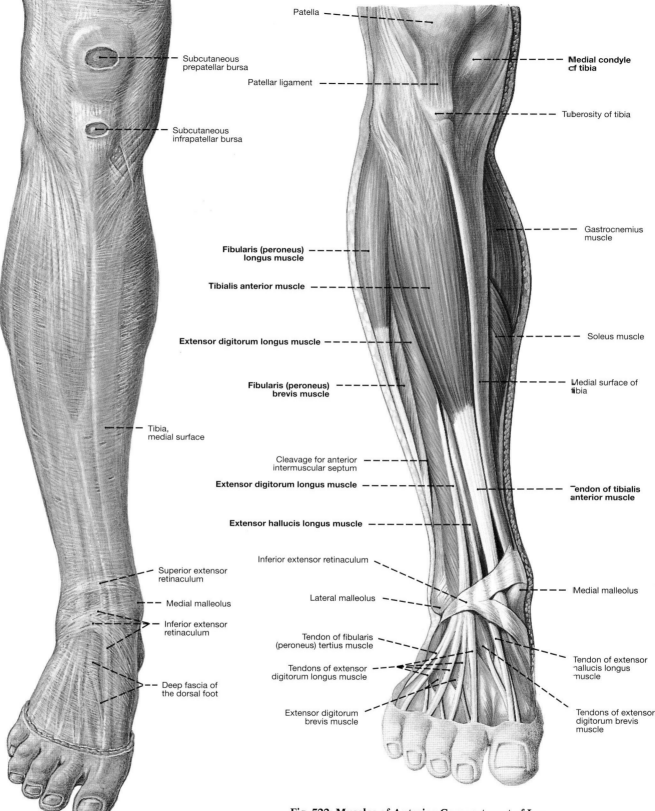

Subcutaneous prepatellar bursa

Subcutaneous infrapatellar bursa

Tibia, medial surface

Superior extensor retinaculum

Medial malleolus

Inferior extensor retinaculum

Deep fascia of the dorsal foot

Patella

Patellar ligament

Fibularis (peroneus) longus muscle

Tibialis anterior muscle

Extensor digitorum longus muscle

Fibularis (peroneus) brevis muscle

Cleavage for anterior intermuscular septum

Extensor digitorum longus muscle

Extensor hallucis longus muscle

Inferior extensor retinaculum

Lateral malleolus

Tendon of fibularis (peroneus) tertius muscle

Tendons of extensor digitorum longus muscle

Extensor digitorum brevis muscle

Medial condyle of tibia

Tuberosity of tibia

Gastrocnemius muscle

Soleus muscle

Medial surface of tibia

Tendon of tibialis anterior muscle

Medial malleolus

Tendon of extensor hallucis longus muscle

Tendons of extensor digitorum brevis muscle

Fig. 522: Muscles of Anterior Compartment of Leg

NOTE: 1)   the medial surface of the tibia separates muscles in the anterior compartment from those of the calf, posteriorly.

2)   the anterior compartment muscles include the **tibialis anterior, extensor hallucis longus, extensor digitorum,** and **fibularis tertius,** which dorsiflex the foot. The long flexors and fibularis tertius also extend the toes (PLATE 345).

Fig. 521: Deep Fascia Investing the Leg and Dorsal Foot

NOTE: the deep fascia binds the muscles and the **superior and inferior extensor retinacula** bind the tendons of the anterior and lateral leg muscles.

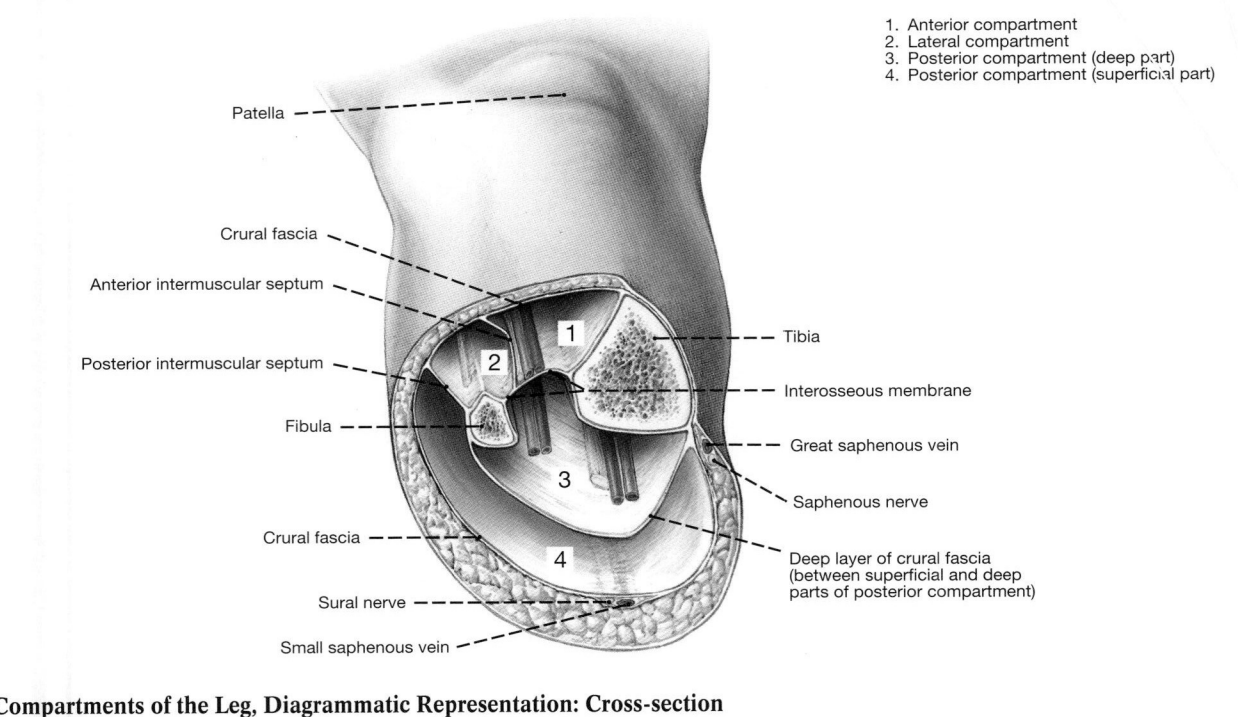

1. Anterior compartment
2. Lateral compartment
3. Posterior compartment (deep part)
4. Posterior compartment (superficial part)

Patella

Crural fascia

Anterior intermuscular septum

Posterior intermuscular septum

Fibula

Crural fascia

Sural nerve

Small saphenous vein

Tibia

Interosseous membrane

Great saphenous vein

Saphenous nerve

Deep layer of crural fascia (between superficial and deep parts of posterior compartment)

Fig. 523: Compartments of the Leg, Diagrammatic Representation: Cross-section
NOTE: this figure shows the compartments of the **left leg** viewed upward from below.

Muscles of the Anterior Compartment of the Leg

Muscle	Origin	Insertion	Innervation	Action
Tibialis Anterior Muscle	Lateral condyle and lateral surface of upper half of the tibia; the interosseous membrane and crural fascia	On the medial and plantar surfaces of the 1st metatarsal bone and the medial cuneiform bone	Deep fibular (peroneal) nerve (L4, L5)	Dorsiflexes the foot at the ankle joint; inverts and adducts the foot at the subtalar and midtarsal joints
Extensor Hallucis Longus Muscle	Medial surface of the fibula; the anterior part of the interosseous membrane and the crural fascia	Dorsal surface of the base of the distal phalanx of the great toe (or hallux)	Deep fibular (peroneal) nerve (L5, S1)	Extends the great toe; dorsiflexes the foot and it tends to invert (supinate) the foot
Extensor Digitorum Longus Muscle	Lateral condyle of tibia; upper ¾ths of anterior surface of the fibula and the interosseous membrane	On the distal phalanges of the four lateral toes	Deep fibular (peroneal) nerve (L5, S1)	Extends the lateral four digits; dorsiflexes the foot and tends to evert (pronate) the foot
Fibularis Tertius Muscle	Distal ⅓rd of the anterior surface of the fibula and the interosseous membrane	Dorsal surface of the base of the 5th metatarsal bone	Deep fibular (peroneal) nerve (L5, S1)	Dorsiflexes the foot and assists in everting (i.e., pronating) the foot

Muscles of the Lateral Compartment of the Leg

Fibularis Longus Muscle	Head and upper ⅔rds of the lateral surface of the body of the fibula	Lateral aspect of the base of the 1st metatarsal bone and the medial cuneiform bone (on the plantar surface of the foot)	Superficial fibular (peroneal) nerve (L4, S1, S2)	Everts the foot (i.e., tends to pronate the foot); it also is a weak plantar flexor of the foot
Fibularis Brevis Muscle	Distal ⅔rds of the lateral surface of the fibula and the intermuscular septum	Lateral surface and base of the 5th metatarsal bone	Superficial fibular (peroneal) nerve (L4, L5, S1)	Everts the foot (i.e., tends to pronate the foot); also acts as a weak plantar flexor of the foot

Fig. 523

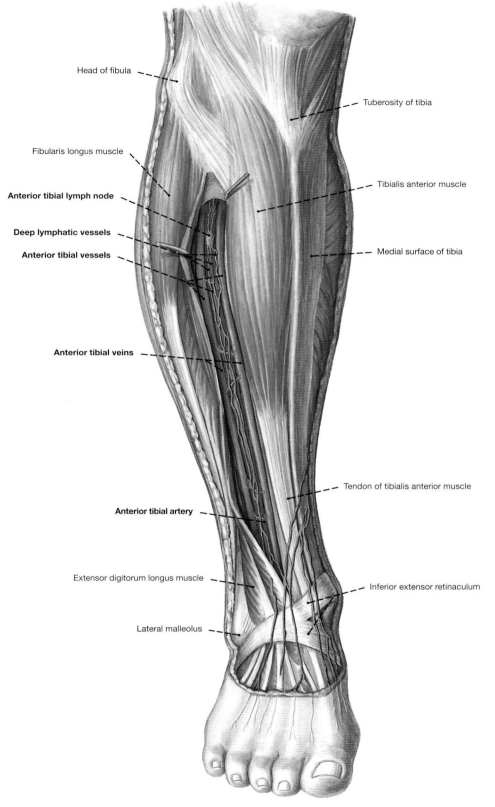

Head of fibula

Tuberosity of tibia

Fibularis longus muscle

Anterior tibial lymph node

Tibialis anterior muscle

Deep lymphatic vessels

Anterior tibial vessels

Medial surface of tibia

Anterior tibial veins

Anterior tibial artery

Tendon of tibialis anterior muscle

Extensor digitorum longus muscle

Inferior extensor retinaculum

Lateral malleolus

Fig. 524: Anterior Tibial Vessels and Lymphatic Channels in the Anterior Compartment

NOTE: 1) by separating the **tibialis anterior muscle** from the other muscles in the anterior compartment, the **anterior tibial artery** is exposed descending in the anterior compartment to the dorsum of the foot.

2) the artery is accompanied by a pair of **anterior tibial veins (venae comitantes)**, which ascend to join the posterior tibial vein posteriorly to help form the popliteal vein.

3) lymphatic channels from the dorsum of the foot course superiorly along the path of these vessels, and at times a lymph node can be found just below the knee.

Fig. 524   **V**

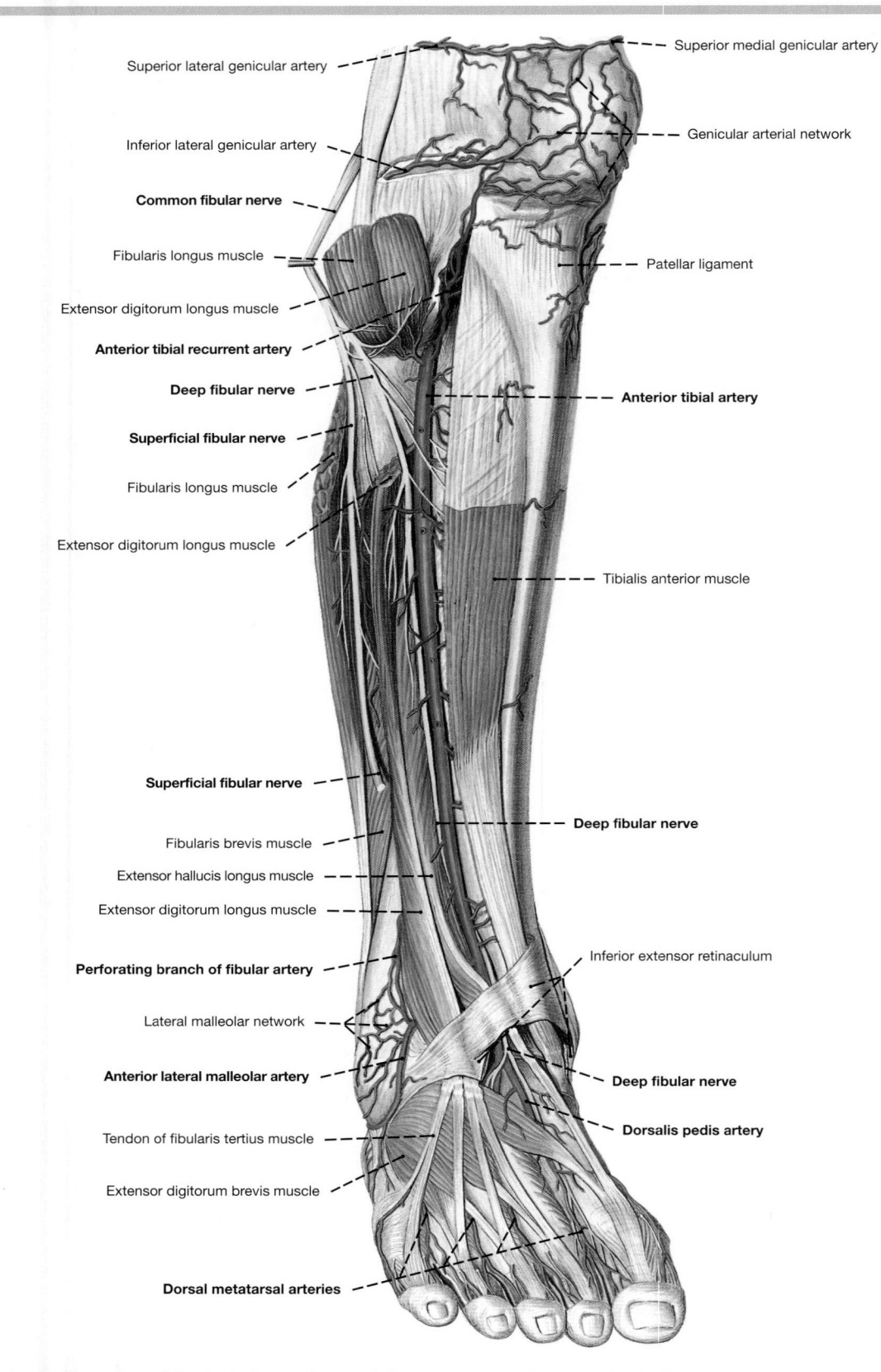

Superior lateral genicular artery

Superior medial genicular artery

Inferior lateral genicular artery

Genicular arterial network

Common fibular nerve

Fibularis longus muscle

Patellar ligament

Extensor digitorum longus muscle

Anterior tibial recurrent artery

Deep fibular nerve

Anterior tibial artery

Superficial fibular nerve

Fibularis longus muscle

Extensor digitorum longus muscle

Tibialis anterior muscle

Superficial fibular nerve

Deep fibular nerve

Fibularis brevis muscle

Extensor hallucis longus muscle

Extensor digitorum longus muscle

Perforating branch of fibular artery

Inferior extensor retinaculum

Lateral malleolar network

Anterior lateral malleolar artery

Deep fibular nerve

Tendon of fibularis tertius muscle

Dorsalis pedis artery

Extensor digitorum brevis muscle

Dorsal metatarsal arteries

Fig. 525: Deep Dissection of the Anterior and Lateral Compartments: Nerves and Arteries
NOTE: 1)   as the **common fibular nerve** courses laterally around the head of the fibula, it divides into the **superficial** and **deep fibular nerves** which innervate the muscles of the lateral and anterior compartments.

   2)   the deep fibular nerve is joined by the **anterior tibial artery**, which descends toward the foot, where it becomes the **dorsalis pedis artery.**

   3)   the superficial fibular nerve becomes cutaneous about 7 inches above the lateral malleolus, while the deep fibular nerve becomes cutaneous between the large and 2nd toes.

Fig. 525

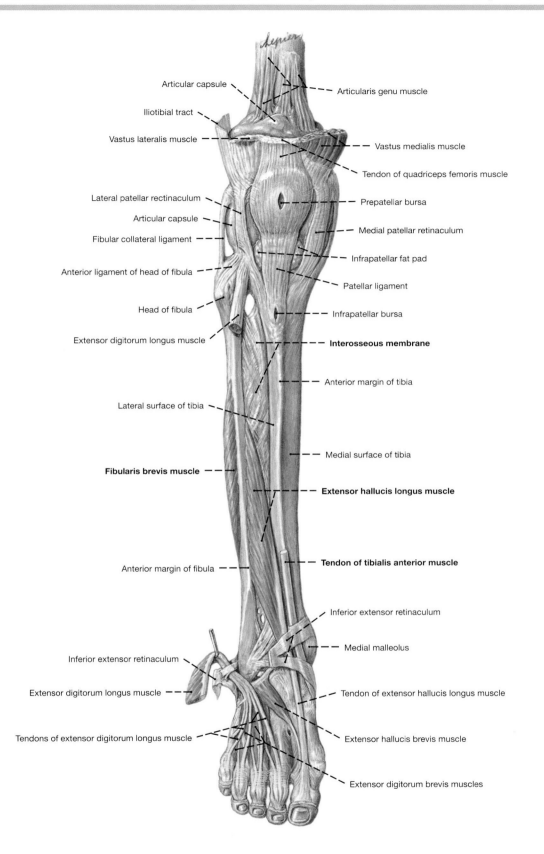

Fig. 526: Deep Dissection of the Anterior and Lateral Compartments: Muscles

NOTE: 1) the bellies of the tibialis anterior and fibularis longus muscles have been removed and the extensor digitorum longus muscle has been reflected. Observe the full extent of the **extensor hallucis longus** and the belly of the **fibularis brevis muscle.**

2) the interosseous membrane between the tibia and the fibula dend the opening above its upper border through which course the anterior tibial vessels.

Fig. 526 V

PLATE 348   Lower Extremity: Lateral Compartment of the Leg (Dissection 6)

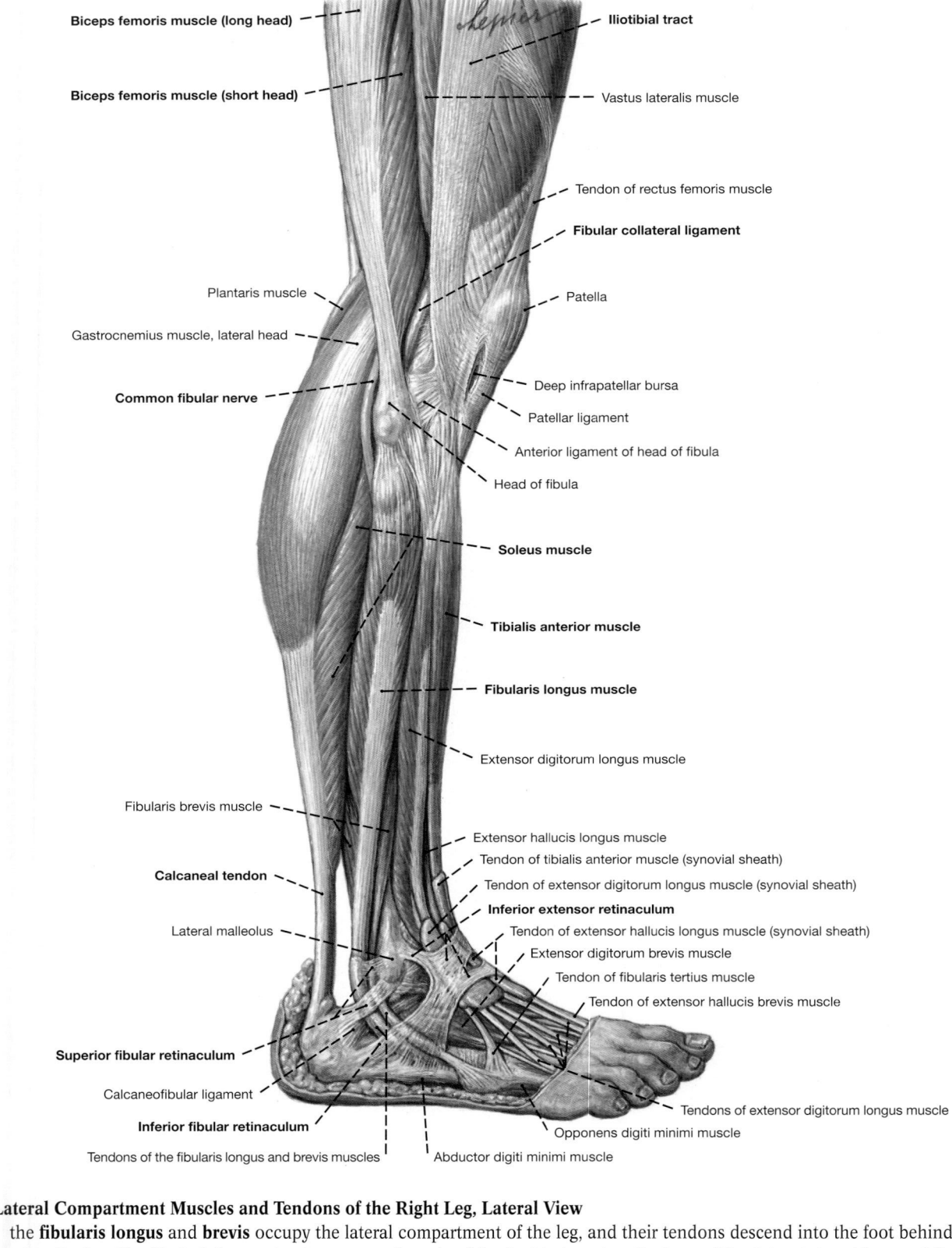

Biceps femoris muscle (long head)

Biceps femoris muscle (short head)

Plantaris muscle

Gastrocnemius muscle, lateral head

Common fibular nerve

Fibularis brevis muscle

Calcaneal tendon

Lateral malleolus

Superior fibular retinaculum

Calcaneofibular ligament

Inferior fibular retinaculum

Tendons of the fibularis longus and brevis muscles

Iliotibial tract

Vastus lateralis muscle

Tendon of rectus femoris muscle

Fibular collateral ligament

Patella

Deep infrapatellar bursa

Patellar ligament

Anterior ligament of head of fibula

Head of fibula

Soleus muscle

Tibialis anterior muscle

Fibularis longus muscle

Extensor digitorum longus muscle

Extensor hallucis longus muscle

Tendon of tibialis anterior muscle (synovial sheath)

Tendon of extensor digitorum longus muscle (synovial sheath)

Inferior extensor retinaculum

Tendon of extensor hallucis longus muscle (synovial sheath)

Extensor digitorum brevis muscle

Tendon of fibularis tertius muscle

Tendon of extensor hallucis brevis muscle

Tendons of extensor digitorum longus muscle

Opponens digiti minimi muscle

Abductor digiti minimi muscle

Fig. 527: Lateral Compartment Muscles and Tendons of the Right Leg, Lateral View

NOTE: 1) the **fibularis longus** and **brevis** occupy the lateral compartment of the leg, and their tendons descend into the foot behind the lateral malleolus. The fibularis longus tendon crosses the sole of the foot to insert on the base of the 1st metatarsal bone, while the fibularis brevis inserts directly onto 5th metatarsal bone.

2) the superficial location of the **head of the fibula** and its relationship to the **common fibular nerve.** Trauma to the lateral side of the leg could cause injury to this nerve resulting in a condition called "foot-drop", because the dorsiflexors would be denervated and the action of the plantar flexors in the posterior compartment would no longer be opposed.

3) the tendons lower the anterior and lateral compartment muscles enter the foot beneath the extensor and fibular retinacula and they are surrounded by tendon sheaths (in blue).

Fig. 527

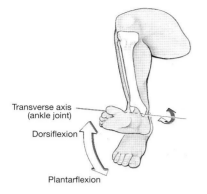

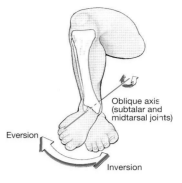

Fig. 528: Dorsiflexion and Plantarflexion of the Foot (at Ankle Joint)

DORSIFLEXION:
1. Attempts to approximate the dorsum of the foot to the anterior leg surface.
2. Is considered as extension at ankle joint.
3. Is performed by muscles in the anterior compartment of the leg.

PLANTARFLEXION:
1. Reverses dorsiflexion and also occurs when one stands on one's toes.
2. Is considered as flexion at ankle joint.
3. Is performed by muscles in the posterior compartment of the leg.

Fig. 529: Inversion and Eversion of the Foot (at Subtalar and Midtarsal Joint)

INVERSION:
1. Attempts to supinate the foot, i.e., to turn the sole medially or inward.
2. Is performed by muscles in the leg that attach medially on the foot (tibialis anterior *and* posterior; extensor *and* flexor hallucis longus).

EVERSION:
1. Attempts to pronate the foot, i.e., to turn the sole laterally or outward.
2. Is performed by muscles in the leg that attach laterally on the foot such as fibularis longus, brevis, and tertius.

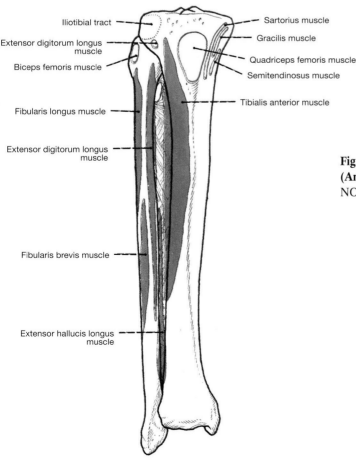

Fig. 530: Muscle Attachments on the Right Tibia and Fibula (Anterior Surface)

NOTE: 1) most of the upper ³/₄ths of the anterior surface of the fibula gives attachment to muscles, while much of the anterior tibia is free of muscle attachments.

2) the only muscle of the anterior and lateral compartments that does **not** arise from the fibula is the tibialis anterior. The only muscle of the thigh that attaches to the fibula is the biceps femoris.

3) portions of the anterior surface of the interosseous membrane are used by all three muscles of the anterior compartment for their origin, whereas neither of the lateral compartment muscles extends that far medially.

4) the sartorius, gracilis, and semitendinosus muscles insert on the medial condyle of the tibia forming a tendinous expansion sometimes called the pes anserinus (goose's foot), while onto the tibial tuberosity inserts the large quadriceps femoris muscle.

5) onto the lateral condyle of the tibia inserts the biceps femoris muscle.

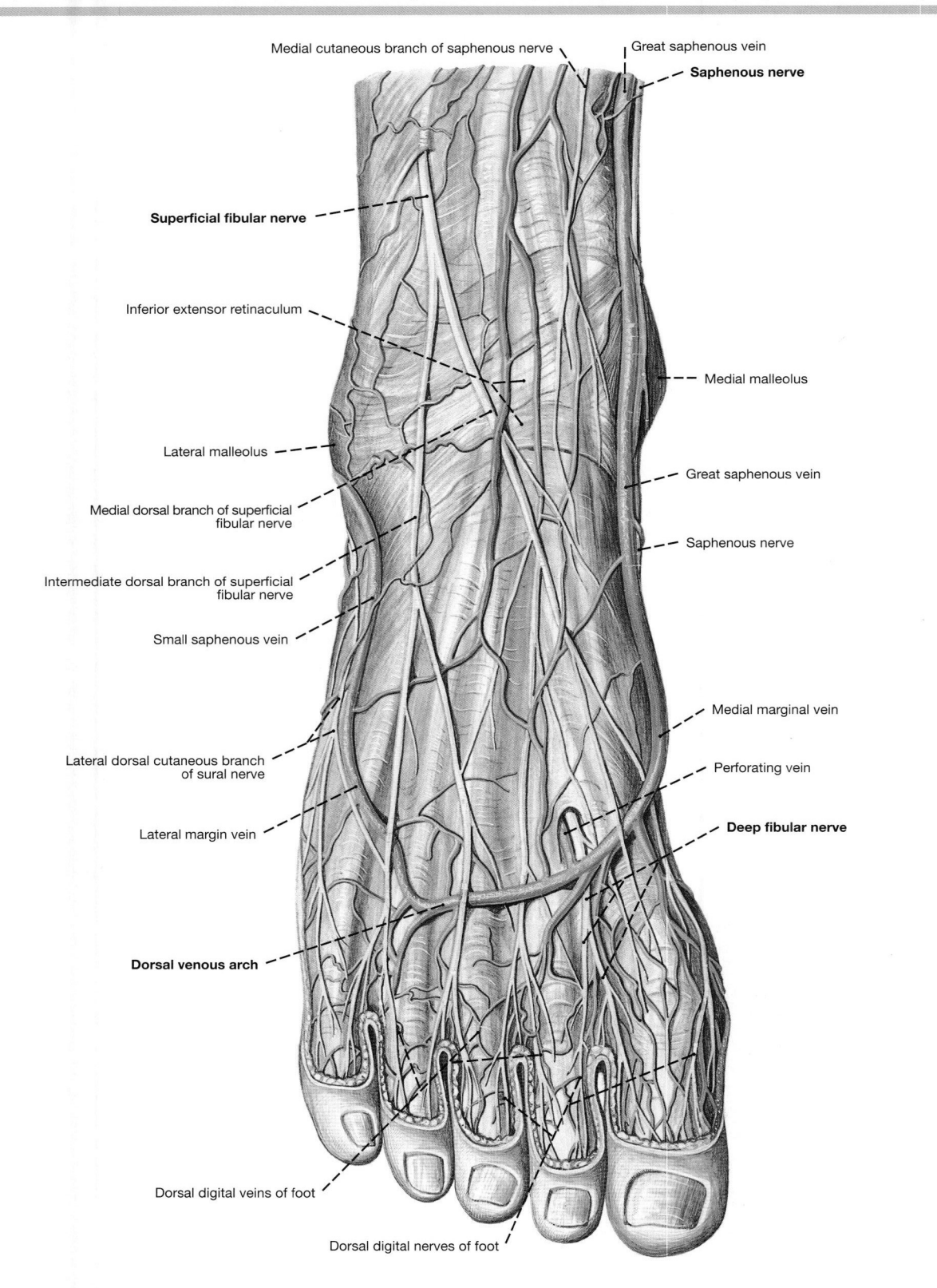

Medial cutaneous branch of saphenous nerve

Great saphenous vein

Saphenous nerve

Superficial fibular nerve

Inferior extensor retinaculum

Medial malleolus

Lateral malleolus

Great saphenous vein

Medial dorsal branch of superficial
fibular nerve

Saphenous nerve

Intermediate dorsal branch of superficial
fibular nerve

Small saphenous vein

Medial marginal vein

Lateral dorsal cutaneous branch
of sural nerve

Perforating vein

Lateral margin vein

Deep fibular nerve

Dorsal venous arch

Dorsal digital veins of foot

Dorsal digital nerves of foot

Fig. 531: Superficial Nerves and Veins of the Dorsal Right Foot

NOTE: 1)   cutaneous innervation of the dorsal foot is supplied principally by the **superficial fibular nerve** (L4, L5, S1). Additionally, the **deep fibular nerve** (L4, L5) supplies the adjacent sides of the 1st and 2nd toes, while the **lateral dorsal cutaneous nerve** (S1, S2; terminal branch of the sural nerve in the foot) supplies the lateral and dorsal aspects of the 5th digit.

2)   the digital and metatarsal veins drain back from the toes to form the dorsal venous arch of the foot. From this arch, the **great saphenous vein** ascends medially and the **small saphenous vein** laterally on the foot dorsum.

3)   the cutaneous branch of the **saphenous nerve** extends downward as far as the ankle joint anteriorly. Medially, the main trunk of the saphenous nerve can extend inferiorly as far as the metatarsophalangeal joint of the large toe.

Fig. 531

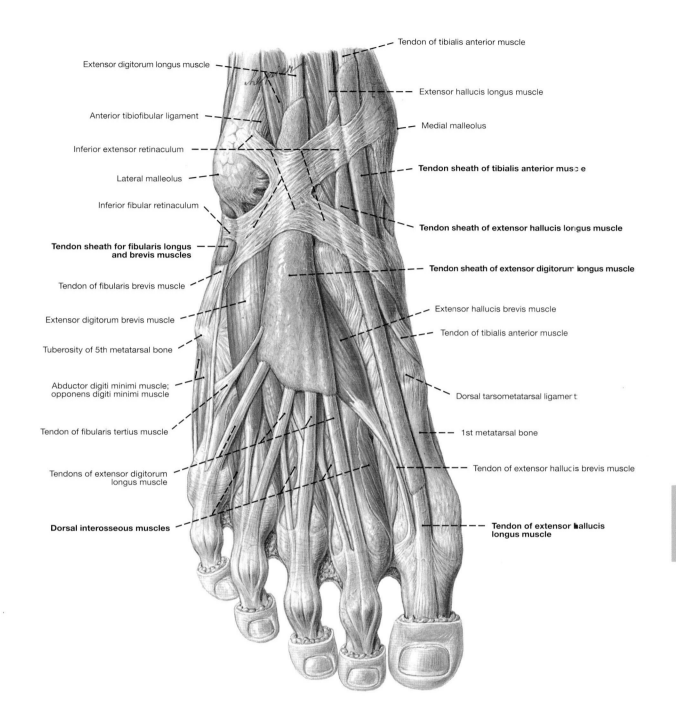

Tendon of tibialis anterior muscle

Extensor digitorum longus muscle

Anterior tibiofibular ligament

Inferior extensor retinaculum

Lateral malleolus

Inferior fibular retinaculum

Tendon sheath for fibularis longus and brevis muscles

Tendon of fibularis brevis muscle

Extensor digitorum brevis muscle

Tuberosity of 5th metatarsal bone

Abductor digiti minimi muscle; opponens digiti minimi muscle

Tendon of fibularis tertius muscle

Tendons of extensor digitorum longus muscle

Dorsal interosseous muscles

Extensor hallucis longus muscle

Medial malleolus

Tendon sheath of tibialis anterior musc e

Tendon sheath of extensor hallucis longus muscle

Tendon sheath of extensor digitorum longus muscle

Extensor hallucis brevis muscle

Tendon of tibialis anterior muscle

Dorsal tarsometatarsal ligamer t

1st metatarsal bone

Tendon of extensor hallucis brevis muscle

Tendon of extensor hallucis longus muscle

Fig. 532: Muscles, Tendons, and Tendon Sheaths of the Dorsal Right Foot (Superficial View)
NOTE: 1) the tendons of the tibialis anterior, extensor hallucis longus, and extensor digitorum longus are bound by the **Y**-shaped (or **X**-shaped) inferior extensor retinaculum as they enter the dorsum of the foot at the level of the ankle joint.
2) the extensor tendons insert onto the dorsal aspect of the distal phalanx of each toe. Additionally, the tendons of the extensor digitorum longus also insert onto the dorsum of the middle phalanx of the four lateral toes.
3) the tendon of the fibularis tertius inserts on the base of the 5th metatarsal bone (and at times the 4th also).
4) separate synovial sheaths (shown in blue) surround the tendons of the tibialis anterior and extensor hallucis longus. Also note the common synovial sheath for the main tendon and the individual digital tendons of the extensor digitorum longus.
5) the tendon sheaths laterally and medially under the two malleoli are shown in Figures 533 and 534.

Fig. 532   **V**

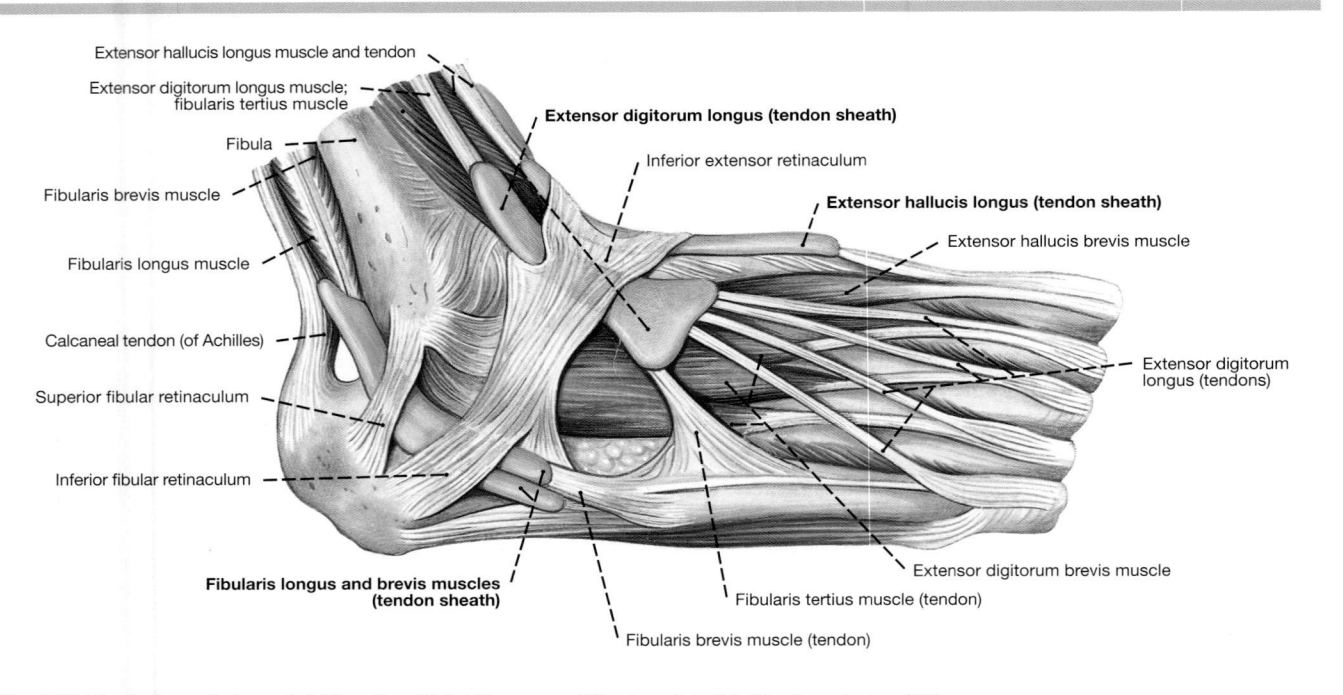

Fig. 533: Tendons and Synovial Sheaths: Right Dorsum of Foot and Ankle Region; Lateral View

NOTE: 1)   similar to the wrist, tendons at the ankle region passing from the leg into the foot are bound by closely investing **retinacula** and are surrounded by **synovial sheaths,** which are indicated in blue in this figure and in Figure 534.

    2)   anterior to the ankle joint and on the dorsum of the foot are three separate synovial sheaths, one that includes the extensor digitorum longus and the fibularis tertius, a 2nd for the extensor hallucis longus and a 3rd for the tibialis anterior (see Figs. 527, 532).

    3)   behind the lateral malleolus is a single tendon sheath for the fibularis longus and brevis muscles, which then splits distally to continue along each individual tendon for some distance.

    4)   the inferior extensor retinaculum and the superior and inferior fibular retinacula, which bind the tendons and their sheaths close to bone.

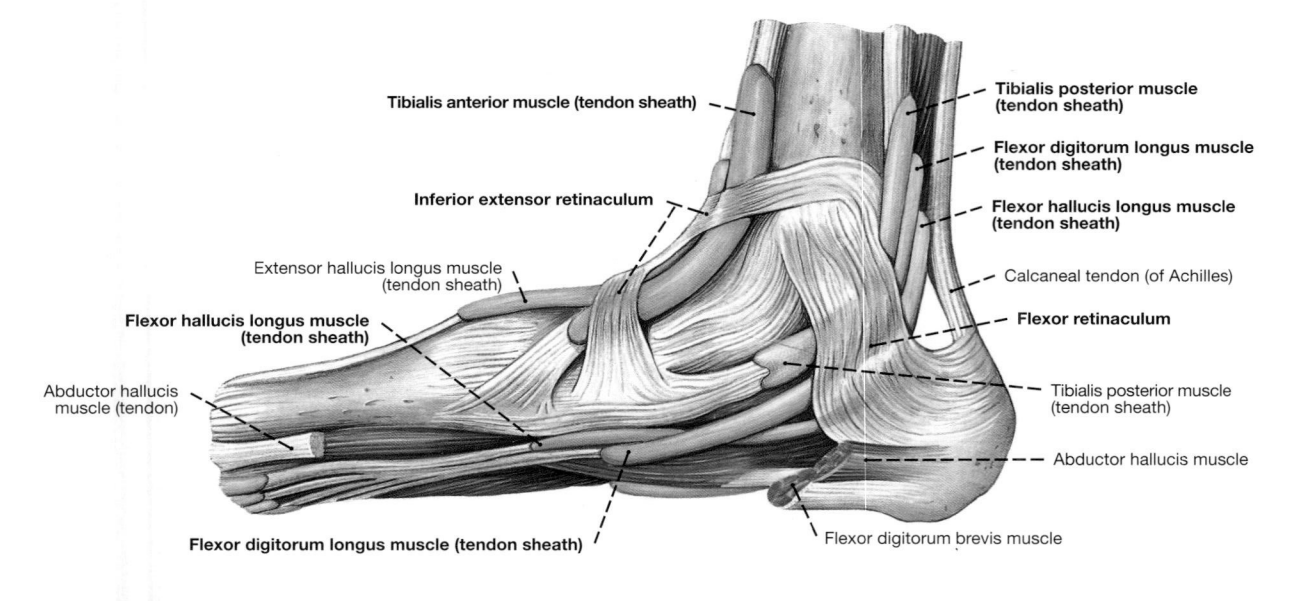

Fig. 534: Tendons and Synovial Sheaths: Right Dorsum of Foot and Ankle Region; Medial View

NOTE: 1)   from this medial view can be seen the synovial sheaths and tendons of the tibialis anterior and extensor hallucis longus on the dorsum of the foot, as well as the three tendons that course beneath the medial malleolus into the plantar aspect of the foot from the posterior compartment: tibialis posterior, the flexor digitorum longus and the flexor hallucis longus.

    2)   the bifurcating nature of the inferior extensor retinaculum, and the manner in which the flexor retinaculum secures the structures beneath the medial malleolus.

Figs. 533, 534

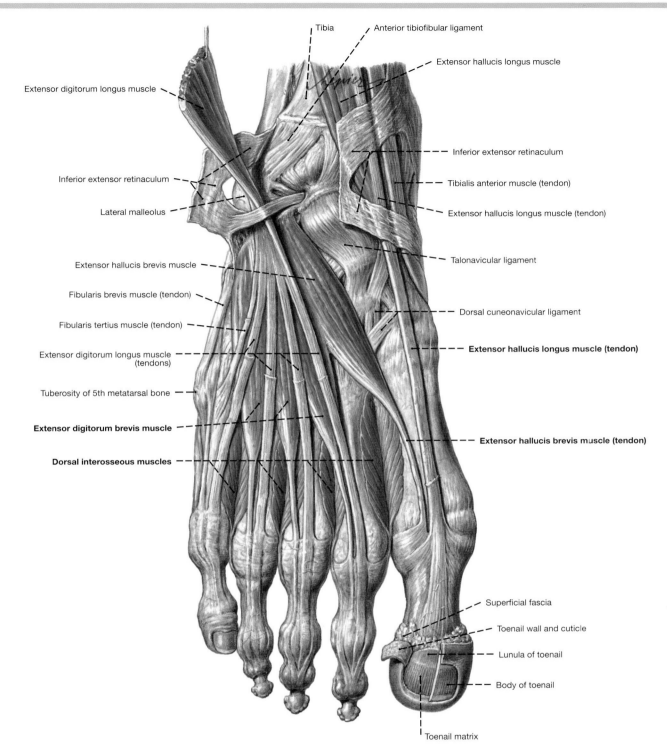

Fig. 535: Muscles and Tendons on the Dorsal Aspect of the Right Foot

Muscles on the Dorsum of the Foot

Muscle	Origin	Insertion	Innervation	Action
Extensor Hallucis Brevis Muscle	Dorsal aspect of the calcaneus bone	Lateral side of the base of the proximal phalanx of the great toe	Deep fibular nerve (L5, S1)	Helps to extend the proximal phalanx of the great toe
Extensor Digitorum Brevis Muscle	Dorsal and lateral aspect of the calcaneus bone	Lateral side of the tendons of the extensor digitorum longus muscle for the 2nd, 3rd and 4th toes	Deep fibular nerve (L5, S1)	Helps to extend the proximal phalanges of the 2nd, 3rd and 4th toes

Fig. 535 **V**

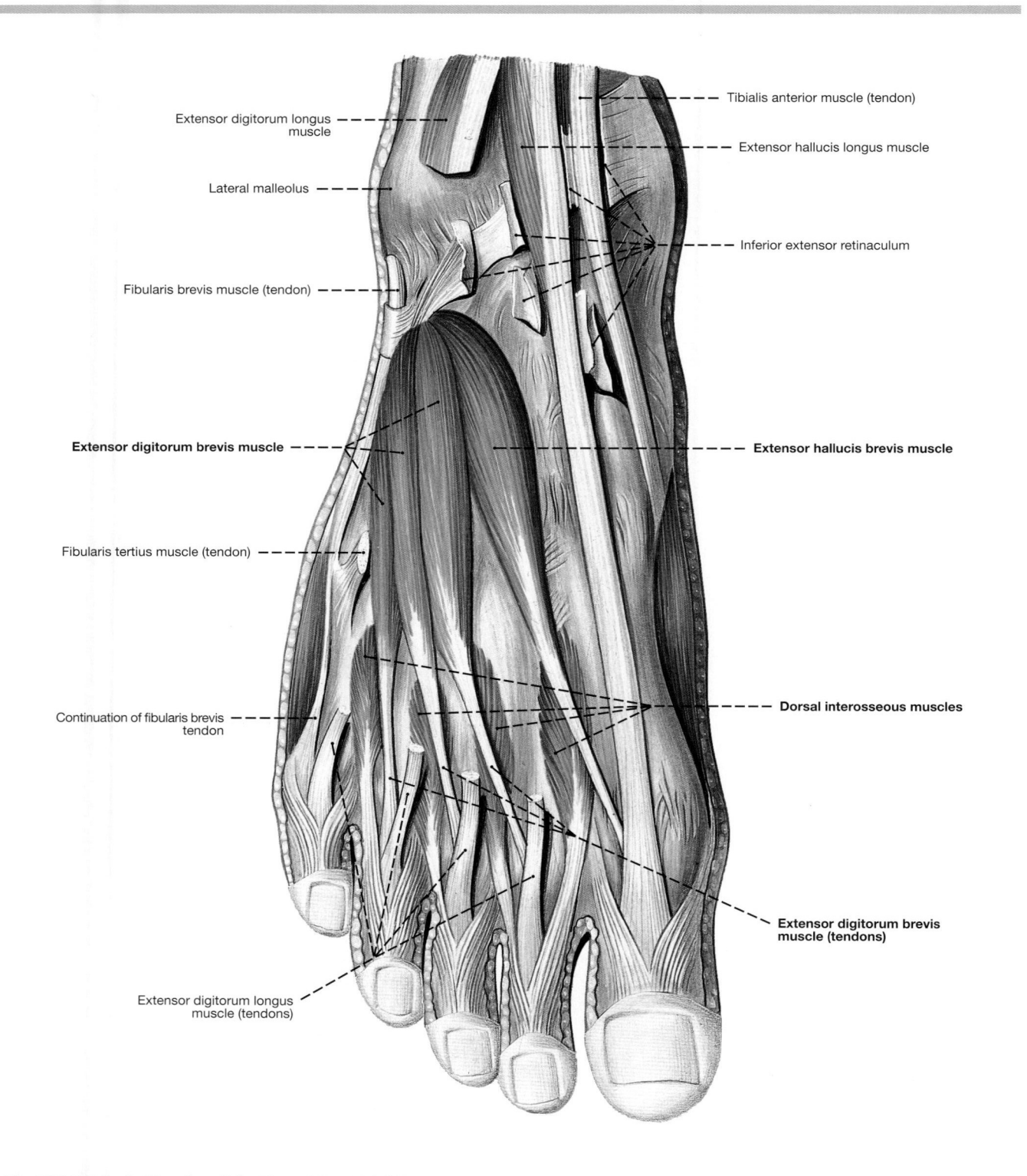

Extensor digitorum longus muscle

Lateral malleolus

Fibularis brevis muscle (tendon)

Extensor digitorum brevis muscle

Fibularis tertius muscle (tendon)

Continuation of fibularis brevis tendon

Extensor digitorum longus muscle (tendons)

Tibialis anterior muscle (tendon)

Extensor hallucis longus muscle

Inferior extensor retinaculum

Extensor hallucis brevis muscle

Dorsal interosseous muscles

Extensor digitorum brevis muscle (tendons)

Fig. 536: Intrinsic Muscles of the Dorsal Foot (right)

NOTE: 1) the inferior extensor retinaculum has been opened and the tendons of the extensor digitorum longus and fibularis tertius muscles have been severed.

    2) the **extensor hallucis brevis muscle** and the three small bellies of the **extensor digitorum brevis.** The delicate tendons of these muscles insert on the proximal phalanx of the medial four toes.

    3) the four **dorsal interosseous muscles.** These muscles abduct the toes from the longitudinal axis of the foot (down the middle of the 2nd toe). The first dorsal interosseous muscle inserts on the medial side of the 2nd toe, while the remaining three insert on the lateral side of the 2nd, 3rd, and 4th toes.

    4) although the dorsal interosseous muscles are usually designated as the deepest layer of muscles on the **plantar** aspect of the foot, they can best be seen on the dorsal surface following reflection of the tendons of the extensor digitorum longus and brevis muscles.

Fig. 536

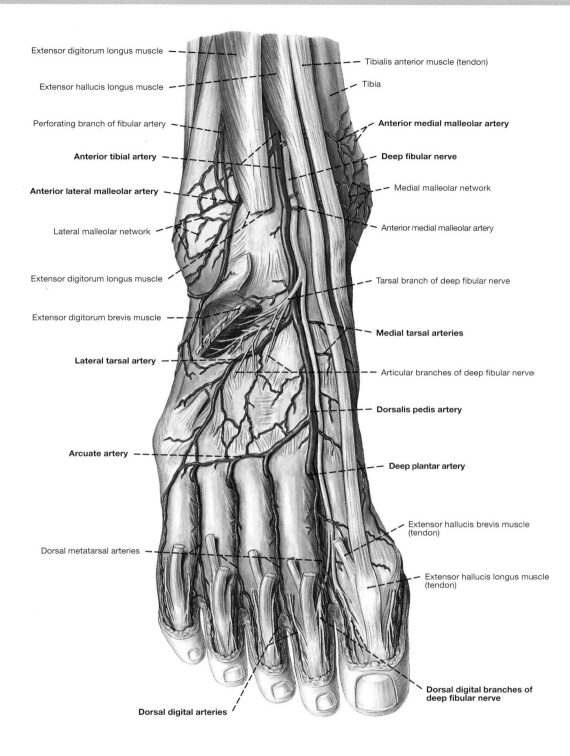

Extensor digitorum longus muscle

Extensor hallucis longus muscle

Perforating branch of fibular artery

Anterior tibial artery

Anterior lateral malleolar artery

Lateral malleolar network

Extensor digitorum longus muscle

Extensor digitorum brevis muscle

Lateral tarsal artery

Arcuate artery

Dorsal metatarsal arteries

Dorsal digital arteries

Tibialis anterior muscle (tendon)

Tibia

Anterior medial malleolar artery

Deep fibular nerve

Medial malleolar network

Anterior medial malleolar artery

Tarsal branch of deep fibular nerve

Medial tarsal arteries

Articular branches of deep fibular nerve

Dorsalis pedis artery

Deep plantar artery

Extensor hallucis brevis muscle (tendon)

Extensor hallucis longus muscle (tendon)

Dorsal digital branches of deep fibular nerve

Fig. 537: Deep Nerves and Arteries of the Dorsal Foot

NOTE: 1) the deeply coursing **anterior tibial artery** and **deep fibular nerve** and their branches have been exposed. They enter the foot between tendons of the extensor hallucis longus and extensor digitorum longus muscles.

2) the anterior tibial artery becomes the **dorsalis pedis artery** below the ankle joint. The **deep plantar artery** branches from the dorsalis pedis and perforates the tissue between the first two metatarsal bones to enter the plantar foot. Note also the **malleolar, tarsal, arcuate, dorsal metatarsal** and **digital arteries.**

3) the **deep fibular nerve** supplies the extensor hallucis and extensor digitorum brevis muscles in the foot and continues distally to terminate as two dorsal digital nerves, which supply sensory innervation to the adjacent sides of the great toe and the 2nd toe. Sensory innervation on the dorsal aspect of the other toes is derived from the **superficial fibular nerve.**

Fig. 537   **V**

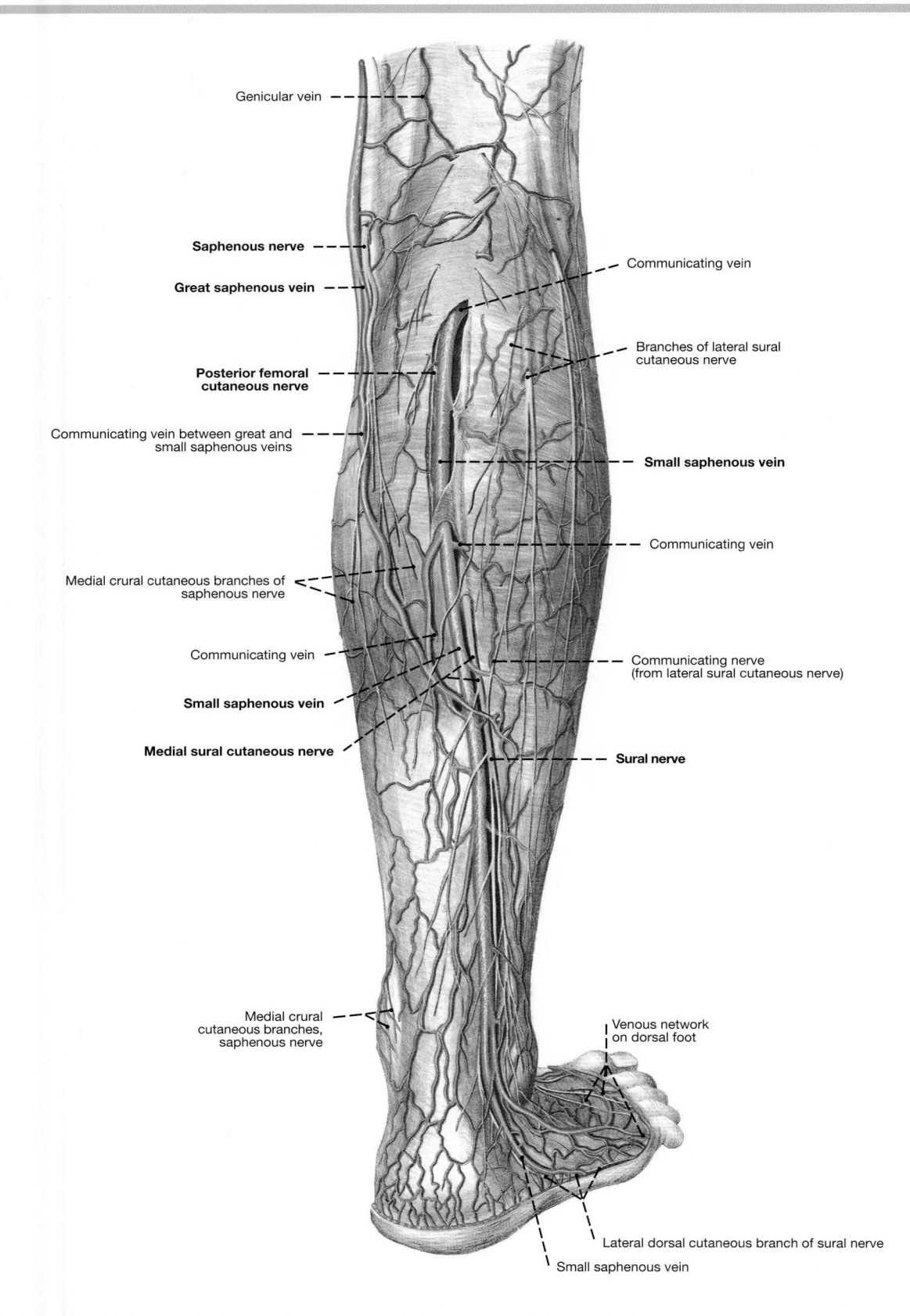

Genicular vein

Saphenous nerve

Great saphenous vein

Posterior femoral
cutaneous nerve

Communicating vein between great and
small saphenous veins

Medial crural cutaneous branches of
saphenous nerve

Communicating vein

Small saphenous vein

Medial sural cutaneous nerve

Medial crural
cutaneous branches,
saphenous nerve

Communicating vein

Branches of lateral sural
cutaneous nerve

Small saphenous vein

Communicating vein

Communicating nerve
(from lateral sural cutaneous nerve)

Sural nerve

Venous network
on dorsal foot

Lateral dorsal cutaneous branch of sural nerve

Small saphenous vein

Fig. 538: Superficial Veins and Cutaneous Nerves of the Posterior Leg and Dorsal Foot
NOTE: 1) the **small saphenous vein** forms on the dorsolateral aspect of the foot and ascends to the popliteal fossa, and superficial
communicating branches interconnect it to the great saphenous vein.

    2) the **sural nerve** is formed by the junction of a large branch, the medial sural cutaneous nerve (from the tibial nerve),
and the lateral sural cutaneous branches from the common fibular nerve. This Nerve supplies most of the posterolateral part of the
leg, and medial crural cutaneous branches of the **saphenous nerve** supply the posteromedial leg.

Fig. 538

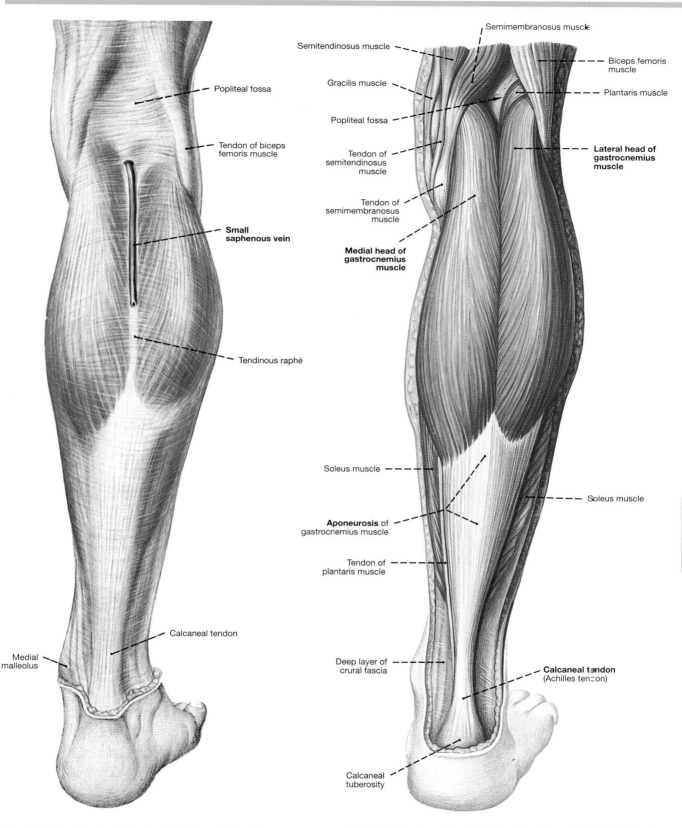

Fig. 539: Deep Fascia of the Leg (the Crural Fascia), Posterior View

NOTE: the deep fascia of the leg closely invests all the muscles between the knee and ankle and forms the fascial covering over the popliteal fossa. It is continuous above with the fascia lata of the thigh and below with the retinacula that bind the tendons close to the bones in the ankle region.

Fig. 540: Muscles of the Posterior Leg: Superficial Calf Muscles

NOTE: 1) the **gastrocnemius muscle** arises by two heads from the condyles and posterior surface of the femur. It inserts by means of the strong **calcaneal tendon** onto the tuberosity of the calcaneus.

2) the gastrocnemius is a strong plantar flexor of the foot and its continued action also flexes the leg at the knee.

PLATE 358   **Knee, Calf, and Foot: Muscles and Tendons, Medial View**

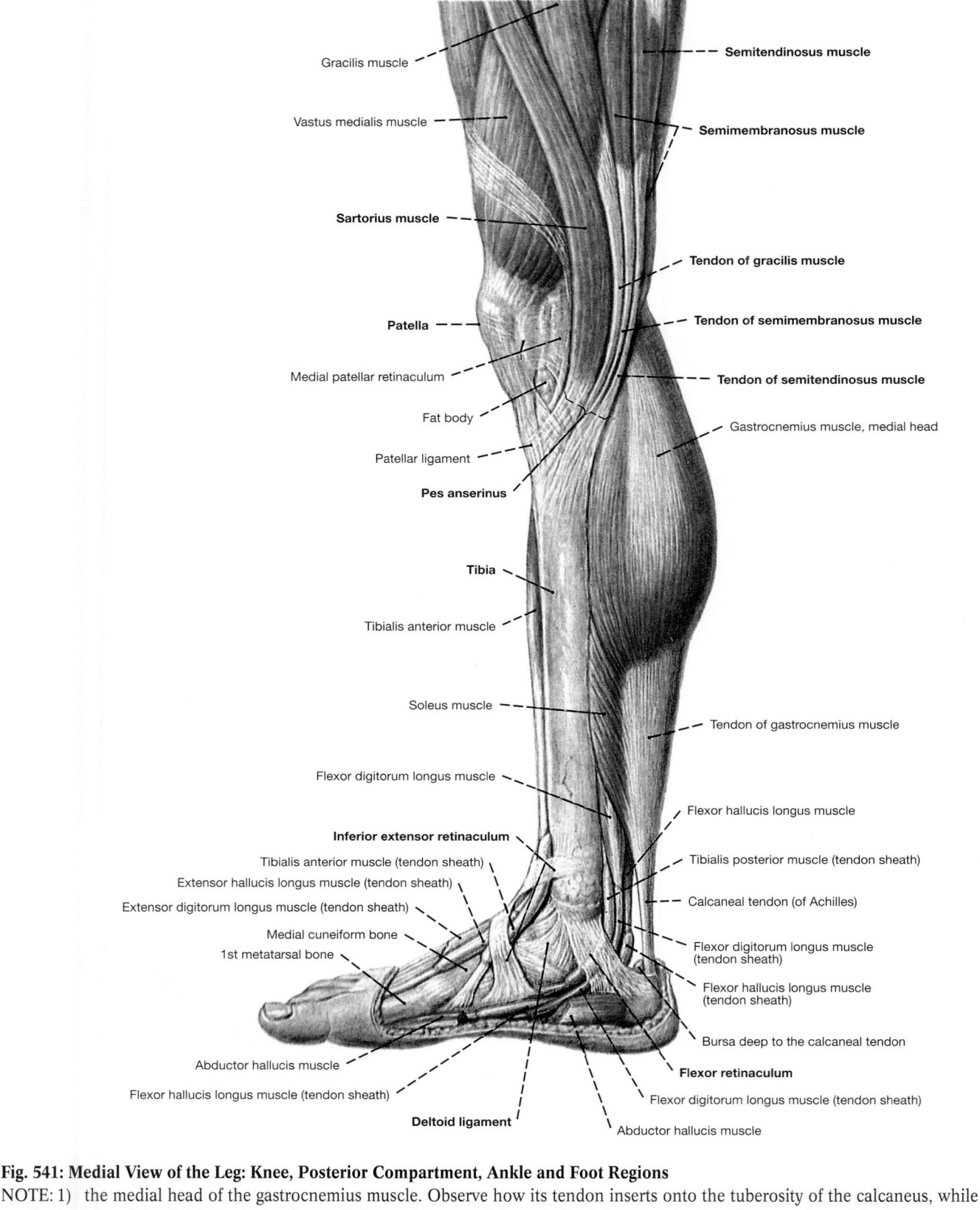

Gracilis muscle

Vastus medialis muscle

Sartorius muscle

Patella

Medial patellar retinaculum

Fat body

Patellar ligament

Pes anserinus

Tibia

Tibialis anterior muscle

Soleus muscle

Flexor digitorum longus muscle

Inferior extensor retinaculum

Tibialis anterior muscle (tendon sheath)

Extensor hallucis longus muscle (tendon sheath)

Extensor digitorum longus muscle (tendon sheath)

Medial cuneiform bone

1st metatarsal bone

Abductor hallucis muscle

Flexor hallucis longus muscle (tendon sheath)

Deltoid ligament

Semitendinosus muscle

Semimembranosus muscle

Tendon of gracilis muscle

Tendon of semimembranosus muscle

Tendon of semitendinosus muscle

Gastrocnemius muscle, medial head

Tendon of gastrocnemius muscle

Flexor hallucis longus muscle

Tibialis posterior muscle (tendon sheath)

Calcaneal tendon (of Achilles)

Flexor digitorum longus muscle
(tendon sheath)

Flexor hallucis longus muscle
(tendon sheath)

Bursa deep to the calcaneal tendon

Flexor retinaculum

Flexor digitorum longus muscle (tendon sheath)

Abductor hallucis muscle

Fig. 541: Medial View of the Leg: Knee, Posterior Compartment, Ankle and Foot Regions
NOTE: 1) the medial head of the gastrocnemius muscle. Observe how its tendon inserts onto the tuberosity of the calcaneus, while the tendons of the tibialis posterior, flexor digitorum longus and flexor hallucis longus enter the plantar surface of the foot.

2) the flexor retinaculum holds these deep posterior compartment muscles close to the bone, thereby increasing their efficiency when they contract. Without these retinacula muscular contraction would result in a bowing of the tendons and a loss of power.

3) the tendons of the sartorius, gracilis, and semitendinosus form the so-called pes anserinus (goose's foot). This tendinous formation helps protect the medial aspect of the knee, while the tendon of the semimembranosus helps reinforce the capsule of the knee joint posteriorly.

Fig. 541

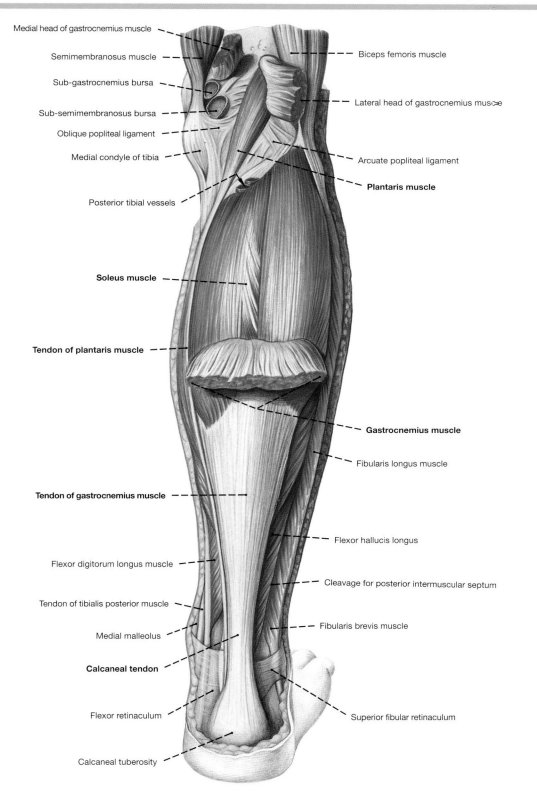

Medial head of gastrocnemius muscle

Semimembranosus muscle

Sub-gastrocnemius bursa

Sub-semimembranosus bursa

Oblique popliteal ligament

Medial condyle of tibia

Posterior tibial vessels

Soleus muscle

Tendon of plantaris muscle

Tendon of gastrocnemius muscle

Flexor digitorum longus muscle

Tendon of tibialis posterior muscle

Medial malleolus

Calcaneal tendon

Flexor retinaculum

Calcaneal tuberosity

Biceps femoris muscle

Lateral head of gastrocnemius muscle

Arcuate popliteal ligament

Plantaris muscle

Gastrocnemius muscle

Fibularis longus muscle

Flexor hallucis longus

Cleavage for posterior intermuscular septum

Fibularis brevis muscle

Superior fibular retinaculum

Fig. 542: Muscles of the Posterior Leg: Soleus and Plantaris Muscles

NOTE: 1)   both heads of the gastrocnemius muscle have been severed. Observe the stumps of their origins from the femur above and the lower flap reflected downward to uncover the **soleus** and **plantaris muscles.**

2)   the soleus muscle is broad and thick and arises from the posterior surface of the fibula, the intermuscular septum and the dorsal aspect of the tibia. Its fibers join the calcaneal tendon and insert in common with the gastrocnemius muscle.

3)   the small plantaris muscle has a long thin tendon that also joins the calcaneal tendon. Although the function of the plantaris is of little significance, its long tendon can be used by surgeons when that type of tissue is required.

Fig. 542   **V**

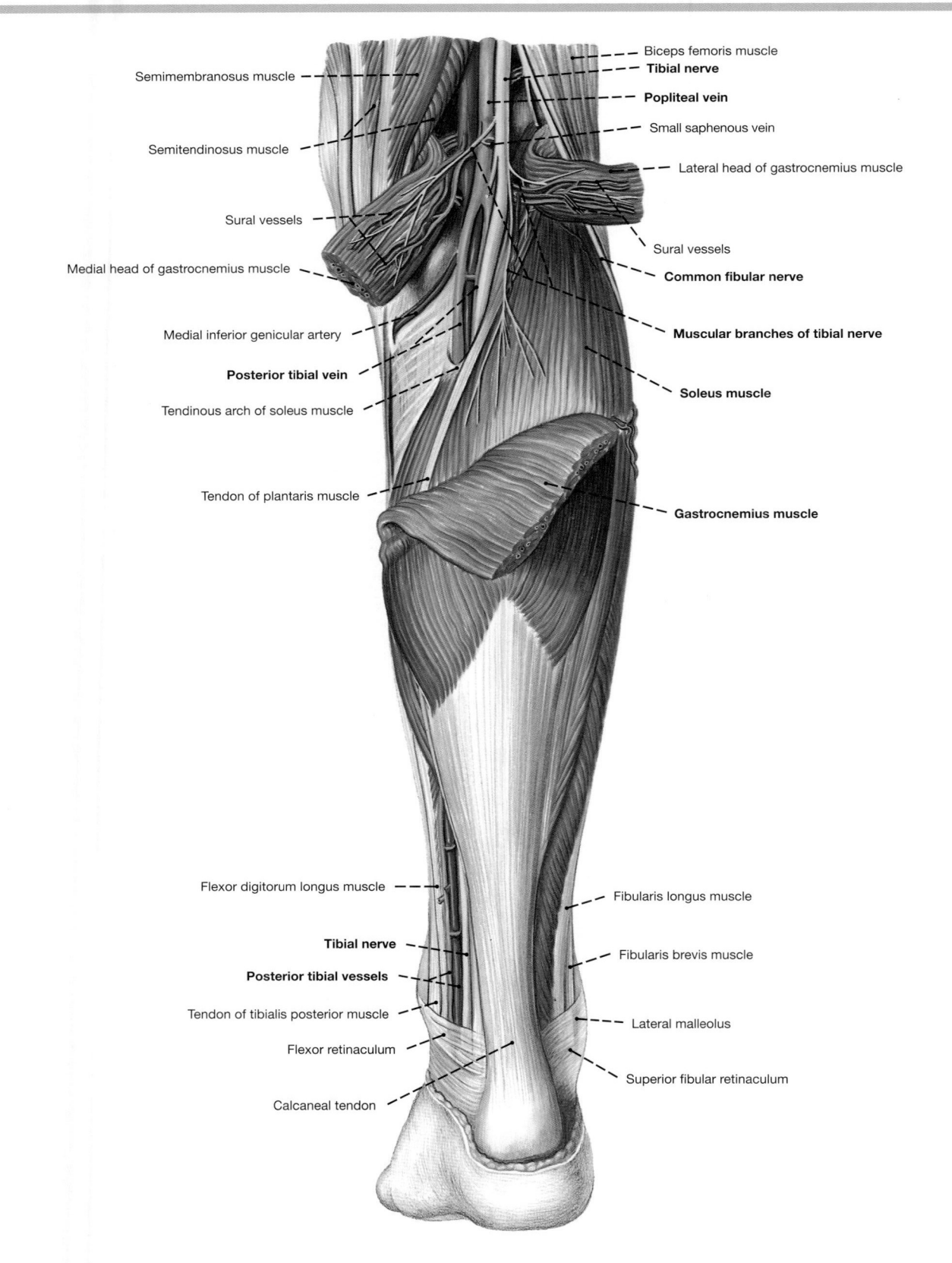

Semimembranosus muscle

Semitendinosus muscle

Sural vessels

Medial head of gastrocnemius muscle

Medial inferior genicular artery

Posterior tibial vein

Tendinous arch of soleus muscle

Tendon of plantaris muscle

Flexor digitorum longus muscle

Tibial nerve

Posterior tibial vessels

Tendon of tibialis posterior muscle

Flexor retinaculum

Calcaneal tendon

Biceps femoris muscle
Tibial nerve
Popliteal vein
Small saphenous vein
Lateral head of gastrocnemius muscle
Sural vessels
Common fibular nerve
Muscular branches of tibial nerve
Soleus muscle
Gastrocnemius muscle
Fibularis longus muscle
Fibularis brevis muscle
Lateral malleolus
Superior fibular retinaculum

Fig. 543: Nerves and Vessels of the Posterior Leg Above and Below the Soleus Muscle

NOTE: 1) the popliteal vessels and tibial nerve, descending from the popliteal fossa into the posterior compartment and the leg, commence to course medially in a gradual manner so that at the ankle they lie behind the medial malleolus.

2) from the popliteal fossa sural branches of the popliteal artery and muscular branches of the tibial nerve descend to supply the gastrocnemius pond soleus muscles. These neurovascular structures course through a tendinous arch in dise soleus muscle and descend deep to the soleus and become superficial again several inches above the medial malleolus.

Fig. 543

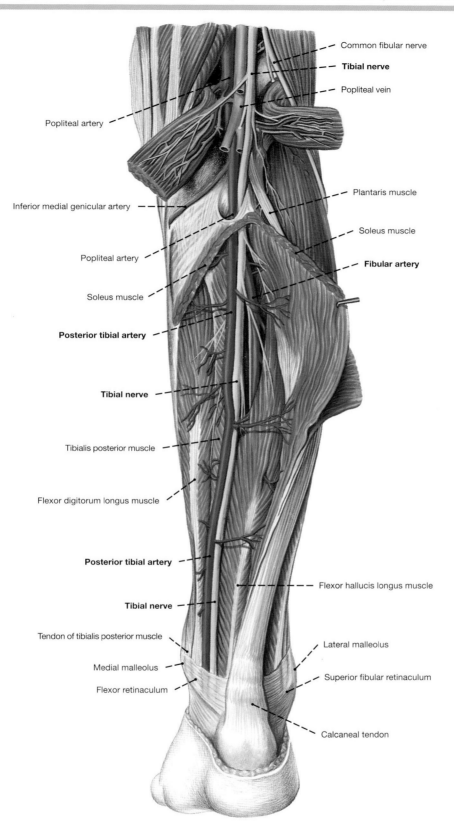

Common fibular nerve

Tibial nerve

Popliteal vein

Popliteal artery

Plantaris muscle

Inferior medial genicular artery

Soleus muscle

Popliteal artery

Fibular artery

Soleus muscle

Posterior tibial artery

Tibial nerve

Tibialis posterior muscle

Flexor digitorum longus muscle

Posterior tibial artery

Flexor hallucis longus muscle

Tibial nerve

Tendon of tibialis posterior muscle

Lateral malleolus

Medial malleolus

Superior fibular retinaculum

Flexor retinaculum

Calcaneal tendon

Fig. 544: Nerves and Vessels of the Right Posterior Leg, Intermediate Dissection

NOTE: 1)   the soleus muscle has been severed and reflected laterally, exposing the course of the tibial artery and posterior tibial nerve
as far as the medial malleolus.

2)   this vessel and nerve descend in the leg between the superficial and deep muscles of the posterior compartment and they
lie between the flexor hallucis longus and the flexor digitorum longus and dorsal to the tibialis posterior muscle.

Fig. 544   **V**

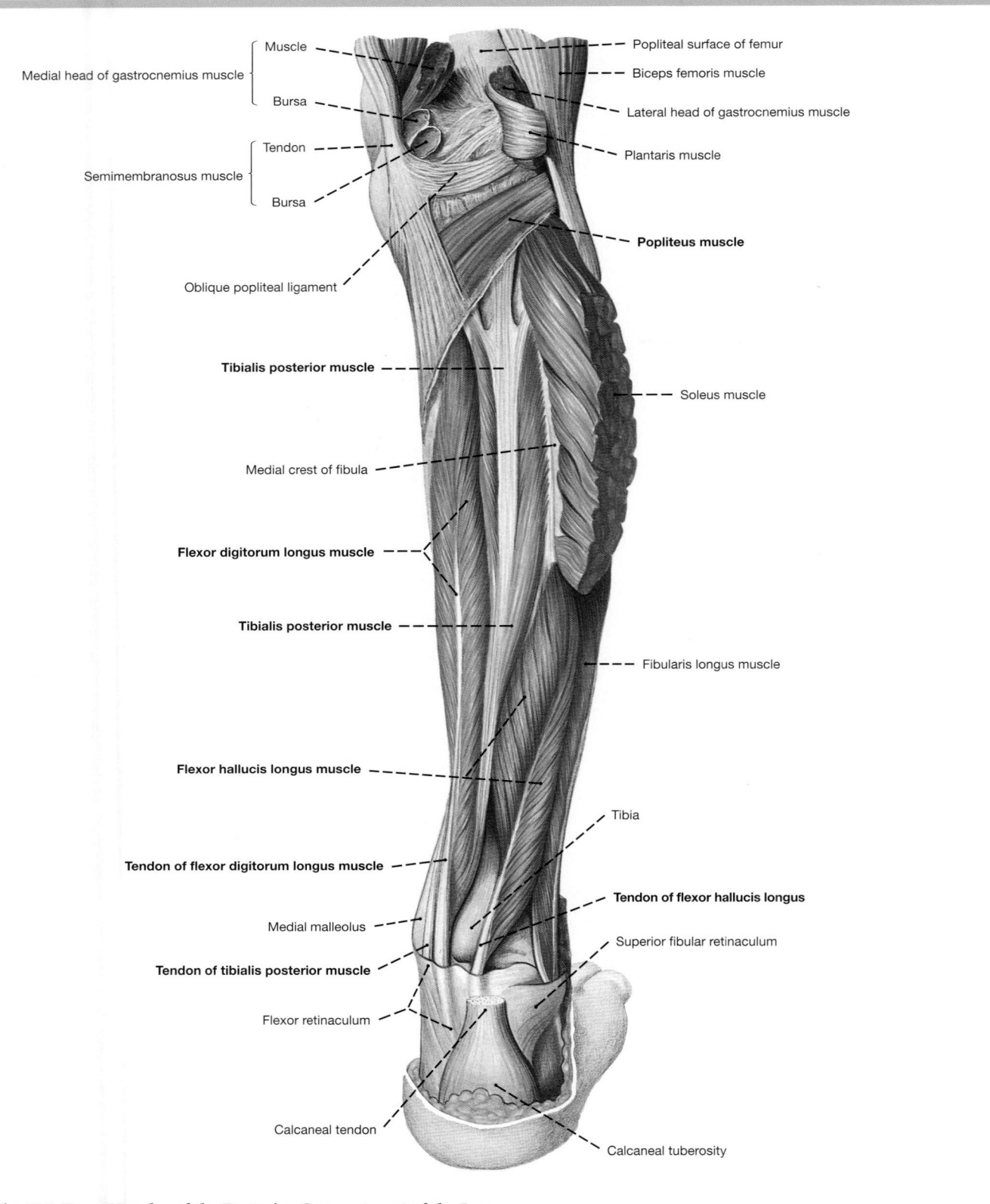

Medial head of gastrocnemius muscle
- Muscle
- Bursa

Semimembranosus muscle
- Tendon
- Bursa

Oblique popliteal ligament

Tibialis posterior muscle

Medial crest of fibula

Flexor digitorum longus muscle

Tibialis posterior muscle

Flexor hallucis longus muscle

Tendon of flexor digitorum longus muscle

Medial malleolus

Tendon of tibialis posterior muscle

Flexor retinaculum

Calcaneal tendon

Popliteal surface of femur

Biceps femoris muscle

Lateral head of gastrocnemius muscle

Plantaris muscle

Popliteus muscle

Soleus muscle

Fibularis longus muscle

Tibia

Tendon of flexor hallucis longus

Superior fibular retinaculum

Calcaneal tuberosity

Fig. 545: Deep Muscles of the Posterior Compartment of the Leg

NOTE: 1)   the four deep posterior compartment muscles are a) the **popliteus,** b) the **flexor digitorum longus,** c) the **tibialis posterior** and d) the **flexor hallucis longus.**

2)   the *popliteus* is a femorotibial muscle and it tends to rotate the leg medially, however, when the tibia is fixed and the knee joint is locked, this muscle rotates the femur laterally on the tibia and thereby it "unlocks" the knee joint.

3)   the other three muscles are cruropedal muscles, and as a group, they invert the foot, flex the toes, and assist in plantarflexion at the ankle joint.

4)   at the ankle region, the tendon of the tibialis posterior is closest to bone behind the medial malleolus. Most lateral is the tendon of the flexor hallucis longus, with the tendon of the flexor digitorum longus in between the other two.

Fig. 545

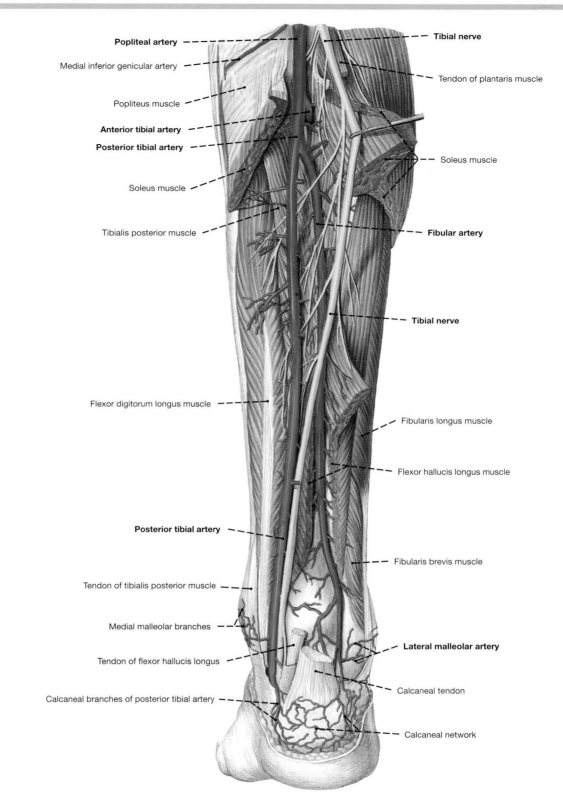

Popliteal artery

Medial inferior genicular artery

Popliteus muscle

Anterior tibial artery

Posterior tibial artery

Soleus muscle

Tibialis posterior muscle

Flexor digitorum longus muscle

Posterior tibial artery

Tendon of tibialis posterior muscle

Medial malleolar branches

Tendon of flexor hallucis longus

Calcaneal branches of posterior tibial artery

Tibial nerve

Tendon of plantaris muscle

Soleus muscle

Fibular artery

Tibial nerve

Fibularis longus muscle

Flexor hallucis longus muscle

Fibularis brevis muscle

Lateral malleolar artery

Calcaneal tendon

Calcaneal network

Fig. 546: Deep Nerves and Arteries of the Posterior Compartment of the Leg

NOTE: 1)   the soleus muscle was resected and the tibial nerve pulled laterally. Observe the branching of the **fibular artery** from the posterior tibial, and its descending course toward the lateral malleolus.

   2)   in the popliteal fossa, the tibial nerve courses superficial to the popliteal artery, whereas at the ankle, the posterior tibial artery is superficial to the tibial nerve.

   3)   behind the medial malleolus, the neurovascular structures are located between the tendons of the flexor digitorum longus and flexor hallucis longus.

Fig. 5-6   **V**

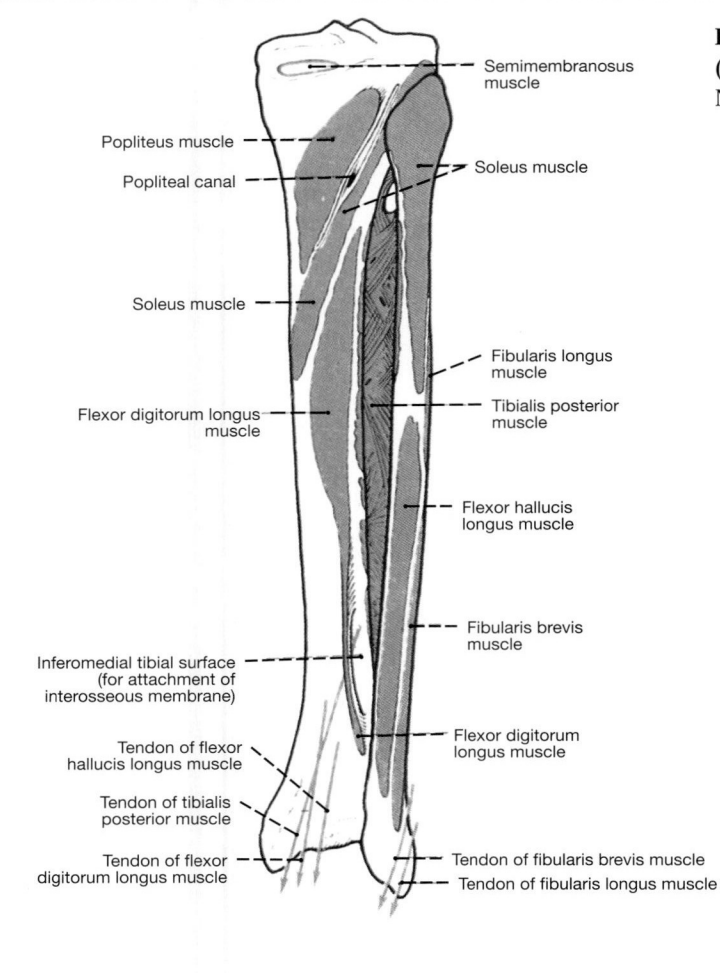

Popliteus muscle

Popliteal canal

Soleus muscle

Flexor digitorum longus
muscle

Inferomedial tibial surface
(for attachment of
interosseous membrane)

Tendon of flexor
hallucis longus muscle

Tendon of tibialis
posterior muscle

Tendon of flexor
digitorum longus muscle

Semimembranosus
muscle

Soleus muscle

Fibularis longus
muscle

Tibialis posterior
muscle

Flexor hallucis
longus muscle

Fibularis brevis
muscle

Flexor digitorum
longus muscle

Tendon of fibularis brevis muscle

Tendon of fibularis longus muscle

Fig. 547: Muscle Attachments on the Right Tibia and Fibula (Posterior Surface)

NOTE: 1) of the posterior compartment muscles, only the gastrocnemius and plantaris do not attach to the posterior surface of the tibia, fibula or interosseous membrane.

2) nearly the entire posterior surface of the fibula serves for the origin of muscles. The **soleus** arises from the upper $1/3$rd of the fibula and along the soleal line of the tibia. Inferior to the soleus the **flexor hallucis longus** arises principally from the fibula, while the **flexor digitorum longus** arises primarily from the tibia.

3) the **tibialis posterior** is interposed between the flexors hallucis longus and digitorum longus and arises, for the most part, from the interosseous membrane.

4) the arrows indicate the course of the tendons into the foot from the posterior surface. The tendon of the tibialis posterior crosses from lateral to medial beneath the tendon of the flexor digitorum longus and enters the foot immediately behind the medial malleolus.

Muscles of the Posterior Compartment of the Leg
Superficial Group

Muscle	Origin	Insertion	Innervation	Action
Gastrocnemius Muscle	MEDIAL HEAD Medial epicondyle of the femur LATERAL HEAD Lateral epicondyle of the femur	Posterior surface of the calcaneus by means of the calcaneal tendon	Tibial nerve (S1, S2)	Plantarflexes the foot; flexes the leg at knee joint; tends to supinate the foot
Soleus Muscle	Posterior surface of head and upper $1/3$rd or body of fibula; soleal line and medial border of tibia	Joins the tendon of the gastrocnemius to insert on the calcaneus by means of calcaneal tendon	Tibial nerve (S1, S2)	Plantarflexes the foot; important as a postural muscle during ordinary standing
Plantaris Muscle	Posterior aspect of lateral epicondyle of femur and from the oblique popliteal ligament	Into the calcaneal tendon with the gastrocnemius and soleus muscles	Tibial nerve (S1, S2)	Assists the gastrocnemius in plantarflexion of the foot and flexing the leg (weak action)

Deep Group

Muscle	Origin	Insertion	Innervation	Action
Popliteus Muscle	Lateral epicondyle of the femur; the lateral meniscus of the knee joint	Posterior surface of the body of the tibia proximal to the soleal line	Tibial nerve (L4, L5, S1)	Flexes and medially rotates the tibia when femur is fixed; laterally rotates the femur to unlock the knee joint when the tibia is fixed
Tibialis Posterior Muscle	Posterior surface of interosseous membrane; posterior surface of tibia and medial surface of the fibula	Tuberosity of the navicular bone; slips to calcaneus, the 3 cuneiforms, the cuboid and the 2nd, 3rd and 4th metatarsal bones	Tibial nerve (L5, S1)	Plantarflexes the foot; inverts and adducts the foot (tends to supinate the foot)

Fig. 547

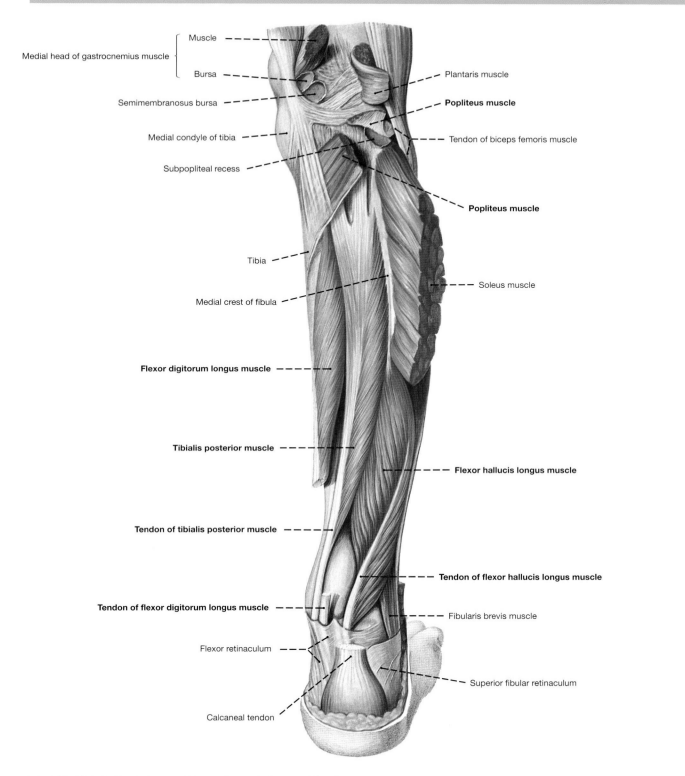

Medial head of gastrocnemius muscle
Muscle
Bursa
Semimembranosus bursa
Medial condyle of tibia
Subpopliteal recess
Tibia
Medial crest of fibula
Flexor digitorum longus muscle
Tibialis posterior muscle
Tendon of tibialis posterior muscle
Tendon of flexor digitorum longus muscle
Flexor retinaculum
Calcaneal tendon

Plantaris muscle
Popliteus muscle
Tendon of biceps femoris muscle
Popliteus muscle
Soleus muscle
Flexor hallucis longus muscle
Tendon of flexor hallucis longus muscle
Fibularis brevis muscle
Superior fibular retinaculum

Fig. 548: Tibialis Posterior and Flexor Hallucis Longus Muscles
Muscles of the Posterior Compartment of the Leg (Cont.)

Muscle	Origin	Insertion	Innervation	Action
Flexor Digitorum Longus Muscle	Posterior surface of tibia and fascia over tibialis posterior	Bases of the distal phalanx of the four lateral toes	Tibial nerve (S1, S2)	Flexes distal phalanx of lateral 4 toes; plantarflexes and supinates the foot
Flexor Hallucis Longus Muscle	Lower $^2/_3$rds of the posterior fibula and lower part of the interosseous membrane	Base of the distal phalanx of the large toe (hallux)	Tibial nerve (S1, S2)	Flexes distal phalanx of large toe; plantarflexes and supinates the foot

Fig. 548   **V**

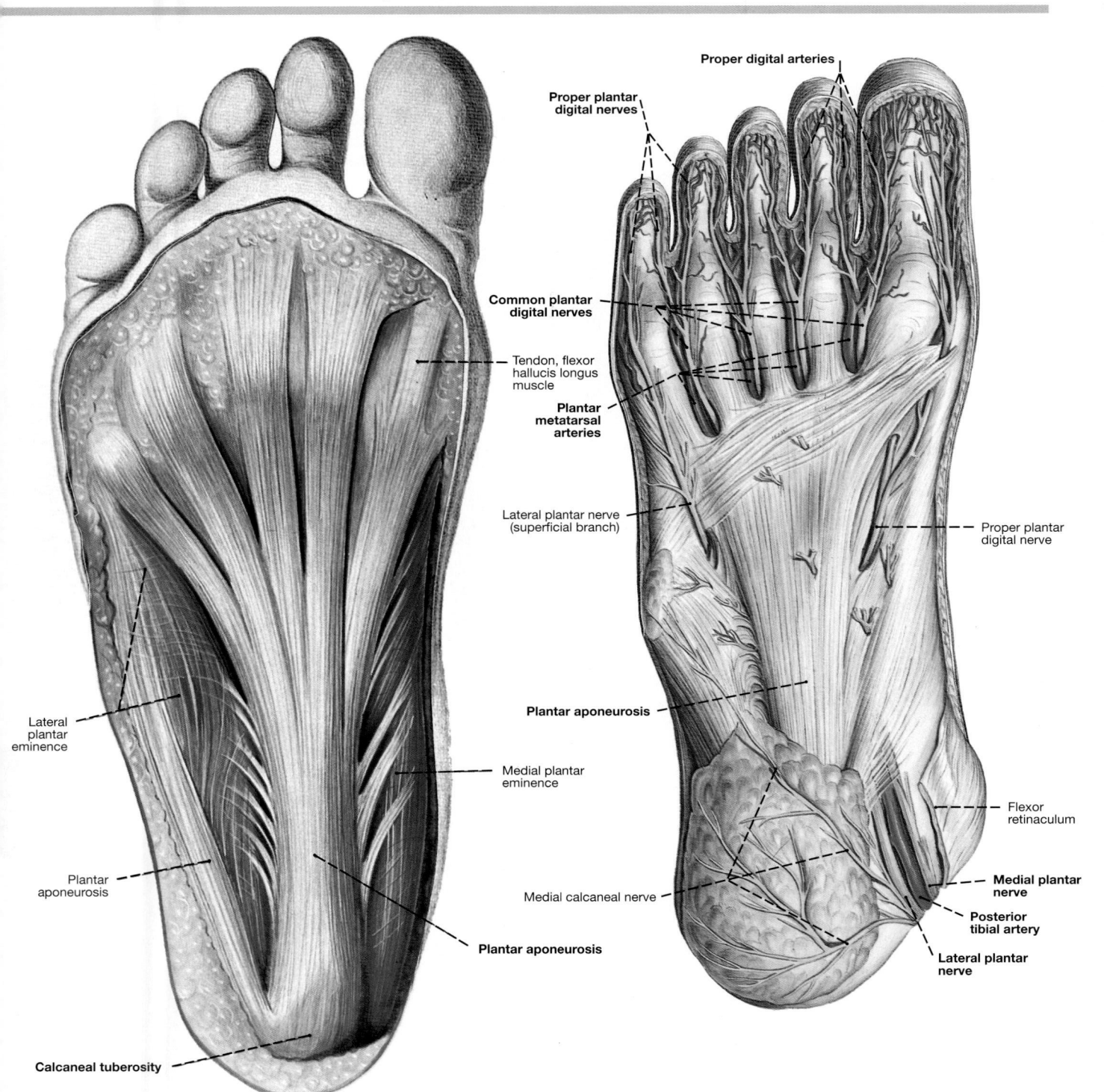

Fig. 549: Sole of the Right Foot: Plantar Aponeurosis
NOTE: 1)   the **plantar aponeurosis** stretching along the sole of the foot. Similar to the palmar aponeurosis in the hand, the plantar aponeurosis is a thickened layer of deep fascia serving a protective function to underlying muscles, vessels and nerves.

2)   the longitudinal orientation of the plantar aponeurosis, and its attachment behind to the calcaneal tuberosity. The aponeurosis divides distally into digital slips, one to each toe. At the margins, fibers partially cover the medial and lateral plantar eminences.

Fig. 550: Sole of the Right Foot: Superficial Nerves and Arteries
NOTE: 1)   the **medial** and **lateral plantar nerves** and **posterior tibial artery** as they enter the foot behind the medial malleolus and then immediately course beneath the plantar aponeurosis toward the digits. Cutaneous branches of the nerves penetrate the aponeurosis to supply the overlying skin and fascia.

2)   between digital slips of the plantar aponeurosis, the vessels and nerves course superficially toward the toes. **Metatarsal arteries** and **common plantar digital nerves** divide to supply adjacent portions of the toes as **proper plantar digital arteries** and **nerves.**

Figs. 549, 550

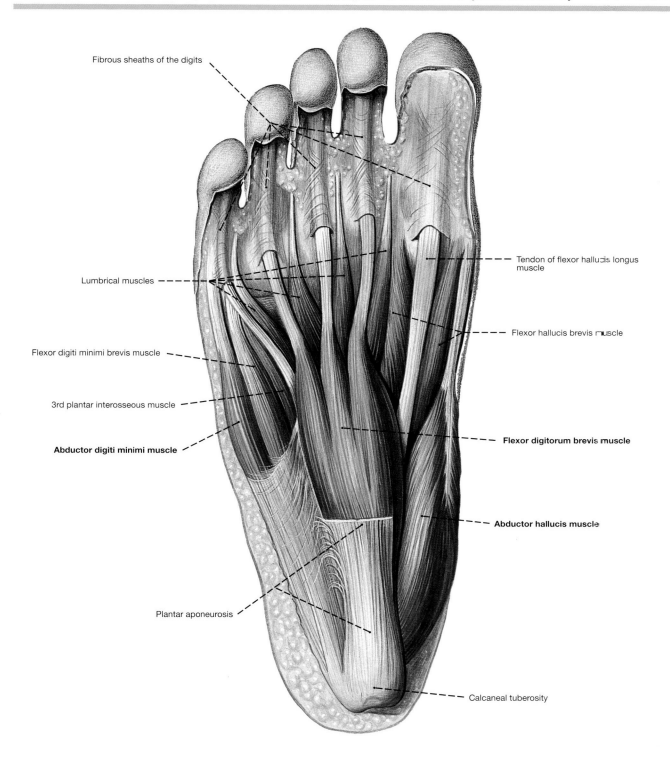

Fibrous sheaths of the digits

Lumbrical muscles

Flexor digiti minimi brevis muscle

3rd plantar interosseous muscle

Abductor digiti minimi muscle

Plantar aponeurosis

Tendon of flexor hallucis longus muscle

Flexor hallucis brevis muscle

Flexor digitorum brevis muscle

Abductor hallucis muscle

Calcaneal tuberosity

Fig. 551: Sole of the Right Foot: First Layer of Plantar Muscles

NOTE: 1)   with most of the plantar aponeurosis removed, three muscles comprising the first layer of plantar muscles are exposed. These are the **abductor hallucis,** the **flexor digitorum brevis,** and the **abductor digiti minimi.**

2)   all three muscles of the first layer arise from the tuberosity of the calcaneus. The abductor hallucis inserts on the proximal phalanx of the large toe. The flexor digitorum brevis separates into four tendons that insert onto the middle phalanges of the four lateral toes. The abductor digiti minimi inserts on the proximal phalanx of the small toe.

3)   the terminal parts of the tendons of the short and long flexors of the toes course within osseous-aponeurotic canals to their insertions on bone.

4)   these canals are covered inferiorly by **digital fibrous sheaths** that arch over the tendons and attach to the sides of the phalanges. Within the canals, **synovial sheaths** are closely reflected around the tendons, which allow for their movement upon muscular contraction.

Fig. 551   **V**

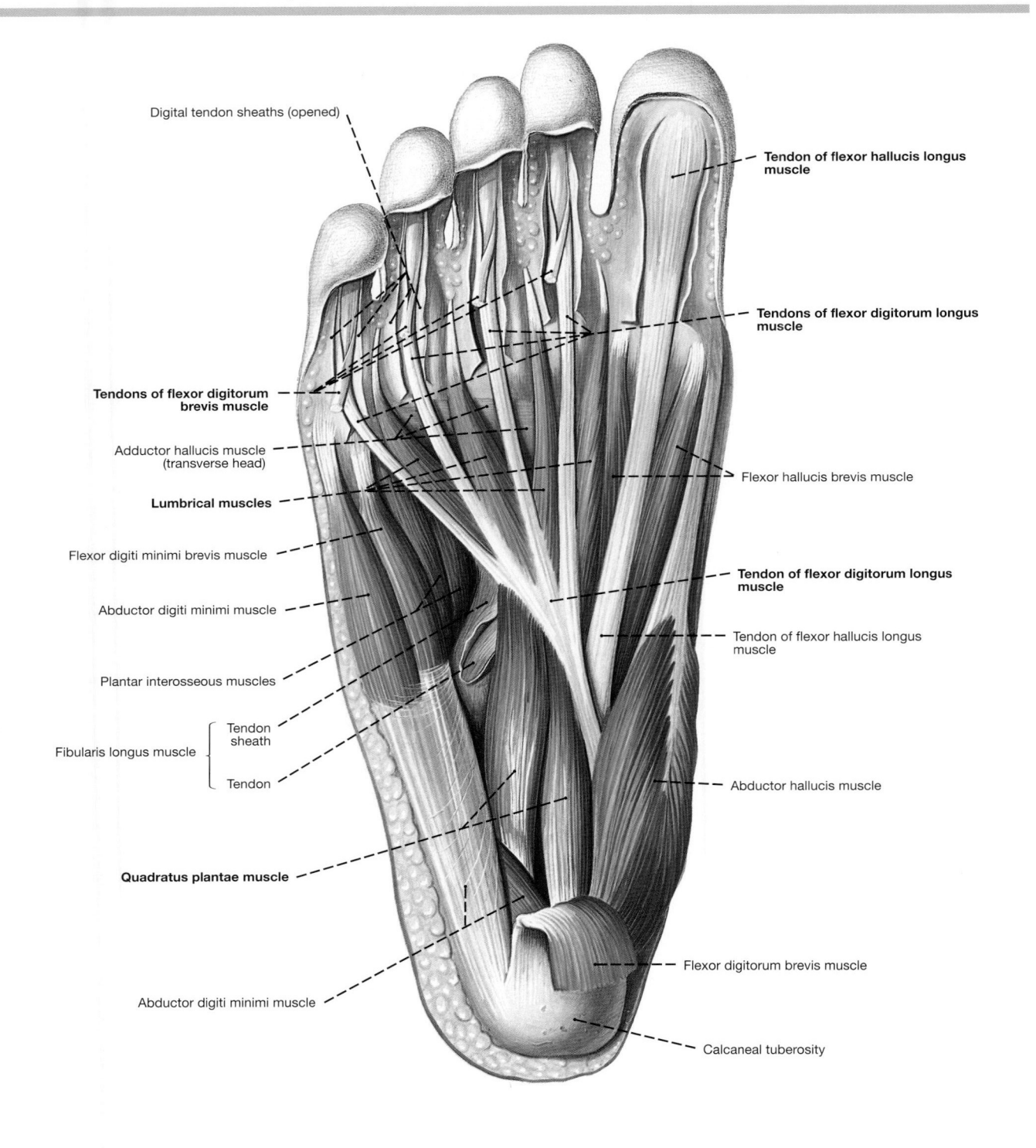

Digital tendon sheaths (opened)

Tendon of flexor hallucis longus muscle

Tendons of flexor digitorum longus muscle

Tendons of flexor digitorum brevis muscle

Adductor hallucis muscle (transverse head)

Flexor hallucis brevis muscle

Lumbrical muscles

Flexor digiti minimi brevis muscle

Tendon of flexor digitorum longus muscle

Abductor digiti minimi muscle

Tendon of flexor hallucis longus muscle

Plantar interosseous muscles

Fibularis longus muscle — Tendon sheath / Tendon

Abductor hallucis muscle

Quadratus plantae muscle

Flexor digitorum brevis muscle

Abductor digiti minimi muscle

Calcaneal tuberosity

Fig. 552: Sole of the Right Foot: Second Layer of Plantar Muscles

NOTE: 1) the tendons of the flexor digitorum brevis muscle were severed and removed, thereby exposing the underlying tendons of the **flexor digitorum longus muscle.**

2) the muscles of the **second layer** in the plantar foot include the **quadratus plantae muscle** and the four **lumbrical muscles.** The quadratus plantae arises by two heads from the calcaneus and inserts into the tendon of the flexor digitorum longus muscle.

3) the four lumbrical muscles arise from the tendons of the flexor digitorum longus muscle. They insert on the medial aspect of the first phalanx of the lateral four toes as well as on the dorsal extensor hoods of the toes.

4) the quadratus plantae muscle helps align the pull of the tendons of the flexor digitorum longus by straightening the diagonal vector of the long tendon.

Fig. 552

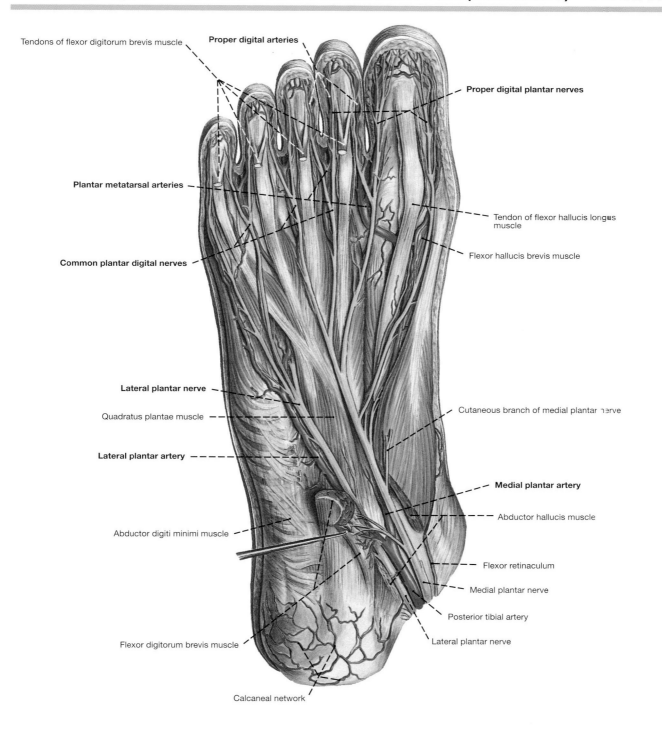

Tendons of flexor digitorum brevis muscle

Proper digital arteries

Proper digital plantar nerves

Plantar metatarsal arteries

Tendon of flexor hallucis longus muscle

Flexor hallucis brevis muscle

Common plantar digital nerves

Lateral plantar nerve

Quadratus plantae muscle

Cutaneous branch of medial plantar nerve

Lateral plantar artery

Medial plantar artery

Abductor hallucis muscle

Abductor digiti minimi muscle

Flexor retinaculum

Medial plantar nerve

Posterior tibial artery

Flexor digitorum brevis muscle

Lateral plantar nerve

Calcaneal network

Fig. 553: Sole of the Right Foot: the Plantar Nerves and Arteries

NOTE: 1)   while the tibial nerve divides into **medial** and **lateral plantar nerves** just below the medial malleolus, the posterior tibial artery enters the plantar surface of the foot as a single vessel and then divides into **medial** and **lateral plantar arteries** beneath or at the medial border of the abductor hallucis muscle.

2)   the lateral plantar nerve supplies the lateral 1½ digits with cutaneous innervation, while the medial plantar nerve supplies the medial 3½ digits. Observe the formation of the **common plantar digital nerves,** which then divide into the **proper plantar digital nerves.**

3)   the main trunks of the plantar vessels and nerves cross the sole of the foot from medial to lateral deep to the flexor digitorum brevis and abductor hallucis muscles (first layer), but superficial to the quadratus plantae and lumbrical muscles (second layer).

Fig. 553   **V**

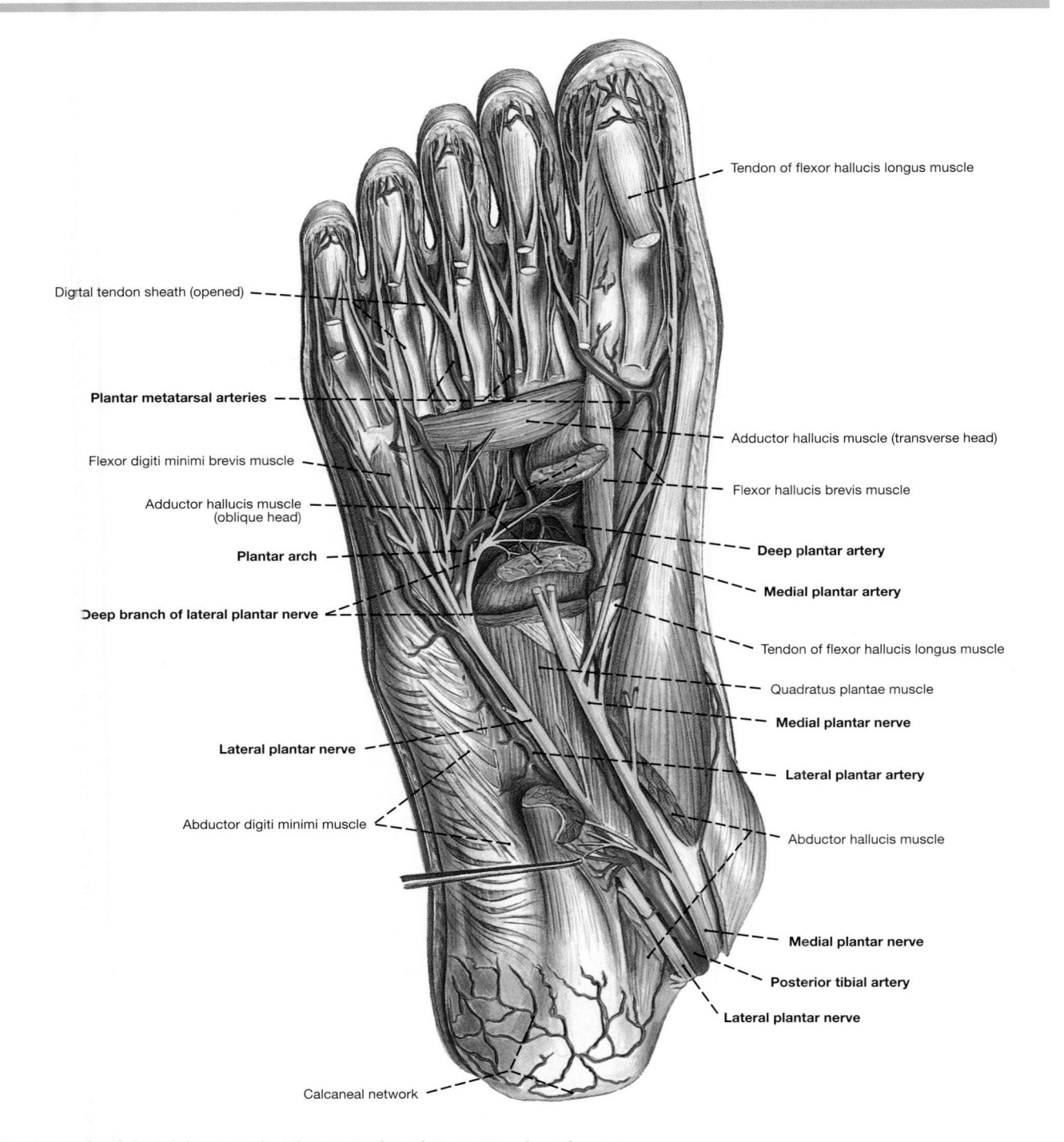

Tendon of flexor hallucis longus muscle

Digital tendon sheath (opened)

Plantar metatarsal arteries

Flexor digiti minimi brevis muscle

Adductor hallucis muscle (oblique head)

Plantar arch

Deep branch of lateral plantar nerve

Lateral plantar nerve

Abductor digiti minimi muscle

Calcaneal network

Adductor hallucis muscle (transverse head)

Flexor hallucis brevis muscle

Deep plantar artery

Medial plantar artery

Tendon of flexor hallucis longus muscle

Quadratus plantae muscle

Medial plantar nerve

Lateral plantar artery

Abductor hallucis muscle

Medial plantar nerve

Posterior tibial artery

Lateral plantar nerve

Fig. 554: Sole of the Right Foot: the Plantar Arch and Deep Vessels and Nerves

NOTE: 1) the formation of the **deep plantar arch** principally from the lateral plantar artery, and the junction of the deep plantar arch with the deep plantar artery from the foot dorsum (see Fig. 537). From the plantar arch branch **plantar metatarsal arteries** that divide into **proper digital arteries**.

2) the muscles of the foot are innervated in the following manner:

	Medial plantar nerve	**Lateral plantar nerve**
1st layer	abductor hallucis flexor digitorum brevis	abductor digiti minimi
2nd layer	1st lumbrical	quadratus plantae 2nd, 3rd and 4th lumbrical
3rd layer	flexor hallucis brevis	adductor hallucis flexor digiti minimi brevis
4th layer		plantar interossei dorsal interossei

Fig. 554

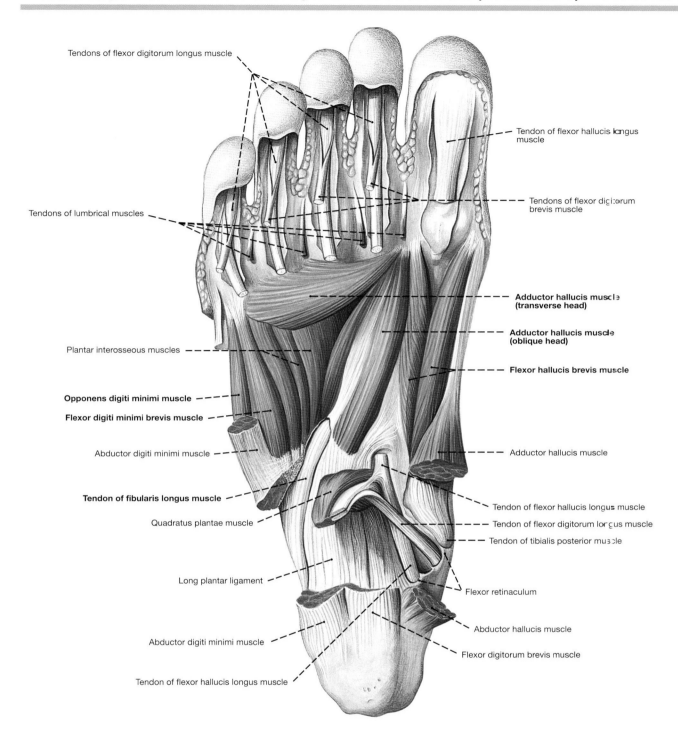

Tendons of flexor digitorum longus muscle

Tendon of flexor hallucis longus muscle

Tendons of lumbrical muscles

Tendons of flexor digitorum brevis muscle

Adductor hallucis muscle (transverse head)

Adductor hallucis muscle (oblique head)

Plantar interosseous muscles

Flexor hallucis brevis muscle

Opponens digiti minimi muscle

Flexor digiti minimi brevis muscle

Abductor digiti minimi muscle

Adductor hallucis muscle

Tendon of fibularis longus muscle

Tendon of flexor hallucis longus muscle

Quadratus plantae muscle

Tendon of flexor digitorum longus muscle

Tendon of tibialis posterior muscle

Long plantar ligament

Flexor retinaculum

Abductor digiti minimi muscle

Abductor hallucis muscle

Flexor digitorum brevis muscle

Tendon of flexor hallucis longus muscle

Fig. 555: Sole of the Right Foot: Third Layer of Plantar Muscles

NOTE: 1)   the third layer of plantar muscles consists of two flexors and an **ad**ductor (with two heads), in contrast to the first layer which contains one flexor and two **ab**ductors. Thus, the **flexor hallucis brevis, flexor digiti minimi brevis,** and the **oblique** and **transverse heads** of the **adductor hallucis** form the third layer of plantar muscles.

2)   at times, those fibers of the flexor digiti minimi brevis that insert on the lateral side of the first phalanx of the 5th toe are referred to as a separate muscle: the **opponens digiti minimi.**

3)   the tendon of the **fibularis longus muscle,** which crosses the plantar aspect of the foot obliquely to insert on the lateral side of the base of the 1st metatarsal and the 1st (medial) cuneiform bone.

Fig. 555   V

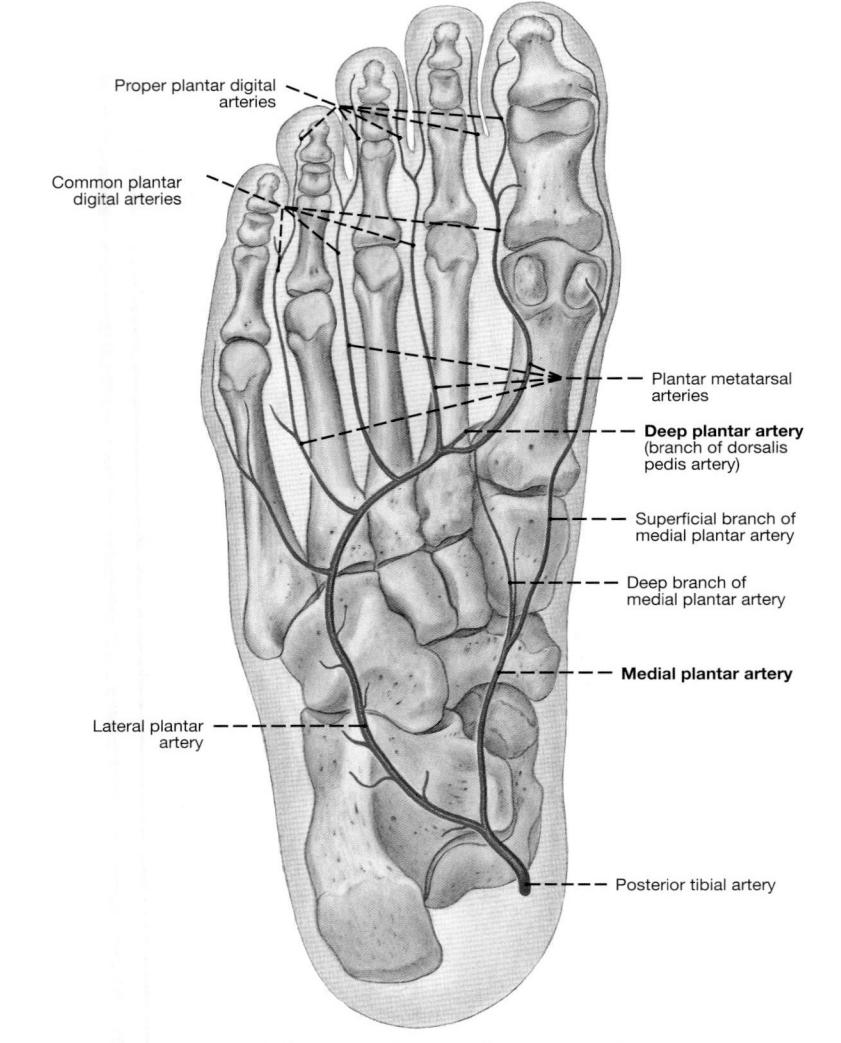

Proper plantar digital arteries

Common plantar digital arteries

Plantar metatarsal arteries

Deep plantar artery (branch of dorsalis pedis artery)

Superficial branch of medial plantar artery

Deep branch of medial plantar artery

Medial plantar artery

Lateral plantar artery

Posterior tibial artery

Fig. 556: Plantar Aspect of the Foot: Diagram of Arteries and Bones
NOTE: the **posterior tibial artery** enters the foot medially behind the medial malleolus, divides into **medial** and **lateral plantar arteries,** and anastomoses with the deep plantar branch of the **dorsalis pedis artery** between the 1st and 2nd digits.

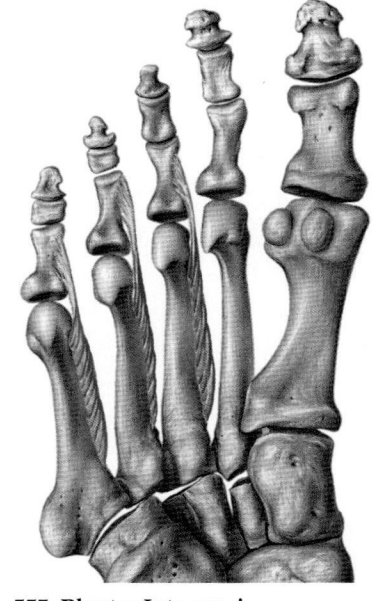

Fig. 557: Plantar Interossei

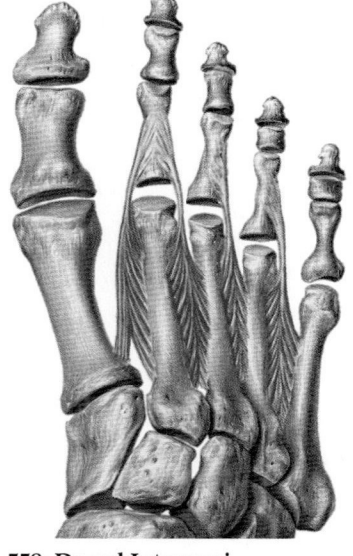

Fig. 558: Dorsal Interossei

Muscles of the Sole of the Foot
1st Layer of Muscles

Muscle	Origin	Insertion	Innervation	Action
Abductor Hallucis Muscle	Flexor retinaculum; medial process of calcaneal tuberosity; plantar aponeurosis	Medial side of the base of the proximal phalanx of the large toe	Medial plantar nerve (L5, S1)	Abducts and flexes the large toe; helps maintain the medial longitudinal arch
Flexor Digitorum Brevis Muscle	Medial process of calcaneal tuberosity; plantar aponeurosis	By four tendons onto the middle phalanx of the lateral four toes	Medial plantar nerve (L5, S1)	Flexes the lateral four toes
Abductor Digiti Minimi Muscle	Medial and lateral processes of the calcaneal tuberosity; plantar aponeurosis	Lateral side of the base of the proximal phalanx of the small toe	Lateral plantar nerve (S2, S3)	Abducts and flexes the little toe

Muscles of the Sole of the Foot (Cont.)
2nd Layer of Muscles

Muscle	Origin	Insertion	Innervation	Action
Quadratus Plantae Muscle	By two heads from the plantar surface of the calcaneus; long plantar ligament	Lateral and deep surfaces of the tendons of the flexor digitorum longus muscle	Lateral plantar nerve (S2, S3)	Assists the flexor digitorum longus; straightens the pull of the flexor digitorum longus along longitudinal axis of foot
Lumbrical Muscles **1st Lumbrical**	Medial side of the 1st tendon (to 2nd toe) of the flexor digitorum longus	Passes along the medial side of 2nd toe and inserts on its dorsal digital expansion	Medial plantar nerve (L5, S1)	Flex the proximal phalanx at the metatarsophalangeal joint; extend the two distal phalanges at the interphalangeal joints
2nd, 3rd and 4th Lumbrical Muscles	Each muscle by two heads from the adjacent surfaces of the 2nd, 3rd and 4th tendons (to the 3rd, 4th and 5th toes) of the flexor digitorum longus muscle	Course along the medial sides of the 3rd, 4th and 5th toes and insert on their respective dorsal digital expansions	Lateral plantar nerve (S2, S3)	

3rd Layer of Muscles

Muscle	Origin	Insertion	Innervation	Action
Flexor Hallucis Brevis Muscle	Plantar surface of cuboid and lateral (3rd) cuneiform bones; tendon of the tibialis posterior	By two tendons onto the sides of the base of the proximal phalanx of the large toe	Medial plantar nerve (L5, S1)	Flexes the proximal phalanx of the large toe at the metatarsophalangeal joint
Flexor Digiti Minimi Muscle	Base of the 5th metatarsal bone; the sheath of the tendon of the fibularis longus	Lateral side of the base of the proximal phalanx of the small toe	Lateral plantar nerve (S2, S3)	Flexes the proximal phalanx of the small toe at the metatarsophalangeal joint
Adductor Hallucis Muscle **TRANSVERSE HEAD**	Plantar metatarso-phalangeal ligaments of 3rd, 4th and 5th toes; deep transverse metatarsal ligaments between the toes	By a common tendon to lateral aspect of the base of the proximal phalanx of the large toe	Lateral plantar nerve (S2, S3)	Adducts large toe; flexes large toe at metatarsophalangeal joint
OBLIQUE HEAD	Bases of the 2nd, 3rd and 4th metatarsal bones; sheath of the tendon of fibularis longus muscle			

4th Layer of Muscles

Muscle	Origin	Insertion	Innervation	Action
Plantar Interossei **(3 Muscles)**	Bases and medial sides of 3rd, 4th and 5th metatarsal bones	Bases of proximal phalanx of 3rd, 4th and 5th toes (medial side); onto the dorsal digital expansions	Lateral plantar nerve (S2, S3)	Adduct 3rd, 4th and 5th toes; flex metatarso-phalangeal joints; extend interphalangeal joints
Dorsal Interossei **(4 Muscles)**	Each by 2 heads from adjacent sides of metatarsal bones	Proximal phalanx and dorsal digital expansions of 2nd, 3rd and 4th toes	Lateral plantar nerve (S2, S3)	Abduct 2nd, 3rd and 4th toes; flex metatarso-phalangeal joints and extend interphalangeal joints

V

PLATE 374   Bones of Lower Limb: Muscle Attachments; Femur (Anterior View)

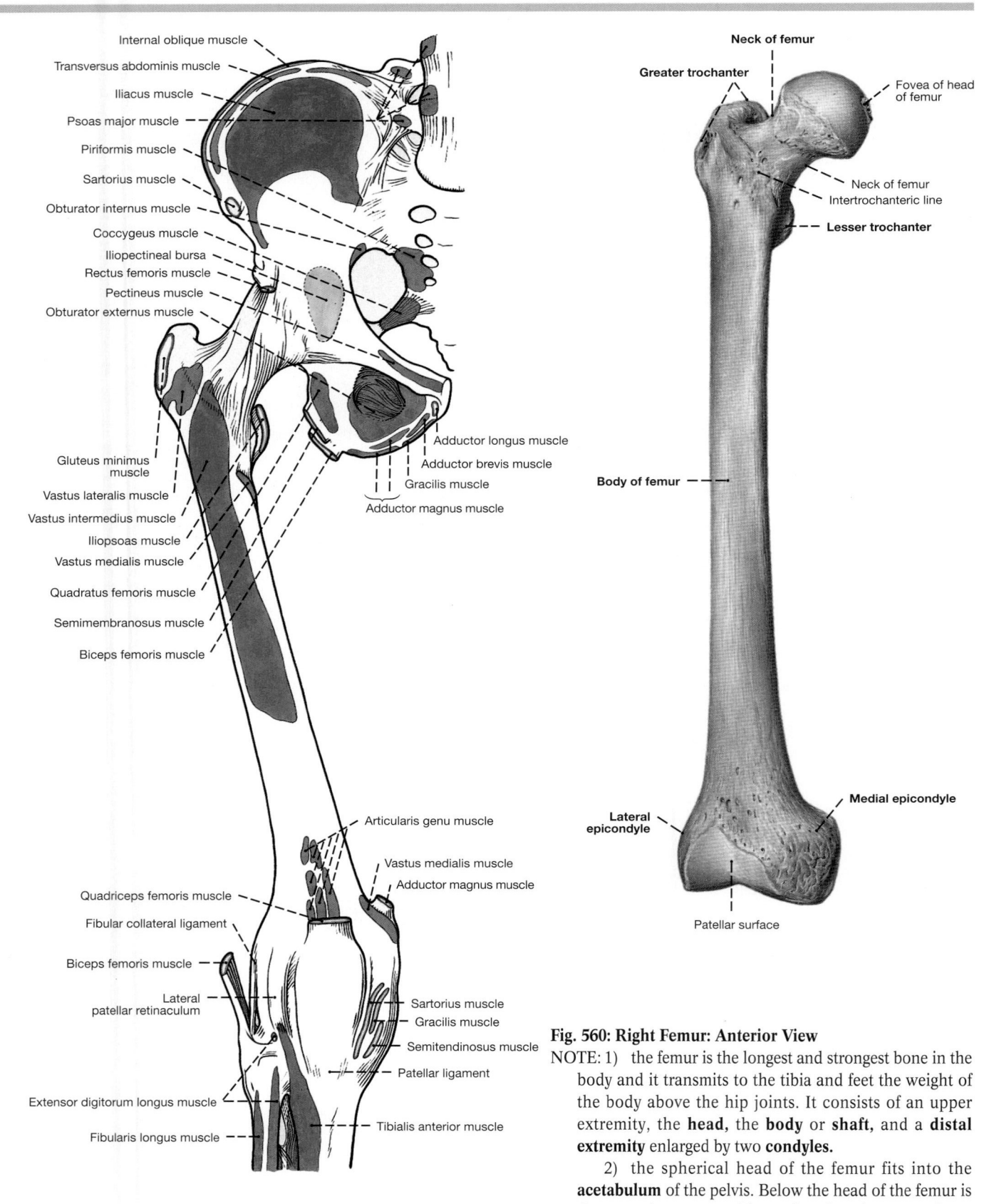

Internal oblique muscle

Transversus abdominis muscle

Iliacus muscle

Psoas major muscle

Piriformis muscle

Sartorius muscle

Obturator internus muscle

Coccygeus muscle

Iliopectineal bursa

Rectus femoris muscle

Pectineus muscle

Obturator externus muscle

Gluteus minimus muscle

Vastus lateralis muscle

Vastus intermedius muscle

Iliopsoas muscle

Vastus medialis muscle

Quadratus femoris muscle

Semimembranosus muscle

Biceps femoris muscle

Adductor longus muscle

Adductor brevis muscle

Gracilis muscle

Adductor magnus muscle

Articularis genu muscle

Vastus medialis muscle

Adductor magnus muscle

Quadriceps femoris muscle

Fibular collateral ligament

Biceps femoris muscle

Lateral patellar retinaculum

Sartorius muscle

Gracilis muscle

Semitendinosus muscle

Patellar ligament

Extensor digitorum longus muscle

Tibialis anterior muscle

Fibularis longus muscle

Neck of femur

Greater trochanter

Fovea of head of femur

Neck of femur

Intertrochanteric line

Lesser trochanter

Body of femur

Lateral epicondyle

Medial epicondyle

Patellar surface

Fig. 560: Right Femur: Anterior View

NOTE: 1) the femur is the longest and strongest bone in the body and it transmits to the tibia and feet the weight of the body above the hip joints. It consists of an upper extremity, the **head,** the **body** or **shaft,** and a **distal extremity** enlarged by two **condyles.**

2) the spherical head of the femur fits into the **acetabulum** of the pelvis. Below the head of the femur is the somewhat narrowed femoral **neck** and two prominent tubercles, the **greater** and **lesser trochanters.**

3) the anterior surface of the body of the femur is smooth and its proximal ²/₃rds gives origin to the vastus intermedius muscle.

Fig. 559: Anterior View of Right Pelvis and Femur Showing Muscle Attachments

Figs. 559, 560

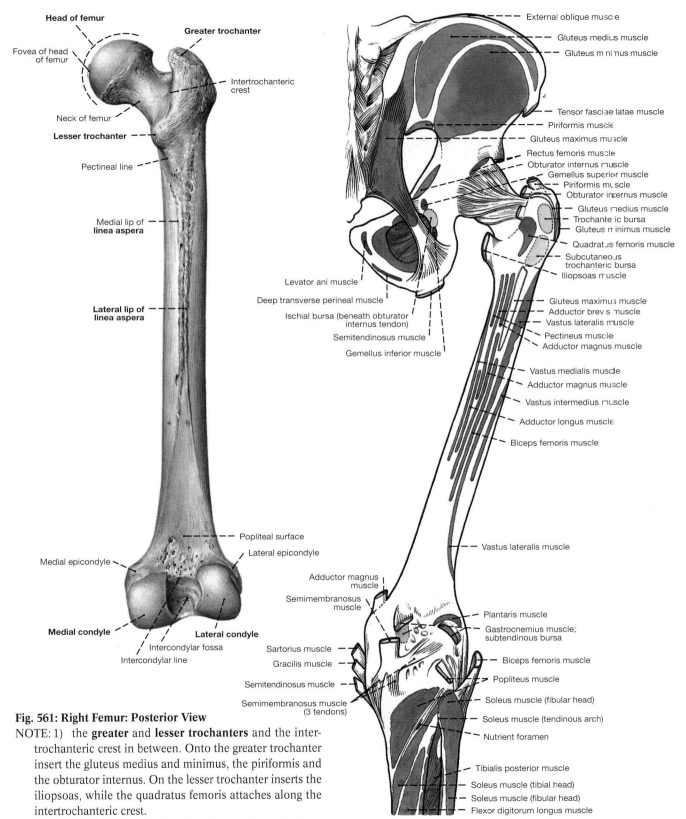

Head of femur

Fovea of head of femur

Greater trochanter

Neck of femur

Intertrochanteric crest

Lesser trochanter

Pectineal line

Medial lip of linea aspera

Lateral lip of linea aspera

Popliteal surface

Lateral epicondyle

Medial epicondyle

Medial condyle

Lateral condyle

Intercondylar fossa

Intercondylar line

External oblique muscle

Gluteus medius muscle

Gluteus minimus muscle

Tensor fasciae latae muscle

Piriformis muscle

Gluteus maximus muscle

Rectus femoris muscle

Obturator internus muscle

Gemellus superior muscle

Piriformis muscle

Obturator internus muscle

Gluteus medius muscle

Trochanteric bursa

Gluteus minimus muscle

Quadratus femoris muscle

Subcutaneous trochanteric bursa

Iliopsoas muscle

Levator ani muscle

Deep transverse perineal muscle

Ischial bursa (beneath obturator internus tendon)

Semitendinosus muscle

Gemellus inferior muscle

Gluteus maximus muscle

Adductor brevis muscle

Vastus lateralis muscle

Pectineus muscle

Adductor magnus muscle

Vastus medialis muscle

Adductor magnus muscle

Vastus intermedius muscle

Adductor longus muscle

Biceps femoris muscle

Vastus lateralis muscle

Adductor magnus muscle

Semimembranosus muscle

Plantaris muscle

Gastrocnemius muscle; subtendinous bursa

Biceps femoris muscle

Popliteus muscle

Soleus muscle (fibular head)

Soleus muscle (tendinous arch)

Nutrient foramen

Sartorius muscle

Gracilis muscle

Semitendinosus muscle

Semimembranosus muscle (3 tendons)

Tibialis posterior muscle

Soleus muscle (tibial head)

Soleus muscle (fibular head)

Flexor digitorum longus muscle

Fig. 561: Right Femur: Posterior View

NOTE: 1) the **greater** and **lesser trochanters** and the intertrochanteric crest in between. Onto the greater trochanter
insert the gluteus medius and minimus, the piriformis and
the obturator internus. On the lesser trochanter inserts the
iliopsoas, while the quadratus femoris attaches along the
intertrochanteric crest.

2) the thick, longitudinally oriented ridge, the **linea
aspera,** along the posterior surface of the body of the femur.
It also serves for muscle attachments.

3) the **medial** and **lateral condyles** and **epicondyles**
inferiorly. The condyles articulate with the tibia and the
intercondyloid fossa affords attachment for the cruciate
ligaments.

**Fig. 562: Posterior View of Right Pelvis and Femur Showing Muscle
Attachments**

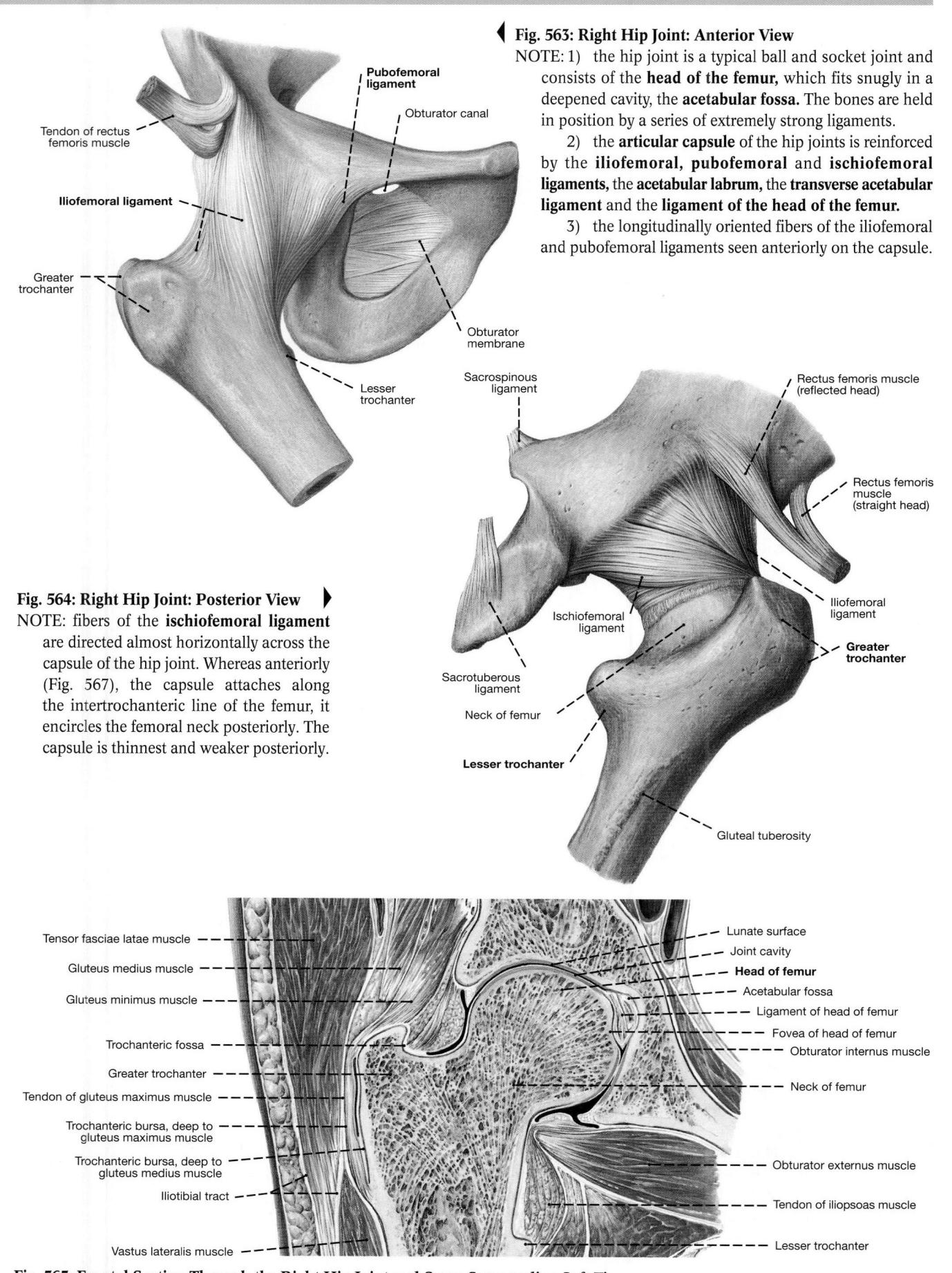

▲ **Fig. 563: Right Hip Joint: Anterior View**
NOTE: 1) the hip joint is a typical ball and socket joint and consists of the **head of the femur,** which fits snugly in a deepened cavity, the **acetabular fossa.** The bones are held in position by a series of extremely strong ligaments.

2) the **articular capsule** of the hip joints is reinforced by the **iliofemoral, pubofemoral** and **ischiofemoral ligaments,** the **acetabular labrum,** the **transverse acetabular ligament** and the **ligament of the head of the femur.**

3) the longitudinally oriented fibers of the iliofemoral and pubofemoral ligaments seen anteriorly on the capsule.

Pubofemoral ligament

Tendon of rectus femoris muscle

Obturator canal

Iliofemoral ligament

Greater trochanter

Obturator membrane

Lesser trochanter

Sacrospinous ligament

Rectus femoris muscle (reflected head)

Rectus femoris muscle (straight head)

Iliofemoral ligament

Fig. 564: Right Hip Joint: Posterior View ▶
NOTE: fibers of the **ischiofemoral ligament** are directed almost horizontally across the capsule of the hip joint. Whereas anteriorly (Fig. 567), the capsule attaches along the intertrochanteric line of the femur, it encircles the femoral neck posteriorly. The capsule is thinnest and weaker posteriorly.

Ischiofemoral ligament

Greater trochanter

Sacrotuberous ligament

Neck of femur

Lesser trochanter

Gluteal tuberosity

Tensor fasciae latae muscle

Gluteus medius muscle

Gluteus minimus muscle

Trochanteric fossa

Greater trochanter

Tendon of gluteus maximus muscle

Trochanteric bursa, deep to gluteus maximus muscle

Trochanteric bursa, deep to gluteus medius muscle

Iliotibial tract

Vastus lateralis muscle

Lunate surface

Joint cavity

Head of femur

Acetabular fossa

Ligament of head of femur

Fovea of head of femur

Obturator internus muscle

Neck of femur

Obturator externus muscle

Tendon of iliopsoas muscle

Lesser trochanter

Fig. 565: Frontal Section Through the Right Hip Joint and Some Surrounding Soft Tissues

Figs. 563, 564, 565

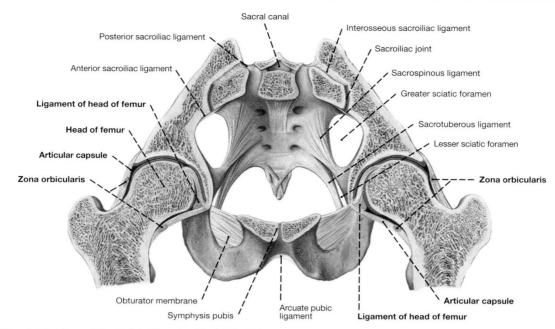

Fig. 566: Frontal Section of the Pelvis Showing Both Hip Joints

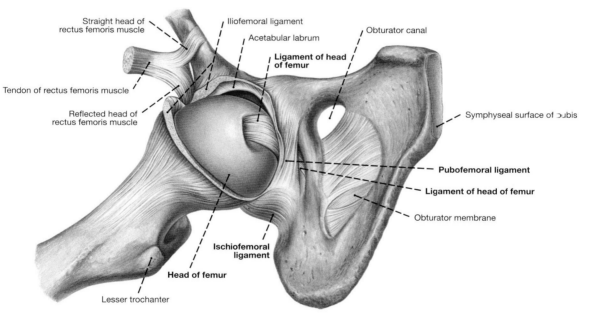

Fig. 567: Anterior Exposure of the Right Hip Joint
NOTE: the articular capsule of the hip joint has been opened near the acetabular labrum. This exposes the cartilage covered head of the femur within the joint cavity. Observe the ligament of the femoral head attached to the femur where cartilage is lacking.

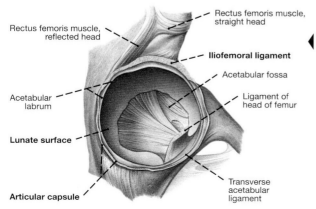

◀ **Fig. 568: Socket of the Right Hip Joint**
NOTE: 1)   the acetabulum is surrounded by a fibrocartilaginous rim, the **acetabular labrum.** This deepens the joint cavity and accommodates enough of the distal head of the femur so that it cannot be pulled from its socket without injuring the acetabular labrum.

2)   the bony acetabulum is incomplete below. Here the acetabular notch is partially covered by the **transverse acetabular ligament.** Through the free portion of the acetabular notch course vessels and nerves that supply the head of the femur.

3)   the **ligament of the head of the femur** attaches the femoral head by two bands to either side of the acetabular notch.

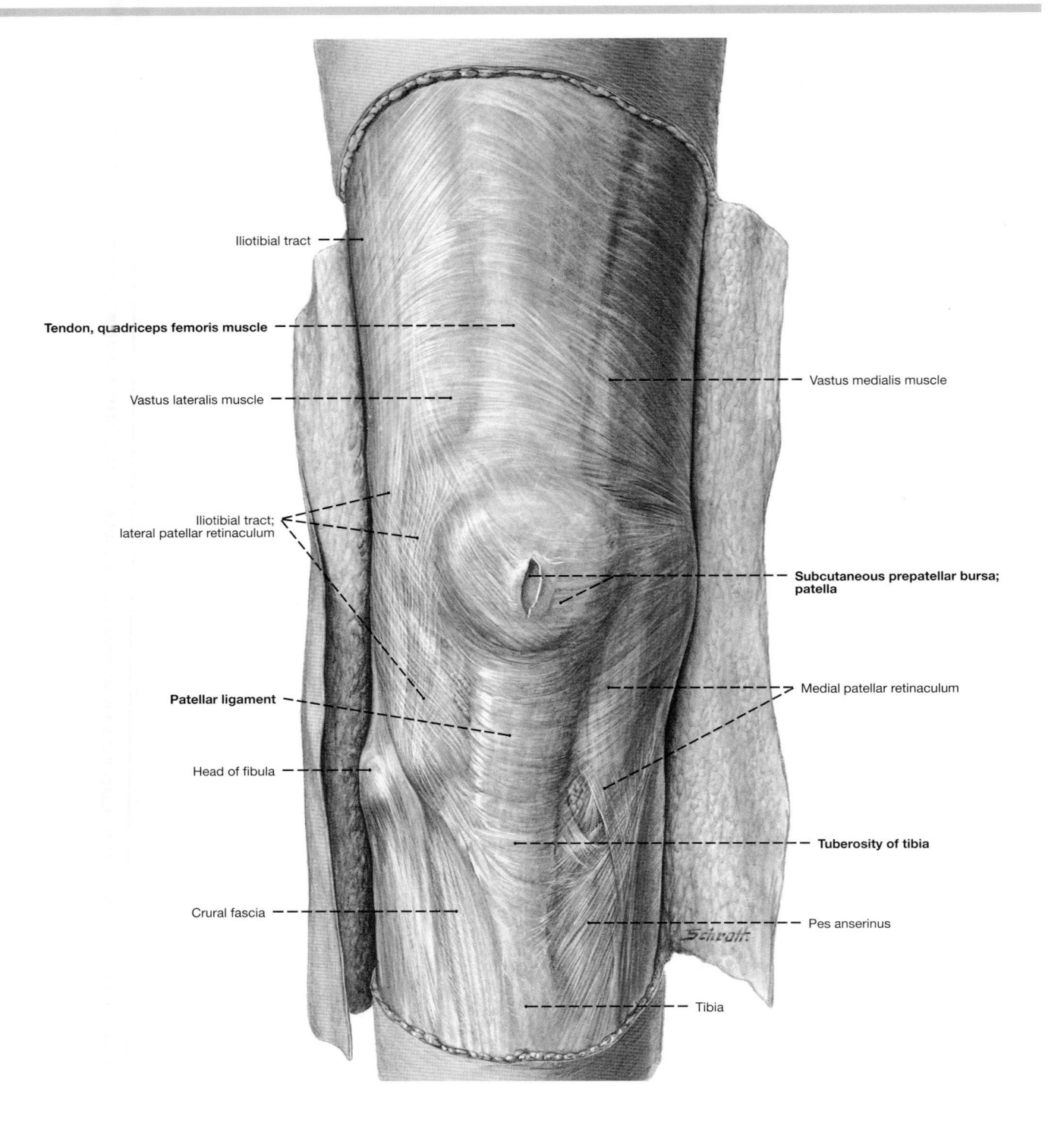

Iliotibial tract

Tendon, quadriceps femoris muscle

Vastus lateralis muscle

Iliotibial tract;
lateral patellar retinaculum

Patellar ligament

Head of fibula

Crural fascia

Vastus medialis muscle

**Subcutaneous prepatellar bursa;
patella**

Medial patellar retinaculum

Tuberosity of tibia

Pes anserinus

Tibia

Fig. 569 Region of the Knee Joint, Anterior View (Superficial Dissection, Right Lower Limb)

NOTE: 1) only the skin and superficial fascia were cut and reflected in this dissection, leaving the lower thigh, upper leg and the intervening structures of the knee joint covered by the closely investing deep fascia of the lower limb.

2) a small longitudinal incision has been made in the deep fascia anterior to the patella, opening the large **subcutaneous prepatellar bursa.**

3) other bursae on the anterior aspect of the knee joint include:
   a) the **subcutaneous infrapatellar bursa** located between the lower part of the tibial tuberosity and the overlying deep fascia,
   b) the **deep infrapatellar bursa** found below the patella between the ligamentum patellae and the upper surface of the tibia,
   c) the **suprapatellar bursa** located above the patella, between the anterior surface of the lower femur and the tendon of the quadriceps femoris muscle (see Fig. 578).

4) these bursae may become inflamed, resulting in the painful condition called bursitis. Often associated with consistent pressure or trauma, prepatellar bursitis (also called "housemaid's knee") is frequently seen in persons who kneel alot or for prolonged periods.

Fig. 569

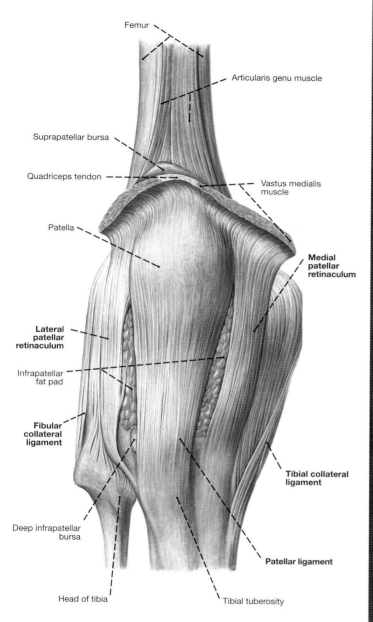

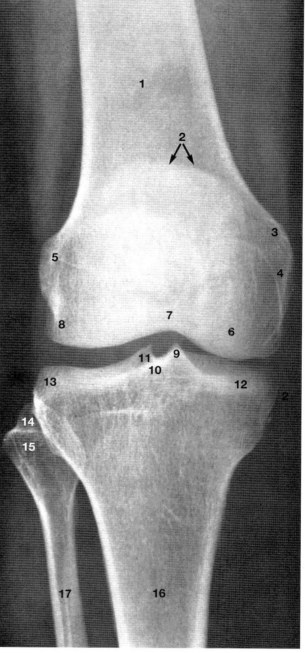

Fig. 570: Right Knee Joint (Anterior View)

NOTE: 1) the deep fascia has been removed and the bellies of the four heads of the quadriceps femoris muscle have been cut to expose the quadriceps tendon, the patella and the patellar ligament.

   2) the **patellar ligament** inserts onto the tibial tuberosity located on the proximal aspect of the anterior tibial surface.

   3) the **medial** and **lateral patellar retinacula.** These structures reinforce the anteromedial and anterolateral parts of the fibrous capsule of the knee joint and often (but not shown in this figure) they are attached to the borders of the patellar ligament and patella.

   4) the **tibial** and **fibular collateral ligaments** and the location of the **deep infrapatellar bursa.**

Fig. 571: Radiograph of the Right Knee (Anterior-Posterior Projection)

NOTE: the following bony structures on the femur, tibia and fibula in the region of the knee.

1. Body of femur
2. Margin of patella
3. Adductor tubercle
4. Medial epicondyle
5. Lateral epicondyle
6. Medial condyle of femur
7. Intercondylar fossa
8. Lateral condyle of femur
9. Medial intercondylar tubercle
10. Anterior intercondylar area
11. Lateral intercondylar tubercle
12. Medial condyle of tibia
13. Lateral condyle of tibia
14. Apex of head of fibula
15. Head of fibula
16. Body of tibia
17. Body of fibula

From Wicke L. Atlas of Radiologic Anatomy, 5th Edition. Philadelphia, Lea and Febiger, 1994.

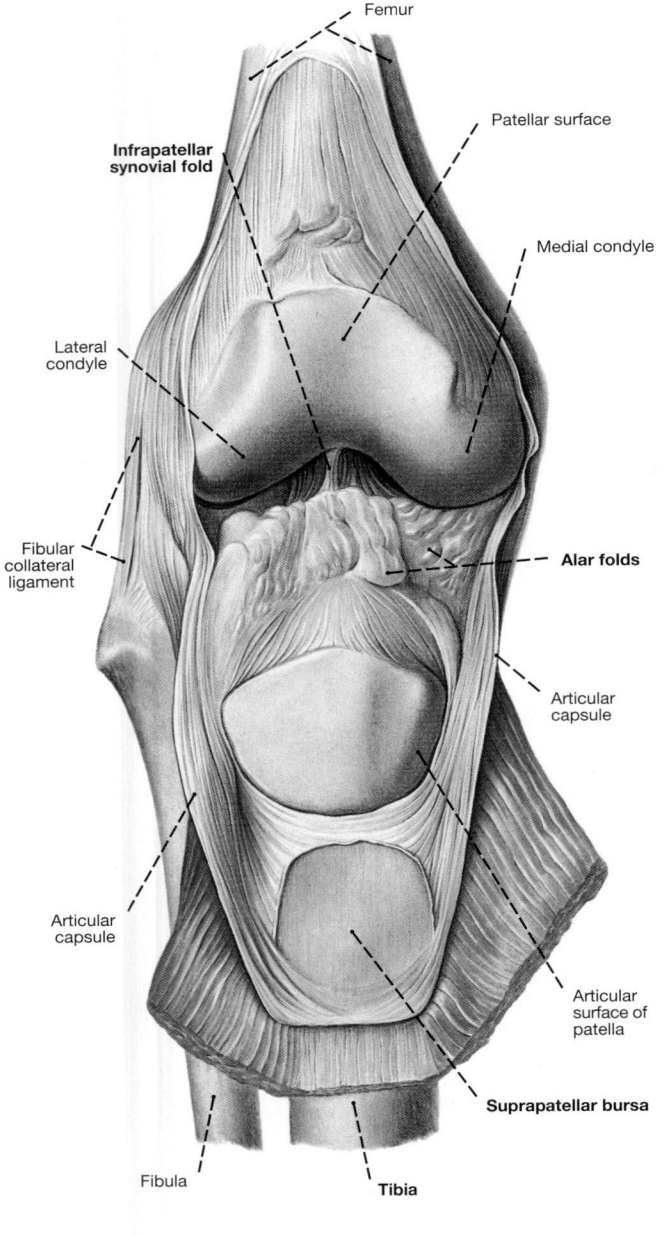

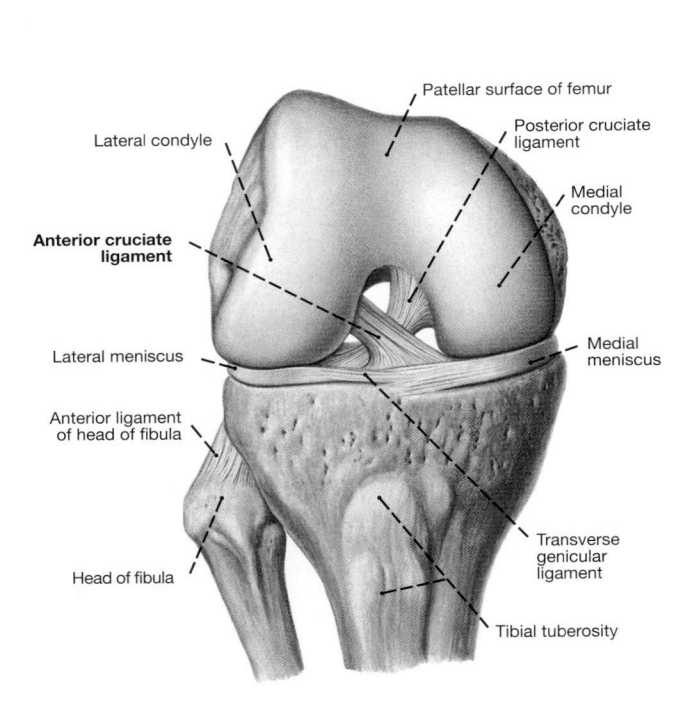

Fig. 572: Knee Joint Opened Anteriorly

NOTE: 1) in this dissection the anterior part of the articular capsule and the quadriceps tendon have been cut and reflected downward along with the **suprapatellar bursa.** The articular surface of the **patella** has also been pulled inferiorly away from its normal position on the femur.

2) from the medial and lateral borders of the patella, the synovial membrane projects as fringe-like **alar folds** on each side. These converge in the midline to form the **infrapatellar synovial fold** which attaches above to the intercondylar fossa of the femur.

3) upon removal of the infrapatellar synovial fold and any fat in the region, the anterior cruciate ligament and the menisci become exposed as seen in Figure 573.

Fig. 573: Flexed Right Knee Joint (Anterior View) Showing the Cruciate Ligaments

NOTE: 1) the **anterior cruciate ligament** is best exposed from this frontal approach. It extends from the posterior part of the medial surface of the lateral femoral condyle to the anterior surface of the tibial plateau.

2) the anterior cruciate ligament helps prevent the posterior, or backward, displacement of the femur on the upper tibial plateau.

3) more importantly, however, the anterior cruciate ligament limits extension of the lateral condyle to which it is attached. When it becomes taut, it causes medial rotation of the femur. This allows the medial condyle, which has a longer and more curved articular surface than the lateral condyle, to reach its full extension, placing the knee joint in a "locked position."

4) thus, the "locked" knee joint is achieved because:

a) the medial condyle has a longer articular surface and a greater curvature than that of the lateral condyle,

b) after the anterior cruciate ligament becomes taut, the lateral condyle can rotate around the "radius of the ligament" and forces the medial condyle to glide backward into its full extension,

c) medial rotation of the femur at the same time causes the oblique popliteal ligament and the medial and lateral collateral ligaments to tighten as well (From Last RJ. Anatomy, Regional and Applied. Edinburgh, Churchill Livingstone, 1978).

Figs. 572, 573

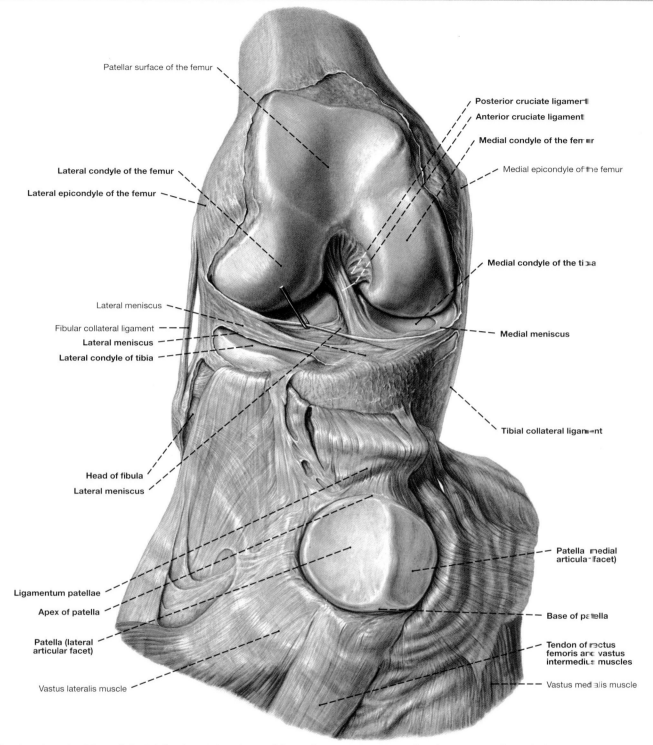

Patellar surface of the femur

Posterior cruciate ligament

Anterior cruciate ligament

Medial condyle of the femur

Medial epicondyle of the femur

Lateral condyle of the femur

Lateral epicondyle of the femur

Medial condyle of the tibia

Lateral meniscus

Fibular collateral ligament

Lateral meniscus

Lateral condyle of tibia

Medial meniscus

Tibial collateral ligament

Head of fibula

Lateral meniscus

Patella (medial articular facet)

Ligamentum patellae

Apex of patella

Base of patella

Patella (lateral articular facet)

Tendon of rectus femoris and vastus intermedius muscles

Vastus lateralis muscle

Vastus medialis muscle

Fig. 574: Anterior View of the Right Knee Joint, Opened from the Front to Expose the Ligaments and Menisci

NOTE: 1)   the bellies of the quadriceps muscle have been severed and reflected downward to expose the inner (posterior) surface of the patella, which is attached above to the joined tendons of the rectus femoris and vastus intermedius and below to the patellar ligament.

2)   the knee joint is a bicondylar synovial joint with a single joint cavity between the condyles of the femur and the condyles of the tibia.

3)   within the notch between the femoral condyles are attached the **posterior** and **anterior cruciate ligaments.** The posterior cruciate ligament is fixed to the medial condyle of the femur, while the anterior cruciate ligament is attached to the lateral condyle of the femur deep in the intercondylar notch.

4)   the attachment of the anterior cruciate ligament onto the anterior part of the tibial plateau is well shown in this figure and the tibial attachment of the posterior cruciate ligament can be seen in Figures 576 and 577. These ligaments are essential for anterior-posterior stability of the knee joint.

Fig. 574   **V**

PLATE 382   Knee Joint: Posterior Superficial View; Internal Ligaments

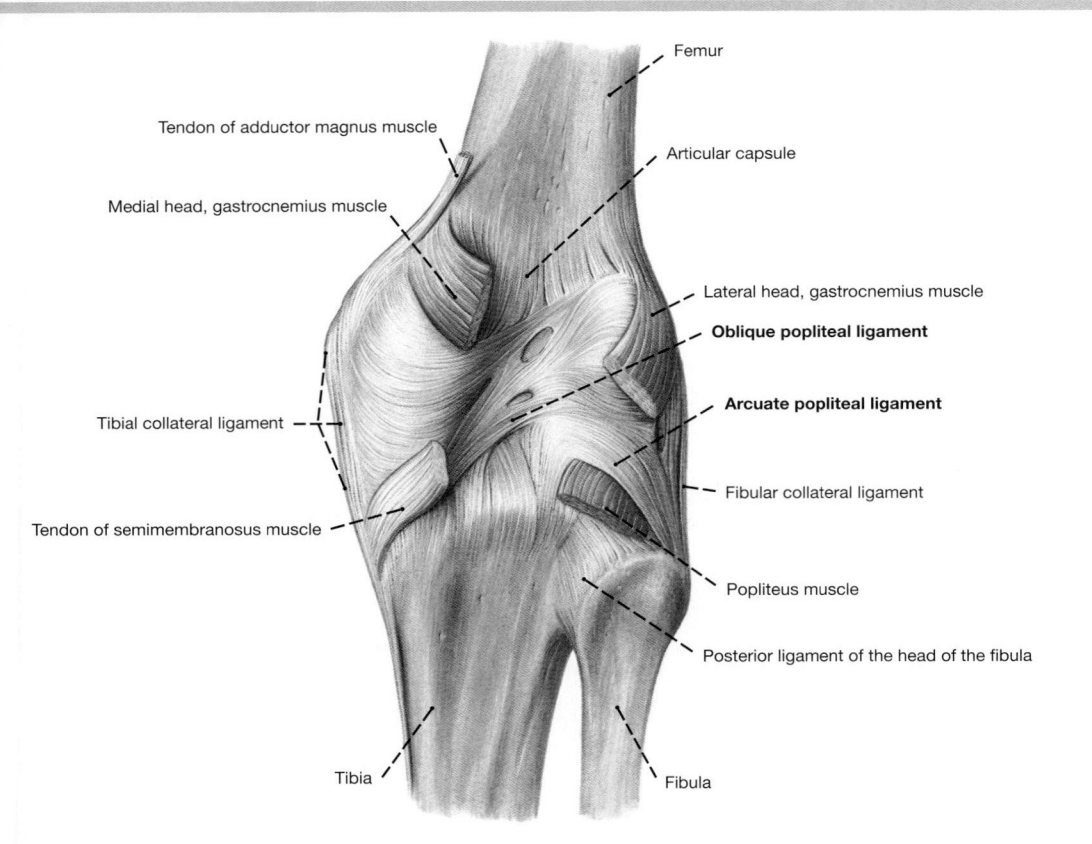

Femur

Tendon of adductor magnus muscle

Articular capsule

Medial head, gastrocnemius muscle

Lateral head, gastrocnemius muscle

Oblique popliteal ligament

Arcuate popliteal ligament

Tibial collateral ligament

Fibular collateral ligament

Tendon of semimembranosus muscle

Popliteus muscle

Posterior ligament of the head of the fibula

Tibia

Fibula

Fig. 575: Knee Joint: Posterior View, Superficial Dissection

NOTE: 1) the posterior aspect of the articular capsule is reinforced by the oblique and arcuate popliteal ligaments and to some extent by the tendons of origin and insertion of muscles.

2) from its insertion, the tendon of the semimembranosus muscle expands upward and laterally across the posterior surface of the articular capsule of the knee joint as the **oblique popliteal ligament.**

3) the **arcuate popliteal ligament** is a band of fibers attached to the head of the fibula and courses superficial to the popliteus muscle to blend with the oblique popliteal ligament and the fibular collateral ligament.

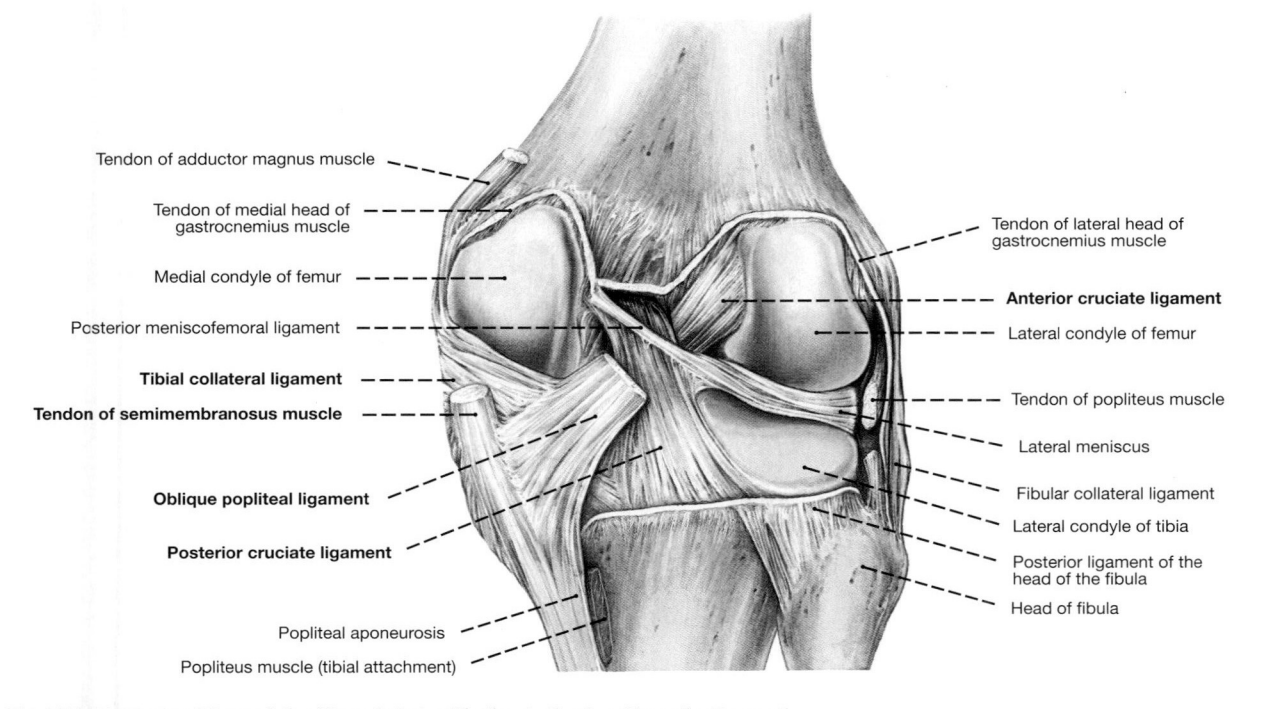

Tendon of adductor magnus muscle

Tendon of medial head of gastrocnemius muscle

Tendon of lateral head of gastrocnemius muscle

Medial condyle of femur

Anterior cruciate ligament

Posterior meniscofemoral ligament

Lateral condyle of femur

Tibial collateral ligament

Tendon of popliteus muscle

Tendon of semimembranosus muscle

Lateral meniscus

Oblique popliteal ligament

Fibular collateral ligament

Lateral condyle of tibia

Posterior cruciate ligament

Posterior ligament of the head of the fibula

Head of fibula

Popliteal aponeurosis

Popliteus muscle (tibial attachment)

Fig. 576: Posterior View of the Knee Joint with the Articular Capsule Opened

NOTE: this more diagrammatic figure should be compared with the dissection in Figure 577.

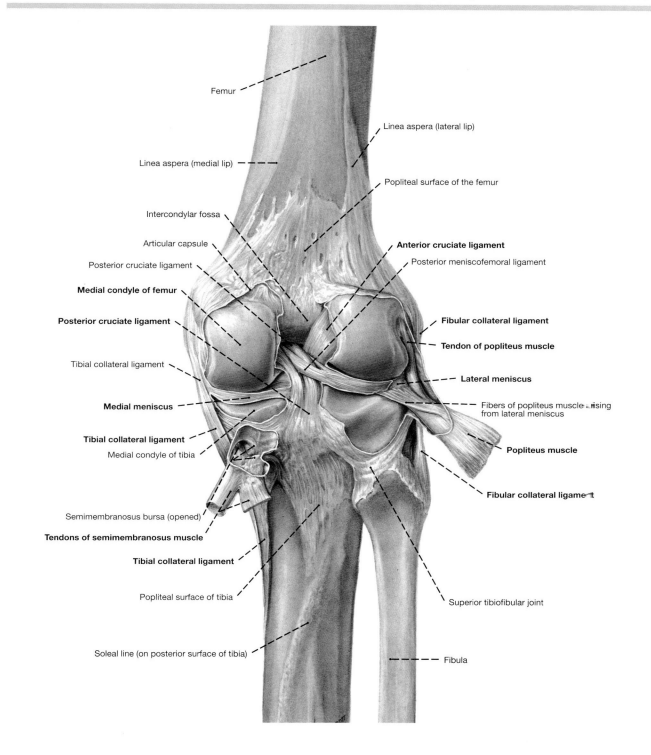

Femur

Linea aspera (lateral lip)

Linea aspera (medial lip)

Popliteal surface of the femur

Intercondylar fossa

Articular capsule

Anterior cruciate ligament

Posterior cruciate ligament

Posterior meniscofemoral ligament

Medial condyle of femur

Posterior cruciate ligament

Fibular collateral ligament

Tendon of popliteus muscle

Tibial collateral ligament

Lateral meniscus

Medial meniscus

Fibers of popliteus muscle arising from lateral meniscus

Tibial collateral ligament

Popliteus muscle

Medial condyle of tibia

Semimembranosus bursa (opened)

Fibular collateral ligament

Tendons of semimembranosus muscle

Tibial collateral ligament

Popliteal surface of tibia

Superior tibiofibular joint

Soleal line (on posterior surface of tibia)

Fibula

Fig. 577: Posterior View of the Right Knee Joint, Opened from Behind to Expose the Ligaments and Menisci

NOTE: 1) the posterior part of the articular capsule has been opened from behind, thereby exposing the femoral condyles, the intercondylar fossa, the anterior and posterior cruciate ligaments, and the medial and lateral menisci.

2) the attachment of the *anterior cruciate ligament* onto the medial aspect of the lateral condyle of the femur and the attachment of the *posterior cruciate ligament* onto the posterior intercondylar surface of the tibia.

3) when the knee joint is flexed and the lower limb is bearing weight, the posterior cruciate ligament prevents the femur from sliding forward along the surface of the tibial plateau. This is especially the case when one walks downhill or descends stairs.

4) the *posterior meniscofemoral ligament*. It courses upward and medially from the posterior part of the lateral meniscus to attach onto the medial condyle of the femur. In this dissection it appears to split and penetrate the fibers of the posterior cruciate ligament.

Fig. 577   **V**

PLATE 384   Knee Joint: Synovial Cavity and Bursae; MRI Section

Fig. 578: Cast of Knee Joint (Distended) Showing Bursae and Joint Cavity (Lateral View)

NOTE: 1) this lateral view of the distended synovial cavity of the right knee joint demonstrates the extensive nature of the synovial membrane of this joint. It is more extensive in this joint than in any other in the body.

2) the synovial membrane reaches *superiorly* above the patella to form a large pouch called the **suprapatellar bursa.** *Laterally,* it courses deep to the popliteus tendon and fibular collateral ligament. *Posteriorly,* it extends above the menisci as high as the origins of the gastrocnemius muscle. *Inferiorly,* the joint cavity descends below both the lateral and medial menisci.

Quadriceps tendon

Suprapatellar synovial bursa

Prepatellar bursa

Joint cavity

Fibular collateral ligament

Joint cavity

Popliteus muscle

Lateral meniscus

Patellar ligament

Deep infrapatellar bursa

Suprapatellar synovial bursa

Medial and lateral menisci

Joint cavity

Fibular collateral ligament

Subpopliteal recess

Joint cavity

Tibial collateral ligament

Popliteus muscle

Fig. 579: Cast of Knee Joint Showing Bursae and Joint Cavity (Posterior View)

NOTE: in this posterior diagram of the right knee joint, the fibrous capsule has been removed to expose the joint cavity. The synovial membrane extends above the menisci, deep to the heads of the gastrocnemius muscle, and below the menisci, deep to the popliteus muscle laterally and the semimembranosus medially.

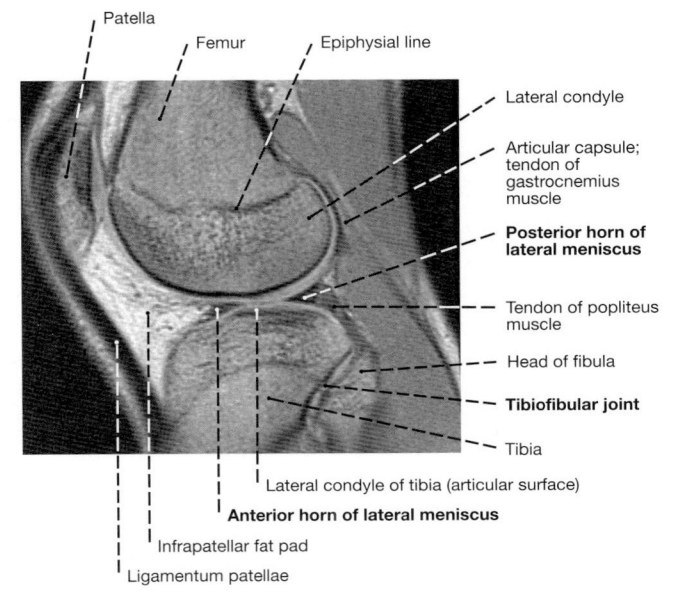

Patella

Femur

Epiphysial line

Lateral condyle

Articular capsule; tendon of gastrocnemius muscle

Posterior horn of lateral meniscus

Tendon of popliteus muscle

Head of fibula

Tibiofibular joint

Tibia

Lateral condyle of tibia (articular surface)

Anterior horn of lateral meniscus

Infrapatellar fat pad

Ligamentum patellae

Fig. 580: Magnetic Resonance Image (MRI) of the Knee Joint, Sagittal Section

NOTE: this sagittal section cuts through the lateral part of the joint and shows the horns of the **lateral meniscus,** the **tendon of the popliteus muscle** and the **superior tibiofibular joint.** Compare this image with Figure 582.

Figs. 578, 579, 580

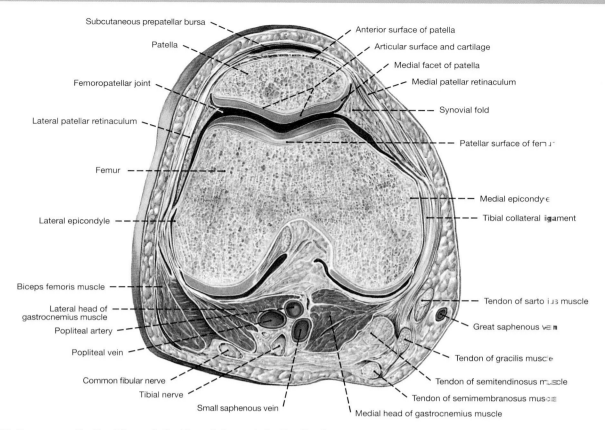

Subcutaneous prepatellar bursa

Patella

Femoropatellar joint

Lateral patellar retinaculum

Femur

Lateral epicondyle

Biceps femoris muscle

Lateral head of
gastrocnemius muscle

Popliteal artery

Popliteal vein

Common fibular nerve

Tibial nerve

Small saphenous vein

Anterior surface of patella

Articular surface and cartilage

Medial facet of patella

Medial patellar retinaculum

Synovial fold

Patellar surface of femur

Medial epicondyle

Tibial collateral ligament

Tendon of sartorius muscle

Great saphenous vein

Tendon of gracilis muscle

Tendon of semitendinosus muscle

Tendon of semimembranosus muscle

Medial head of gastrocnemius muscle

Fig. 581: Transverse Section Through the Knee Joint and the Popliteal Fossa
NOTE: the relationship of the muscles, vessels and nerves in the popliteal fossa to the bony structures of the knee joint.

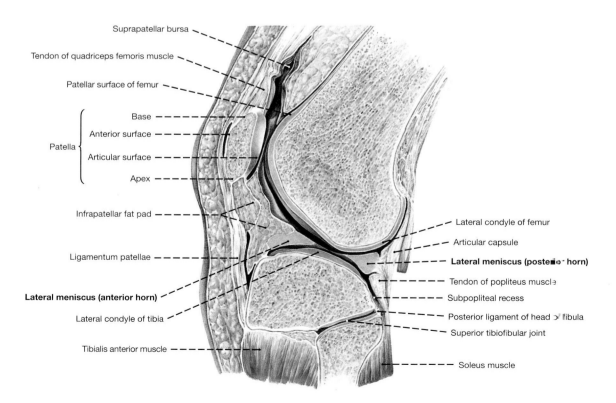

Suprapatellar bursa

Tendon of quadriceps femoris muscle

Patellar surface of femur

Patella {
Base
Anterior surface
Articular surface
Apex
}

Infrapatellar fat pad

Ligamentum patellae

Lateral meniscus (anterior horn)

Lateral condyle of tibia

Tibialis anterior muscle

Lateral condyle of femur

Articular capsule

Lateral meniscus (posterior horn)

Tendon of popliteus muscle

Subpopliteal recess

Posterior ligament of head of fibula

Superior tibiofibular joint

Soleus muscle

Fig. 582: Sagittal Section Through the Lateral Part of the Knee Joint
NOTE: the horns of the lateral meniscus, the tendon of the popliteus muscle, and the superior tibiofibular joint and then compare these structures in this drawing with those in the MRI section seen in Figure 580.

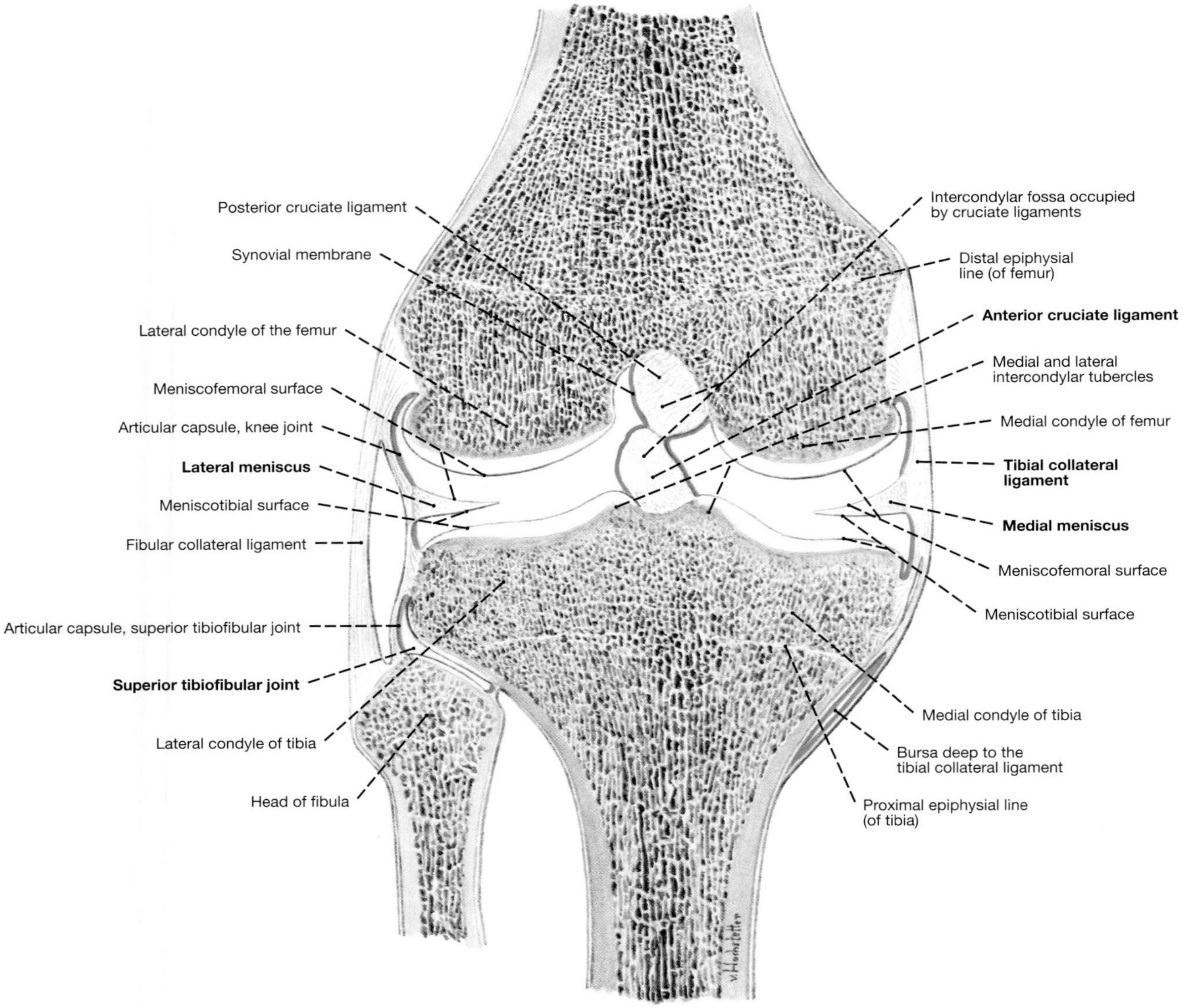

PLATE 386   Knee Joint: Frontal Section and MRI

Posterior cruciate ligament

Synovial membrane

Lateral condyle of the femur

Meniscofemoral surface

Articular capsule, knee joint

Lateral meniscus

Meniscotibial surface

Fibular collateral ligament

Articular capsule, superior tibiofibular joint

Superior tibiofibular joint

Lateral condyle of tibia

Head of fibula

Intercondylar fossa occupied
by cruciate ligaments

Distal epiphysial
line (of femur)

Anterior cruciate ligament

Medial and lateral
intercondylar tubercles

Medial condyle of femur

**Tibial collateral
ligament**

Medial meniscus

Meniscofemoral surface

Meniscotibial surface

Medial condyle of tibia

Bursa deep to the
tibial collateral ligament

Proximal epiphysial line
(of tibia)

Fig. 583: Frontal Section of the Right Knee Joint and the Superior Tibiofibular Joint
NOTE: the **synovial membrane,** enclosing the synovial cavity, is outlined in **green.** Observe that the cruciate ligaments and the menisci
are outside the synovial cavity of the knee joint even though they are inside the articular capsule of the joint. The tibial and fibular
collateral ligaments also are outside the synovial cavity.

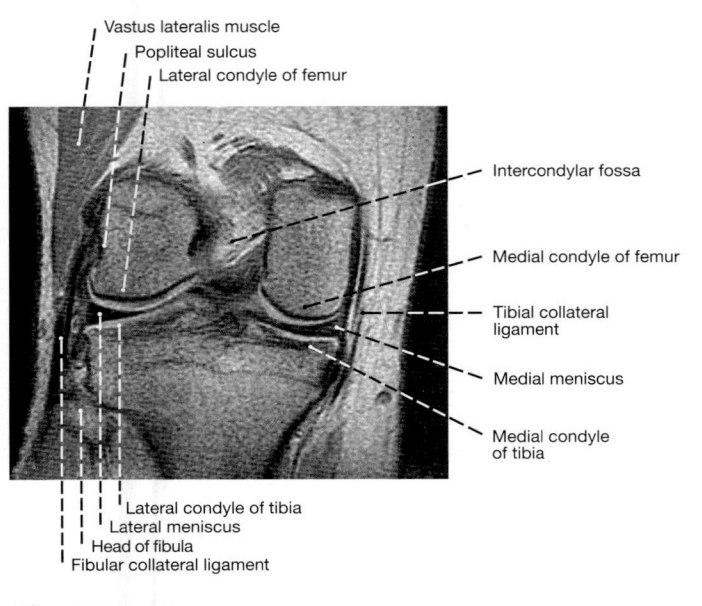

Vastus lateralis muscle
Popliteal sulcus
Lateral condyle of femur

Intercondylar fossa

Medial condyle of femur

Tibial collateral
ligament

Medial meniscus

Medial condyle
of tibia

Lateral condyle of tibia
Lateral meniscus
Head of fibula
Fibular collateral ligament

**Fig. 584: Magnetic Resonance Image (MRI) of the
Knee Joint, Frontal Section**
NOTE: this MRI frontal section cuts through the intercondylar
eminence of the tibia (not labelled) and the intercondylar
fossa of the femur. Observe the menisci, which in this frontal
section, have a triangular shape.

Fig. 585: Condyles of the Right Tibia (from Above), Showing the ▶ Menisci and the Attachments on the Tibia of the Cruciate Ligaments

NOTE: 1) the C-shaped menisci lie above the condyles of the tibia; they are triangular in cross-section and composed of fibrous connective tissue and NOT cartilage.

2) the **medial meniscus** is larger and has a more open curve than that of the **lateral meniscus.** Both menisci are attached at their anterior and posterior horns to the tibial surface.

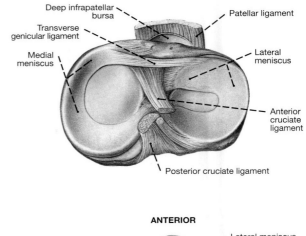

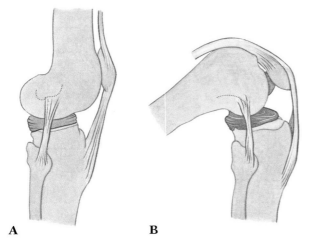

A   **B**

Fig. 586: Lateral Views of the Right Knee Joint ◢

NOTE: in **A** the knee joint is extended, while in **B** it is flexed. When greater flexion at the knee joint occurs, the menisci (especially the lateral meniscus) are pulled posteriorly on the tibial plateau (see Figure 587).

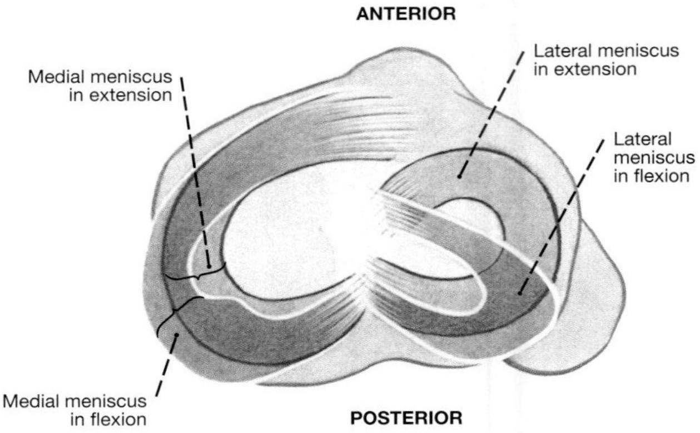

Fig. 587: Superior View of the Right Tibial Surface Showing Positions of the Menisci During Extension and Flexion

MORE ABOUT THE MENISCI:

1) the **lateral meniscus** receives a flat tendon of insertion from the upper fibers of the **popliteus muscle,** and this muscle comes into action during "unlocking" of the knee joint by slightly rotating the femur laterally in preparation to taking a step. In addition these fibers draw the posterior convexity of the lateral meniscus backward "out of harm's way" during flexion of the tibia at the knee joint.

2) in addition to its attachment on the tibia, the **medial meniscus** is securely attached to the tibial collateral ligament and is frequently injured in athletes when

    a) the foot of the victim is planted firmly on the ground and the knee is semi-flexed

    b) and the victim is hit from behind ("clipping" in football) causing the weight of the body to severely rotate the femur medially.

Thus, the leg is abducted and the tibial collateral ligament can be torn along with the medial meniscus.

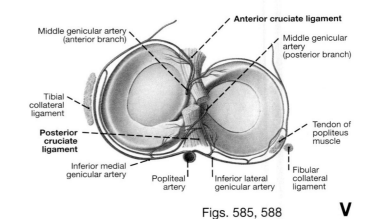

Fig. 588: Arterial Supply of the Menisci, Right Knee ▶

NOTE: the **medial** and **lateral genicular arteries** encircle the tibia and supply the menisci. The **middle genicular artery** supplies the cruciate ligaments. (From Sick H, Koriké JG. Z Anat Entwickl-Gesch 1969; 129: 359–379).

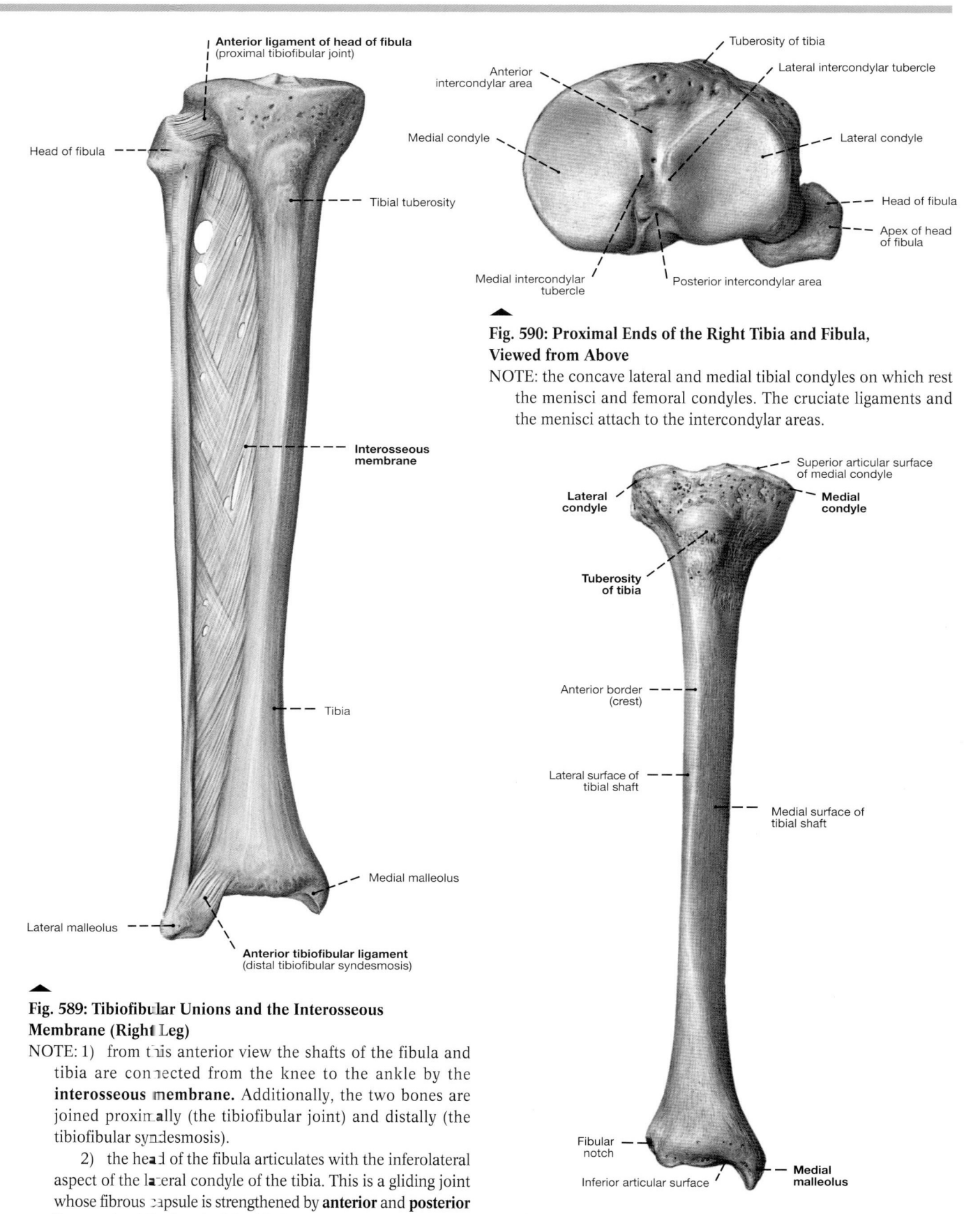

Anterior ligament of head of fibula
(proximal tibiofibular joint)

Head of fibula

Tibial tuberosity

Interosseous membrane

Tibia

Medial malleolus

Lateral malleolus

Anterior tibiofibular ligament
(distal tibiofibular syndesmosis)

Tuberosity of tibia

Anterior intercondylar area

Lateral intercondylar tubercle

Medial condyle

Lateral condyle

Head of fibula

Apex of head of fibula

Medial intercondylar tubercle

Posterior intercondylar area

Fig. 590: Proximal Ends of the Right Tibia and Fibula, Viewed from Above
NOTE: the concave lateral and medial tibial condyles on which rest the menisci and femoral condyles. The cruciate ligaments and the menisci attach to the intercondylar areas.

Superior articular surface of medial condyle

Lateral condyle

Medial condyle

Tuberosity of tibia

Anterior border (crest)

Lateral surface of tibial shaft

Medial surface of tibial shaft

Fibular notch

Inferior articular surface

Medial malleolus

Fig. 589: Tibiofibular Unions and the Interosseous Membrane (Right Leg)
NOTE: 1) from this anterior view the shafts of the fibula and tibia are connected from the knee to the ankle by the **interosseous membrane.** Additionally, the two bones are joined proximally (the tibiofibular joint) and distally (the tibiofibular syndesmosis).

    2) the head of the fibula articulates with the inferolateral aspect of the lateral condyle of the tibia. This is a gliding joint whose fibrous capsule is strengthened by **anterior** and **posterior ligaments of the head of the fibula.**

    3) the syndesmosis between the distal ends of the fibula and tibia is bound by anterior and posterior tibiofibular ligaments.

Fig. 591: Right Tibia, Anterior View ▲
NOTE: the proximal extremity is marked by the tibial condyles and the tibial tuberosity. The medial aspect of the distal extremity forms the medial malleolus.

Figs. 592 and 593: Right Fibula, Medial and Lateral Views ▶

NOTE: 1) the fibula is a long slender bone situated lateral to the tibia to which it articulates proximally and distally. The fibula expands inferiorly to form the **lateral malleolus.** The medial aspect of its inferior articular surface participates with the tibia to form the **talocrural joint (ankle joint).**

2) although the fibula does not bear any weight of the trunk (not participating in the knee joint), it is important since numerous muscles attach to its surface (see Figs. 529 and 547) and because it helps form the ankle joint.

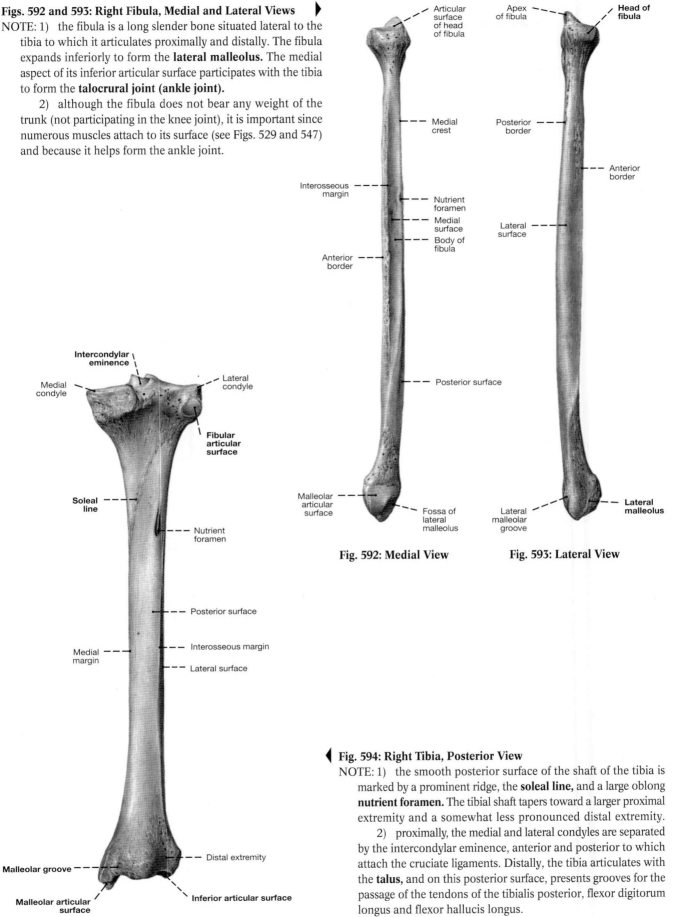

Fig. 592: Medial View   **Fig. 593: Lateral View**

◀ **Fig. 594: Right Tibia, Posterior View**

NOTE: 1) the smooth posterior surface of the shaft of the tibia is marked by a prominent ridge, the **soleal line,** and a large oblong **nutrient foramen.** The tibial shaft tapers toward a larger proximal extremity and a somewhat less pronounced distal extremity.

2) proximally, the medial and lateral condyles are separated by the intercondylar eminence, anterior and posterior to which attach the cruciate ligaments. Distally, the tibia articulates with the **talus,** and on this posterior surface, presents grooves for the passage of the tendons of the tibialis posterior, flexor digitorum longus and flexor hallucis longus.

PLATE 390   Bones of the Foot and Muscle Attachments (Dorsal View)

Fig. 595: Dorsal Aspect of the Bones of the Right Foot Showing the Attachments of Muscles

Red = origin; Blue = insertion

NOTE: 1) the insertion of the **calcaneal tendon** (of Achilles) on the posterior surface of the calcaneus. This tendon is the strongest in the body and a bursa is interposed between the bone and the tendon.

2) the only other muscle that attaches to the tarsal bones on this dorsal aspect is the **extensor digitorum brevis,** which arises from the dorsolateral surface of the calcaneus, distal to its articulation with the talus. Its medial part inserts on the proximal phalanx of the large toe while its other 3 tendons insert on the middle phalanx of the 2nd, 3rd and 4th toes.

3) the insertions of the **fibularis brevis** and **tertius** onto the base of the 5th metatarsal.

4) the 4 dorsal interosseous muscles, two of which insert on the 2nd toe and the 3rd and 4th insert on the dorsolateral aspect of the 3rd and 4th toes.

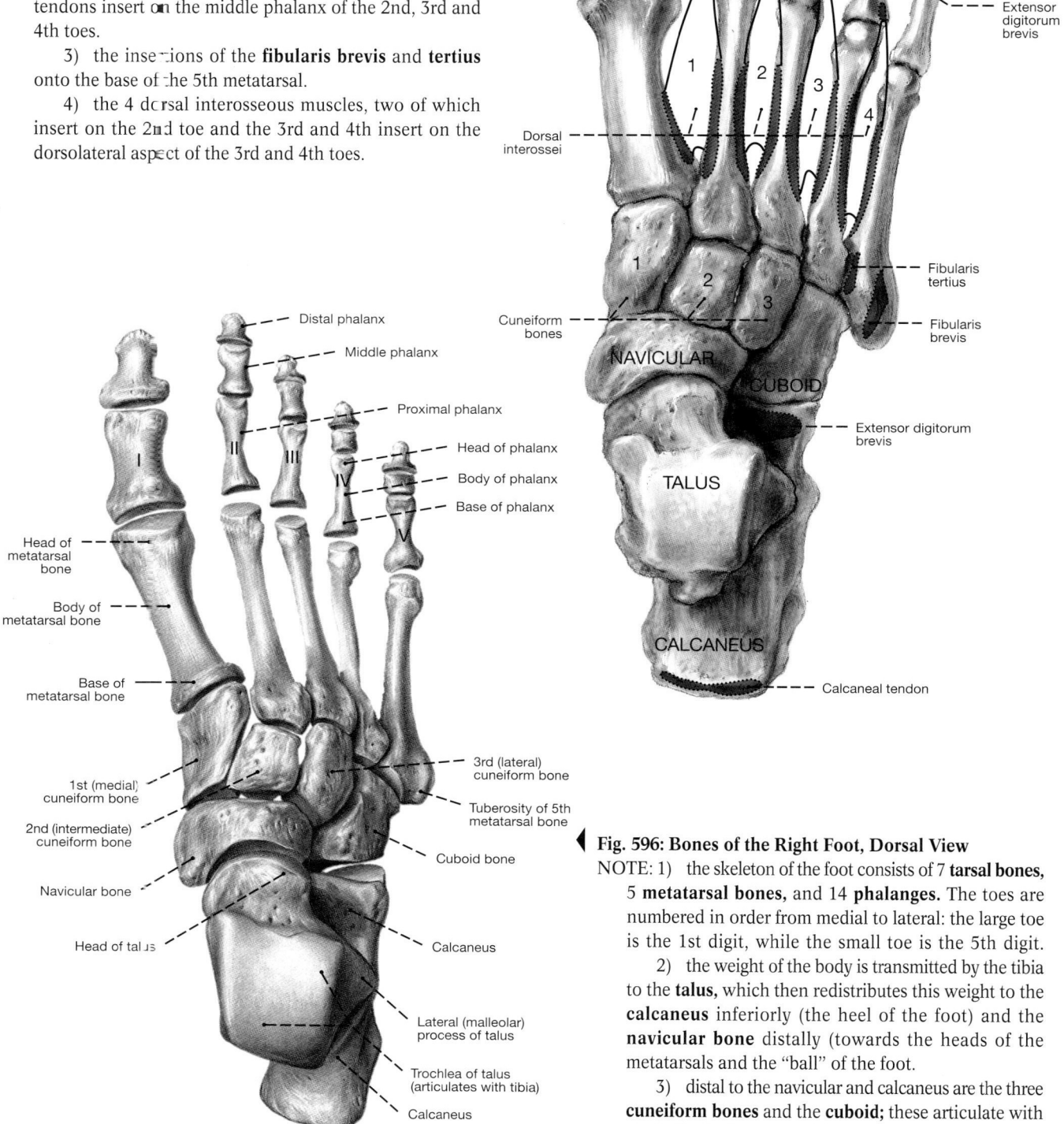

Fig. 596: Bones of the Right Foot, Dorsal View

NOTE: 1) the skeleton of the foot consists of 7 **tarsal bones,** 5 **metatarsal bones,** and 14 **phalanges.** The toes are numbered in order from medial to lateral: the large toe is the 1st digit, while the small toe is the 5th digit.

2) the weight of the body is transmitted by the tibia to the **talus,** which then redistributes this weight to the **calcaneus** inferiorly (the heel of the foot) and the **navicular bone** distally (towards the heads of the metatarsals and the "ball" of the foot.

3) distal to the navicular and calcaneus are the three **cuneiform bones** and the **cuboid;** these articulate with the individual metatarsal bones of the digits.

Figs. 595, 596

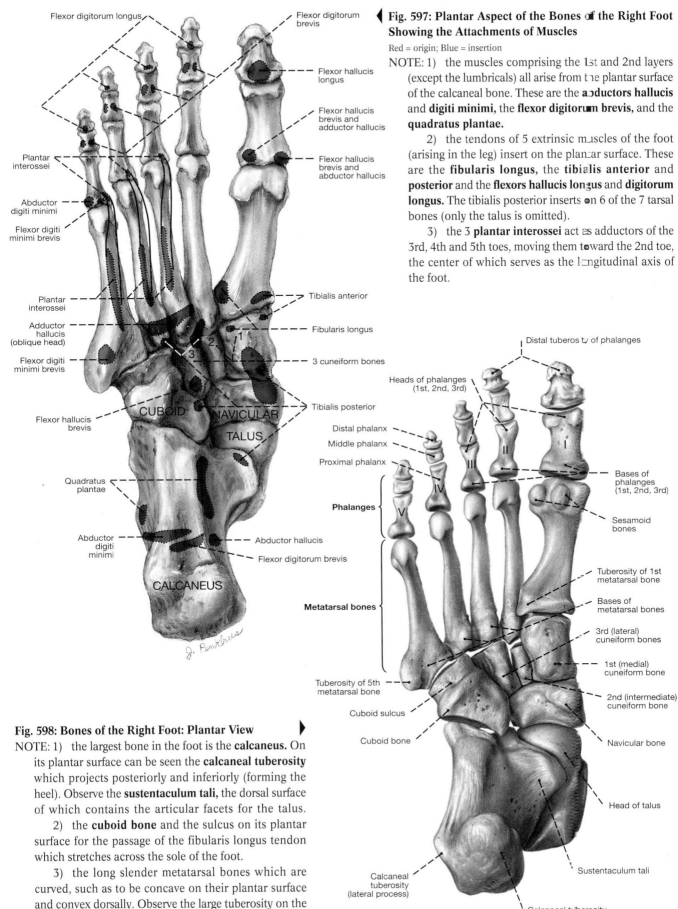

Fig. 597: Plantar Aspect of the Bones of the Right Foot Showing the Attachments of Muscles

Red = origin; Blue = insertion

NOTE: 1) the muscles comprising the 1st and 2nd layers (except the lumbricals) all arise from the plantar surface of the calcaneal bone. These are the **abductors hallucis** and **digiti minimi,** the **flexor digitorum brevis,** and the **quadratus plantae.**

2) the tendons of 5 extrinsic muscles of the foot (arising in the leg) insert on the plantar surface. These are the **fibularis longus,** the **tibialis anterior** and **posterior** and the **flexors hallucis longus** and **digitorum longus.** The tibialis posterior inserts on 6 of the 7 tarsal bones (only the talus is omitted).

3) the 3 **plantar interossei** act as adductors of the 3rd, 4th and 5th toes, moving them toward the 2nd toe, the center of which serves as the longitudinal axis of the foot.

Fig. 598: Bones of the Right Foot: Plantar View ▶

NOTE: 1) the largest bone in the foot is the **calcaneus.** On its plantar surface can be seen the **calcaneal tuberosity** which projects posteriorly and inferiorly (forming the heel). Observe the **sustentaculum tali,** the dorsal surface of which contains the articular facets for the talus.

2) the **cuboid bone** and the sulcus on its plantar surface for the passage of the fibularis longus tendon which stretches across the sole of the foot.

3) the long slender metatarsal bones which are curved, such as to be concave on their plantar surface and convex dorsally. Observe the large tuberosity on the lateral side of the base of the 5th metatarsal bone.

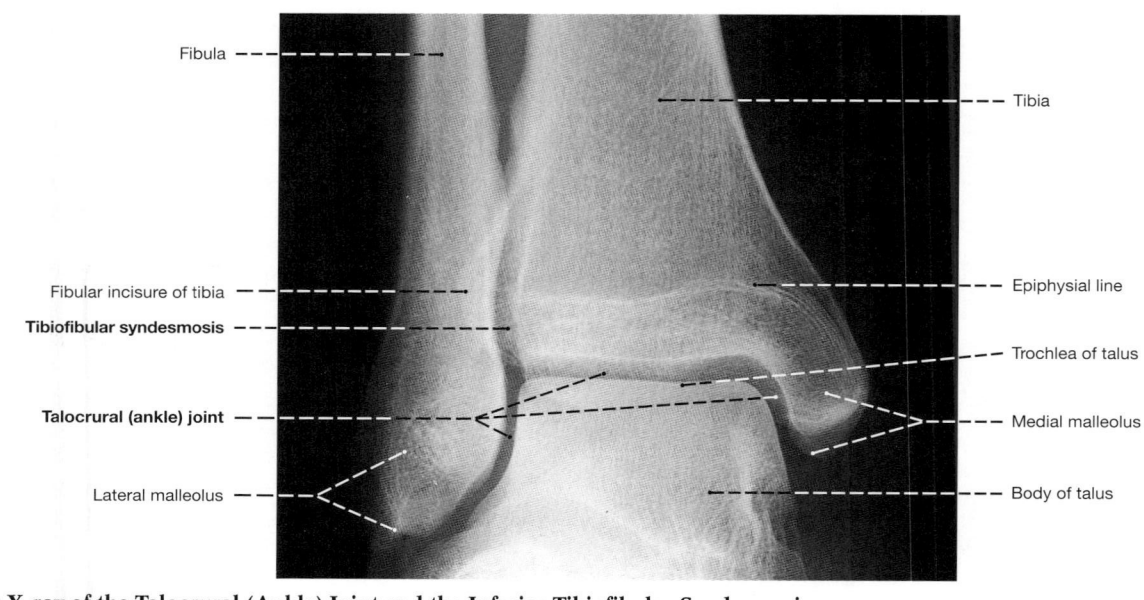

Fibula

Tibia

Fibular incisure of tibia

Epiphysial line

Tibiofibular syndesmosis

Trochlea of talus

Talocrural (ankle) joint

Medial malleolus

Lateral malleolus

Body of talus

Fig. 599: X-ray of the Talocrural (Ankle) Joint and the Inferior Tibiofibular Syndesmosis

NOTE: 1)   this is an AP radiograph showing both the ankle joint and the tibiofibular syndesmosis.

2)   the ankle joint is a ginglymus or hinge joint. The bony structures participating in this joint superiorly are the distal end of the **tibia** and its **medial malleolus,** and the distal **fibula** and its **lateral malleolus.** Together these structures form a concave receptacle for the convex proximal surface of the **talus.**

3)   the inferior tibiofibular joint connects the convex or medial side of the lower part of the fibular with the concavity of the fibular notch of the tibia. These surfaces are separated by the upward prolongation (4 to 5 mm) of the synovial membrane of the talocrural joint. The part of the articulation that is fibrous is called **tibiofibular syndesmosis.**

Tibia

Epiphysial line

Tibiofibular syndesmosis

Talocrural (ankle) joint

Medial malleolus of tibia

Epiphysial line

Body of talus

Deltoid ligament (posterior tibiotalar part)

Lateral malleolus of fibula

Flexor retinaculum

Posterior talofibular ligament

Tendon and sheath of tibialis posterior muscle

Calcaneofibular ligament

Tendon and sheath of flexor digitorum longus muscle

Subtalar joint (talocalcaneal joint)

Interosseous talocalcaneal ligament

Superior fibular retinaculum

Subtalar joint (talocalcaneal joint)

Tendon of fibularis brevis muscle

Medial plantar vessels and nerve

Tendon sheath of fibularis muscles

Quadratus plantae muscle

Tendon of fibularis longus muscle

Inferior fibular retinaculum

Abductor hallucis muscle

Calcaneus

Lateral plantar vessels and nerve

Abductor digiti minimi muscle

Plantar aponeurosis

Flexor digitorum brevis muscle

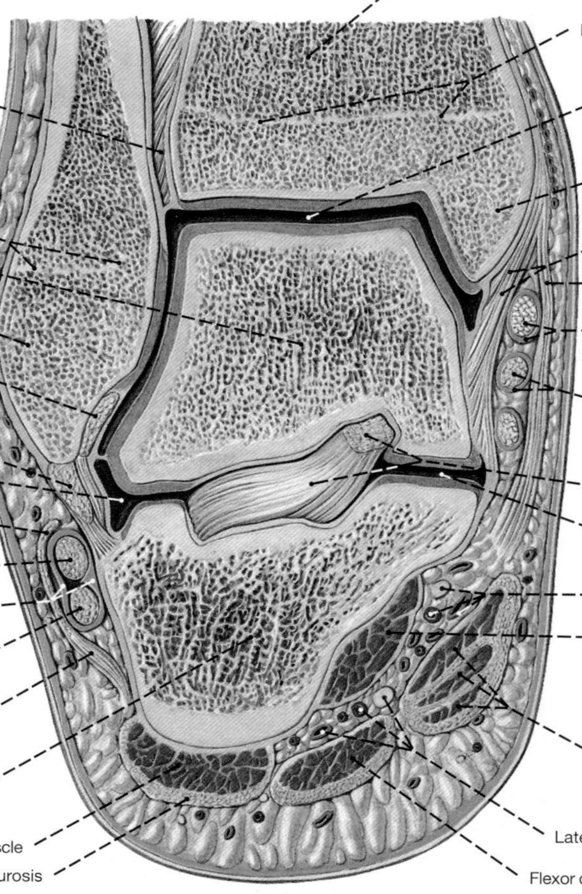

Fig. 600: Coronal Section Through the Talocrural (Ankle) and Subtalar Joints and the Tibiofibular Syndesmosis

Figs. 599, 600

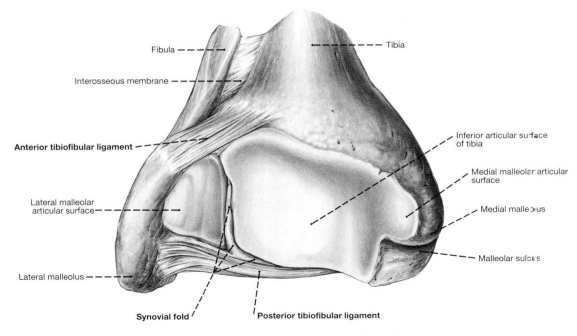

Fibula

Tibia

Interosseous membrane

Inferior articular surface of tibia

Anterior tibiofibular ligament

Medial malleolar articular surface

Lateral malleolar articular surface

Medial malleolus

Medial malleolar articular surface

Malleolar sulcus

Lateral malleolus

Synovial fold

Posterior tibiofibular ligament

Fig. 601: Inferior Articular Surface of the Tibia and Fibula at the Talocrural (Ankle) Joint

NOTE: 1) the medial and lateral sides of the upper part of the talocrural (ankle) joint are formed by the articular surfaces of the medial malleolus (tibia) and lateral malleolus (fibula). These grasp the sides of the talus.

2) the inferior articular surface of the tibia is wider anteriorly than posteriorly to accommodate the broader anterior surface of the talus. In full dorsiflexion, the ankle joint is very stable and does not allow any side to side movement, but in full plantarflexion a degree of side to side movement can occur.

3) the synovial fold of the ankle joint that extends upward between the inferior surfaces of the fibula and tibia.

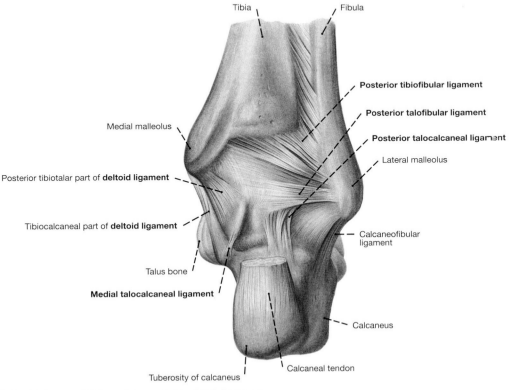

Tibia

Fibula

Posterior tibiofibular ligament

Posterior talofibular ligament

Posterior talocalcaneal ligament

Medial malleolus

Lateral malleolus

Posterior tibiotalar part of **deltoid ligament**

Tibiocalcaneal part of **deltoid ligament**

Calcaneofibular ligament

Talus bone

Medial talocalcaneal ligament

Calcaneus

Tuberosity of calcaneus

Calcaneal tendon

Fig. 602: Ankle Joint (Talocrural) Viewed from Behind (Right Foot)

NOTE: 1) the posterior aspect of the articular capsule is somewhat strengthened by the posterior talofibular and posterior tibiofibular ligaments. Laterally, the calcaneofibular ligament and medially, the strong deltoid ligament assist in protecting this joint.

2) the ligamentous bands that help stabilize the talocalcaneal articulation posteriorly: the posterior and medial talocalcaneal ligaments.

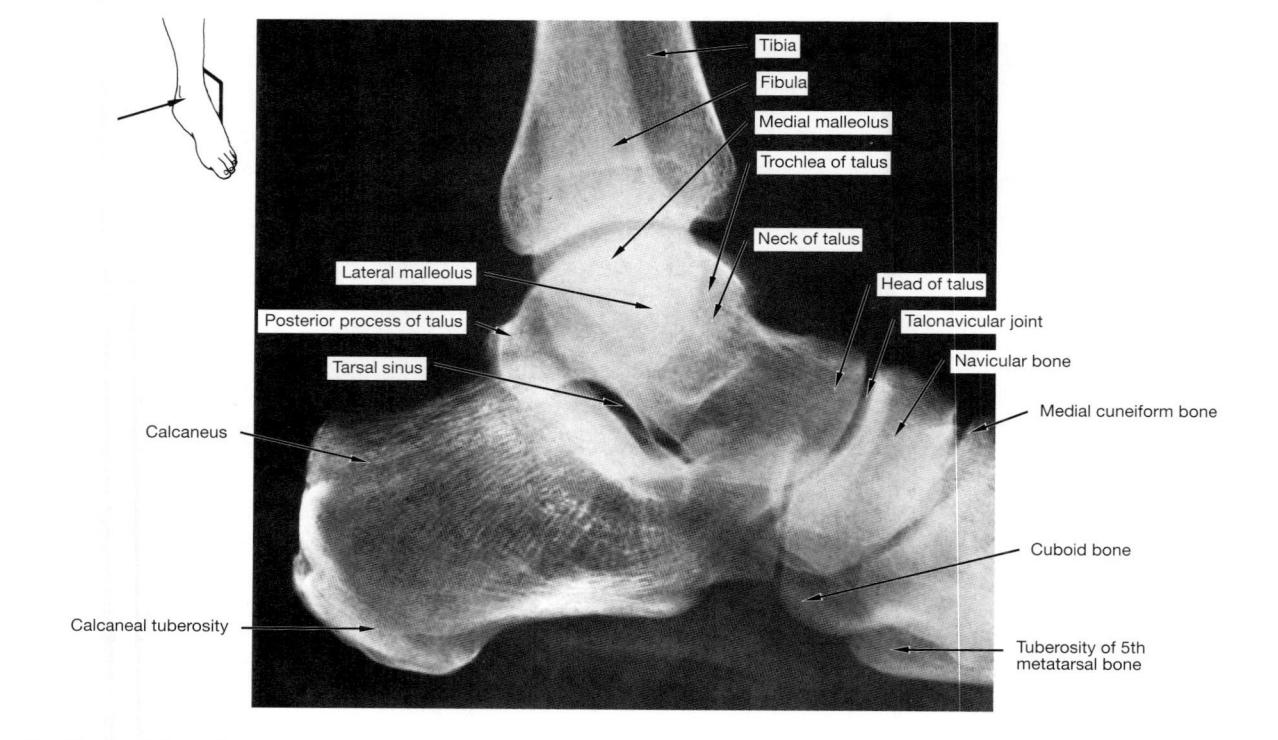

Fig. 603: X-ray of the Talocrural (Ankle) Joint, Lateral View

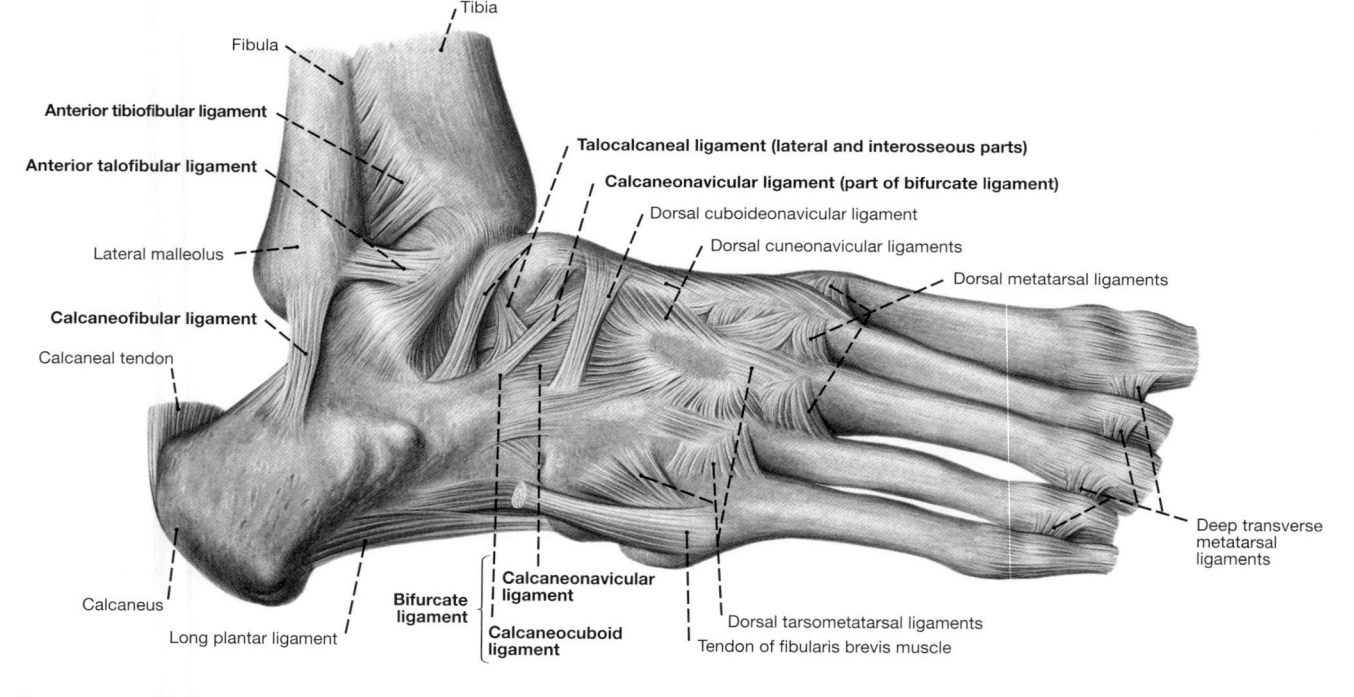

Fig. 604: Lateral Ligaments of the Ankle Joint and of the Dorsolateral Foot (Right)

NOTE: 1)   the fibula is attached to the tibia distally by the **anterior (inferior) tibiofibular ligament.** Additionally, the lateral malleolus of the fibula is attached to the talus by the relatively weak **anterior talofibular ligament** and the much stronger **posterior talofibular ligament** (Fig. 602). The fibula is attached to the calcaneus by the **calcaneofibular ligament.** Together these latter three bands constitute the lateral ligament of the ankle.

   2)   the **interosseous talocalcaneal ligament,** which is the principal ligament that strengthens the **subtalar joint** (between talus and calcaneus), the **lateral talocalcaneal ligament** also helps strengthen this joint as does the **medial talocalcaneal ligament,** which blends with the deltoid ligament (not shown).

   3)   the (dorsal) **calcaneonavicular ligament,** part of the **bifurcate ligament,** which attaches the dorsolateral aspect of the navicular bone with bone the calcaneus. Along with this (dorsal) calcaneonavicular ligament, the (dorsal) calcaneocuboid ligament constitutes the **"bifurcate" ligament.**

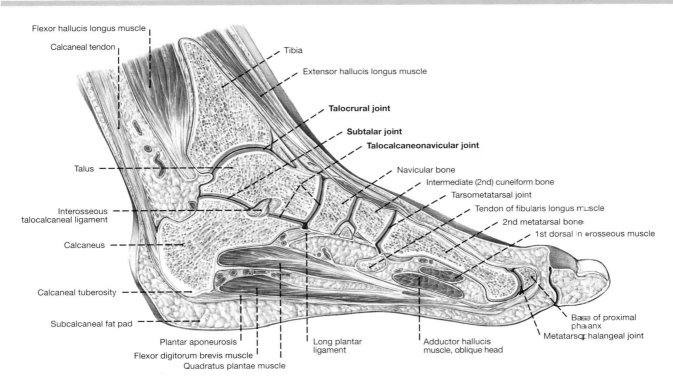

Flexor hallucis longus muscle

Calcaneal tendon

Tibia

Extensor hallucis longus muscle

Talocrural joint

Subtalar joint

Talocalcaneonavicular joint

Talus

Navicular bone

Intermediate (2nd) cuneiform bone

Tarsometatarsal joint

Tendon of fibularis longus muscle

Interosseous talocalcaneal ligament

2nd metatarsal bone

1st dorsal interosseous muscle

Calcaneus

Calcaneal tuberosity

Subcalcaneal fat pad

Base of proximal phalanx

Metatarsophalangeal joint

Plantar aponeurosis

Long plantar ligament

Adductor hallucis muscle, oblique head

Flexor digitorum brevis muscle

Quadratus plantae muscle

Fig. 605: Sagittal Section of Foot Showing Talocrural, Subtalar and Talocalcaneonavicular Joints

NOTE: 1) this sagittal section, viewed from the medial aspect, cuts through the trochlea, neck and head of the talus.

2) the joint between the talus and calcaneus, the **subtalar joint,** is strengthened principally by the **interosseous talocalcaneal ligament** (see also Fig. 600).

3) the **talocalcaneonavicular joint** anteriorly is of important clinical significance because the weight of the body tends to push the head of the talus downward between the navicular and calcaneus. This results in flat feet.

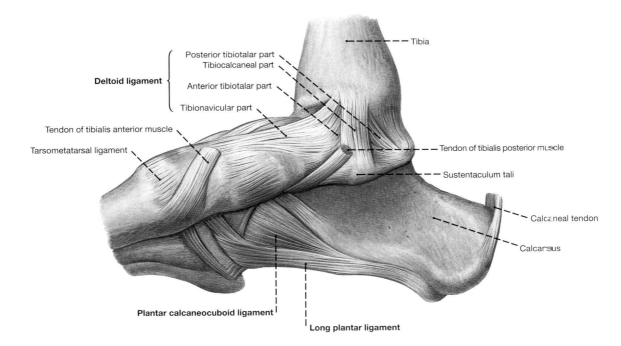

Deltoid ligament

Posterior tibiotalar part

Tibiocalcaneal part

Anterior tibiotalar part

Tibionavicular part

Tendon of tibialis anterior muscle

Tarsometatarsal ligament

Tibia

Tendon of tibialis posterior muscle

Sustentaculum tali

Calcaneal tendon

Calcaneus

Plantar calcaneocuboid ligament

Long plantar ligament

Fig. 606: Ligaments of the Ankle and Foot: Medial View (Right Foot)

NOTE: 1) the medial aspect of the ankle joint is protected by the triangular **deltoid ligament** which connects the tibia to the navicular, calcaneus and talus. The deltoid ligament has four parts: (a) an anterior **tibionavicular part** that attaches the medial malleolus to the navicular, (b) a superficial **tibiocalcaneal part** attaching the malleolus to the sustentaculum tali of the calcaneus, and (c and d) the **anterior** and **posterior tibiotalar parts** that lie more deeply and attach the malleolus to the adjacent talus.

2) the insertions of the tendons of the tibialis anterior and posterior muscles attach on this medial aspect of the foot. Observe also the **long plantar** and **plantar calcaneocuboid ligaments** on the plantar surface.

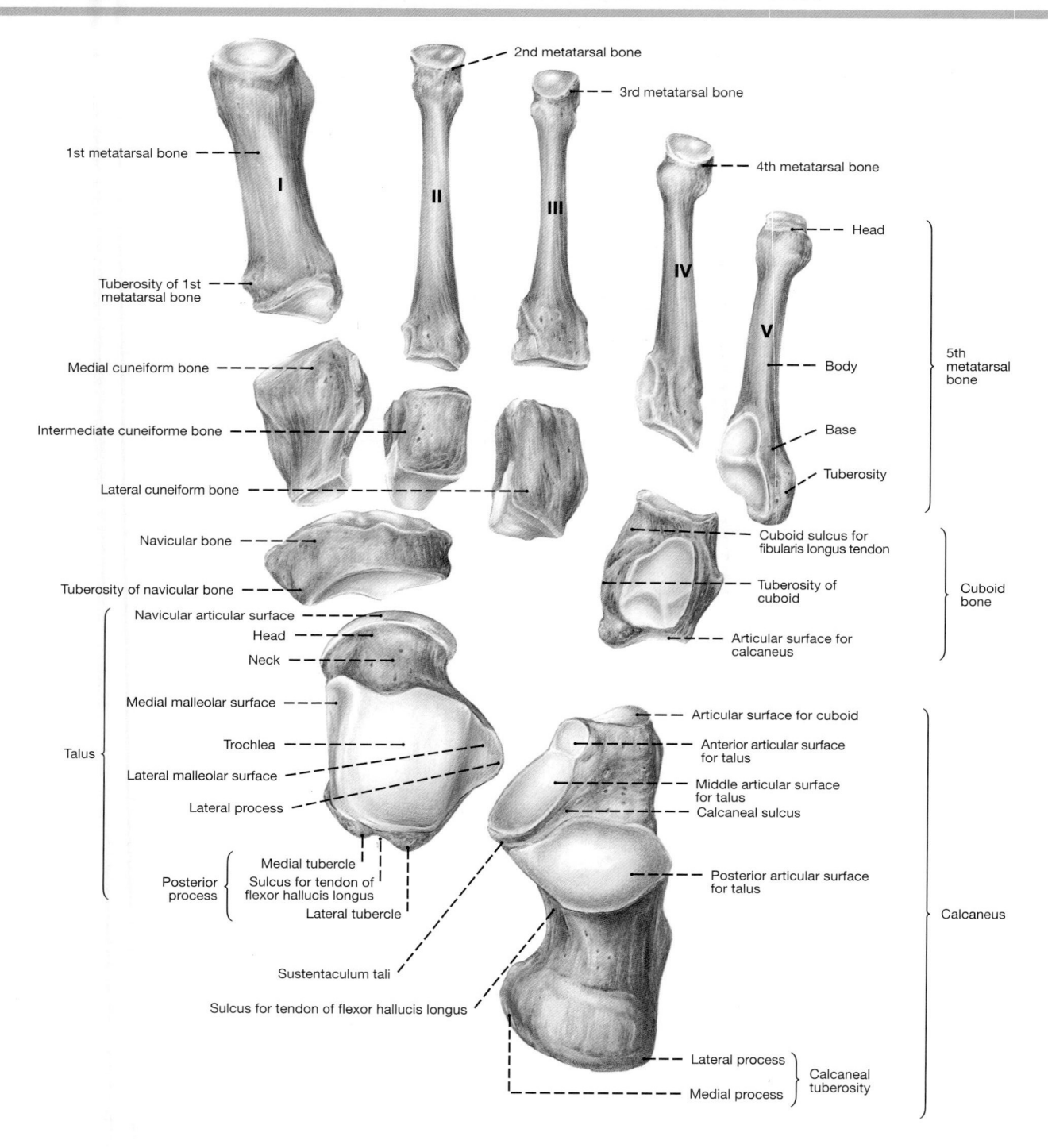

Fig. 607: Tarsal and Metatarsal Bones of the Right Foot

NOTE: 1)   in this dorsal view (except for the cuboid bone, which has been rotated so that its medial surface is presented dorsally) are depicted the **seven tarsal bones** and the **five metatarsal bones;** the phalanges are not shown.

    2)   the tarsal bones, although homologues of the carpal bones, are of greater size and strength than the bones of the wrist because they function to support the weight of the body in standing.

    3)   of the seven tarsal bones, the **talus** and **calcaneus** comprise the proximal row and the **three cuneiforms** and the **cuboid,** the distal row. Interposed between the talus and the cuneiforms medially is the **navicular bone,** while the calcaneus and cuboid articulate directly.

    4)   the **five metatarsal bones** interconnect the tarsal bones with the phalanges (not shown), and they are numbered from medial to lateral. The medial cuneiform articulates distally Lilith the 1st metatarsal, the intermediate cuneiform with the 2nd metatarsal, and the lateral cuneiform with the 3rd metatarsal. The cuboid articulates distally with both the 4th and 5th metatarsal bones.

Fig. 607

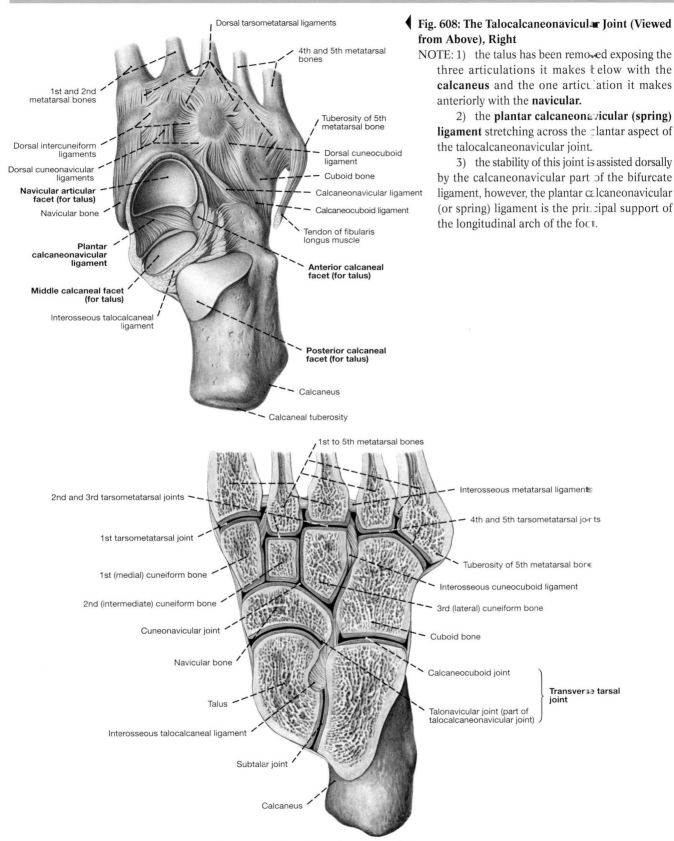

Dorsal tarsometatarsal ligaments

4th and 5th metatarsal bones

1st and 2nd metatarsal bones

Dorsal intercuneiform ligaments

Dorsal cuneonavicular ligaments

Navicular articular facet (for talus)

Navicular bone

Plantar calcaneonavicular ligament

Middle calcaneal facet (for talus)

Interosseous talocalcaneal ligament

Tuberosity of 5th metatarsal bone

Dorsal cuneocuboid ligament

Cuboid bone

Calcaneonavicular ligament

Calcaneocuboid ligament

Tendon of fibularis longus muscle

Anterior calcaneal facet (for talus)

Posterior calcaneal facet (for talus)

Calcaneus

Calcaneal tuberosity

Fig. 608: The Talocalcaneonavicular Joint (Viewed from Above), Right

NOTE: 1) the talus has been removed exposing the three articulations it makes below with the **calcaneus** and the one articulation it makes anteriorly with the **navicular.**

2) the **plantar calcaneonavicular (spring) ligament** stretching across the plantar aspect of the talocalcaneonavicular joint.

3) the stability of this joint is assisted dorsally by the calcaneonavicular part of the bifurcate ligament, however, the plantar calcaneonavicular (or spring) ligament is the principal support of the longitudinal arch of the foot.

1st to 5th metatarsal bones

2nd and 3rd tarsometatarsal joints

1st tarsometatarsal joint

1st (medial) cuneiform bone

2nd (intermediate) cuneiform bone

Cuneonavicular joint

Navicular bone

Talus

Interosseous talocalcaneal ligament

Subtalar joint

Calcaneus

Interosseous metatarsal ligament

4th and 5th tarsometatarsal joints

Tuberosity of 5th metatarsal bone

Interosseous cuneocuboid ligament

3rd (lateral) cuneiform bone

Cuboid bone

Calcaneocuboid joint

Talonavicular joint (part of talocalcaneonavicular joint)

Transverse tarsal joint

Fig. 609: Intertarsal and Tarsometatarsal Joints (Horizontal Section of the Right Foot)

NOTE: 1) the **transverse tarsal joint (midtarsal joint)** extends across the foot and actually is formed by two separate joint cavities, the **calcaneocuboid joint** laterally and the **talonavicular** part of the talocalcaneonavicular joint medially. These two joints allow some eversion and inversion movements of the foot.

2) the joints in the foot reflect a natural division of the bones into a *medial group* (talus, navicular, the three cuneiforms and the medial three metatarsals and phalanges) and a *lateral group* (calcaneus, cuboid and the lateral two metatarsals and phalanges).

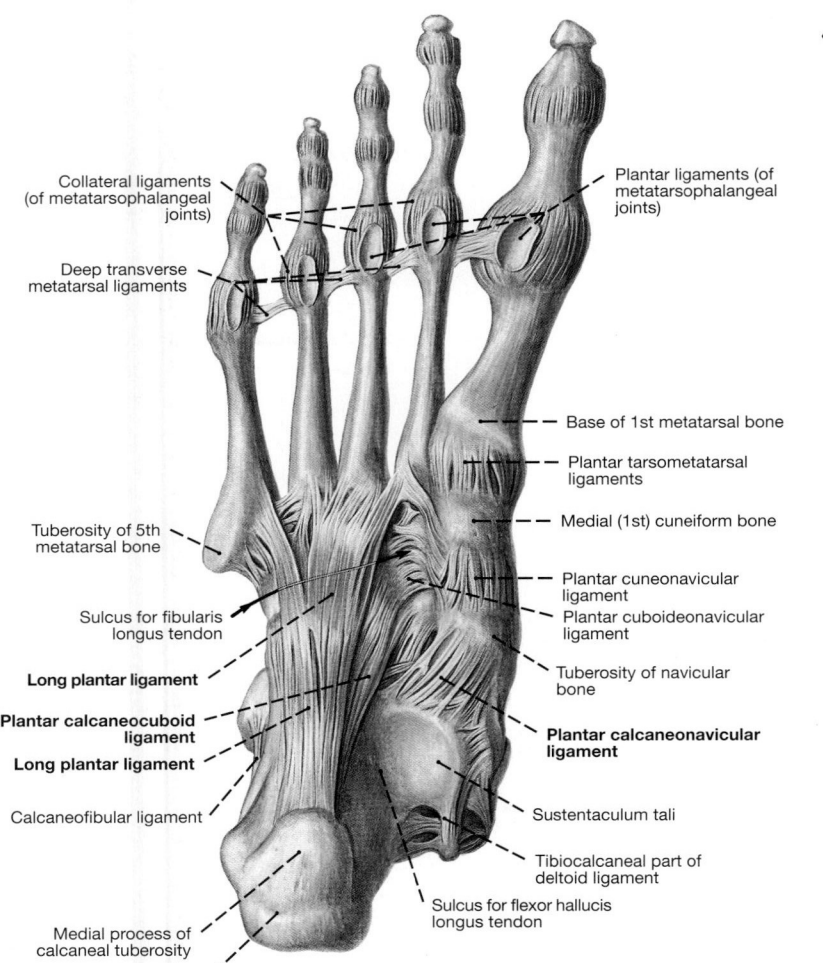

Collateral ligaments
(of metatarsophalangeal
joints)

Plantar ligaments (of
metatarsophalangeal
joints)

Deep transverse
metatarsal ligaments

Base of 1st metatarsal bone

Plantar tarsometatarsal
ligaments

Tuberosity of 5th
metatarsal bone

Medial (1st) cuneiform bone

Plantar cuneonavicular
ligament

Sulcus for fibularis
longus tendon

Plantar cuboideonavicular
ligament

Long plantar ligament

Tuberosity of navicular
bone

**Plantar calcaneocuboid
ligament**

**Plantar calcaneonavicular
ligament**

Long plantar ligament

Calcaneofibular ligament

Sustentaculum tali

Tibiocalcaneal part of
deltoid ligament

Medial process of
calcaneal tuberosity

Sulcus for flexor hallucis
longus tendon

Tuberosity of calcaneus

Fig. 610: Ligaments on the Plantar Surface of the Right Foot (Superficial)

NOTE: 1) the **long plantar ligament** is the longest and most superficial of the plantar tarsal ligaments. It stretches from the calcaneus posteriorly to an oblique ridge on the plantar surface of the cuboid, where most of its fibers terminate.

2) the superficial fibers of the long plantar ligament pass over the cuboid to insert on the bases of the lateral three metatarsal bones, thereby forming a tunnel for the **fibularis longus tendon.**

3) the **plantar calcaneocuboid** or **short plantar ligament** is very strong and lies deep to the long plantar ligament and closer to the bones.

4) identify the **plantar calcaneonavicular (spring) ligament** medially. It is attached to the sustentaculum tali of the calcaneus and extends along the entire inferior surface of the navicular bone. It is important for the support of the medial arch of the foot.

Fig. 611: Plantar Calcaneonavicular Ligament and the Insertions of Three Tendons (Right Foot)

NOTE: 1) the metatarsal extensions of the long plantar ligament have been cut away to reveal the groove for the tendon of the fibularis longus muscle. This tendon inserts onto the base of the 1st metatarsal bone and the 1st (medial) cuneiform bone.

2) two other tendons insert on the medial side of the plantar surface: the tibialis anterior and posterior tendons.

3) the fibers of the calcaneocuboid (short plantar) and calcaneonavicular (spring) ligaments all stem from the calcaneus and then diverge in a radial manner toward the medial side of the foot.

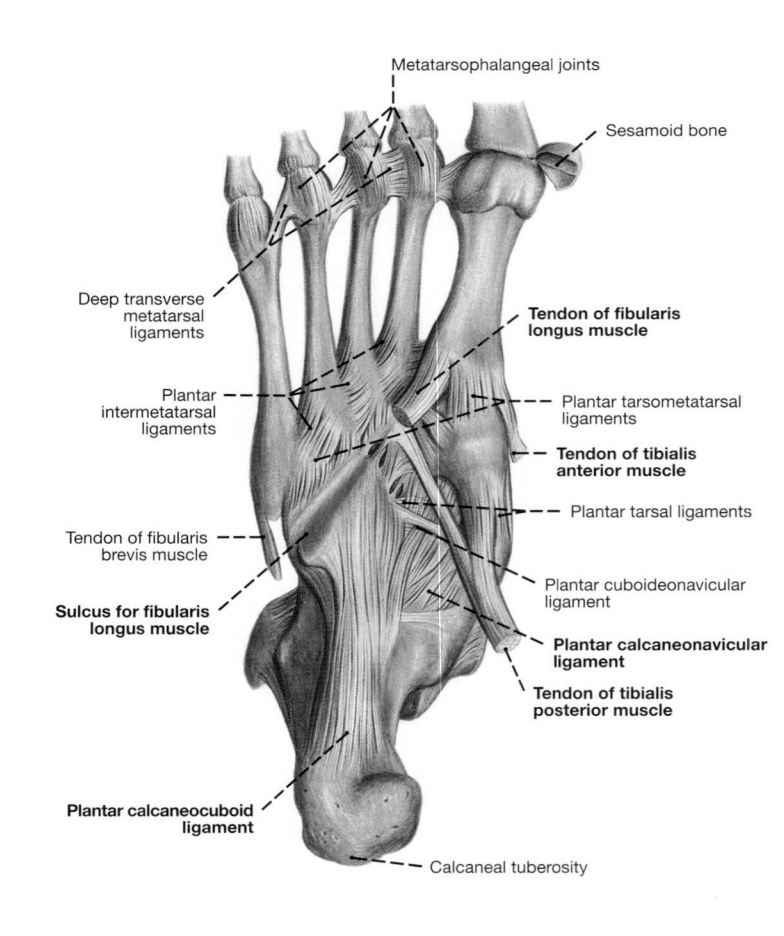

Metatarsophalangeal joints

Sesamoid bone

Deep transverse
metatarsal
ligaments

**Tendon of fibularis
longus muscle**

Plantar
intermetatarsal
ligaments

Plantar tarsometatarsal
ligaments

**Tendon of tibialis
anterior muscle**

Plantar tarsal ligaments

Tendon of fibularis
brevis muscle

Plantar cuboideonavicular
ligament

**Sulcus for fibularis
longus muscle**

**Plantar calcaneonavicular
ligament**

**Tendon of tibialis
posterior muscle**

**Plantar calcaneocuboid
ligament**

Calcaneal tuberosity

Fig. 612: Skeleton of the Foot, Showing the ▶ Arches: Medial View

NOTE: 1)   this figure demonstrates that the weight of the body is transmitted from the tibia to the talus along the mechanical axis (a–b). From the talus the weight is buttressed behind to the calcaneus (b–d) and anteriorly to the heads of the metatarsal bones (b–c). The arch formed between these two points (c–d) is the **medial longitudinal arch.**

2)   the **transverse arch** (e–f) of the foot is formed by the naviular, the three cuneiforms, the cuboid, and the bases of the five metatarsal bones. The transverse arch is maintained by the ligaments, which interconnect the cuneiforms and the bases of the metatarsal bones. The tendon of the fibularis longus muscle is also important in maintaining the transverse arch.

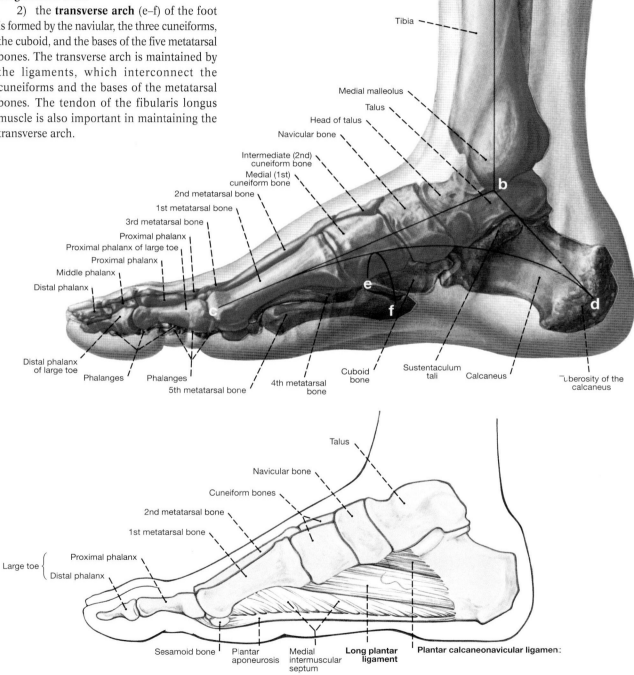

Red = tibia and tibial row
Blue = fibula and fibular row
    of tarsal bones

Fig. 613: Longitudinal Arch of the Foot: Underlying Support Structures

NOTE: 1)   the medial longitudinal arch of the foot is formed by the calcaneus, talus, navicular, the three cuneiform bones and the medial three metatarsal bones. Observe the arched nature of the medial margin of the foot.

2)   the integrity of the medial longitudinal arch depends on structures underlying the talocalcaneonavicular septum, but much more important are the **long plantar ligament** and especially the **plantar calcaneonavicular ligament.**

PLATE 400   Cross-sections of the Thigh and Leg

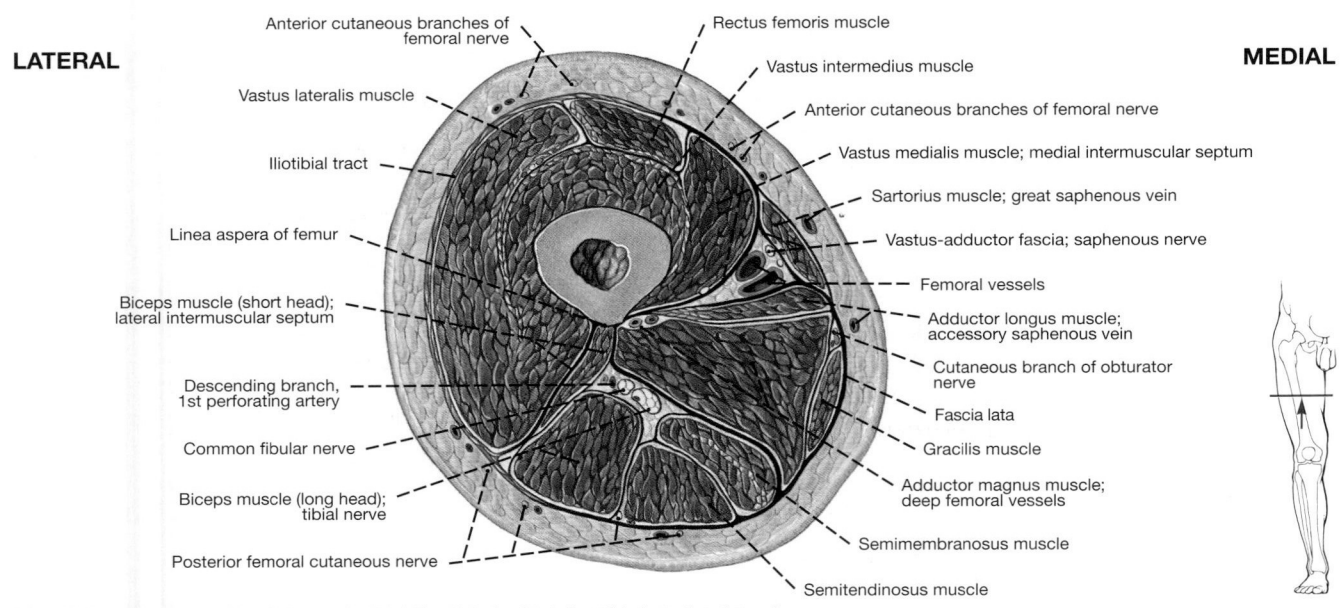

LATERAL

MEDIAL

Anterior cutaneous branches of femoral nerve

Rectus femoris muscle

Vastus lateralis muscle

Vastus intermedius muscle

Iliotibial tract

Anterior cutaneous branches of femoral nerve

Linea aspera of femur

Vastus medialis muscle; medial intermuscular septum

Biceps muscle (short head); lateral intermuscular septum

Sartorius muscle; great saphenous vein

Vastus-adductor fascia; saphenous nerve

Descending branch, 1st perforating artery

Femoral vessels

Common fibular nerve

Adductor longus muscle; accessory saphenous vein

Cutaneous branch of obturator nerve

Biceps muscle (long head); tibial nerve

Fascia lata

Gracilis muscle

Posterior femoral cutaneous nerve

Adductor magnus muscle; deep femoral vessels

Semimembranosus muscle

Semitendinosus muscle

Fig. 614:   Cross-section Through Middle Third of Right Thigh (Distal Surface)

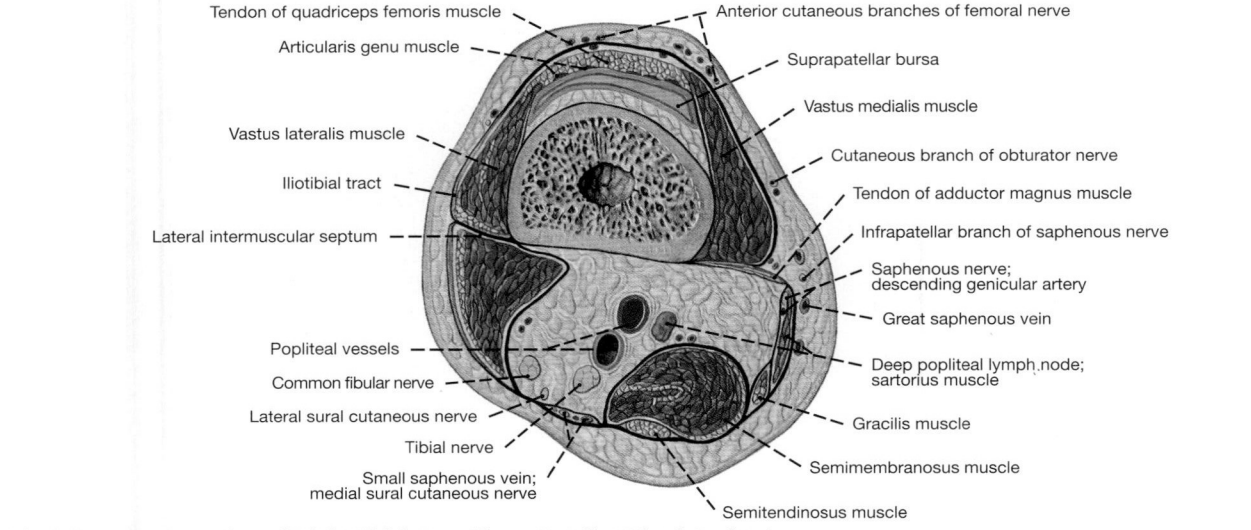

Tendon of quadriceps femoris muscle

Anterior cutaneous branches of femoral nerve

Articularis genu muscle

Suprapatellar bursa

Vastus lateralis muscle

Vastus medialis muscle

Iliotibial tract

Cutaneous branch of obturator nerve

Lateral intermuscular septum

Tendon of adductor magnus muscle

Infrapatellar branch of saphenous nerve

Saphenous nerve; descending genicular artery

Great saphenous vein

Popliteal vessels

Common fibular nerve

Deep popliteal lymph node; sartorius muscle

Lateral sural cutaneous nerve

Gracilis muscle

Tibial nerve

Semimembranosus muscle

Small saphenous vein; medial sural cutaneous nerve

Semitendinosus muscle

Fig. 615:   Cross-section of Right Thigh Just Above Patella (Distal Surface)

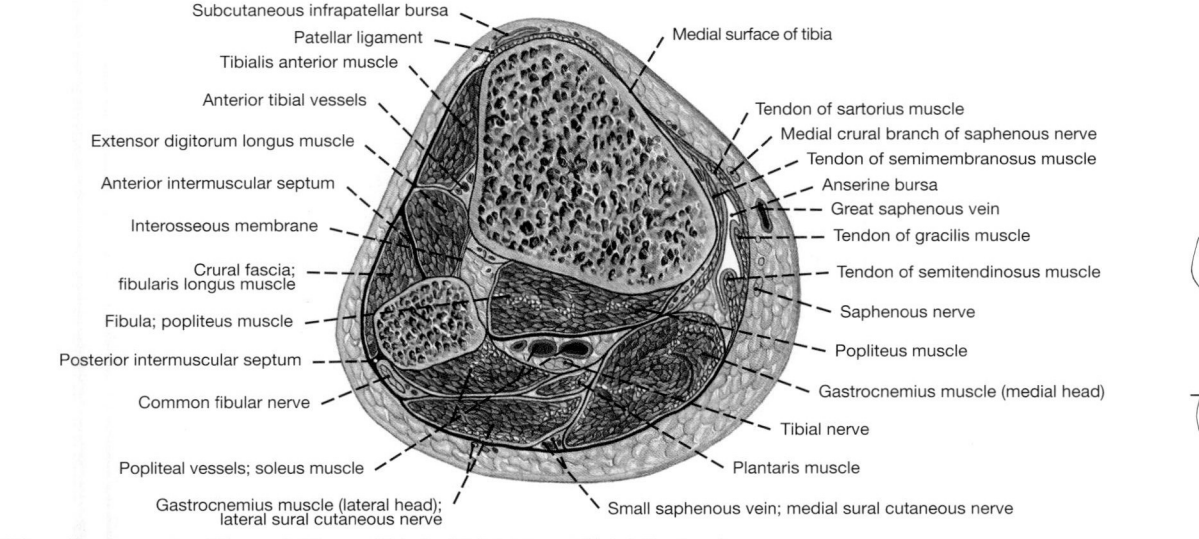

Subcutaneous infrapatellar bursa

Patellar ligament

Medial surface of tibia

Tibialis anterior muscle

Anterior tibial vessels

Tendon of sartorius muscle

Extensor digitorum longus muscle

Medial crural branch of saphenous nerve

Tendon of semimembranosus muscle

Anterior intermuscular septum

Anserine bursa

Interosseous membrane

Great saphenous vein

Crural fascia; fibularis longus muscle

Tendon of gracilis muscle

Tendon of semitendinosus muscle

Fibula; popliteus muscle

Saphenous nerve

Posterior intermuscular septum

Popliteus muscle

Common fibular nerve

Gastrocnemius muscle (medial head)

Tibial nerve

Popliteal vessels; soleus muscle

Plantaris muscle

Gastrocnemius muscle (lateral head); lateral sural cutaneous nerve

Small saphenous vein; medial sural cutaneous nerve

Fig. 616:   Cross-section Through Upper Third of Right Leg (Distal Surface)

Figs. 614, 615, 616

LATERAL

MEDIAL

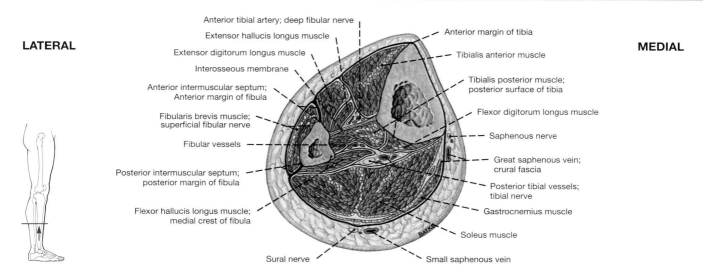

Anterior tibial artery; deep fibular nerve

Extensor hallucis longus muscle

Extensor digitorum longus muscle

Interosseous membrane

Anterior intermuscular septum;
Anterior margin of fibula

Fibularis brevis muscle;
superficial fibular nerve

Fibular vessels

Posterior intermuscular septum;
posterior margin of fibula

Flexor hallucis longus muscle;
medial crest of fibula

Sural nerve

Anterior margin of tibia

Tibialis anterior muscle

Tibialis posterior muscle;
posterior surface of tibia

Flexor digitorum longus muscle

Saphenous nerve

Great saphenous vein;
crural fascia

Posterior tibial vessels;
tibial nerve

Gastrocnemius muscle

Soleus muscle

Small saphenous vein

Fig. 617:   Cross-section Through the Middle of Right Leg (Distal Surface)

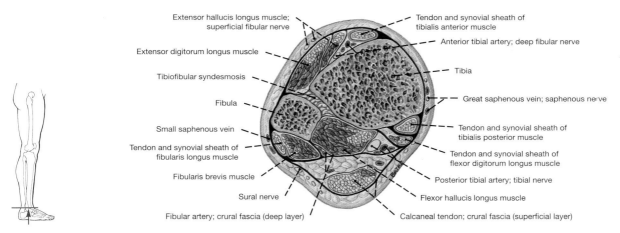

Extensor hallucis longus muscle;
superficial fibular nerve

Extensor digitorum longus muscle

Tibiofibular syndesmosis

Fibula

Small saphenous vein

Tendon and synovial sheath of
fibularis longus muscle

Fibularis brevis muscle

Sural nerve

Fibular artery; crural fascia (deep layer)

Tendon and synovial sheath of
tibialis anterior muscle

Anterior tibial artery; deep fibular nerve

Tibia

Great saphenous vein; saphenous nerve

Tendon and synovial sheath of
tibialis posterior muscle

Tendon and synovial sheath of
flexor digitorum longus muscle

Posterior tibial artery; tibial nerve

Flexor hallucis longus muscle

Calcaneal tendon; crural fascia (superficial layer)

Fig. 618:   Cross-section Through the Right Leg Just Above the Malleoli (Distal Surface)

DORSAL

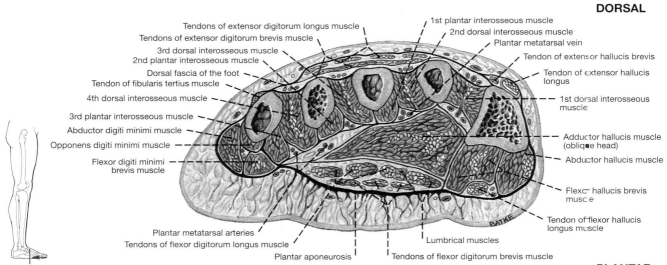

Tendons of extensor digitorum longus muscle

Tendons of extensor digitorum brevis muscle

3rd dorsal interosseous muscle

2nd plantar interosseous muscle

Dorsal fascia of the foot

Tendon of fibularis tertius muscle

4th dorsal interosseous muscle

3rd plantar interosseous muscle

Abductor digiti minimi muscle

Opponens digiti minimi muscle

Flexor digiti minimi
brevis muscle

1st plantar interosseous muscle

2nd dorsal interosseous muscle

Plantar metatarsal vein

Tendon of extensor hallucis brevis

Tendon of extensor hallucis
longus

1st dorsal interosseous
muscle

Adductor hallucis muscle
(oblique head)

Abductor hallucis muscle

Flexor hallucis brevis
muscle

Tendon of flexor hallucis
longus muscle

Plantar metatarsal arteries

Tendons of flexor digitorum longus muscle

Plantar aponeurosis

Lumbrical muscles

Tendons of flexor digitorum brevis muscle

PLANTAR

Fig. 619:   Cross-section of the Right Foot Through the Metatarsal Bones (Distal Surface)

PLATE 402   MRIs of Thigh and Leg

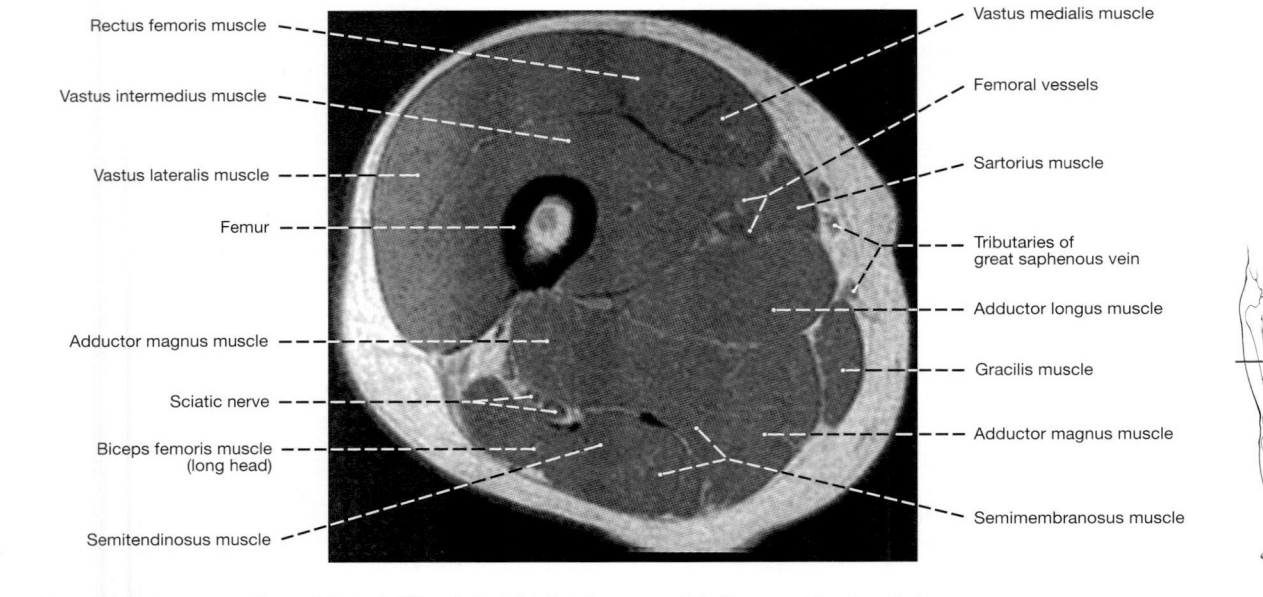

Rectus femoris muscle

Vastus intermedius muscle

Vastus lateralis muscle

Femur

Adductor magnus muscle

Sciatic nerve

Biceps femoris muscle
(long head)

Semitendinosus muscle

Vastus medialis muscle

Femoral vessels

Sartorius muscle

Tributaries of
great saphenous vein

Adductor longus muscle

Gracilis muscle

Adductor magnus muscle

Semimembranosus muscle

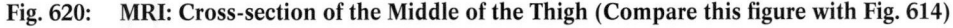

Fig. 620:   MRI: Cross-section of the Middle of the Thigh (Compare this figure with Fig. 614)

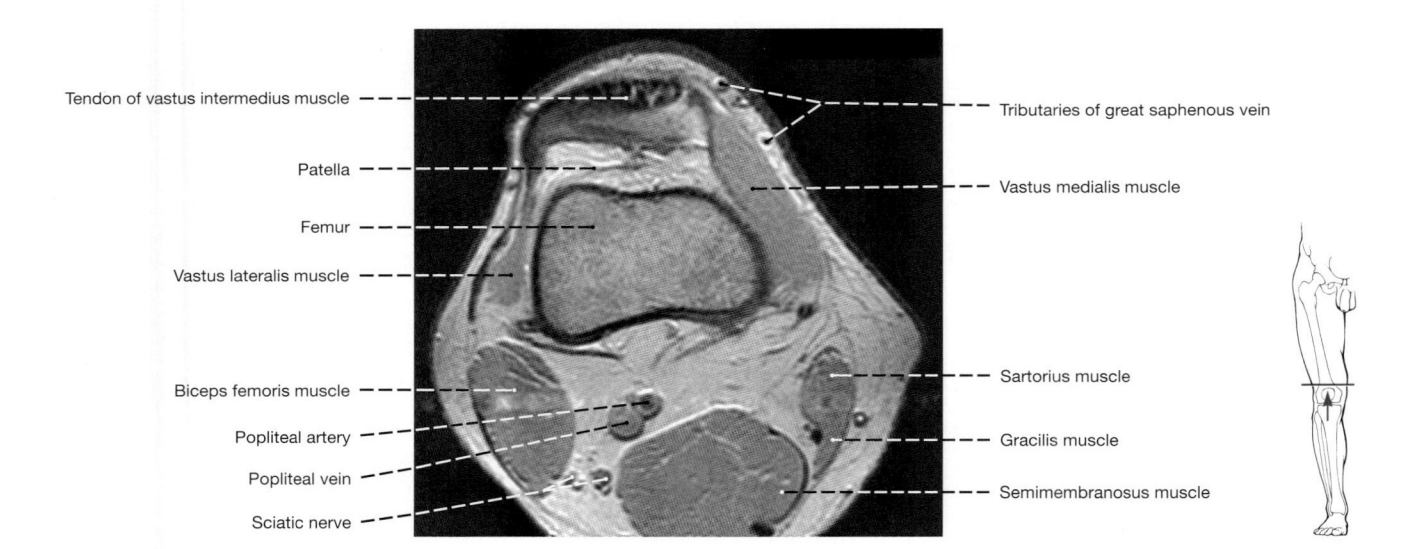

Tendon of vastus intermedius muscle

Patella

Femur

Vastus lateralis muscle

Biceps femoris muscle

Popliteal artery

Popliteal vein

Sciatic nerve

Tributaries of great saphenous vein

Vastus medialis muscle

Sartorius muscle

Gracilis muscle

Semimembranosus muscle

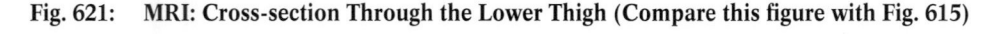

Fig. 621:   MRI: Cross-section Through the Lower Thigh (Compare this figure with Fig. 615)

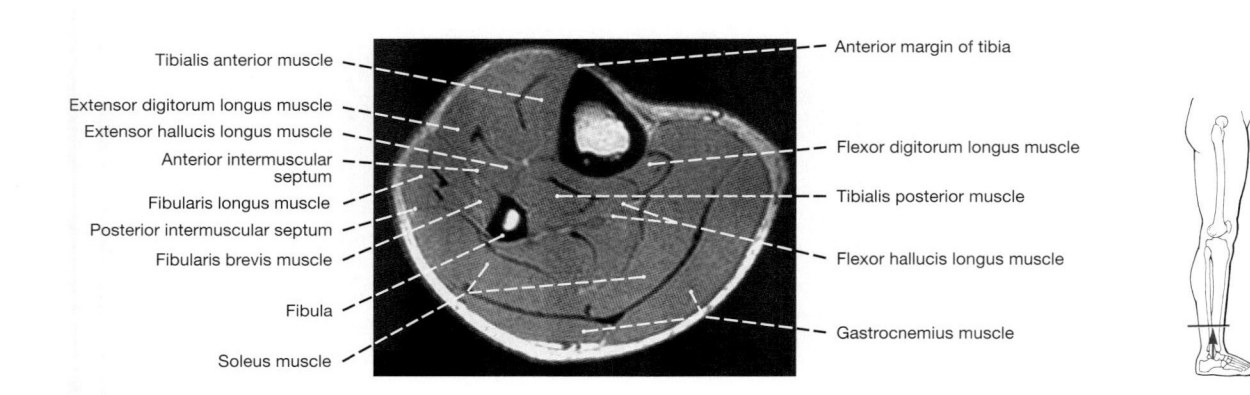

Tibialis anterior muscle

Extensor digitorum longus muscle
Extensor hallucis longus muscle
Anterior intermuscular
septum
Fibularis longus muscle
Posterior intermuscular septum
Fibularis brevis muscle

Fibula

Soleus muscle

Anterior margin of tibia

Flexor digitorum longus muscle

Tibialis posterior muscle

Flexor hallucis longus muscle

Gastrocnemius muscle

Fig. 622:   MRI: Cross-section Through the Lower Leg

PART VI
THE BACK, VERTEBRAL COLUMN, AND SPINAL CORD

(PLATES 403–434 – FIGURES 623–690)

PART VI The Back, Vertebral Column and Spinal Cord

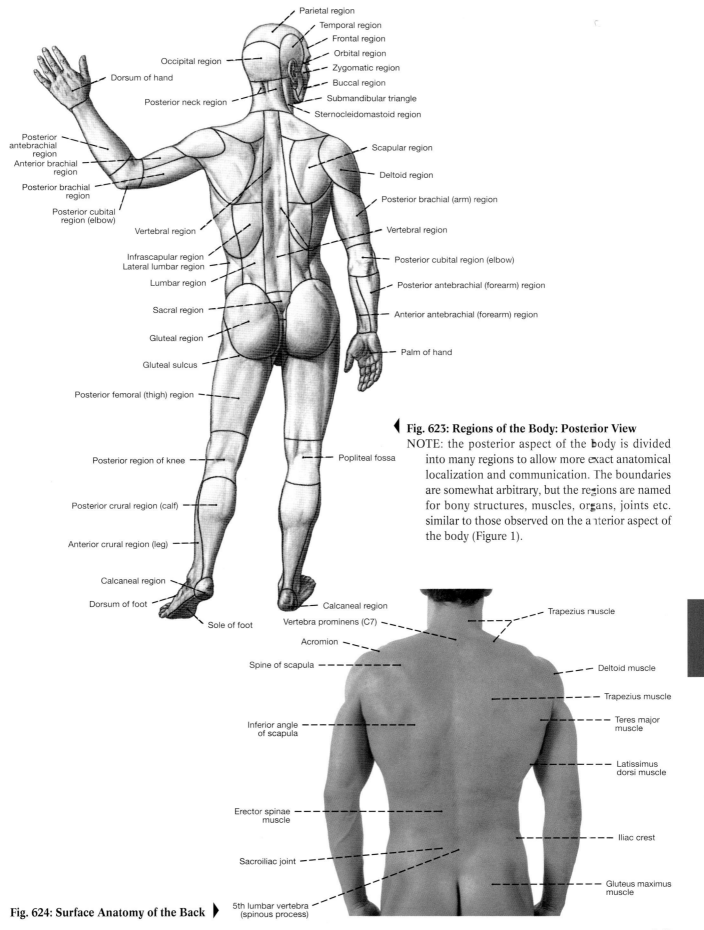

Parietal region
Temporal region
Frontal region
Orbital region
Occipital region
Zygomatic region
Dorsum of hand
Buccal region
Posterior neck region
Submandibular triangle
Sternocleidomastoid region
Scapular region
Posterior antebrachial region
Anterior brachial region
Deltoid region
Posterior brachial region
Posterior brachial (arm) region
Posterior cubital region (elbow)
Vertebral region
Vertebral region
Infrascapular region
Lateral lumbar region
Posterior cubital region (elbow)
Lumbar region
Posterior antebrachial (forearm) region
Sacral region
Anterior antebrachial (forearm) region
Gluteal region
Gluteal sulcus
Palm of hand
Posterior femoral (thigh) region

Fig. 623: Regions of the Body: Posterior View

NOTE: the posterior aspect of the body is divided into many regions to allow more exact anatomical localization and communication. The boundaries are somewhat arbitrary, but the regions are named for bony structures, muscles, organs, joints etc. similar to those observed on the anterior aspect of the body (Figure 1).

Posterior region of knee
Popliteal fossa
Posterior crural region (calf)
Anterior crural region (leg)
Calcaneal region
Dorsum of foot
Calcaneal region
Sole of foot
Vertebra prominens (C7)
Trapezius muscle
Acromion
Spine of scapula
Deltoid muscle
Trapezius muscle
Teres major muscle
Inferior angle of scapula
Latissimus dorsi muscle
Erector spinae muscle
Iliac crest
Sacroiliac joint
Gluteus maximus muscle

Fig. 624: Surface Anatomy of the Back ▶

5th lumbar vertebra (spinous process)

PLATE 404   The Back: Dermatomes and Cutaneous Nerves

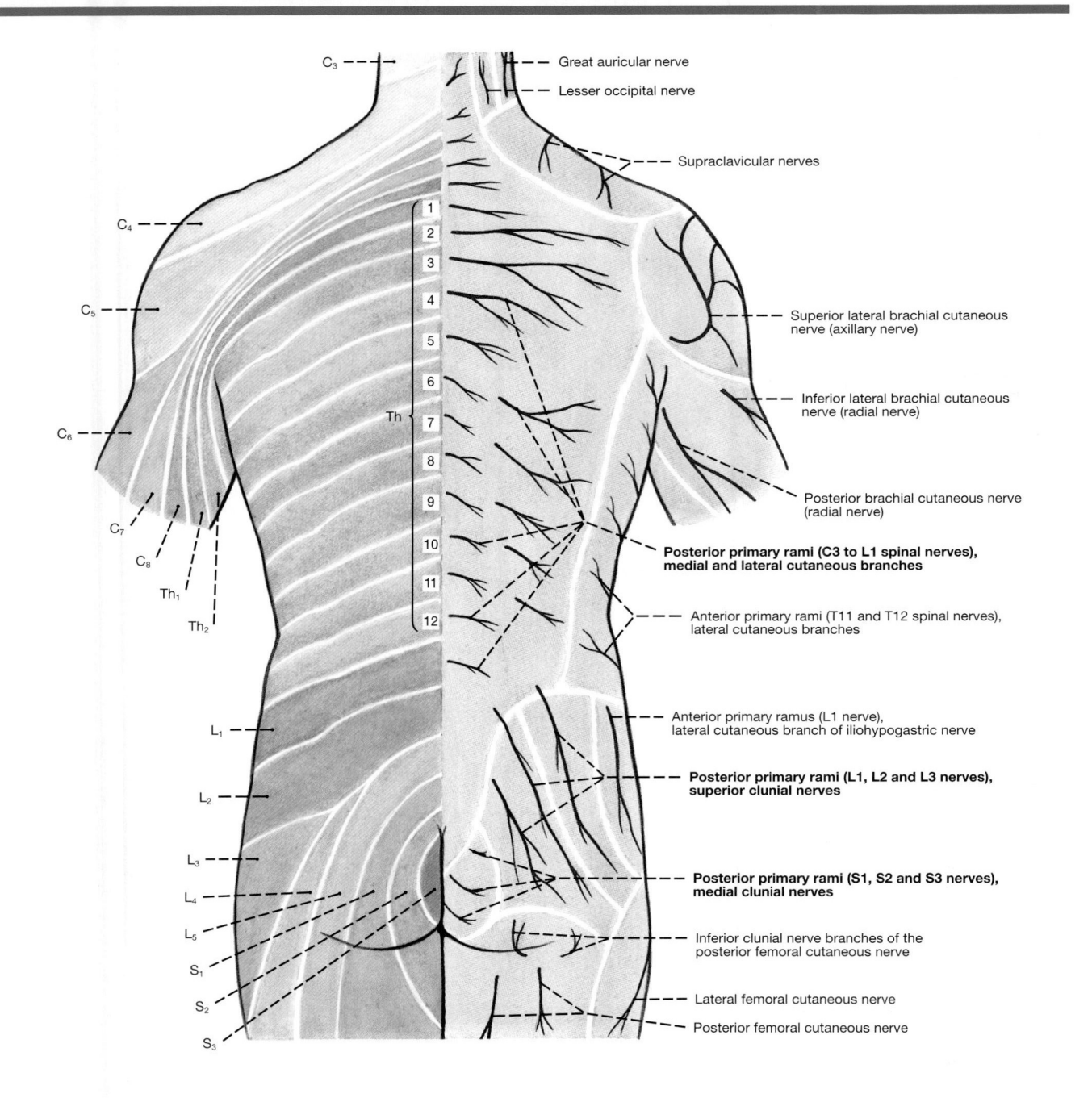

Fig. 625: Dermatomes and Cutaneous Nerve Distribution: Posterior Aspect of the Body

NOTE: 1)   **dermatomes** are shown on the left and the **cutaneous nerve** distribution and surface areas for the dorsum of the trunk are shown on the right.

2)   an area of skin supplied by the cutaneous branches of a single nerve is called a dermatome. There is considerable overlap between adjacent segmental nerves and, although the loss of a single spinal nerve produces an area of altered sensation, it does not result in total sensory loss.

3)   destruction of at least three consecutive spinal nerves is required to produce a total sensory loss of the dermatome supplied by the middle nerve of the three.

4)   mapping of skin areas affected by herpes zoster (shingles) has added to our knowledge of dermatome distribution. Another experimental procedure is that of "remaining sensibility." In the latter, dermatome areas are established in animals after severence of several roots above and below the intact root whose dermatome is being studied.

5)   the posterior primary rami of spinal nerves C3 through L1 (bold face) supply the posterior skin of the trunk, while the lateral neck, upper limb, and lateral trunk are supplied by anterior primary rami.

6)   the posterior primary rami (bold face) of L1, L2, and L3 (superior clunial nerves) as well as the posterior primary rami (bold face) of S1, S2, and S3 (medial clunial nerves) supply the gluteal and sacral regions. The remaining nerves of the posterior lower trunk and limbs are from anterior primary rami.

Fig. 625

Fig. 626: Branching of a Typical Spinal Nerve

NOTE: 1)   fibers from both dorsal and motor roots join to form a spinal nerve that soon divides into a **posterior** and an **anterior primary ramus.** The posterior primary ramus courses dorsally to innervate the muscles and skin of the back. The anterior primary ramus courses laterally and anteriorly around the body to innervate the rest of the segment.

2)   the posterior primary rami of typical spinal nerves are smaller in diameter than the anterior rami, and each usually divides into medial and lateral branches which contain both motor and sensory fibers innervating structures in the back.

3)   unlike anterior primary rami which join to form the cervical, brachial and lumbosacral plexuses, the peripheral nerves derived from the posterior rami do not, as a rule, intercommunicate and form plexuses. There is, however, some segmental overlap of peripheral sensory fields as seen with the anterior rami.

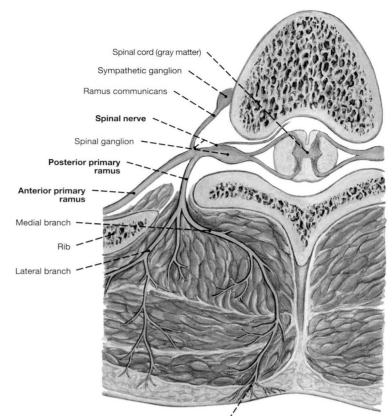

Spinal cord (gray matter)
Sympathetic ganglion
Ramus communicans
Spinal nerve
Spinal ganglion
Posterior primary ramus
Anterior primary ramus
Medial branch
Rib
Lateral branch
Medial cutaneous branch

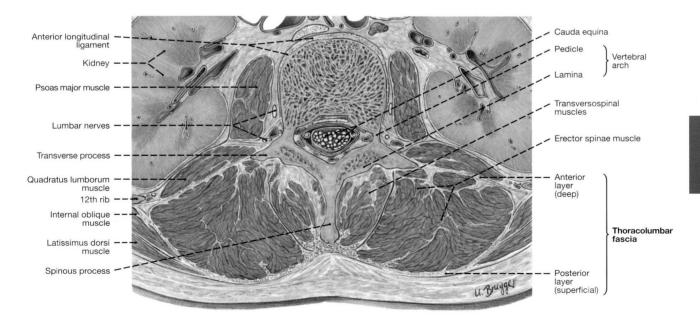

Anterior longitudinal ligament
Kidney
Psoas major muscle
Lumbar nerves
Transverse process
Quadratus lumborum muscle
12th rib
Internal oblique muscle
Latissimus dorsi muscle
Spinous process

Cauda equina
Pedicle
Lamina
} Vertebral arch
Transversospinal muscles
Erector spinae muscle
Anterior layer (deep)
Posterior layer (superficial)
Thoracolumbar fascia

Fig. 627: Cross-section L2 Vertebral Level: Deep Back Muscles and Thoracolumbar Fascia

NOTE: 1)   this cross-section of the deep back shows the lumbar part of the thoracolumbar fascia as it encloses the divisions of the erector spinae and transversospinal muscles. The fascia is formed by a posterior (superficial) layer and an anterior (deep) layer.

2)   medially, the layers of the thoracolumbar fascia attach to the spinous and transverse processes of the lumbar vertebrae and laterally they become continuous with the aponeuroses and fascias of the latissimus dorsi and anterior abdominal muscles.

3)   the quadratus lumborum and psoas major muscles located deep to the erector spinae. Observe the relationship of the kidneys anterior to the quadratus lumborum muscles.

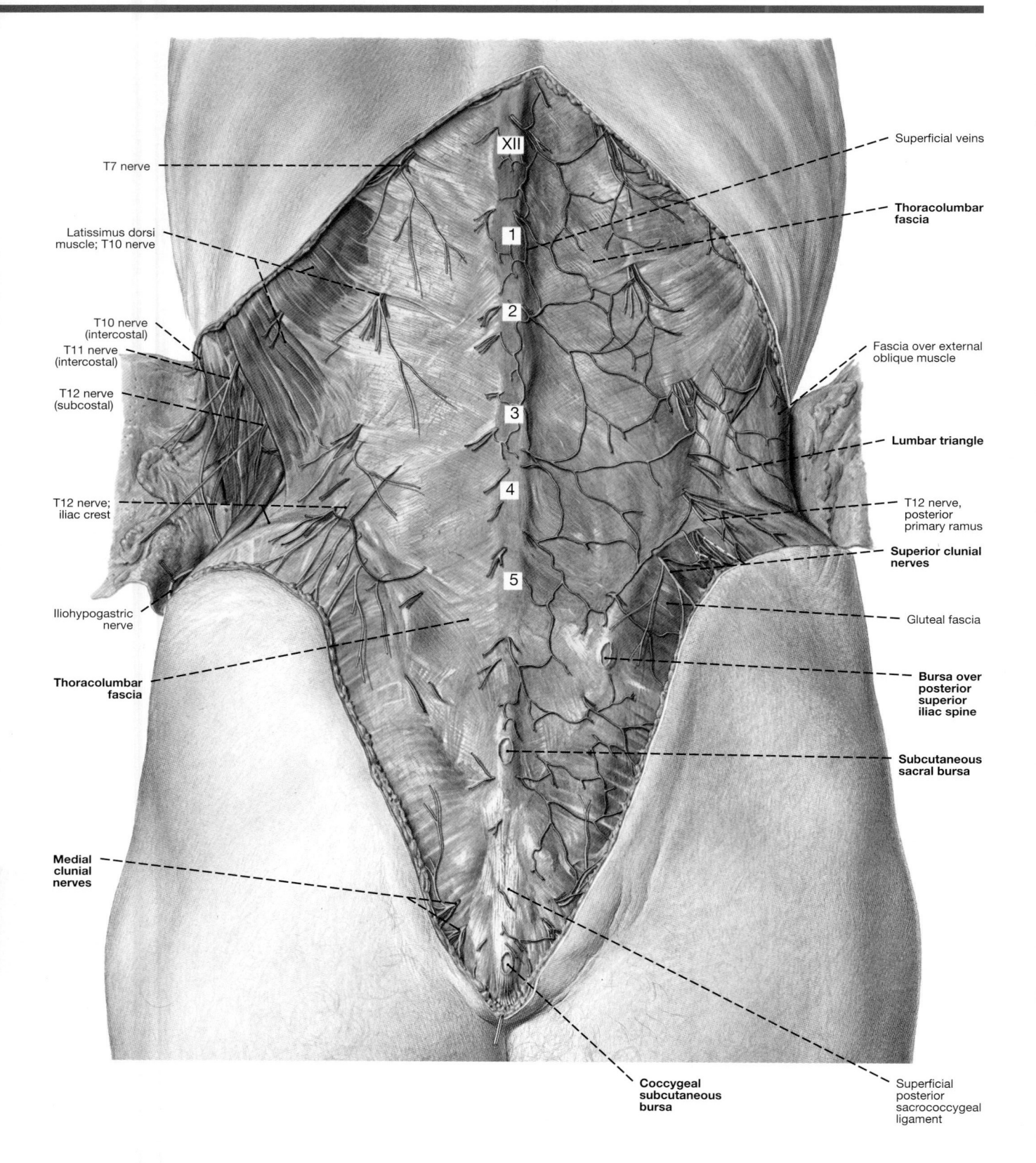

T7 nerve

Latissimus dorsi muscle; T10 nerve

T10 nerve (intercostal)

T11 nerve (intercostal)

T12 nerve (subcostal)

T12 nerve; iliac crest

Iliohypogastric nerve

Thoracolumbar fascia

Medial clunial nerves

XII

1

2

3

4

5

Superficial veins

Thoracolumbar fascia

Fascia over external oblique muscle

Lumbar triangle

T12 nerve, posterior primary ramus

Superior clunial nerves

Gluteal fascia

Bursa over posterior superior iliac spine

Subcutaneous sacral bursa

Coccygeal subcutaneous bursa

Superficial posterior sacrococcygeal ligament

Fig. 628: The Lumbosacral Region of the Back: Superficial Dissection

NOTE: 1)   the spinous processes of the T12 and five lumbar vertebrae are numbered and the superficial vessels and the cutaneous branches of the posterior primary rami of the spinal nerves penetrate the thoracolumbar fascia.

2)   the **lumbar triangle** (labelled on the right) is bounded by the crest of the ilium, the external oblique muscle and the latissimus dorsi muscle. Surgeons frequently approach the kidney through this triangle.

3)   the **superior clunial nerves** (posterior primary rami of L1, L2, L3) supply the skin over the gluteal region and the **medial clunial nerves** (posterior primary rami of S1, S2, S3) supply the dorsal sacral region.

Fig. 628

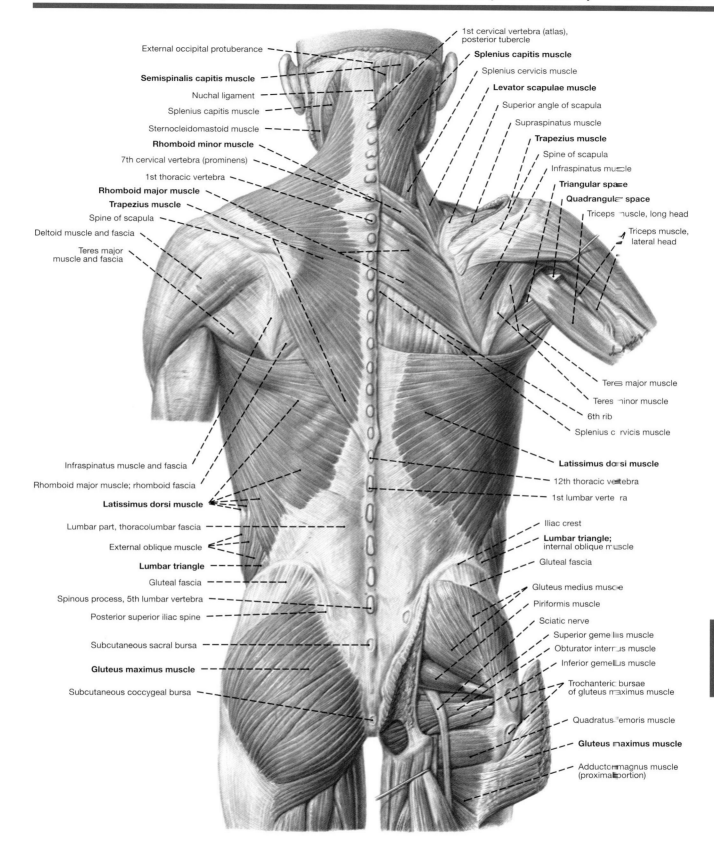

Fig. 629: Muscles of the Posterior Neck, Shoulder, Back, and Gluteal Region

NOTE: the most superficial layer of back muscles includes the **latissimus dorsi** and the **trapezius.** Beneath the trapezius, the **levator scapulae** and **rhomboid major** and **minor muscles** attach along the vertebral border of the scapula. In the neck, the **splenius capitis** and **semispinalis capitis** lie directly under the trapezius.

Fig. 629   **VI**

PLATE 408   The Back: Intermediate and Deep Back Muscles

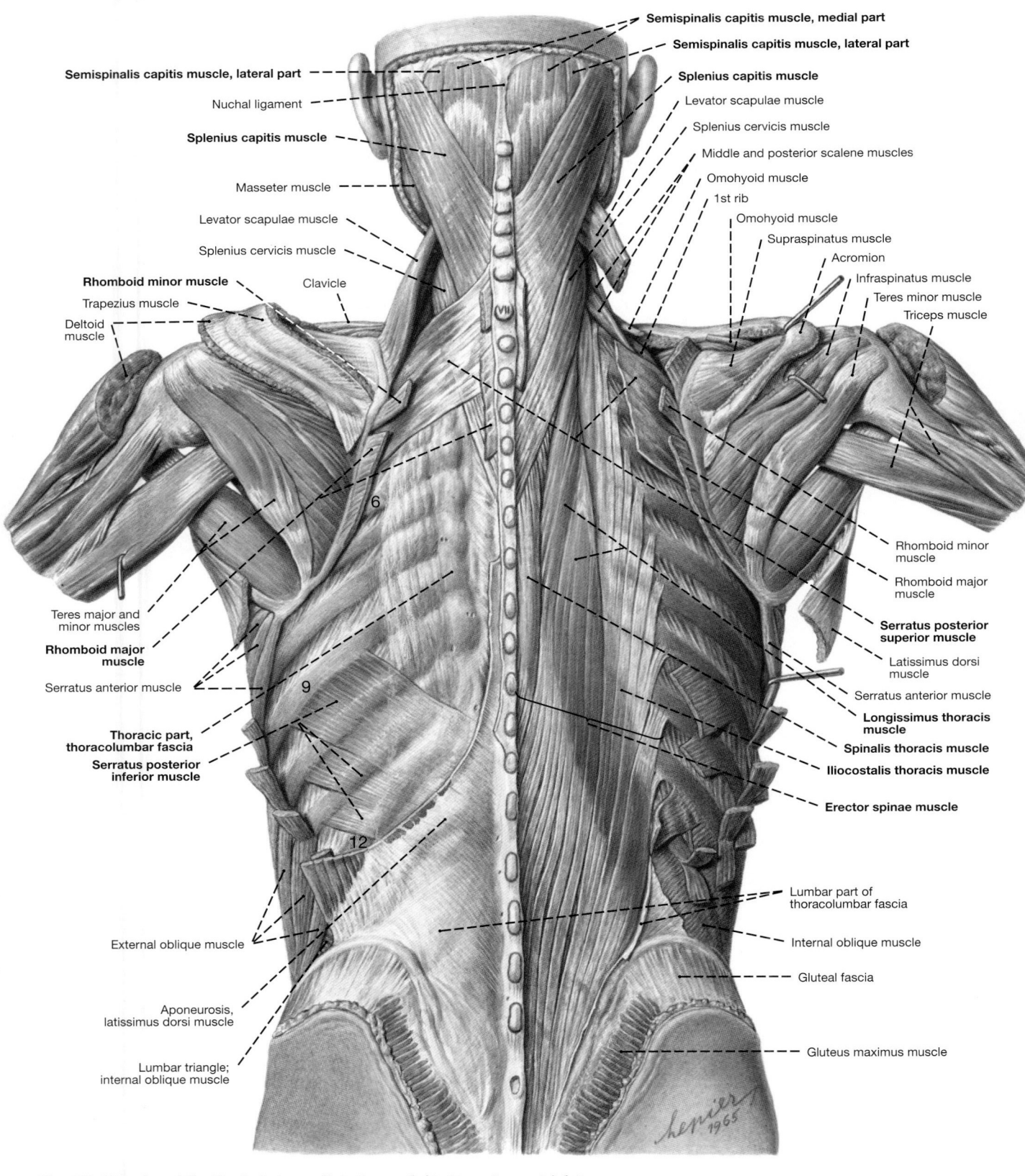

Fig. 630: Muscles of the Back: Intermediate Layer (left), Deep Layer (right)

NOTE: 1) **on the left side,** the superficial back muscles (trapezius and latissimus dorsi) have been cut as have the rhomboids, which attach the vertebral border of the scapula to the vertebral column. Observe the underlying serratus posterior superior and inferior muscles.

2) **on the right side,** the serratus posterior muscles and the thoracolumbar fascia have been removed, exposing the erector spinae muscle (formerly called sacrospinalis muscle).

3) **in the neck,** the splenius cervicis, splenius capitis and semispinalis capitis underlie the trapezius.

Fig. 630

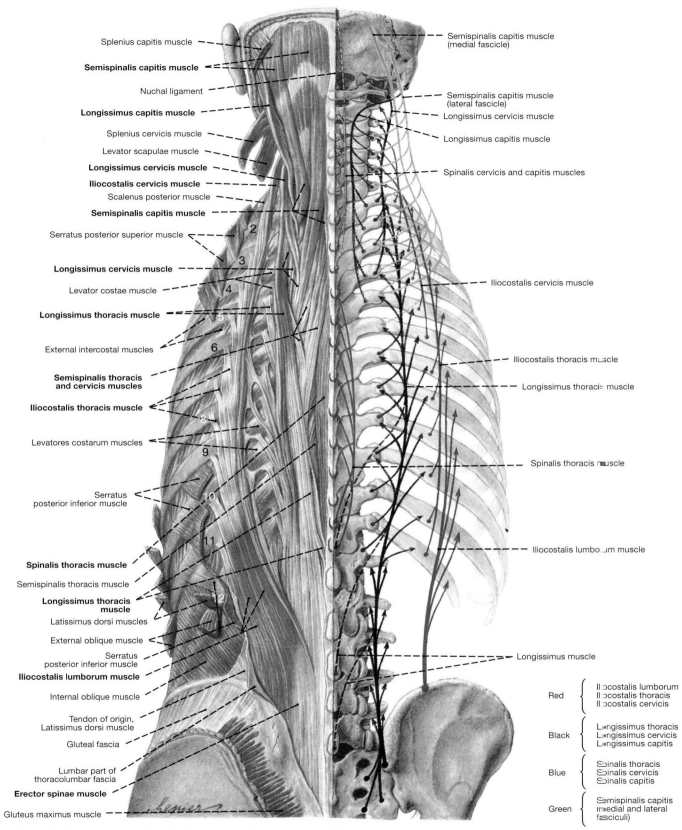

Splenius capitis muscle

Semispinalis capitis muscle

Nuchal ligament

Longissimus capitis muscle

Splenius cervicis muscle

Levator scapulae muscle

Longissimus cervicis muscle

Iliocostalis cervicis muscle

Scalenus posterior muscle

Semispinalis capitis muscle

Serratus posterior superior muscle

Longissimus cervicis muscle

Levator costae muscle

Longissimus thoracis muscle

External intercostal muscles

Semispinalis thoracis and cervicis muscles

Iliocostalis thoracis muscle

Levatores costarum muscles

Serratus posterior inferior muscle

Spinalis thoracis muscle

Semispinalis thoracis muscle

Longissimus thoracis muscle

Latissimus dorsi muscles

External oblique muscle

Serratus posterior inferior muscle

Iliocostalis lumborum muscle

Internal oblique muscle

Tendon of origin, Latissimus dorsi muscle

Gluteal fascia

Lumbar part of thoracolumbar fascia

Erector spinae muscle

Gluteus maximus muscle

Semispinalis capitis muscle (medial fascicle)

Semispinalis capitis muscle (lateral fascicle)

Longissimus cervicis muscle

Longissimus capitis muscle

Spinalis cervicis and capitis muscles

Iliocostalis cervicis muscle

Iliocostalis thoracis muscle

Longissimus thoracis muscle

Spinalis thoracis muscle

Iliocostalis lumborum muscle

Longissimus muscle

Red	Iliocostalis lumborum Iliocostalis thoracis Iliocostalis cervicis
Black	Longissimus thoracis Longissimus cervicis Longissimus capitis
Blue	Spinalis thoracis Spinalis cervicis Spinalis capitis
Green	Semispinalis capitis medial and lateral fasciculi)

Fig. 631: Deep Muscles of the Back and Neck: Erector Spinae Muscle

NOTE: 1) **on the left,** the erector spinae (sacrospinalis) muscle is separated into iliocostalis, longissimus, and spinalis parts. **In the neck,** observe the semispinalis capitis, which has both medial and lateral fascicles. The semispinalis cervicis and thoracis extend inferiorly from above and lie deep to the sacrospinalis layer of musculature.

2) **on the right,** all of the muscles have been removed and their attachments have been diagrammed by means of colored lines and arrows.

Fig. 631   VI

PLATE 410   The Back: Chart of Superficial and Intermediate Back Muscles

Superficial Muscles of the Back

Muscle	Origin	Insertion	Innervation	Action
Trapezius Muscle	Medial third of the superior nuchal line; external occipital protuberance; ligamentum nuchae; spinous process of C7 and T1 to T12 vertebrae	Lateral third of the clavicle; medial margin of acromion; spine of the scapula	Motor fibers from spinal part of the accessory nerve (XI); sensory fibers from C3, C4	Assists serratus anterior in rotating the scapula during abduction of the humerus between 90 and 180 degrees; upper fibers elevate the scapula; lower fibers depress the scapula; middle fibers adduct the scapula; occipital fibers draw the head laterally
Latissimus Dorsi Muscle	Thoracolumbar fascia; spinous processes of lower 6 thoracic vertebrae and 5 lumbar vertebrae and the sacrum; iliac crest; lower 3 or 4 ribs	Floor of the intertubercular sulcus of the humerus	Thoracodorsal nerve from the posterior cord of the brachial plexus (C6, C7, C8)	Extends, adducts and medially rotates humerus; with insertion fixed, it elevates the trunk to the arms, as in climbing

Intermediate Muscles of the Back

Muscle	Origin	Insertion	Innervation	Action
Rhomboid Major Muscle	Spinous processes of T2 to T5 thoracic vertebrae	Medial border of scapula between the scapular spine and inferior angle	Dorsal scapular nerve (C5)	Adducts the scapula by pulling it medially toward the vertebral column; rotates the scapula by depressing the lateral angle; helps fix scapula to thoracic wall
Rhomboid Minor Muscle	Spinous process of C7 and T1 vertebrae	Medial border of scapula at the level of the spine of the scapula	Dorsal scapular nerve (C5)	Assists the rhomboid major muscle
Levator Scapulae Muscle	Transverse processes of atlas and axis and the posterior tubercles of the transverse processes of C3 and C4 vertebrae	Superior angle and upper medial border of scapula	C3 and C4 nerves and the dorsal scapular nerve (C5)	Elevates superior border of scapula; rotates scapula laterally thereby tilting the glenoid cavity downward
Serratus Posterior Superior	Spinous processes of C7 and T1 to T3 thoracic vertebrae	Onto the upper borders of the 2nd, 3rd, 4th and 5th ribs	Ventral primary rami of T1 to T4 spinal nerves	Elevates the 2nd to the 5th ribs
Serratus Posterior Inferior	Spinous processes of T11, T12 and upper 3 lumbar vertebrae	Onto the inferior border of the lower 4 ribs	Ventral primary rami of T9, T10, T11 and T12 spinal nerves	Draws the lower 4 ribs downward and backward

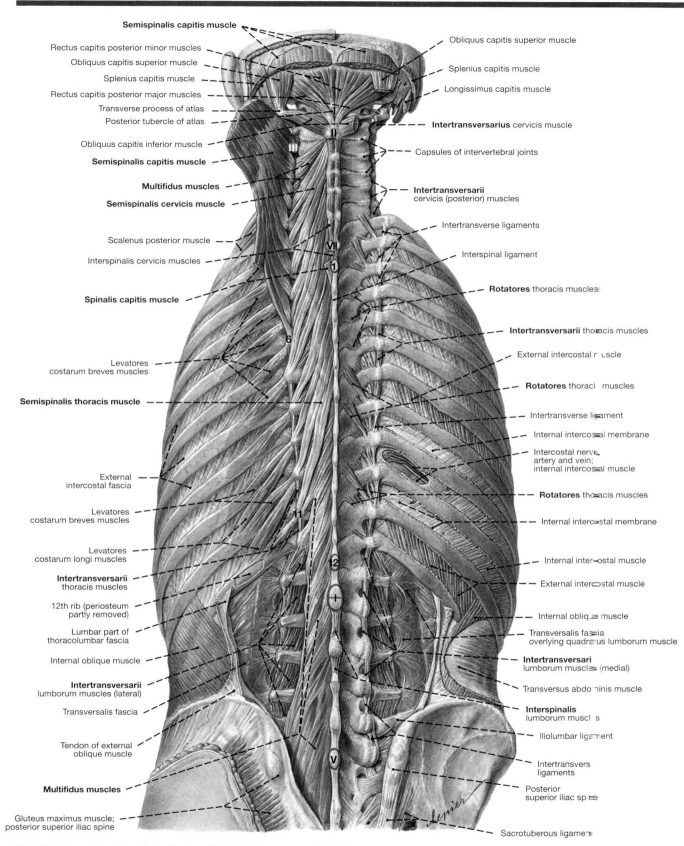

Fig. 632: Deep Muscles of the Back and Neck: Transversospinal Group

NOTE: 1) the **transversospinal** groups of muscles lie deep to the **erector spinae** and they extend between the transverse processes of the vertebrae to the spinous processes of higher vertebrae. These muscles are extensors of the vertebral column or acting individually and on one side, they bend and rotate the vertebrae of that side.

    2) within this group of muscles are the **semispinalis** (thoracis, cervicis and capitis), the **multifidus,** the **rotatores** (lumborum, thoracis, cervicis), the **interspinales** (lumborum, thoracis, cervicis), and the **intertransversarii.**

Fig. 632 **VI**

PLATE 412   The Back: Chart of Deep Back Muscles

Deep Muscles of the Back

ERECTOR SPINAE MUSCLE

Muscle	Origin	Insertion	Innervation	Action
ILIOCOSTALIS MUSCLE (Lateral column)				
Iliocostalis Lumborum Muscle	Posteromedial part of the iliac crest and from the most lateral part of the common tendon of the erector spinae muscle	By 6 or 7 muscle fascicles onto the inferior borders of the lower 6 or 7 ribs at their angles	Dorsal primary rami of lower thoracic and upper lumbar nerves	Extends, laterally flexes and assists in rotation of the vertebral column; can depress the ribs
Iliocostalis Thoracis Muscle	Upper borders of the lower 6 ribs at their angles	Upper borders of the first 6 ribs at their angles and on the transverse process of the 7th cervical vertebra	Dorsal primary rami of the C8 and upper 6 thoracic spinal nerves	Extends, laterally flexes and assists in rotation of the thoracic vertebrae
Iliocostalis Cervicis Muscle	Angles of the 3rd, 4th, 5th and 6th ribs	Posterior tubercles of transverse processes of 4th, 5th and 6th cervical vertebrae	Dorsal primary rami of the lower cervical and upper thoracic spinal nerves	Extends, laterally flexes and assists in rotation of lower cervical and upper thoracic vertebrae
LONGISSIMUS MUSCLE (Intermediate column)				
Longissimus Thoracis Muscle	Intermediate continuation of the erector spinae muscle; transverse processes of the lumbar vertebrae	Onto the tips of transverse processes of all thoracic vertebrae; onto the lower 9 or 10 ribs between their tubercles and angles	Dorsal primary rami of the thoracic and lumbar spinal nerves	Extends and laterally flexes the vertebral column; also able to depress the ribs
Longissimus Cervicis Muscle	Tips of transverse processes of upper 4 or 5 thoracic vertebrae	Posterior tubercles of transverse processes of C2 to C6 cervical vertebrae	Dorsal primary rami of upper thoracic and lower cervical spinal nerves	Extends vertebral column and bends it to one side
Longissimus Capitis Muscle	From transverse processes of upper 4 or 5 thoracic vertebrae; articular processes of lower 3 or 4 cervical vertebrae	Posterior margin of the mastoid process of the temporal bone	Dorsal primary rami of middle and lower cervical spinal nerves	Extends the head; muscle of one side bends head to the same side and turns face to that side
SPINALIS MUSCLE (Medial column)				
Spinalis Thoracis Muscle	From spinous processes of T11, T12, L1 and L2 vertebrae	Spinous processes of upper 4 to 8 thoracic vertebrae	Dorsal primary rami of thoracic spinal nerves	Extends vertebral column
Spinalis Cervicis Muscle	Spinous processes of C7, T1 and T2 vertebrae and ligamentum nuchae	Spinous process of the axis and those of the C3 and C4	Dorsal primary rami of lower cervical spinal nerves	Extends the cervical vertebrae
Spinalis Capitis Muscle	Spinous processes of lower cervical and upper thoracic vertebrae	Inserts with the semispinalis capitis muscle between the superior and inferior nuchal lines of the occipital bone	Dorsal primary rami of upper cervical spinal nerves	Extends the head
TRANSVERSOSPINALIS GROUP OF MUSCLES				
SEMISPINALIS MUSCLES				
Semispinalis Thoracis Muscle	Transverse processes of the 6th to 10th thoracic vertebrae	Spinous processes of C7, C8 and upper 4 thoracic vertebrae	Dorsal primary rami of lower cervical and upper thoracic spinal nerves	Extends vertebral column and rotates it to the opposite side
Semispinalis Cervicis Muscle	Transverse processes of upper 5 or 6 thoracic vertebrae	Spinous processes of the axis and 3rd, 4th and 5th cervical vertebrae	Dorsal primary rami of the middle cervical spinal nerves	Extends cervical spinal column; rotates vertebrae to opposite side
Semispinalis Capitis Muscle	Tips of transverse processes of the C7 and upper 6 or 7 thoracic vertebrae	Between the superior and inferior nuchal lines on the occipital bone	Dorsal primary rami of the cervical spinal nerves	Extends the head and rotates it such that the face is turned to the opposite side

Deep Muscles of the Back (cont.)

Muscle	Origin	Insertion	Innervation	Action
MULTIFIDUS MUSCLES	From the back of the sacrum; mamillary processes of lumbar vertebrae; transverse processes of all thoracic vertebrae; articular processes of lower 4 cervical vertebrae	Onto the spinous processes of higher vertebrae; each multifidus muscle spans two to four vertebrae	Supplied segmentally by dorsal primary rami of the lumbar, thoracic spinal nerves	Bends or laterally flexes the vertebral column and rotates it to the opposite side; both multifidi columns acting together extend the vertebral column
ROTATORES MUSCLES **Rotatores Thoracis Muscles**	From transverse processes of thoracic vertebrae deep to the multifidus muscles	On the base of the spine of thoracic vertebra above the origin or the one above that	Dorsal primary rami of the thoracic spinal nerves	Extend the vertebral column and bend it toward the opposite side
Rotatores Cervicis Muscles **(These are less well defined)**	From the articular processes of the cervical vertebrae	To the base of the spines of the cervical vertebra immediately above	Dorsal primary rami of cervical spinal nerves	Extend cervical vertebrae and bend them to the opposite side
Rotatores Lumborum Muscles **(These are less well defined)**	From the mamillary processes of the lumbar vertebrae	To the base of the spines of the lumbar vertebra immediately above	Dorsal primary rami of lumbar spinal nerves	Extend lumbar vertebrae and bend them to the opposite side

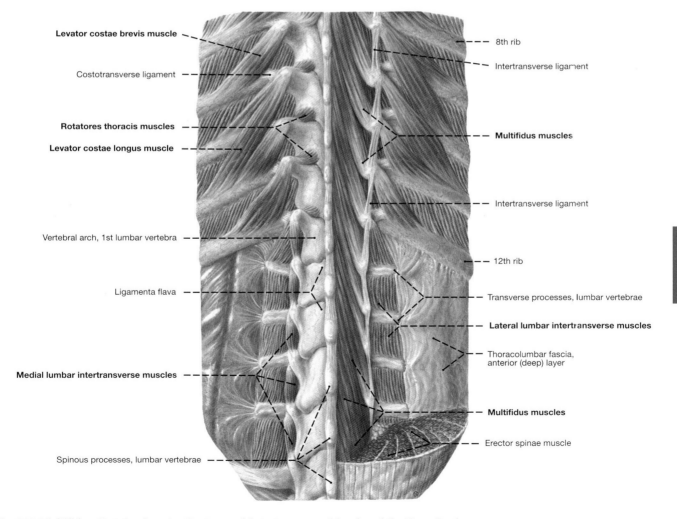

Fig. 633: Multifidus, Rotator, Levator Costae, and Intertransverse Muscles of the Deep Back
NOTE: the erector spinae and semispinalis muscles have been removed.

Fig. 633   **VI**

PLATE 414   The Back: Superficial Vessels and Nerves

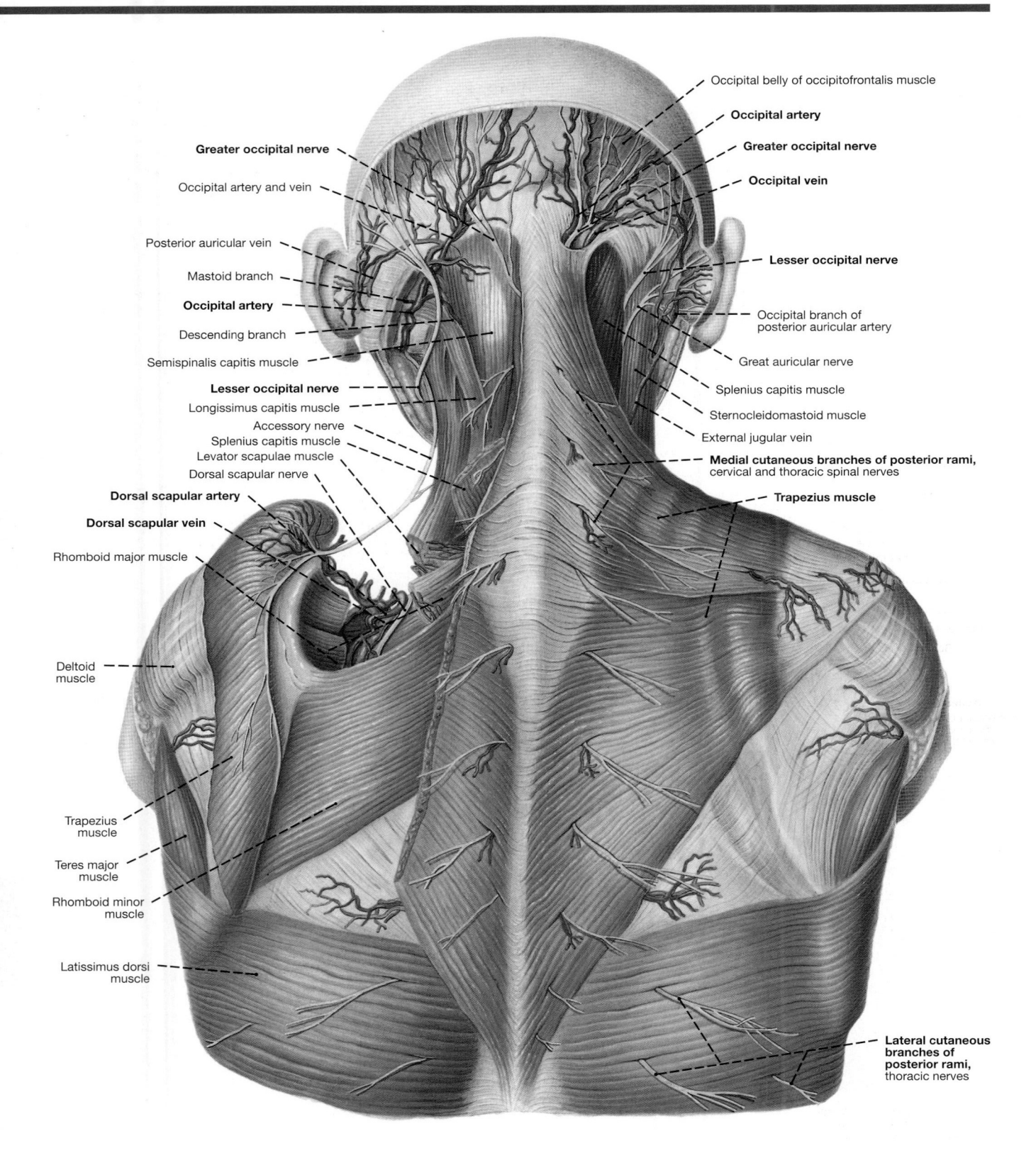

Occipital belly of occipitofrontalis muscle

Occipital artery

Greater occipital nerve

Occipital vein

Lesser occipital nerve

Occipital branch of
posterior auricular artery

Great auricular nerve

Splenius capitis muscle

Sternocleidomastoid muscle

External jugular vein

Medial cutaneous branches of posterior rami,
cervical and thoracic spinal nerves

Trapezius muscle

Greater occipital nerve

Occipital artery and vein

Posterior auricular vein

Mastoid branch

Occipital artery

Descending branch

Semispinalis capitis muscle

Lesser occipital nerve

Longissimus capitis muscle

Accessory nerve

Splenius capitis muscle

Levator scapulae muscle

Dorsal scapular nerve

Dorsal scapular artery

Dorsal scapular vein

Rhomboid major muscle

Deltoid
muscle

Trapezius
muscle

Teres major
muscle

Rhomboid minor
muscle

Latissimus dorsi
muscle

**Lateral cutaneous
branches of
posterior rami,**
thoracic nerves

Fig. 634: Nerves and Vessels of the Superficial and Intermediate Muscle Layers of the Upper Back and Posterior Neck

NOTE: 1)   the cutaneous branches of the **posterior primary rami** of the cervical and thoracic spinal nerves supplying the posterior neck and back segmentally. Observe the **accessory nerve (XI)** as it descends to supply the trapezius and sternocleidomastoid muscles.

2)   the **greater occipital nerve,** a sensory nerve from the posterior primary ramus of the C2 spinal nerve. It is accompanied by the occipital vessels. Observe also the **lesser occipital nerve,** which courses to the skin of the lateral posterior scalp and arises from the **anterior primary ramus** of C2.

3)   the **dorsal scapular nerve** and **vessels** that course beneath the **levator sacpulae** and **rhomboid muscles.**

Fig. 634

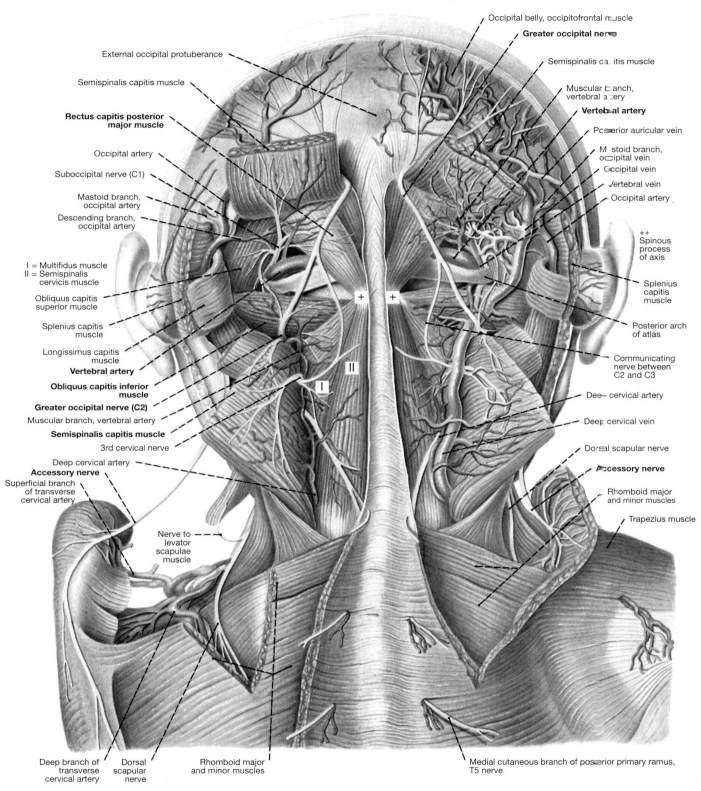

Fig. 635: Deep Vessels and Nerves of the Suboccipital Region and Upper Back; Suboccipital Triangle

NOTE: 1) the **suboccipital triangle** lies deep to the semispinalis muscle and is bounded by the **rectus capitis posterior major, obliquus capitis superior,** and **obliquus capitis inferior.**

2) the **vertebral artery** crosses the base of the suboccipital triangle, while the **suboccipital nerve** (posterior primary ramus of C1) courses **through** the triangle to supply motor innervation to the three muscles that bound the triangle as well as the rectus capitis posterior minor and the overlying semispinalis capitis muscle.

3) the **greater occipital nerve** (posterior primary ramus of C2), a sensory nerve, emerges below the obliquus capitis inferior and then courses medially and superiorly to become subcutaneous just lateral and below the external occipital protuberance.

Fig 635   **VI**

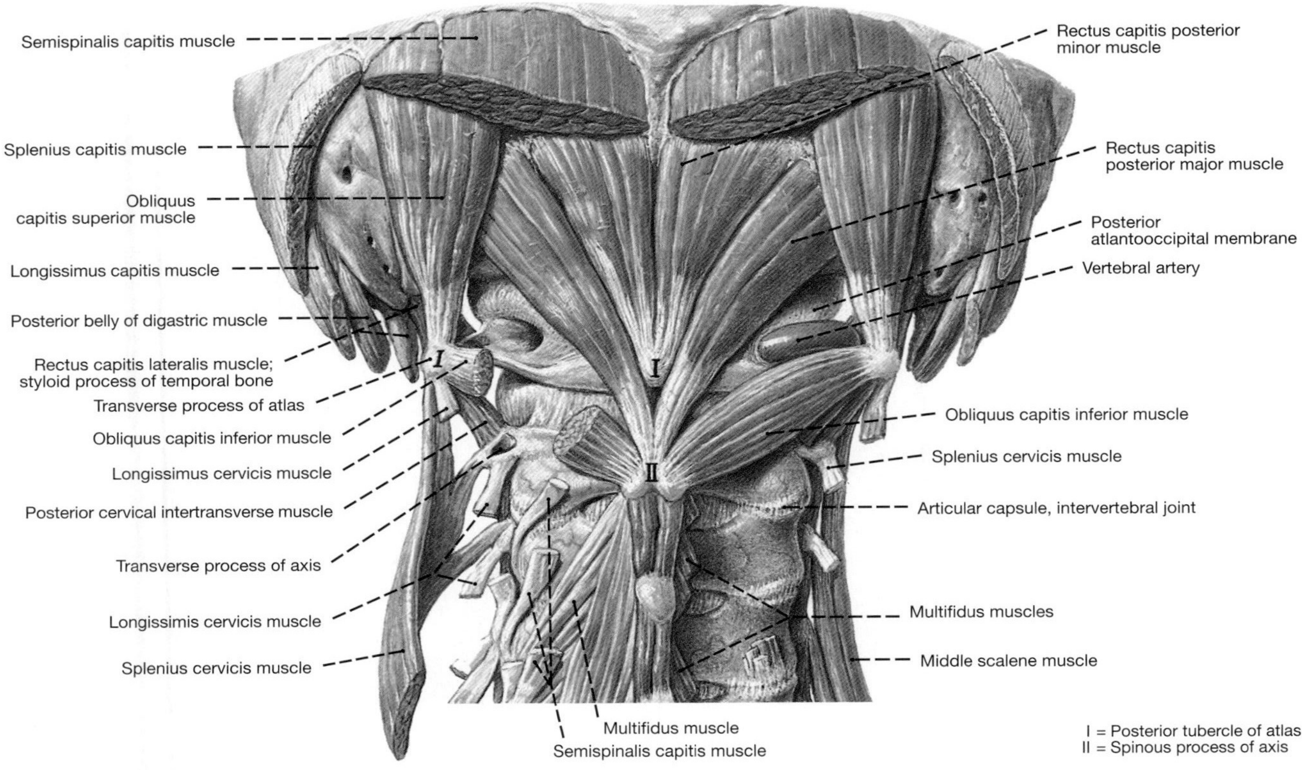

PLATE 416   Suboccipital Region: Muscles, Vessels, Nerves

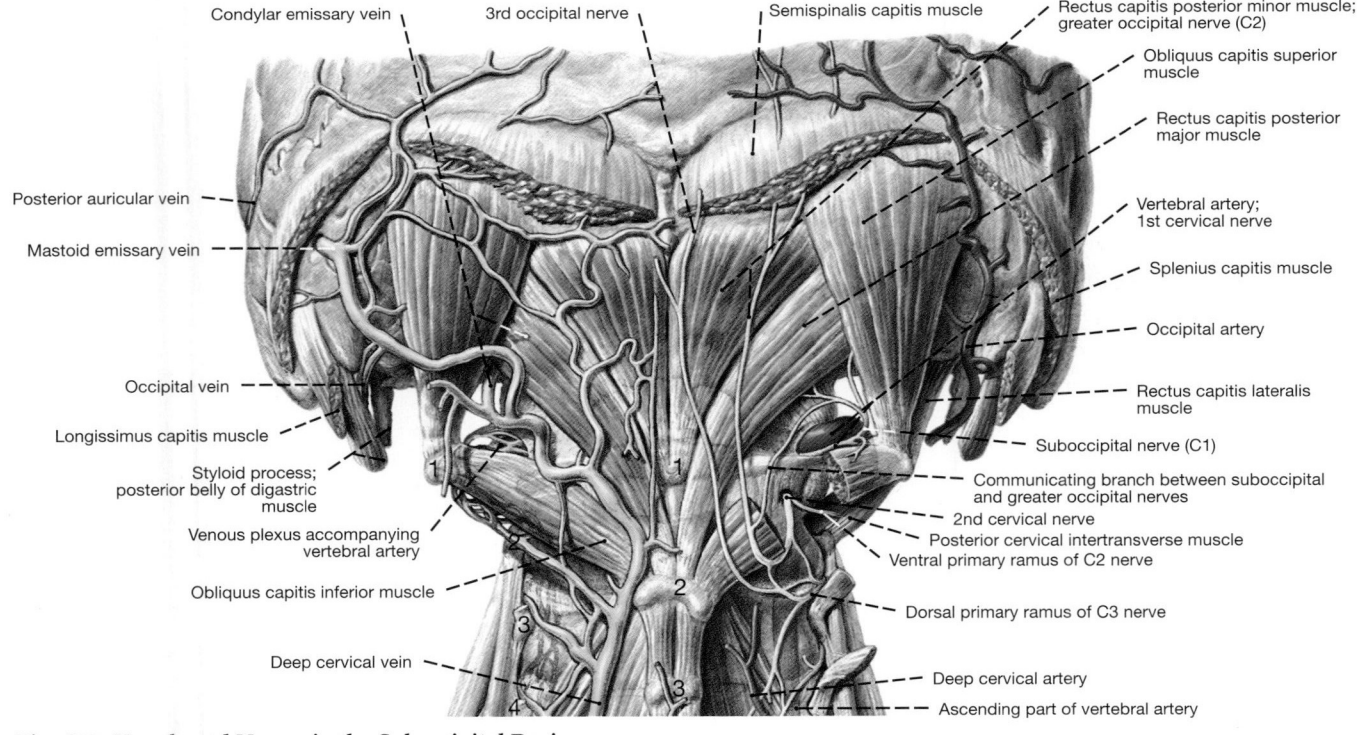

Semispinalis capitis muscle

Splenius capitis muscle

Obliquus capitis superior muscle

Longissimus capitis muscle

Posterior belly of digastric muscle

Rectus capitis lateralis muscle; styloid process of temporal bone

Transverse process of atlas

Obliquus capitis inferior muscle

Longissimus cervicis muscle

Posterior cervical intertransverse muscle

Transverse process of axis

Longissimis cervicis muscle

Splenius cervicis muscle

Rectus capitis posterior minor muscle

Rectus capitis posterior major muscle

Posterior atlantooccipital membrane

Vertebral artery

Obliquus capitis inferior muscle

Splenius cervicis muscle

Articular capsule, intervertebral joint

Multifidus muscles

Middle scalene muscle

Multifidus muscle
Semispinalis capitis muscle

I = Posterior tubercle of atlas
II = Spinous process of axis

Fig. 636: Muscles of the Suboccipital Triangle
NOTE: 1)   the **obliquus capitis inferior, obliquus capitis superior,** and **rectus capitis posterior major muscles** outline the **suboccipital triangle.**

2)   the **vertebral artery** crosses the floor of the triangle and penetrates the posterior atlantooccipital membrane to enter the foramen magnum. There the two vertebral arteries join to form the **basilar artery** on the ventral aspect of the brain stem.

Condylar emissary vein

3rd occipital nerve

Semispinalis capitis muscle

Rectus capitis posterior minor muscle; greater occipital nerve (C2)

Obliquus capitis superior muscle

Rectus capitis posterior major muscle

Posterior auricular vein

Mastoid emissary vein

Vertebral artery; 1st cervical nerve

Splenius capitis muscle

Occipital artery

Occipital vein

Rectus capitis lateralis muscle

Longissimus capitis muscle

Suboccipital nerve (C1)

Styloid process; posterior belly of digastric muscle

Communicating branch between suboccipital and greater occipital nerves

2nd cervical nerve
Posterior cervical intertransverse muscle
Ventral primary ramus of C2 nerve

Venous plexus accompanying vertebral artery

Obliquus capitis inferior muscle

Dorsal primary ramus of C3 nerve

Deep cervical vein

Deep cervical artery

Ascending part of vertebral artery

Fig. 637: Vessels and Nerves in the Suboccipital Region
NOTE: 1)   the **vertebral, occipital** and **deep cervical arteries** (right) and **veins** (left).

2)   the **suboccipital nerve** (C1, principally motor) and the **greater occipital** and **3rd occipital nerves** (posterior primary rami of C2 and C3 nerves, respectively).

Fig. 636, 637

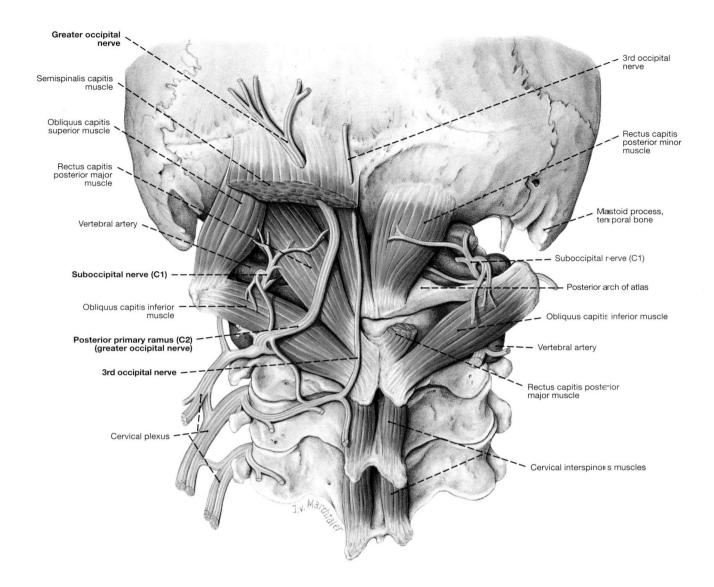

Greater occipital nerve

Semispinalis capitis muscle

Obliquus capitis superior muscle

Rectus capitis posterior major muscle

Vertebral artery

Suboccipital nerve (C1)

Obliquus capitis inferior muscle

Posterior primary ramus (C2) (greater occipital nerve)

3rd occipital nerve

Cervical plexus

3rd occipital nerve

Rectus capitis posterior minor muscle

Mastoid process, temporal bone

Suboccipital nerve (C1)

Posterior arch of atlas

Obliquus capitis inferior muscle

Vertebral artery

Rectus capitis posterior major muscle

Cervical interspinous muscles

J.v. Marchialer

Fig. 638: Nerves of the Suboccipital Region

NOTE: 1) the **suboccipital nerve (C1),** primarily a motor nerve, emerges from the spinal cord **above** the atlas courses **through** the suboccipital triangle and supplies motor innervation to all four suboccipital muscles.

2) the **greater occipital (C2)** and **3rd occipital nerves (C3)** branch from the posterior primary rami of those segments. After passing through the deep muscles of the back, they become purely sensory to supply the skin on the posterior scalp and neck.

Muscles of the Suboccipital Region

Muscle	Origin	Insertion	Innervation	Action
Rectus Capitis Posterior Major Muscle	Spinous process of axis	Lateral part of inferior nuchal line of occipital bone	Suboccipital nerve (dorsal ramus of C1)	Extends the head and rotates it to the same side
Rectus Capitis Posterior Minor Muscle	Tubercle on the posterior arch of the atlas	Medial part of inferior nuchal line of occipital bone	Suboccipital nerve (dorsal ramus of C1)	Extends the head
Obliquus Capitis Superior Muscle	Upper surface of transverse process of the atlas	Onto occipital bone between superior and inferior nuchal lines	Suboccipital nerve (dorsal ramus of C1)	Extends the head and bends it laterally
Obliquus Capitis Inferior Muscle	Apex of spinous process of axis	Inferior and dorsal part of transverse process of the atlas	Suboccipital nerve (dorsal ramus of C1)	Rotates the atlas and thereby turns the face toward the same side

Fig. 638   **VI**

PLATE 418   Cervical Vertebrae

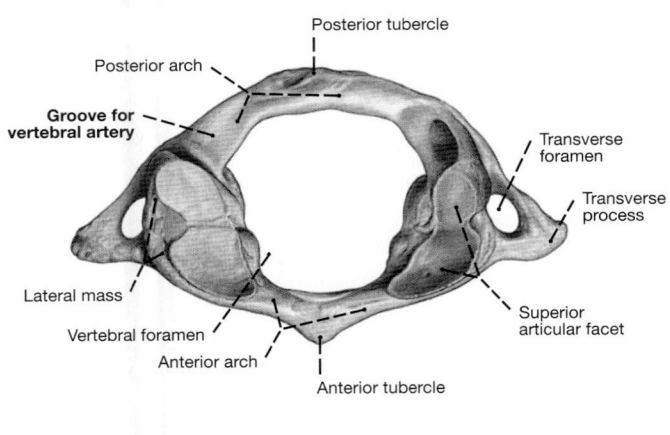

Fig. 639: Atlas, Viewed from Above

NOTE: the superior articular facets are the sites of the occipitoatlantal joints behind which are the grooves for the vertebral arteries.

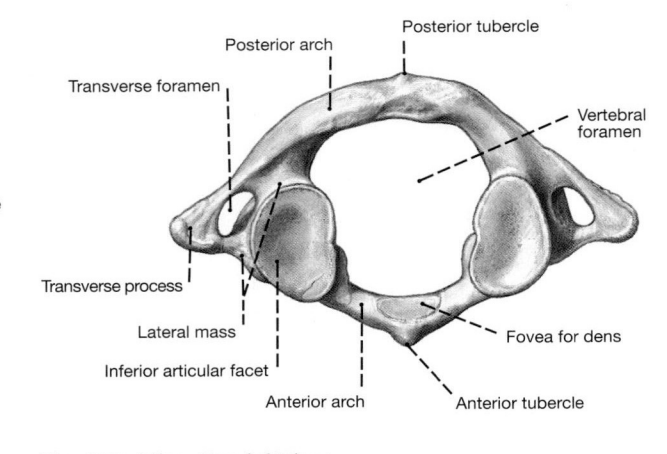

Fig. 640: Atlas, Caudal View

NOTE: the inferior articular facets on the inferior surface of the lateral mass articulate with the axis below.

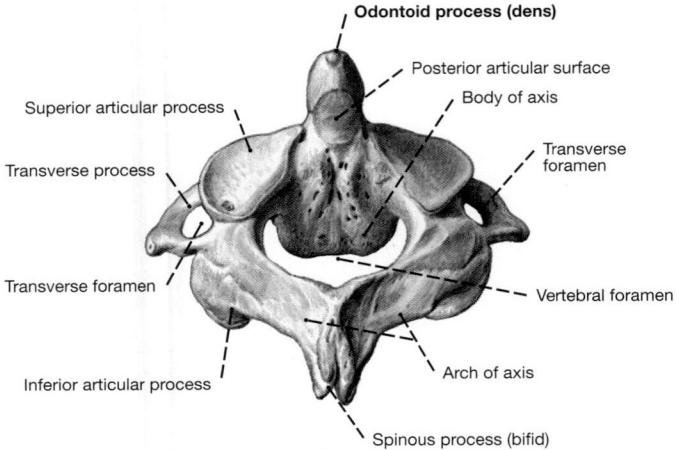

Fig. 641: Posterior View of the Axis

NOTE: the large body and the odontoid process of the axis and the posterior articular facet which articulates with the anterior arch of the atlas.

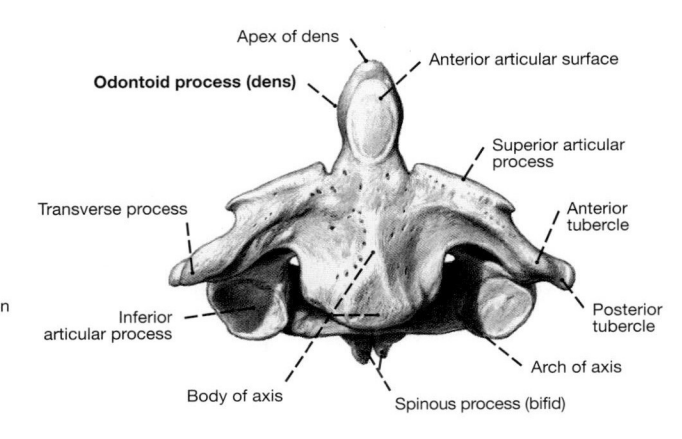

Fig. 642: Anterior View of the Axis

NOTE: the articular facet on the anterior surface of the odontoid process behind (posterior) which extends the transverse ligament of the atlas.

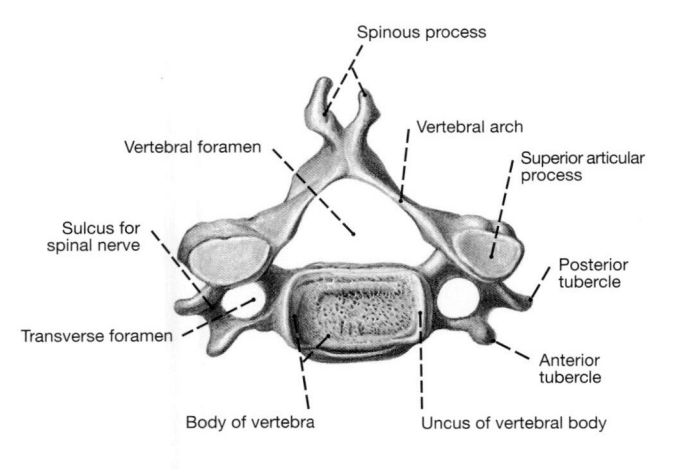

Fig. 643: Fifth Cervical Vertebra (from Above)

NOTE: the 5th cervical vertebra is typical of 3rd, 4th and 6th cervical vertebrae, and different from the 1st (atlas), 2nd (axis) and 7th which present special features. Also note the delicate structure of this vertebra.

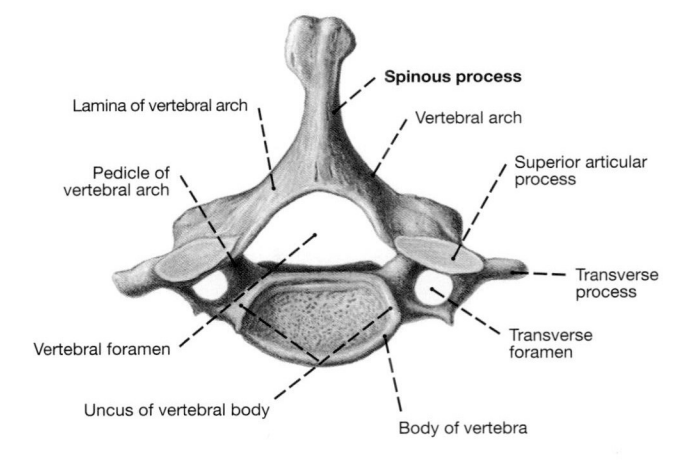

Fig. 644: Seventh Cervical Vertebra (from Above)

NOTE: the 7th cervical vertebra, being transitional between cervical and thoracic vertebrae, has a transverse foramen similar to the cervical and a large spinous process similar to the thoracic. The latter gives it the name **vertebra prominens.**

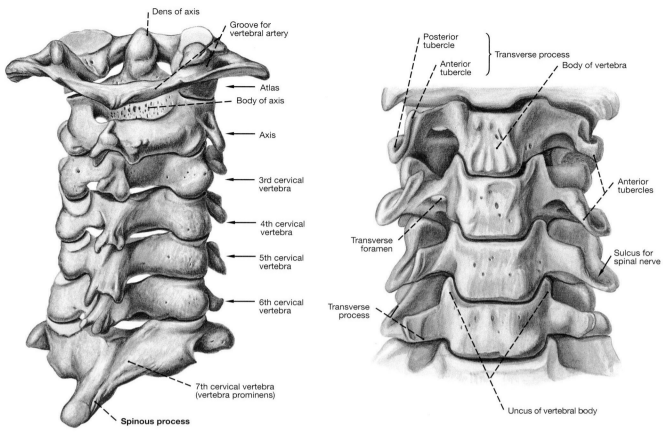

Fig. 645: Cervical Spinal Column (Dorsal)
NOTE: while flexion and extension of the head are performed at the atlantooccipital joint, turning of the head to the left or right is the result of rotation of the atlas on the axis.

Fig. 646: Cervical Vertebrae (Ventral View)
NOTE: only a small part of the 2nd to 7th cervical vertebrae are shown above and below the convex anterior surfaces of the bodies of the 3rd to 6th vertebrae.

◀ **Fig. 647: Atlantooccipital and Atlantoaxial Joints (Posterior View)**
NOTE: from the posterior margin of the foramen magnum to the upper border of the posterior arch of the atlas stretches the posterior atlantooccipital membrane.

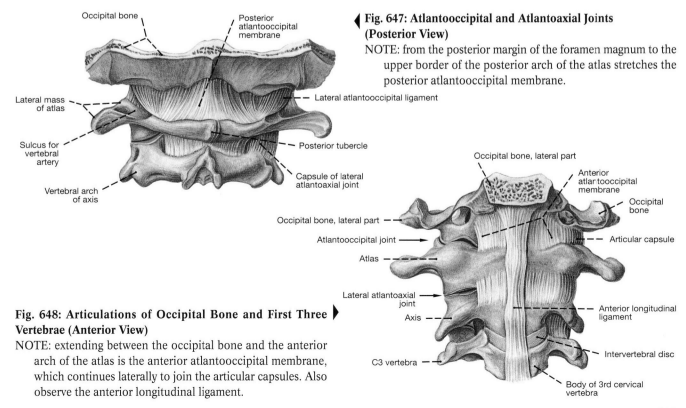

Fig. 648: Articulations of Occipital Bone and First Three ▶ Vertebrae (Anterior View)
NOTE: extending between the occipital bone and the anterior arch of the atlas is the anterior atlantooccipital membrane, which continues laterally to join the articular capsules. Also observe the anterior longitudinal ligament.

PLATE 420   **Craniovertebral Joints and Ligaments**

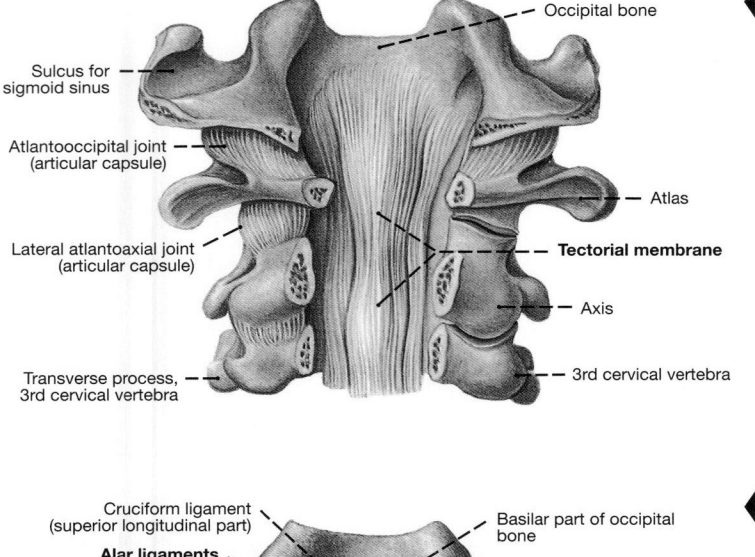

Occipital bone

Sulcus for
sigmoid sinus

Atlantooccipital joint
(articular capsule)

Lateral atlantoaxial joint
(articular capsule)

Atlas

Tectorial membrane

Axis

Transverse process,
3rd cervical vertebra

3rd cervical vertebra

Fig. 649: Tectorial Membrane, Dorsal View

NOTE: the tectorial membrane is a broadened upward extension of the posterior longitudinal ligament and attaches the axis to the occipital bone (see also Fig. 653). It covers the posterior surface of the odontoid process and lies dorsal to the cruciform ligament, covering it as well.

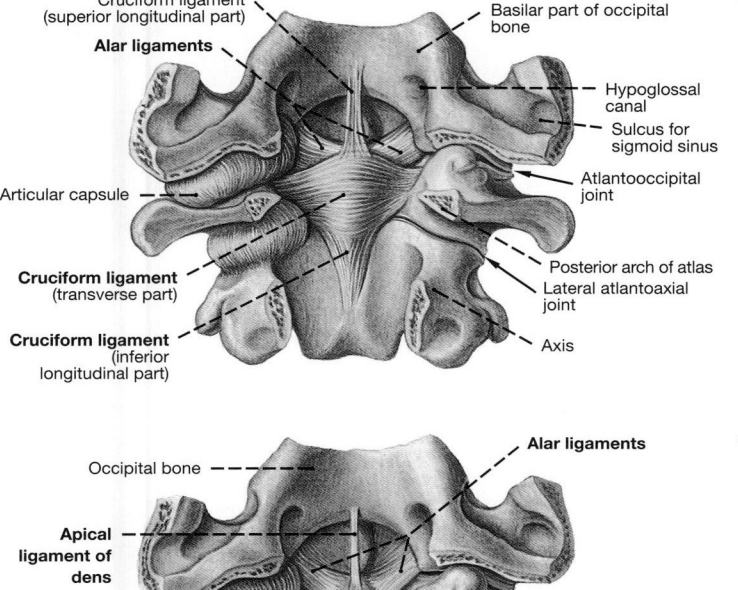

Cruciform ligament
(superior longitudinal part)

Alar ligaments

Basilar part of occipital
bone

Hypoglossal
canal

Sulcus for
sigmoid sinus

Articular capsule

Atlantooccipital
joint

Cruciform ligament
(transverse part)

Posterior arch of atlas

Lateral atlantoaxial
joint

Cruciform ligament
(inferior
longitudinal part)

Axis

Fig. 650: Atlantooccipital and Atlantoaxial Joints Showing the Cruciform Ligament (Posterior View)

NOTE: the posterior arches of the atlas and axis have been removed and the cruciform ligament is seen from this posterior view. It consists of the transverse ligament (see Fig. 652) and the longitudinal fascicles that extend superiorly and inferiorly.

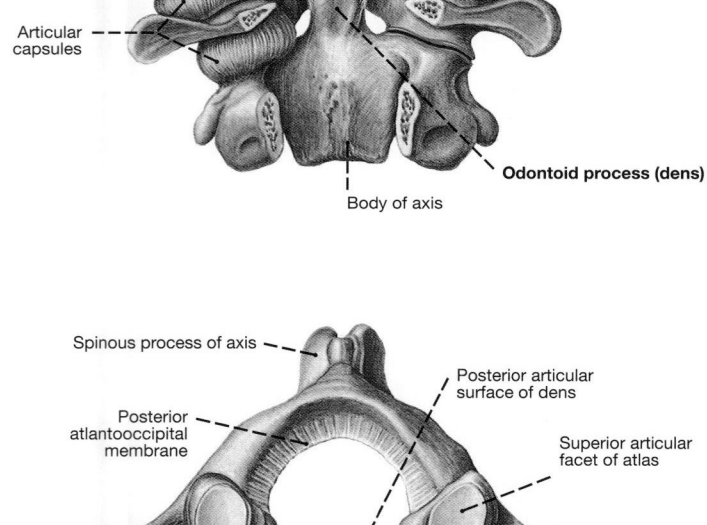

Occipital bone

Alar ligaments

**Apical
ligament of
dens**

Articular
capsules

Odontoid process (dens)

Body of axis

Fig. 651: Alar and Apical Ligaments (Posterior View)

NOTE: this figure is oriented the same as Fig. 650. The cruciform ligament has been removed to reveal the odontoid process of the axis. This is attached superiorly to the occipital bone by the two alar ligaments and the apical ligament of the dens. These ligaments tend to limit lateral rotation of the skull.

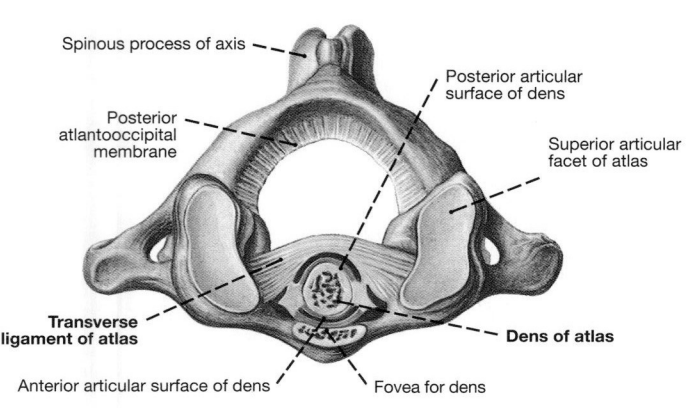

Spinous process of axis

Posterior articular
surface of dens

Posterior
atlantooccipital
membrane

Superior articular
facet of atlas

**Transverse
ligament of atlas**

Dens of atlas

Anterior articular surface of dens

Fovea for dens

Fig. 652: Median Atlantoaxial Joint (from Above)

NOTE: the odontoid process of the axis articulates with the anterior arch of the atlas, thereby forming the median atlantoaxial joint, and the thick and strong transverse ligament (part of the cruciform) of the atlas retains the dens on its posterior surface.

Figs. 649–652

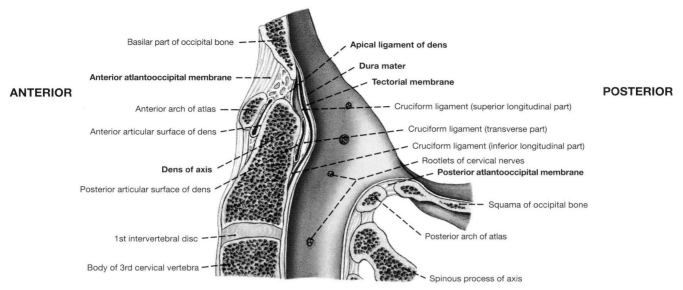

ANTERIOR

POSTERIOR

Basilar part of occipital bone

Apical ligament of dens

Dura mater

Anterior atlantooccipital membrane

Tectorial membrane

Anterior arch of atlas

Cruciform ligament (superior longitudinal part)

Anterior articular surface of dens

Cruciform ligament (transverse part)

Cruciform ligament (inferior longitudinal part)

Rootlets of cervical nerves

Dens of axis

Posterior atlantooccipital membrane

Posterior articular surface of dens

Squama of occipital bone

1st intervertebral disc

Posterior arch of atlas

Body of 3rd cervical vertebra

Spinous process of axis

Fig. 653: Median Sagittal Section of Atlantooccipital and Atlantoaxial Regions

NOTE: the relationships from anterior to posterior of the following structures: the anterior arch of the atlas, the joint between the atlas and the odontoid process (median atlantoaxial joint), the "joint" between the odontoid process and the transverse ligament of the atlas, the tectorial membrane and finally, the dura mater covering the spinal cord.

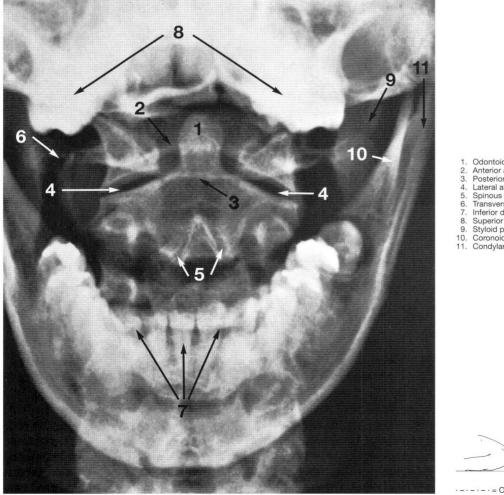

= Orbito-meatal line

1. Odontoid process of axis
2. Anterior arch of atlas (inferior margin)
3. Posterior arch of atlas (inferior margin)
4. Lateral atlantoaxial joints
5. Spinous process of axis (bifid)
6. Transverse process of atlas
7. Inferior dental arch
8. Superior dental arch
9. Styloid process of temporal bone
10. Coronoid process of mandible
11. Condylar process of mandible

Fig. 654: X-ray of the Odontoid Process and the Atlantoaxial Joints

NOTE: this is an AP projection taken through the oral cavity as shown in diagram.

PLATE 422   Vertebral Column

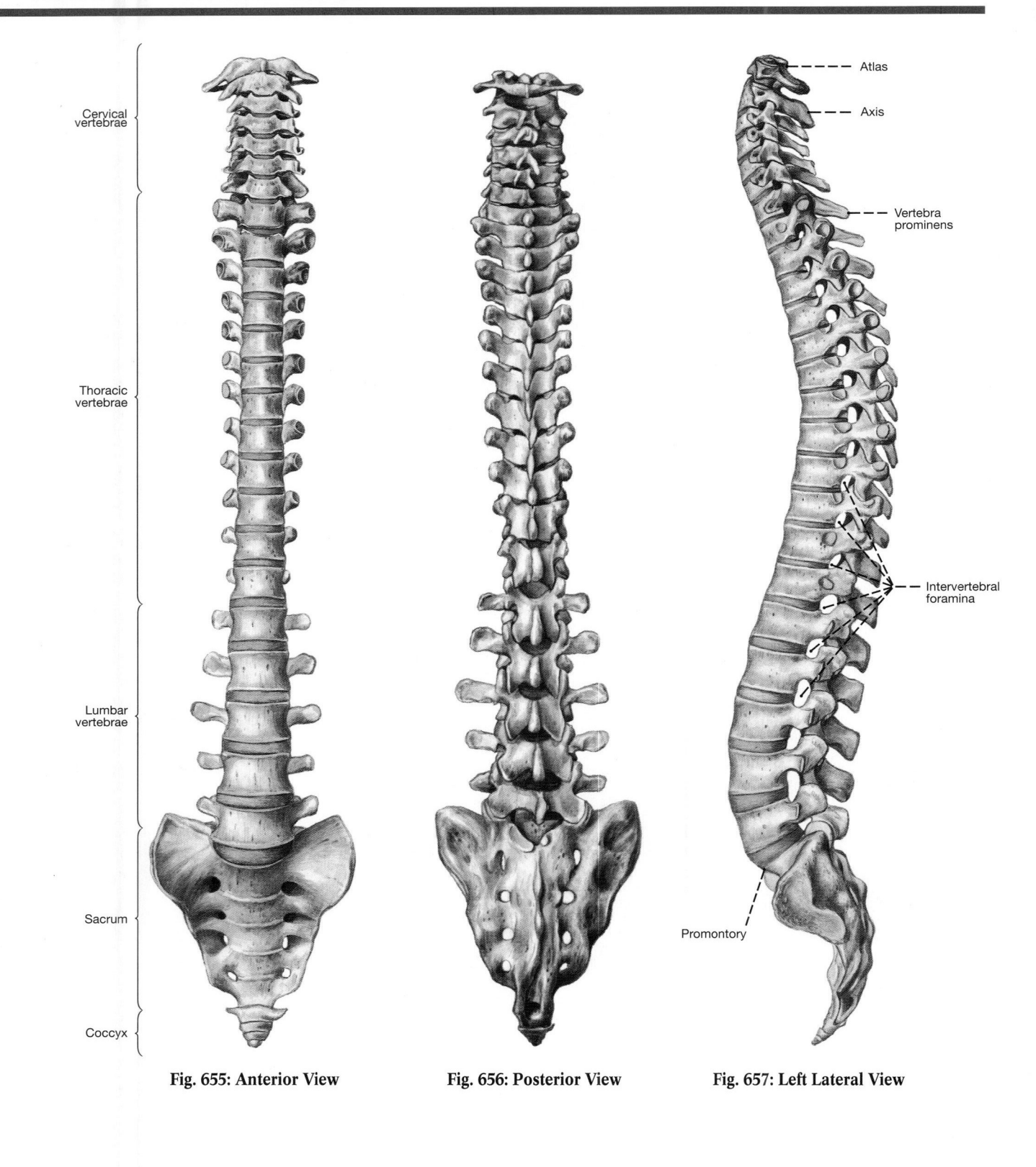

Cervical vertebrae

Thoracic vertebrae

Lumbar vertebrae

Sacrum

Coccyx

Atlas

Axis

Vertebra prominens

Intervertebral foramina

Promontory

Fig. 655: Anterior View   **Fig. 656: Posterior View**   **Fig. 657: Left Lateral View**

Figs. 655, 656 and 657: Vertebral Column, Including the Sacrum and Coccyx

NOTE: 1)   the vertebral column normally consists of 7 **cervical,** 12 **thoracic,** and 5 **lumbar** vertebrae and the **sacrum** and **coccyx.** Its principal functions are to assist in the maintenance of the erect posture in humans, to encase and protect the spinal cord, and to allow attachments of the musculature important for movements of the head and trunk.

2)   from a dorsal or ventral view, the normal spinal column is straight. When viewed from the side, the vertebral column presents two ventrally convex curvatures (cervical and lumbar) and two dorsally convex curvatures (thoracic and sacral).

Figs. 655, 656, 657

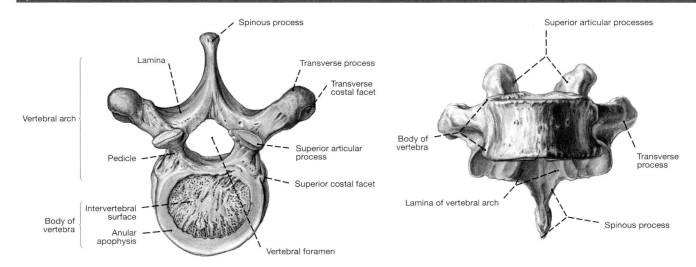

Fig. 658: Sixth Thoracic Vertebra (from Above)

Fig. 659: Tenth Thoracic Vertebra (Ventral View)

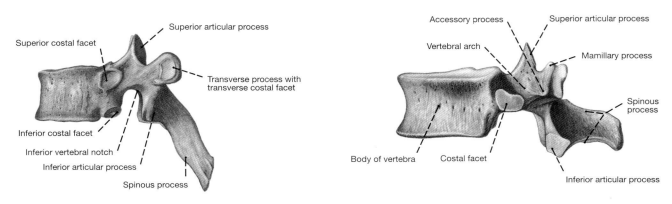

Fig. 660: Sixth Thoracic Vertebra (from Left Lateral Side)

Fig. 661: Twelfth Thoracic Vertebra, Lateral View

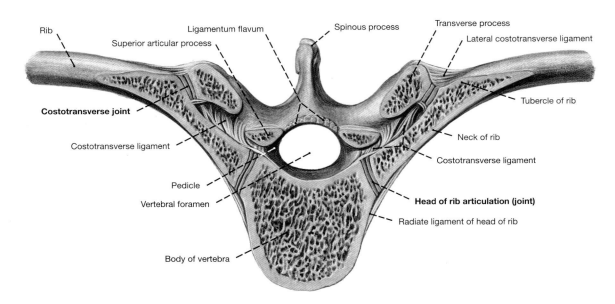

Fig. 662: Costovertebral Joints, Transverse Section as Seen From Above
NOTE: each rib articulates with the thoracic vertebrae at two places:
    a) the **head of the rib** articulates with the **vertebral body** and,
    b) the **tubercle** on the **neck of the rib** articulates with the **transverse process** of the vertebra.

PLATE 424   **Costovertebral Joints and Ligaments**

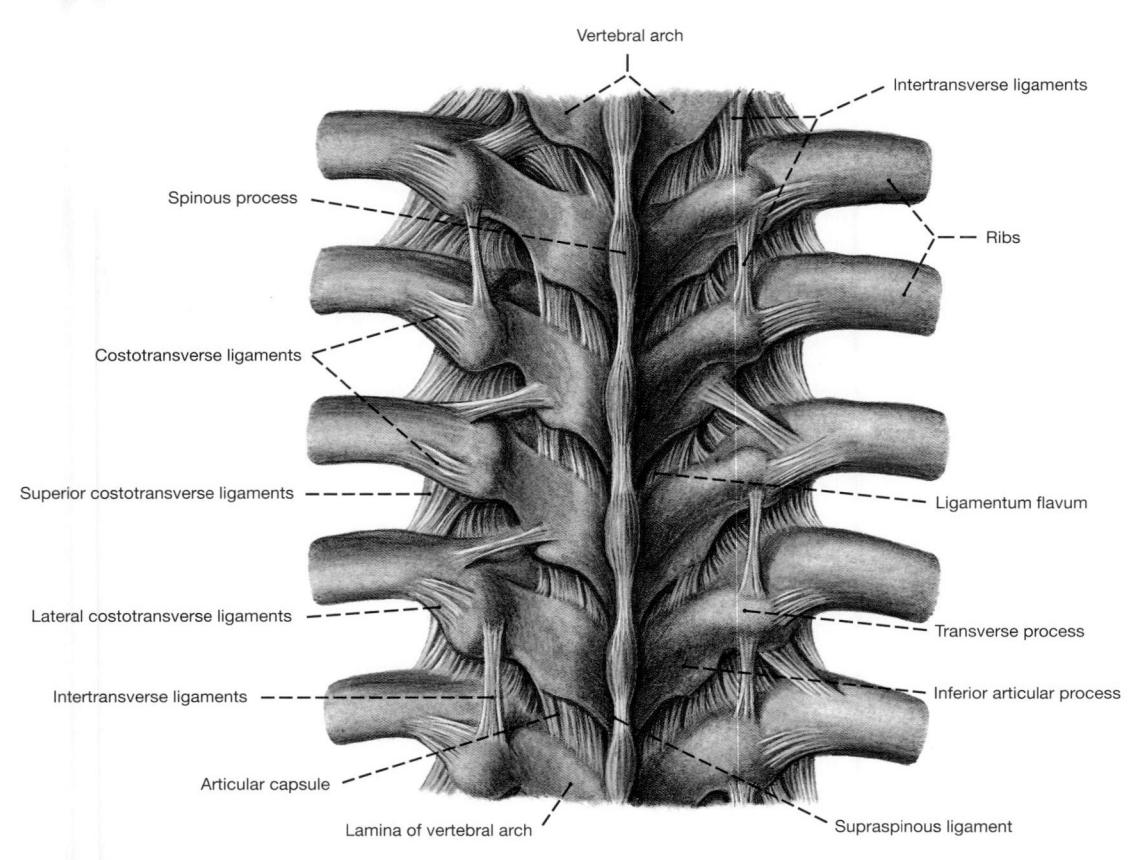

Fig. 663: Lower Costovertebral Joints (Posterior View)

NOTE: 1)   five pairs of costovertebral joints, viewed from behind, show to advantage the articulations between the necks and tubercles of the ribs and the transverse processes of the thoracic vertebrae.

2)   the ligaments that connect these gliding joints are the **costotransverse, lateral costotransverse,** and **superior costotransverse ligaments.**

3)   the costotransverse joints (neck of rib with transverse process) are not to be confused with the joints between the heads of the ribs and the bodies of the vertebrae.

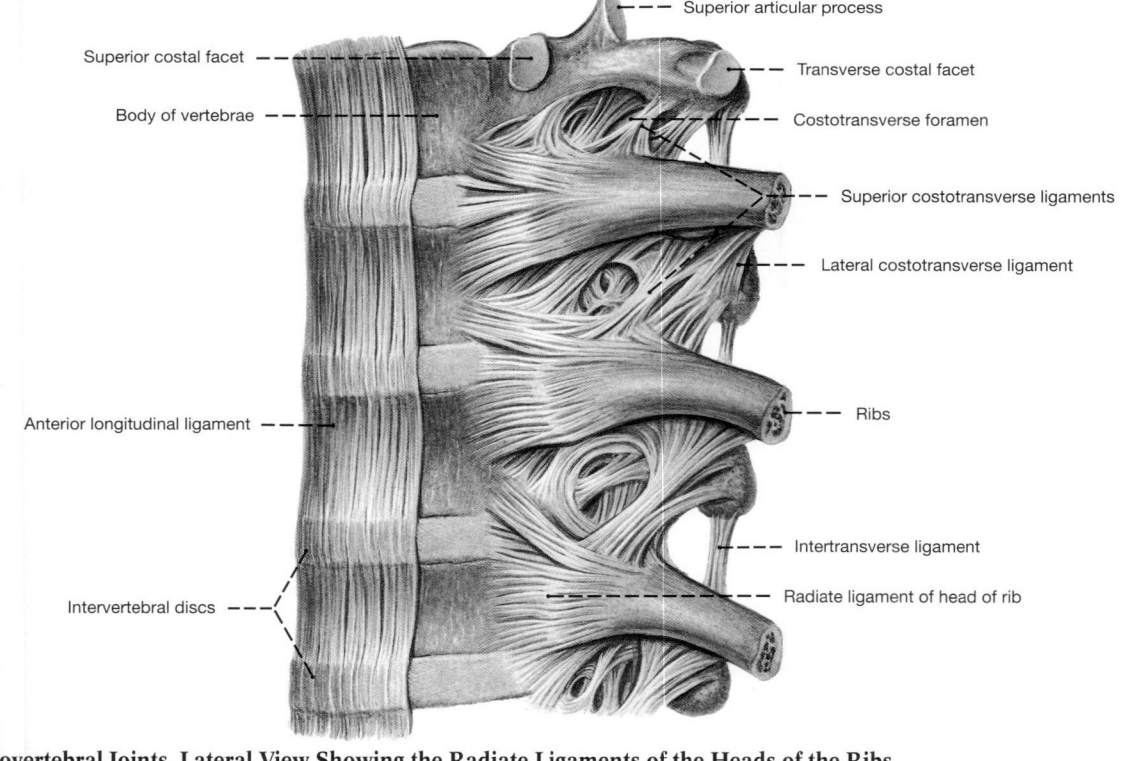

Fig. 664: Costovertebral Joints, Lateral View Showing the Radiate Ligaments of the Heads of the Ribs

Figs. 663, 664

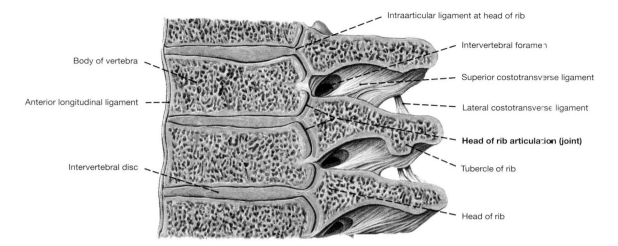

Intraarticular ligament at head of rib

Intervertebral foramen

Body of vertebra

Superior costotransverse ligament

Anterior longitudinal ligament

Lateral costotransverse ligament

Head of rib articulation (joint)

Intervertebral disc

Tubercle of rib

Head of rib

Fig. 665: Sagittal Section Through the Spinal Column Showing the Costovertebral Joints
NOTE: the following important structures: the intervertebral discs, the intraarticular and costotransverse ligaments, and the intervertebral foramina which transmit the spinal nerves and their accompanying vessels.

Fig. 666: Anterior Longitudinal Ligament (Ventral View)
NOTE: the **anterior longitudinal ligament** extends from the axis to the sacrum along the anterior aspect of the bodies of the vertebrae and the intervertebral discs to which it is firmly attached. Its fibers are white and glistening and can readily be identified.

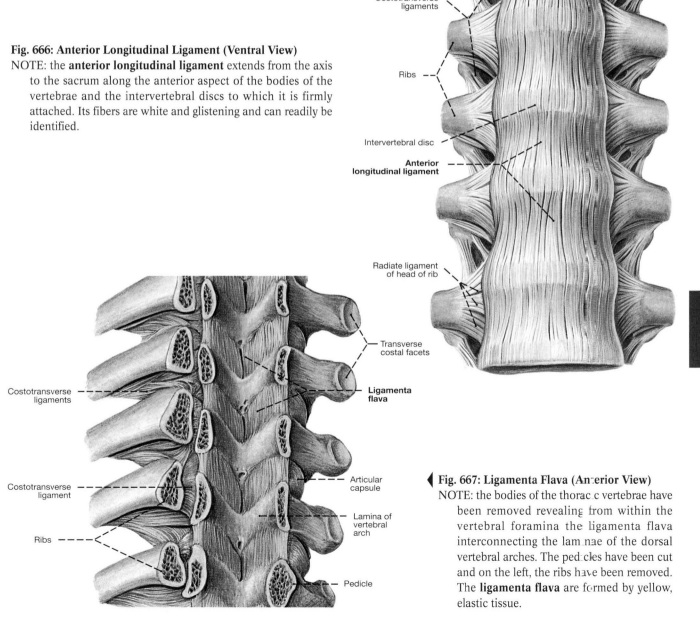

Costotransverse ligaments

Ribs

Intervertebral disc

Anterior longitudinal ligament

Radiate ligament of head of rib

Transverse costal facets

Ligamenta flava

Costotransverse ligaments

Articular capsule

Costotransverse ligament

Lamina of vertebral arch

Ribs

Pedicle

Fig. 667: Ligamenta Flava (Anterior View)
NOTE: the bodies of the thoracic vertebrae have been removed revealing from within the vertebral foramina the ligamenta flava interconnecting the laminae of the dorsal vertebral arches. The pedicles have been cut and on the left, the ribs have been removed. The **ligamenta flava** are formed by yellow, elastic tissue.

PLATE 426   Lumbar Vertebrae

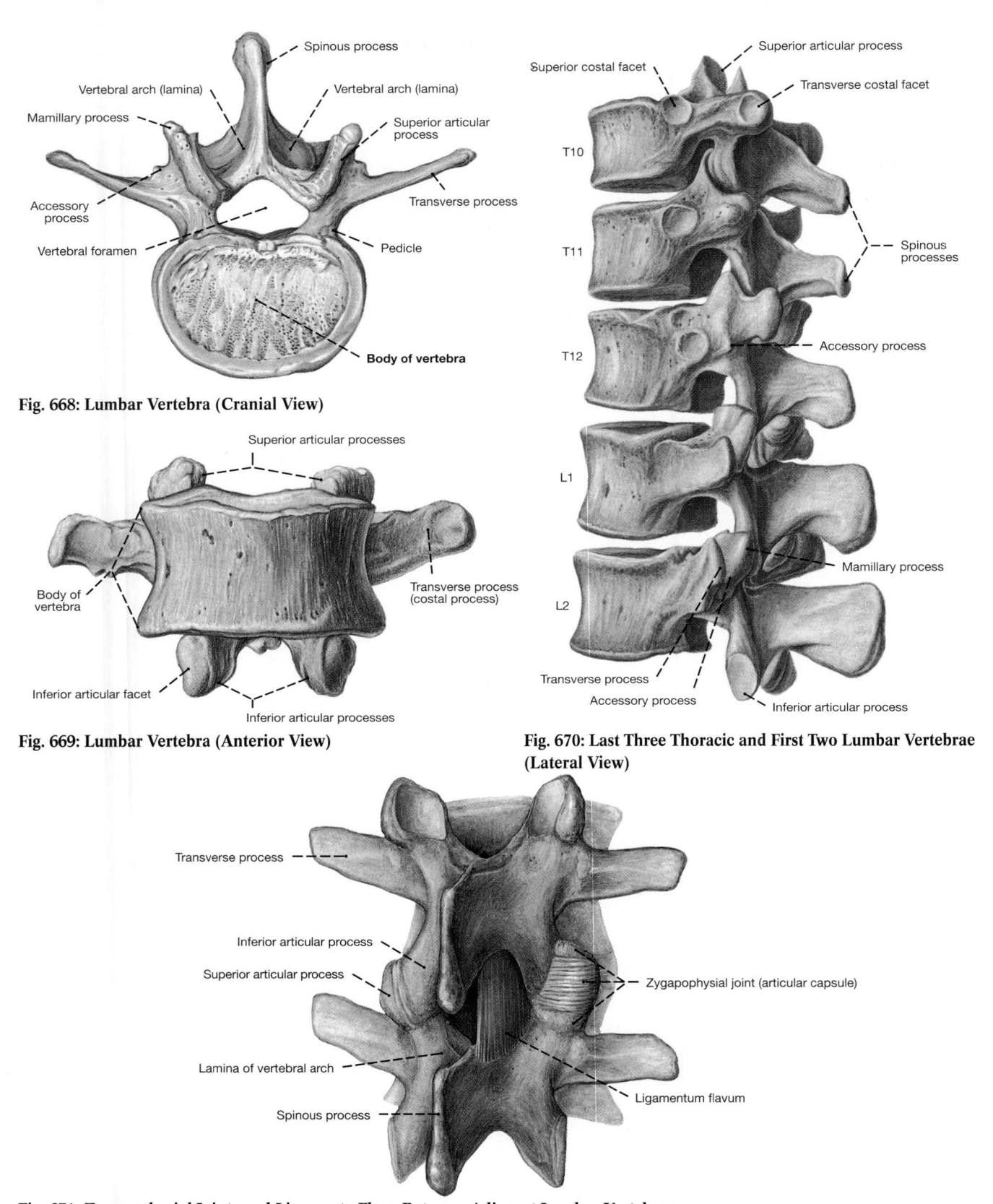

Fig. 668: Lumbar Vertebra (Cranial View)

Fig. 669: Lumbar Vertebra (Anterior View)

Fig. 670: Last Three Thoracic and First Two Lumbar Vertebrae (Lateral View)

Fig. 671: Zygapophysial Joints and Ligamenta Flava Between Adjacent Lumbar Vertebrae

NOTE: 1) in this posterior view, the articular capsule of the zygapophysial joint (between the articular processes) and the ligamentum flavum have been removed on the left side.

2) each ligamentum flavum is attached to the anterior surface of the lamina above and to the posterior surface of the lamina below. They are elastic and permit separation of the laminae during flexion of the spine and they inhibit abrupt and extreme movements of the vertebral column, thus protecting the intervertebral discs (see also Fig. 667).

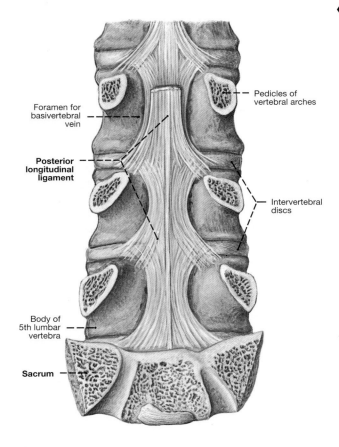

Pedicles of vertebral arches

Foramen for basivertebral vein

Posterior longitudinal ligament

Intervertebral discs

Body of 5th lumbar vertebra

Sacrum

Fig. 672: Posterior Longitudinal Ligament and Intervertebral Discs, Lumbosacral Region

NOTE: 1)   this dorsal view of the spinal column shows the pedicles of the lumbar vertebrae severed to expose the posterior longitudinal ligament.

2)   this ligament courses along the posterior aspect of the bodies of the vertebrae within the vertebral canal, and it extends from the axis (where it joins the tectorial membrane) to the sacrum, which is shown in this figure.

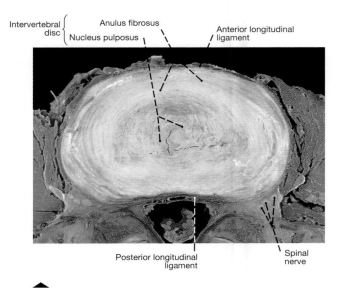

Intervertebral disc
{ Anulus fibrosus
Nucleus pulposus }

Anterior longitudinal ligament

Posterior longitudinal ligament

Spinal nerve

Fig. 673: Lumbar Intervertebral Disc (Viewed from Above)

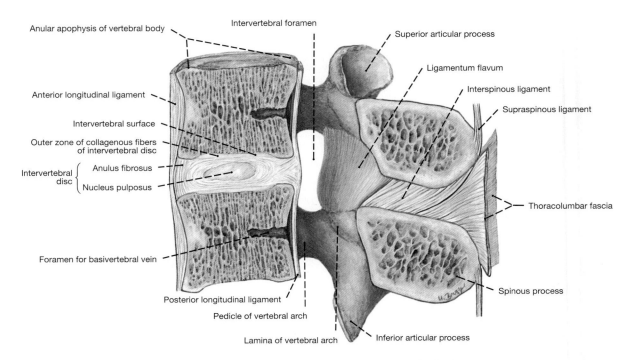

Anular apophysis of vertebral body

Intervertebral foramen

Superior articular process

Anterior longitudinal ligament

Ligamentum flavum

Interspinous ligament

Intervertebral surface

Supraspinous ligament

Outer zone of collagenous fibers of intervertebral disc

Intervertebral disc
{ Anulus fibrosus
Nucleus pulposus }

Thoracolumbar fascia

Foramen for basivertebral vein

Spinous process

Posterior longitudinal ligament

Pedicle of vertebral arch

Lamina of vertebral arch

Inferior articular process

Fig. 674: Median Sagittal Section Through Two Lumbar Vertebrae and an Intervertebral Disc

NOTE: 1)   the anterior and posterior longitudinal ligaments ventral and dorsal to the bodies of the lumbar vertebrae.

2)   the ligamentum flavum forms an important ligamentous connection between the laminae of adjacent vertebral arches on the dorsal aspect of the vertebral canal.

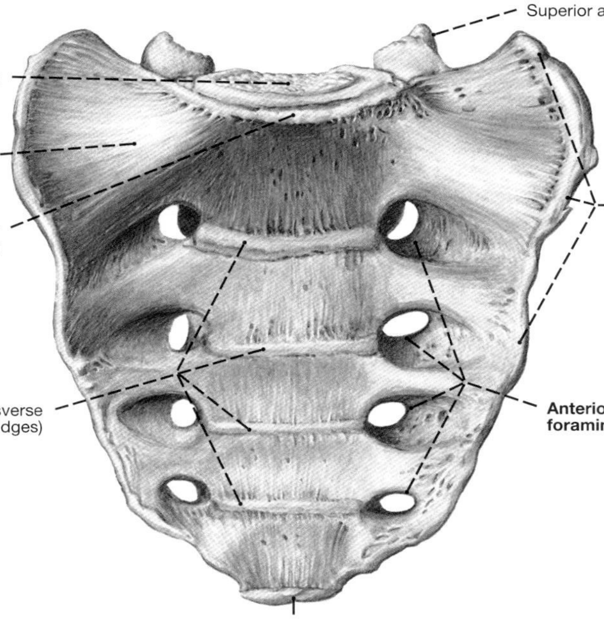

PLATE 428   **Sacrum and Coccyx**

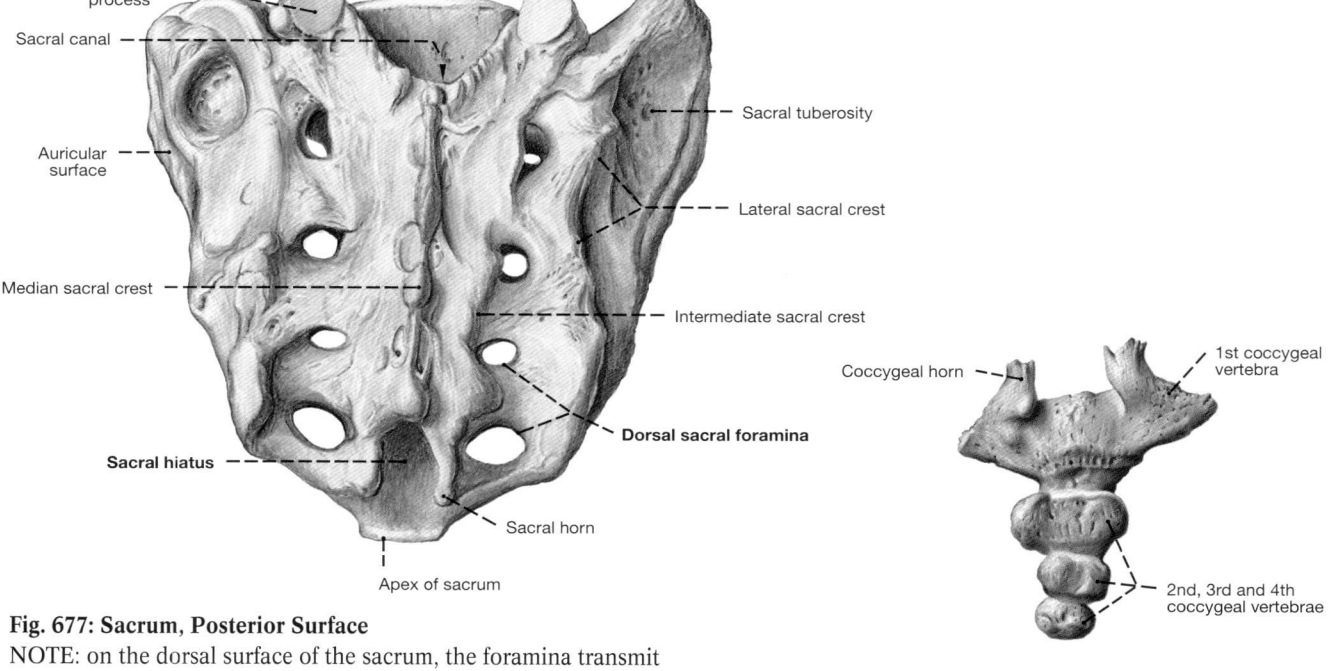

Superior articular process

Base of sacrum

Anterior aspect
of sacral wings
(ala)

Promontory
of sacrum

Lateral part

Transverse
lines (ridges)

**Anterior sacral
foramina**

Apex of sacrum

Fig. 675: Sacrum, Anterior or Pelvic Surface

NOTE: 1)   the sacrum is a large triangular bone formed by the fusion
of five sacral vertebrae, and it is wedged between the two hip
bones with which it articulates laterally.

2)   superiorly, the sacrum articulates with the 5th lumbar
vertebra, and inferiorly with the coccyx.

3)   the anterior (pelvic) surface of the sacrum is concave
and shows four pelvic foramina on each side. These transmit the
ventral rami of the upper four sacral nerves.

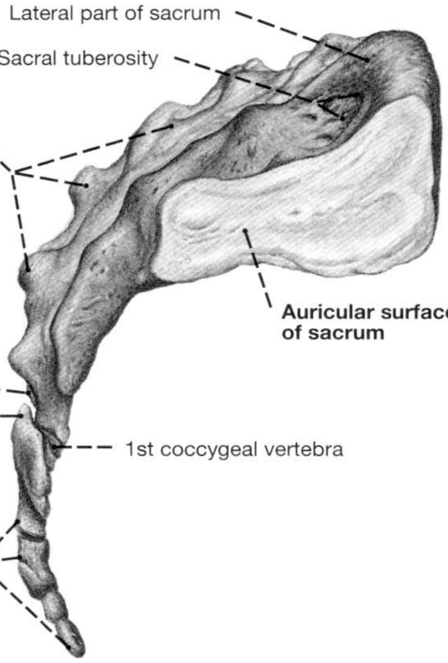

Lateral part of sacrum

Sacral tuberosity

Median
sacral crest

**Auricular surface
of sacrum**

Sacral horn

Coccygeal horn

1st coccygeal vertebra

Coccyx

Fig. 676: Sacrum and Coccyx, Lateral View

NOTE: the auricular (ear-shaped) surface of the sacrum
articulates with the iliac portion of the pelvis.
Inferiorly, the sacral apex joins the coccyx.

Superior articular
process

Sacral canal

Auricular
surface

Median sacral crest

Sacral hiatus

Sacral tuberosity

Lateral sacral crest

Intermediate sacral crest

Dorsal sacral foramina

Sacral horn

Apex of sacrum

Coccygeal horn

1st coccygeal
vertebra

2nd, 3rd and 4th
coccygeal vertebrae

Fig. 677: Sacrum, Posterior Surface

NOTE: on the dorsal surface of the sacrum, the foramina transmit
the dorsal rami of the sacral nerves. The dorsal laminae of the 5th
sacral vertebra fails to fuse, thereby leaving a midline opening into
the sacral canal called the sacral hiatus.

Fig. 678: Coccyx, Dorsal View

NOTE: this coccyx has four segments, but in many
people there are three or five.

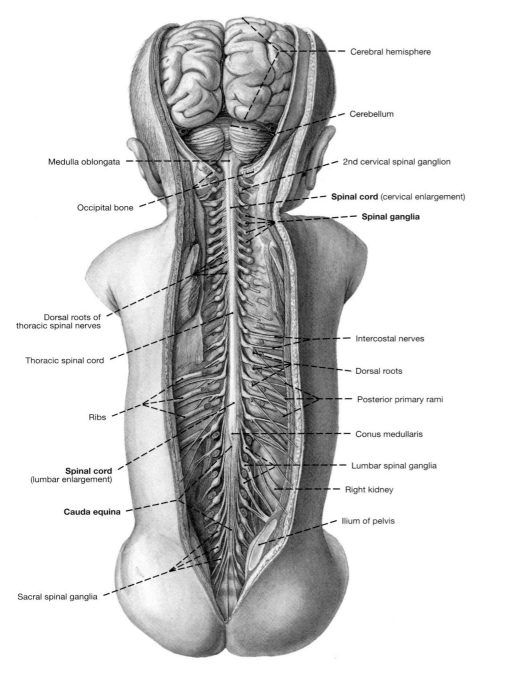

Cerebral hemisphere

Cerebellum

Medulla oblongata

2nd cervical spinal ganglion

Occipital bone

Spinal cord (cervical enlargement)

Spinal ganglia

Dorsal roots of thoracic spinal nerves

Intercostal nerves

Thoracic spinal cord

Dorsal roots

Posterior primary rami

Ribs

Conus medullaris

Spinal cord (lumbar enlargement)

Lumbar spinal ganglia

Right kidney

Cauda equina

Ilium of pelvis

Sacral spinal ganglia

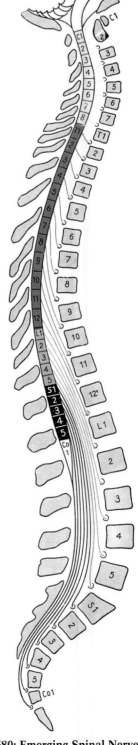

Fig. 679: Spinal Cord and Brain of a Newborn Child (Posterior View)

NOTE: 1) the central nervous system has been exposed by the removal of the dorsal part of the spinal column and of the dorsal cranium. The spinal ganglia have been dissected as have their corresponding spinal nerves.

2) although in this dissection it appears as though the substance of the spinal cord terminates at about L1, it is more usual in the newborn for the cord to end at about L3 or L4, thereby filling the spinal canal more completely than in the adult.

3) the dorsal root ganglion of the 1st cervical nerve may be very small and often absent (see small ganglion above that of C2). Both anterior and posterior primary rami of C1 are principally motor, although from time to time C1 will have a small cutaneous branch.

Fig. 680: Emerging Spinal Nerves and Segments in the Adult

Yellow: Cervical segments (C1–C8)
Red: Thoracic segments (T1–T12)
Blue: Lumbar segments (L1–L5)
Black: Sacral segments (S1–S5)
White: Coccygeal segments (C1–C2)
NOTE: many spinal nerves travel long distances before they leave the vertebral canal in the adult.

PLATE 430   **Spinal Cord: Dorsal and Ventral Views**

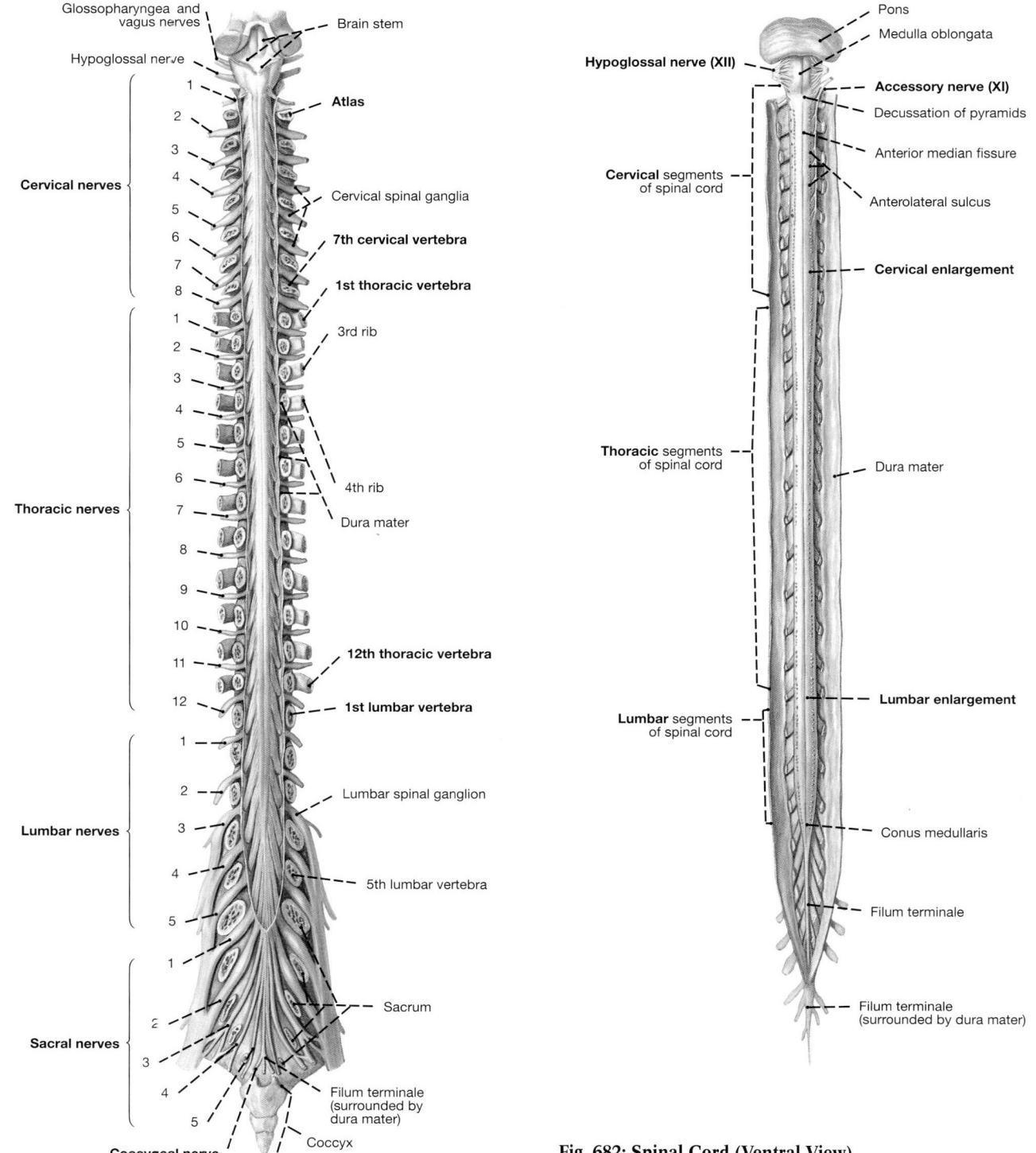

Fig. 681: Spinal Cord Within the Vertebral Canal (Dorsal View)

NOTE: 1) the 1st cervical nerve emerges above the first vertebra and the 8th cervical nerve emerges below the 7th vertebra.

2) the cervical spinal cord is continuous above with the medulla oblongata of the brain stem.

3) each spinal nerve is formed by the union of the dorsal and ventral roots of that segment and it emerges between the two adjacent vertebrae through the intervertebral foramen.

Fig. 682: Spinal Cord (Ventral View)

NOTE: 1) the origin of the spinal portion of the accessory nerve (XI) arising from the cervical spinal cord and ascending to join the bulbar portion of that nerve.

2) the alignment of the rootlets of the hypoglossal nerve (XII) with the ventral roots of the spinal cord.

3) the anterior median fissure is located in the longitudinal midline of the spinal cord. Within this fissure courses the anterior spinal artery (see Fig. 683).

4) the cervical and lumbar enlargements caused by the large numbers of sensory and motor neurons located in these regions that are required to supply innervation to the upper and lower limbs.

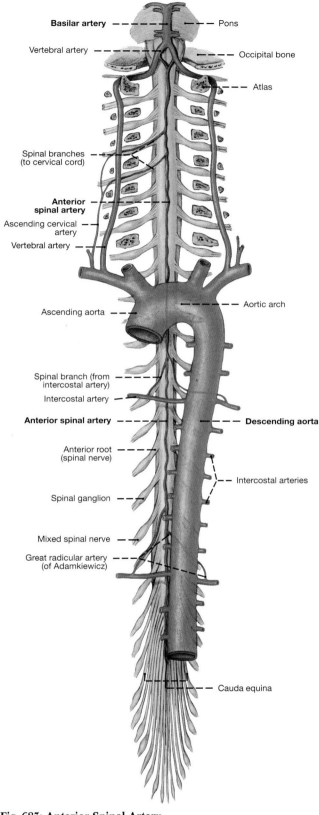

Basilar artery — Pons

Vertebral artery — Occipital bone

Atlas

Spinal branches (to cervical cord)

Anterior spinal artery

Ascending cervical artery

Vertebral artery

Ascending aorta — Aortic arch

Spinal branch (from intercostal artery)

Intercostal artery

Anterior spinal artery — **Descending aorta**

Anterior root (spinal nerve)

Intercostal arteries

Spinal ganglion

Mixed spinal nerve

Great radicular artery (of Adamkiewicz)

Cauda equina

Fig. 683: Anterior Spinal Artery

NOTE: the anterior spinal artery is formed by vessels from the vertebral arteries. It receives anastomotic branches from certain cervical, thoracic, and lumbar segmental arteries along the spinal roots. An especially large branch (artery of Adamkiewicz) arises in the lower thoracic or upper lumbar region.

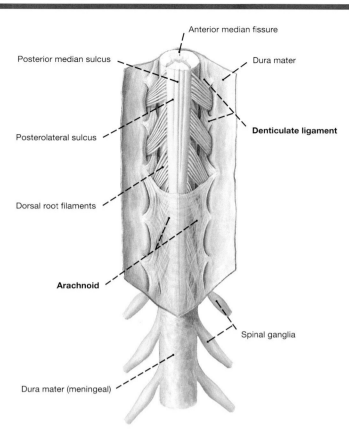

Anterior median fissure

Posterior median sulcus — Dura mater

Posterolateral sulcus — **Denticulate ligament**

Dorsal root filaments

Arachnoid

Spinal ganglia

Dura mater (meningeal)

Fig. 684: Spinal Cord with Dura Mater Dissected Open (Dorsal View)

NOTE: extensions of the pia mater to the meningeal dura mater between the roots of the spinal nerves are called **denticulate ligaments.** The arachnoid sends fine attachments to both the pia and dura.

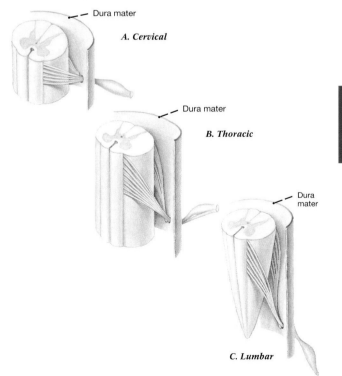

Dura mater

A. Cervical

Dura mater

B. Thoracic

Dura mater

C. Lumbar

Fig. 685A–C: Relationship of the Dorsal and Ventral Roots to the Dura Mater (Various Spinal Levels)

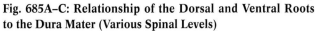

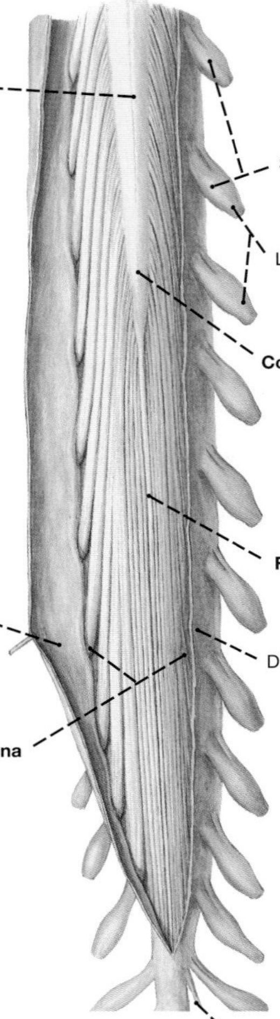

PLATE 432   Spinal Cord: Cauda Equina

Anterior median fissure

Spinal ganglia

Lumbar spinal nerves

Conus medullaris

Filum terminale

Dura mater

Dura mater

Cauda equina

Coccygeal nerve

Fig. 686: Conus Medullaris and Cauda Equina (Ventral)
NOTE: 1) the termination of the neural part of the spinal cord at the conus medullaris. Its membranous continuation as the filum terminale measures about 20 cm and extends as far as the coccyx.

2) the cauda equina refers to the roots of the spinal nerves below the conus and these are seen to surround the filum.

3) prolongations of the dura continue to cover the spinal nerves for some distance as they enter the intervertebral foramen.

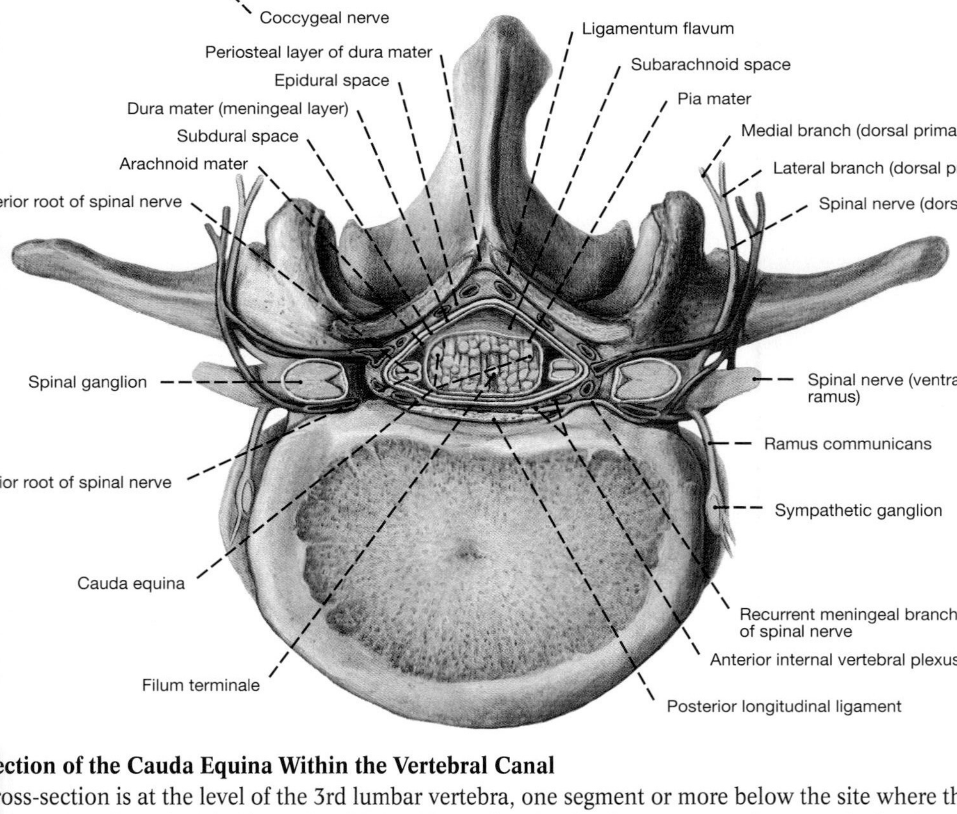

Periosteal layer of dura mater

Epidural space

Dura mater (meningeal layer)

Subdural space

Arachnoid mater

Posterior root of spinal nerve

Ligamentum flavum

Subarachnoid space

Pia mater

Medial branch (dorsal primary ramus)

Lateral branch (dorsal primary ramus)

Spinal nerve (dorsal primary ramus)

Spinal ganglion

Spinal nerve (ventral primary ramus)

Ramus communicans

Sympathetic ganglion

Anterior root of spinal nerve

Cauda equina

Recurrent meningeal branch of spinal nerve

Anterior internal vertebral plexus

Filum terminale

Posterior longitudinal ligament

Fig. 687: Cross-section of the Cauda Equina Within the Vertebral Canal
NOTE: 1) this cross-section is at the level of the 3rd lumbar vertebra, one segment or more below the site where the spinal cord ends.

2) specimens of cerebrospinal fluid may be obtained by performing lumbar punctures between the laminae or spines of the 3rd and 4th or 4th and 5th lumbar vertebrae.

Figs. 686, 687

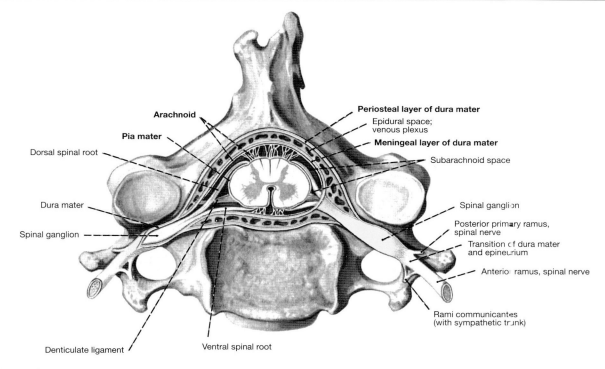

Fig. 688: Meninges of the Spinal Cord Shown at Cervical Level (Transverse Section)

NOTE: 1) the meningeal dura mater (inner layer of yellow) surrounds the spinal cord and continues along the spinal nerve through the intervertebral foramen. Its outer periosteal layer is formed of connective tissue that closely adheres to the bone of the vertebrae forming the vertebral canal.

2) the delicate film-like arachnoid, which lies between the meningeal layer of the dura mater and the vascularized pia mater, which is closely applied to the cord.

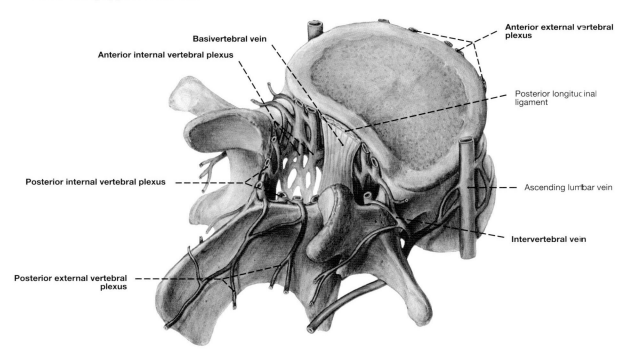

Fig. 689: Veins of the Vertebral Column

NOTE: 1) the veins drain blood from the vertebrae and the contents of the spinal canal form plexuses that extend the entire length of the spinal column (Batson's veins).

2) the plexuses are grouped according to whether they lie external or within the vertebral canal. Thus, they include **external vertebral, internal vertebral, basivertebral, intervertebral** and **veins of the spinal cord.**

3) the basivertebral veins drain the bodies of the vertebrae and may flow into anterior external or anterior internal vertebral plexuses.

PLATE 434   Vertebral Column and Spinal Cord: Anterior View

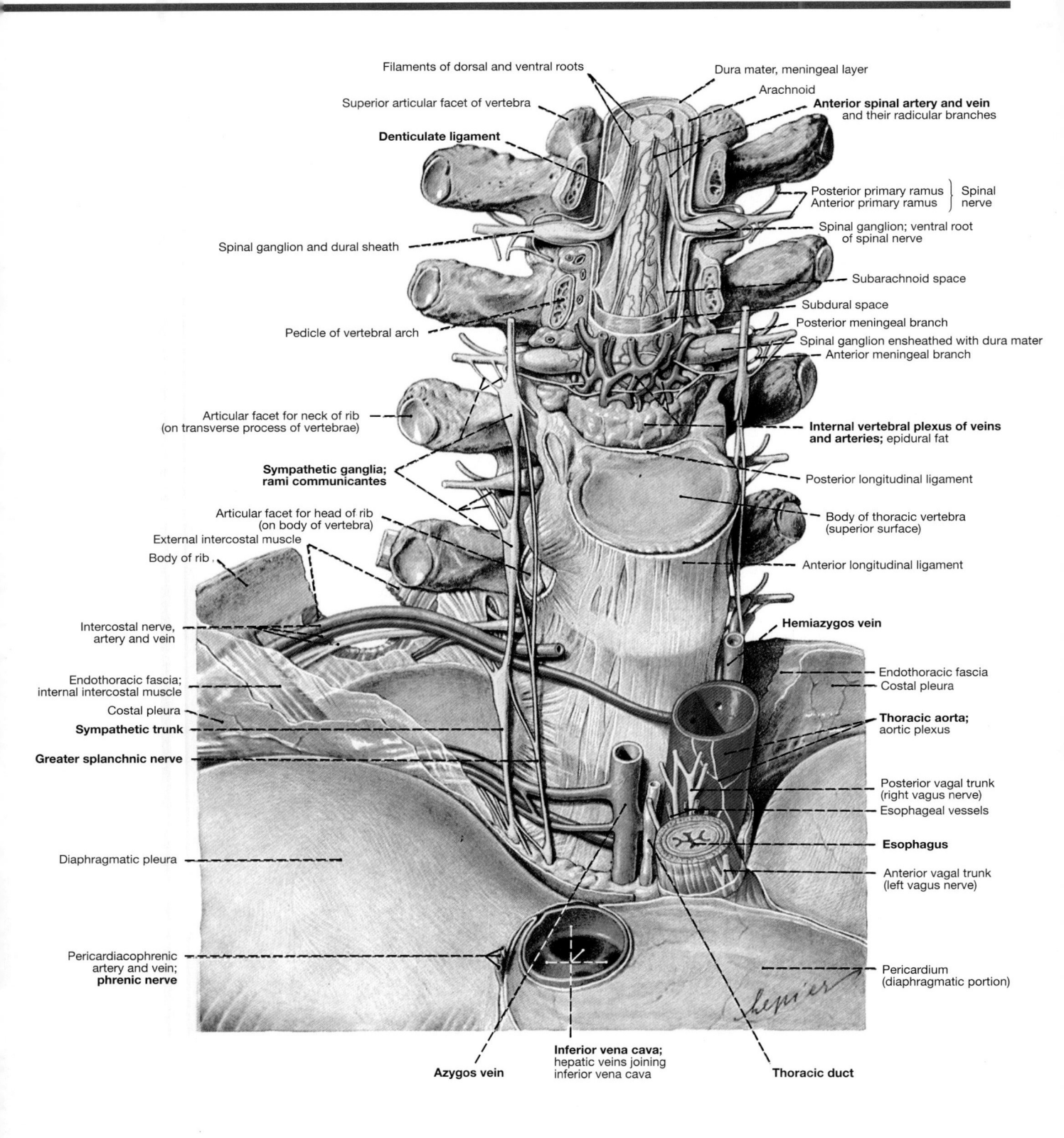

Filaments of dorsal and ventral roots

Superior articular facet of vertebra

Denticulate ligament

Spinal ganglion and dural sheath

Pedicle of vertebral arch

Articular facet for neck of rib
(on transverse process of vertebrae)

**Sympathetic ganglia;
rami communicantes**

Articular facet for head of rib
(on body of vertebra)
External intercostal muscle
Body of rib

Intercostal nerve,
artery and vein

Endothoracic fascia;
internal intercostal muscle
Costal pleura
Sympathetic trunk

Greater splanchnic nerve

Diaphragmatic pleura

Pericardiacophrenic
artery and vein;
phrenic nerve

Dura mater, meningeal layer
Arachnoid
Anterior spinal artery and vein
and their radicular branches

Posterior primary ramus ⎫ Spinal
Anterior primary ramus ⎭ nerve

Spinal ganglion; ventral root
of spinal nerve

Subarachnoid space

Subdural space
Posterior meningeal branch
Spinal ganglion ensheathed with dura mater
Anterior meningeal branch

**Internal vertebral plexus of veins
and arteries;** epidural fat

Posterior longitudinal ligament

Body of thoracic vertebra
(superior surface)

Anterior longitudinal ligament

Hemiazygos vein

Endothoracic fascia
Costal pleura

Thoracic aorta;
aortic plexus

Posterior vagal trunk
(right vagus nerve)
Esophageal vessels

Esophagus

Anterior vagal trunk
(left vagus nerve)

Pericardium
(diaphragmatic portion)

Azygos vein

Inferior vena cava;
hepatic veins joining
inferior vena cava

Thoracic duct

Fig. 690: Anterior Dissection of Vertebral Column, Spinal Cord and Prevertebral Structures at a Lower Thoracic Level

NOTE: 1) the internal vertebral plexus of veins and arteries which lie in the epidural space, where also is found the epidural fat. These should not be confused with the spinal vessels, which are situated in the pia mater and which are seen to be intimately applied to the spinal cord tissue.

2) the ganglionated sympathetic chain observable here in the thoracic region receiving and giving communicating rami with the spinal nerves. Note also the formation of the greater splanchnic nerve and its descent prevertebrally into the abdomen.

3) the aorta, inferior vena cava, azygos and hemiazygos veins, esophagus, and thoracic duct all lying anterior or somewhat to the left of the vertebral column and passing through the diaphragm.

Figs. 690

PART VII
THE NECK AND HEAD

(PLATES 435–576 – FIGURES 691–940)

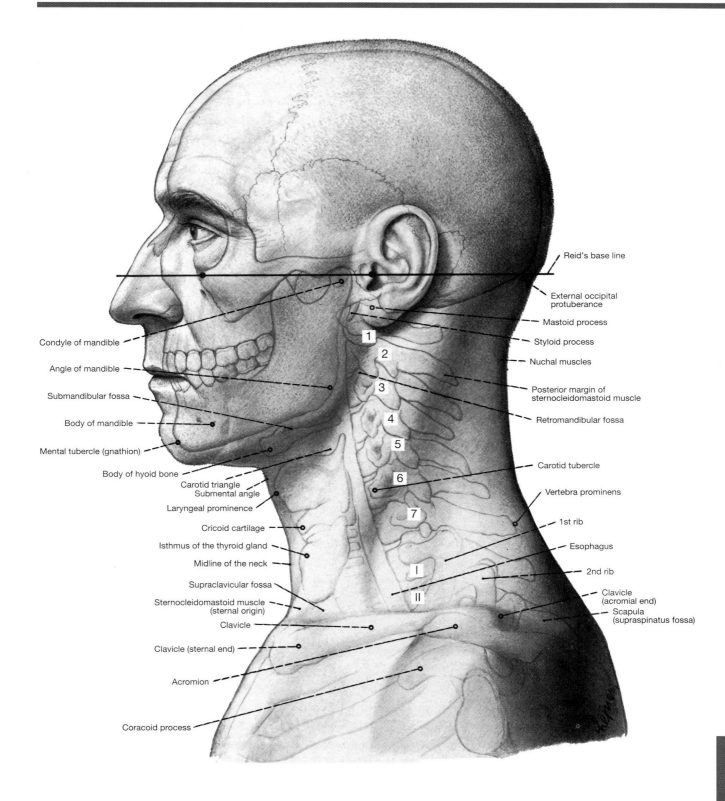

Reid's base line

External occipital protuberance

Mastoid process

Styloid process

Nuchal muscles

Posterior margin of sternocleidomastoid muscle

Retromandibular fossa

Carotid tubercle

Vertebra prominens

1st rib

Esophagus

2nd rib

Clavicle (acromial end)

Scapula (supraspinatus fossa)

Condyle of mandible

Angle of mandible

Submandibular fossa

Body of mandible

Mental tubercle (gnathion)

Body of hyoid bone

Carotid triangle
Submental angle

Laryngeal prominence

Cricoid cartilage

Isthmus of the thyroid gland

Midline of the neck

Supraclavicular fossa

Sternocleidomastoid muscle (sternal origin)

Clavicle

Clavicle (sternal end)

Acromion

Coracoid process

Fig. 691: External Features of the Neck Shown in Relation to Underlying Skeletal and Visceral Structures

NOTE: 1)   the palpable bony points are indicated by open circles at the end of certain leader lines.

2)   the seven cervical and two upper thoracic vertebrae as well as the prominent skeletal features of the pectoral girdle. Observe the laryngeal cartilages and hyoid bone in the anterior neck and their respective vertebral planes.

3)   a horizontal line (Reid's base line), drawn from the inferior margin of the orbit through the center of the external auditory canal and continuing backward to the center of the occipital bone, is frequently used for cranial topography and cephalometric studies.

Fig. 691   **VII**

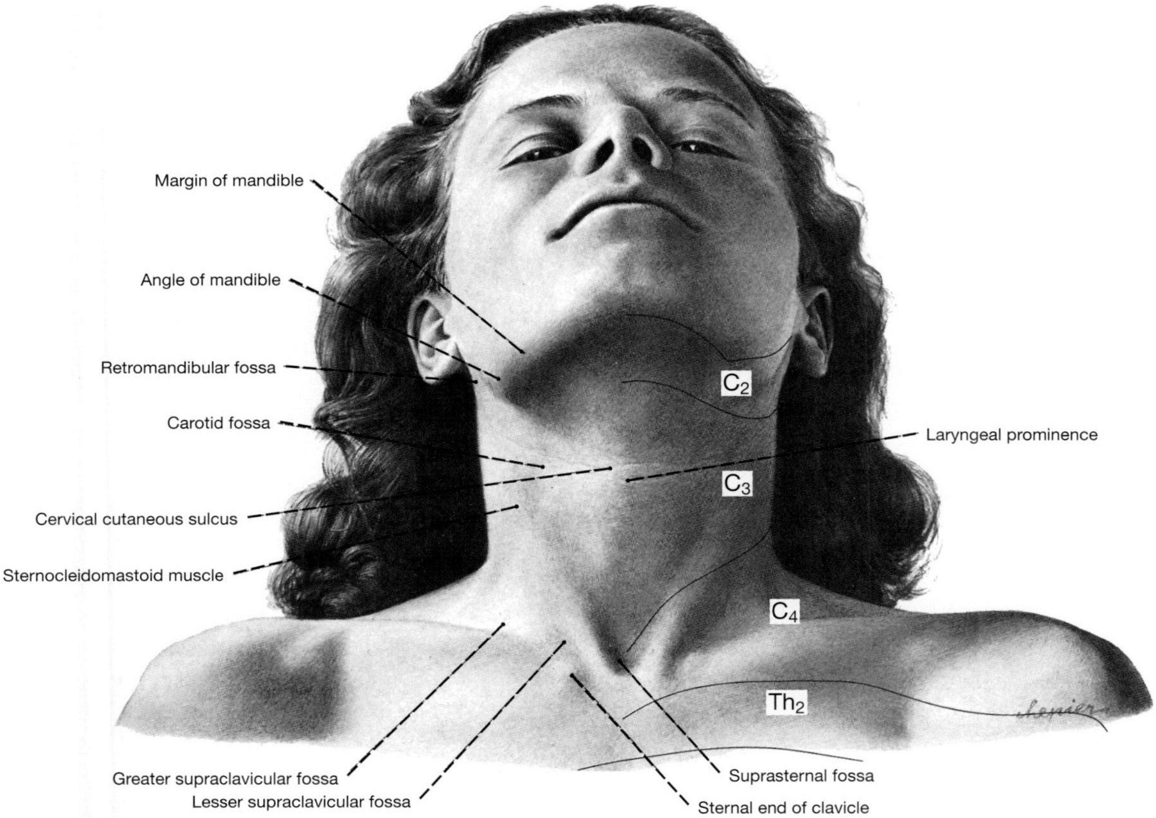

PLATE 436   Neck: Surface Anatomy; Triangles

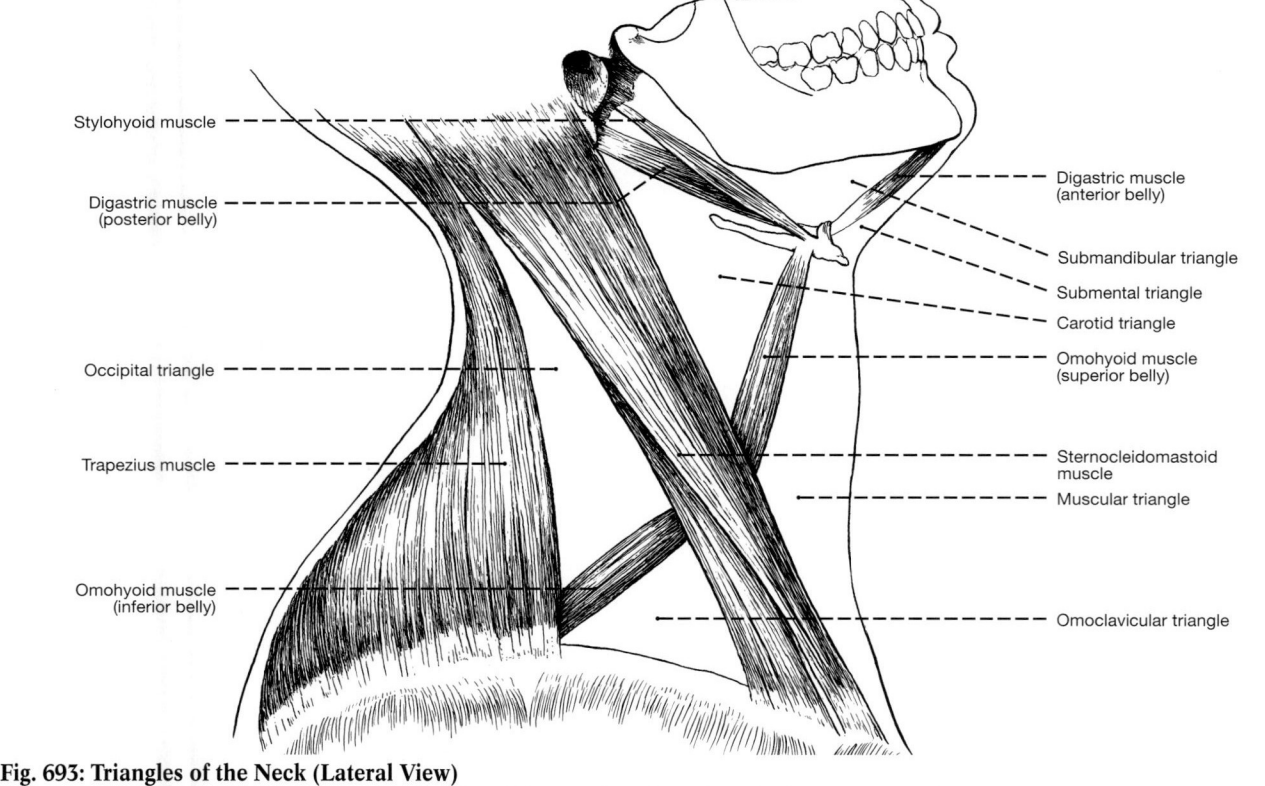

Margin of mandible

Angle of mandible

Retromandibular fossa

Carotid fossa

Cervical cutaneous sulcus

Sternocleidomastoid muscle

C₂

C₃

C₄

Th₂

Laryngeal prominence

Greater supraclavicular fossa

Lesser supraclavicular fossa

Suprasternal fossa

Sternal end of clavicle

Fig. 692: Surface Anatomy and Dermatomes of the Neck, Anterior View
NOTE: the sequence of cervical dermatomes of the neck is interrupted below C4 because segments C5, C6, C7, C8 and Th1 serve the upper limb and are not represented in the neck.

Stylohyoid muscle

Digastric muscle (posterior belly)

Occipital triangle

Trapezius muscle

Omohyoid muscle (inferior belly)

Digastric muscle (anterior belly)

Submandibular triangle

Submental triangle

Carotid triangle

Omohyoid muscle (superior belly)

Sternocleidomastoid muscle

Muscular triangle

Omoclavicular triangle

Fig. 693: Triangles of the Neck (Lateral View)
NOTE: the triangles of the neck are useful in describing the location of cervical organs and other structures. The entire area *anterior* to the sternocleidomastoid muscle is called the **anterior triangle,** while the area *posterior* to this muscle is the **posterior triangle** (from Clemente CD. Gray's Anatomy, 30th Edition. Lea & Febiger, Philadelphia, PA).

Figs. 692, 693

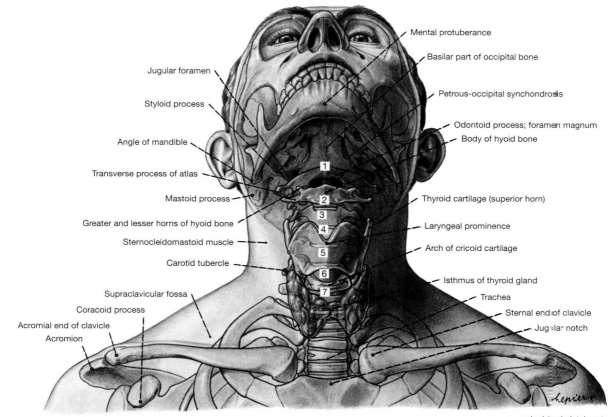

Mental protuberance

Basilar part of occipital bone

Petrous-occipital synchondrosis

Odontoid process; foramen magnum

Body of hyoid bone

Thyroid cartilage (superior horn)

Laryngeal prominence

Arch of cricoid cartilage

Isthmus of thyroid gland

Trachea

Sternal end of clavicle

Jugular notch

Jugular foramen

Styloid process

Angle of mandible

Transverse process of atlas

Mastoid process

Greater and lesser horns of hyoid bone

Sternocleidomastoid muscle

Carotid tubercle

Supraclavicular fossa

Coracoid process

Acromial end of clavicle

Acromion

• = palpable skeletal parts
1–7 = cervical vertebrae

Fig. 694: Surface Projection of the Thyroid Gland and Skeletal Structures in the Neck and the Thoracic Inlet (Anterior View)
NOTE: 1)   the anterior aspect of the bodies of the cervical vertebrae have been numbered sequentially.

2)   the hyoid bone lies at about the upper level of the 3rd cervical vertebra; the thyroid cartilage at the level of C4 and C5, and the cricoid cartilage at C6. Below this are two inches of trachea in the neck (C7 and T1) and (not shown) two inches of trachea in the thorax (T2 and T3) before the trachea bifurcates at T4.

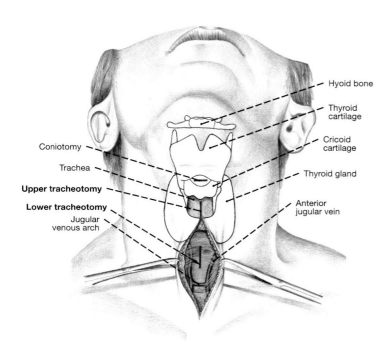

Hyoid bone

Thyroid cartilage

Cricoid cartilage

Thyroid gland

Anterior jugular vein

Coniotomy

Trachea

Upper tracheotomy

Lower tracheotomy
Jugular venous arch

Fig. 695: Projection of Larynx and Trachea Showing Sites for Entry into the Respiratory Pathway
NOTE: 1)   the hyoid bone, laryngeal cartilages (thyroid and cricoid), thyroid gland and tracheal region of the anterior neck are projected to the surface, as have three sites where entrance into the respiratory tract may be achieved readily (in red).

2)   the upper transverse incision cuts through the cricothyroid ligament and conus elasticus and can be called a **coniotomy,** while the **upper tracheotomy** and **lower tracheotomy** can be made in the trachea above or below the thyroid gland.

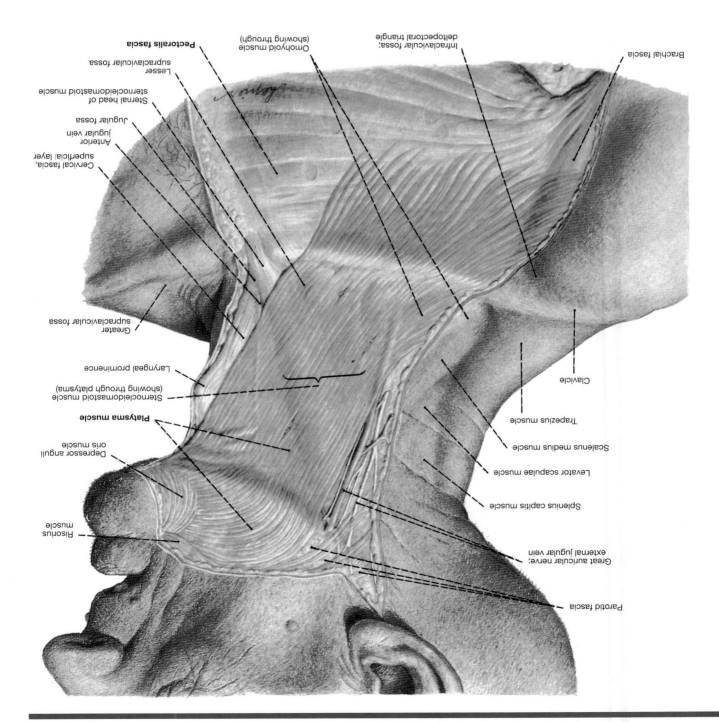

PLATE 438   The Neck: The Platysma Muscle

Fig. 696: Right Platysma Muscle and Pectoral Fascia

NOTE: 1) the **platysma muscle** is a broad, thin quadrangular muscle located in the superficial fascia and extends from the angle of the mouth and chin downward across the clavicle to the upper part of the thorax and anterior shoulder.

2) the platysma is considered a muscle of facial expression, many of which do not attach to bony structures, but arise and insert within the superficial fascia.

3) upon concentration, the platysma tends to depress the angle of the mouth and wrinkle the skin of the neck, thereby participating in the formation of facial expressions of anxiety, sadness, dissatisfaction and suffering.

4) similar to other muscles of facial expression, the platysma is innervated by the **facial nerve (cervical branch),** the 7th cranial nerve (VII).

5) overlying the pectoralis major is the well-developed pectoralis fascia, which extends from the midline in the thorax laterally to the axilla. Observe the external jugular vein and great auricular nerve exposed in the upper lateral aspect of the neck.

Labels (clockwise):

Brachial fascia

Infraclavicular fossa; deltopectoral triangle

Omohyoid muscle (showing through)

Pectoralis fascia

Lesser supraclavicular fossa

Sternal head of sternocleidomastoid muscle

Jugular fossa

Anterior jugular vein

Cervical fascia, superficial layer

Greater supraclavicular fossa

Laryngeal prominence

Sternocleidomastoid muscle (showing through platysma)

Platysma muscle

Depressor anguli oris muscle

Risorius muscle

Parotid fascia

Great auricular nerve; external jugular vein

Splenius capitis muscle

Levator scapulae muscle

Scalenus medius muscle

Trapezius muscle

Clavicle

Fig. 696

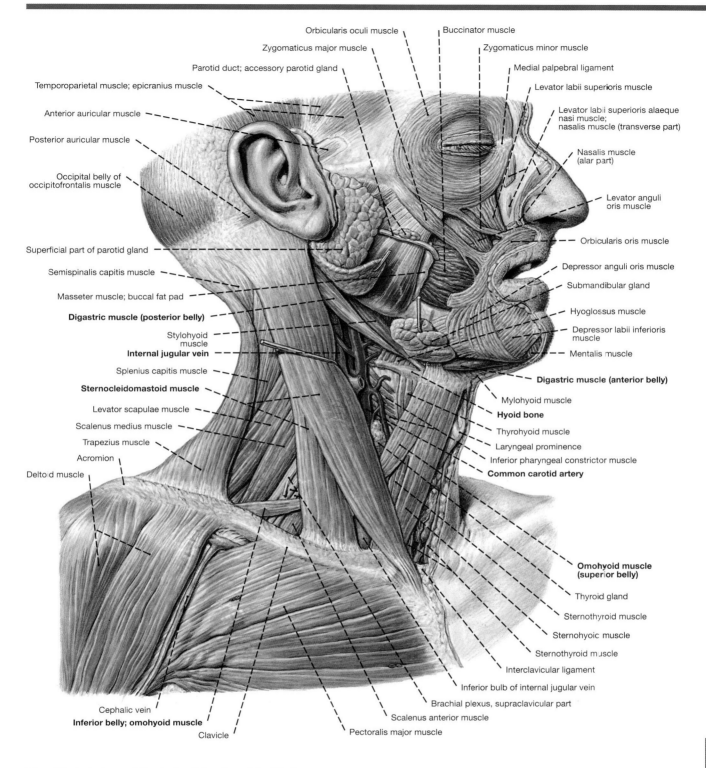

Orbicularis oculi muscle
Buccinator muscle
Zygomaticus major muscle
Zygomaticus minor muscle
Parotid duct; accessory parotid gland
Medial palpebral ligament
Temporoparietal muscle; epicranius muscle
Levator labii superioris muscle
Anterior auricular muscle
Levator labii superioris alaeque nasi muscle; nasalis muscle (transverse part)
Posterior auricular muscle
Nasalis muscle (alar part)
Occipital belly of occipitofrontalis muscle
Levator anguli oris muscle
Superficial part of parotid gland
Orbicularis oris muscle
Semispinalis capitis muscle
Depressor anguli oris muscle
Masseter muscle; buccal fat pad
Submandibular gland
Digastric muscle (posterior belly)
Hyoglossus muscle
Stylohyoid muscle
Depressor labii inferioris muscle
Internal jugular vein
Mentalis muscle
Splenius capitis muscle
Digastric muscle (anterior belly)
Sternocleidomastoid muscle
Mylohyoid muscle
Levator scapulae muscle
Hyoid bone
Scalenus medius muscle
Thyrohyoid muscle
Trapezius muscle
Laryngeal prominence
Acromion
Inferior pharyngeal constrictor muscle
Deltoid muscle
Common carotid artery
Omohyoid muscle (superior belly)
Thyroid gland
Sternothyroid muscle
Sternohyoic muscle
Sternothyroid muscle
Interclavicular ligament
Inferior bulb of internal jugular vein
Cephalic vein
Brachial plexus, supraclavicular part
Inferior belly; omohyoid muscle
Scalenus anterior muscle
Clavicle
Pectoralis major muscle

Fig. 697: Anterior and Posterior Triangles of the Neck

NOTE: 1) the **anterior triangle** of the neck is bounded by the midline of the neck, the anterior border of the sternocleidomastoid muscle and the mandible. This area is further subdivided by the superior belly of the omohyoid muscle and the two bellies of the digastric into:

    a) **muscular triangle** (midline, superior belly of omohyoid and sternocleidomastoid);

    b) **carotid triangle** (superior belly of omohyoid, sternocleidomastoid muscle, and posterior belly of digastric);

    c) **submandibular triangle** (anterior and posterior bellies of digastric, and the inferior margin of the mandible);

    d) **submental triangle** (midline, anterior belly of digastric, and hyoid bone).

  2) the **posterior triangle** of the neck is bounded by the posterior border of the sternocleidomastoid muscle, the trapezius and the clavicle. This area is further subdivided into the **occipital triangle** above and the **omoclavicular triangle** below by the inferior belly of the omohyoid.

Fig. 697   **VII**

PLATE 440   The Neck: Vessels and Nerves, Platysma Level (Dissection 1)

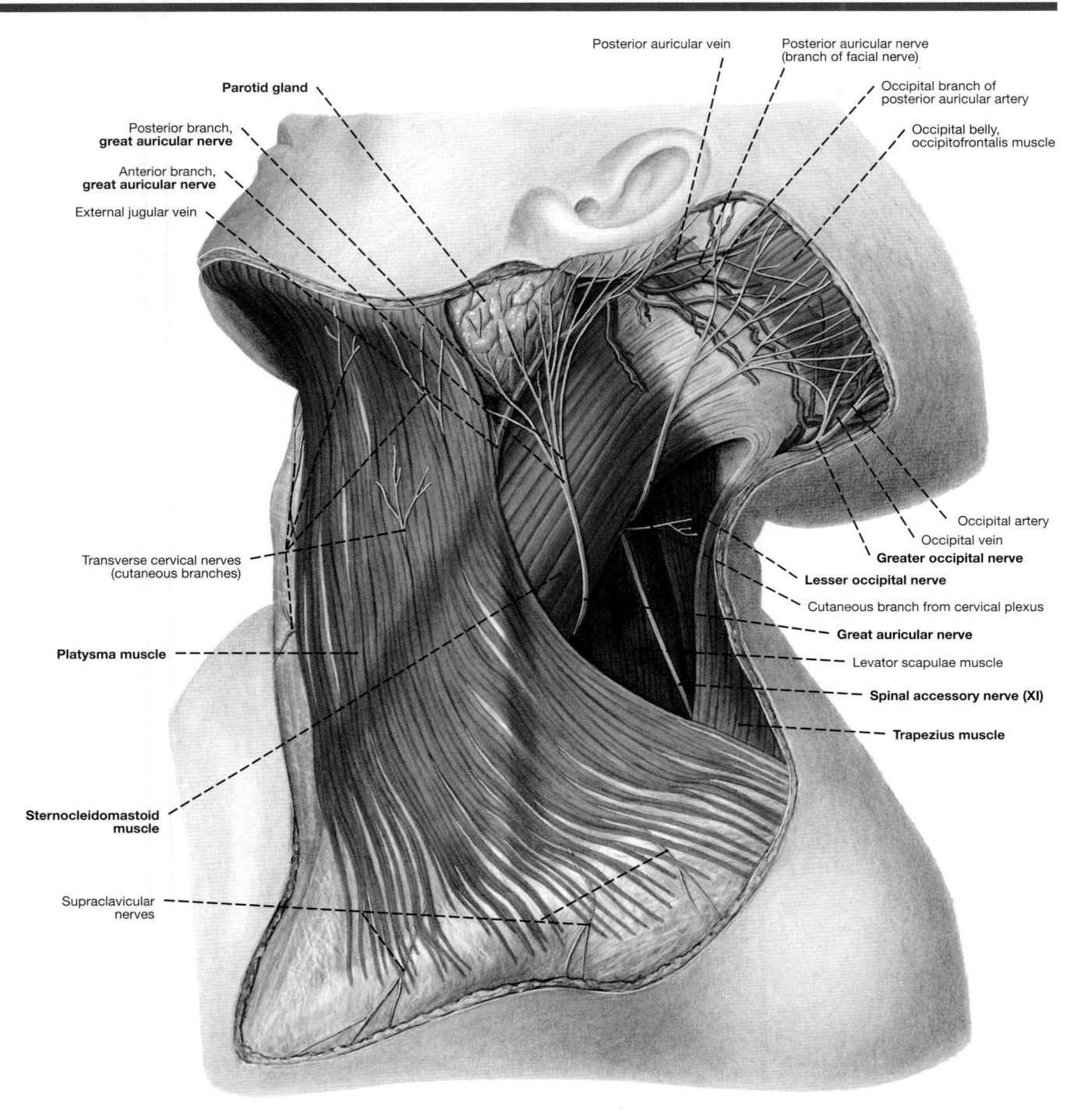

Fig. 698: Nerves and Blood Vessels of the Neck, Stage 1: Platysma Layer

NOTE: 1) the skin has been removed from both the anterior and posterior triangle areas to reveal the platysma muscle. Observe the cutaneous branches of the **transverse cervical nerves,** derived from the cervical plexus and penetrating through the platysma and superficial fascia to reach the skin of the anterolateral aspect of the neck.

2) four other nerves: the **great auricular (C2, C3);** the **lesser occipital (C2);** the **greater occipital (C2);** and the **accessory (XI).**

3) after it has supplied the sternocleidomastoid muscle, the accessory nerve (XI) descends in the posterior triangle to reach the trapezius muscle which it also supplies.

4) the **supraclavicular nerves.** These descend in the neck under cover of the deep fascia and platysma muscle. They become superficial just above the clavicle and then cross that bone as the anterior (medial), middle (intermediate) and posterior (lateral) supraclavicular nerves (see also Fig. 699). They derive from the 3rd and 4th cervical nerves, and supply skin over the clavicle, the upper trunk (down to the 2nd rib) and the shoulder from the acromion laterally to the midline anteriorly.

Fig. 698

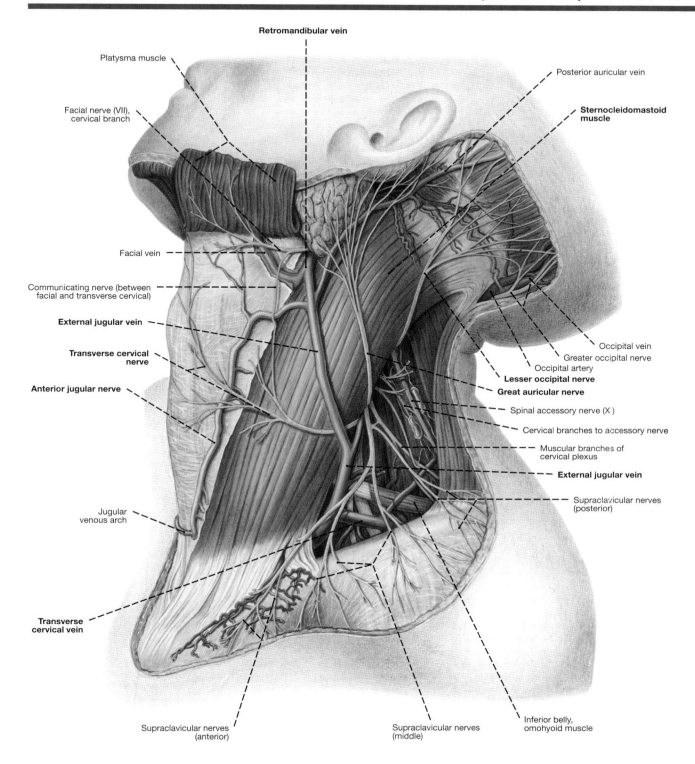

Retromandibular vein

Platysma muscle

Posterior auricular vein

Facial nerve (VII),
cervical branch

**Sternocleidomastoid
muscle**

Facial vein

Communicating nerve (between
facial and transverse cervical)

External jugular vein

**Transverse cervical
nerve**

Anterior jugular nerve

Occipital vein
Greater occipital nerve
Occipital artery
Lesser occipital nerve
Great auricular nerve

Spinal accessory nerve (X)

Cervical branches to accessory nerve

Muscular branches of
cervical plexus

External jugular vein

Supraclavicular nerves
(posterior)

Jugular
venous arch

**Transverse
cervical vein**

Supraclavicular nerves
(anterior)

Supraclavicular nerves
(middle)

Inferior belly,
omohyoid muscle

Fig. 699: Nerves and Blood Vessels of the Neck, Stage 2: Sternocleidomastoid Layer

NOTE: 1)   with the platysma muscle reflected upward, the full extent of the sternocleidomastoid muscle is exposed.

2)   the nerves of the cervical plexus diverge at the posterior border of the sternocleidomastoid muscle: the **great auricular** and **lesser occipital** ascend to the head, the **transverse cervical** (transverse colli) course across the neck, while the **supraclavicular nerves** descend over the clavicle.

3)   the **external jugular vein** formed by the junction of the **retromandibular** and **posterior auricular veins.** The external jugular crosses the sternocleidomastoid muscle obliquely and receives tributaries from the anterior jugular, posterior external jugular (not shown), transverse cervical and suprascapular vein (not shown) before it ends in the subclavian vein.

4)   the cervical branch of the **facial (VII) nerve** supplying the inner surface of the platysma muscle with motor innervation.

Fig. 699   **VII**

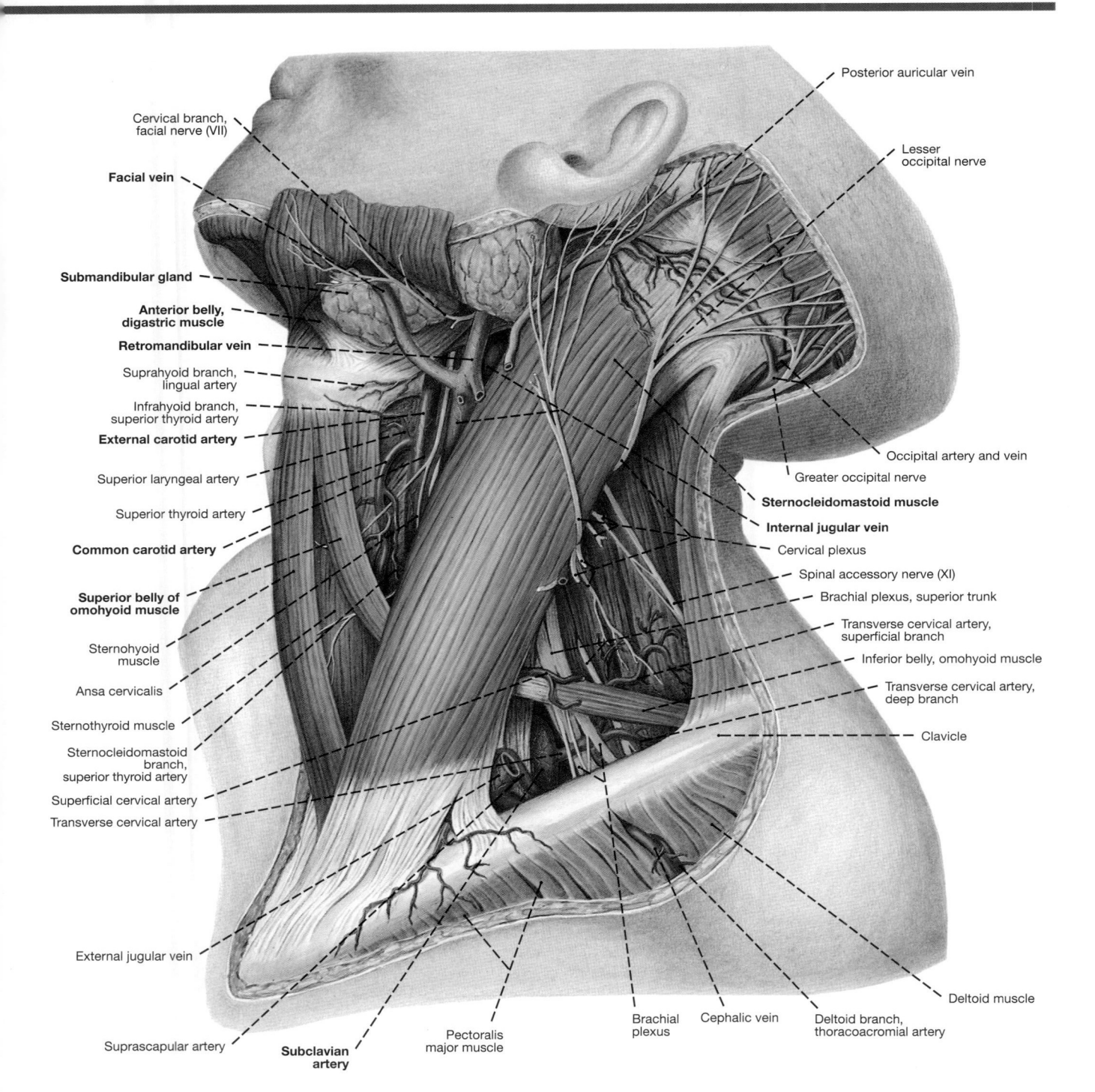

Posterior auricular vein

Cervical branch, facial nerve (VII)

Lesser occipital nerve

Facial vein

Submandibular gland

Anterior belly, digastric muscle

Retromandibular vein

Suprahyoid branch, lingual artery

Infrahyoid branch, superior thyroid artery

External carotid artery

Superior laryngeal artery

Superior thyroid artery

Common carotid artery

Superior belly of omohyoid muscle

Sternohyoid muscle

Ansa cervicalis

Sternothyroid muscle

Sternocleidomastoid branch, superior thyroid artery

Superficial cervical artery

Transverse cervical artery

External jugular vein

Suprascapular artery

Subclavian artery

Pectoralis major muscle

Brachial plexus

Cephalic vein

Deltoid branch, thoracoacromial artery

Occipital artery and vein

Greater occipital nerve

Sternocleidomastoid muscle

Internal jugular vein

Cervical plexus

Spinal accessory nerve (XI)

Brachial plexus, superior trunk

Transverse cervical artery, superficial branch

Inferior belly, omohyoid muscle

Transverse cervical artery, deep branch

Clavicle

Deltoid muscle

Fig. 700: Nerves and Blood Vessels of the Neck, Stage 3: the Anterior Triangle

NOTE: 1) with the investing layer of fascia removed, the outlines of the muscular, carotid, and submandibular triangles within the anterior region of the neck are revealed.

2) the infrahyoid (strap) muscles which cover the thyroid gland and the lateral aspect of the larynx in the **muscular triangle.** This is bounded by the sternocleidomastoid, the midline and the superior belly of the digastric muscle.

3) the carotid vessels and internal jugular vein can be seen in the **carotid triangle** which is bounded by the superior belly of the omohyoid, posterior belly of the digastric (not labelled) and the sternocleidomastoid.

4) with the platysma muscle cut and reflected upward, the submandibular gland is seen in the **submandibular triangle,** between the anterior and posterior bellies of the digastric and the inferior border of the mandible.

5) the spinal accessory nerve descending in the posterior triangle from beneath the sternocleidomastoid Dhich it supplies, to reach the trapezius muscle (not labelled), which it also supplies with motor innervation.

Fig. 700

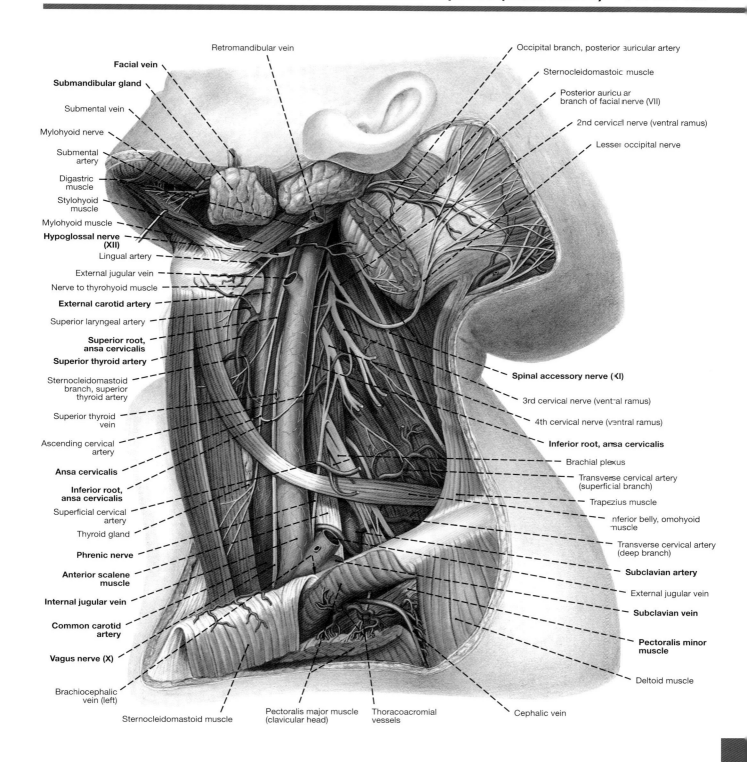

Retromandibular vein

Facial vein

Submandibular gland

Submental vein

Mylohyoid nerve

Submental artery

Digastric muscle

Stylohyoid muscle

Mylohyoid muscle

Hypoglossal nerve (XII)

Lingual artery

External jugular vein

Nerve to thyrohyoid muscle

External carotid artery

Superior laryngeal artery

Superior root, ansa cervicalis

Superior thyroid artery

Sternocleidomastoid branch, superior thyroid artery

Superior thyroid vein

Ascending cervical artery

Ansa cervicalis

Inferior root, ansa cervicalis

Superficial cervical artery

Thyroid gland

Phrenic nerve

Anterior scalene muscle

Internal jugular vein

Common carotid artery

Vagus nerve (X)

Brachiocephalic vein (left)

Sternocleidomastoid muscle

Pectoralis major muscle (clavicular head)

Thoracoacromial vessels

Cephalic vein

Occipital branch, posterior auricular artery

Sternocleidomastoid muscle

Posterior auricular branch of facial nerve (VII)

2nd cervical nerve (ventral ramus)

Lesser occipital nerve

Spinal accessory nerve (XI)

3rd cervical nerve (ventral ramus)

4th cervical nerve (ventral ramus)

Inferior root, ansa cervicalis

Brachial plexus

Transverse cervical artery (superficial branch)

Trapezius muscle

Inferior belly, omohyoid muscle

Transverse cervical artery (deep branch)

Subclavian artery

External jugular vein

Subclavian vein

Pectoralis minor muscle

Deltoid muscle

Fig. 701: Nerves and Blood Vessels of the Neck, Stage 4: Large Vessels

NOTE: 1)   the sternocleidomastoid and the superficial veins and nerves have been removed to expose the **carotid arteries, internal jugular vein, omohyoid muscle, vagus nerve,** and **ansa cervicalis.**

2)   superiorly, the facial vein has been cut and the submandibular gland has been elevated, thereby exposing the **hypoglossal nerve (XII).**

3)   nerve fibers, originating from C1 and travelling for a short distance with the hypoglossal nerve, leave that nerve to descend in the neck. They form the **superior root of the ansa cervicalis** and are joined by other descending fibers from C2 and C3 which are called the **inferior root of the ansa cervicalis.** The ansa cervicalis supplies motor innervation for a number of the strap muscles.

4)   the **common carotid artery, internal jugular vein,** and **vagus nerve.** These form a vertically oriented neurovascular bundle in the neck that is normally surrounded by the carotid sheath of deep fascia. The common carotid artery bifurcates at about the level of the hyoid bone to form the **external** and **internal carotid arteries.**

Fig. 701   **VII**

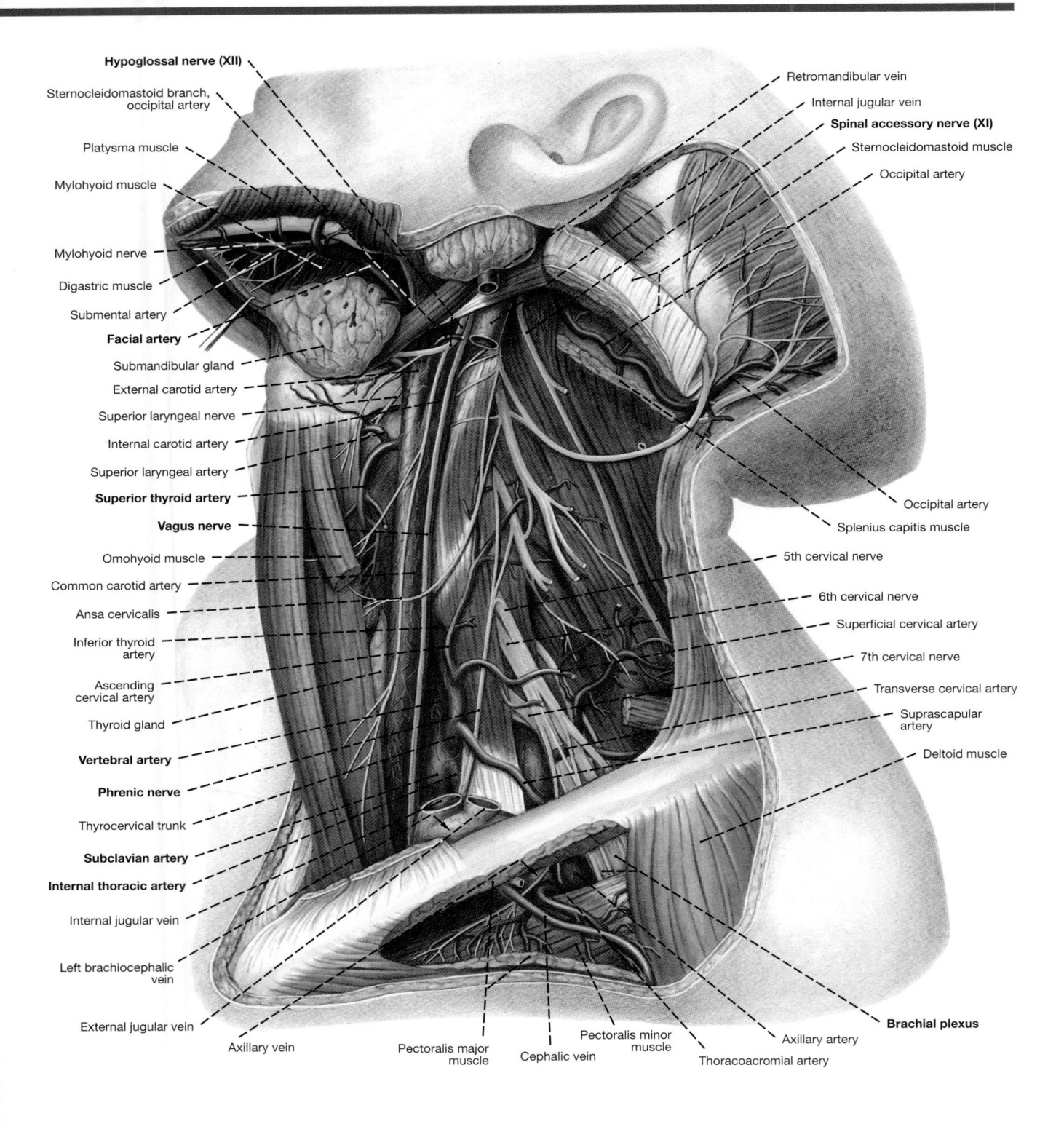

Hypoglossal nerve (XII)
Sternocleidomastoid branch, occipital artery
Platysma muscle
Mylohyoid muscle
Mylohyoid nerve
Digastric muscle
Submental artery
Facial artery
Submandibular gland
External carotid artery
Superior laryngeal nerve
Internal carotid artery
Superior laryngeal artery
Superior thyroid artery
Vagus nerve
Omohyoid muscle
Common carotid artery
Ansa cervicalis
Inferior thyroid artery
Ascending cervical artery
Thyroid gland
Vertebral artery
Phrenic nerve
Thyrocervical trunk
Subclavian artery
Internal thoracic artery
Internal jugular vein
Left brachiocephalic vein
External jugular vein

Retromandibular vein
Internal jugular vein
Spinal accessory nerve (XI)
Sternocleidomastoid muscle
Occipital artery
Occipital artery
Splenius capitis muscle
5th cervical nerve
6th cervical nerve
Superficial cervical artery
7th cervical nerve
Transverse cervical artery
Suprascapular artery
Deltoid muscle

Axillary vein
Pectoralis major muscle
Cephalic vein
Pectoralis minor muscle
Thoracoacromial artery
Axillary artery
Brachial plexus

Fig. 702: Nerves and Blood Vessels of the Neck, Stage 5: Subclavian Artery
NOTE: 1)   with the internal and external jugular veins removed, the subclavian artery is exposed as it ascends from the thorax and loops within the subclavian triangle of the neck to descend beneath the clavicle into the axilla. Observe its **vertebral, thyrocervical** and **internal thoracic** branches.

2)   the **transverse cervical artery** comes off separately from the subclavian in this dissection and it divides into an ascending (superficial) branch and a descending (deep) branch (neither of which are labelled in this figure).

3)   the **vagus nerve** coursing with the internal and common carotid arteries, and the **phrenic nerve** descending in the neck along the surface of the anterior scalene muscle.

4)   the **superior thyroid, facial** and **occipital** branches of the external carotid artery. The occipital artery courses posteriorly, deep to the sternocleidomastoid and splenius capitis muscles, and it becomes superficial on the posterior aspect of the scalp.

Fig. 702

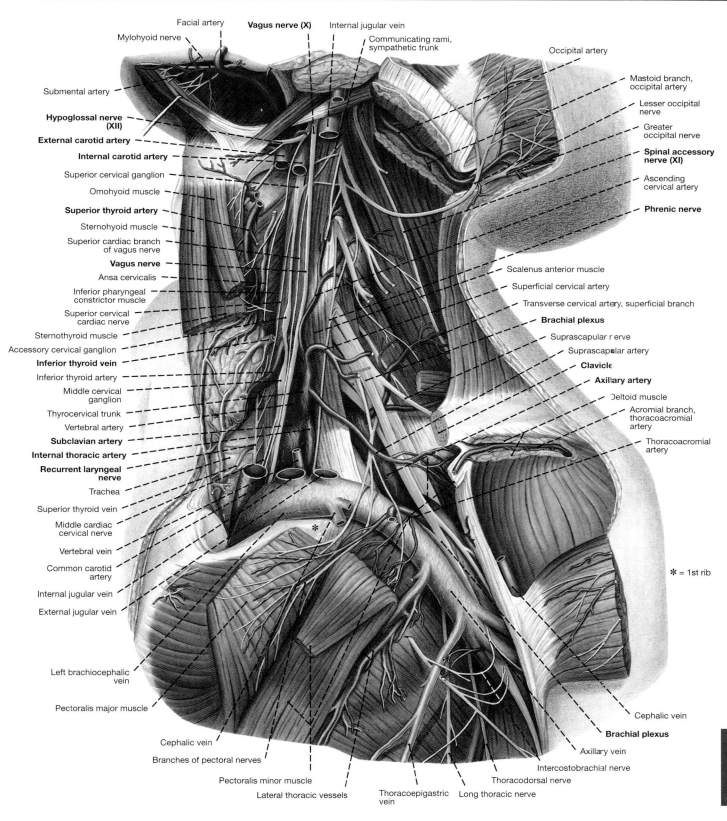

Fig. 703: Nerves and Blood Vessels of the Neck, Stage 6: Brachial Plexus

NOTE: 1)   with the carotid arteries, jugular veins and clavicle removed, the roots and trunks of the **brachial plexus** are exposed as they divide into cords that surround the axillary artery in the axilla.

2)   the **sympathetic trunk** lying deep to the carotid arteries and coursing with the **vagus nerve** and the superior cardiac branch of the vagus nerve.

3)   the **thyroid gland, superior** and **inferior thyroid arteries** and the **thyroid veins.** Note also the proximity of the **recurrent laryngeal nerve** to the thyroid gland.

Fig. 703   **VII**

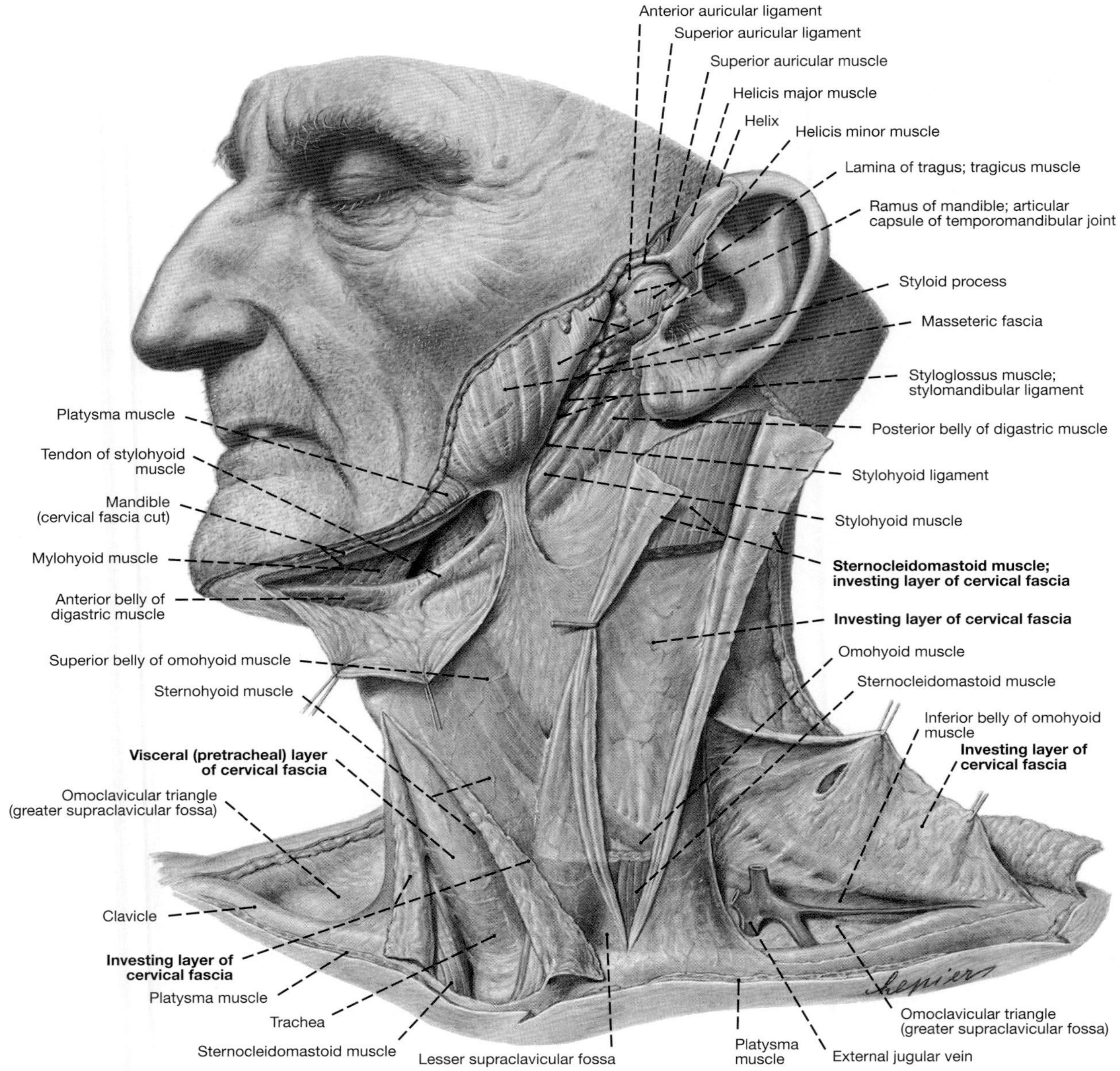

PLATE 446   The Neck: Cervical Fascial Layers

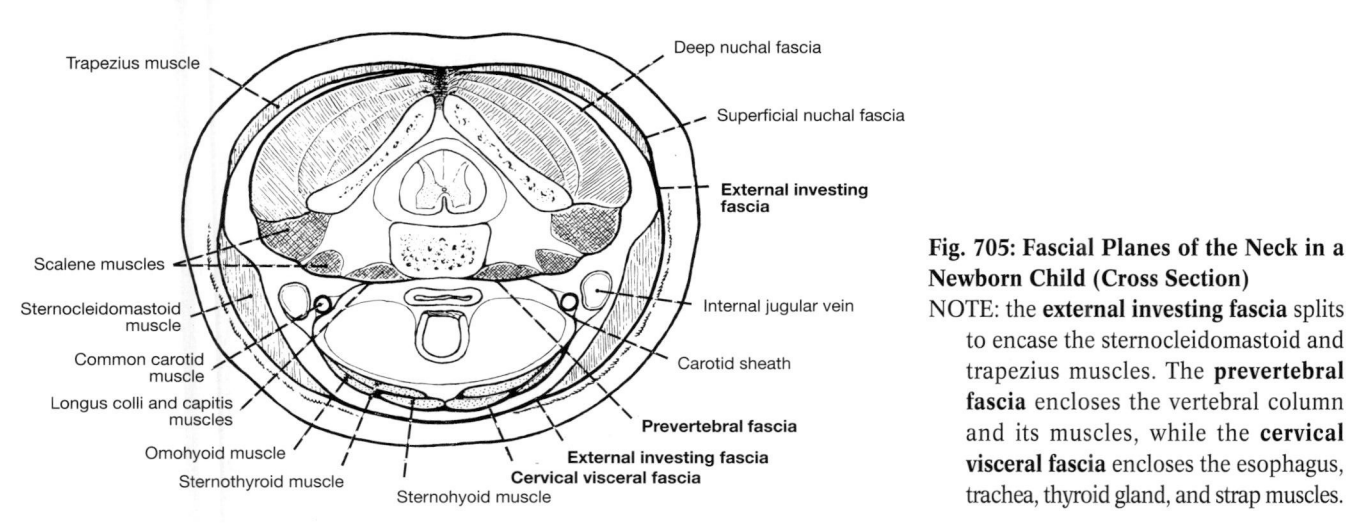

Anterior auricular ligament
Superior auricular ligament
Superior auricular muscle
Helicis major muscle
Helix   Helicis minor muscle
Lamina of tragus; tragicus muscle
Ramus of mandible; articular capsule of temporomandibular joint
Styloid process
Masseteric fascia
Styloglossus muscle; stylomandibular ligament
Posterior belly of digastric muscle
Stylohyoid ligament
Stylohyoid muscle
Sternocleidomastoid muscle; investing layer of cervical fascia
Investing layer of cervical fascia
Omohyoid muscle
Sternocleidomastoid muscle
Inferior belly of omohyoid muscle
Investing layer of cervical fascia
Omoclavicular triangle (greater supraclavicular fossa)
External jugular vein
Platysma muscle
Lesser supraclavicular fossa
Sternocleidomastoid muscle
Trachea
Platysma muscle
Investing layer of cervical fascia
Clavicle
Omoclavicular triangle (greater supraclavicular fossa)
Visceral (pretracheal) layer of cervical fascia
Sternohyoid muscle
Superior belly of omohyoid muscle
Anterior belly of digastric muscle
Mylohyoid muscle
Mandible (cervical fascia cut)
Tendon of stylohyoid muscle
Platysma muscle

Fig. 704: External Investing and Cervical Visceral (Pretracheal) Fascial Layers of the Neck
NOTE: the **external investing layer** of deep fascia is seen surrounding the sternocleidomastoid muscle, while the **cervical visceral layer** of deep fascia (also called **pretracheal layer**) is located deep to the investing layer enclosing the strap muscles.

Trapezius muscle
Deep nuchal fascia
Superficial nuchal fascia
External investing fascia
Internal jugular vein
Carotid sheath
Scalene muscles
Sternocleidomastoid muscle
Common carotid muscle
Longus colli and capitis muscles
Omohyoid muscle
Sternothyroid muscle
Sternohyoid muscle
Prevertebral fascia
External investing fascia
Cervical visceral fascia

Fig. 705: Fascial Planes of the Neck in a Newborn Child (Cross Section)
NOTE: the **external investing fascia** splits to encase the sternocleidomastoid and trapezius muscles. The **prevertebral fascia** encloses the vertebral column and its muscles, while the **cervical visceral fascia** encloses the esophagus, trachea, thyroid gland, and strap muscles.

Fig. 704, 705

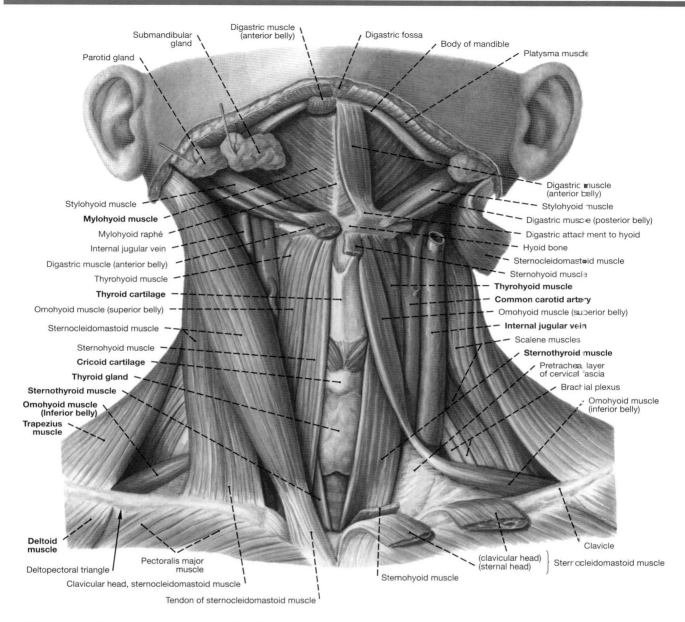

Parotid gland
Submandibular gland
Digastric muscle (anterior belly)
Digastric fossa
Body of mandible
Platysma muscle

Stylohyoid muscle
Mylohyoid muscle
Mylohyoid raphé
Internal jugular vein
Digastric muscle (anterior belly)
Thyrohyoid muscle
Thyroid cartilage
Omohyoid muscle (superior belly)
Sternocleidomastoid muscle
Sternohyoid muscle
Cricoid cartilage
Thyroid gland
Sternothyroid muscle
Omohyoid muscle (Inferior belly)
Trapezius muscle

Deltoid muscle
Deltopectoral triangle
Pectoralis major muscle
Clavicular head, sternocleidomastoid muscle
Tendon of sternocleidomastoid muscle

Digastric muscle (anterior belly)
Stylohyoid muscle
Digastric muscle (posterior belly)
Digastric attachment to hyoid
Hyoid bone
Sternocleidomastoid muscle
Sternohyoid muscle
Thyrohyoid muscle
Common carotid artery
Omohyoid muscle (superior belly)
Internal jugular vein
Scalene muscles
Sternothyroid muscle
Pretracheal layer of cervical fascia
Brachial plexus
Omohyoid muscle (inferior belly)

Clavicle
(clavicular head) (sternal head) } Sternocleidomastoid muscle
Sternohyoid muscle

Fig. 706: Anterior View of the Musculature of the Neck

NOTE: 1)   the right superior belly of the digastric muscle was removed and the submandibular gland elevated to show the mylohyoid muscle. On the left side (reader's right), the sternocleidomastoid and sternohyoid muscles have been transected and the submandibular gland removed.

2)   the relationship of the strap muscles to the thyroid gland and realize that below the thyroid gland and above the suprasternal notch, the trachea lies immediately under the skin.

Muscle	Origin	Insertion	Innervation	Action
Sternocleidomastoid Muscle	**STERNAL HEAD** Upper part of the ventral surface of the manubrium of the sternum **CLAVICULAR HEAD** Upper border and anterior surface of the medial ⅓rd of the clavicle	Lateral surface of the mastoid process and the lateral half of the superior nuchal line	*Motor fibers:* Accessory nerve *Sensory fibers:* Anterior rami of C2 and C3 nerves	*When one side acts:* Bends the head laterally toward the shoulder of the same side; rotates the head, turning the face upward, directing it to the opposite side *When both sides act:* Flexes the head and neck

Fig. 706   **VII**

PLATE 448   Anterior (Strap) Muscles of the Neck; Muscle Chart

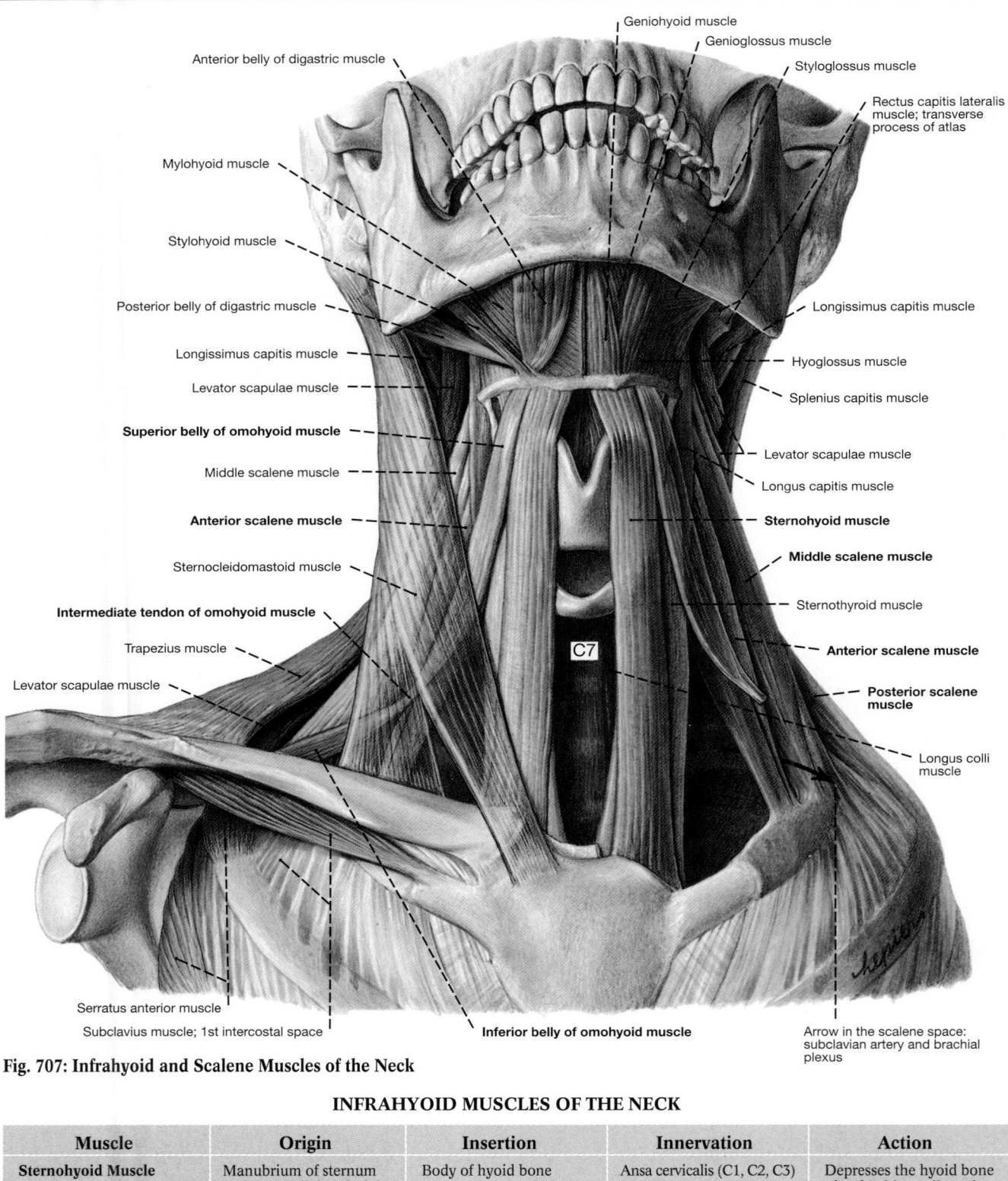

Geniohyoid muscle

Genioglossus muscle

Anterior belly of digastric muscle

Styloglossus muscle

Rectus capitis lateralis muscle; transverse process of atlas

Mylohyoid muscle

Stylohyoid muscle

Posterior belly of digastric muscle

Longissimus capitis muscle

Longissimus capitis muscle

Hyoglossus muscle

Levator scapulae muscle

Splenius capitis muscle

Superior belly of omohyoid muscle

Levator scapulae muscle

Middle scalene muscle

Longus capitis muscle

Anterior scalene muscle

Sternohyoid muscle

Sternocleidomastoid muscle

Middle scalene muscle

Intermediate tendon of omohyoid muscle

Sternothyroid muscle

Trapezius muscle

Anterior scalene muscle

Levator scapulae muscle

Posterior scalene muscle

C7

Longus colli muscle

Serratus anterior muscle

Subclavius muscle; 1st intercostal space

Inferior belly of omohyoid muscle

Arrow in the scalene space: subclavian artery and brachial plexus

Fig. 707: Infrahyoid and Scalene Muscles of the Neck

INFRAHYOID MUSCLES OF THE NECK

Muscle	Origin	Insertion	Innervation	Action
Sternohyoid Muscle	Manubrium of sternum and the medial end of the clavicle	Body of hyoid bone	Ansa cervicalis (C1, C2, C3)	Depresses the hyoid bone after food is swallowed
Sternothyroid Muscle	Posterior surface of the manubrium of the sternum	Oblique line on the lamina of the thyroid cartilage	Ansa cervicalis (C1, C2, C3)	Depresses the hyoid bone and the larynx
Thyrohyoid Muscle	Oblique line on the lamina of the thyroid cartilage	Lower border of the greater horn of the hyoid bone	Fibers from the C1 spinal nerve that course for a short distance with XII	Depresses the hyoid bone or elevates the larynx
Omohyoid Muscle	Upper border of the scapula near the suprascapular notch	Lower border of the body of the hyoid bone	Ansa cervicalis (C1, C2, C3)	Depresses and helps stabilize the hyoid bone

Fig. 707

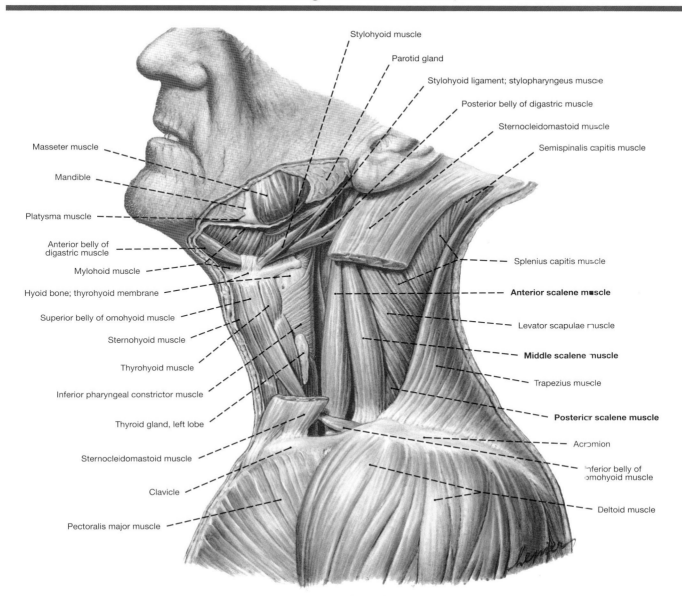

Stylohyoid muscle

Parotid gland

Stylohyoid ligament; stylopharyngeus muscle

Posterior belly of digastric muscle

Sternocleidomastoid muscle

Semispinalis capitis muscle

Masseter muscle

Mandible

Platysma muscle

Anterior belly of digastric muscle

Mylohoid muscle

Hyoid bone; thyrohyoid membrane

Superior belly of omohyoid muscle

Sternohyoid muscle

Thyrohyoid muscle

Inferior pharyngeal constrictor muscle

Thyroid gland, left lobe

Sternocleidomastoid muscle

Clavicle

Pectoralis major muscle

Splenius capitis muscle

Anterior scalene muscle

Levator scapulae muscle

Middle scalene muscle

Trapezius muscle

Posterior scalene muscle

Acromion

Inferior belly of omohyoid muscle

Deltoid muscle

Fig. 708: Muscular Floor of the Posterior Triangle of the Neck and the Scalene Muscles

MUSCLES OF THE POSTERIOR TRIANGLE OF THE NECK

LEVATOR SCAPULAE described on PLATE 410
SEMISPINALIS CAPITIS described on PLATE 413

Muscle	Origin	Insertion	Innervation	Action
Anterior Scalene Muscle	By four tendons, each one from the transverse processes of the 3rd, 4th, 5th and 6th cervical vertebrae	Onto the scalene tubercle of the 1st rib	Anterior rami of the (4th), 5th and 6th cervical spinal nerves	*When neck is fixed:* elevates the 1st rib *When 1st rib is fixed:* bends neck forward and laterally, and rotates it to the opposite side
Middle Scalene Muscle	Transverse processes of C2 to C7 vertebrae (often also from the atlas)	Superior surface of 1st rib between the tubercle and groove for subclavian artery	Anterior rami of the 3rd through the 8th cervical nerves	Same as anterior scalene muscle
Posterior Scalene Muscle	Transverse processes of 4th, 5th and 6th cervical vertebrae	Outer surface of the 2nd rib	Anterior rami of the C6, C7 and C8 spinal nerves	Raises the 2nd rib; or, bends and rotates the neck
Splenius Capitis Muscle	Caudal half of the ligamentum nuchae; spinous processes of C7, and upper 4 thoracic vertebrae	Lateral 1/3 rd of the superior nuchal line and onto the mastoid process of the temporal bone	Dorsal rami of the middle cervical spinal nerves	Laterally flexes head; rotates head and neck to same side; when both muscles act they extend head and neck

Fig. 708   **VII**

PLATE 450   **The Neck: Jugular System of Veins**

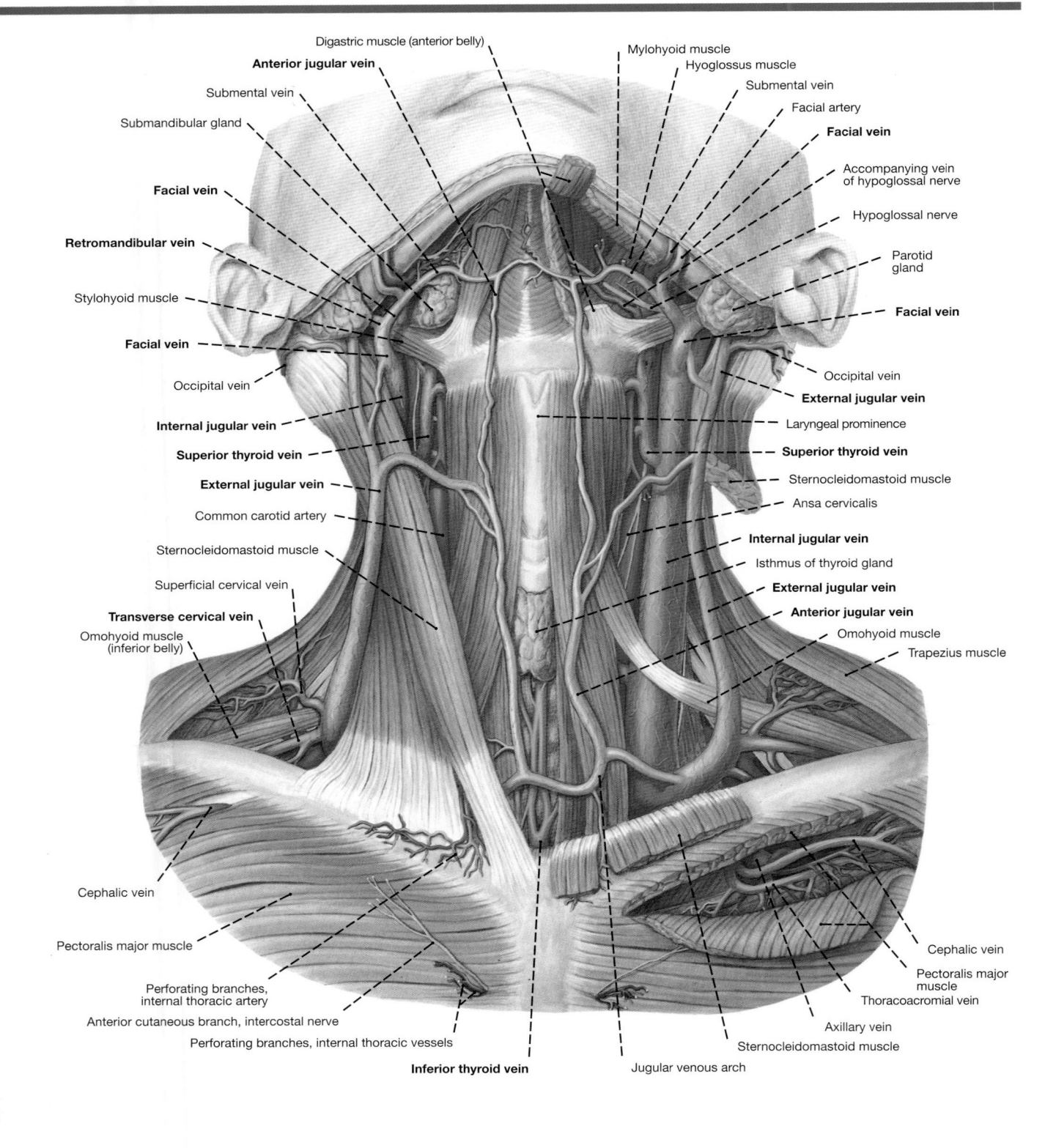

Fig. 709: Veins of the Neck and Infraclavicular Region

NOTE: 1) the **jugular system of veins** consists of anterior, external and internal jugular veins, all shown on the left side where the sternocleidomastoid muscle was removed.

2) the **anterior jugular** descends close to the midline, is frequently small and drains laterally into the external jugular. The **external jugular** courses along the surface of the sternocleidomastoid muscle. It forms within the parotid gland and enlarges because of its occipital, retromandibular and facial tributaries. The external jugular flows into the subclavian vein after it receives tributaries from the scapular and clavicular regions.

3) the **internal jugular** is large and collects blood from the brain, face and neck. At its junction with the subclavian, the **brachiocephalic vein** is formed.

Fig. 709

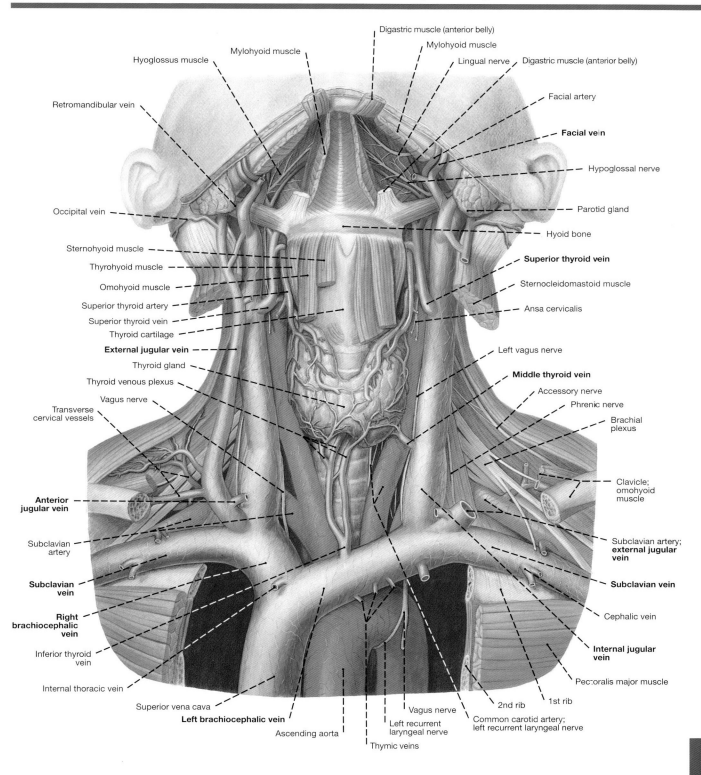

Digastric muscle (anterior belly)
Mylohyoid muscle
Mylohyoid muscle
Hyoglossus muscle
Lingual nerve
Digastric muscle (anterior belly)
Facial artery
Retromandibular vein
Facial vein
Hypoglossal nerve
Occipital vein
Parotid gland
Hyoid bone
Sternohyoid muscle
Superior thyroid vein
Thyrohyoid muscle
Sternocleidomastoid muscle
Omohyoid muscle
Ansa cervicalis
Superior thyroid artery
Superior thyroid vein
Thyroid cartilage
Left vagus nerve
External jugular vein
Thyroid gland
Middle thyroid vein
Thyroid venous plexus
Accessory nerve
Vagus nerve
Phrenic nerve
Transverse cervical vessels
Brachial plexus
Clavicle; omohyoid muscle
Anterior jugular vein
Subclavian artery; **external jugular vein**
Subclavian artery
Subclavian vein
Subclavian vein
Cephalic vein
Right brachiocephalic vein
Internal jugular vein
Inferior thyroid vein
Pectoralis major muscle
Internal thoracic vein
Superior vena cava
2nd rib
1st rib
Left brachiocephalic vein
Vagus nerve
Common carotid artery; left recurrent laryngeal nerve
Ascending aorta
Left recurrent laryngeal nerve
Thymic veins

Fig. 710: Deep Arteries and Veins of the Neck and Great Vessels of the Thorax

NOTE: 1) the sternocleidomastoid and strap muscles have been removed from the neck, thereby exposing the carotid arteries, internal jugular veins, and thyroid gland.

2) the middle portion of the anterior thoracic wall has been resected to show the aortic arch and its branches, the brachiocephalic veins and their tributaries, the superior vena cava and the vagus nerves.

3) in the submandibular region, the mylohyoid and anterior digastric muscles have been cut, revealing the lingual and hypoglossal nerves.

Fig. 710   **VII**

PLATE 452   The Neck: Deep Vessels and Nerves; Thyroid Gland

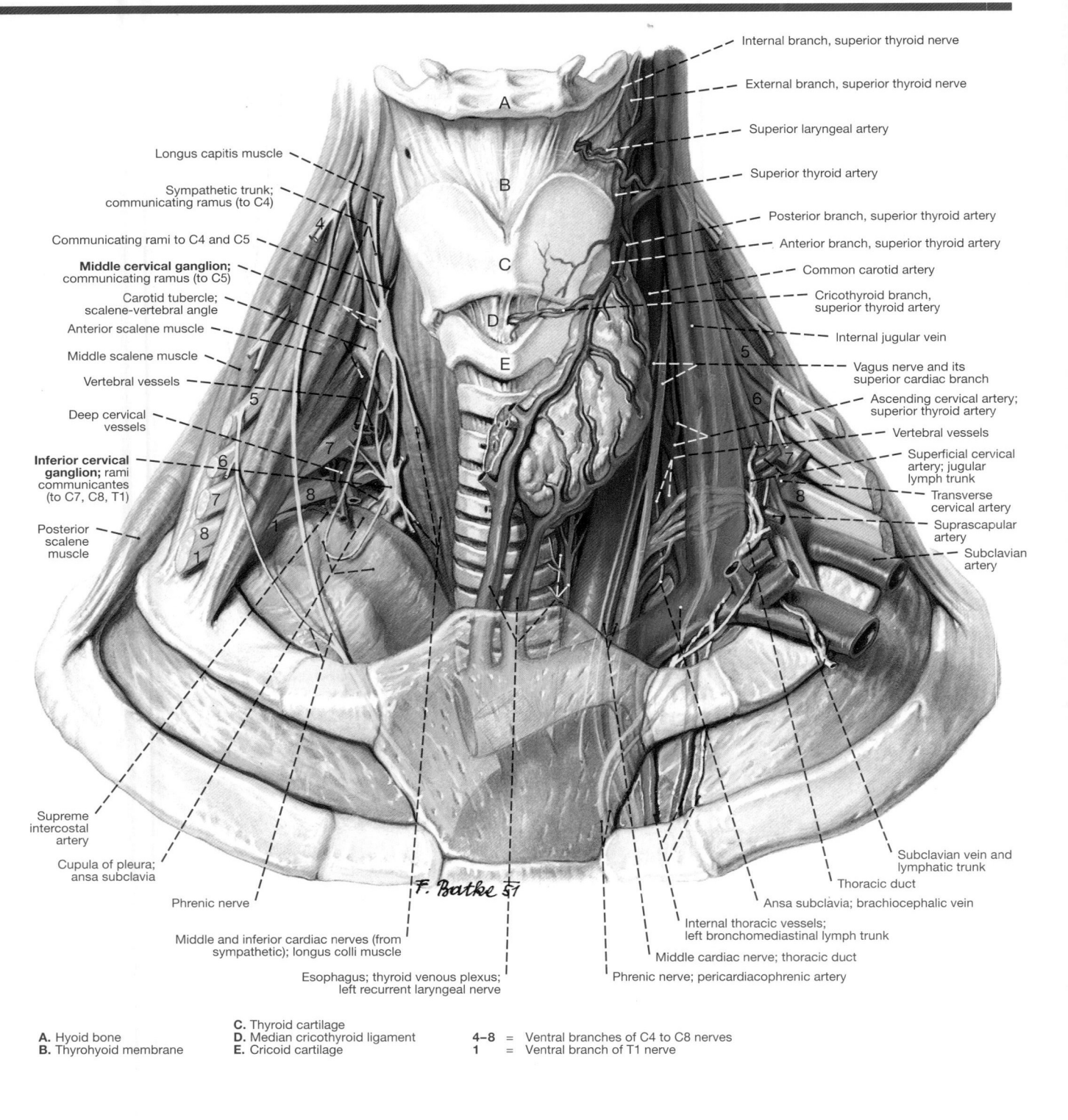

Internal branch, superior thyroid nerve

External branch, superior thyroid nerve

Superior laryngeal artery

Superior thyroid artery

Posterior branch, superior thyroid artery

Anterior branch, superior thyroid artery

Common carotid artery

Cricothyroid branch, superior thyroid artery

Internal jugular vein

Vagus nerve and its superior cardiac branch

Ascending cervical artery; superior thyroid artery

Vertebral vessels

Superficial cervical artery; jugular lymph trunk

Transverse cervical artery

Suprascapular artery

Subclavian artery

Longus capitis muscle

Sympathetic trunk; communicating ramus (to C4)

Communicating rami to C4 and C5

Middle cervical ganglion; communicating ramus (to C5)

Carotid tubercle; scalene-vertebral angle

Anterior scalene muscle

Middle scalene muscle

Vertebral vessels

Deep cervical vessels

Inferior cervical ganglion; rami communicantes (to C7, C8, T1)

Posterior scalene muscle

Supreme intercostal artery

Cupula of pleura; ansa subclavia

Phrenic nerve

Middle and inferior cardiac nerves (from sympathetic); longus colli muscle

Esophagus; thyroid venous plexus; left recurrent laryngeal nerve

Subclavian vein and lymphatic trunk

Thoracic duct

Ansa subclavia; brachiocephalic vein

Internal thoracic vessels; left bronchomediastinal lymph trunk

Middle cardiac nerve; thoracic duct

Phrenic nerve; pericardiacophrenic artery

F. Batke 51

A. Hyoid bone
B. Thyrohyoid membrane

C. Thyroid cartilage
D. Median cricothyroid ligament
E. Cricoid cartilage

4–8 = Ventral branches of C4 to C8 nerves
1   = Ventral branch of T1 nerve

Fig. 711: Vessels, Nerves and Viscera of the Anterior and Posterior Cervical Regions
NOTE: 1) the sternocleidomastoid and strap muscles have been removed. **On the right side** (reader's left), the large vessels, vagus nerve and right lobe of the thyroid gland have been resected to reveal the scalene muscles, the roots of the brachial plexus, the inferior and middle cervical ganglia and cupula of the right pleura.

2) **on the left side,** the course of the vagus nerve and its recurrent laryngeal branch. Observe also the thoracic duct as it ascends into the root of the neck to open into the venous system at the junction of the left internal jugular and subclavian veins.

3) the course of the phrenic nerves. They are derived from the 3rd, 4th and 5th cervical nerves, lie along the ventral surface of the anterior scalene muscle and enter the thorax deep to the sternocostal joint of the first rib.

4) the cupula of the pleura over the apex of each lung. These project 3 to 5 cm above the sternal angle of the 1st rib and are unprotected by bone.

Fig. 711

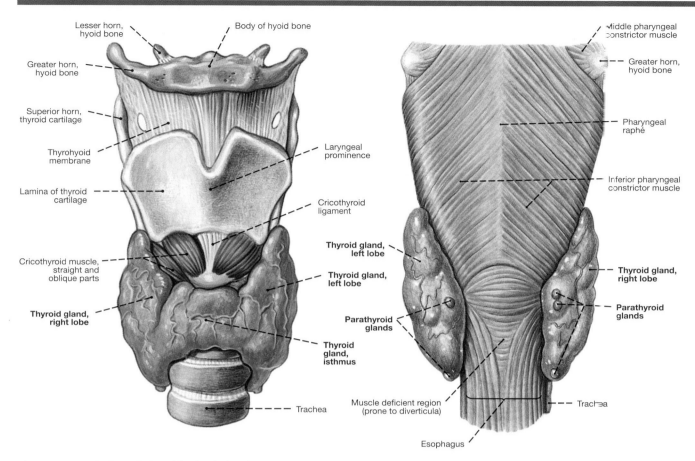

Fig. 712: Ventral View of Thyroid Gland Showing Relation to Larynx and Trachea

Fig. 713: Dorsal View of Thyroid Gland Showing Relation to Pharynx and Parathyroids

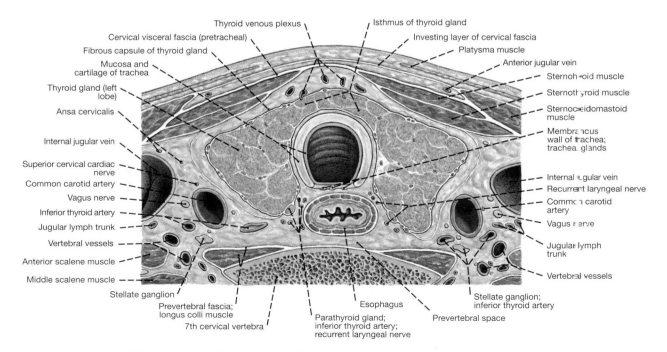

Fig. 714: Cross-section of the Anterior Neck at the Level of the C7 Vertebra

NOTE: the relationship of the isthmus and lobes of the thyroid gland to the trachea. Also observe the location of the parathyroid glands, the recurrent laryngeal nerves and the inferior thyroid arteries along the posteromedial border of the thyroid gland.

PLATE 454   The Neck: Thyroid Gland, Vessels and Adjacent Deep Nerves

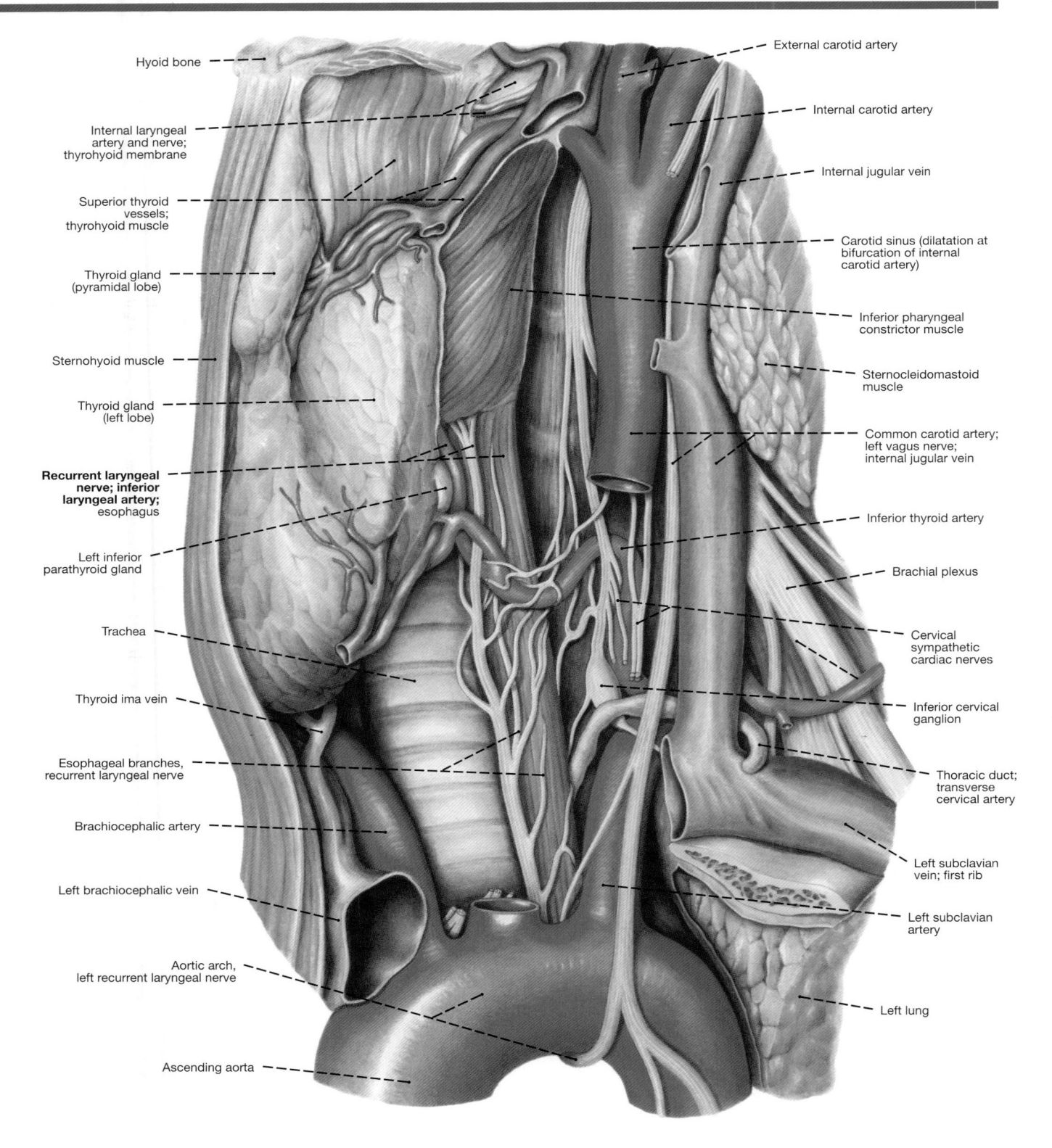

Hyoid bone

Internal laryngeal artery and nerve; thyrohyoid membrane

Superior thyroid vessels; thyrohyoid muscle

Thyroid gland (pyramidal lobe)

Sternohyoid muscle

Thyroid gland (left lobe)

Recurrent laryngeal nerve; inferior laryngeal artery; esophagus

Left inferior parathyroid gland

Trachea

Thyroid ima vein

Esophageal branches, recurrent laryngeal nerve

Brachiocephalic artery

Left brachiocephalic vein

Aortic arch, left recurrent laryngeal nerve

Ascending aorta

External carotid artery

Internal carotid artery

Internal jugular vein

Carotid sinus (dilatation at bifurcation of internal carotid artery)

Inferior pharyngeal constrictor muscle

Sternocleidomastoid muscle

Common carotid artery; left vagus nerve; internal jugular vein

Inferior thyroid artery

Brachial plexus

Cervical sympathetic cardiac nerves

Inferior cervical ganglion

Thoracic duct; transverse cervical artery

Left subclavian vein; first rib

Left subclavian artery

Left lung

Fig. 715: Nerves and Vessels in the Deep Part of the Lower Neck; Relation of Thyroid Gland to Cervical Vessels and Nerves
NOTE: 1)   this anterolateral view of the **left side** of the lower neck shows the lateral aspect of the left lobe of the thyroid gland and the vessels entering and leaving the gland. These are the superior and inferior thyroid arteries and veins and the thyroid ima vein. Observe a parathyroid gland located behind the thyroid adjacent to the inferior thyroid vessels.

2)   the left vagus nerve with its recurrent laryngeal branch exposed. Obseve the surgically important relationship between the two terminal branches of the inferior thyroid artery and the recurrent laryngeal nerve. This nerve courses between these two branches (as shown here) about 33% of the time. The nerve ascends deep to these vessels about 55% of dee time and superficial to the vessels about 11% of the time (from Hollinshead WH. Surg Clin North Amer 32: 1115, 1952).

Fig. 715

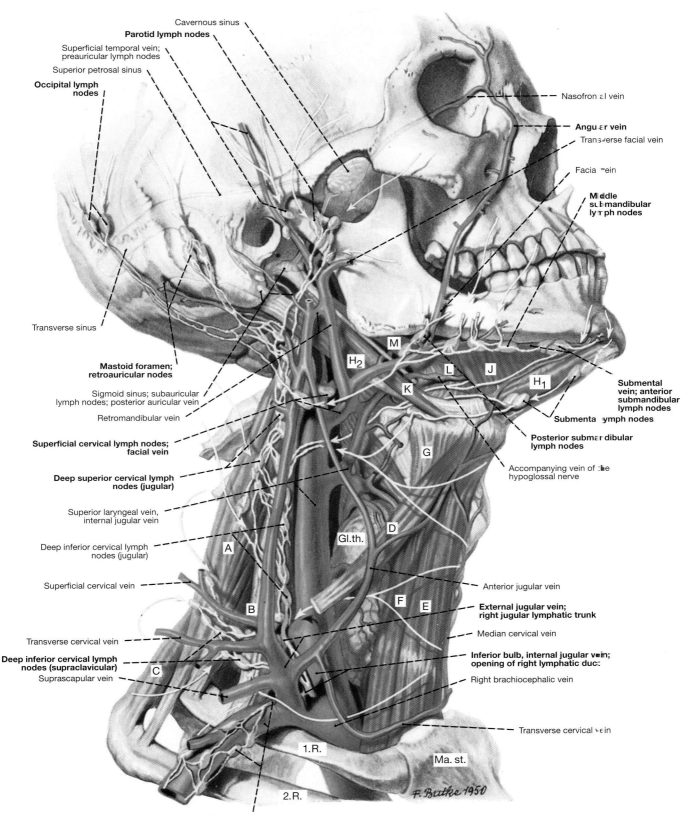

Cavernous sinus

Parotid lymph nodes

Superficial temporal vein;
preauricular lymph nodes

Superior petrosal sinus

Occipital lymph nodes

Transverse sinus

**Mastoid foramen;
retroauricular nodes**

Sigmoid sinus; subauricular
lymph nodes; posterior auricular vein

Retromandibular vein

**Superficial cervical lymph nodes;
facial vein**

**Deep superior cervical lymph
nodes (jugular)**

Superior laryngeal vein,
internal jugular vein

Deep inferior cervical lymph
nodes (jugular)

Superficial cervical vein

Transverse cervical vein

**Deep inferior cervical lymph
nodes (supraclavicular)**

Suprascapular vein

Nasofrontal vein

Angular vein

Transverse facial vein

Facial vein

**Middle
submandibular
lymph nodes**

**Submental
vein; anterior
submandibular
lymph nodes**

Submental lymph nodes

**Posterior submandibular
lymph nodes**

Accompanying vein of the
hypoglossal nerve

Anterior jugular vein

**External jugular vein;
right jugular lymphatic trunk**

Median cervical vein

**Inferior bulb, internal jugular vein;
opening of right lymphatic duct**

Right brachiocephalic vein

Transverse cervical vein

1. R.

Ma. st.

2. R.

F. Batke 1950

Subclavian lymphatic trunk; subclavian vein; apical lymph nodes

Fig. 716: Lymph Nodes, Lymphatic Channels and Veins of the Face, Lower Head and Neck (Right Lateral View)
NOTE: superficial lymph channels of the face and temporal and occipital regions drain downward and backward to cervical nodes
along the internal jugular vein. These in turn drain into the jugular lymphatic trunk which enters the brachiocephalic vein.

A = Middle scalene muscle
B = Anterior scalene muscle
C = Posterior scalene muscle
D = Omohyoid muscle

E = Sternohyoid muscle
F = Sternothyroid muscle
G = Thyrohyoid muscle
Gl. th. = Thyroid gland

H_1 = Digastric muscle (anterior belly)
H_2 = Digastric muscle (posterior belly)
J = Mylohyoid muscle
K = Stylohyoid muscle

L = Hyoglossus muscle
M = Styloglossus muscle
Ma. st. = Manubrium sterni
1., 2. R. = 1st and 2nd ribs

Fig. 716   **VII**

PLATE 456   The Neck: Anterior Vertebral Muscles

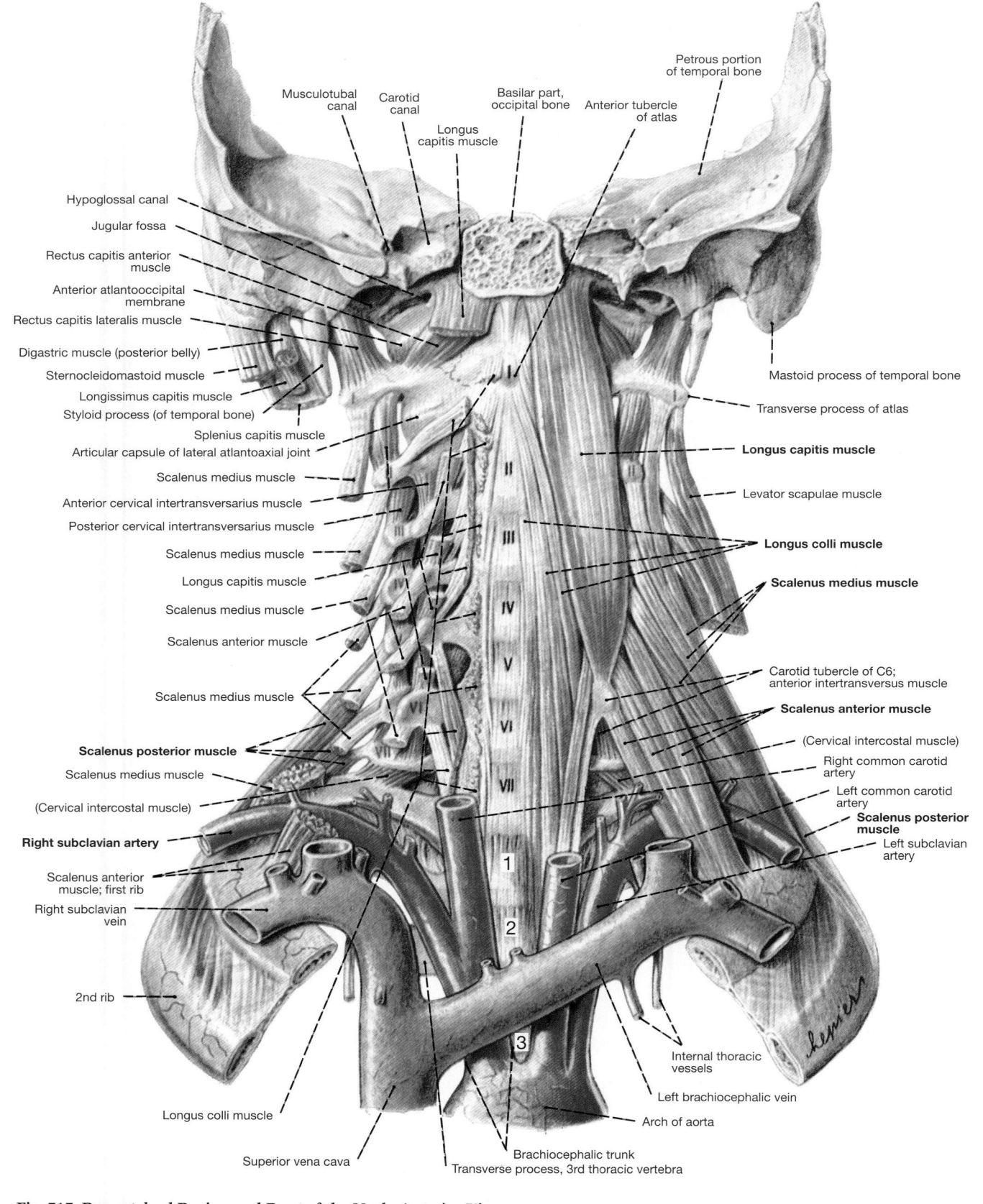

Musculotubal canal

Carotid canal

Longus capitis muscle

Basilar part, occipital bone

Anterior tubercle of atlas

Petrous portion of temporal bone

Anterior tubercle of atlas

Hypoglossal canal

Jugular fossa

Rectus capitis anterior muscle

Anterior atlantooccipital membrane

Rectus capitis lateralis muscle

Digastric muscle (posterior belly)

Sternocleidomastoid muscle

Longissimus capitis muscle

Styloid process (of temporal bone)

Splenius capitis muscle

Articular capsule of lateral atlantoaxial joint

Scalenus medius muscle

Anterior cervical intertransversarius muscle

Posterior cervical intertransversarius muscle

Scalenus medius muscle

Longus capitis muscle

Scalenus medius muscle

Scalenus anterior muscle

Scalenus medius muscle

Scalenus posterior muscle

Scalenus medius muscle

(Cervical intercostal muscle)

Right subclavian artery

Scalenus anterior muscle; first rib

Right subclavian vein

2nd rib

Longus colli muscle

Superior vena cava

Mastoid process of temporal bone

Transverse process of atlas

Longus capitis muscle

Levator scapulae muscle

Longus colli muscle

Scalenus medius muscle

Carotid tubercle of C6; anterior intertransversus muscle

Scalenus anterior muscle

(Cervical intercostal muscle)

Right common carotid artery

Left common carotid artery

Scalenus posterior muscle

Left subclavian artery

Internal thoracic vessels

Left brachiocephalic vein

Arch of aorta

Brachiocephalic trunk

Transverse process, 3rd thoracic vertebra

Fig. 717: Prevertebral Region and Root of the Neck, Anterior View

NOTE: 1)   on the specimen's right, the longus colli, longus capitis and the scalene muscles have been removed, exposing the transverse processes of the cervical vertebrae onto which these muscles are seen to attach.

2)   there are two long (longus colli and longus capitis) and two short (rectus capitis anterior and lateralis) prevertebral muscles. These flex the head and neck forward and bend the head and neck laterally.

Fig. 717

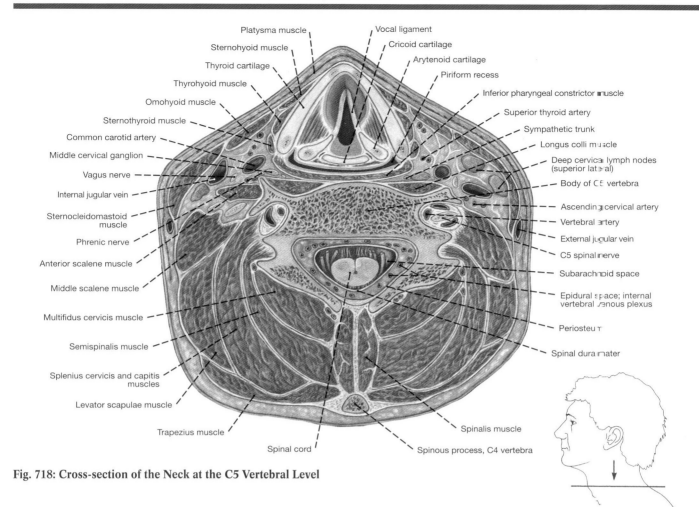

Platysma muscle
Sternohyoid muscle
Thyroid cartilage
Thyrohyoid muscle
Omohyoid muscle
Sternothyroid muscle
Common carotid artery
Middle cervical ganglion
Vagus nerve
Internal jugular vein
Sternocleidomastoid muscle
Phrenic nerve
Anterior scalene muscle
Middle scalene muscle
Multifidus cervicis muscle
Semispinalis muscle
Splenius cervicis and capitis muscles
Levator scapulae muscle
Trapezius muscle
Spinal cord

Vocal ligament
Cricoid cartilage
Arytenoid cartilage
Piriform recess
Inferior pharyngeal constrictor muscle
Superior thyroid artery
Sympathetic trunk
Longus colli muscle
Deep cervical lymph nodes (superior lateral)
Body of C5 vertebra
Ascending cervical artery
Vertebral artery
External jugular vein
C5 spinal nerve
Subarachnoid space
Epidural space; internal vertebral venous plexus
Periosteum
Spinal dura mater
Spinalis muscle
Spinous process, C4 vertebra

Fig. 718: Cross-section of the Neck at the C5 Vertebral Level

ANTERIOR VERTEBRAL MUSCLES

Muscle	Origin	Insertion	Innervation	Action
Longus Colli Muscle	**SUPERIOR OBLIQUE PART** Anterior tubercles of transverse processes of 3rd, 4th and 5th cervical vertebrae	Tubercle of the anterior arch of the atlas	Ventral rami of the C2 to C6 spinal nerves	Weak flexor of the neck; slightly rotates and bends neck laterally
	INFERIOR OBLIQUE PART Anterior surface of the bodies of the first two or three thoracic vertebrae	Anterior tubercles of the transverse processes of the 5th and 6th cervical vertebrae		
	VERTICAL PART Anterolateral surfaces of the last 3 cervical and upper 3 thoracic vertebrae	Anterior surfaces of the bodies of 2nd, 3rd and 4th cervical vertebrae		
Longus Capitis Muscle	By tendinous slips from the transverse processes of the 3rd, 4th, 5th and 6th cervical vertebrae	Inferior surface of the basilar part of the occipital bone	Branches from the anterior rami of C1, C2 and C3 nerves	Flexes the head and the upper cervical spine
Rectus Capitis Anterior	Anterior surface of the lateral mass of the atlas and its transverse process	Inferior surface of the basilar part of the occipital bone	Fibers from the anterior rami of C1 and C2	Flexes the head and helps stabilize the atlantooccipital joint
Rectus Capitis Lateralis	Superior surface of the transverse process of the atlas	Inferior surface of the jugular process of the occipital bone	Anterior rami of the C1 and C2 nerves	Bends the head laterally to the same side

Fig. 718   **VII**

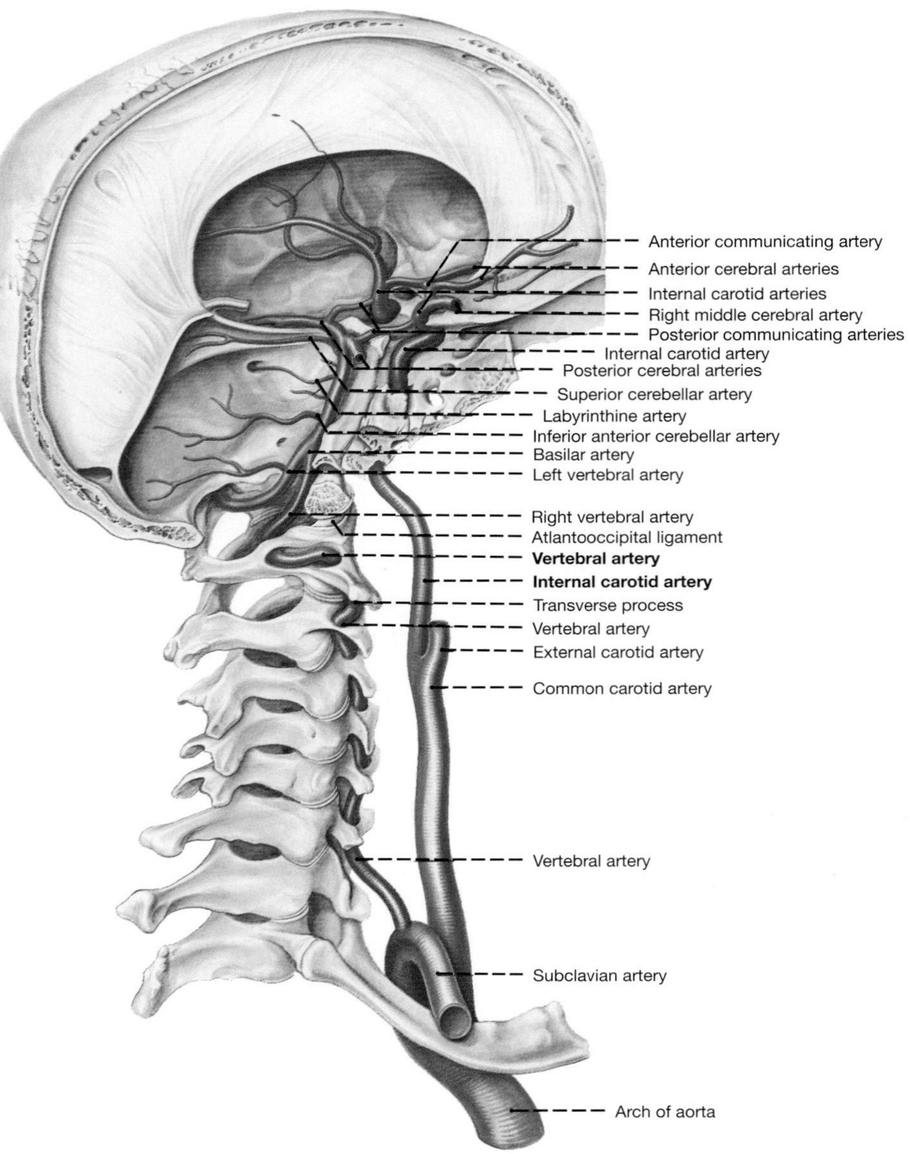

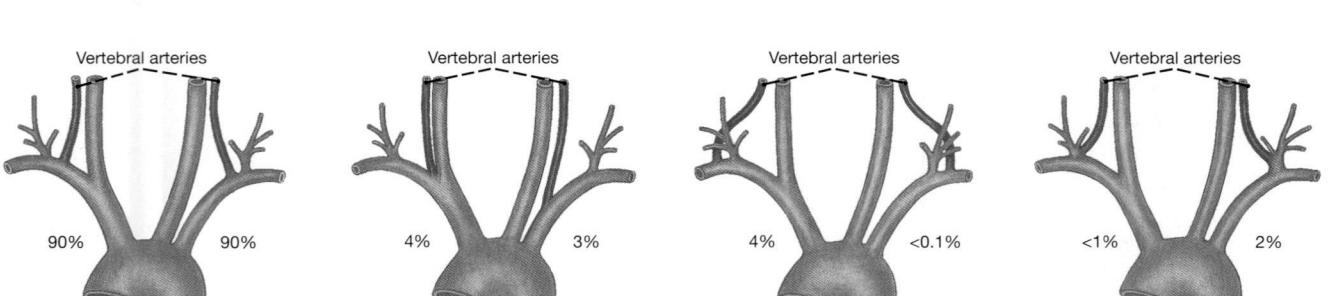

Anterior communicating artery
Anterior cerebral arteries
Internal carotid arteries
Right middle cerebral artery
Posterior communicating arteries
Internal carotid artery
Posterior cerebral arteries
Superior cerebellar artery
Labyrinthine artery
Inferior anterior cerebellar artery
Basilar artery
Left vertebral artery

Right vertebral artery
Atlantooccipital ligament
Vertebral artery
Internal carotid artery
Transverse process
Vertebral artery
External carotid artery
Common carotid artery

Vertebral artery

Subclavian artery

Arch of aorta

Fig. 719: Vertebral and Internal Carotid Arteries

NOTE: 1)   both the internal carotid and vertebral arteries ascend in the neck to enter the cranial cavity to supply blood to the brain. Although the vertebral arteries give off some spinal and muscular branches in the neck prior to entering the skull, the internal carotid arteries do not have branches in the neck.

2)   the origin of the **vertebral artery** from the subclavian, and its ascent in the neck through the foramina in the transverse processes of the cervical vertebrae.

3)   the two vertebral arteries join to form the **basilar artery.** This vessel courses along the ventral aspect of the brainstem.

4)   the **internal carotid artery** begins at the bifurcation of the common carotid, and ascends to its entrance in the carotid canal in the petrous part of the temporal bone. After a somewhat tortuous course, it enters the cranial cavity.

Vertebral arteries	Vertebral arteries	Vertebral arteries	Vertebral arteries
90% 90%	4% 3%	4% <0.1%	<1% 2%
a	b	c	d

Fig. 720: Variations (and Percentages) in the Origin of the Vertebral Arteries

Figs. 719, 720

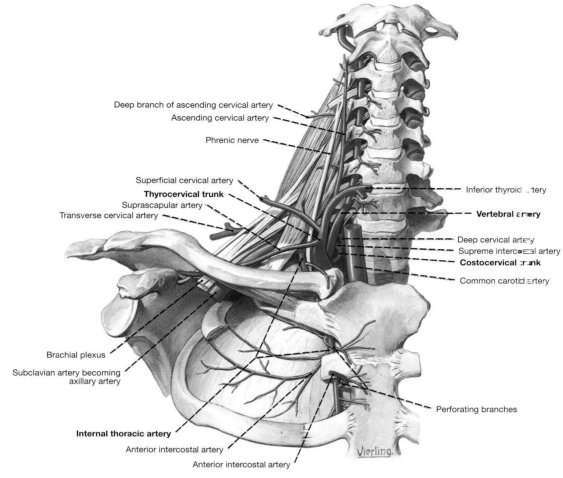

Fig. 721: Right Subclavian Artery and Its Branches

NOTE: 1) the right subclavian artery arises from the brachiocephalic trunk, although on the left it branches from the aorta. It ascends into the root of the neck, arches laterally and then descends between the 1st rib and clavicle to become the axillary artery.

2) the subclavian artery generally has four major branches and sometimes five. These are the **vertebral artery,** the **internal thoracic artery,** the **thyrocervical trunk,** and the **costocervical trunk.**

3) in about 40% of bodies, there is also a **transverse cervical artery** arising directly from the subclavian. Thus, in this region there is considerable variation in the origin of vessels such as the suprascapular artery, the transverse cervical artery and this latter vessel's superficial and deep branches, the superficial cervical artery and the descending scapular artery (for a complete description of these vessels see: Clemente CD, Editor. Gray's Anatomy of the Human Body, 30th Ed. Phila, Lea & Febiger, 1985; 703–709).

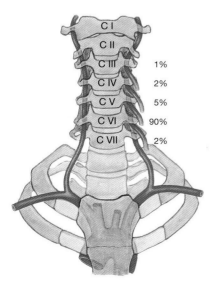

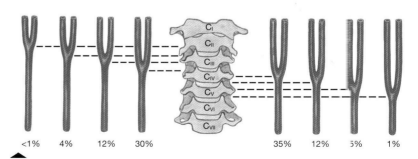

Fig. 722: Variations in the Vertebral Level at Which the Common Carotid Artery Divides

◀ Fig. 723: Variations in the Level of Entry of the Vertebral Artery Into the Transverse Foramina of Cervical Vertebrae

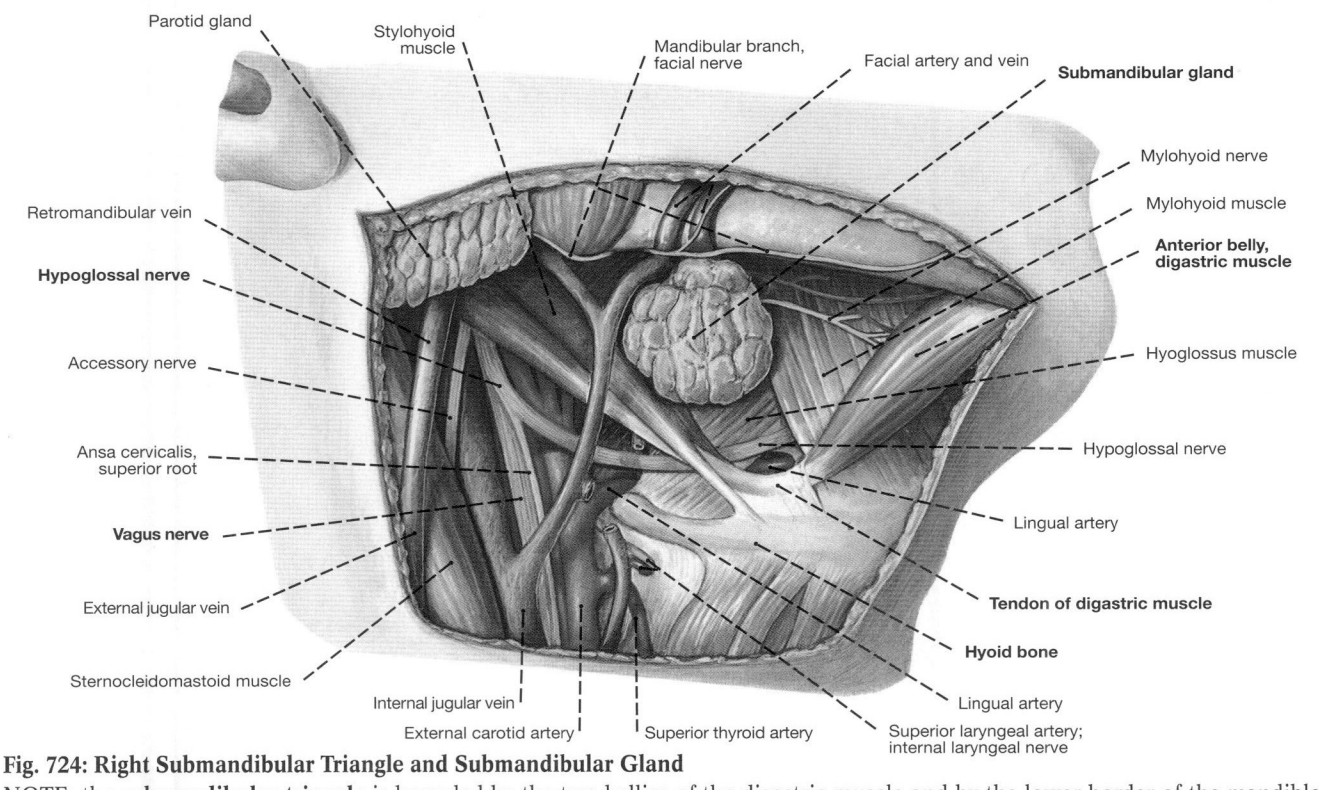

Fig. 724: Right Submandibular Triangle and Submandibular Gland
NOTE: the **submandibular triangle** is bounded by the two bellies of the digastric muscle and by the lower border of the mandible. The floor of the triangle is formed by the mylohyoid and hyoglossus muscles, between which the **hypoglossal nerve** enters the oral cavity.

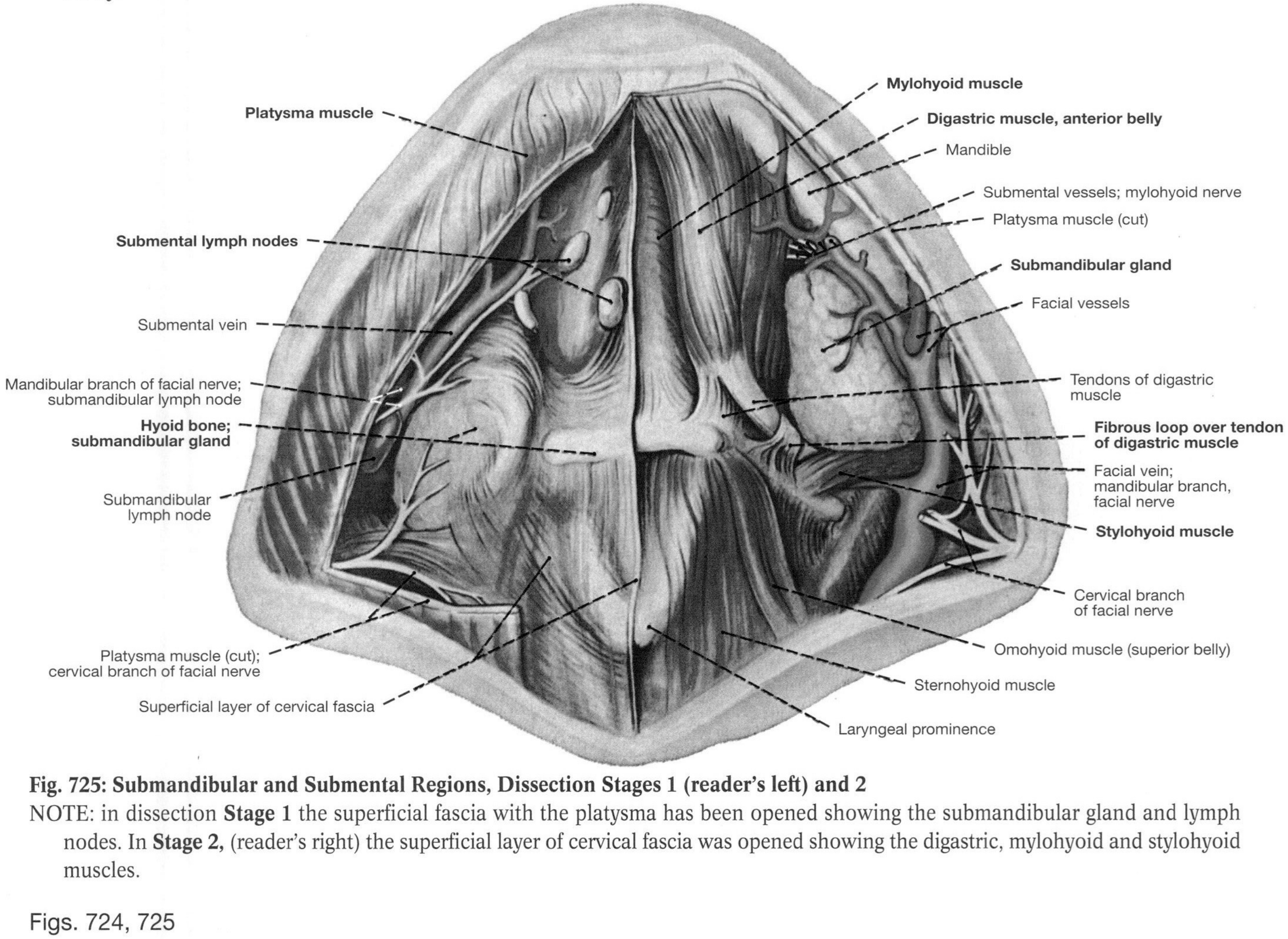

Fig. 725: Submandibular and Submental Regions, Dissection Stages 1 (reader's left) and 2
NOTE: in dissection **Stage 1** the superficial fascia with the platysma has been opened showing the submandibular gland and lymph nodes. In **Stage 2,** (reader's right) the superficial layer of cervical fascia was opened showing the digastric, mylohyoid and stylohyoid muscles.

Figs. 724, 725

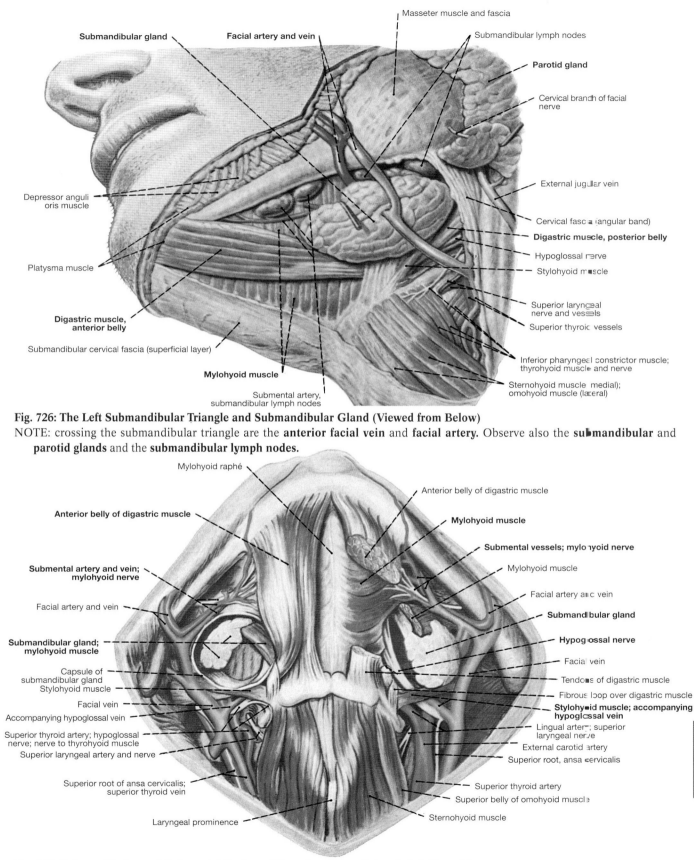

Fig. 726: The Left Submandibular Triangle and Submandibular Gland (Viewed from Below)
NOTE: crossing the submandibular triangle are the **anterior facial vein** and **facial artery.** Observe also the **submandibular** and **parotid glands** and the **submandibular lymph nodes.**

Fig. 727: Submandibular and Submental Regions, Dissection Stages 3 (reader's left) and 4
NOTE: in dissection **Stage 3** much of the submandibular gland has been removed revealing the **submental nerve** and **mylohyoid nerve.** In **Stage 4** (reader's right) the anterior digastric and part of the mylohyoid were removed, exposing the **hypoglossal nerve** and **accompanying vein.**

PLATE 462   The Face: Superficial Muscles, Anterior View

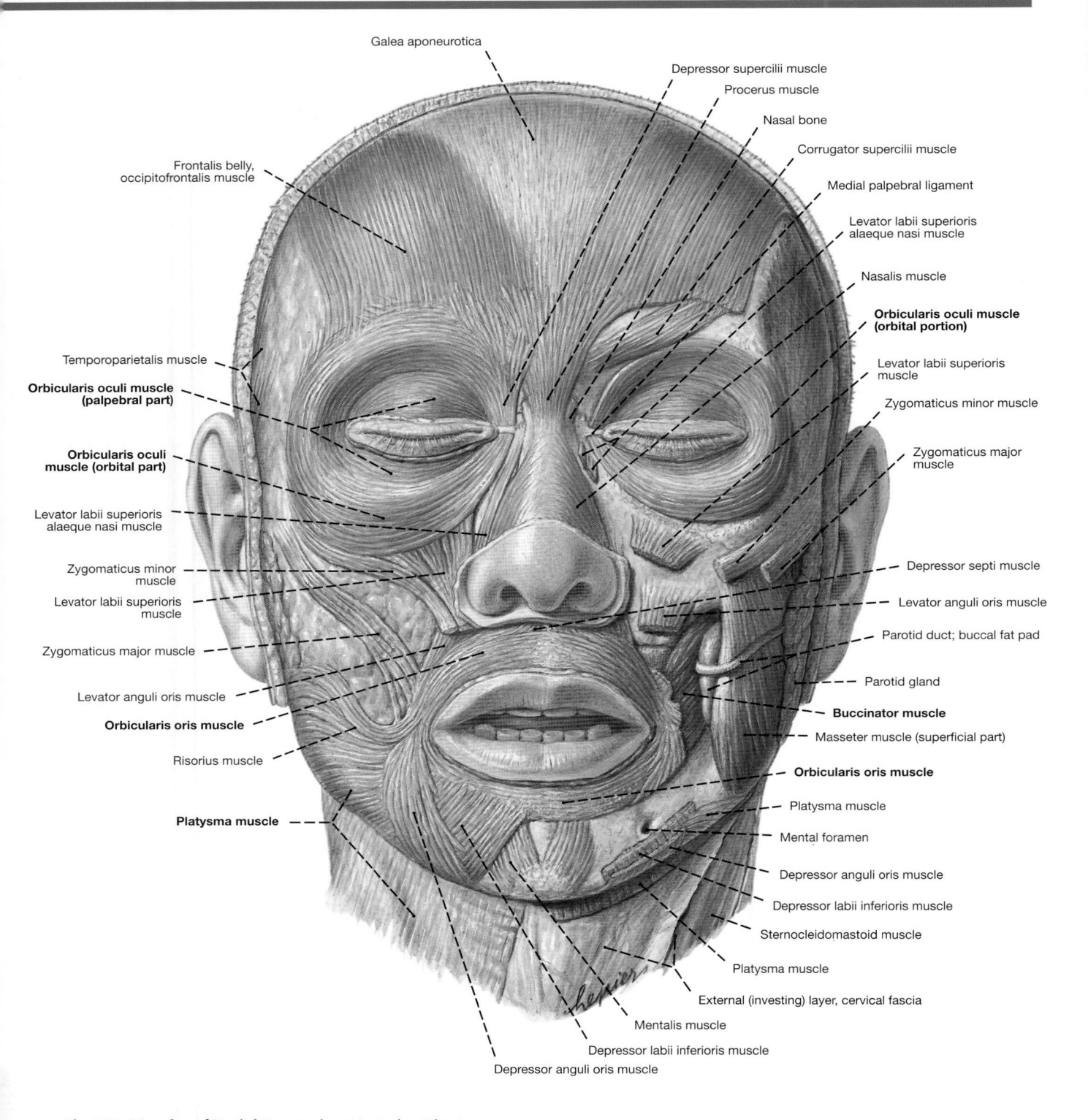

Galea aponeurotica

Depressor supercilii muscle

Procerus muscle

Nasal bone

Corrugator supercilii muscle

Medial palpebral ligament

Levator labii superioris alaeque nasi muscle

Nasalis muscle

Orbicularis oculi muscle (orbital portion)

Levator labii superioris muscle

Zygomaticus minor muscle

Zygomaticus major muscle

Depressor septi muscle

Levator anguli oris muscle

Parotid duct; buccal fat pad

Parotid gland

Buccinator muscle

Masseter muscle (superficial part)

Orbicularis oris muscle

Platysma muscle

Mental foramen

Depressor anguli oris muscle

Depressor labii inferioris muscle

Sternocleidomastoid muscle

Platysma muscle

External (investing) layer, cervical fascia

Mentalis muscle

Depressor labii inferioris muscle

Depressor anguli oris muscle

Frontalis belly, occipitofrontalis muscle

Temporoparietalis muscle

Orbicularis oculi muscle (palpebral part)

Orbicularis oculi muscle (orbital part)

Levator labii superioris alaeque nasi muscle

Zygomaticus minor muscle

Levator labii superioris muscle

Zygomaticus major muscle

Levator anguli oris muscle

Orbicularis oris muscle

Risorius muscle

Platysma muscle

Fig. 728: Muscles of Facial Expression (Anterior View)

NOTE: 1) the muscles of facial expression are located within the layers of superficial fascia. Having developed from the mesoderm of the **2nd branchial arch,** they are innervated by the nerve of that arch, the seventh cranial or **facial nerve.**

2) facial muscles may be grouped into: a) muscles of the **scalp,** b) muscles of the **external ear,** c) muscles of the **eyelid,** d) the **nasal muscles** and e) the **oral muscles.** The borders of some facial muscles are not easily defined. The **platysma muscle** also belongs to the facial group, even though it extends over the neck.

3) the circular muscles surrounding the eyes (**orbicularis oculi**) and the mouth (**orbicularis oris**) assist in closure of the orbital and oral apertures, and thus contribute to functions such as closing the eyes and the ingestion of liquids and food.

4) since facial muscles respond to thoughts and emotions, they aid in communication.

5) the **buccinator muscles** are flat and are situated on the lateral aspects of the oral cavity. They assist in mastication by pressing the cheeks against the teeth, preventing food from accumulating in the oral vestibule.

Fig. 728

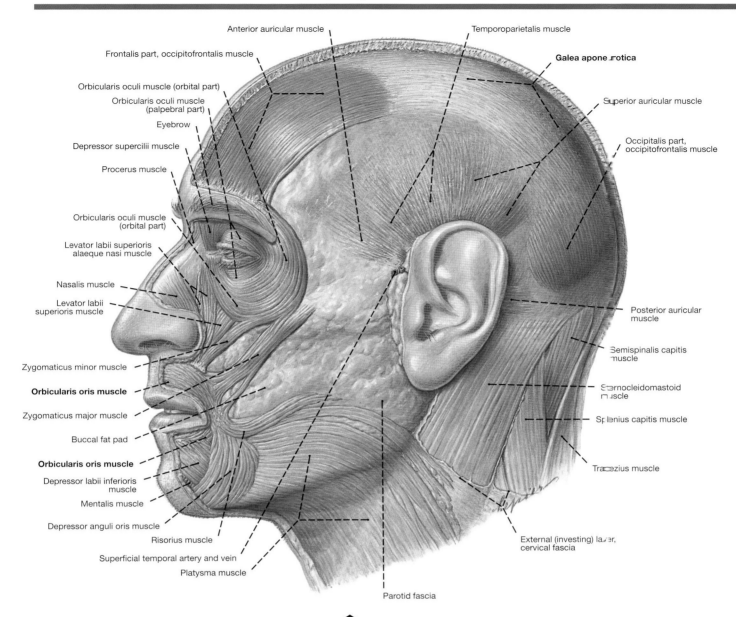

Anterior auricular muscle

Frontalis part, occipitofrontalis muscle

Orbicularis oculi muscle (orbital part)

Orbicularis oculi muscle (palpebral part)

Eyebrow

Depressor supercilii muscle

Procerus muscle

Orbicularis oculi muscle (orbital part)

Levator labii superioris alaeque nasi muscle

Nasalis muscle

Levator labii superioris muscle

Zygomaticus minor muscle

Orbicularis oris muscle

Zygomaticus major muscle

Buccal fat pad

Orbicularis oris muscle

Depressor labii inferioris muscle

Mentalis muscle

Depressor anguli oris muscle

Risorius muscle

Superficial temporal artery and vein

Platysma muscle

Parotid fascia

Temporoparietalis muscle

Galea aponeurotica

Superior auricular muscle

Occipitalis part, occipitofrontalis muscle

Posterior auricular muscle

Semispinalis capitis muscle

Sternocleidomastoid muscle

Splenius capitis muscle

Trapezius muscle

External (investing) layer, cervical fascia

Fig. 729: Muscles of Facial Expression and the Superficial Posterior Cervical Muscles

NOTE: 1) the **frontalis** and **occipitalis** portions of the occipito-frontalis muscle are continuous with an epicranial aponeurosis called the **galea aponeurotica.**

    2) the **orbicularis oculi** consists of orbital, palpebral and lacrimal (not shown) portions.

    3) into the **orbicularis oris** merge a number of facial muscles in a somewhat radial manner.

Fig. 730: Branches of the Facial Nerve Supplying the Superficial ▶ Facial Muscles

NOTE: all the muscles of facial expression are innervated by branches of the 7th cranial nerve, the **facial nerve.** These branches are the **temporal, zygomatic, buccal, mandibular, cervical** and **posterior auricular** nerves.

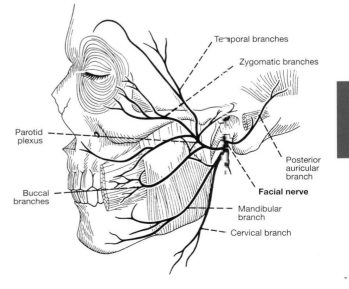

Temporal branches

Zygomatic branches

Parotid plexus

Buccal branches

Posterior auricular branch

Facial nerve

Mandibular branch

Cervical branch

SUPRAHYOID MUSCLES

Muscle	Origin	Insertion	Innervation	Action
Digastric Muscle	ANTERIOR BELLY Digastric fossa on inner aspect of lower border of mandible POSTERIOR BELLY Mastoid notch of the temporal bone	Ends by an intermediate tendon between the two bellies which attaches to the hyoid bone	ANTERIOR BELLY Mylohyoid branch of trigeminal nerve (V) POSTERIOR BELLY Digastric branch of the facial nerve (VII)	Opens the mouth by depressing the mandible; elevates the hyoid bone
Stylohyoid Muscle	Posterior and lateral surface of styloid process of temporal bone	Body of the hyoid bone near the greater horn	Stylohyoid branch of the facial nerve (VII)	Elevates, fixes and retracts the hyoid bone
Mylohyoid Muscle The two mylohyoid muscles form the floor of the oral cavity	Entire length of the mylohyoid line of the mandible	POSTERIOR FIBERS Into body of the hyoid bone MIDDLE and ANTERIOR FIBERS The median raphé between the muscles of both sides	Mylohyoid branch of the trigeminal nerve (V)	During swallowing both muscles raise floor of mouth; elevate hyoid bone; depress mandible in opening the mouth
Geniohyoid Muscle	Inferior mental spine on the inner surface of the symphysis menti	Anterior surface of the body of hyoid bone	1st cervical nerve carried along the hypoglossal nerve	Elevates and draws hyoid bone forward; when hyoid is fixed, it retracts and depresses mandible

SUPERFICIAL MUSCLES OF THE FACE AND HEAD
MUSCLES OF THE SCALP

Muscle	Origin	Insertion	Innervation	Action
Occipitofrontalis Muscle	OCCIPITAL BELLY Lateral ²/₃rds of superior nuchal line on occipital bone and mastoid part of temporal bone	Into the galea aponeurotica	Posterior auricular branch of the facial nerve (VII)	Draws scalp back; raises eyebrow and wrinkles forehead in expression of surprise
	FRONTAL BELLY Fibers continuous with those of procerus medially and orbicularis oculi laterally	Into the galea aponeurotica	Temporal branch of the facial nerve (VII)	
Temporoparietalis Muscle	From temporal fascia above and in front of auricle of ear	Onto the temporal fascia and skin on the side of the head	Temporal branch of the facial nerve (VII)	Tightens the scalp and draws back the skin of the temples

EXTRINSIC MUSCLES OF THE EAR

Muscle	Origin	Insertion	Innervation	Action
Anterior Auricular Muscle	Anterior part of the temporal fascia	Onto the spine of the helix	Temporal branch of the facial nerve (VII)	Draws auricle of ear forward and upward (minimal action)
Superior Auricular Muscle	Epicranial aponeurosis on the side of the head	Upper part of the cranial surface of auricle of ear	Temporal branch of the facial nerve (VII)	Draws the auricle of the ear upward (minimal action)
Posterior Auricular Muscle	Mastoid process of the temporal bone	Medial surface of auricle at convexity of concha	Posterior auricular branch of the facial nerve (VII)	Draws the auricle backward (minimal action)

MUSCLES OF THE EYELIDS

Muscle	Origin	Insertion	Innervation	Action
Orbicularis Oculi Muscle Palpebral Part	Medial palpebral ligament	Cross the eyelids and interlace to form the lateral palpebral raphé	Temporal and zygomatic branches of the facial nerve (VII)	Closes the eyelids gently as in sleeping and blinking
Orbital Part	Nasal part of frontal bone; frontal process of the maxilla; medial palpebral ligament	Forms ellipse around orbit without being interrupted on the lateral side	Temporal and zygomatic branches of the facial nerve (VII)	Closes the eyelids when a more forceful contraction is necessary as in winking one eye
Corrugator Supercilii Muscle	Medial end of the superciliary arch	Deep surface of the skin above the middle of the supraorbital margin	Temporal branch of the facial nerve (VII)	Draws the eyebrow medially and down

SUPERFICIAL MUSCLES OF THE FACE AND HEAD (Cont.)
MUSCLES OF THE NOSE

Muscle	Origin	Insertion	Innervation	Action
Procerus Muscle	From fascia over the lower of the nasal bone	Into the skin of the lower part of the forehead between the eyebrows	Buccal branch of the facial nerve (VII)	Draws down the medial angle of the eyebrow such as in frowning or concentration
Nasalis Muscle	TRANSVERSE PART From the maxilla lateral to the nasal notch	Ascends to bridge of nose; meshes with opposite insertion	Buccal branch of the facial nerve (VII)	Compresses the nasal aperture
	ALAR PART From the maxilla above the lateral incisor tooth	Attaches to the cartilaginous ala of the nose	Buccal branch of the facial nerve (VII)	Assists in opening the nasal aperture in deep inspiration
Depressor Septi Muscle	From the maxilla above the medial incisor	Into the mobile part of the nasal septum	Buccal branch of the facial nerve (VII)	Assists alar part of nasalis muscle in widening nares

MUSCLES OF THE MOUTH

Muscle	Origin	Insertion	Innervation	Action
Levator Labii Superioris Muscle	Along lower part of orbit from maxilla and zygomatic bones	Upper lip between levators anguli oris and labii superioris alaeque nasi	Buccal branch of the facial nerve (VII)	Raises the upper lip and carries it forward
Levator Labii Superioris Alaeque Nasi Muscle	Upper part of the frontal process of the maxilla	Inserts by 2 slips: into alar cartilage and into upper lip with levator labii superioris	Buccal branch of the facial nerve (VII)	Raises the upper lip and dilates the nostril
Levator Anguli Oris Muscle	Canine fossa of the maxilla just below the infraorbital foramen	Into angle of mouth merging with orbicularis oris, depressor anguli oris and zygomaticus major	Buccal branch of the facial nerve (VII)	Raises the angle of the mouth and forms the nasolabial furrow
Zygomaticus Minor Muscle	Lateral surface of the zygomatic bone	Upper lip between levator labii superioris and zygomaticus major	Buccal branch of the facial nerve (VII)	Elevates the upper lip and helps form the nasolabial furrow
Zygomaticus Major Muscle	From the zygomatic bone in front of the zygomaticotemporal suture	Into angle of mouth with levator and depressor anguli oris and orbicularis oris muscles	Buccal branch of the facial nerve (VII)	Draws the angle of the mouth upward and backward as in laughing
Risorius Muscle	From parotid fascia over masseter muscle	Into the skin at the angle of the mouth	Buccal branch of the facial nerve (VII)	Retracts the angle of the mouth
Depressor Labii Inferioris Muscle	Oblique line of mandible between symphysis menti and the mental foramen	Into lower lip and at midline blending with muscle from other side	Mandibular branch of facial nerve (VII)	Draws the lower lip downward and a bit laterally
Depressor Anguli Oris Muscle	From oblique line of mandible, lateral and below depressor labii inferioris	Into the angle of the mouth blending with orbicularis oris and risorius	Mandibular branch of the facial nerve (VII)	Draws angle of mouth down and laterally as in expression of sadness
Mentalis Muscle	From the incisive fossa of the mandible	Into the skin of the chin	Mandibular branch of the facial nerve (VII)	Raises and protrudes lower lip; wrinkles chin in expression of doubt or disdain
Orbicularis Oris Muscle	Fibers derived from other facial muscles (buccinator, levators and depressors of lips and angles, zygomatic muscles) pass into lips; also some intrinsic muscle fibers make up orbicularis oris	Several strata of muscle fibers form a sphincter-like muscle with fibers that decussate at the angles of the mouth	Buccal branch of the facial nerve (VII)	Closes the lips and its deep fibers can press the lips against the teeth; also it protrudes the lips and is important in speech
Buccinator Muscle	Alveolar processes of mandible and maxilla opposite upper and lower molar teeth; posteriorly, it arises from the pterygomandibular raphé opposite superior constrictor	Fibers course forward to blend into the formation of the orbicularis oris, decussating at the angles of the mouth	Buccal branch of the facial nerve (VII)	Compresses the cheeks during chewing; also compresses the distended cheeks as in blowing on a horn

PLATE 466   The Face: Muscles of Mastication; Parotid Gland

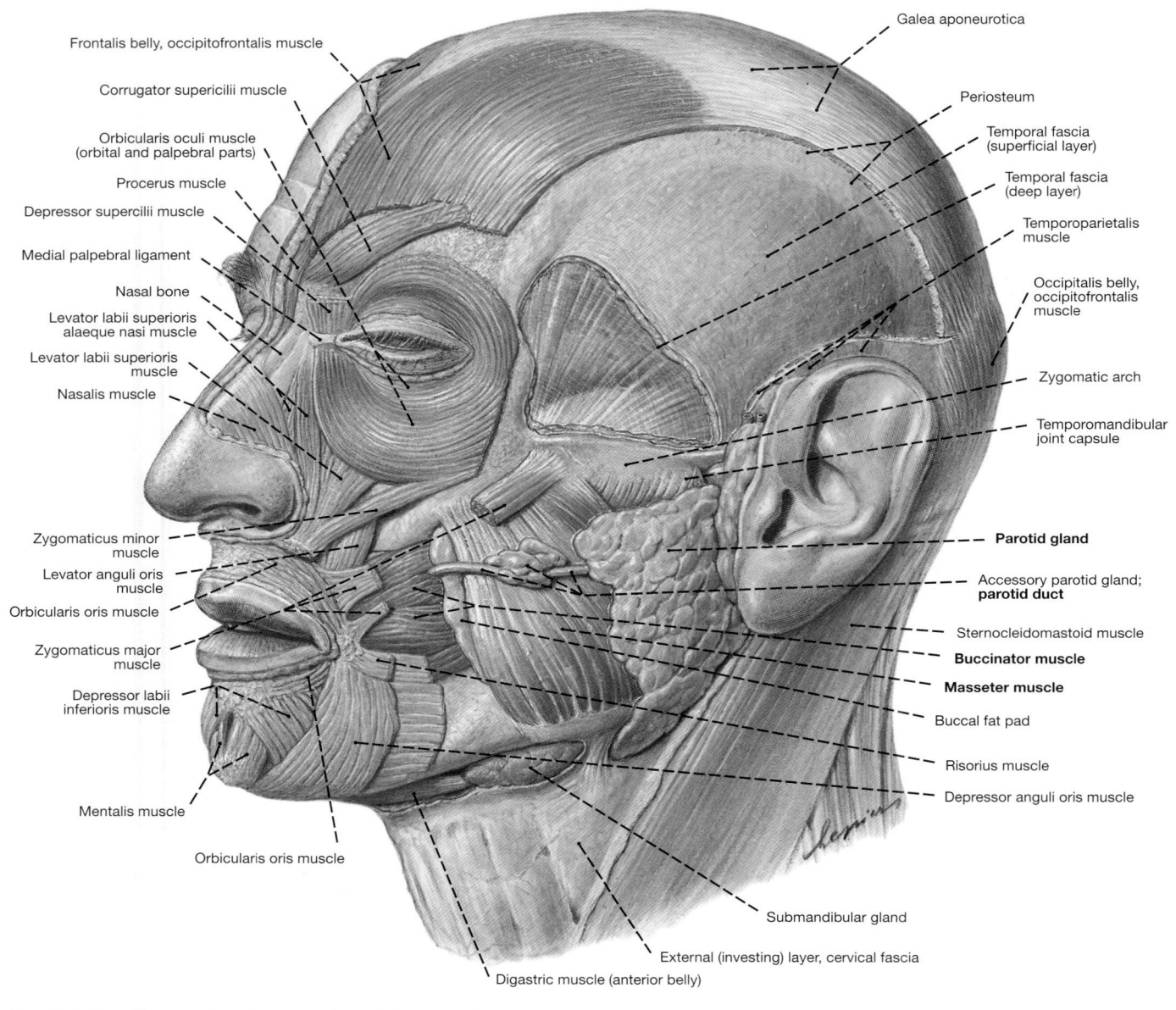

Galea aponeurotica

Periosteum

Temporal fascia (superficial layer)

Temporal fascia (deep layer)

Temporoparietalis muscle

Occipitalis belly, occipitofrontalis muscle

Zygomatic arch

Temporomandibular joint capsule

Parotid gland

Accessory parotid gland; **parotid duct**

Sternocleidomastoid muscle

Buccinator muscle

Masseter muscle

Buccal fat pad

Risorius muscle

Depressor anguli oris muscle

Submandibular gland

External (investing) layer, cervical fascia

Digastric muscle (anterior belly)

Frontalis belly, occipitofrontalis muscle

Corrugator supericilii muscle

Orbicularis oculi muscle (orbital and palpebral parts)

Procerus muscle

Depressor supercilii muscle

Medial palpebral ligament

Nasal bone

Levator labii superioris alaeque nasi muscle

Levator labii superioris muscle

Nasalis muscle

Zygomaticus minor muscle

Levator anguli oris muscle

Orbicularis oris muscle

Zygomaticus major muscle

Depressor labii inferioris muscle

Mentalis muscle

Orbicularis oris muscle

Fig. 731: Parotid Gland and Duct and the Masseter Muscle

NOTE: 1)   the **parotid gland** extends from the zygomatic arch to below the angle of the mandible. It lies anterior to the ear and superficial to the **masseter muscle.** It is enclosed in a tight fascial sheath, and its duct courses medially across the face to enter the oral cavity through the fibers of the **buccinator muscle.**

2)   the masseter muscle extends from the zygomatic bone to the ramus, angle and body of the mandible. It elevates the mandible (closes the mouth) and is supplied by the trigeminal nerve.

Fig. 732: Parasympathetic Innervation of the Parotid Gland ▶

NOTE: 1)   preganglionic parasympathetic fibers that innervate the parotid gland emerge from the brain stem in the 9th (glossopharyngeal) nerve.

2)   these fibers then travel along the **tympanic nerve** to the middle ear, and then form the **lesser petrosal nerve** that joins the **otic ganglion.**

3)   postganglionic fibers then travel within the **auriculotemporal nerve** to reach the parotid gland.

Inferior salivatorius nucleus

Lesser petrosal nerve

Tympanic branch of glossopharyngeal nerve

Otic ganglion

Auriculotemporal nerve

Figs. 731, 732

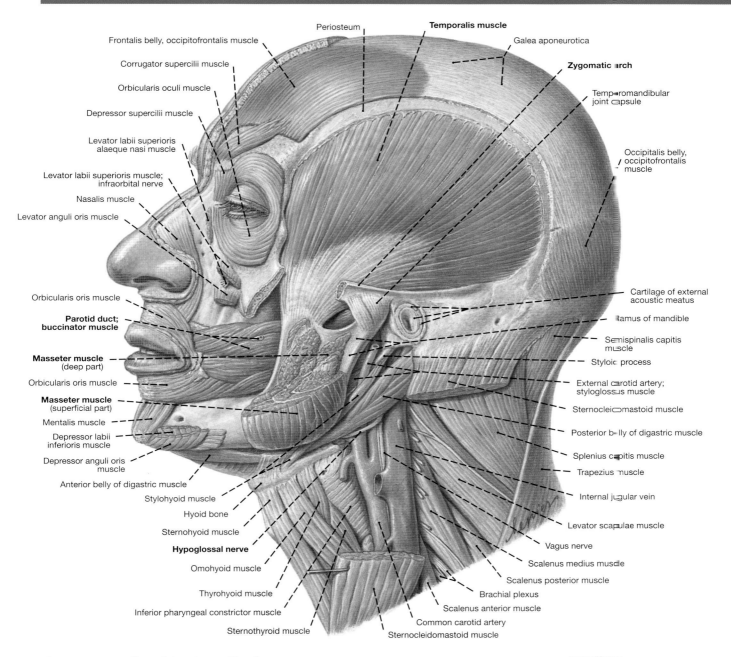

Periosteum
Temporalis muscle
Galea aponeurotica
Frontalis belly, occipitofrontalis muscle
Corrugator supercilii muscle
Zygomatic arch
Orbicularis oculi muscle
Temporomandibular joint capsule
Depressor supercilii muscle
Levator labii superioris alaeque nasi muscle
Occipitalis belly, occipitofrontalis muscle
Levator labii superioris muscle; infraorbital nerve
Nasalis muscle
Levator anguli oris muscle
Cartilage of external acoustic meatus
Orbicularis oris muscle
Ramus of mandible
Parotid duct; buccinator muscle
Semispinalis capitis muscle
Styloid process
Masseter muscle (deep part)
External carotid artery; styloglossus muscle
Orbicularis oris muscle
Masseter muscle (superficial part)
Sternocleidomastoid muscle
Mentalis muscle
Posterior belly of digastric muscle
Depressor labii inferioris muscle
Splenius capitis muscle
Depressor anguli oris muscle
Trapezius muscle
Anterior belly of digastric muscle
Internal jugular vein
Stylohyoid muscle
Hyoid bone
Levator scapulae muscle
Sternohyoid muscle
Vagus nerve
Hypoglossal nerve
Scalenus medius muscle
Omohyoid muscle
Scalenus posterior muscle
Thyrohyoid muscle
Brachial plexus
Inferior pharyngeal constrictor muscle
Scalenus anterior muscle
Sternothyroid muscle
Common carotid artery
Sternocleidomastoid muscle

Fig. 733: Temporalis and Buccinator Muscles

NOTE: 1) the external ear and zygomatic arch have been removed along with most of the masseter muscle to demonstrate the origin of the temporalis muscle from the temporal fossa and its insertion on the coronoid process of the mandible. Similar to the masseter, the temporalis is innervated by the mandibular branch of the trigeminal nerve.

2) the various fiber bundles of the buccinator muscle as they extend directly into the orbicularis oris at both the upper and lower lips. Similar to the other facial muscles, the buccinator is supplied by the facial nerve (VII, buccal branch).

Fig. 734: Cutaneous Nerve Patterns (Dermatomes) of the Head and Neck

NOTE: 1) the anterior and lateral surfaces of the head and face are supplied by the divisions of the trigeminal nerve.

2) the posterior and lateral surfaces of the head and neck are supplied by the cervical nerves. Small areas of skin around the ear are innervated by the facial (VII), glossopharyngeal (IX) and vagus (X) nerves.

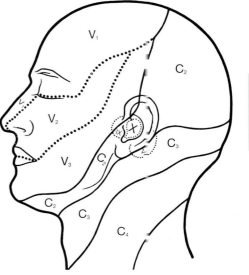

PLATE 468   The Face: Superficial Vessels and Nerves (Dissection 1)

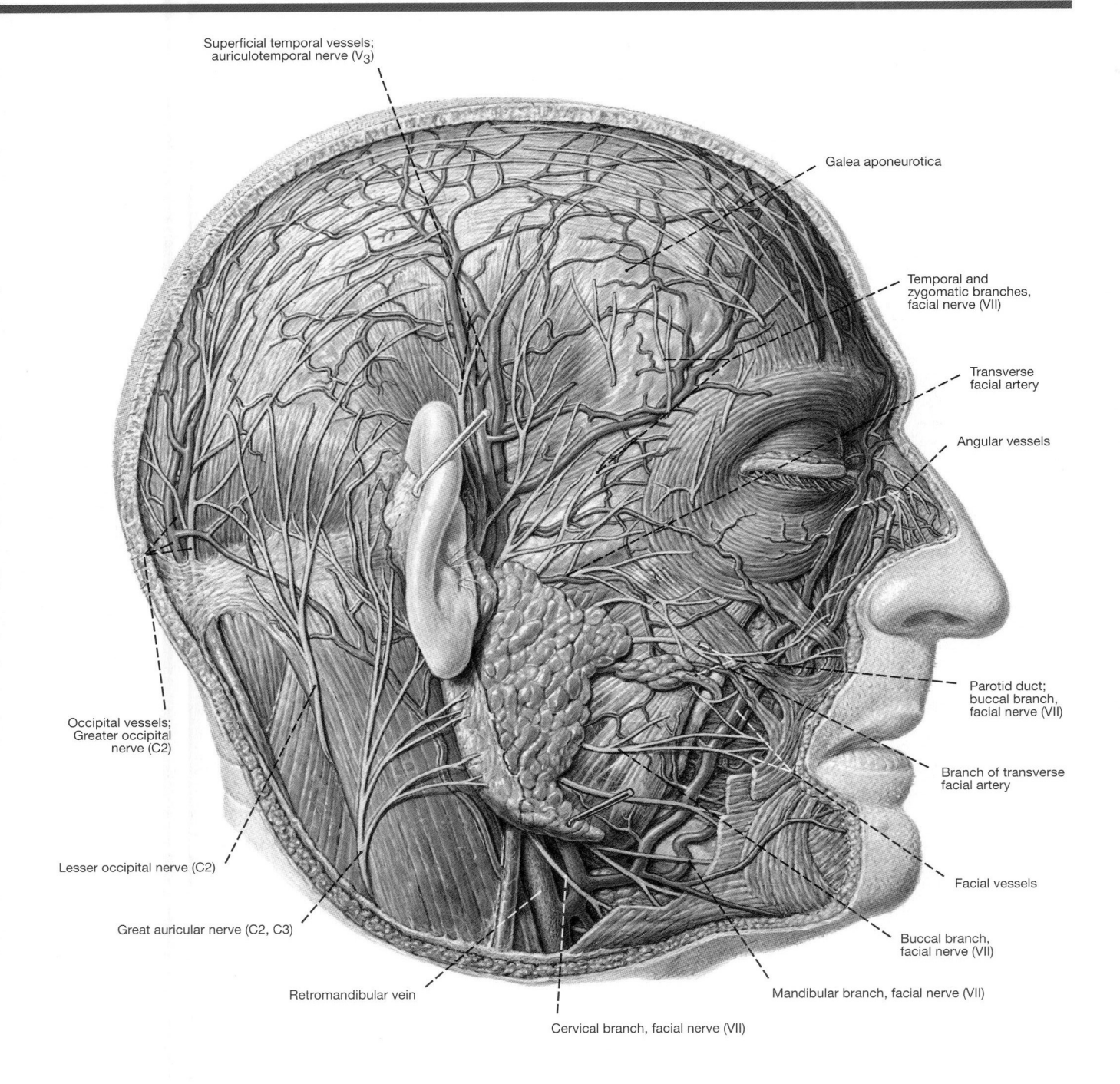

Superficial temporal vessels;
auriculotemporal nerve (V₃)

Galea aponeurotica

Temporal and
zygomatic branches,
facial nerve (VII)

Transverse
facial artery

Angular vessels

Parotid duct;
buccal branch,
facial nerve (VII)

Branch of transverse
facial artery

Facial vessels

Buccal branch,
facial nerve (VII)

Mandibular branch, facial nerve (VII)

Cervical branch, facial nerve (VII)

Retromandibular vein

Great auricular nerve (C2, C3)

Lesser occipital nerve (C2)

Occipital vessels;
Greater occipital
nerve (C2)

Fig. 735: Superficial Dissection of the Face: Vessels and Nerves (1)

NOTE: 1)   in this dissection the capsule of the parotid gland has been opened to reveal the substance of the gland and the branches of
the **facial nerve** that emerge from under its borders. These cross the face to supply the muscles of facial expression (see Fig. 736)
for a more complete view of the facial branches.

2)   the cervical nerves. The **greater occipital nerve** is a sensory nerve from the *posterior* primary ramus of C2 and it courses
upward with the occipital vessels to supply the posterior scalp. The **lesser occipital (C2)** and **great auricular (C2, C3) nerves** are
from the *anterior* primary rami and are also sensory nerves. They supply the posterolateral neck region and the lateral scalp behind
the ear.

3)   the course of the **facial artery and vein** is partially covered by the muscles of facial expression. These vessels have been
exposed to demonstrate their ascent lateral to the nose to reach the medial side of the orbit where they are called the **angular artery
and vein.**

Fig. 735

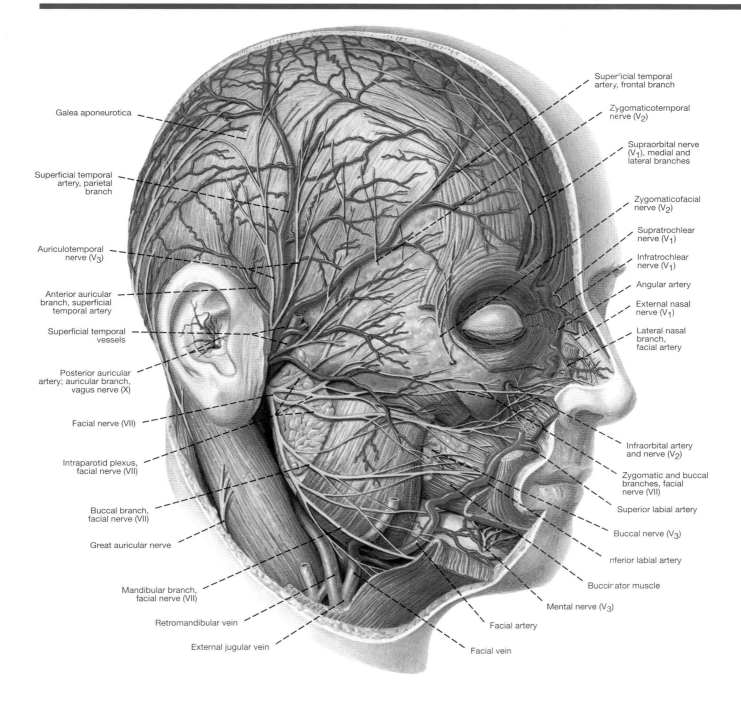

Galea aponeurotica

Superficial temporal artery, parietal branch

Auriculotemporal nerve (V₃)

Anterior auricular branch, superficial temporal artery

Superficial temporal vessels

Posterior auricular artery; auricular branch, vagus nerve (X)

Facial nerve (VII)

Intraparotid plexus, facial nerve (VII)

Buccal branch, facial nerve (VII)

Great auricular nerve

Mandibular branch, facial nerve (VII)

Retromandibular vein

External jugular vein

Superficial temporal artery, frontal branch

Zygomaticotemporal nerve (V₂)

Supraorbital nerve (V₁), medial and lateral branches

Zygomaticofacial nerve (V₂)

Supratrochlear nerve (V₁)

Infratrochlear nerve (V₁)

Angular artery

External nasal nerve (V₁)

Lateral nasal branch, facial artery

Infraorbital artery and nerve (V₂)

Zygomatic and buccal branches, facial nerve (VII)

Superior labial artery

Buccal nerve (V₃)

nferior labial artery

Buccirator muscle

Mental nerve (V₃)

Facial artery

Facial vein

Fig. 736: Superficial Dissection of the Face: Vessels and Nerves (2)

NOTE: 1)   the superficial part of the parotid gland has been removed to show the branches of the **facial nerve** which emerge from the substance of the gland. Identify the **temporal, zygomatic, buccal, mandibular** and **cervical** branches. The **posterior auricular** branch is not shown.

2)   the superficial sensory branches of the **trigeminal nerve:**

a)   from the **ophthalmic division:** the supraorbital, supratrochlear, the ascending and descending branches of the infratrochlear and the external nasal.

b)   from the **maxillary division:** the zygomaticotemporal, zygomaticofacial and the infraorbital.

c)   from the **mandibular division:** the buccal, mental and auriculotemporal.

3)   the general distribution of **superficial temporal artery.** Observe also the course of the **facial artery** across the face to become the **angular artery.** Among other structures, the facial artery supplies the chin and the upper and lower lips and it anastomoses with vessels emerging from the orbit.

Fig. 736   **VII**

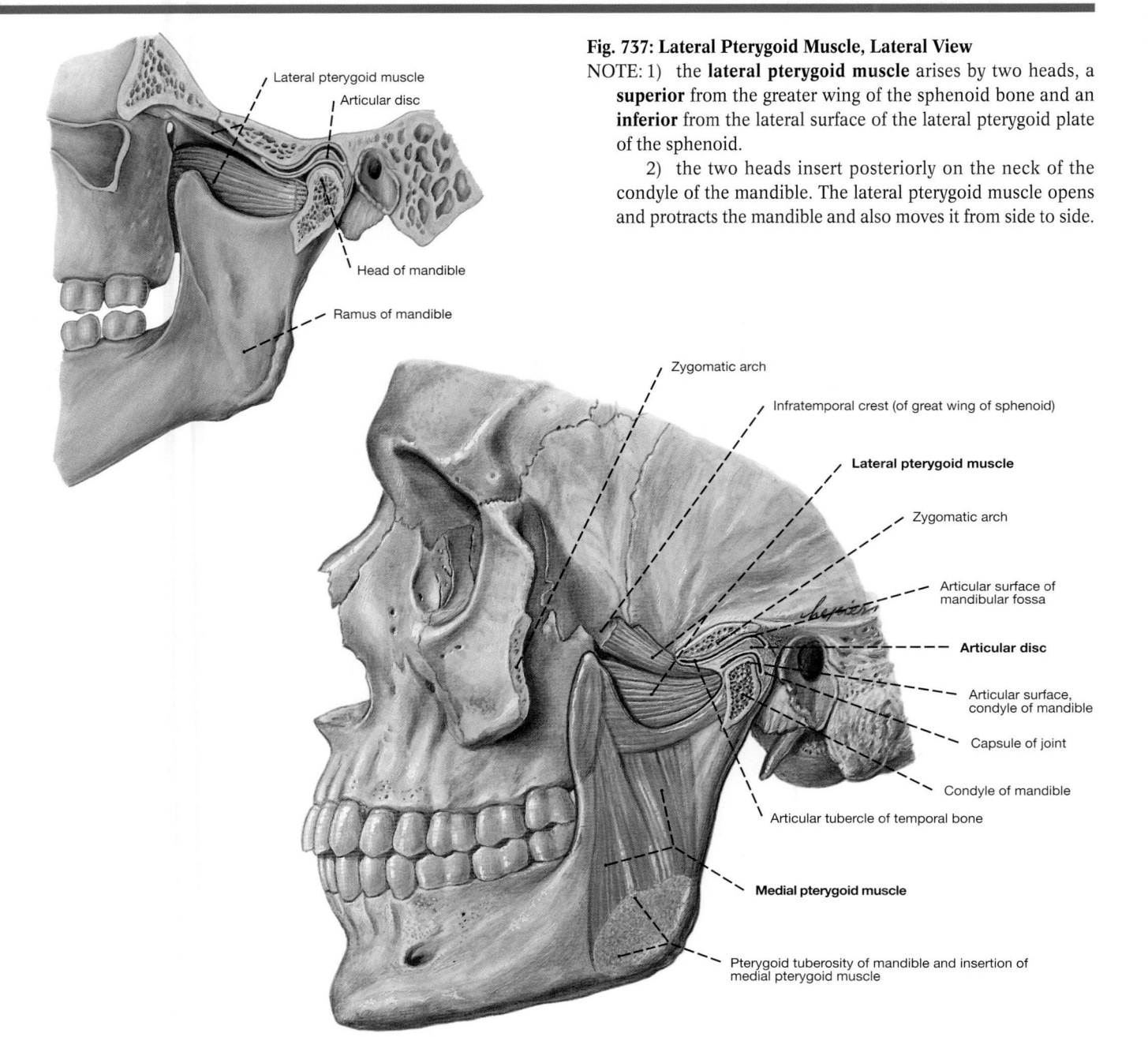

Lateral pterygoid muscle

Articular disc

Head of mandible

Ramus of mandible

Fig. 737: Lateral Pterygoid Muscle, Lateral View
NOTE: 1) the **lateral pterygoid muscle** arises by two heads, a **superior** from the greater wing of the sphenoid bone and an **inferior** from the lateral surface of the lateral pterygoid plate of the sphenoid.

2) the two heads insert posteriorly on the neck of the condyle of the mandible. The lateral pterygoid muscle opens and protracts the mandible and also moves it from side to side.

Zygomatic arch

Infratemporal crest (of great wing of sphenoid)

Lateral pterygoid muscle

Zygomatic arch

Articular surface of mandibular fossa

Articular disc

Articular surface, condyle of mandible

Capsule of joint

Condyle of mandible

Articular tubercle of temporal bone

Medial pterygoid muscle

Pterygoid tuberosity of mandible and insertion of medial pterygoid muscle

Fig. 738: Medial and Lateral Pterygoid Muscles (Lateral View)
NOTE: 1) the left zygomatic arch has been removed. Posteriorly, the bone has been cut through the **temporomandibular joint,** revealing the articular disc. The medial pterygoid muscle and part of the lateral pterygoid muscle on the inner aspect of the mandible is represented as though the bone were transparent.

2) the **medial pterygoid muscle** arises from the medial surface of the lateral pterygoid plate of the sphenoid as well as from the palatine bone, and inserts on the medial surface of the ramus and angle of the mandible. It assists the masseter and temporalis in closing the jaw.

MUSCLES OF MASTICATION

Muscle	Origin	Insertion	Innervation	Action
Masseter Muscle	Zygomatic surface of maxilla and the zygomatic arch	Lateral surface of ramus of mandible and the coronoid process of mandible	Masseteric branch of mandibular nerve	Closes the jaw by elevating the mandible
Temporalis Muscle	Temporal fossa and deep surface of the temporal fascia	Medial surface of anterior border of coronoid process; anterior border of ramus of mandible	Deep temporal branches of the mandibular nerve	Elevates mandible and closes the jaw; posterior fibers retract mandible

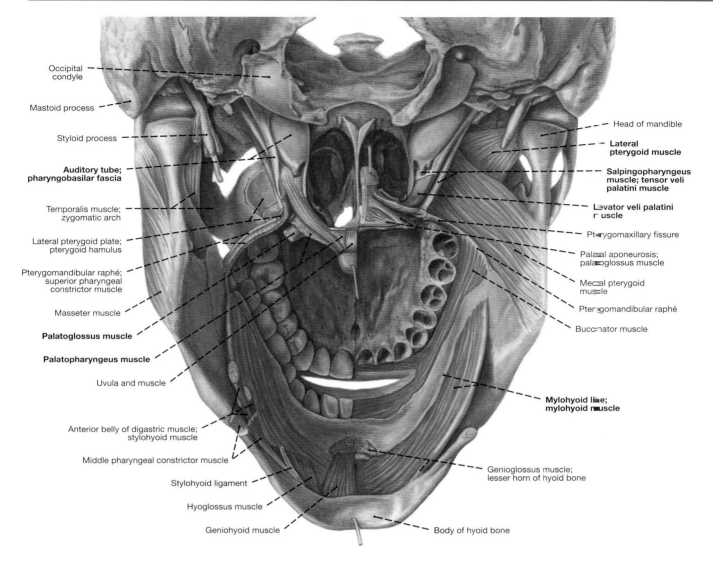

Occipital condyle

Mastoid process

Styloid process

Auditory tube; pharyngobasilar fascia

Temporalis muscle; zygomatic arch

Lateral pterygoid plate; pterygoid hamulus

Pterygomandibular raphé; superior pharyngeal constrictor muscle

Masseter muscle

Palatoglossus muscle

Palatopharyngeus muscle

Uvula and muscle

Anterior belly of digastric muscle; stylohyoid muscle

Middle pharyngeal constrictor muscle

Stylohyoid ligament

Hyoglossus muscle

Geniohyoid muscle

Head of mandible

Lateral pterygoid muscle

Salpingopharyngeus muscle; tensor veli palatini muscle

Levator veli palatini muscle

Pterygomaxillary fissure

Palatal aponeurosis; palatoglossus muscle

Medial pterygoid muscle

Pterygomandibular raphé

Buccinator muscle

Mylohyoid line; mylohyoid muscle

Genioglossus muscle; lesser horn of hyoid bone

Body of hyoid bone

Fig. 739: Pterygoid, Mylohyoid and Geniohyoid Muscles as Seen from Below and Behind
NOTE: 1) a muscular sling is formed around the ramus of mandible to its angle by the insertions of the **medial pterygoid** (seen on the right) and **masseter muscles** (seen on the left). The medial pterygoid muscle descends to attach along the medial aspect of the mandible, while the masseter courses down to insert on the outer aspect of the jaw.

2) the fibers of the lateral pterygoid (right side) course principally in the horizontal plane. The **mylohyoid** and **geniohyoid muscles** attach the mandible to the hyoid bone. Other muscles shown are the **tensor** and **levator veli palatini muscles.**

MUSCLES OF MASTICATION (Cont.)

Muscle	Origin	Insertion	Innervation	Action
Lateral Pterygoid Muscle	SUPERIOR HEAD Infratemporal crest and lateral surface of greater wing of sphenoid bone INFERIOR HEAD Lateral surface of lateral pterygoid plate of sphenoid	Neck of condyle of mandible; articular disc and capsule of temporomandibular joint	Lateral pterygoid branch of mandibular nerve	Opens mouth by drawing condyle and disc forward; *Acting together:* protrudes mandible *Acting alternately:* grinding action
Medial Pterygoid Muscle	DEEP HEAD Medial surface of lateral pterygoid plate of sphenoid; pyramidal process of palatine bone SUPERFICIAL HEAD Pyramidal process of palatine bone; tuberosity of maxilla	Lower and posterior part of medial surface of ramus and angle of mandible	Medial pterygoid branch of mandibular nerve	Elevates mandible closing jaw; *Acting together:* protrudes mandible *Acting alone:* protrudes one side *Acting alternately:* grinding action

Fig. 739   **VII**

PLATE 472   **Temporomandibular Joint and Mandibular Ligaments**

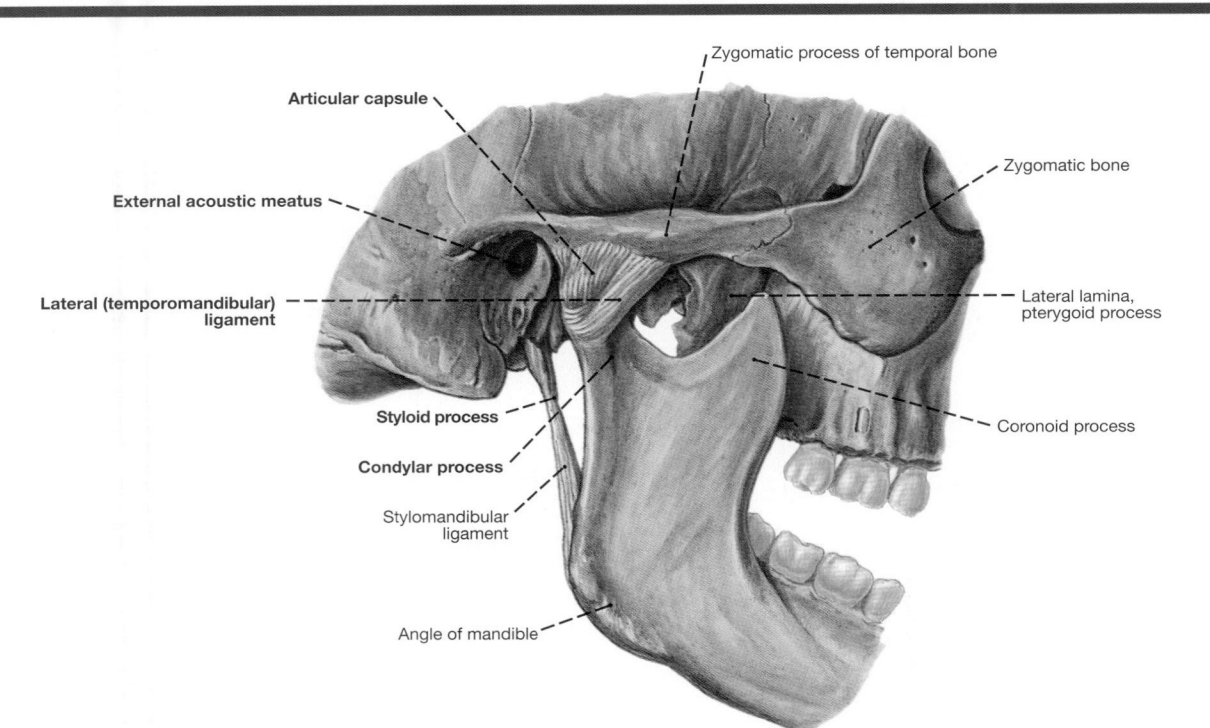

Fig. 740: Right Temporomandibular Joint (Lateral View)

NOTE: 1) the articular capsule and the **lateral** (temporomandibular) **ligament** which extend between the zygomatic process of the temporal bone above to the neck of the condylar process of the mandibular ramus below.

2) the articular capsule is a loose sac that is fused anteriorly and laterally with the **lateral ligament.** Note also the **stylomandibular ligament** extending from the tip of the styloid process to the angle and posterior border of the mandible.

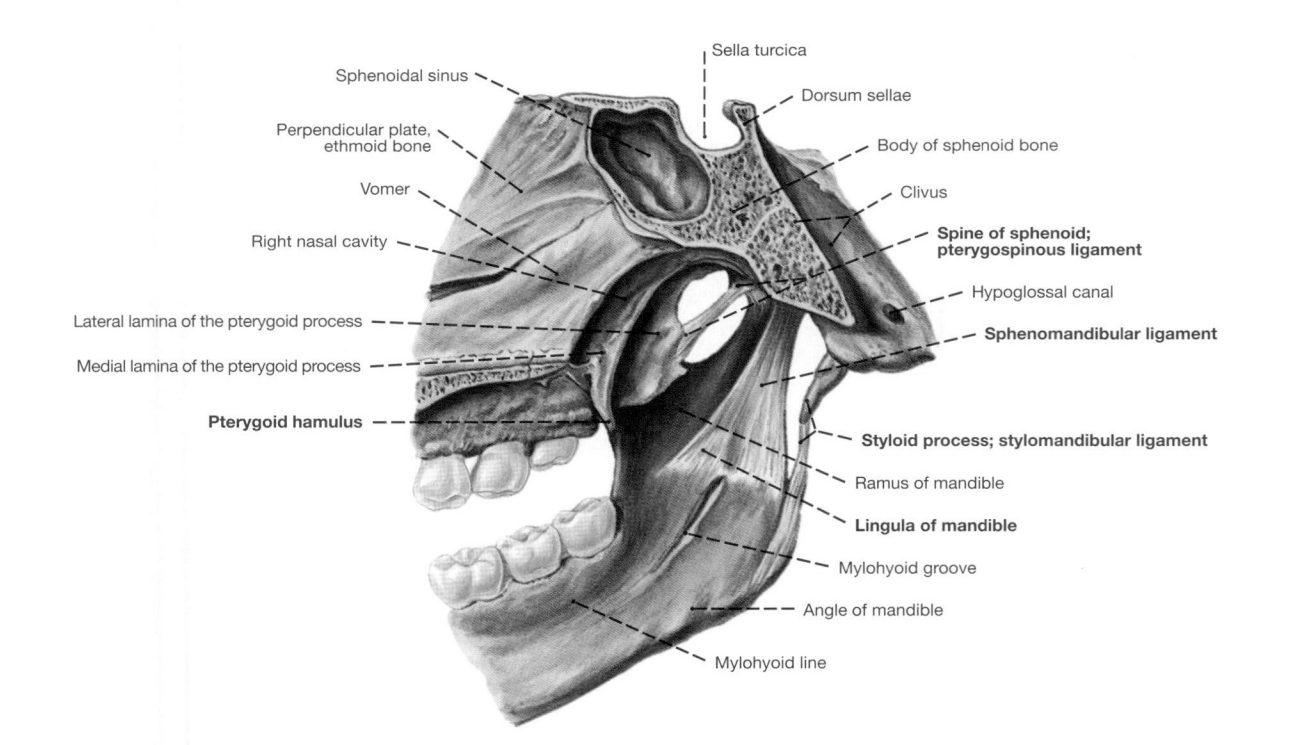

Fig. 741: Right Temporomandibular Region (Medial View)

NOTE: medial to the temporomandibular joint, the **pterygospinous ligament** extends from the sphenoidal spine to the posterior margin of the lateral pterygoid plate. The **sphenomandibular ligament** descends from the sphenoidal spine to the lingula of the mandible.

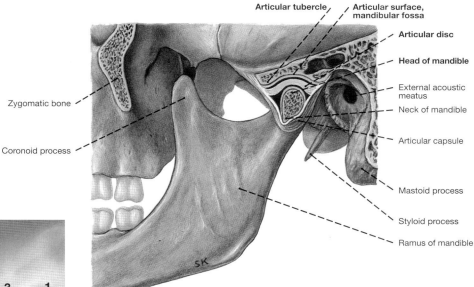

Fig. 742: Sagittal Section of the Temporomandibular Joint With the Jaw Closed
NOTE: 1) an **articular disc** is interposed between the mandibular fossa of the temporal bone and the mandibular condyle, creating two joint cavities.
2) with the jaw closed, the head of the condyle of the mandible and the articular disc lie totally within the mandibular fossa.

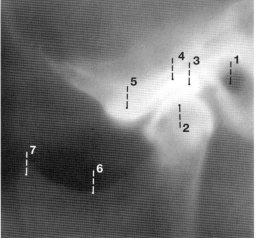

◀ Fig. 743: Arthrograph of the Temporomandibular Joint With the Jaw Closed

For Figs. 743 and 745
1. External acoustic meatus
2. Condylar process
3. Articular disc
4. Mandibular fossa, temporal bone
5. Articular tubercle, temporal bone
6. Mandibular notch
7. Coronoid process

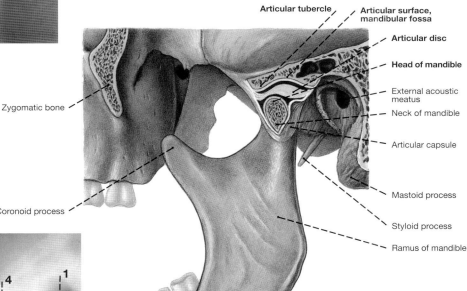

Fig. 744: Sagittal Section of the Temporomandibular Joint With the Jaw Opened
NOTE: when the jaw is opened, the condyle **glides forward** within the joint capsule to lie opposite the **articular tubercle** of the temporal bone.

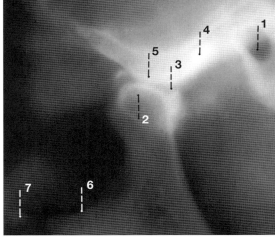

◀ Fig. 745: Arthrograph of the Temporomandibular Joint With the Jaw Opened
NOTE: the mandibular condyle moves forward significantly when the jaw is opened. In Figures 743 and 745 compare the distance between the condyle (2) and the external acoustic meatus (1).

PLATE 474   The Face: Superficial and Deep Arteries

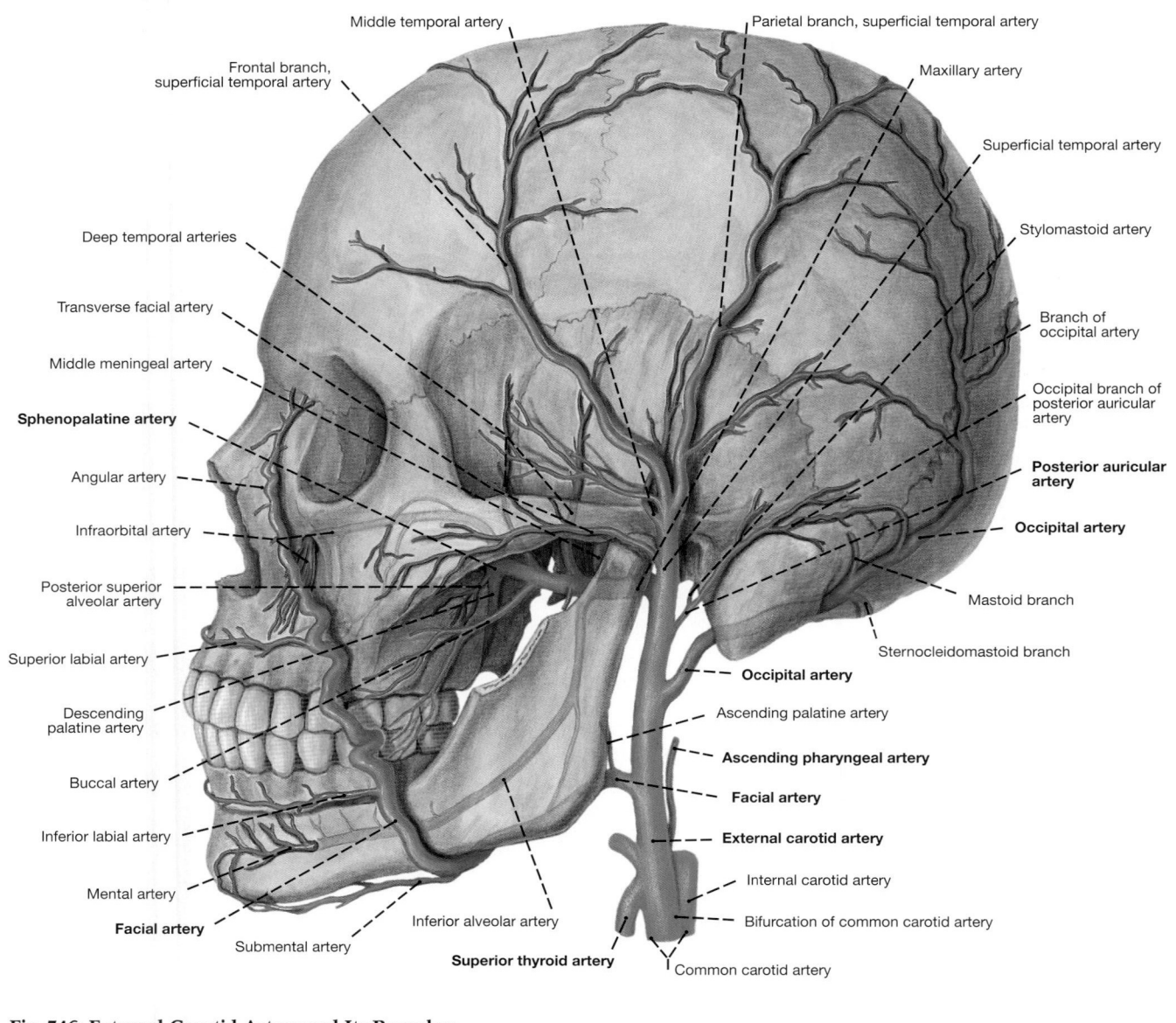

Middle temporal artery

Frontal branch,
superficial temporal artery

Deep temporal arteries

Transverse facial artery

Middle meningeal artery

Sphenopalatine artery

Angular artery

Infraorbital artery

Posterior superior
alveolar artery

Superior labial artery

Descending
palatine artery

Buccal artery

Inferior labial artery

Mental artery

Facial artery

Submental artery

Inferior alveolar artery

Superior thyroid artery

Parietal branch, superficial temporal artery

Maxillary artery

Superficial temporal artery

Stylomastoid artery

Branch of
occipital artery

Occipital branch of
posterior auricular
artery

**Posterior auricular
artery**

Occipital artery

Mastoid branch

Sternocleidomastoid branch

Occipital artery

Ascending palatine artery

Ascending pharyngeal artery

Facial artery

External carotid artery

Internal carotid artery

Bifurcation of common carotid artery

Common carotid artery

Fig. 746: External Carotid Artery and Its Branches

NOTE: 1) the **external carotid artery** branches from the common carotid and is the principal artery that supplies the anterior neck, the face, the scalp, the walls of the oral and nasal cavities, the bones of the skull and the dura mater, but not the orbit or brain.

2) its main branches from inferior to superior are:

a) the **superior thyroid** which courses downward to supply the thyroid gland. It also supplies the sternocleidomastoid and infrahyoid muscles and the inner aspect of the larynx by way of the **superior laryngeal artery.**

b) the **ascending pharyngeal** which ascends to supply the pharyngeal constrictor muscles and other small branches to the prevertebral muscles, middle ear and dura mater.

c) the **lingual** which is the principal artery of the tongue. It also gives branches to suprahyoid muscles and the sublingual gland.

d) the **facial** which ascends to supply the anteromedial aspect of the face. It also sends branches to the palatine tonsil, the submandibular gland and on the face, to both lips and the nose. It ends as the **angular artery** which anastomoses with the infraorbital.

e) the **occipital** which courses to the back of the head to supply the scalp. On its way it sends branches to the sternocleidomastoid and other muscles and to the dura mater.

f) the **posterior auricular** which courses behind the external ear. It helps supply the scalp, the middle ear and the external auricle.

g) the **superficial temporal** which supplies the side of the head and gives off the **transverse facial artery** which courses across the face.

h) the **maxillary** which is the principal artery of the deep face. It has three parts and many branches. It supplies the tympanic membrane, gives rise to the **middle meningeal artery,** supplies the muscles of mastication, all lower and some upper teeth, the infraorbital region, the hard and soft palate, and the walls of the nasal cavity.

Fig. 746

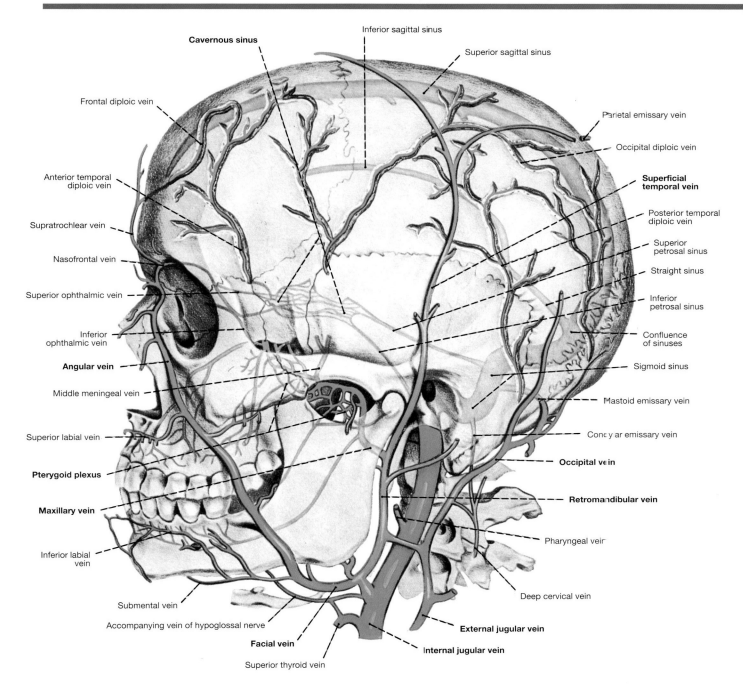

Fig. 747: Principal Superficial Veins of the Face and Head, Showing Connections to Deeper Veins

NOTE: 1) the **angular vein** is formed at the root of the nose and courses inferolaterally to become the **facial vein.** The angular-facial trunk communicates by way of deeper vessels with the **cavernous sinus** within the cranial cavity and with the **pterygoid plexus** of veins in the infratemporal fossa.

2) the **superficial temporal vein** which drains the lateral aspect of the superficial head and the **maxillary vein** which drains the deep face. They join to form the **retromandibular vein.**

3) the **occipital vein** which forms on the posterolateral aspect of the scalp and which courses downward into the **external jugular vein.** The diploic veins and the various emissary veins (condylar, mastoid and parietal veins) interconnect the superficial veins with the **dural sinuses.**

4) within the cranial cavity, the **sigmoid sinus,** draining most of the other dural sinuses, terminates at the jugular foramen. Just below this foramen, the sigmoid sinus becomes the **internal jugular vein** which descends in the neck to the thorax.

Fig. 747   **VII**

PLATE 476   The Face: Deep Vessels and Nerves (Dissection 1)

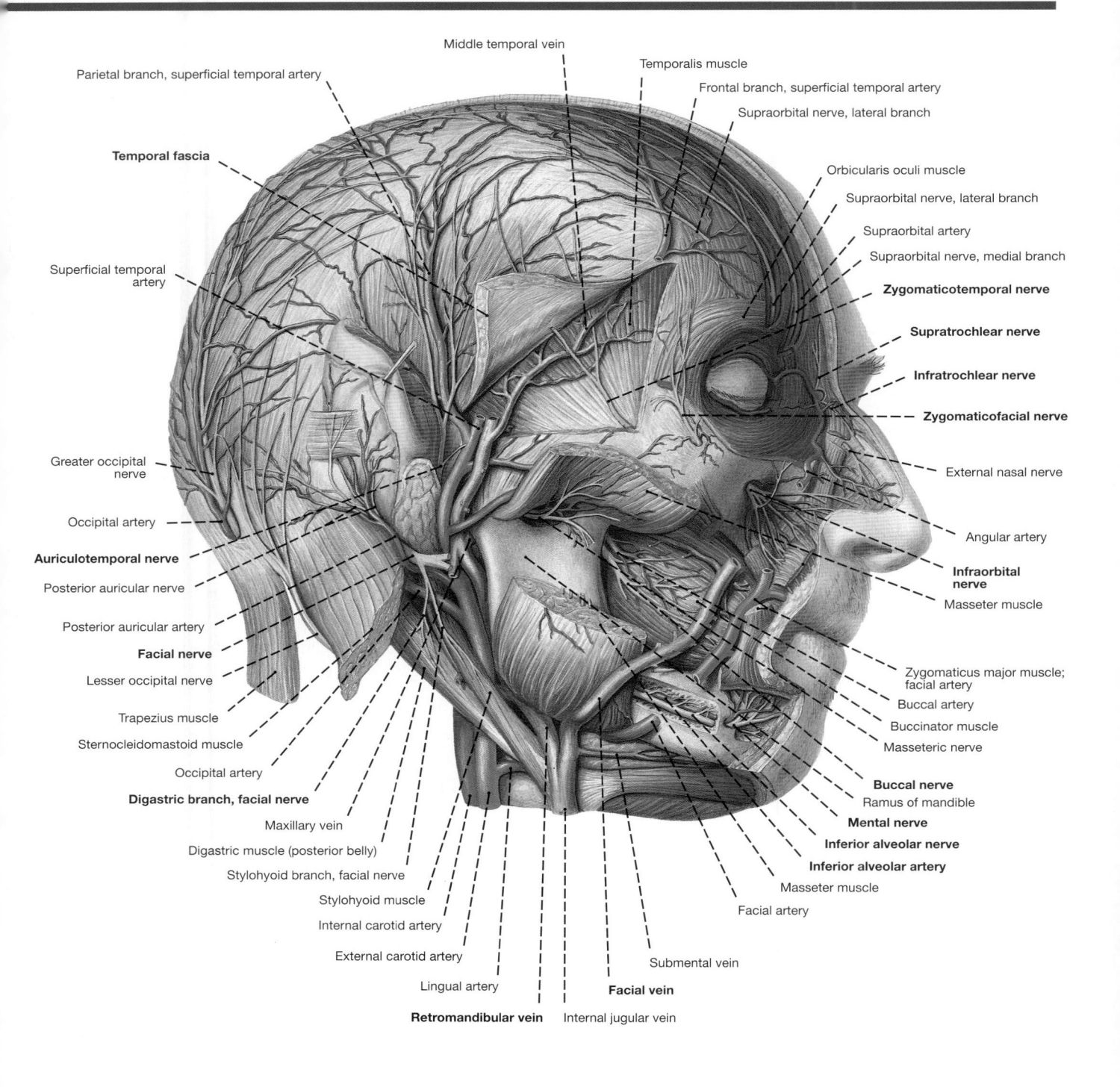

Middle temporal vein
Temporalis muscle
Parietal branch, superficial temporal artery
Frontal branch, superficial temporal artery
Supraorbital nerve, lateral branch
Temporal fascia
Orbicularis oculi muscle
Supraorbital nerve, lateral branch
Supraorbital artery
Supraorbital nerve, medial branch
Superficial temporal artery
Zygomaticotemporal nerve
Supratrochlear nerve
Infratrochlear nerve
Zygomaticofacial nerve
Greater occipital nerve
External nasal nerve
Occipital artery
Angular artery
Auriculotemporal nerve
Infraorbital nerve
Posterior auricular nerve
Masseter muscle
Posterior auricular artery
Facial nerve
Zygomaticus major muscle; facial artery
Lesser occipital nerve
Buccal artery
Trapezius muscle
Buccinator muscle
Masseteric nerve
Sternocleidomastoid muscle
Occipital artery
Buccal nerve
Ramus of mandible
Digastric branch, facial nerve
Mental nerve
Maxillary vein
Inferior alveolar nerve
Digastric muscle (posterior belly)
Inferior alveolar artery
Stylohyoid branch, facial nerve
Masseter muscle
Stylohyoid muscle
Facial artery
Internal carotid artery
External carotid artery
Lingual artery
Submental vein
Facial vein
Retromandibular vein   Internal jugular vein

Fig. 748: Vessels and Nerves of the Deep Face (Dissection 1)

NOTE: 1) the temporal fascia has been cut and partially reflected. The superficial muscles on the side of the face and the parotid gland have been removed. The main trunk of the facial nerve has been cut and its branches across the face removed. The masseter muscle was severed and reflected upward to show the masseteric artery and nerve.

   2) the following branches of the **trigeminal nerve:**
      a) **ophthalmic division:** supraorbital, supratrochlear, infratrochlear, and external nasal branches.
      b) **maxillary division:** zygomaticotemporal, zygomaticofacial, and infraorbital branches.
      c) **mandibular division:** auriculotemporal, masseteric, buccal, inferior alveolar, and mental branches.

   3) the posterior auricular, digastric, and stylohyoid branches of the facial nerve, which arise from the facial nerve trunk prior to its division within the parotid gland.

   4) the anastomosis of arteries above and at the medial aspect of the orbit. The vessels involved include the frontal branch of the superficial temporal, the supraorbital, supratrochlear and angular arteries and their branches.

Fig. 748

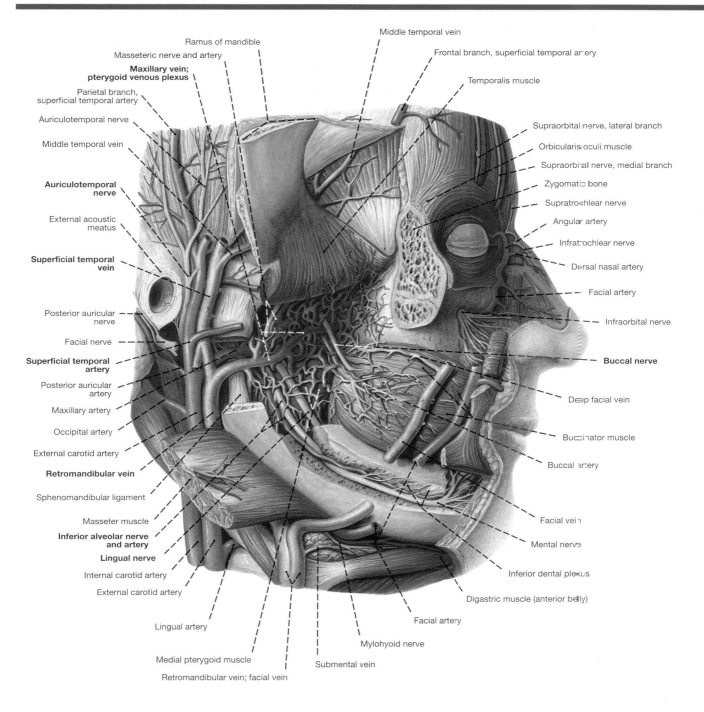

Middle temporal vein

Ramus of mandible

Masseteric nerve and artery

Frontal branch, superficial temporal artery

Maxillary vein; pterygoid venous plexus

Temporalis muscle

Parietal branch, superficial temporal artery

Supraorbital nerve, lateral branch

Auriculotemporal nerve

Orbicularis oculi muscle

Middle temporal vein

Supraorbital nerve, medial branch

Auriculotemporal nerve

Zygomatic bone

Supratrochlear nerve

External acoustic meatus

Angular artery

Infratrochlear nerve

Superficial temporal vein

Dorsal nasal artery

Facial artery

Posterior auricular nerve

Facial nerve

Infraorbital nerve

Superficial temporal artery

Buccal nerve

Posterior auricular artery

Maxillary artery

Deep facial vein

Occipital artery

Buccinator muscle

External carotid artery

Buccal artery

Retromandibular vein

Sphenomandibular ligament

Facial vein

Masseter muscle

Mental nerve

Inferior alveolar nerve and artery

Lingual nerve

Inferior dental plexus

Internal carotid artery

Digastric muscle (anterior belly)

External carotid artery

Lingual artery

Facial artery

Medial pterygoid muscle

Mylohyoid nerve

Retromandibular vein; facial vein

Submental vein

Fig. 749: Infratemporal Region of the Deep Face (Dissection 2)

NOTE: 1) the zygomatic arch has been cut and reflected upward along with the insertion of the temporalis muscle. A portion of the mandible has also been removed to show the course of the **maxillary vein** and **artery** deep to the mandible. The branches of the artery in the infratemporal region can better be seen in Figure 750.

2) the maxillary vein forms from the **pterygoid plexus** of veins which lies adjacent to the pterygoid muscles and which anastomoses with the facial vein by way of the **deep facial vein.** This plexus also anastomoses with the cavernous sinus through communicating veins in the foramen lacerum and foramen ovale and by way of the inferior ophthalmic vein.

3) the body of the mandible has been opened to expose the course of the inferior alveolar artery and nerve.

Fig. 749   **VII**

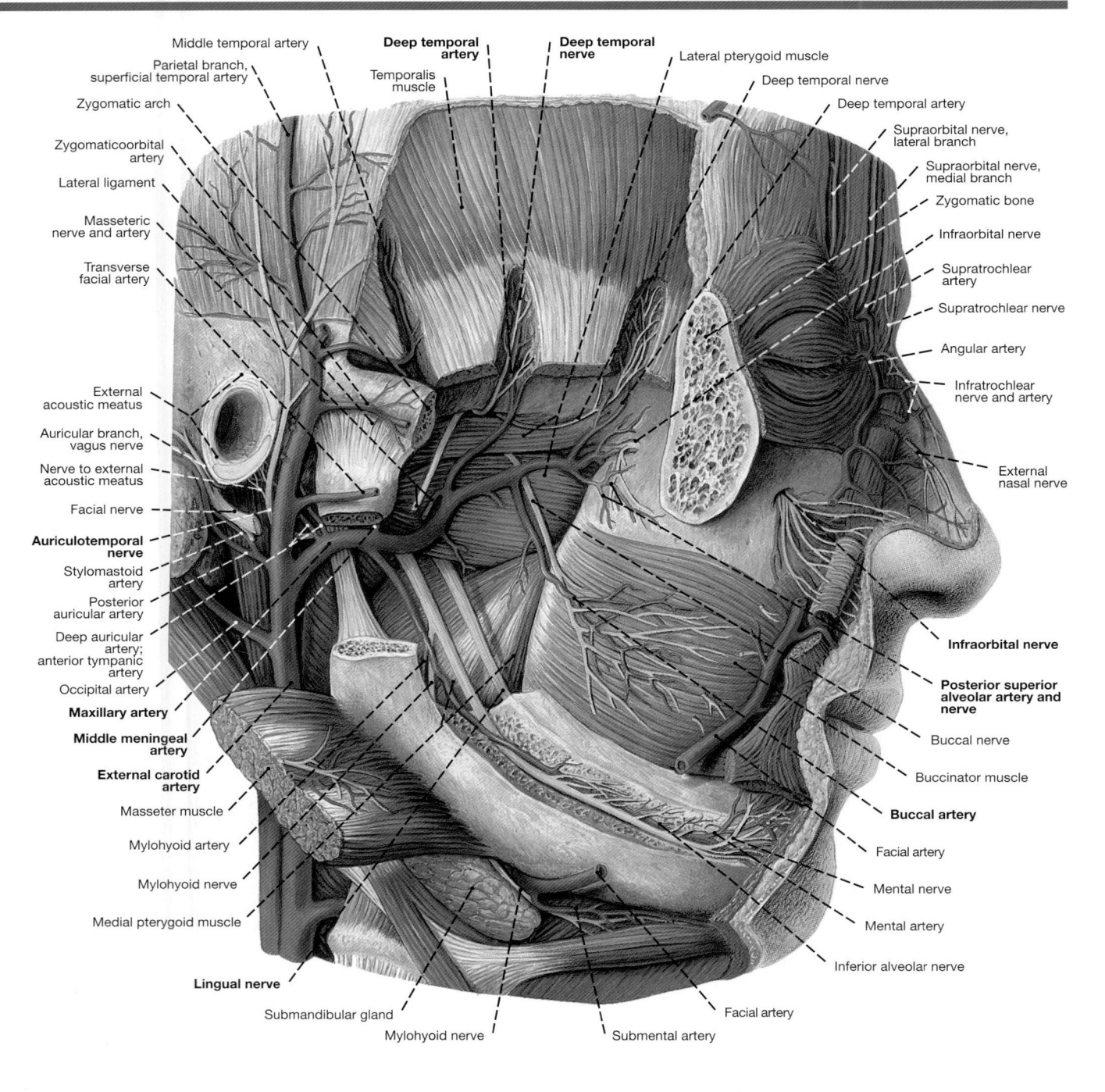

Fig. 750: Infratemporal Region of the Deep Face: Maxillary Artery (Dissection 3)

NOTE: 1) the **infratemporal fossa** has been opened from laterally to show the pterygoid muscles, the maxillary artery and its branches and some of the branches of the mandibular division of the trigeminal nerve.

2) in this dissection, the following branches of the **maxillary artery** are shown:

a) deep auricular, b) anterior tympanic, c) inferior alveolar, d) middle meningeal, e) masseteric (cut), f) deep temporal, g) pterygoid (not labelled), h) buccal, i) posterior superior alveolar, and j) infraorbital. **NOT** shown in this view are the greater palatine branch, the artery of the pterygoid canal, and the pharyngeal and sphenopalatine branches.

3) the following branches of the **mandibular division** of the **trigeminal nerve**:

a) auriculotemporal, b) lingual, c) inferior alveolar, d) mylohyoid, e) masseteric, and e) deep temporal. Observe the course of the inferior alveolar nerve, accompanied by the inferior alveolar artery within the mandible.

Fig. 750

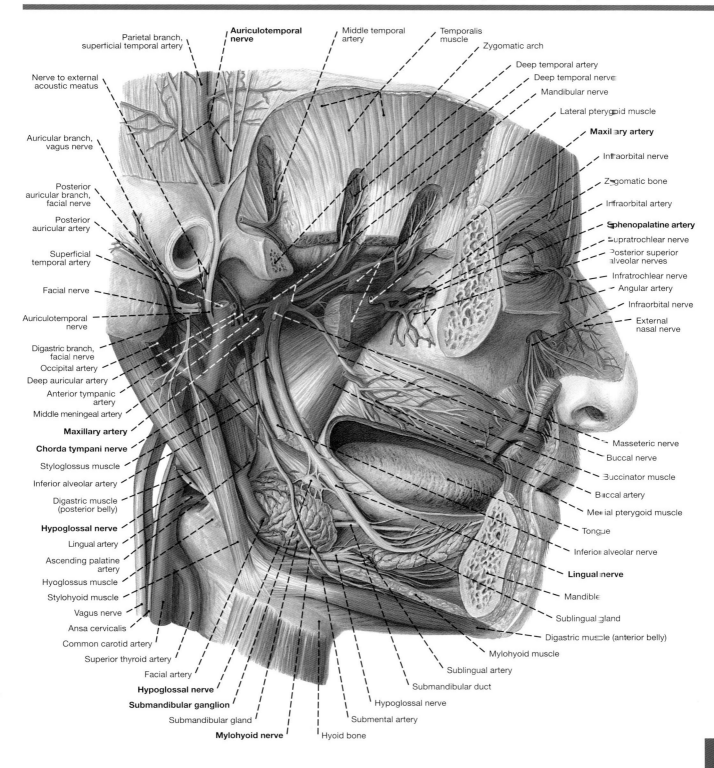

Parietal branch, superficial temporal artery

Auriculotemporal nerve

Middle temporal artery

Temporalis muscle

Zygomatic arch

Deep temporal artery

Deep temporal nerve

Mandibular nerve

Lateral pterygoid muscle

Maxillary artery

Infraorbital nerve

Zygomatic bone

Infraorbital artery

Sphenopalatine artery

Supratrochlear nerve

Posterior superior alveolar nerves

Infratrochlear nerve

Angular artery

Infraorbital nerve

External nasal nerve

Nerve to external acoustic meatus

Auricular branch, vagus nerve

Posterior auricular branch, facial nerve

Posterior auricular artery

Superficial temporal artery

Facial nerve

Auriculotemporal nerve

Digastric branch, facial nerve

Occipital artery

Deep auricular artery

Anterior tympanic artery

Middle meningeal artery

Maxillary artery

Chorda tympani nerve

Styloglossus muscle

Inferior alveolar artery

Digastric muscle (posterior belly)

Hypoglossal nerve

Lingual artery

Ascending palatine artery

Hyoglossus muscle

Stylohyoid muscle

Vagus nerve

Ansa cervicalis

Common carotid artery

Superior thyroid artery

Facial artery

Hypoglossal nerve

Submandibular ganglion

Submandibular gland

Mylohyoid nerve

Hyoid bone

Submental artery

Hypoglossal nerve

Submandibular duct

Sublingual artery

Mylohyoid muscle

Digastric muscle (anterior belly)

Sublingual gland

Mandible

Lingual nerve

Inferior alveolar nerve

Tongue

Medial pterygoid muscle

Buccal artery

Buccinator muscle

Buccal nerve

Masseteric nerve

Fig. 751: Infratemporal Region of the Deep Face: Mandibular Nerve Branches (Dissection 4)

NOTE: 1) the zygomatic arch, much of the right mandible and the lateral pterygoid muscle have been removed in this dissection. Also, a portion of the maxillary artery has been cut away along with the distal part of the inferior alveolar nerve beyond the point where the mylohyoid nerve branches.

2) the **lingual nerve** coursing to the tongue. High in the infratemporal fossa, the **chorda tympani nerve** (a branch of the facial) joins the lingual. The chorda tympani carries both special sensory **taste** fibers from the anterior two-thirds of the tongue and **preganglionic parasympathetic** fibers from the facial to the **submandibular ganglion.**

3) the distal part of the maxillary artery as it courses toward the sphenopalatine foramen. After giving off the infraorbital artery, the sphenopalatine branch enters the nasal cavity through the foramen and serves as the principal vessel to the nasal mucosa.

Fig. 751   **VII**

PLATE 480   Skull and Orbital Cavity: Anterior View

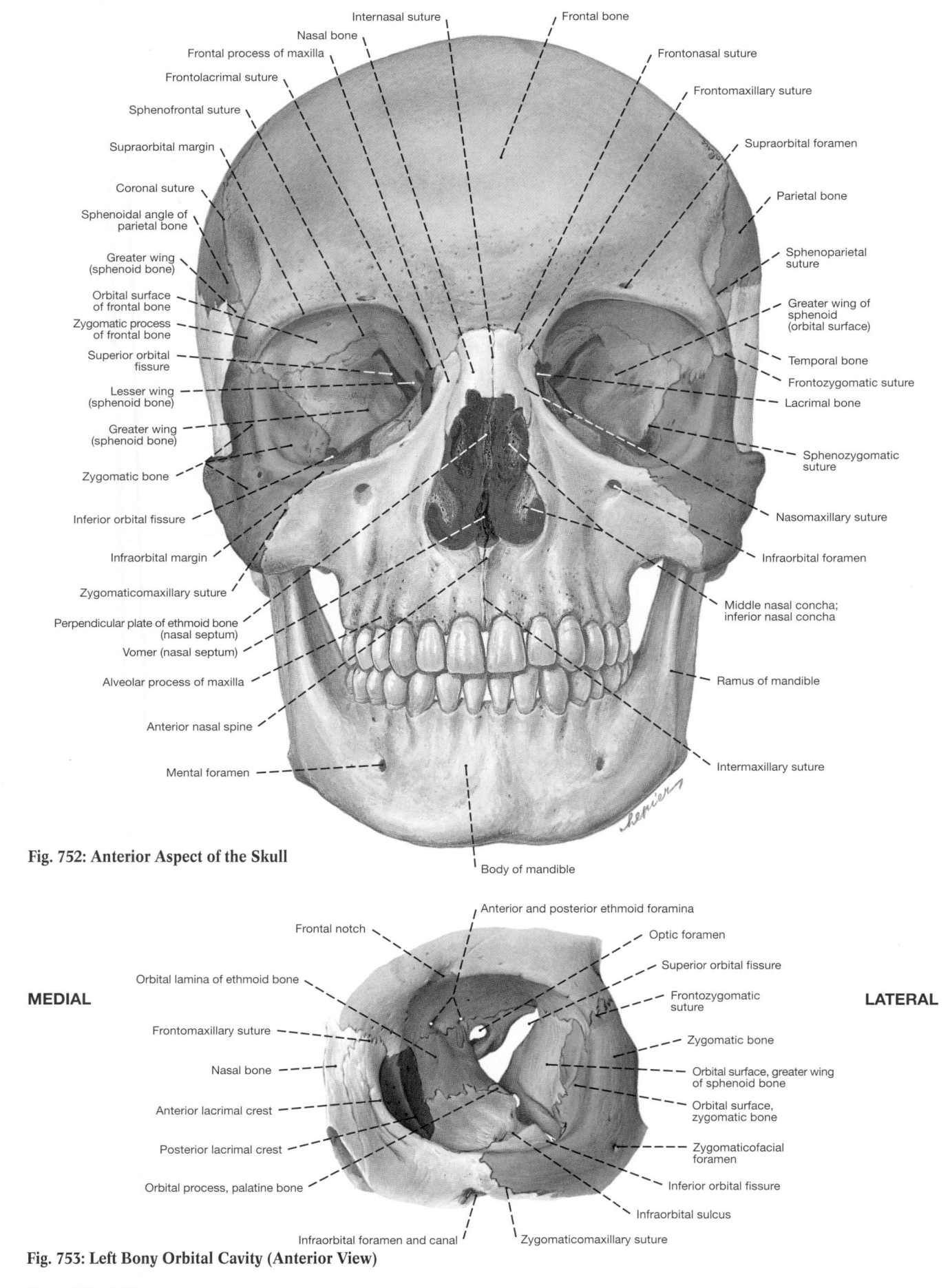

Internasal suture

Nasal bone

Frontal process of maxilla

Frontolacrimal suture

Sphenofrontal suture

Supraorbital margin

Coronal suture

Sphenoidal angle of parietal bone

Greater wing (sphenoid bone)

Orbital surface of frontal bone

Zygomatic process of frontal bone

Superior orbital fissure

Lesser wing (sphenoid bone)

Greater wing (sphenoid bone)

Zygomatic bone

Inferior orbital fissure

Infraorbital margin

Zygomaticomaxillary suture

Perpendicular plate of ethmoid bone (nasal septum)

Vomer (nasal septum)

Alveolar process of maxilla

Anterior nasal spine

Mental foramen

Frontal bone

Frontonasal suture

Frontomaxillary suture

Supraorbital foramen

Parietal bone

Sphenoparietal suture

Greater wing of sphenoid (orbital surface)

Temporal bone

Frontozygomatic suture

Lacrimal bone

Sphenozygomatic suture

Nasomaxillary suture

Infraorbital foramen

Middle nasal concha; inferior nasal concha

Ramus of mandible

Intermaxillary suture

Body of mandible

Fig. 752: Anterior Aspect of the Skull

Anterior and posterior ethmoid foramina

Frontal notch

Optic foramen

Orbital lamina of ethmoid bone

Superior orbital fissure

Frontozygomatic suture

MEDIAL

LATERAL

Frontomaxillary suture

Zygomatic bone

Nasal bone

Orbital surface, greater wing of sphenoid bone

Anterior lacrimal crest

Orbital surface, zygomatic bone

Posterior lacrimal crest

Zygomaticofacial foramen

Orbital process, palatine bone

Inferior orbital fissure

Infraorbital sulcus

Infraorbital foramen and canal

Zygomaticomaxillary suture

Fig. 753: Left Bony Orbital Cavity (Anterior View)

Figs. 752, 753

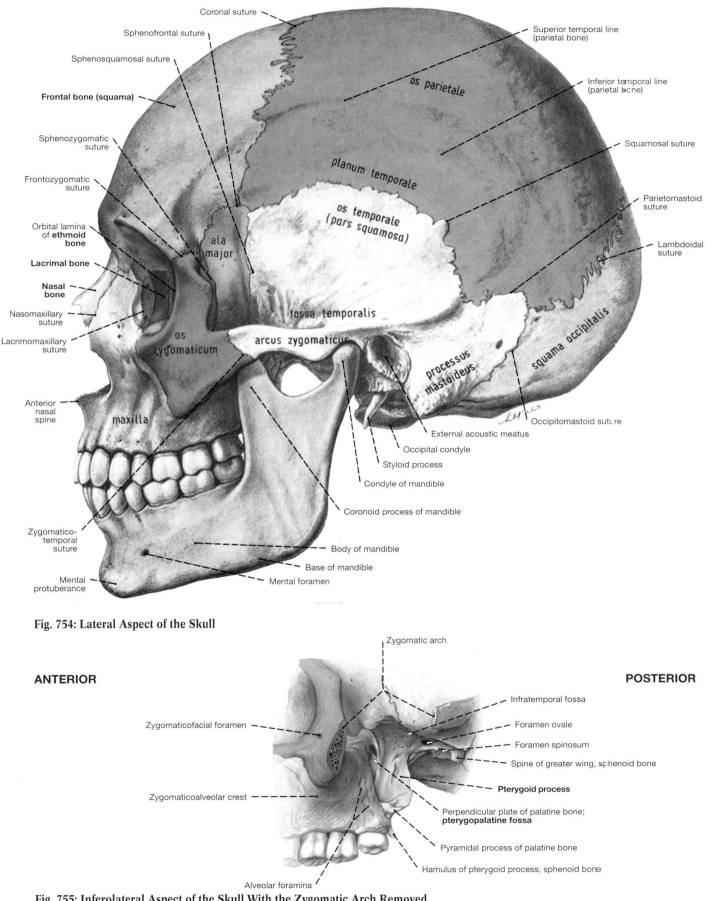

Coronal suture

Sphenofrontal suture

Sphenosquamosal suture

Frontal bone (squama)

Sphenozygomatic suture

Frontozygomatic suture

Orbital lamina of **ethmoid bone**

Lacrimal bone

Nasal bone

Nasomaxillary suture

Lacrimomaxillary suture

Anterior nasal spine

Zygomatico-temporal suture

Mental protuberance

Superior temporal line (parietal bone)

Inferior temporal line (parietal bone)

Squamosal suture

Parietomastoid suture

Lambdoidal suture

Occipitomastoid suture

External acoustic meatus

Occipital condyle

Styloid process

Condyle of mandible

Coronoid process of mandible

Body of mandible

Base of mandible

Mental foramen

os parietale

planum temporale

os temporale (pars squamosa)

fossa temporalis

arcus zygomaticus

processus mastoideus

squama occipitalis

ala major

os zygomaticum

maxilla

Fig. 754: Lateral Aspect of the Skull

ANTERIOR

POSTERIOR

Zygomatic arch

Zygomaticofacial foramen

Zygomaticoalveolar crest

Alveolar foramina

Infratemporal fossa

Foramen ovale

Foramen spinosum

Spine of greater wing, sphenoid bone

Pterygoid process

Perpendicular plate of palatine bone; **pterygopalatine fossa**

Pyramidal process of palatine bone

Hamulus of pterygoid process, sphenoid bone

Fig. 755: Inferolateral Aspect of the Skull With the Zygomatic Arch Removed
NOTE: the pterygopalatine fossa and the pterygoid process of the sphenoid bone.

PLATE 482   **Calvaria From Above; the Occipital Bone, Posterior View**

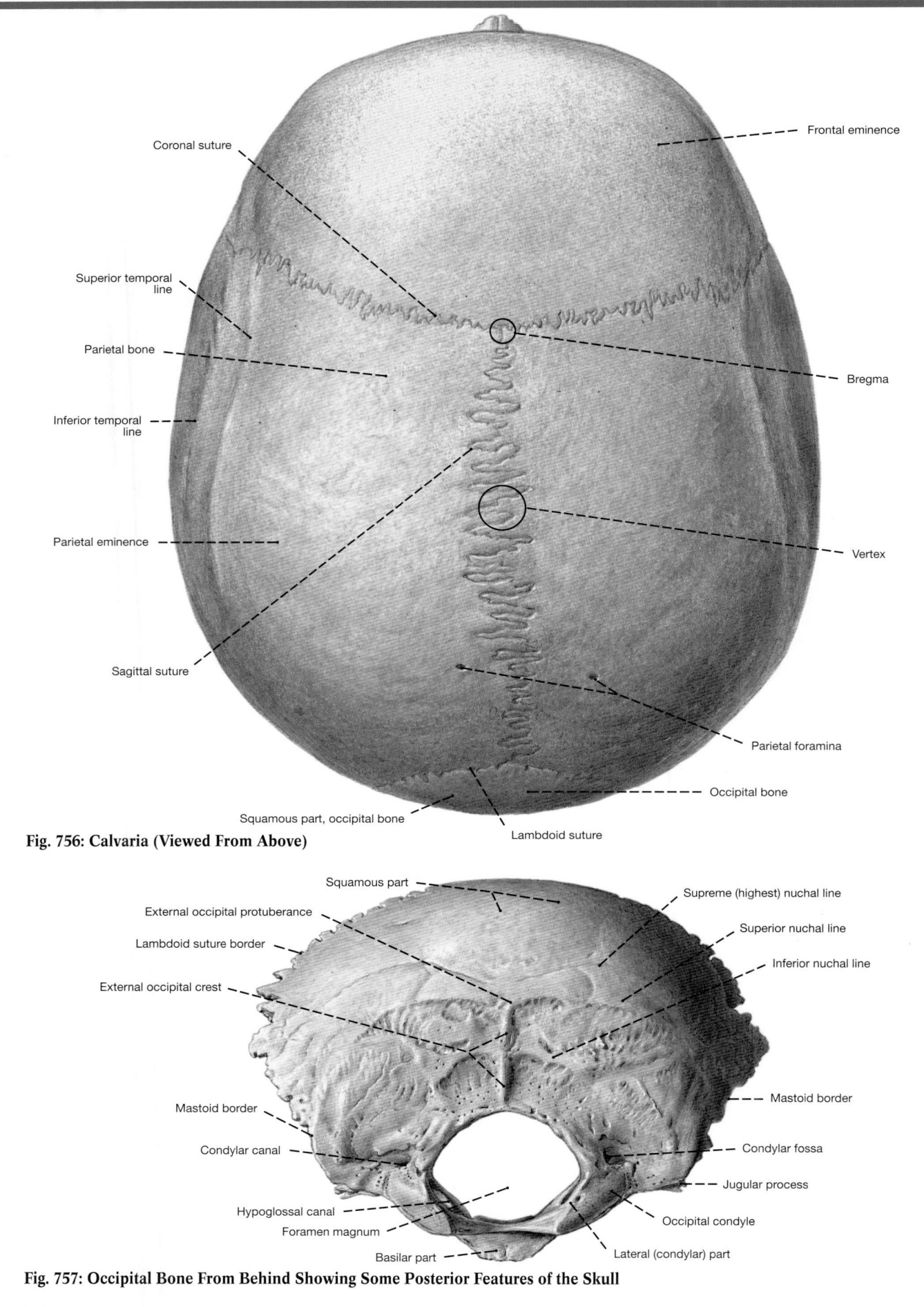

Coronal suture

Frontal eminence

Superior temporal line

Parietal bone

Bregma

Inferior temporal line

Parietal eminence

Vertex

Sagittal suture

Parietal foramina

Occipital bone

Squamous part, occipital bone

Lambdoid suture

Fig. 756: Calvaria (Viewed From Above)

Squamous part

Supreme (highest) nuchal line

External occipital protuberance

Superior nuchal line

Lambdoid suture border

Inferior nuchal line

External occipital crest

Mastoid border

Condylar fossa

Mastoid border

Jugular process

Condylar canal

Hypoglossal canal

Occipital condyle

Foramen magnum

Lateral (condylar) part

Basilar part

Fig. 757: Occipital Bone From Behind Showing Some Posterior Features of the Skull

Figs. 756, 757

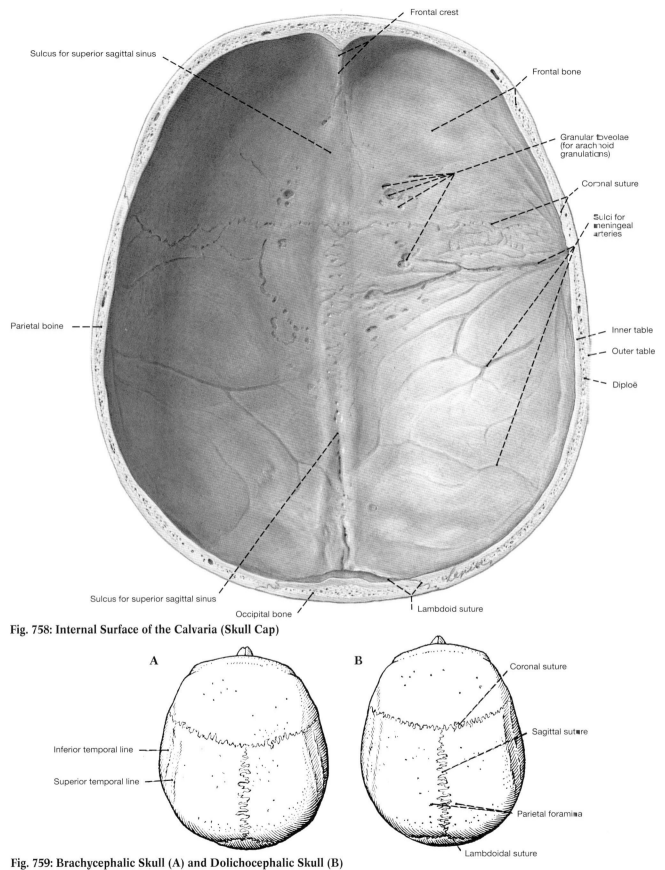

Frontal crest

Sulcus for superior sagittal sinus

Frontal bone

Granular foveolae (for arachnoid granulations)

Coronal suture

Sulci for meningeal arteries

Parietal boine

Inner table

Outer table

Diploë

Sulcus for superior sagittal sinus

Occipital bone

Lambdoid suture

Fig. 758: Internal Surface of the Calvaria (Skull Cap)

A

B

Coronal suture

Sagittal suture

Inferior temporal line

Superior temporal line

Parietal foramina

Lambdoidal suture

Fig. 759: Brachycephalic Skull (A) and Dolichocephalic Skull (B)
NOTE: skulls are classified by comparing their width to length. When the greatest width exceeds 80% of the length, the skull is more round and called **brachycephalic (A).** When the width is less than 75% of length, the more oblong skull is called **dolichocephalic (B).** When the comparison is between 75% and 80%, the skull is classified as **mesaticephalic.**

PLATE 484   Newborn Skull: Anterior and Lateral Views

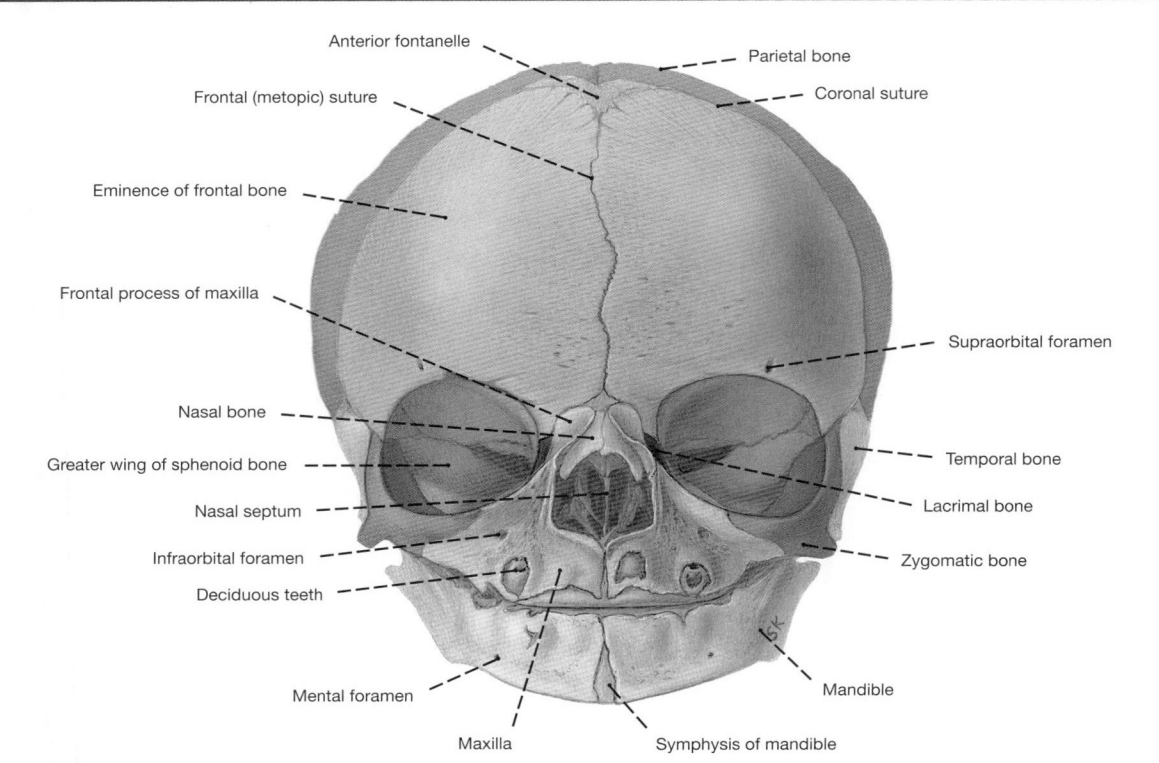

Anterior fontanelle
Parietal bone
Frontal (metopic) suture
Coronal suture
Eminence of frontal bone
Frontal process of maxilla
Supraorbital foramen
Nasal bone
Greater wing of sphenoid bone
Temporal bone
Nasal septum
Lacrimal bone
Infraorbital foramen
Zygomatic bone
Deciduous teeth
Mental foramen
Mandible
Maxilla
Symphysis of mandible

Fig. 760: Skull at Birth (Frontal View)

NOTE: 1)   the bones that enclose the cranial cavity (neurocranium) include the **frontal, parietal, occipital, temporal** and **sphenoid bones** and the **cribriform plate** of the **ethmoid bone.**

2)   the bones that form the face and hard palate and enclose the nasal cavity are the **mandible, maxilla, zygomatic, lacrimal, nasal** and **palatine bones,** the **inferior concha,** most of the **ethmoid bone** and the **vomer.**

3)   the skull at birth is large in comparison to the size of the rest of the body because of the precocious growth of the brain, the facial bones, however, are still not well developed.

4)   the maxilla and mandible are rudimentary at birth and the teeth have yet to erupt. Additionally, the maxillary sinuses and nasal cavity are small as are the frontal, ethmoid and sphenoid sinuses.

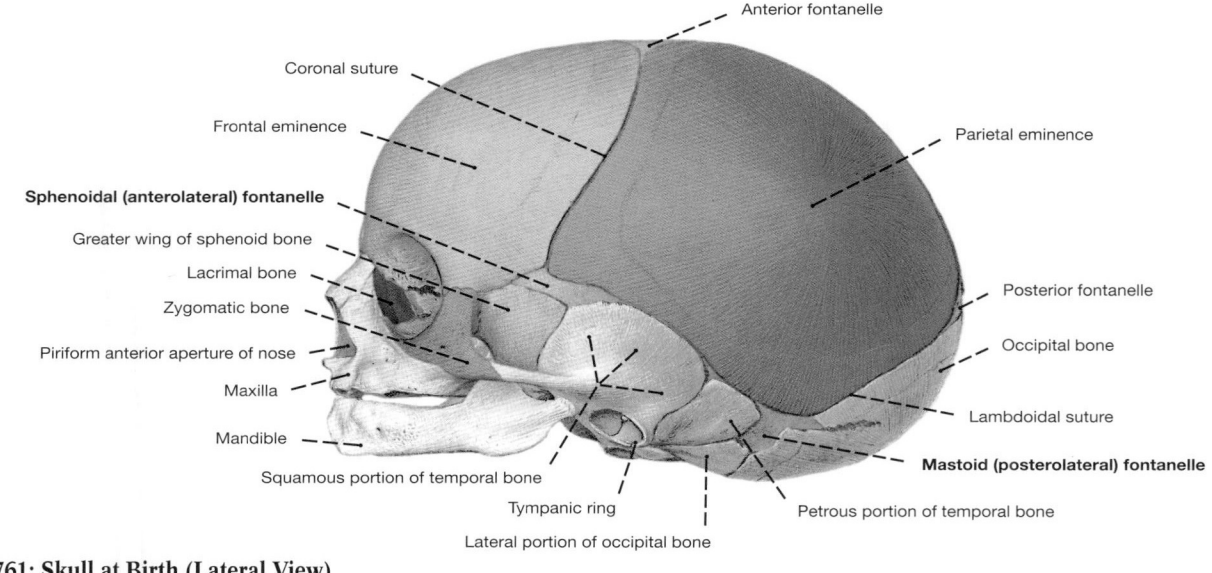

Anterior fontanelle
Coronal suture
Frontal eminence
Parietal eminence
Sphenoidal (anterolateral) fontanelle
Greater wing of sphenoid bone
Lacrimal bone
Zygomatic bone
Posterior fontanelle
Piriform anterior aperture of nose
Occipital bone
Maxilla
Lambdoidal suture
Mandible
Mastoid (posterolateral) fontanelle
Squamous portion of temporal bone
Tympanic ring
Petrous portion of temporal bone
Lateral portion of occipital bone

Fig. 761: Skull at Birth (Lateral View)

NOTE: 1)   ossification of the maturing *flat bones of the skull* is accomplished by the intramembranous process of bone formation. At birth this process is incomplete, thereby leaving soft membranous sites between the growing bones. Bones forming the base of the cranial cavity develop by ossification in cartilage.

2)   the incompletely ossified nature of the skull just prior to birth is of some benefit, however, since the mobility of the bones permits changes in skull shape, as may be required during the birth process.

3)   the **sphenoidal** (or anterolateral) fontanelle located at the pterion and the **mastoid** (or posterolateral) found at the asterion.

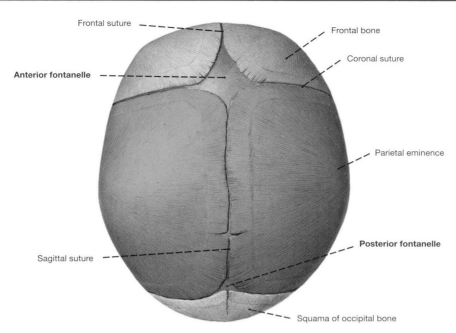

Frontal suture
Frontal bone
Anterior fontanelle
Coronal suture
Parietal eminence
Posterior fontanelle
Sagittal suture
Squama of occipital bone

Fig. 762: Skull at Birth (Seen from Above)

NOTE: 1)   the soft sites on the skull of the newborn infant are called **fontanelles.** From this superior view can be seen the **anterior** and **posterior fontanelles.**

2)   the largest of the fontanelles at birth is the **anterior fontanelle** located at the bregma and interconnecting the frontal and parietal bones. It is approximately diamond shaped and is situated at the junction of the coronal and sagittal sutures.

3)   by following the sagittal suture to its junction with the occipital bone will locate the **posterior fontanelle** (at the lambda). This is generally triangular in shape and is small at birth.

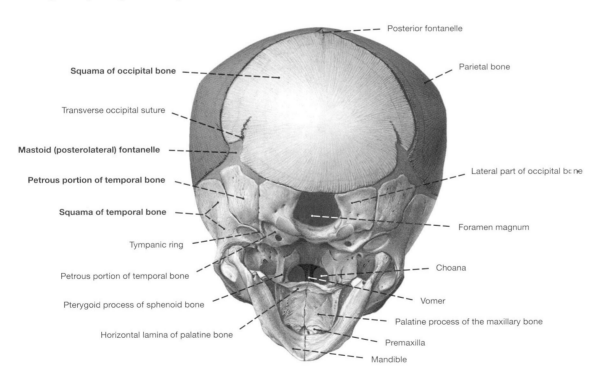

Posterior fontanelle
Squama of occipital bone
Parietal bone
Transverse occipital suture
Mastoid (posterolateral) fontanelle
Petrous portion of temporal bone
Lateral part of occipital bone
Squama of temporal bone
Foramen magnum
Tympanic ring
Petrous portion of temporal bone
Choana
Pterygoid process of sphenoid bone
Vomer
Horizontal lamina of palatine bone
Palatine process of the maxillary bone
Premaxilla
Mandible

Fig. 763: Skull at Birth (Posterior-Inferior View)

NOTE: 1)   the separate ossification of the petrous and squamous portions of the temporal bone as well as the basilar and squamous parts of the occipital bone.

2)   the **mastoid** (posterolateral) **fontanelles** are found at the articulation of the occipital, temporal, and parietal bones.

3)   growth and ossification of the bones that encase the brain are more precocious than the bones that form the facial skeleton. Facial bones continue growth through puberty. This differential accounts for the marked differences in facial features seen in a 4- or 5-year-old child with that same person at 15 or 16 years of age.

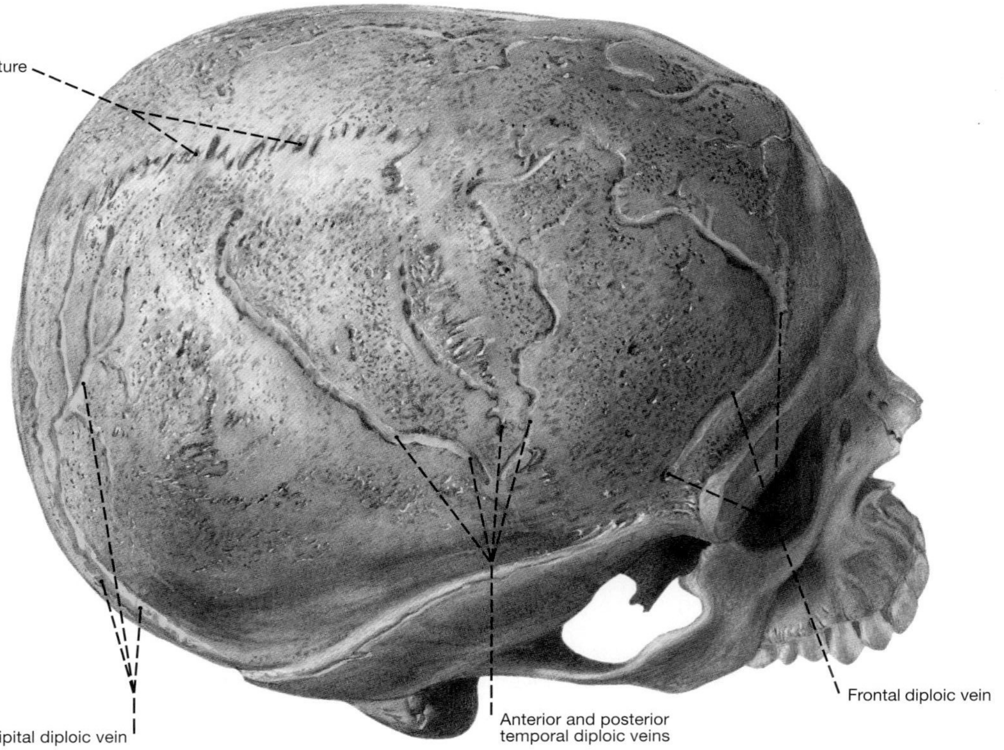

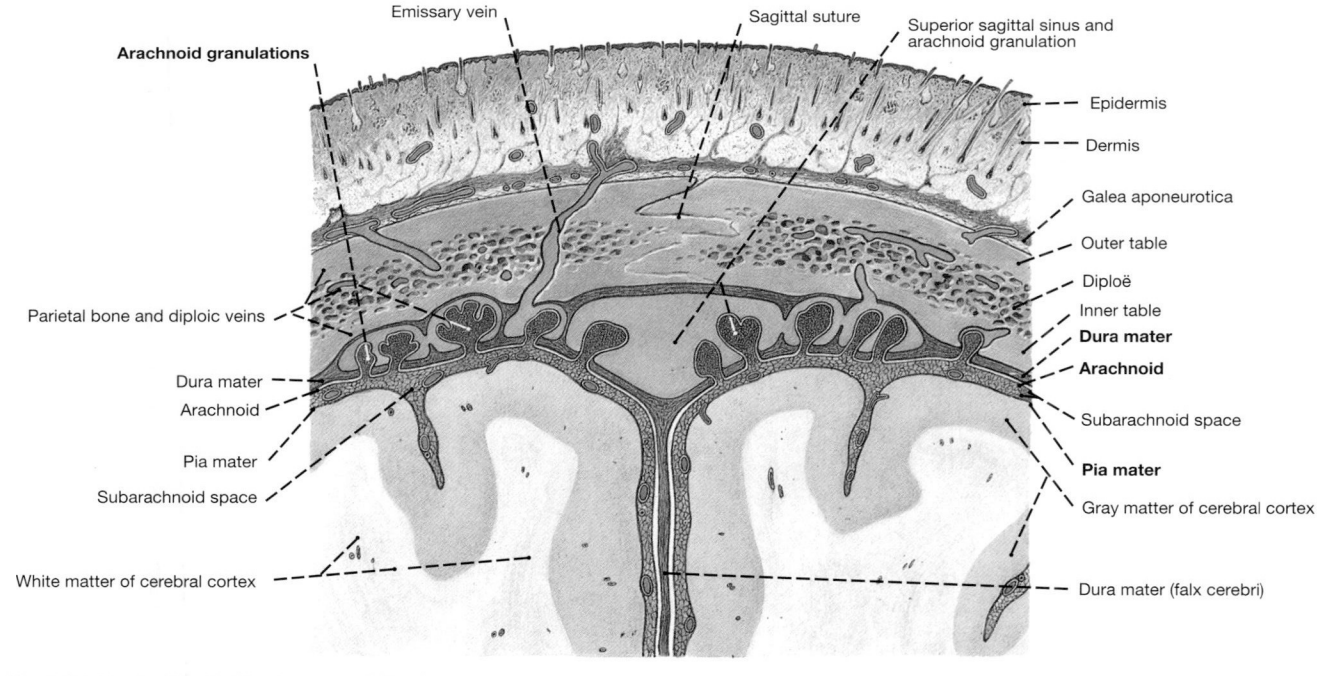

Sagittal suture

Occipital diploic vein

Anterior and posterior
temporal diploic veins

Frontal diploic vein

Fig. 764: Diploic Veins

NOTE: 1)   by removal of the outermost table of compact bone, a more spongy layer of bone is encountered. Within this latter layer course venous channels called the **diploic veins.** These veins communicate with the scalp on the exterior and the dural sinuses within the skull.

  2)   the diploic veins are named according to their location: **frontal, temporal,** and **occipital.**

Emissary vein

Arachnoid granulations

Sagittal suture

Superior sagittal sinus and
arachnoid granulation

Epidermis

Dermis

Galea aponeurotica

Outer table

Diploë

Inner table

Dura mater

Arachnoid

Parietal bone and diploic veins

Dura mater

Arachnoid

Pia mater

Subarachnoid space

Subarachnoid space

Pia mater

Gray matter of cerebral cortex

White matter of cerebral cortex

Dura mater (falx cerebri)

Fig. 765: Scalp, Skull, Meninges and Brain

NOTE: 1)   this is a frontal section through the cranium and upper cerebrum and shows the bony and soft coverings of the brain. The veins and dural sinuses are colored in blue while the bone is light brown.

  2)   superficial to the dura mater, arachnoid and pia mater which encase the neural tissue of the brain are found the bony skull and the layers of the scalp.

  3)   the **arachnoid granulations.** Tufts of arachnoid (sometime called arachnoid villi) lie next to the endothelium of the sinuses and allow passage of the cerebrospinal fluid from the subarachnoid space into the venous system.

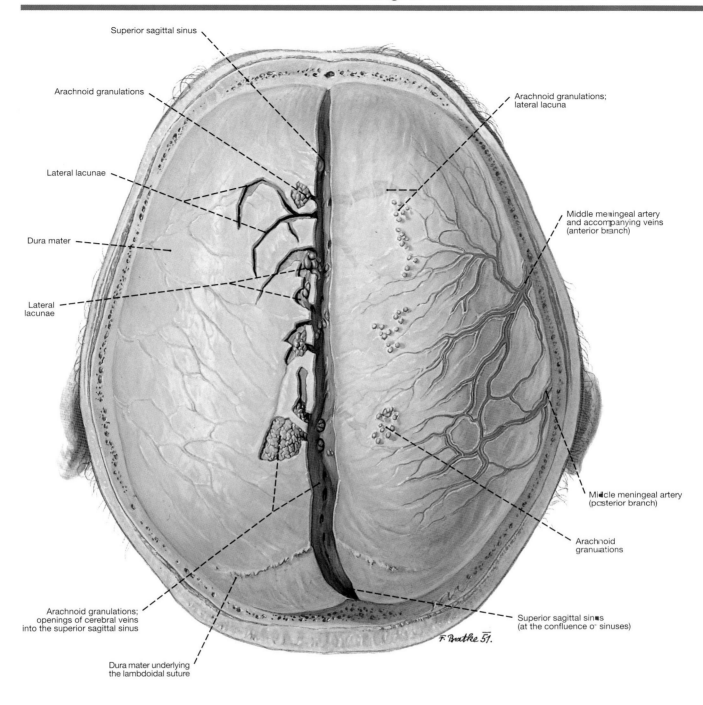

Superior sagittal sinus

Arachnoid granulations

Lateral lacunae

Dura mater

Lateral lacunae

Arachnoid granulations; openings of cerebral veins into the superior sagittal sinus

Dura mater underlying the lambdoidal suture

Arachnoid granulations; lateral lacuna

Middle meningeal artery and accompanying veins (anterior branch)

Middle meningeal artery (posterior branch)

Arachnoid granulations

Superior sagittal sinus (at the confluence of sinuses)

F. Batke 51.

Fig. 766: Surface of the Dura Mater with the Superior Sagittal Sinus Opened; Viewed From Above

NOTE: 1)   the skull cap (also called **calvaria**) has been removed, leaving the **dura mater** intact. The dura is a two-layered structure (an inner **meningeal layer** and an outer **periosteal layer**), but these layers are inseparably fused throughout much of their expanse. In this dissection the "two layers" were stripped from the skull as a single membrane.

2)   in some regions the meningeal and periosteal layers are separated to form the cavities for the **venous sinuses** in the dura mater. In this dissection the longitudinally oriented **superior sagittal sinus** has been opened as have a number of lateral venous lacunae that communicate with this sinus.

3)   the **arachnoid granulations.** These are elevated bulbous protrusions of the arachnoid into the dura mater and, since they grow in size from infancy through childhood, they eventually form pits on the inner surface of the skull (see Fig. 758).

4)   the projections from the arachnoid are called **archnoid villi** and appear as diverticula of the subarachnoid space into the venous sinuses. Cerebrospinal fluid passes from the subarachnoid space through the arachnoid villi into the venous blood of the dural sinus (see also Fig. 765).

Fig. 766   **VII**

PLATE 488   **Dura Mater and Dural Venous Sinuses, Lateral View**

x = Pituitary gland
+ = Optic nerve
✳ = Internal carotid artery

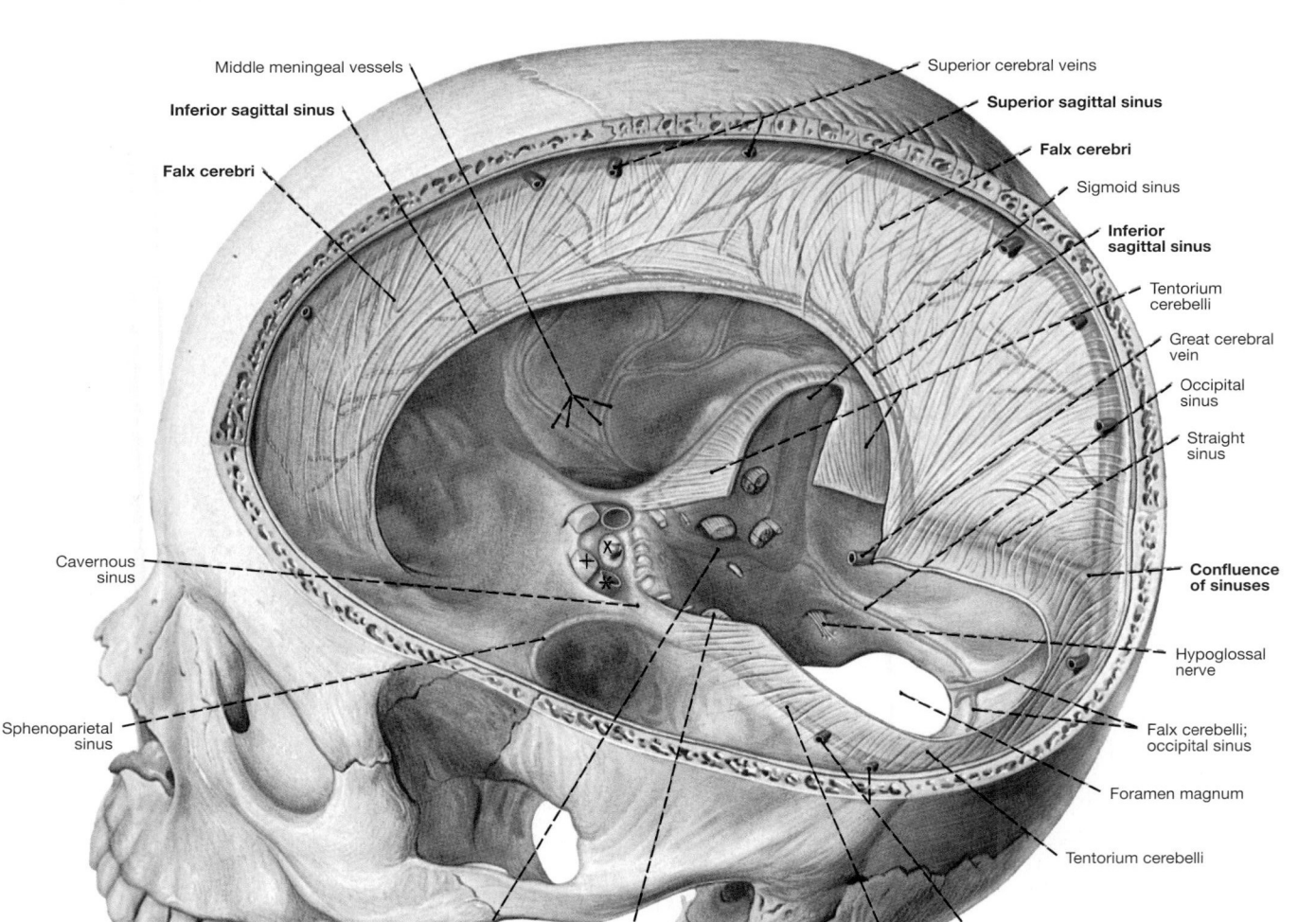

Middle meningeal vessels

Inferior sagittal sinus

Falx cerebri

Superior cerebral veins

Superior sagittal sinus

Falx cerebri

Sigmoid sinus

Inferior sagittal sinus

Tentorium cerebelli

Great cerebral vein

Occipital sinus

Straight sinus

Cavernous sinus

Confluence of sinuses

Hypoglossal nerve

Sphenoparietal sinus

Falx cerebelli; occipital sinus

Foramen magnum

Tentorium cerebelli

Inferior cerebral veins

Inferior petrosal sinus   Trigeminal nerve   Superior petrosal sinus

Fig. 767: Intracranial Dura Mater and the Dural Sinuses

NOTE: 1) with the skull opened and the brain removed, the reflections of the dura mater are exposed. The sinuses are colored blue, the arteries red. Most of the left **tentorium cerebelli** and part of the right were cut away to open the posterior cranial fossa.

2) the five **unpaired sinuses:** the **superior** and **inferior sagittal sinuses** and the **straight sinus.** Two other unpaired sinuses (not labelled) at the base of the skull are the **intercavernous** and **basilar sinuses.** These can be seen in Figure 768.

3) the seven **paired sinuses:** transverse sinus, **sigmoid sinus, occipital sinus, superior** and **inferior petrosal sinuses, cavernous sinus** and the **sphenoparietal sinus.** The dural sinuses consist of spaces between the two layers of dura, which drain the cerebral blood, returning it to the **internal jugular vein.**

4) the *sphenoparietal sinuses* course near the posterior margin of the lesser wings of the sphenoid bone and help form the boundary between the anterior and middle cranial fossae. Similarly, the *superior petrosal sinuses* course along the superior margins of the petrous parts of the temporal bone at the boundary between the middle and posterior cranial fossae.

5) the sickle-shaped **falx cerebri.** This double-layered, midline reflection of dura mater extends from the crista galli anteriorly to the tentorium cerebelli posteriorly. It also extends vertically between the two cerebral hemispheres. Within the layers of the falx, observe the *superior* and *inferior sagittal sinuses* and the *straight sinus,* all of which flow into the *transverse sinus* or the *confluence of sinuses.*

6) the **tentorium cerebelli** is a tent-like reflection of dura mater which forms a partition between the occipital lobes of the cerebral cortex and the cerebellum. The **falx cerebelli** extends vertically between the two cerebellar hemispheres.

Fig. 767

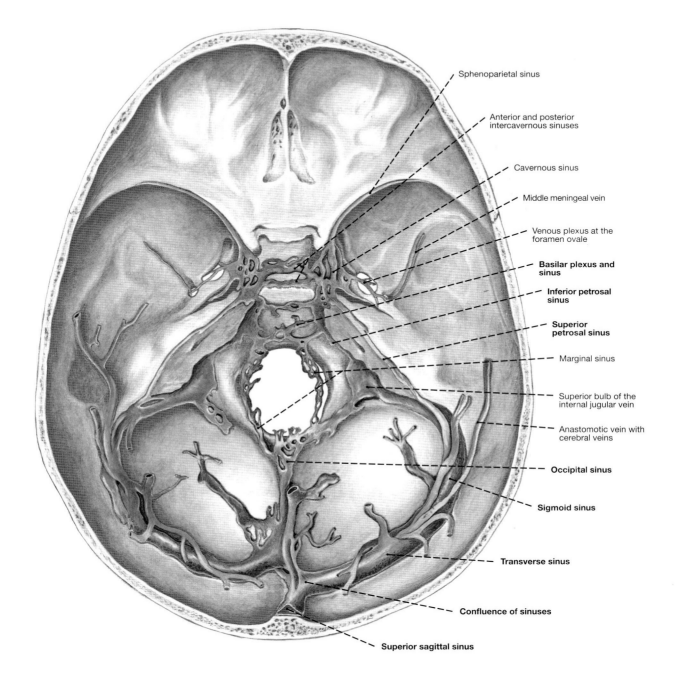

Sphenoparietal sinus

Anterior and posterior intercavernous sinuses

Cavernous sinus

Middle meningeal vein

Venous plexus at the foramen ovale

Basilar plexus and sinus

Inferior petrosal sinus

Superior petrosal sinus

Marginal sinus

Superior bulb of the internal jugular vein

Anastomotic vein with cerebral veins

Occipital sinus

Sigmoid sinus

Transverse sinus

Confluence of sinuses

Superior sagittal sinus

Fig. 768: Dural Sinuses at the Base of the Cranial Cavity Seen From Above
NOTE: 1) the falx cerebri and the tentorium cerebelli and other dural reflections at the base of the cranial cavity have been removed to expose the venous sinuses from above.

2) on both sides, the **transverse sinus** courses laterally from the **confluence of sinuses** and then continues as the **sigmoid sinus.** Just above the jugular foramen, the sigmoid sinus enlarges as the **superior bulb of the internal jugular vein.** Below the jugular foramen it becomes the **internal jugular vein** (see Fig. 747).

3) venous blood also flows to the transverse-sigmoid sinus from the **occipital sinus** and the **superior** and **inferior petrosal sinuses.** Additionally, the **cavernous, intercavernous** and **basilar sinuses** adjacent to the body of the sphenoid bone and the basilar part of the occipital bone also drain posteriorly and laterally into the sigmoid sinus at the jugular foramen.

4) anastomoses between these internal sinuses and the external veins occur through the various foramina, such as the superior orbital fissure (with the ophthalmic veins) and through the foramen lacerum and the foramen ovale (with the pterygoid plexus of veins). Other anastomoses occur with the cerebral veins, the meningeal veins and emissary veins.

Fig. 768   **VII**

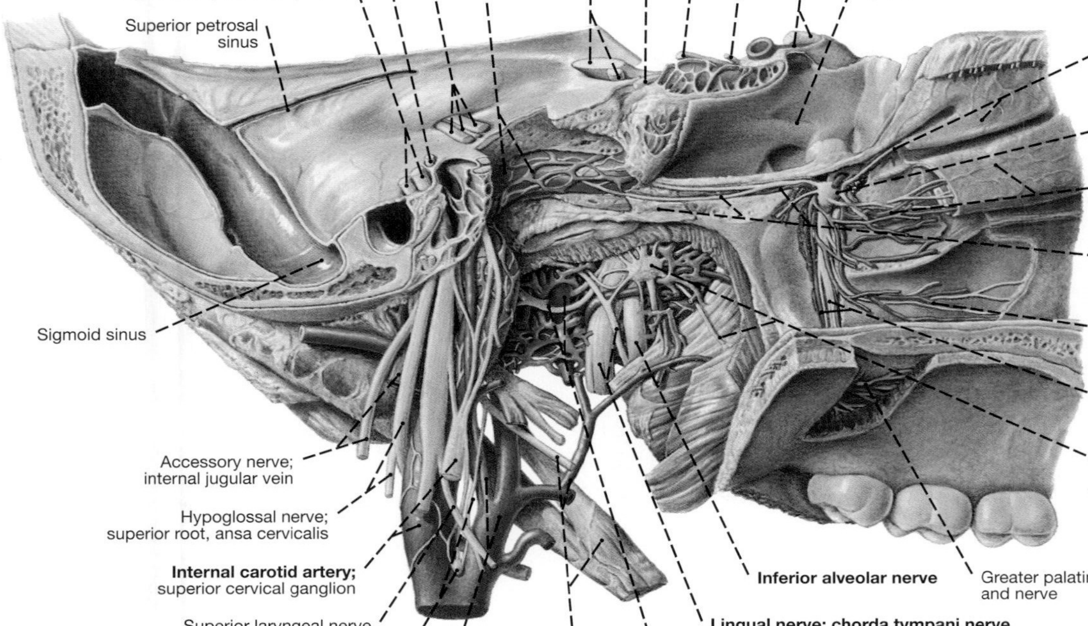

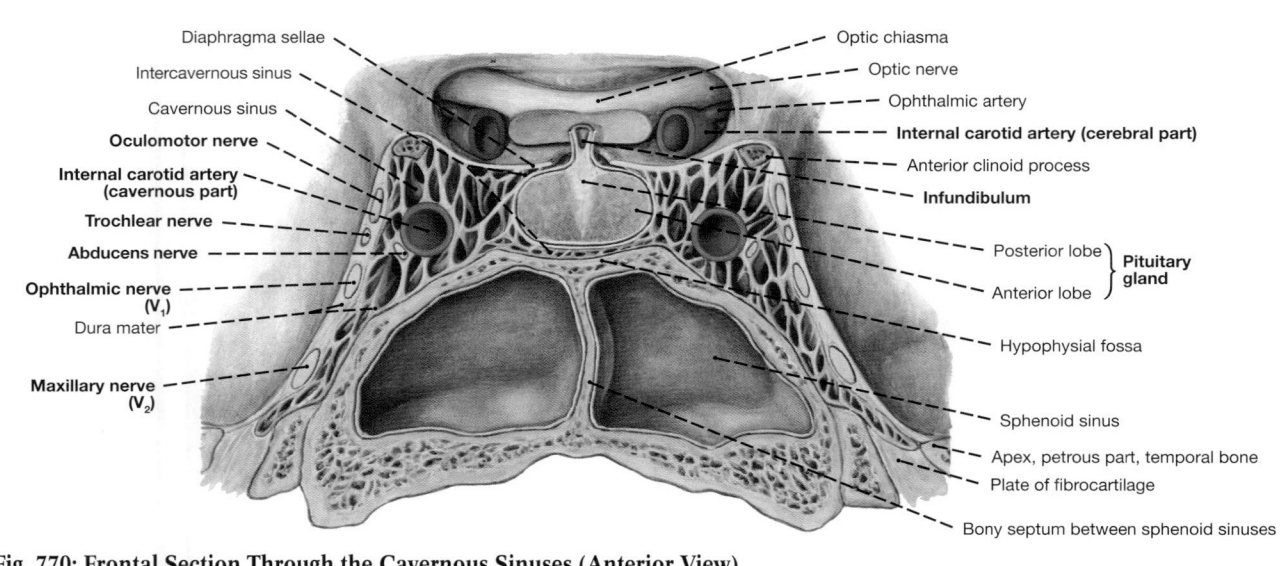

Internal carotid artery; internal carotid plexus

Vestibulocochlear nerve; facial nerve

Glossopharyngeal nerve

Vagus nerve; accessory nerve

Superior petrosal sinus

Trigeminal nerve

Abducens nerve

Oculomotor nerve

Trochlear nerve

Ophthalmic artery; optic nerve

Sphenoid sinus

Superior nasal concha; posterior superior lateral nasal nerve

Pterygopalatine ganglion

Middle nasal concha; posterior superior lateral nasal vessels

Artery and nerve of pterygoid canal; plate of fibrocartilage

Posterior inferior lateral nasal vessels and nerves

Descending palatine vessels and nerves

Otic ganglion; nerve to tensor veli palatini muscle

Sigmoid sinus

Accessory nerve; internal jugular vein

Hypoglossal nerve; superior root, ansa cervicalis

Internal carotid artery; superior cervical ganglion

Superior laryngeal nerve

Carotid body and nerve

External carotid artery; ascending pharyngeal artery

Inferior alveolar nerve

Greater palatine vessels and nerve

Lingual nerve; chorda tympani nerve

Middle meningeal artery; auriculotemporal nerve

Stylohyoid muscle; glossopharyngeal nerve; ascending palatine artery

Fig. 769: Internal Carotid Artery: Petrous and Cavernous Parts

NOTE: 1)   in this preparation the skull was initially bisected and the **medial surface** of the **left half** dissected. The carotid canal in the petrous part of the temporal bone has been opened to show the ascent of the internal carotid artery.

    2)   the **petrous part** of the internal carotid artery at first ascends vertically in the carotid canal and then it curves forward and medially. Upon leaving the carotid canal it continues medially across the foramen lacerum where it overlies the fibrocartilaginous plate of that foramen. It then curves on itself in an S-shaped manner within the cavernous sinus which it leaves to open at the base of the skull (see Figs. 771, 773).

    3)   the pterygopalatine fossa has been approached from its medial side and the greater palatine canal to the oral cavity opened. Note also the otic ganglion, branches of the mandibular nerve and the chorda tympani nerve exposed in the infratemporal fossa.

Diaphragma sellae

Intercavernous sinus

Cavernous sinus

Oculomotor nerve

Internal carotid artery (cavernous part)

Trochlear nerve

Abducens nerve

Ophthalmic nerve (V₁)

Dura mater

Maxillary nerve (V₂)

Optic chiasma

Optic nerve

Ophthalmic artery

Internal carotid artery (cerebral part)

Anterior clinoid process

Infundibulum

Posterior lobe ⎫ Pituitary
Anterior lobe ⎭ gland

Hypophysial fossa

Sphenoid sinus

Apex, petrous part, temporal bone

Plate of fibrocartilage

Bony septum between sphenoid sinuses

Fig. 770: Frontal Section Through the Cavernous Sinuses (Anterior View)

NOTE: the internal carotid artery (which is seen to have turned back on itself above) and the oculomotor, trochlear, V_1, V_2, and abducens nerves traverse the cavernous sinus.

Figs. 769, 770

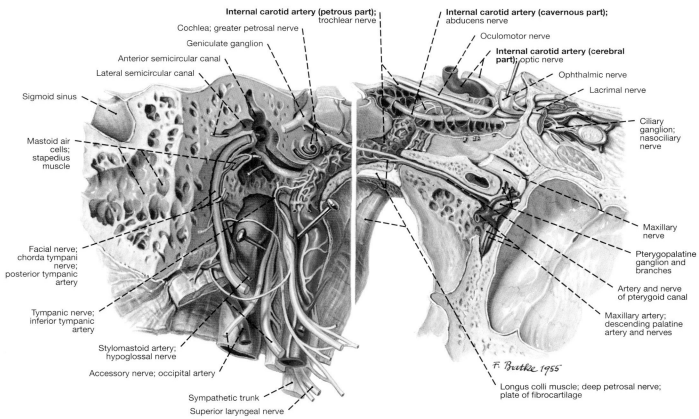

Internal carotid artery (petrous part);
trochlear nerve

Cochlea; greater petrosal nerve

Geniculate ganglion

Anterior semicircular canal

Lateral semicircular canal

Sigmoid sinus

Mastoid air
cells;
stapedius
muscle

Facial nerve;
chorda tympani
nerve;
posterior tympanic
artery

Tympanic nerve;
inferior tympanic
artery

Stylomastoid artery;
hypoglossal nerve

Accessory nerve; occipital artery

Sympathetic trunk

Superior laryngeal nerve

Internal carotid artery (cavernous part);
abducens nerve

Oculomotor nerve

Internal carotid artery (cerebral
part); optic nerve

Ophthalmic nerve

Lacrimal nerve

Ciliary
ganglion;
nasociliary
nerve

Maxillary
nerve

Pterygopalatine
ganglion and
branches

Artery and nerve
of pterygoid canal

Maxillary artery;
descending palatine
artery and nerves

Longus colli muscle; deep petrosal nerve;
plate of fibrocartilage

F. Batke 1955

Fig. 771: Internal Carotid Artery: Petrous and Cavernous Parts

NOTE: 1) in this dissection the **right** temporal bone has been opened and this lateral view shows a vertical section along the superior margin of that bone. The carotid and facial canals have been opened along with the internal ear. More anteriorly, the section goes through the sphenoid bone, opening its pterygoid canal and meeting the petrous section in a V-shaped manner.

2) surrounded by a plexus of veins and sympathetic fibers, the **cavernous part** of the artery ascends into the cavernous sinus and curves forward in the carotid sulcus along the side of the body of the sphenoid bone. It then curves upward to perforate the dura mater just lateral to the optic nerve where this **cerebral part** divides into its terminal branches.

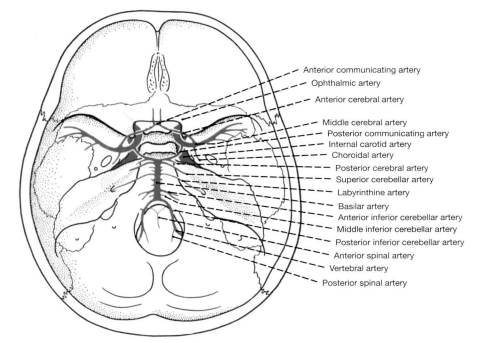

Anterior communicating artery

Ophthalmic artery

Anterior cerebral artery

Middle cerebral artery

Posterior communicating artery

Internal carotid artery

Choroidal artery

Posterior cerebral artery

Superior cerebellar artery

Labyrinthine artery

Basilar artery

Anterior inferior cerebellar artery

Middle inferior cerebellar artery

Posterior inferior cerebellar artery

Anterior spinal artery

Vertebral artery

Posterior spinal artery

Fig. 772: Cerebral Part of the Internal Carotid Artery and Other Vessels at Base of Brain

NOTE: the two internal carotid arteries (cerebral parts) and the basilar artery (formed by the two vertebral arteries) give rise to all the **named vessels** in this figure (see also Fig. 775).

PLATE 492   Base of the Cranial Cavity: Blood Vessels and Nerves

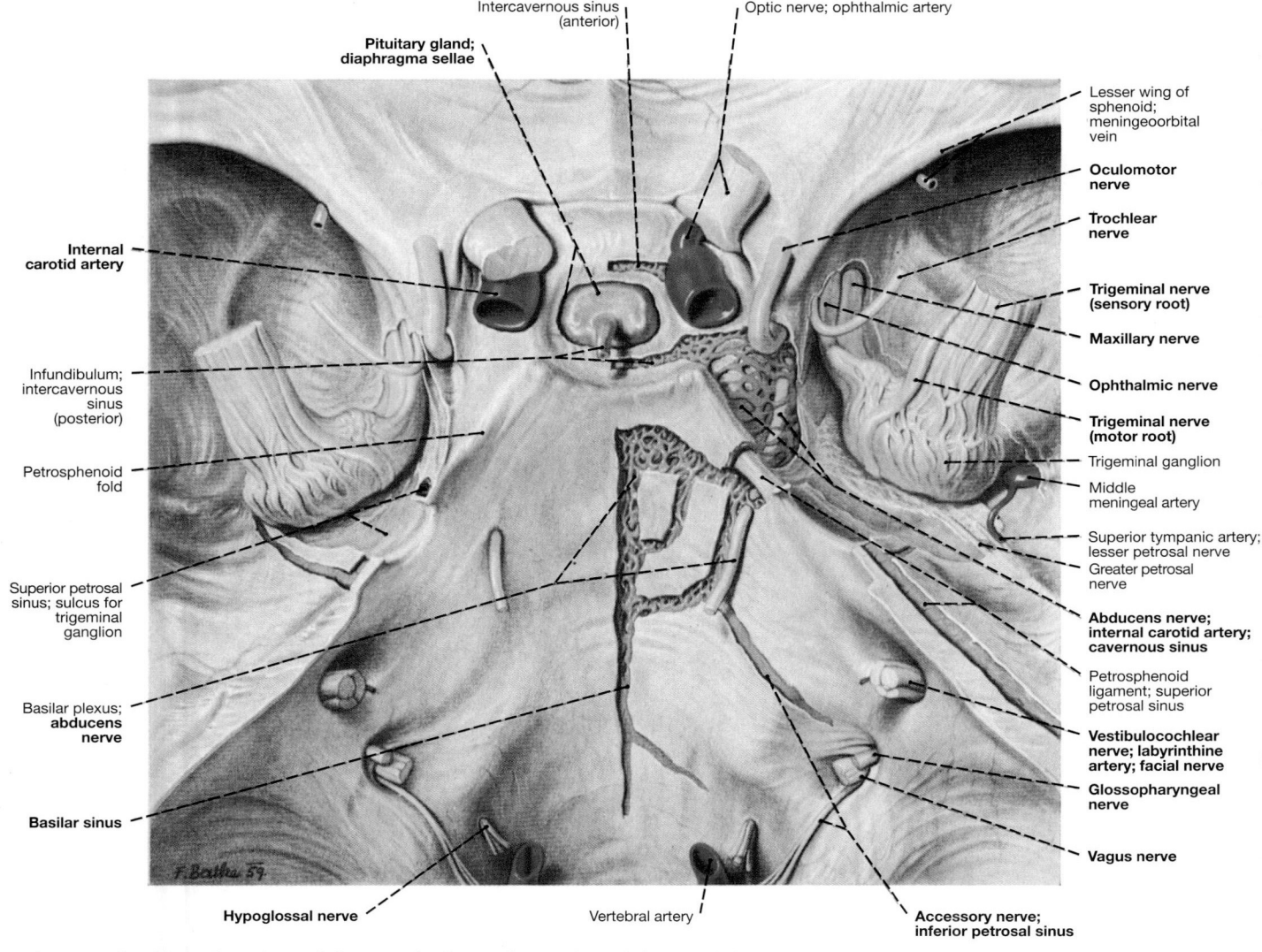

Intercavernous sinus (anterior)

Pituitary gland; diaphragma sellae

Optic nerve; ophthalmic artery

Lesser wing of sphenoid; meningeoorbital vein

Oculomotor nerve

Trochlear nerve

Internal carotid artery

Trigeminal nerve (sensory root)

Maxillary nerve

Ophthalmic nerve

Infundibulum; intercavernous sinus (posterior)

Trigeminal nerve (motor root)

Trigeminal ganglion

Petrosphenoid fold

Middle meningeal artery

Superior tympanic artery; lesser petrosal nerve

Greater petrosal nerve

Superior petrosal sinus; sulcus for trigeminal ganglion

Abducens nerve; internal carotid artery; cavernous sinus

Petrosphenoid ligament; superior petrosal sinus

Basilar plexus; abducens nerve

Vestibulocochlear nerve; labyrinthine artery; facial nerve

Glossopharyngeal nerve

Basilar sinus

Vagus nerve

Hypoglossal nerve

Vertebral artery

Accessory nerve; inferior petrosal sinus

Fig. 773: Blood Vessels and Cranial Nerves in the Basilar Region of the Cranial Cavity
NOTE: 1) the dura mater has been opened to expose the right cavernous sinus, the anterior and posterior intercavernous sinuses, the basilar plexus of veins and the right superior and inferior petrosal sinuses.

2) stumps of the oculomotor, trochlear and trigeminal nerves have been pulled forward; also the right optic nerve has been elevated to reveal the origin of the ophthalmic artery from the cerebral part of the internal carotid artery.

3) the infundibulum, or stalk, of the pituitary gland by which the gland was attached to the hypothalamus. Note also the stumps of all the cranial nerves (except the olfactory).

Dorsum sellae

Posterior intercavernous sinus

Posterior lobe (neurohypophysis)

Infundibulum

Pars tuberalis

Diaphragma sellae

Pars intermedia

Anterior lobe (adenohypophysis)

Optic nerve

Pars distalis

Anterior intercavernous sinus

Sella turcica (hypophysial fossa)

Sphenoid sinus

Sphenoid bone

Fig. 774: Median Sagittal Section Through the Pituitary Gland and the Sella Turcica of the Sphenoid Bone
NOTE: the **sella turcica** (hypophysial fossa) in the sphenoid bone is lined and covered (**diaphragma sellae**) by dura mater. The anterior and posterior lobes form a single organ that lies below and slightly behind the optic chiasma.

Figs. 773, 774

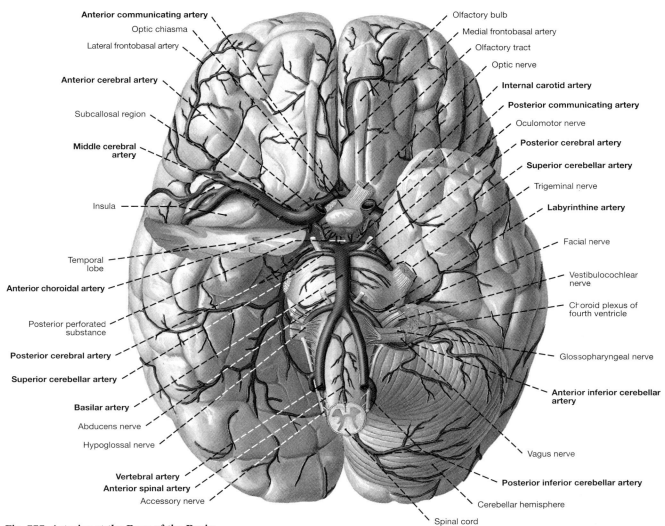

Fig. 775: Arteries at the Base of the Brain

NOTE: 1)   branches of the **vertebral arteries** form the anterior spinal artery *medially* and the posterior inferior cerebellar arteries *laterally.*

2)   the **basilar artery** is formed near the pontomedullary junction and gives off the anterior inferior cerebellar, labyrinthine, pontine (not labelled), superior cerebellar and posterior cerebral arteries successively as it ascends.

3)   the **internal carotid arteries** connect with the posterior cerebral by way of the posterior communicating arteries, and then give off the middle and anterior cerebral arteries. The anterior cerebral arteries are joined by the anterior communicating artery.

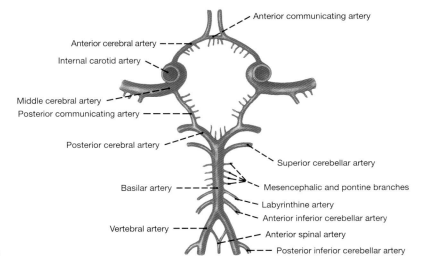

Fig. 776: Circle of Willis

NOTE: the circle of Willis is formed by the **posterior cerebral, posterior communicating, internal carotid, anterior cerebral,** and **anterior communicating arteries.**

PLATE 494   Base of the Skull (Inner Surface): Cranial Nerves and Vessels

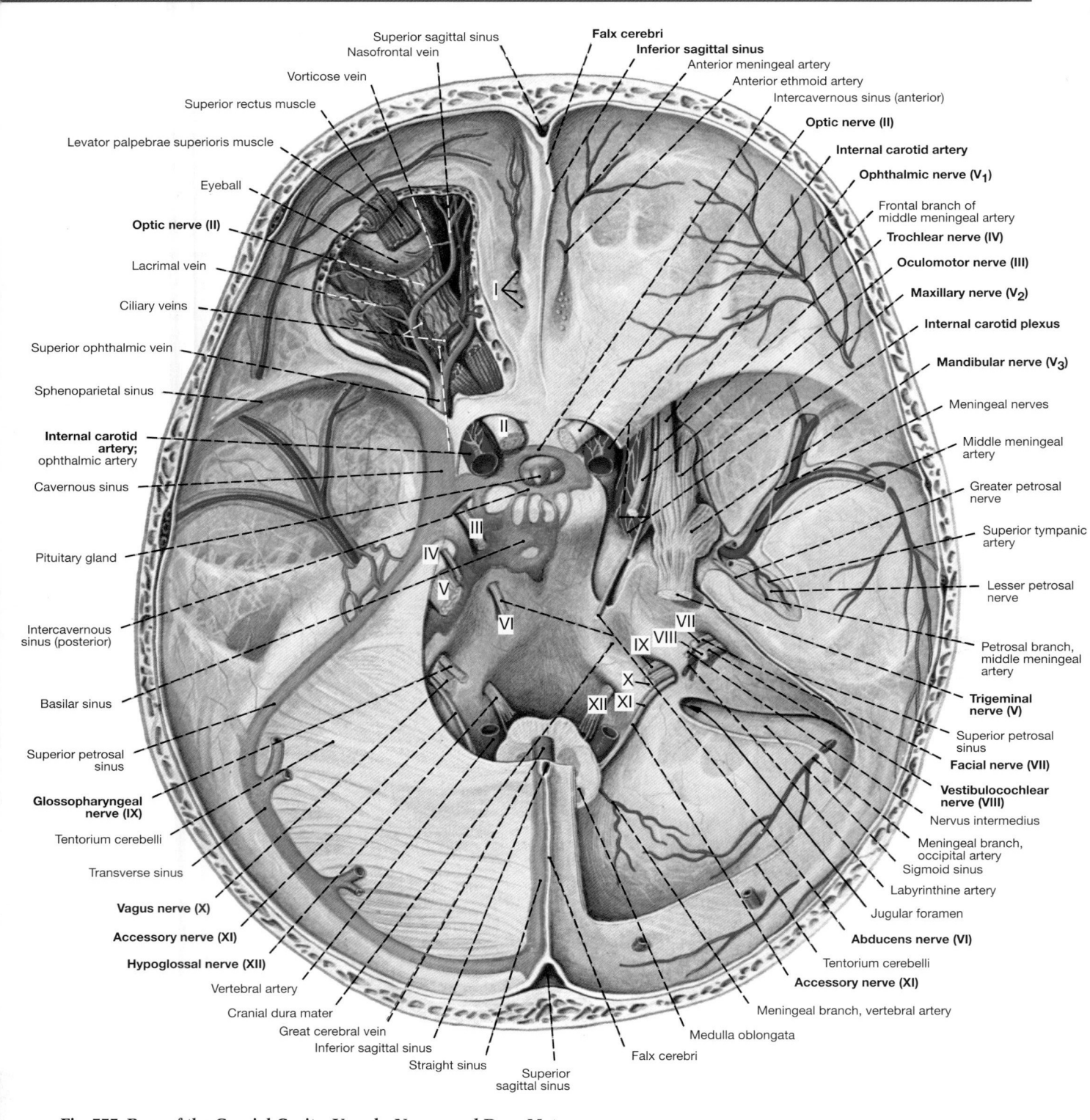

Superior sagittal sinus
Nasofrontal vein
Vorticose vein
Superior rectus muscle
Levator palpebrae superioris muscle
Eyeball
Optic nerve (II)
Lacrimal vein
Ciliary veins
Superior ophthalmic vein
Sphenoparietal sinus
Internal carotid artery; ophthalmic artery
Cavernous sinus
Pituitary gland
Intercavernous sinus (posterior)
Basilar sinus
Superior petrosal sinus
Glossopharyngeal nerve (IX)
Tentorium cerebelli
Transverse sinus
Vagus nerve (X)
Accessory nerve (XI)
Hypoglossal nerve (XII)
Vertebral artery
Cranial dura mater
Great cerebral vein
Inferior sagittal sinus
Straight sinus
Superior sagittal sinus

Falx cerebri
Inferior sagittal sinus
Anterior meningeal artery
Anterior ethmoid artery
Intercavernous sinus (anterior)
Optic nerve (II)
Internal carotid artery
Ophthalmic nerve (V₁)
Frontal branch of middle meningeal artery
Trochlear nerve (IV)
Oculomotor nerve (III)
Maxillary nerve (V₂)
Internal carotid plexus
Mandibular nerve (V₃)
Meningeal nerves
Middle meningeal artery
Greater petrosal nerve
Superior tympanic artery
Lesser petrosal nerve
Petrosal branch, middle meningeal artery
Trigeminal nerve (V)
Superior petrosal sinus
Facial nerve (VII)
Vestibulocochlear nerve (VIII)
Nervus intermedius
Meningeal branch, occipital artery
Sigmoid sinus
Labyrinthine artery
Jugular foramen
Abducens nerve (VI)
Tentorium cerebelli
Accessory nerve (XI)
Meningeal branch, vertebral artery
Medulla oblongata
Falx cerebri

Fig. 777: Base of the Cranial Cavity: Vessels, Nerves and Dura Mater

NOTE: 1)   the anterior, middle, and posterior **cranial fossae** in the floor of the cranial cavity. In the anterior fossae rest the **frontal lobes** of the brain, while the **temporal lobes** lie in the middle fossae and the **brainstem** and **cerebellum** rest in the posterior fossa.

2)   the dura mater and the orbital plate of the frontal bone have been removed to expose the left orbit from above. The **superior ophthalmic vein** drains posteriorly into the cavernous sinus and the **optic nerve** is seen to course from the orbit through the optic canal.

3)   the medial aspect of the middle fossa shows the cavernous sinus, the internal carotid artery, the 3rd, 4th, 5th and 6th cranial nerves coursing toward the orbit or the face and the middle meningeal artery traversing the foramen spinosum.

4)   the foramina for the last six pairs of cranial nerves in the posterior fossa. The 7th and 8th nerves pass through the internal acoustic meatus, while the 9th, 10th and 11th nerves traverse the jugular foramen and the 12th nerve traverses at the hypoglossal canal.

Fig. 777

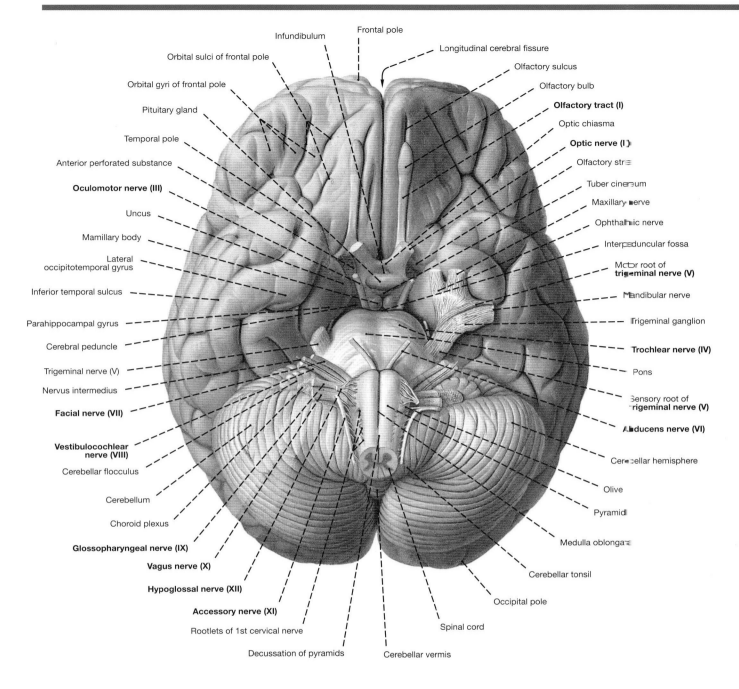

Infundibulum

Frontal pole

Orbital sulci of frontal pole

Longitudinal cerebral fissure

Olfactory sulcus

Orbital gyri of frontal pole

Olfactory bulb

Olfactory tract (I)

Pituitary gland

Optic chiasma

Optic nerve (II)

Temporal pole

Olfactory stria

Anterior perforated substance

Tuber cinereum

Oculomotor nerve (III)

Maxillary nerve

Uncus

Ophthalmic nerve

Mamillary body

Interpeduncular fossa

Lateral
occipitotemporal gyrus

Motor root of
trigeminal nerve (V)

Inferior temporal sulcus

Mandibular nerve

Parahippocampal gyrus

Trigeminal ganglion

Cerebral peduncle

Trochlear nerve (IV)

Trigeminal nerve (V)

Pons

Nervus intermedius

Sensory root of
trigeminal nerve (V)

Facial nerve (VII)

Abducens nerve (VI)

**Vestibulocochlear
nerve (VIII)**

Cerebellar hemisphere

Cerebellar flocculus

Olive

Cerebellum

Pyramid

Choroid plexus

Medulla oblongata

Glossopharyngeal nerve (IX)

Vagus nerve (X)

Cerebellar tonsil

Hypoglossal nerve (XII)

Occipital pole

Accessory nerve (XI)

Rootlets of 1st cervical nerve

Spinal cord

Decussation of pyramids

Cerebellar vermis

Fig. 778: Ventral View of the Brain Showing the Origins of the Cranial Nerves
NOTE: 1) the cranial nerves attach to the base of the brain. The **olfactory tracts** and **optic nerves (I and II)** subserve receptors of special sense in the nose and eye, and as cranial nerve trunks attach to the base of the forebrain in contrast to all other cranial nerves which attach to the midbrain, pons or medulla of the brainstem.

2) the **oculomotor (III), trochlear (IV)** and **abducens (VI) nerves** are motor nerves to the extraocular muscles. The **trigeminal nerve (V)** is the largest of the cranial nerves and the trochlear is the smallest. The abducens nerve attaches to the brainstem at the junction of the pons and medulla (pontomedullary junction) medial to the attachments of the **facial (VII)** and **vestibulocochlear (VIII) nerves.**

3) the **glossopharyngeal (IX)** and **vagus (X) nerves** emerge from the medulla laterally in a line comparable to the spinal and medullary parts of the **accessory nerve (XI)**. In contrast, the **hypoglossal nerve (XII)** rootlets emerge from the ventral medulla in a line consistent with the ventral rootlets of the cervical nerves of the spinal cord.

Fig. 778   **VII**

PLATE 496   Base of the Skull: Cranial Fossae

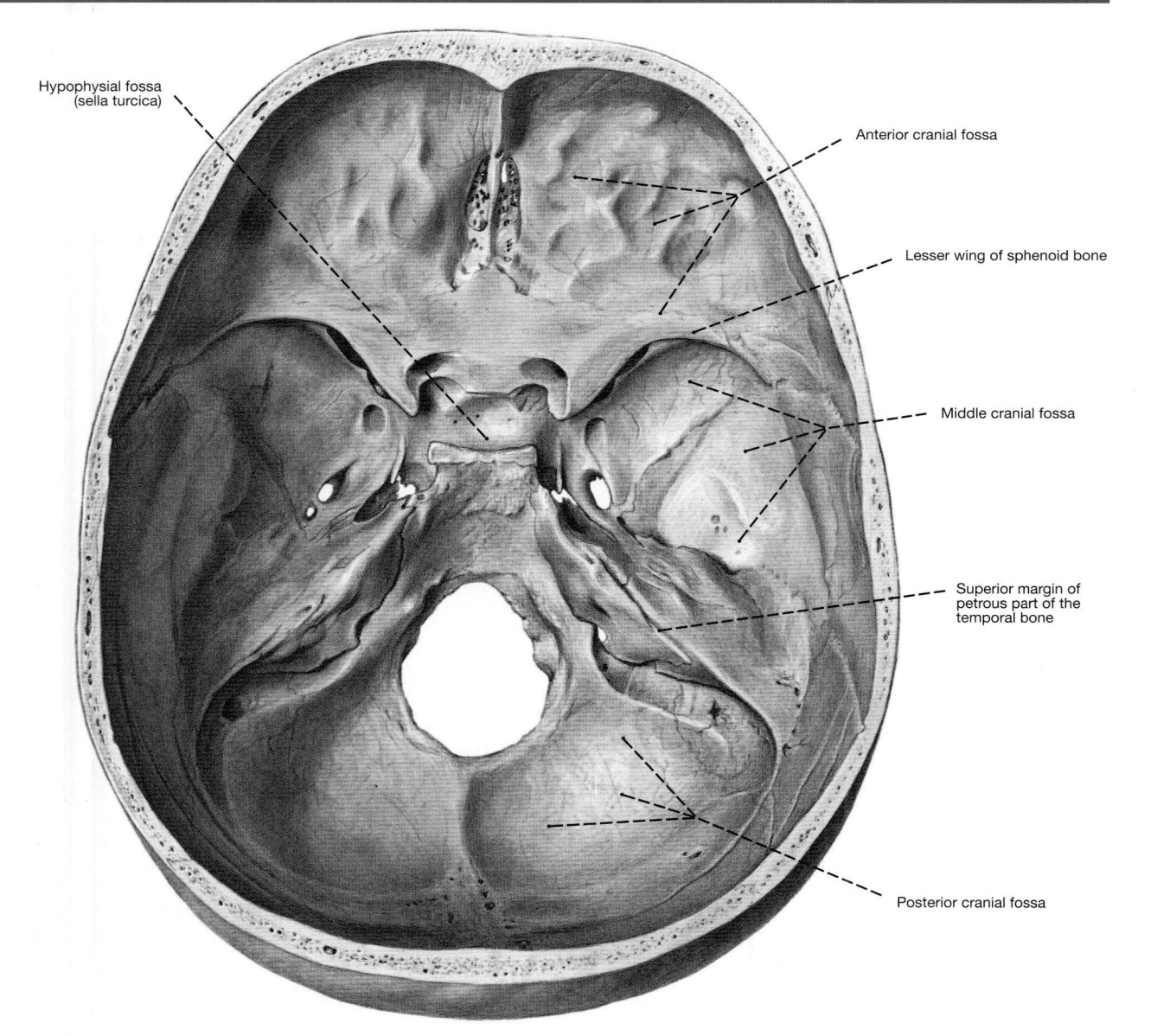

Hypophysial fossa
(sella turcica)

Anterior cranial fossa

Lesser wing of sphenoid bone

Middle cranial fossa

Superior margin of
petrous part of the
temporal bone

Posterior cranial fossa

Fig. 779: Interior of the Base of the Skull (From Above)

NOTE: 1)   the **anterior cranial fossa** extends from the inner surface of the frontal bone to the lesser wing of the sphenoid bone.

2)   the **middle cranial fossa** extends from the lesser wing of the sphenoid bone to the superior margin of the petrous part of the temporal bone.

3)   the **posterior cranial fossa** extends from the superior margin of the petrous part of the temporal bone backward to the posterior limit of the skull (occipital bone).

Fig. 780: Base of the Skull: Internal Aspect (Superior View)

NOTE: there are important structures that traverse the foramina at the base of the skull.

1)   **ANTERIOR CRANIAL FOSSA:**
   a)   **Foramen cecum:** a small vein
   b)   **Cribriform plate:** filaments of olfactory receptor neurons to the olfactory bulb
   c)   **Anterior ethmoid foramen:** anterior ethmoidal vessels and nerve
   d)   **Posterior ethmoid foramen:** posterior ethmoidal vessels and nerve

2)   **MIDDLE CRANIAL FOSSA:**
   a)   **Optic foramen:** optic nerve; ophthalmic artery
   b)   **Superior orbital fissure:** oculomotor nerve; trochlear nerve; ophthalmic nerve; abducens nerve; sympathetic nerve fibers; superior ophthalmic vein; orbital branch of middle meningeal artery; dural recurrent branch of the lacrimal artery
   c)   **Foramen rotundum:** maxillary nerve

Fig. 779

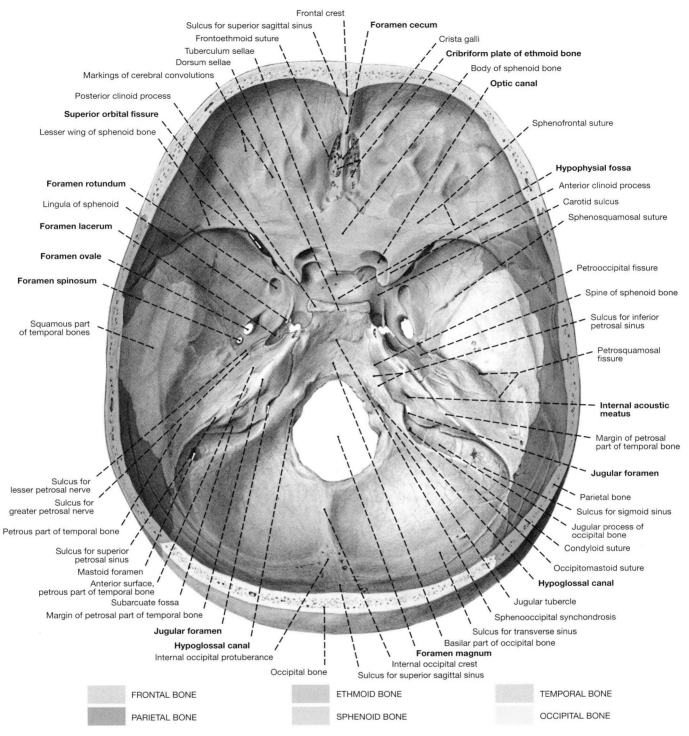

Frontal crest
Sulcus for superior sagittal sinus
Frontoethmoid suture
Tuberculum sellae
Dorsum sellae
Markings of cerebral convolutions
Posterior clinoid process
Superior orbital fissure
Lesser wing of sphenoid bone
Foramen rotundum
Lingula of sphenoid
Foramen lacerum
Foramen ovale
Foramen spinosum
Squamous part of temporal bones
Sulcus for lesser petrosal nerve
Sulcus for greater petrosal nerve
Petrous part of temporal bone
Sulcus for superior petrosal sinus
Mastoid foramen
Anterior surface, petrous part of temporal bone
Subarcuate fossa
Margin of petrosal part of temporal bone
Jugular foramen
Hypoglossal canal
Internal occipital protuberance
Occipital bone

Foramen cecum
Crista galli
Cribriform plate of ethmoid bone
Body of sphenoid bone
Optic canal
Sphenofrontal suture
Hypophysial fossa
Anterior clinoid process
Carotid sulcus
Sphenosquamosal suture
Petrooccipital fissure
Spine of sphenoid bone
Sulcus for inferior petrosal sinus
Petrosquamosal fissure
Internal acoustic meatus
Margin of petrosal part of temporal bone
Jugular foramen
Parietal bone
Sulcus for sigmoid sinus
Jugular process of occipital bone
Condyloid suture
Occipitomastoid suture
Hypoglossal canal
Jugular tubercle
Sphenooccipital synchondrosis
Sulcus for transverse sinus
Basilar part of occipital bone
Foramen magnum
Internal occipital crest
Sulcus for superior sagittal sinus

| FRONTAL BONE | ETHMOID BONE | TEMPORAL BONE |
| PARIETAL BONE | SPHENOID BONE | OCCIPITAL BONE |

   d) **Foramen ovale:** mandibular nerve; accessory meningeal artery
   e) **Foramen spinosum:** middle meningeal artery; a recurrent dural branch of mandibular nerve
   f) **Foramen lacerum:** the internal carotid artery passes across the foramen above the fibrocartilaginous plate but does *not* traverse it. The nerve of the pterygoid canal emerges from the foramen to enter the pterygoid canal. The meningeal branch of the ascending pharyngeal artery actually traverses the foramen.

3) **POSTERIOR CRANIAL FOSSA:**
   a) **Internal acoustic meatus:** facial nerve; vestibulocochlear nerve; labyrinthine artery
   b) **Jugular foramen:** sigmoid sinus which becomes internal jugular vein; meningeal branches of occipital and ascending pharyngeal arteries; glossopharyngeal nerve; vagus nerve; accessory nerve
   c) **Hypoglossal canal:** hypoglossal nerve
   d) **Foramen magnum:** spinal cord; spinal part of accessory nerve; anterior and posterior spinal arteries; vertebral arteries; tectorial membrane

Fig. 780   **VII**

PLATE 498   Base of Skull: Inferior Surface, Foramina and Markings

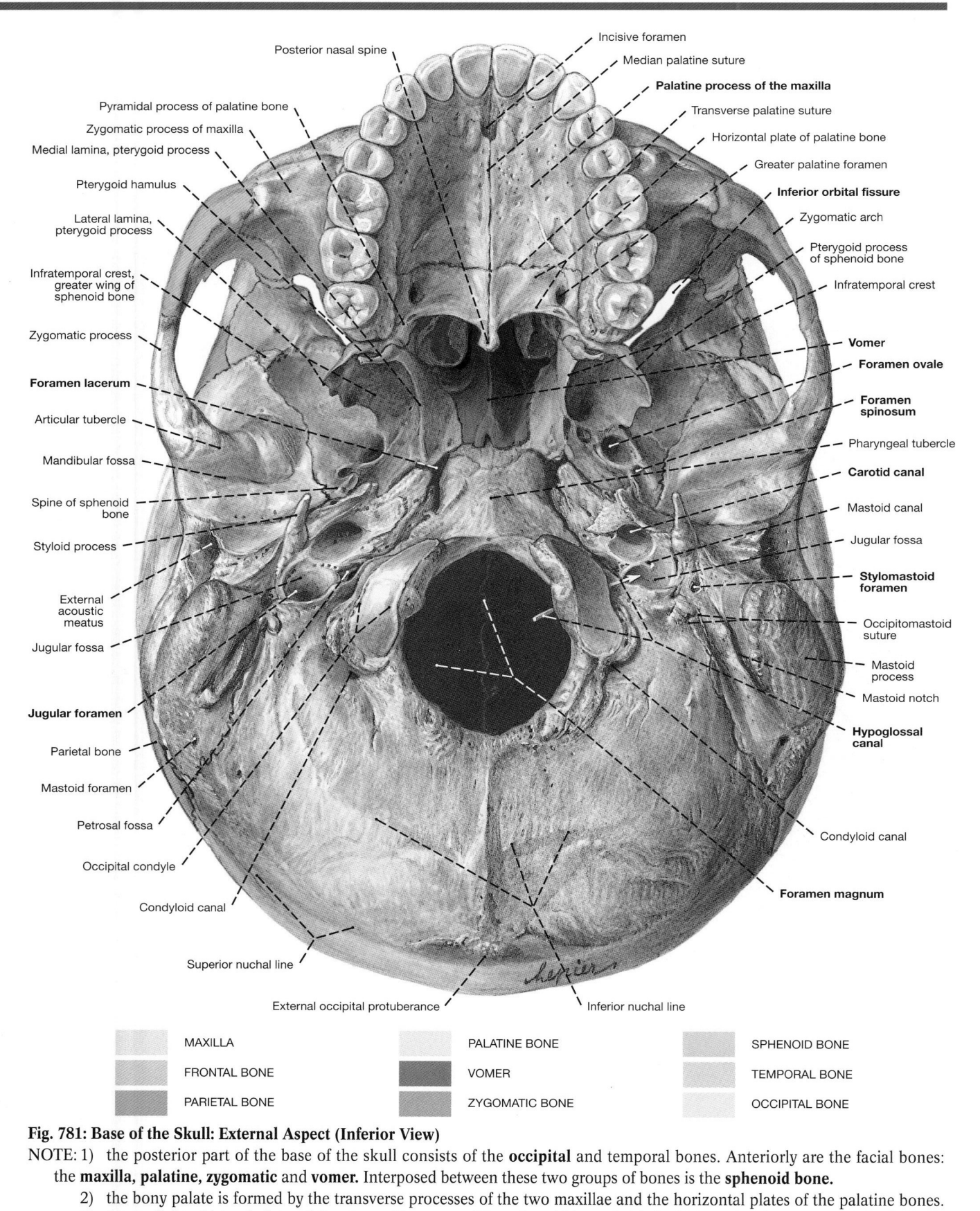

Posterior nasal spine
Incisive foramen
Median palatine suture
Palatine process of the maxilla
Pyramidal process of palatine bone
Transverse palatine suture
Zygomatic process of maxilla
Horizontal plate of palatine bone
Medial lamina, pterygoid process
Greater palatine foramen
Pterygoid hamulus
Inferior orbital fissure
Lateral lamina, pterygoid process
Zygomatic arch
Infratemporal crest, greater wing of sphenoid bone
Pterygoid process of sphenoid bone
Zygomatic process
Infratemporal crest
Foramen lacerum
Vomer
Articular tubercle
Foramen ovale
Mandibular fossa
Foramen spinosum
Spine of sphenoid bone
Pharyngeal tubercle
Styloid process
Carotid canal
External acoustic meatus
Mastoid canal
Jugular fossa
Jugular fossa
Jugular foramen
Stylomastoid foramen
Parietal bone
Occipitomastoid suture
Mastoid foramen
Mastoid process
Petrosal fossa
Mastoid notch
Occipital condyle
Hypoglossal canal
Condyloid canal
Superior nuchal line
Condyloid canal
External occipital protuberance
Foramen magnum
Inferior nuchal line

MAXILLA
PALATINE BONE
SPHENOID BONE
FRONTAL BONE
VOMER
TEMPORAL BONE
PARIETAL BONE
ZYGOMATIC BONE
OCCIPITAL BONE

Fig. 781: Base of the Skull: External Aspect (Inferior View)

NOTE: 1) the posterior part of the base of the skull consists of the **occipital** and temporal bones. Anteriorly are the facial bones: the **maxilla, palatine, zygomatic** and **vomer.** Interposed between these two groups of bones is the **sphenoid bone.**

2) the bony palate is formed by the transverse processes of the two maxillae and the horizontal plates of the palatine bones.

3) the medial and lateral plates of the pterygoid process of the sphenoid bone, behind which are the foramen ovale and foramen spinosum in the greater wings of the sphenoid.

4) the **foramen lacerum, carotid canal, jugular foramen, styloid process** (of temporal bone), **hypoglossal canal** (arrow), and the **foramen magnum.**

Fig. 781

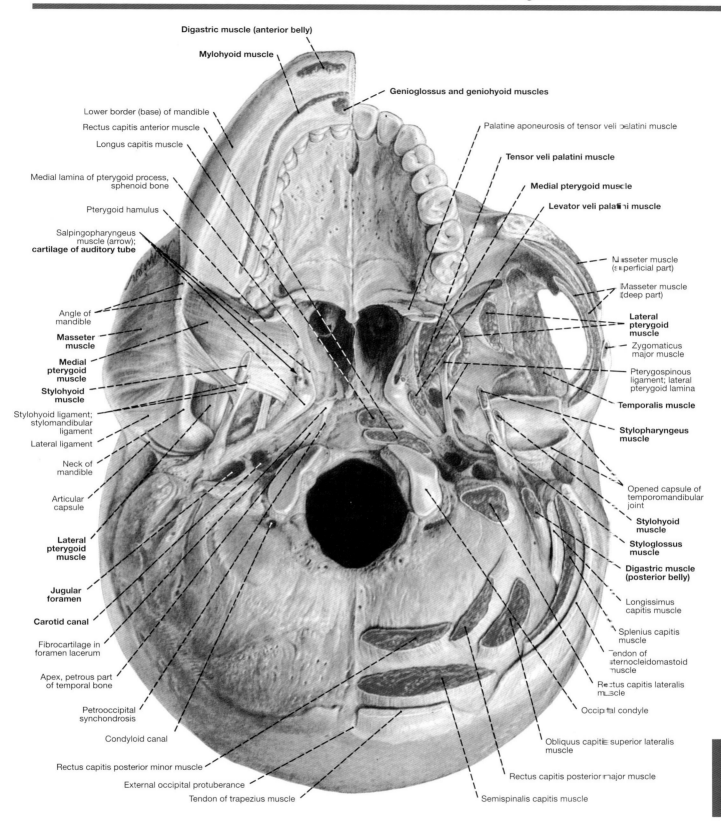

Digastric muscle (anterior belly)

Mylohyoid muscle

Genioglossus and geniohyoid muscles

Lower border (base) of mandible

Rectus capitis anterior muscle

Longus capitis muscle

Palatine aponeurosis of tensor veli palatini muscle

Tensor veli palatini muscle

Medial lamina of pterygoid process, sphenoid bone

Medial pterygoid muscle

Pterygoid hamulus

Levator veli palatini muscle

Salpingopharyngeus muscle (arrow); **cartilage of auditory tube**

Masseter muscle (superficial part)

Masseter muscle (deep part)

Angle of mandible

Lateral pterygoid muscle

Masseter muscle

Zygomaticus major muscle

Medial pterygoid muscle

Pterygospinous ligament; lateral pterygoid lamina

Stylohyoid muscle

Temporalis muscle

Stylohyoid ligament; stylomandibular ligament

Stylopharyngeus muscle

Lateral ligament

Neck of mandible

Opened capsule of temporomandibular joint

Articular capsule

Stylohyoid muscle

Lateral pterygoid muscle

Styloglossus muscle

Digastric muscle (posterior belly)

Jugular foramen

Longissimus capitis muscle

Carotid canal

Splenius capitis muscle

Fibrocartilage in foramen lacerum

Tendon of sternocleidomastoid muscle

Apex, petrous part of temporal bone

Rectus capitis lateralis muscle

Petrooccipital synchondrosis

Occipital condyle

Condyloid canal

Rectus capitis posterior minor muscle

Obliquus capitis superior lateralis muscle

External occipital protuberance

Rectus capitis posterior major muscle

Tendon of trapezius muscle

Semispinalis capitis muscle

Fig. 782: Muscle Origins and Other Structures on the Base of the Skull

NOTE: 1)   the left mandible and muscles of mastication (reader's right) have been removed. Observe the attachments of the superficial and deep parts of the **masseter muscle,** the **temporalis muscle,** the 2 heads of the **lateral pterygoid muscle** and the **medial pterygoid.**

2)   the **levator veli palatini muscle** arises from the inferior surface of the apex of the temporal bone, anterior to the opening of the carotid canal. The **tensor veli palatini muscle** lies lateral and anterior to the levator, and it arises from the scaphoid fossa at the base of the medial pterygoid plate, from the sphenoidal spine and from the lateral aspect of the cartilaginous auditory tube.

3) the cartilage of the **auditory tube** as it opens inferomedially in the lateral wall of the nasopharynx.

Fig. 782   **VII**

PLATE 500   The Eye: Surface Anatomy (Anterior View)

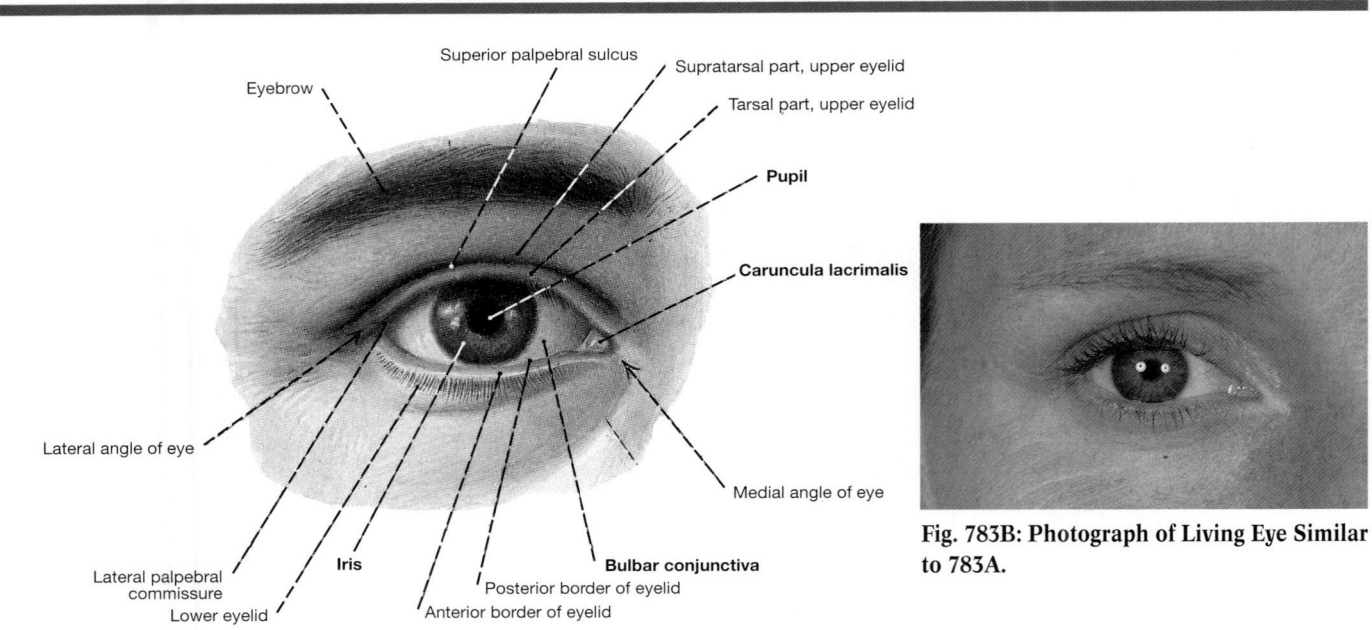

Fig. 783B: Photograph of Living Eye Similar to 783A.

Fig. 783A: Right Eye and Eyelids

NOTE: 1) the eyeball, protected in front by two movable and thin **eyelids** or **palpebrae,** is covered by a transparent mucous membrane, the **conjunctiva,** which reflects along the inner surface of both eyelids as the **palpebral conjunctiva.**

2) at the medial angle of the eye is located a small, reddish island of tissue called the **caruncula lacrimalis.**

3) the **pupil** is the opening in the **iris.** Constriction and dilatation of the pupil is controlled autonomically. Parasympathetic fibers in the oculomotor nerve innervate the constrictor muscle of the pupil, while sympathetic fibers from the superior cervical ganglion supply the pupillary dilator muscle.

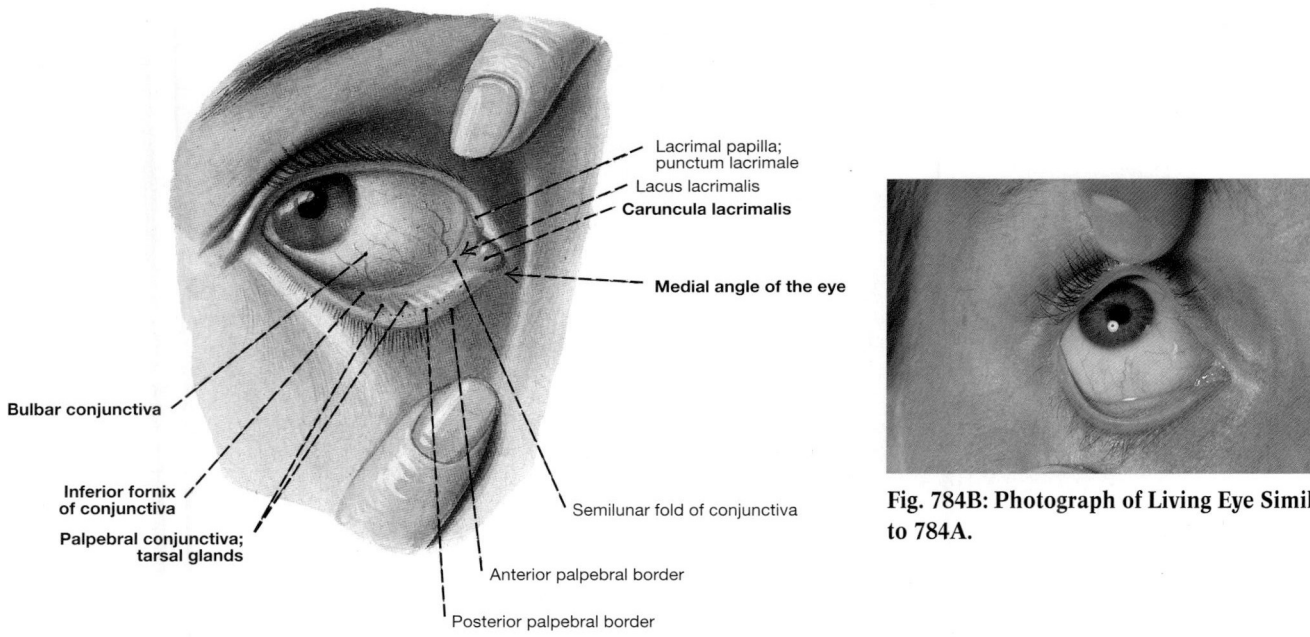

Fig. 784B: Photograph of Living Eye Similar to 784A.

Fig. 784A: Right Lower Eyelid and Medial Angle

NOTE: 1) the right lower eyelid has been pulled downward to show the inner surface of the lower lid (i.e., the palpebral conjunctiva) and to enlarge the exposure of the medial angle (also called the **medial canthus**).

2) the conjunctiva is highly vascular and its bulbar part (over the eyeball) and inferior palpebral part (on the inner surface of the lower eyelid) are continuous along a line of reflection called the **inferior conjunctival fornix.** A similar reflection line, the **superior conjunctival fornix,** lies between the eyeball and the upper eyelid.

3) when the medial angle is more completely exposed, a pair of small openings, the **puncta lacrimalia,** can be found located above and below the caruncula lacrimalis. These openings lead into small **lacrimal canals** through which tears enter the **lacrimal sac.**

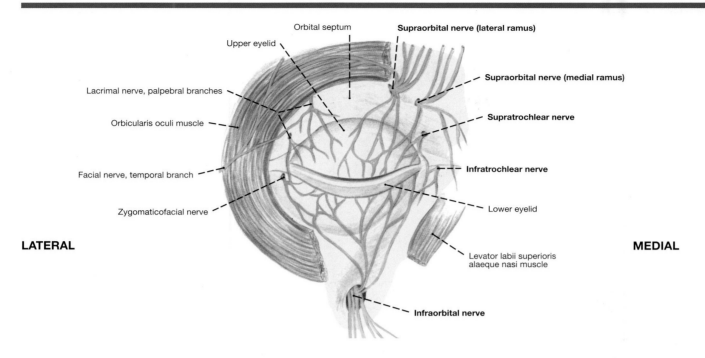

Fig. 785: Innervation of the Eyelids; Anterior View, Right Eye

NOTE: 1)   the rich cutaneous innervation found around the anterior orbit is derived from the ophthalmic and maxillary divisions of the trigeminal nerve, which achieve the anterior orbital region through foramina in the frontal, zygomatic, and maxillary bones.

2)   superomedially are found the large rami of the **supraorbital** branch of the frontal nerve (V_1), which emerges through the supraorbital foramen or notch. Also note the **supratrochlear** branch of the frontal nerve, which appears through a small foramen above the trochlea of the superior oblique muscle.

3)   the **infratrochlear nerve.** This is a terminal branch of the nasociliary nerve (V_1) that becomes superficial below the trochlea of the superior oblique. Along with palpebral branches of the **infraorbital nerve** (V_2), it sends fibers to the lower eyelid.

4)   the **lacrimal nerve** (V_1) superolaterally, supplying the upper eyelid; the **zygomaticofacial nerve** (V_2) to the lower eyelid and skin over the cheek bone; the **temporal branch of the facial nerve** which is a motor nerve to the orbicularis oculi muscle.

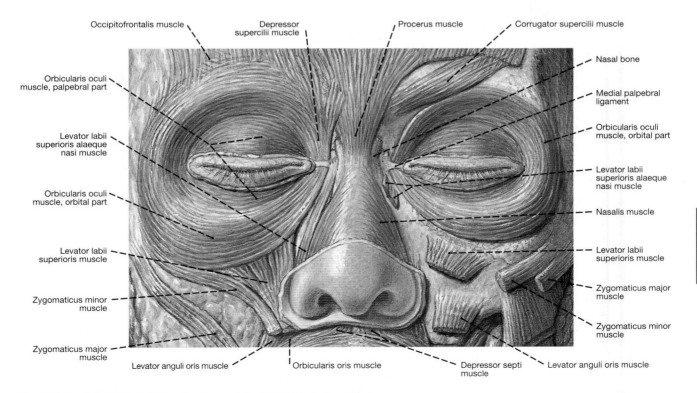

Fig. 786: Superficial Facial Muscles Around the Orbit (Anterior View)

PLATE 502   The Bony Orbit: Anterior View and Frontal Section

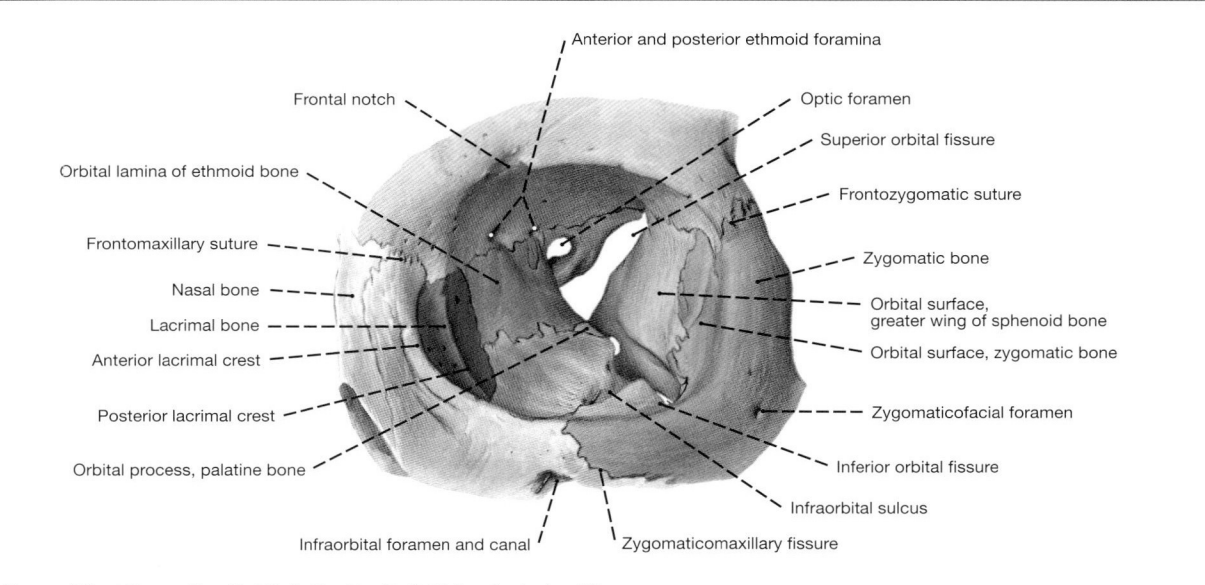

Anterior and posterior ethmoid foramina

Frontal notch

Optic foramen

Superior orbital fissure

Orbital lamina of ethmoid bone

Frontozygomatic suture

Frontomaxillary suture

Zygomatic bone

Nasal bone

Lacrimal bone

Orbital surface, greater wing of sphenoid bone

Anterior lacrimal crest

Orbital surface, zygomatic bone

Posterior lacrimal crest

Zygomaticofacial foramen

Orbital process, palatine bone

Inferior orbital fissure

Infraorbital sulcus

Infraorbital foramen and canal

Zygomaticomaxillary fissure

Fig. 787: Bones That Form the Orbital Cavity; Left Side, Anterior View

NOTE: 1) the bony structure of the orbit is composed of parts of seven bones: the **maxilla, zygomatic, frontal, lacrimal, palatine, ethmoid,** and **sphenoid.**

2) the **roof** of the orbit is formed by the orbital plate of the *frontal bone;* the **floor** consists of the orbital plate of the *maxilla,* the *palatine* and the *zygomatic bones;* the **medial wall** is thin and delicate and is formed by the frontal process of the *maxilla,* the orbital lamina of the *ethmoid* and the *lacrimal bone;* the strong **lateral wall** consists of the orbital processes of the *sphenoid* and *zygomatic bones.*

3) the **optic foramen,** the **superior** and **inferior orbital fissures** and the **anterior** and **posterior ethmoid foramina.**

	NASAL BONE		VOMER		TEMPORAL BONE
	FRONTAL BONE		ZYGOMATIC BONE		INFERIOR NASAL CONCHA
	PALATINE BONE		MAXILLA		SPHENOID BONE
	ETHMOID BONE				LACRIMAL BONE

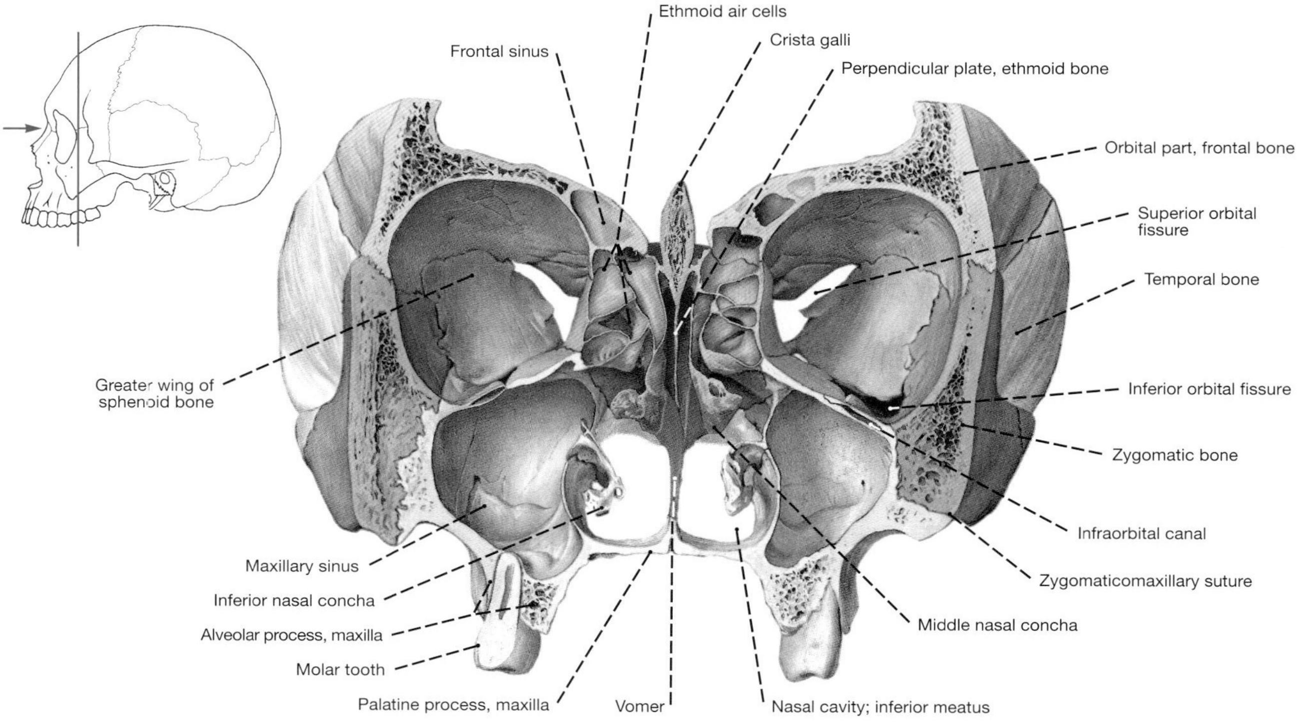

Ethmoid air cells

Crista galli

Frontal sinus

Perpendicular plate, ethmoid bone

Orbital part, frontal bone

Superior orbital fissure

Temporal bone

Greater wing of sphenoid bone

Inferior orbital fissure

Zygomatic bone

Infraorbital canal

Maxillary sinus

Zygomaticomaxillary suture

Inferior nasal concha

Alveolar process, maxilla

Middle nasal concha

Molar tooth

Palatine process, maxilla

Vomer

Nasal cavity; inferior meatus

Fig. 788: Frontal Section Through the Orbital and Nasal Cavities and the Maxillary Sinus

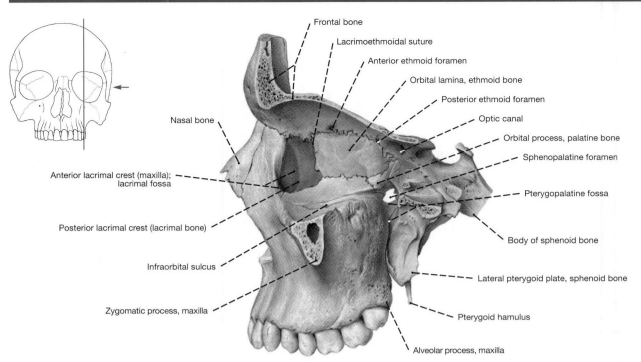

Fig. 789: Medial Wall of the Left Orbital Cavity and a Lateral View of the Pterygopalatine Fossa

NOTE: 1)   anteriorly on the thin medial wall of the orbital cavity is found the **lacrimal fossa** for the **lacrimal sac.** The fossa is
limited in front by the anterior lacrimal crest of the maxilla and behind by the posterior lacrimal crest of the lacrimal bone.

2)   the medial wall is formed by the orbital lamina of the **ethmoid bone** and the **lacrimal bone.** The **maxilla** inferiorly and the
sphenoid and **palatine bones** posteriorly also contribute to this wall. Observe also the **anterior** and **posterior ethmoidal foramina.**

FRONTAL BONE	NASAL BONE	MAXILLA
LACRIMAL BONE	PALATINE BONE	TEMPORAL BONE
SPHENOID BONE	ETHMOID BONE	ZYGOMATIC BONE

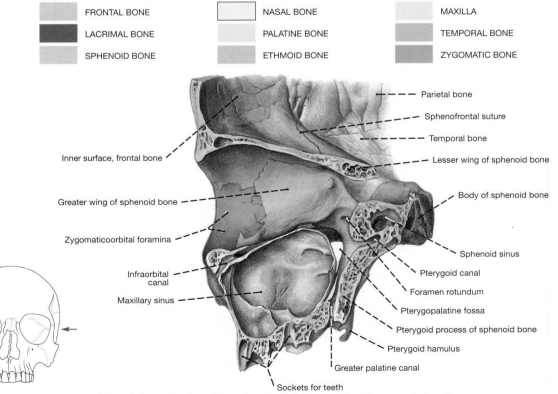

Fig. 790: The Lateral Wall of the Right Orbital Cavity and a Medial View of the Pterygopalatine Fossa

NOTE: 1)   the lateral wall of the orbit is formed by the orbital surface of the greater wing of the **sphenoid bone** and the frontal
process of the **zygomatic bone.** Note the small zygomaticoorbital foramina through which course the **zygomaticofacial** and
zygomaticotemporal branches of the maxillary nerve (sensory nerves).

2)   the **foramen rotundum** and the **infraorbital canal** for the **maxillary nerve.** Also note the **maxillary sinus** below the orbit
and the **pterygopalatine fossa** and **greater palatine canal** behind the maxillary sinus and below the apex of the orbit.

PLATE 504   The Eye: Anterior Approach to the Orbit (Dissections 1 and 2)

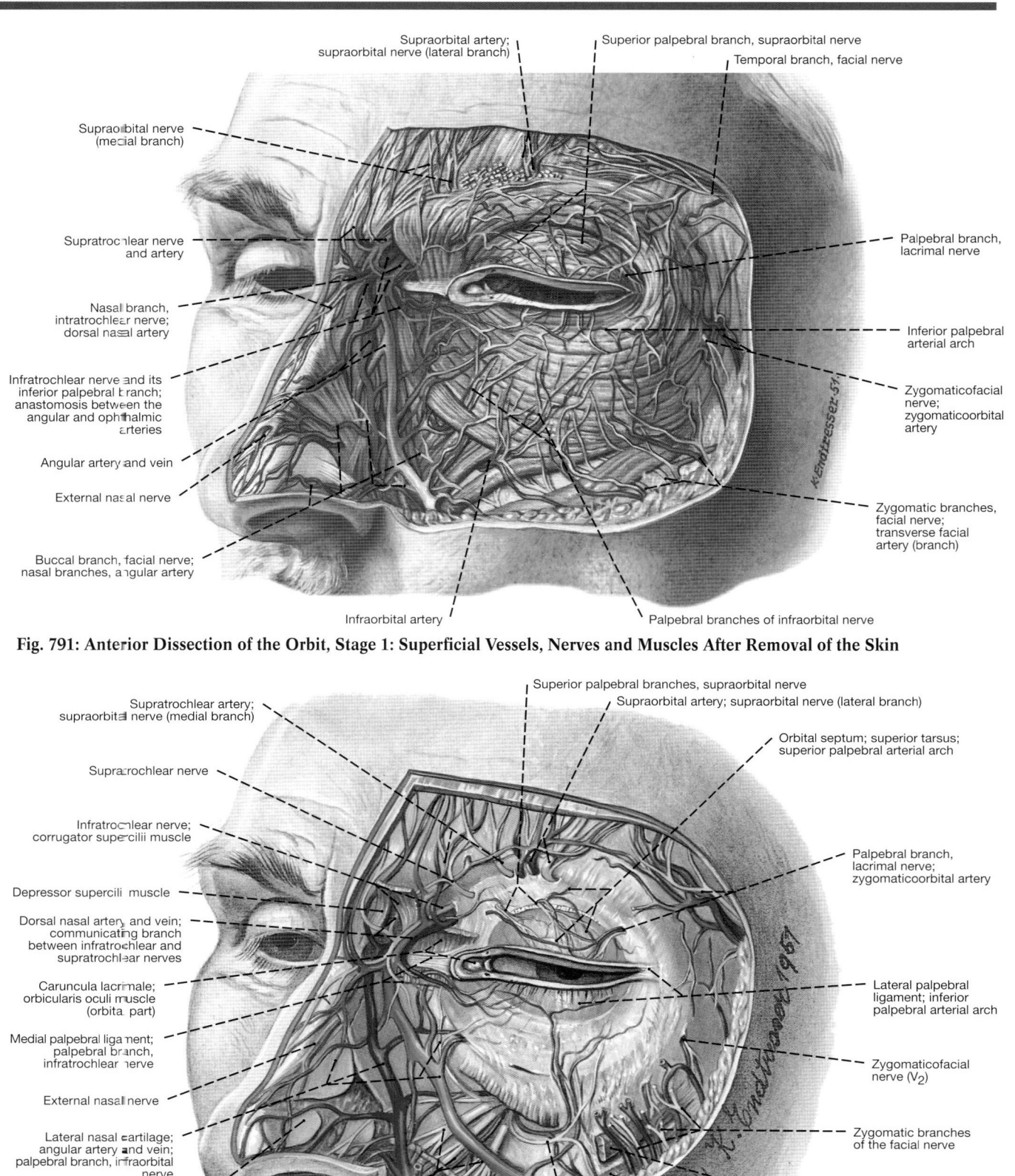

Supraorbital artery;
supraorbital nerve (lateral branch)

Superior palpebral branch, supraorbital nerve

Temporal branch, facial nerve

Supraorbital nerve
(medial branch)

Supratrochlear nerve
and artery

Nasal branch,
intratrochlear nerve;
dorsal nasal artery

Infratrochlear nerve and its
inferior palpebral branch;
anastomosis between the
angular and ophthalmic
arteries

Angular artery and vein

External nasal nerve

Buccal branch, facial nerve;
nasal branches, angular artery

Infraorbital artery

Palpebral branches of infraorbital nerve

Palpebral branch,
lacrimal nerve

Inferior palpebral
arterial arch

Zygomaticofacial
nerve;
zygomaticoorbital
artery

Zygomatic branches,
facial nerve;
transverse facial
artery (branch)

Fig. 791: Anterior Dissection of the Orbit, Stage 1: Superficial Vessels, Nerves and Muscles After Removal of the Skin

Superior palpebral branches, supraorbital nerve

Supraorbital artery; supraorbital nerve (lateral branch)

Supratrochlear artery;
supraorbital nerve (medial branch)

Supratrochlear nerve

Infratrochlear nerve;
corrugator supercilii muscle

Depressor supercilii muscle

Dorsal nasal artery and vein;
communicating branch
between infratrochlear and
supratrochlear nerves

Caruncula lacrimale;
orbicularis oculi muscle
(orbital part)

Medial palpebral ligament;
palpebral branch,
infratrochlear nerve

External nasal nerve

Lateral nasal cartilage;
angular artery and vein;
palpebral branch, infraorbital
nerve

Greater alar cartilage of
the nose

Infraorbital artery and nerve

Buccal branch, facial nerve

Orbital septum; superior tarsus;
superior palpebral arterial arch

Palpebral branch,
lacrimal nerve;
zygomaticoorbital artery

Lateral palpebral
ligament; inferior
palpebral arterial arch

Zygomaticofacial
nerve (V$_2$)

Zygomatic branches
of the facial nerve

Zygomaticus minor muscle

Zygomaticus major muscle

Palpebral branch, infraorbital nerve;
levator anguli oris muscle

Fig. 792: Anterior Dissection of the Orbit, Stage 2: Vessels and Nerves After Removal of the Orbicularis Oculi and Other Superficial Muscles

Figs. 791, 792

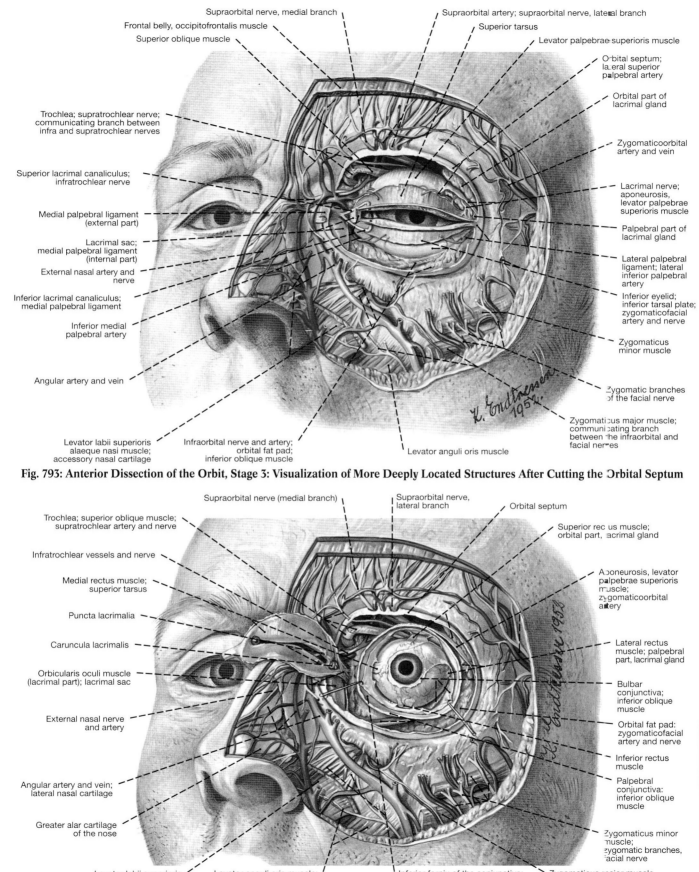

Fig. 793: Anterior Dissection of the Orbit, Stage 3: Visualization of More Deeply Located Structures After Cutting the Orbital Septum

Fig. 794: Anterior Dissection of the Orbit, Stage 4: Exposure of the Eyeball After Cutting the Lateral Palpebral Ligament and Reflecting the Eyelids Medially

PLATE 506   The Orbital Septum, Eyelids and Tarsal Plates

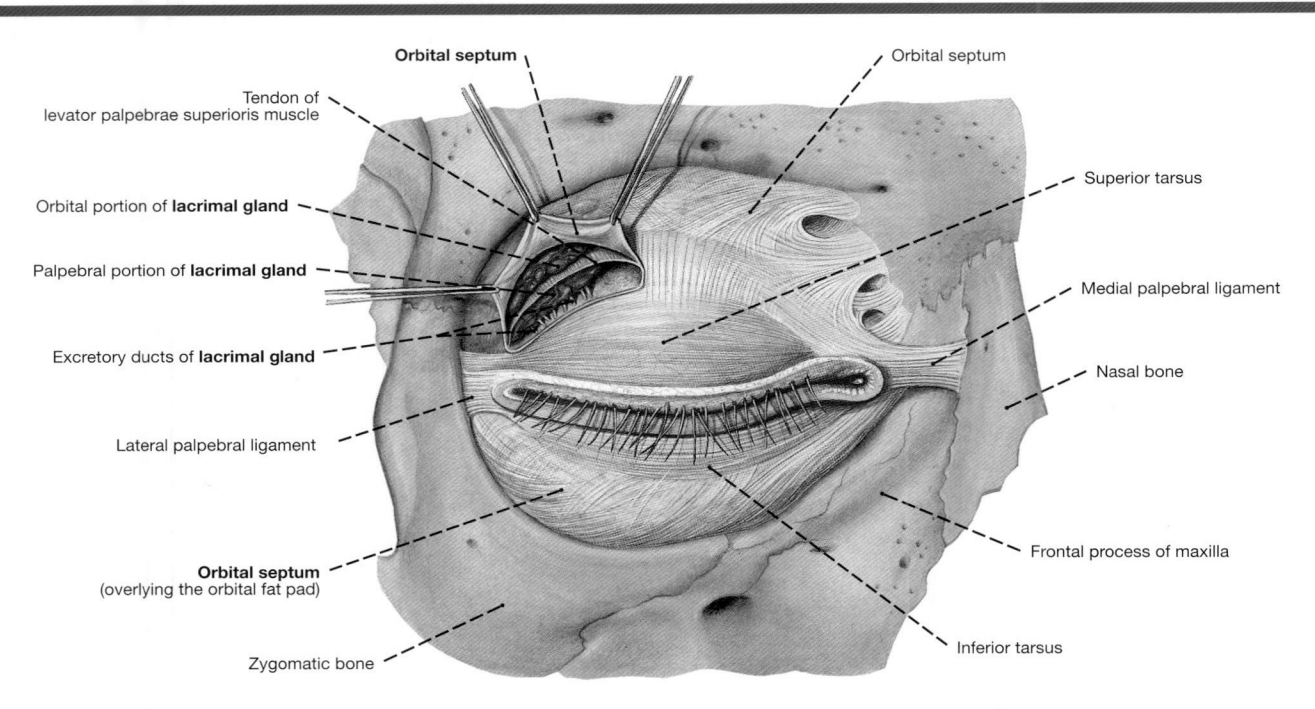

Orbital septum

Tendon of
levator palpebrae superioris muscle

Orbital portion of **lacrimal gland**

Palpebral portion of **lacrimal gland**

Excretory ducts of **lacrimal gland**

Lateral palpebral ligament

Orbital septum
(overlying the orbital fat pad)

Zygomatic bone

Orbital septum

Superior tarsus

Medial palpebral ligament

Nasal bone

Frontal process of maxilla

Inferior tarsus

Fig. 795: Orbital Septum, Lacrimal Gland, and Tarsi of the Right Eye
NOTE: 1) with the skin, superficial fascia and orbicularis oculi muscle removed, the orbital septum has been exposed anteriorly. The
septum attaches to the periosteum of the bone peripherally around the orbit and to the tarsi of the eyelids centrally.
    2) the lacrimal gland and its excretory ducts in the upper lateral aspect of the anterior orbit lying just beneath the orbital septum.

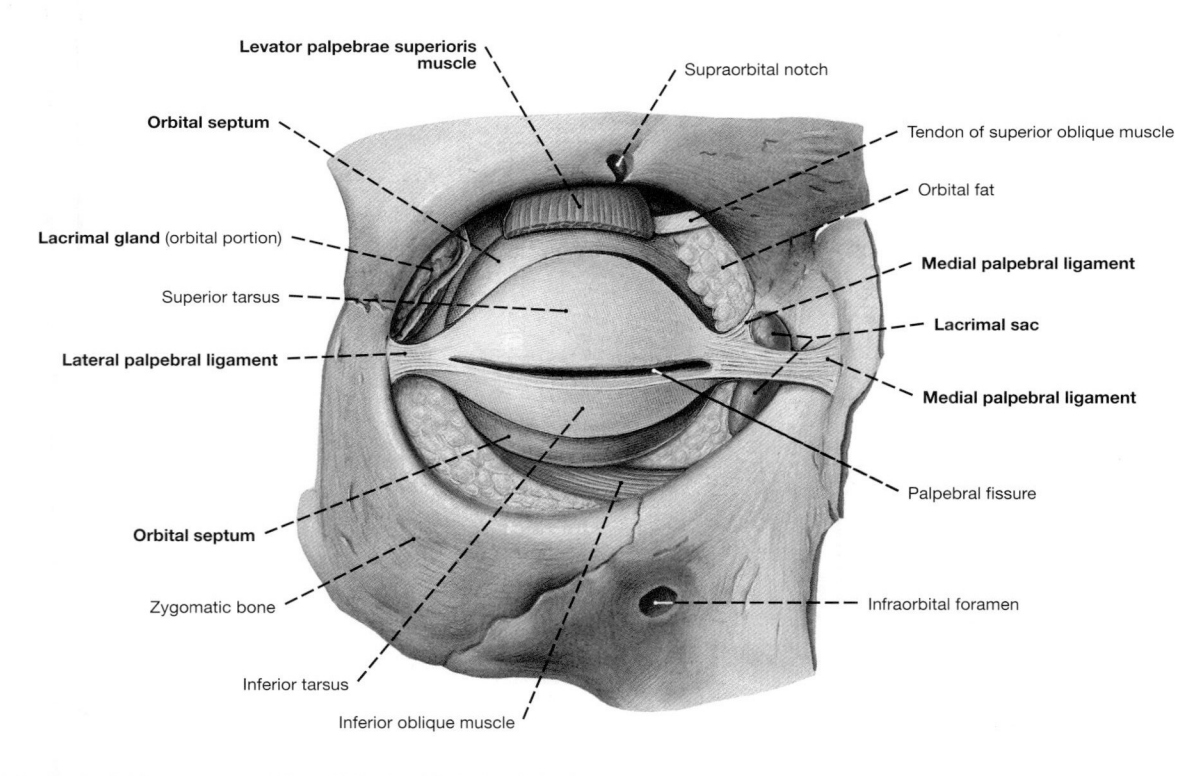

**Levator palpebrae superioris
muscle**

Orbital septum

Lacrimal gland (orbital portion)

Superior tarsus

Lateral palpebral ligament

Orbital septum

Zygomatic bone

Inferior tarsus

Inferior oblique muscle

Supraorbital notch

Tendon of superior oblique muscle

Orbital fat

Medial palpebral ligament

Lacrimal sac

Medial palpebral ligament

Palpebral fissure

Infraorbital foramen

Fig. 796: Palpebral Ligaments and Tarsal Plates (Anterior View)
NOTE: 1) the superficial structures of the orbit have been removed along with the orbital septum and the tendon of the levator palpebrae
superioris muscle.
    2) the lateral and medial margins of the tarsal plates are attached to the lateral and medial palpebral ligaments which in turn
are attached to bone. The medial ligament is located just anterior to the lacrimal sac.
    3) from this anterior view, both the tendon of the superior oblique muscle Iand the inferior oblique muscle can be visualized.
Note also the location of the orbital portion of the lacrimal gland in the upper lateral part of the orbit.

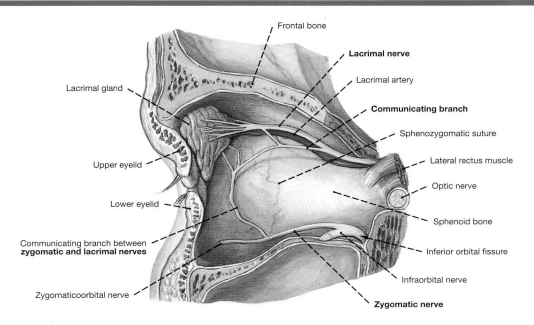

Fig. 797: Innervation of the Lacrimal Gland

NOTE: 1)   the lacrimal gland is supplied by the lacrimal artery which is a thin, tortuous branch of the ophthalmic artery that courses anteriorly in the orbital cavity.

2)   the lacrimal gland receives postganglionic parasympathetic fibers that are secretomotor in type. Preganglionic fibers are said to emerge from the brain in the nervus intermedius part of the facial nerve (VII). These fibers then synapse with the cell bodies of the postganglionic neurons in the pterygopalatine ganglion.

3)   the preganglionic parasympathetic fibers reach the pterygopalatine ganglion by way of the greater petrosal nerve which then becomes part of the nerve of the pterygoid canal. The postganglionic fibers leave the ganglion and travel for a short distance with the zygomatic nerve, a branch of the infraorbital nerve. From this nerve, in the inferior part of the orbit, the parasympathetic fibers, by way of a communicating branch to the lacrimal nerve, travel to the lacrimal gland.

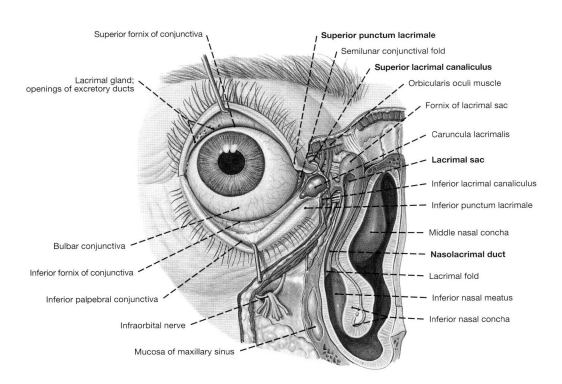

Fig. 798: Lacrimal Canaliculi, Lacrimal Sac, and Nasolacrimal Duct

NOTE: from the ducts of the lacrimal gland, tears moisten the surface of the eyeball and drain medially through the lacrimal canaliculi to the lacrimal sac and then descend to the nasal cavity by way of the nasolacrimal duct.

PLATE 508   Lacrimal Apparatus

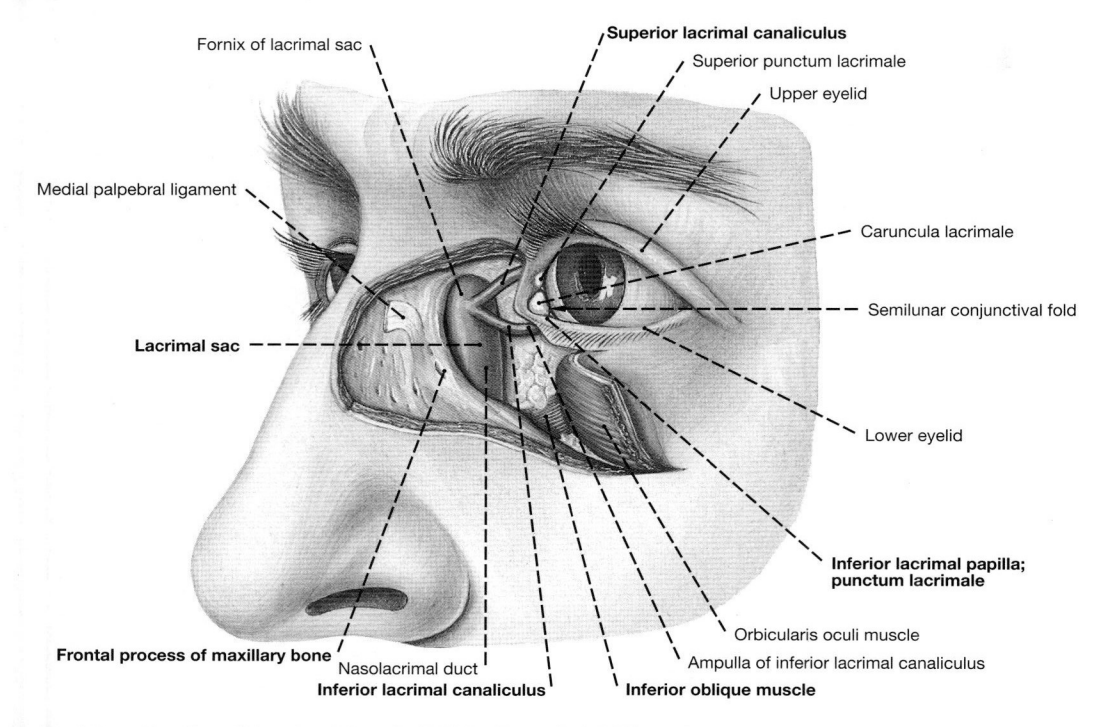

Fig. 799: Lacrimal Canaliculi and Lacrimal Sac: Left Side, Superficial Dissection

NOTE: 1)   the skin and superficial fascia have been removed over the medial angle of the orbit. Observe the cut orbicularis oculi muscle and medial palpebral ligament. The latter structure is still attached to the frontal process of the maxilla.

2)   severence of the medial palpebral ligament exposes the underlying lacrimal sac which is located in a small fossa formed by the maxilla and lacrimal bone. This sac receives a lacrimal canaliculus from each eyelid, and these two ducts are each about 1 cm long.

Fig. 800: Lacrimal Canaliculi, Lacrimal Sac and Nasolacrimal Duct: Left Side, Deep Dissection

NOTE: 1)   at the medial edge of both eyelids are found single minute orifices (puncta lacrimalia) of the lacrimal canaliculi which lead from the eyelids to the lacrimal sac.

2)   the lacrimal sac forms the upper end of the nasolacrimal duct which then extends about $3\frac{1}{2}$ inches into the inferior meatus of the nasal cavity.

3)   lacrimal secretions pass across the surface of the eyeball toward the canaliculi and then are transported to the nasal cavity by the nasolacrimal duct. Excessive secretions, as in crying, roll over the edge of the lower eyelid as tears.

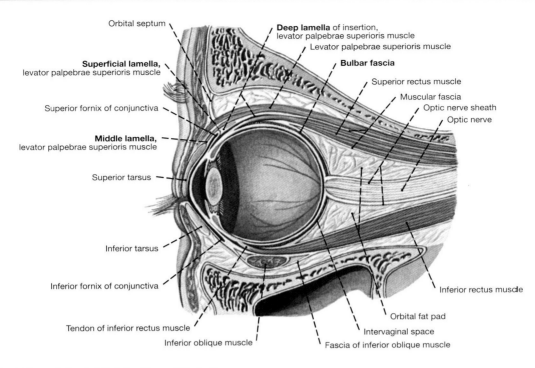

Orbital septum

Deep lamella of insertion,
levator palpebrae superioris muscle

Levator palpebrae superioris muscle

Superficial lamella,
levator palpebrae superioris muscle

Bulbar fascia

Superior rectus muscle

Superior fornix of conjunctiva

Muscular fascia

Optic nerve sheath

Optic nerve

Middle lamella,
levator palpebrae superioris muscle

Superior tarsus

Inferior tarsus

Inferior fornix of conjunctiva

Inferior rectus muscle

Tendon of inferior rectus muscle

Orbital fat pad

Intervaginal space

Inferior oblique muscle

Fascia of inferior oblique muscle

Fig. 801: Sagittal View of the Orbital Cavity and Eyeball

NOTE: 1) the **bulbar fascia** is a thin membrane that encloses the posterior ³/₄ths of the eyeball and separates the eyeball from the orbital fat and other contents of the orbital cavity.

2) the bulbar fascia is prolonged over the bellies of the ocular muscles but then is pierced by the tendons of these muscles as they insert on the outer coat of the eyeball.

3) the insertion of the **levator palpebrae superioris** is trilaminar. The superficial layer inserts into the upper eyelid, the middle into the superior tarsus and the deep layer inserts into the superior fornix of the conjunctiva.

4) the palpebral **conjunctiva** is a thin transparent mucous membrane on the innermost aspect of the eyelid. At the conjunctival angle (fornix), it reflects over the eyeball as far as the sclerocorneal junction.

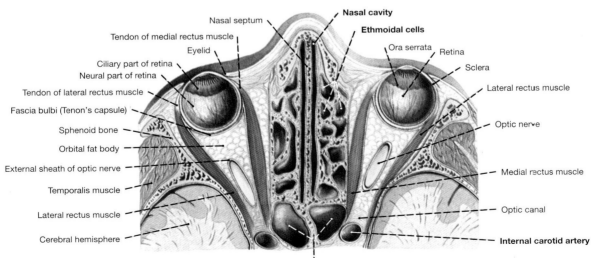

Nasal septum

Nasal cavity

Ethmoidal cells

Tendon of medial rectus muscle

Eyelid

Ora serrata

Retina

Ciliary part of retina

Sclera

Neural part of retina

Tendon of lateral rectus muscle

Lateral rectus muscle

Fascia bulbi (Tenon's capsule)

Sphenoid bone

Optic nerve

Orbital fat body

External sheath of optic nerve

Medial rectus muscle

Temporalis muscle

Lateral rectus muscle

Optic canal

Cerebral hemisphere

Internal carotid artery

Sphenoid sinus

Fig. 802: Horizontal Section Through Both Orbits at the Level of the Sphenoid Sinus

NOTE: 1) between the orbital cavities is situated the **ethmoid bone** containing the ethmoidal air sinuses (air cells). The vertically oriented perpendicular plate of the ethmoid serves as part of the nasal septum, and it subdivides the nasal cavity into two chambers.

2) the posterior portion of the orbits are separated by the **sphenoid sinuses,** located within the body of the sphenoid bone. These sinuses frequently are not symmetrical.

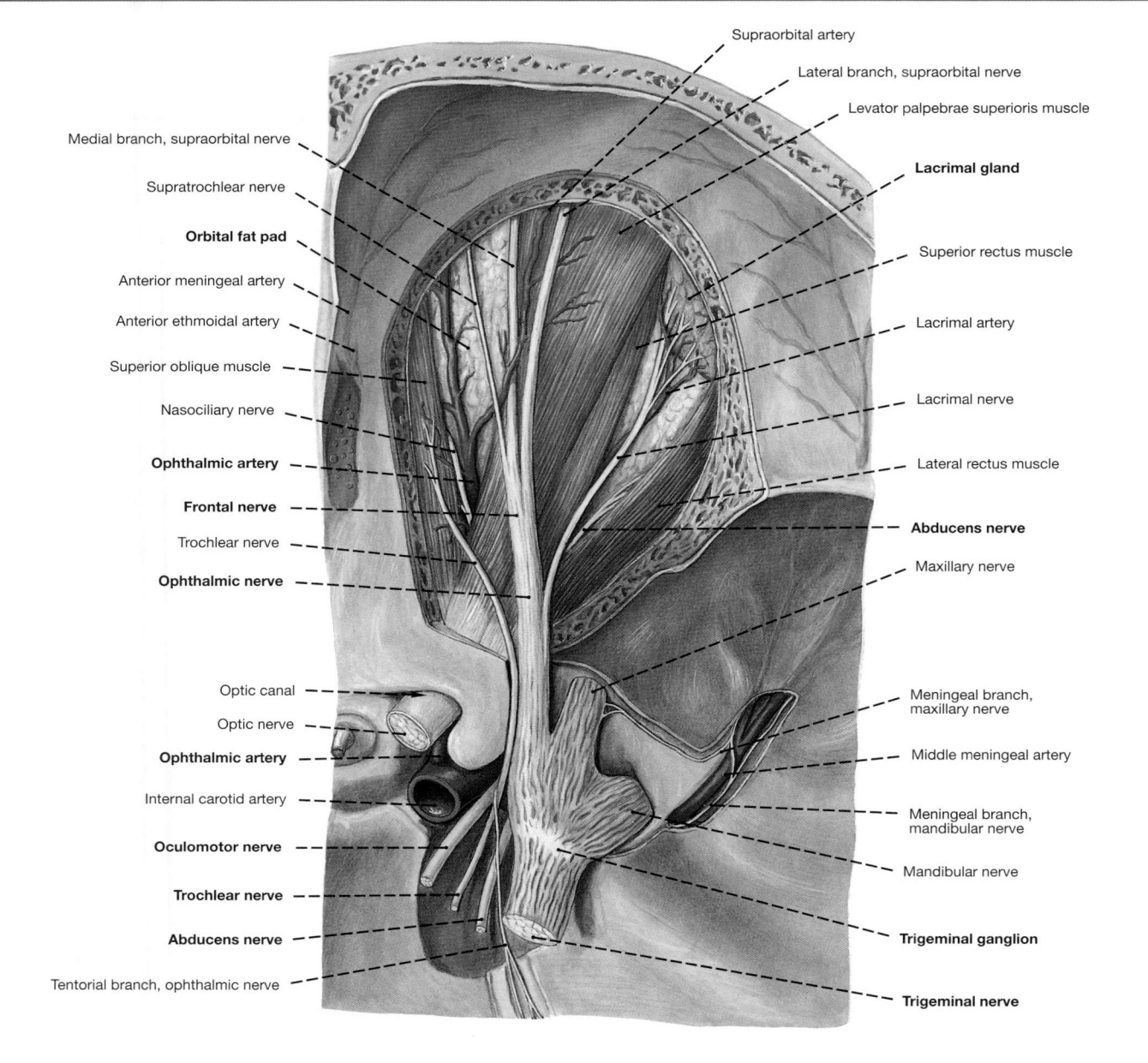

Supraorbital artery

Lateral branch, supraorbital nerve

Levator palpebrae superioris muscle

Lacrimal gland

Medial branch, supraorbital nerve

Supratrochlear nerve

Orbital fat pad

Anterior meningeal artery

Anterior ethmoidal artery

Superior oblique muscle

Nasociliary nerve

Ophthalmic artery

Frontal nerve

Trochlear nerve

Ophthalmic nerve

Superior rectus muscle

Lacrimal artery

Lacrimal nerve

Lateral rectus muscle

Abducens nerve

Maxillary nerve

Optic canal

Optic nerve

Ophthalmic artery

Internal carotid artery

Oculomotor nerve

Trochlear nerve

Abducens nerve

Tentorial branch, ophthalmic nerve

Meningeal branch, maxillary nerve

Middle meningeal artery

Meningeal branch, mandibular nerve

Mandibular nerve

Trigeminal ganglion

Trigeminal nerve

Fig. 803: Nerves and Arteries of the Orbit (Stage 1), Superior View: Ophthalmic Nerve and Artery

NOTE: 1) the orbital plate of the frontal bone has been removed and the superior orbital fissure opened to expose the structures of the right orbit from above. The ophthalmic division of the trigeminal nerve divides into **lacrimal, frontal** and **nasociliary branches.**

2) the **lacrimal nerve** courses anteriorly and laterally in the orbit and accompanies the lacrimal branch of the ophthalmic artery to supply the lacrimal gland.

3) the **frontal nerve** overlies the levator palpebrae superioris muscle and soon divides into a delicate **supratrochlear branch** and larger medial and lateral **supraorbital branches.** These course to the front of the orbit where they emerge on the forehead.

4) the **nasociliary nerve** crosses the orbit from lateral to medial, deep to the superior rectus muscle, and accompanies the ophthalmic artery for a short distance.

5) the **trochlear nerve** enters the orbit medial to the ophthalmic nerve to supply the superior oblique muscle.

6) the **optic nerve** leaves the orbit and enters the cranial cavity just medial to the internal carotid artery and the ophthalmic artery enters the orbit through the optic canal.

Fig. 803

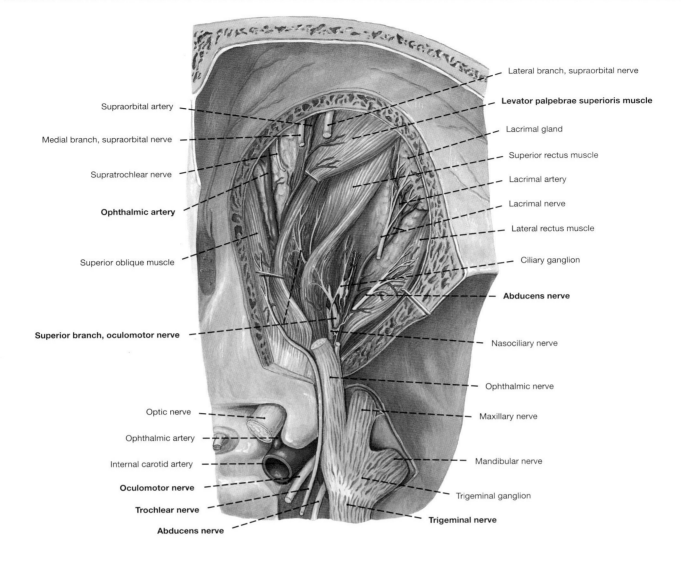

Lateral branch, supraorbital nerve

Supraorbital artery

Levator palpebrae superioris muscle

Medial branch, supraorbital nerve

Lacrimal gland

Supratrochlear nerve

Superior rectus muscle

Ophthalmic artery

Lacrimal artery

Lacrimal nerve

Lateral rectus muscle

Superior oblique muscle

Ciliary ganglion

Abducens nerve

Superior branch, oculomotor nerve

Nasociliary nerve

Ophthalmic nerve

Optic nerve

Maxillary nerve

Ophthalmic artery

Internal carotid artery

Mandibular nerve

Oculomotor nerve

Trochlear nerve

Trigeminal ganglion

Abducens nerve

Trigeminal nerve

Fig. 804: Nerves and Arteries of the Orbit (Stage 2), Superior View: Trochlear and Abducens Nerves

NOTE: 1) with the right orbit opened from above, the ophthalmic division of the trigeminal nerve and its lacrimal, supratrochlear and frontal branches have been cut. The levator palpebrae superioris and superior rectus muscles have been pulled medially to reveal their inferior surfaces where filaments from the **superior branch of the oculomotor nerve** innervate the two muscles.

2) the **nasociliary branch** of the ophthalmic nerve is still intact as it is seen turning medially deep to the superior rectus muscle. Note also that a fine communicating filament containing sensory fibers interconnects the ciliary ganglion and nasociliary nerve.

3) the **trochlear nerve** supplying the superior oblique muscle along its upper surface. If this nerve is injured, a patient has difficulty turning the eyeball laterally and down; when asked to look inferolaterally, the affected eye rotates medially, resulting in double vision or diplopia.

4) the **abducens nerve** supplying the lateral rectus muscle along its medial surface. After emerging from the brainstem at the pontomedullary junction, this nerve follows a long course in the floor of the cranial cavity and enters the orbit through the superior orbital fissure.

5) injury to the abducens nerve produces a diminished ability to move the eyeball laterally. From the resulting medial or convergent gaze of the affected eyeball, the patient complains of diplopia (double vision).

Fig. 804   **VII**

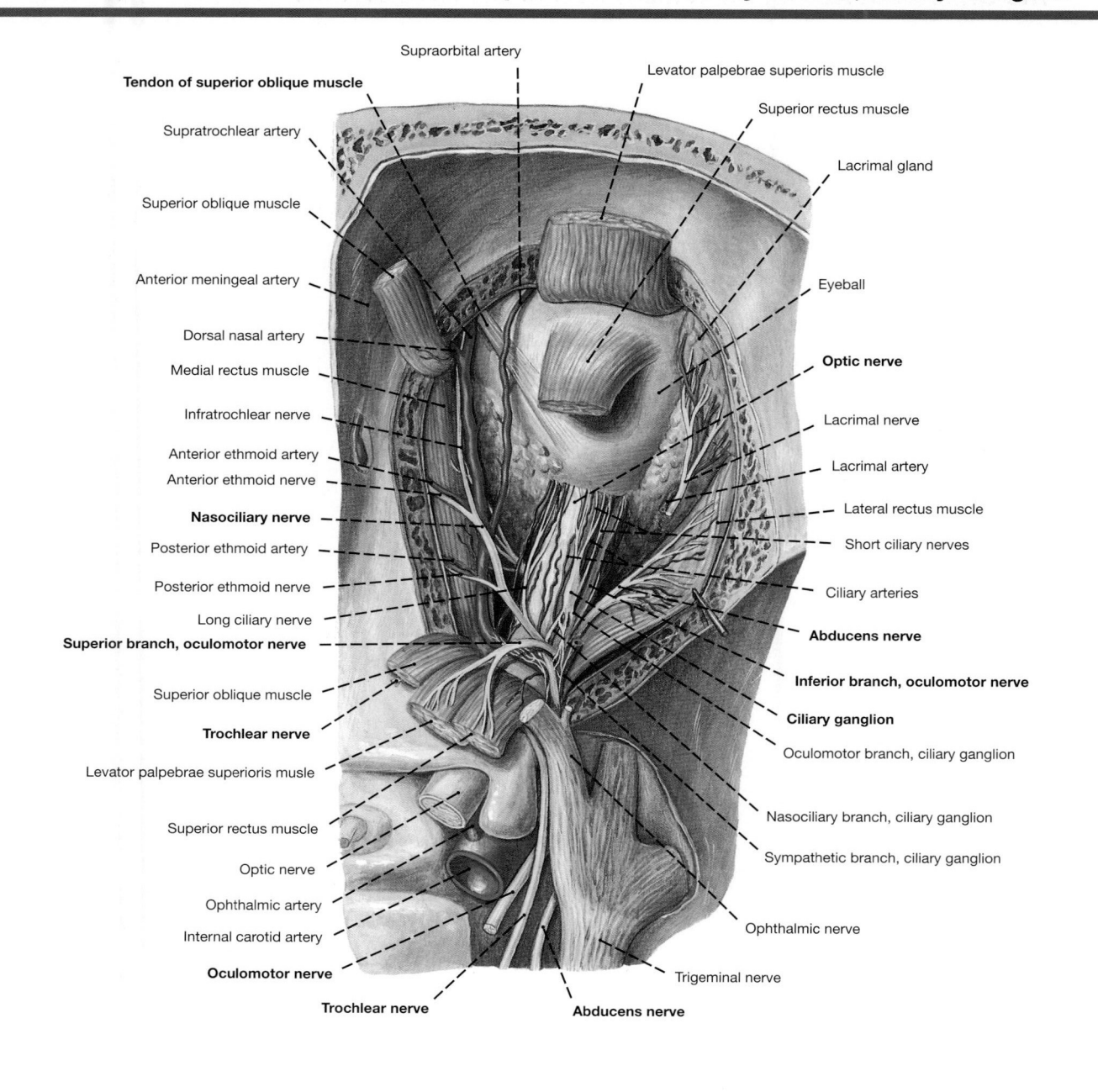

Supraorbital artery

Tendon of superior oblique muscle

Levator palpebrae superioris muscle

Supratrochlear artery

Superior rectus muscle

Superior oblique muscle

Lacrimal gland

Anterior meningeal artery

Dorsal nasal artery

Eyeball

Medial rectus muscle

Optic nerve

Infratrochlear nerve

Lacrimal nerve

Anterior ethmoid artery

Lacrimal artery

Anterior ethmoid nerve

Nasociliary nerve

Lateral rectus muscle

Posterior ethmoid artery

Short ciliary nerves

Posterior ethmoid nerve

Ciliary arteries

Long ciliary nerve

Abducens nerve

Superior branch, oculomotor nerve

Inferior branch, oculomotor nerve

Superior oblique muscle

Ciliary ganglion

Trochlear nerve

Oculomotor branch, ciliary ganglion

Levator palpebrae superioris musle

Nasociliary branch, ciliary ganglion

Superior rectus muscle

Sympathetic branch, ciliary ganglion

Optic nerve

Ophthalmic artery

Ophthalmic nerve

Internal carotid artery

Oculomotor nerve

Trigeminal nerve

Trochlear nerve

Abducens nerve

Fig. 805: Nerves and Arteries of the Orbit (Stage 3), Superior View: Optic Nerve and Ciliary Ganglion

NOTE: 1) with the levator palpebrae superioris, superior rectus and superior oblique muscles cut and reflected, the **nasociliary nerve** and **ophthalmic artery** are seen crossing over the **optic nerve** from lateral to medial.

2) the relationship to the optic nerve of the longitudinally oriented **long ciliary arteries** (from the ophthalmic) and the **long ciliary nerves** (2 or 3 branches from the nasociliary nerve).

3) the **ciliary ganglion** lies lateral to the optic nerve. Its **parasympathetic root** comes from the oculomotor nerve and its **sensory root** from the nasociliary nerve. Postganglionic parasympathetic fibers reach the eyeball by the **short ciliary nerves.**

4) postganglionic parasympathetic nerve fibers supply the **sphincter of the pupil** and the muscle responsible for accommodation of the lens, the **ciliaris muscle.**

5) some **sympathetic fibers** that arrive in the orbit along the ophthalmic artery also course through the ciliary ganglion. These are principally vasoconstrictor fibers to arteries that supply the eyeball. Sympathetic fibers that supply the **dilator of the pupil** course to the posterior pole of the eyeball by way of the **long ciliary nerves.**

6) although the supratrochlear nerve is derived from the frontal branch of the ophthalmic nerve, the **infratrochlear nerve** (as well as the **anterior** and **posterior ethmoid nerves**) is derived from the nasociliary branch of the ophthalmic nerve.

Fig. 805

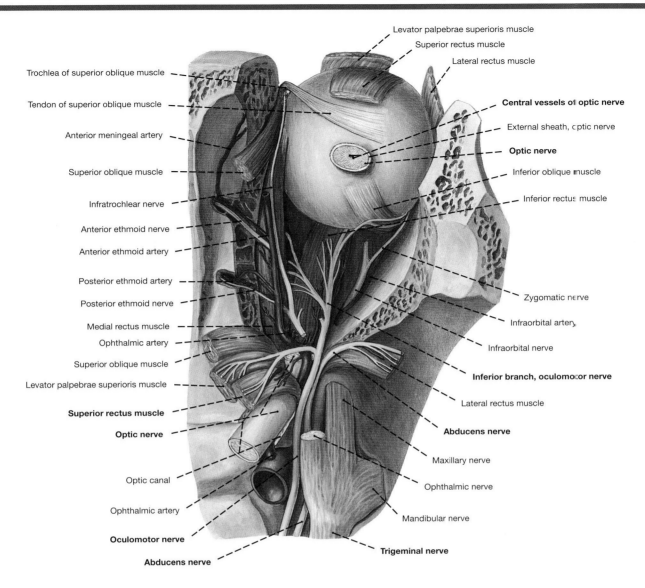

Levator palpebrae superioris muscle

Superior rectus muscle

Lateral rectus muscle

Trochlea of superior oblique muscle

Tendon of superior oblique muscle

Anterior meningeal artery

Superior oblique muscle

Infratrochlear nerve

Anterior ethmoid nerve

Anterior ethmoid artery

Posterior ethmoid artery

Posterior ethmoid nerve

Medial rectus muscle

Ophthalmic artery

Superior oblique muscle

Levator palpebrae superioris muscle

Superior rectus muscle

Optic nerve

Optic canal

Ophthalmic artery

Oculomotor nerve

Abducens nerve

Central vessels of optic nerve

External sheath, optic nerve

Optic nerve

Inferior oblique muscle

Inferior rectus muscle

Zygomatic nerve

Infraorbital artery

Infraorbital nerve

Inferior branch, oculomotor nerve

Lateral rectus muscle

Abducens nerve

Maxillary nerve

Ophthalmic nerve

Mandibular nerve

Trigeminal nerve

Fig. 806: Nerves and Arteries of the Orbit (Stage 4), Superior View: Oculomotor Nerve (Inferior Branch)
NOTE: 1) the levator palpebrae superioris, superior rectus, superior oblique and lateral rectus muscles have been cut and reflected; the optic nerve has also been severed. The anterior half of the eyeball has been depressed and its posterior pole directed upward. Observe the **central vessels of the optic nerve,** as well as the insertions of the superior oblique and inferior oblique muscles.

2) the **oculomotor nerve** courses through the superior orbital fissure and the common tendinous ring. It quickly gives off its **superior branch** which courses upward in the orbit to supply the levator palpebrae superioris and superior rectus muscles. The **inferior branch** of the oculomotor nerve courses anteriorly in the deep part of the orbit to supply the inferior rectus, medial rectus and inferior oblique muscles.

3) the anterior and posterior ethmoid arteries and nerves and the infratrochlear nerve all located medially in the orbit. Note also the **infraorbital nerve** and **artery** in the infraorbital groove more laterally.

4) the **ophthalmic artery** is the first branch of the internal carotid artery within the cranial cavity; it immediately enters the orbit through the optic canal with the optic nerve. Probably, the most important of the branches of the ophthalmic artery is the **central artery of the optic nerve (or retina)** which courses with its **vein** within the optic nerve.

5) the central artery is the **only** source of blood to the neural retina and an increase in pressure on the posterior part of the orbital cavity or edema of the optic nerve caused by an inflammatory process can seriously compromise vision either by blockage of the artery or by diminishing the flow in the **central retinal vein.**

Fig. 806   **VII**

PLATE 514   The Orbit: Muscles and Other Structures (Lateral View)

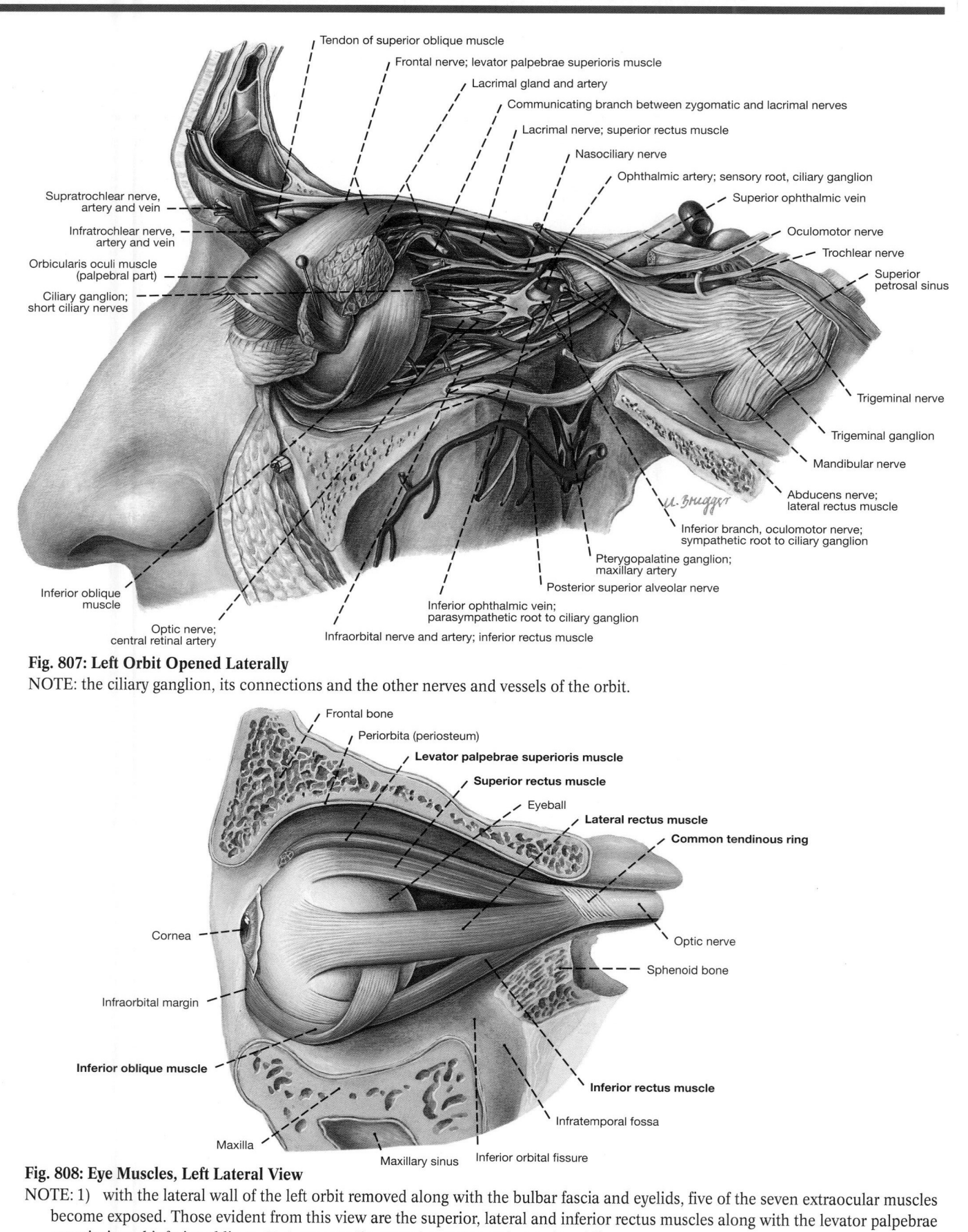

Tendon of superior oblique muscle

Frontal nerve; levator palpebrae superioris muscle

Lacrimal gland and artery

Communicating branch between zygomatic and lacrimal nerves

Lacrimal nerve; superior rectus muscle

Nasociliary nerve

Ophthalmic artery; sensory root, ciliary ganglion

Superior ophthalmic vein

Oculomotor nerve

Trochlear nerve

Superior petrosal sinus

Trigeminal nerve

Trigeminal ganglion

Mandibular nerve

Abducens nerve; lateral rectus muscle

Inferior branch, oculomotor nerve; sympathetic root to ciliary ganglion

Pterygopalatine ganglion; maxillary artery

Posterior superior alveolar nerve

Inferior ophthalmic vein; parasympathetic root to ciliary ganglion

Infraorbital nerve and artery; inferior rectus muscle

Optic nerve; central retinal artery

Inferior oblique muscle

Ciliary ganglion; short ciliary nerves

Orbicularis oculi muscle (palpebral part)

Infratrochlear nerve, artery and vein

Supratrochlear nerve, artery and vein

Fig. 807: Left Orbit Opened Laterally

NOTE: the ciliary ganglion, its connections and the other nerves and vessels of the orbit.

Frontal bone

Periorbita (periosteum)

Levator palpebrae superioris muscle

Superior rectus muscle

Eyeball

Lateral rectus muscle

Common tendinous ring

Optic nerve

Sphenoid bone

Inferior orbital fissure

Inferior orbital fissure

Inferior rectus muscle

Inferior oblique muscle

Infraorbital margin

Cornea

Maxilla

Maxillary sinus

Infratemporal fossa

Fig. 808: Eye Muscles, Left Lateral View

NOTE: 1) with the lateral wall of the left orbit removed along with the bulbar fascia and eyelids, five of the seven extraocular muscles become exposed. Those evident from this view are the superior, lateral and inferior rectus muscles along with the levator palpebrae superioris and inferior oblique. Not seen are the superior rectus and superior oblique.

2) of the seven muscles, all except the levator palpebrae superioris and the inferior oblique take origin from the common tendinous ring which surrounds the optic nerve.

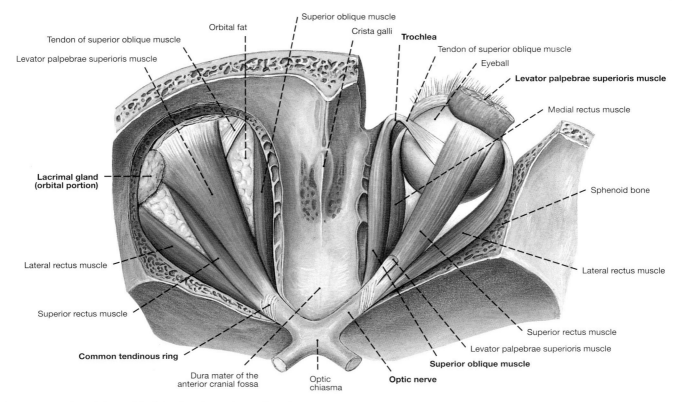

Fig. 809: Muscles of the Orbital Cavity (Seen From above)

NOTE: 1)   the orbital plates of the frontal bones have been removed from within the cranial cavity. On the **left side** only the bony roof of the orbit has been opened and the muscles, orbital fat and lacrimal gland have been left intact.

2)   on the **right side** the levator palpebrae superioris muscle has been resected and the orbital fat removed to expose the ocular muscles.

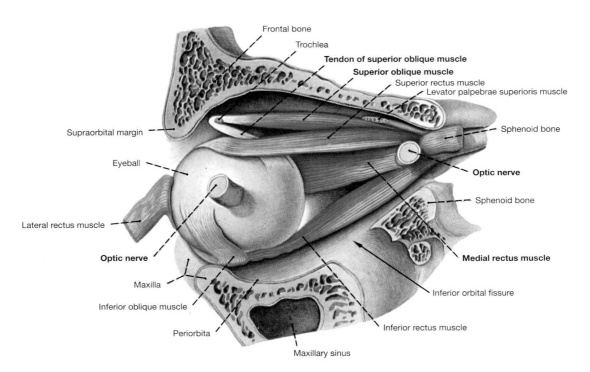

Fig. 810: Eye Muscles, Left Lateral View (Lateral Rectus Muscle and Optic Nerve Cut)

NOTE: the eyeball has been rotated 90° such that its posterior pole is directed laterally. This reveals to advantage the medial rectus muscle and the superior oblique muscle and tendon as it bends around the trochlea to insert on the eyeball.

PLATE 516   **The Orbit: Extraocular Muscles, Insertions and Actions**

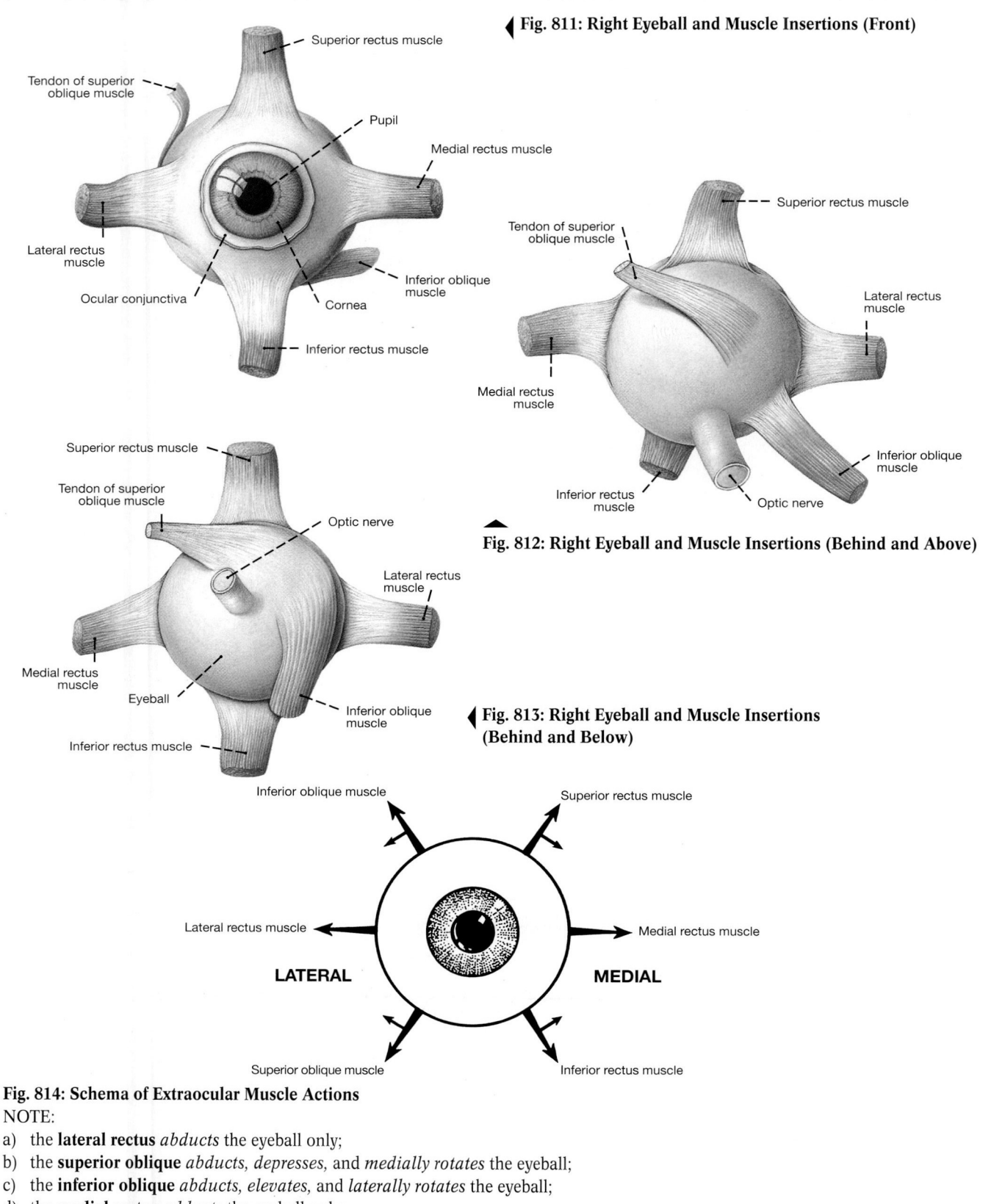

Fig. 811: Right Eyeball and Muscle Insertions (Front)

Fig. 812: Right Eyeball and Muscle Insertions (Behind and Above)

Fig. 813: Right Eyeball and Muscle Insertions (Behind and Below)

Fig. 814: Schema of Extraocular Muscle Actions
NOTE:
a) the **lateral rectus** *abducts* the eyeball only;
b) the **superior oblique** *abducts, depresses,* and *medially rotates* the eyeball;
c) the **inferior oblique** *abducts, elevates,* and *laterally rotates* the eyeball;
d) the **medial rectus** *adducts* the eyeball only;
e) the **inferior rectus** *adducts, depresses,* and *laterally rotates* the eyeball;
f) the **superior rectus** *adducts, elevates,* and *medially rotates* the eyeball.
NOTE: the following muscle innervations:
a) the **oculomotor nerve (III):** levator palpebrae superioris, superior rectus, medial rectus, inferior rectus and inferior oblique muscles;
b) the **trochlear nerve (IV):** superior oblique muscle;
c) the **abducens nerve (VI):** lateral rectus muscle.

Figs. 811– 814

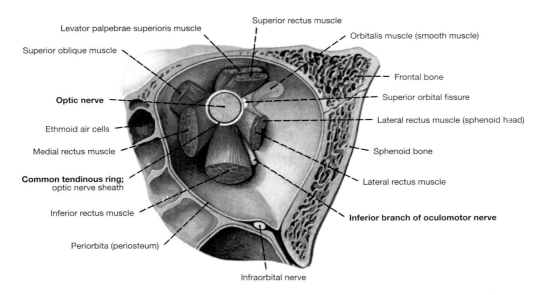

Levator palpebrae superioris muscle
Superior rectus muscle
Superior oblique muscle
Orbitalis muscle (smooth muscle)
Frontal bone
Optic nerve
Superior orbital fissure
Ethmoid air cells
Lateral rectus muscle (sphenoid head)
Medial rectus muscle
Sphenoid bone
Common tendinous ring;
optic nerve sheath
Lateral rectus muscle
Inferior rectus muscle
Inferior branch of oculomotor nerve
Periorbita (periosteum)
Infraorbital nerve

Fig. 815: Origins of the Ocular Muscles, Apex of Left Orbit

NOTE: 1)   this anterior view of the apex of the left orbit shows the stumps of the ocular muscles which have been cut close to their origins.

2)   the four rectus muscles **arise** from a tendinous ring surrounding the optic canal. The levator palpebrae superioris and superior oblique **arise** from the sphenoid bone close to the tendinous ring, while the inferior oblique (not shown here, see Fig. 796) **arises** from the orbital surface of the maxilla.

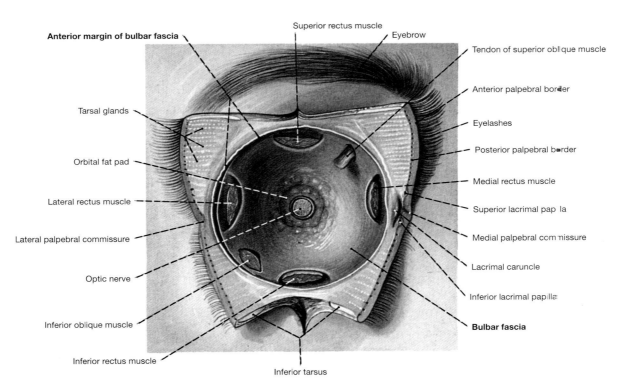

Anterior margin of bulbar fascia
Superior rectus muscle
Eyebrow
Tendon of superior oblique muscle
Anterior palpebral border
Tarsal glands
Eyelashes
Orbital fat pad
Posterior palpebral border
Lateral rectus muscle
Medial rectus muscle
Superior lacrimal papilla
Lateral palpebral commissure
Medial palpebral commissure
Optic nerve
Lacrimal caruncle
Inferior lacrimal papilla
Inferior oblique muscle
Bulbar fascia
Inferior rectus muscle
Inferior tarsus

Fig. 816: Bulbar Fascia (Capsule of Tenon), Right Eye

NOTE: 1)   longitudinal incisions have been made down the middle of each eyelid and the flaps have been reflected to expose the orbital cavity anteriorly.

2)   the **optic nerve** has been severed at the optic disc, and the eyeball along with the insertions of the ocular muscles, have been removed from the orbital cavity.

3)   the **bulbar fascia**, which envelopes the posterior aspect of the eyeball (from the sclerocorneal junction to the optic nerve), has been left within the orbit. Observe how the bulbar fascia is perforated by the tendons of the ocular muscles. It is also pierced from behind by the ciliary vessels and nerves.

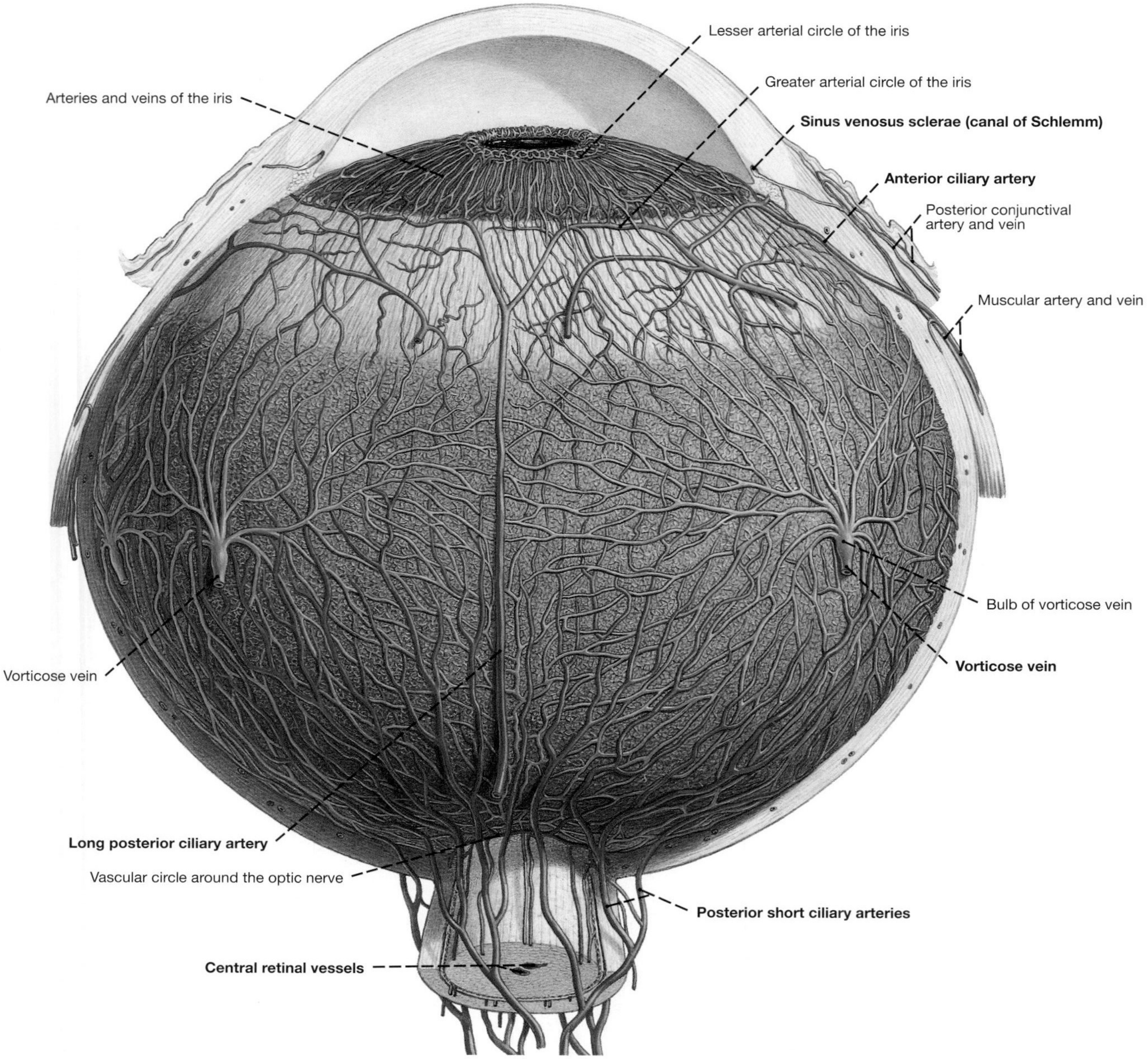

PLATE 518   **The Eyeball: Vascular Tunic (Chorioid); Optic Disc**

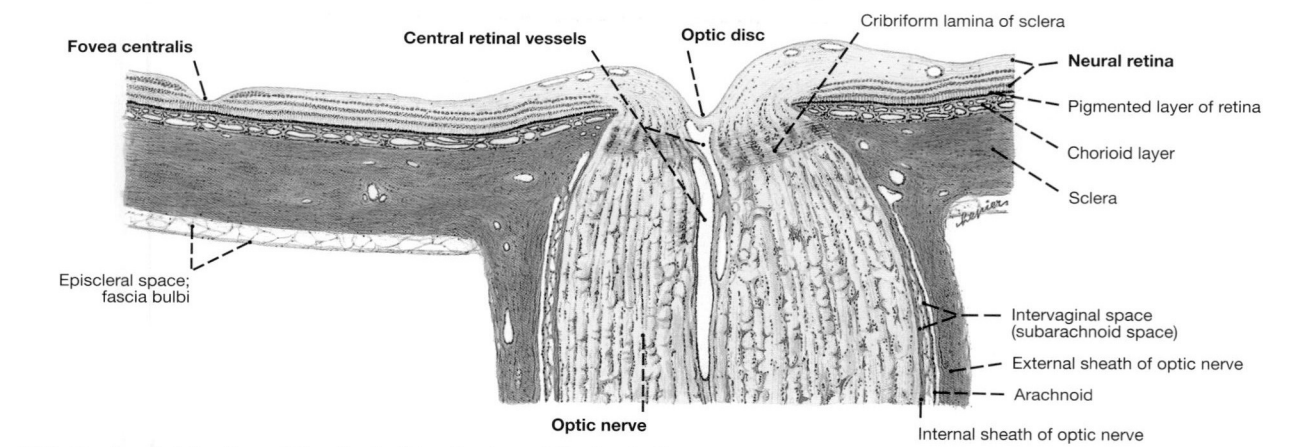

Lesser arterial circle of the iris

Greater arterial circle of the iris

Sinus venosus sclerae (canal of Schlemm)

Anterior ciliary artery

Posterior conjunctival artery and vein

Muscular artery and vein

Arteries and veins of the iris

Bulb of vorticose vein

Vorticose vein

Vorticose vein

Long posterior ciliary artery

Vascular circle around the optic nerve

Posterior short ciliary arteries

Central retinal vessels

Fig. 817: Chorioid or Vascular Tunic of the Eyeball
NOTE: the **chorioid** consists of a dense vascular plexus derived from **long (2) and short (5 to 7) posterior ciliary arteries** and several **anterior ciliary arteries.** These drain into the **vorticose veins,** tributaries of the ophthalmic veins.

Fovea centralis

Central retinal vessels

Optic disc

Cribriform lamina of sclera

Neural retina

Pigmented layer of retina

Chorioid layer

Sclera

Episcleral space; fascia bulbi

Intervaginal space (subarachnoid space)

External sheath of optic nerve

Arachnoid

Internal sheath of optic nerve

Optic nerve

Fig. 818: Horizontal Section of the Optic Disc Region of Tune Eyeball
NOTE: the axons of the optic nerve leave the eyeball at the **optic disc,** or blind spot where there are no visual receptors.

Figs. 817, 818

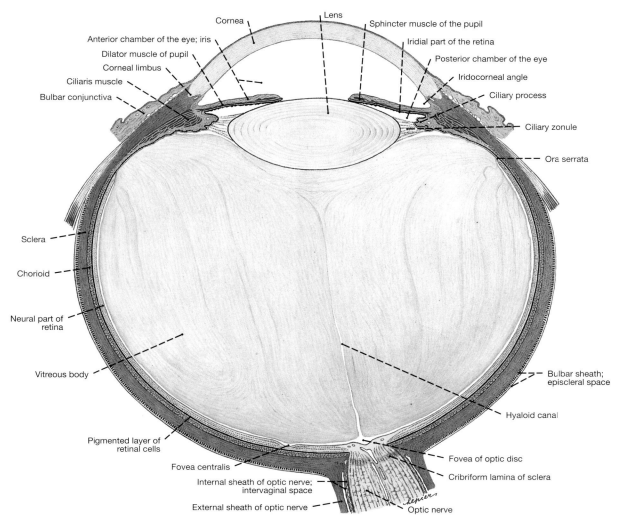

Fig. 819: Horizontal Section of the Left Eyeball Through the Optic Disc and Optic Nerve
NOTE: the eyeball is composed of three concentric layers or tunics:
    a)   an **outer fibrous tunic** (red), which consists of the **sclera** posteriorly and the translucent **cornea** anteriorly;
    b)   the **middle vascular tunic** (blue), which consists of the **chorioid** posteriorly and the **ciliary body** and **iris** anteriorly;
    c)   the **inner neural tunic** (yellow), which is the **retina.** It consists of a *neural* part posteriorly and a *non-neural* part that
         underlies the ciliary body and the iris. The junction between the neural and non-neural parts is called the **ora serrata.**

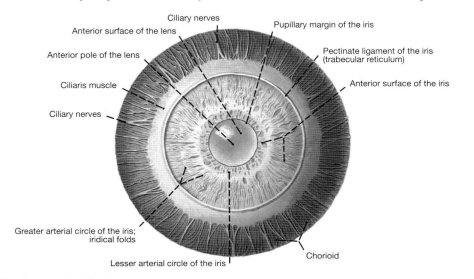

Fig. 820: Iris and Pupil (Anterior View)
NOTE: behind the iris is located the anterior pole of the lens.

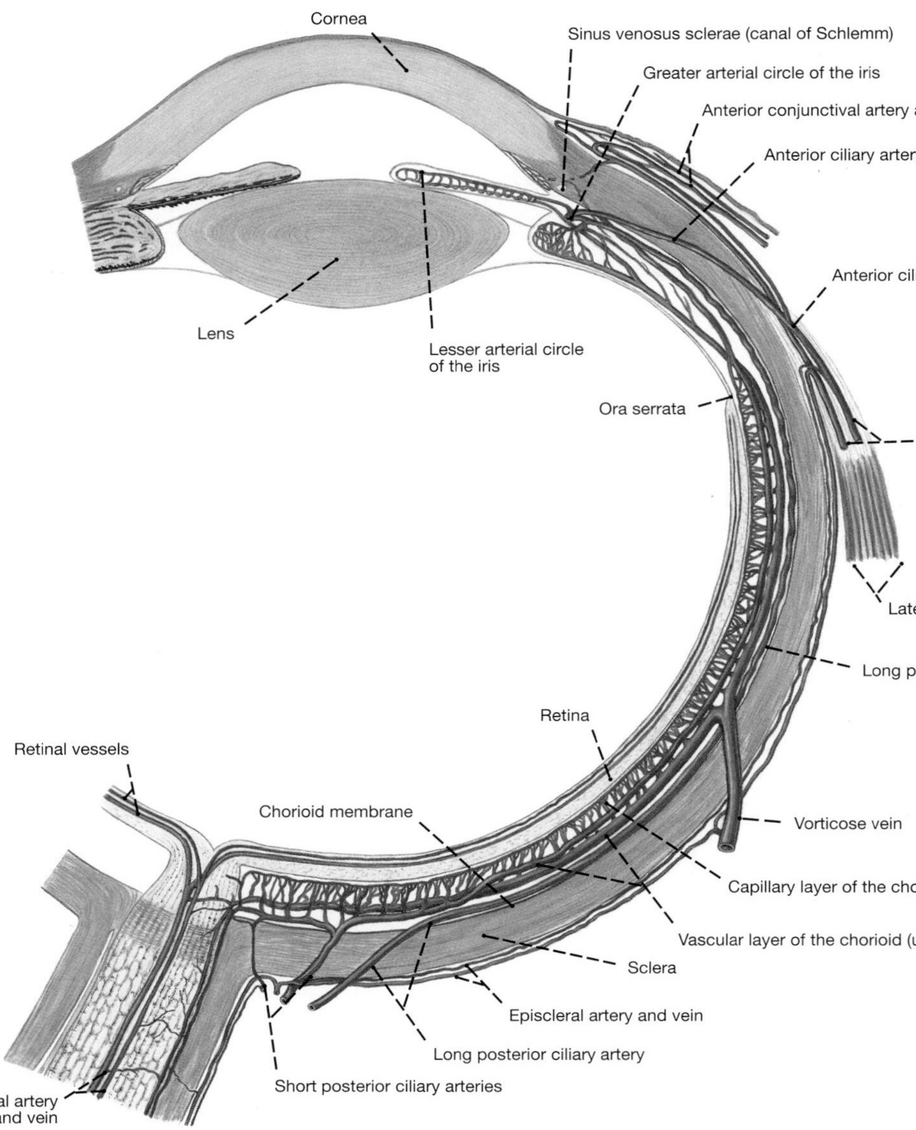

PLATE 520   The Eyeball: Arteries and Veins

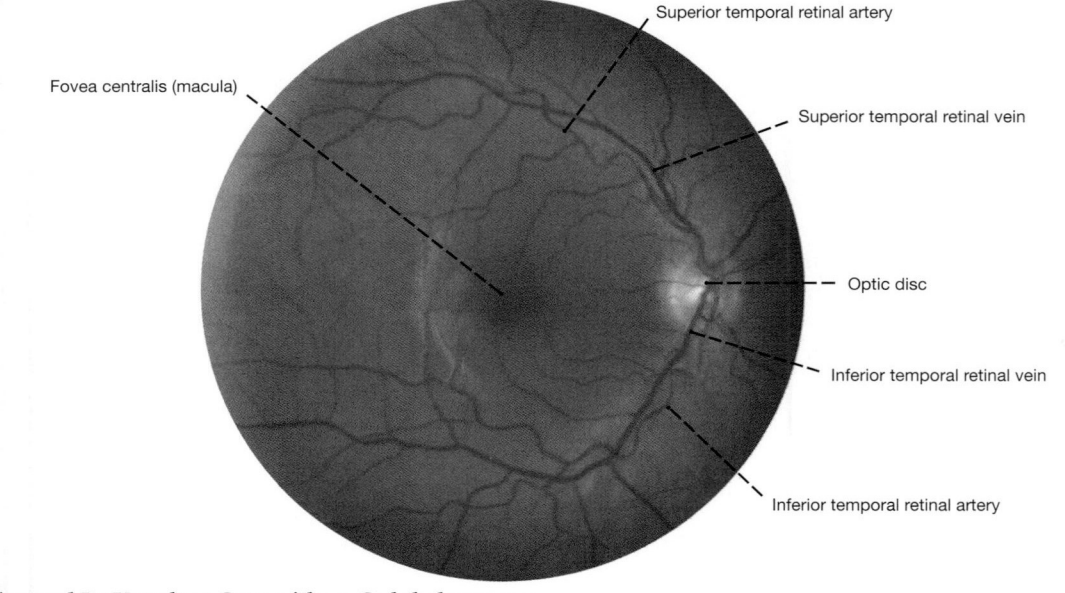

Cornea

Sinus venosus sclerae (canal of Schlemm)

Greater arterial circle of the iris

Anterior conjunctival artery and vein

Anterior ciliary artery

Anterior ciliary artery

Anterior ciliary vessels

Lens

Lesser arterial circle of the iris

Ora serrata

Lateral rectus muscle

Long posterior ciliary artery

Retina

Retinal vessels

Chorioid membrane

Vorticose vein

Capillary layer of the chorioid

Vascular layer of the chorioid (uvea)

Sclera

Episcleral artery and vein

Long posterior ciliary artery

Short posterior ciliary arteries

Central retinal artery and vein

Fig. 821: Horizontal Section Through the Eyeball Showing the Blood Supply to Its Three Layers

Superior temporal retinal artery

Fovea centralis (macula)

Superior temporal retinal vein

Optic disc

Inferior temporal retinal vein

Inferior temporal retinal artery

Fig. 822: Retina and Its Vessels as Seen with an Ophthalmoscope
NOTE: this shows the fundus of the eye with the **retinal vessels** passing through the optic disc.

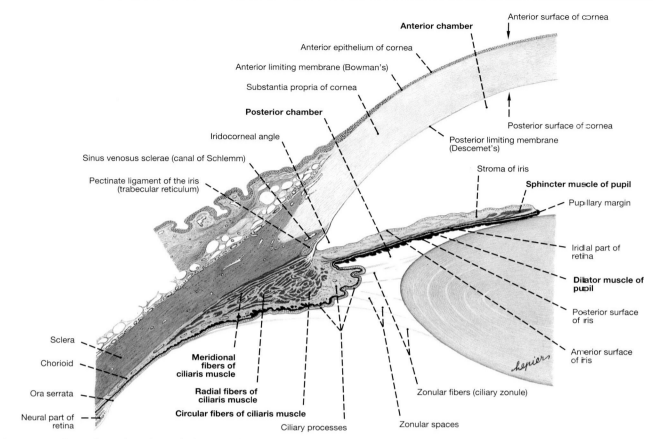

Fig. 823: Horizontal Section Through the Anterior Part of the Eyeball

NOTE: 1) the **iris** is the anterior continuation of the ciliary body and chorioid and it separates the anterior chamber from the posterior chamber.

    2) the **ciliary body** contains the **ciliaris muscle** and its fibers are oriented in radial, circular, and meridional (longitudinal) directions. When the eye needs to focus on a near object (accommodation), the ciliary muscle contracts and this pulls the ciliary body and chorioid forward, thereby relieving tension produced by the zonular fibers. The lens becomes thicker and increases its convexity. Parasympathetic fibers supply this muscle.

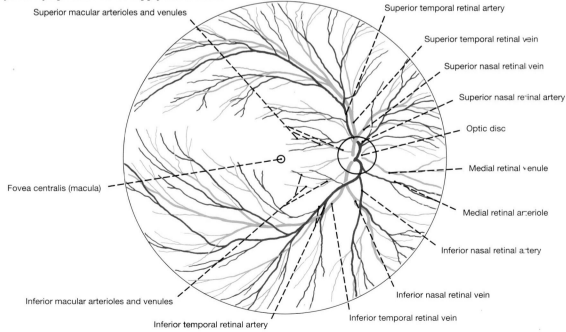

Fig. 824: Schematic Drawing of the Retinal Vessels

NOTE: the central retinal artery initially divides into **superior and inferior branches.** Each of these subdivide into **nasal and temporal branches,** supplying the four retinal quadrants.

PLATE 522   External Nose; Lateral Wall of the Nasal Cavity

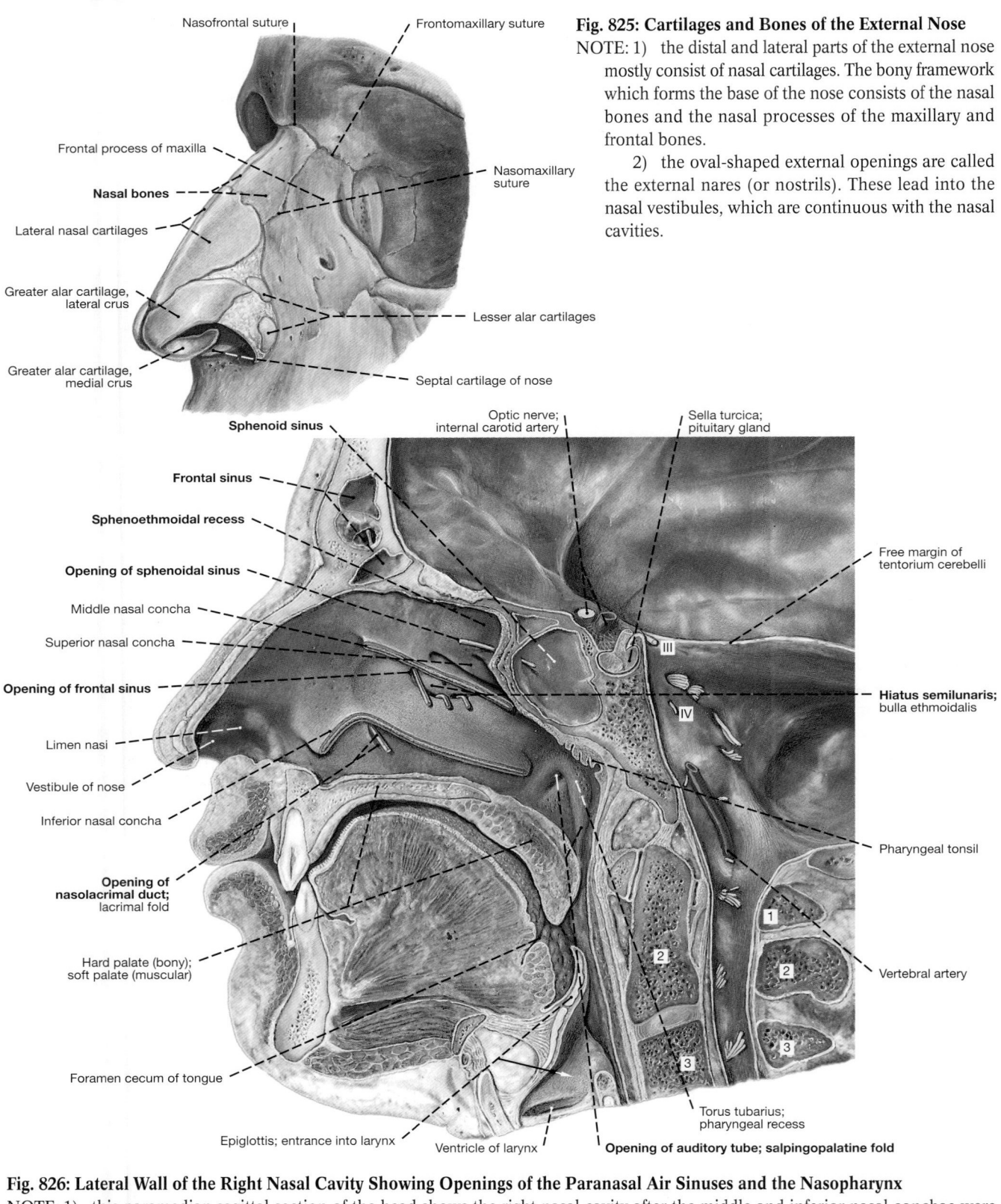

Nasofrontal suture

Frontomaxillary suture

Frontal process of maxilla

Nasal bones

Lateral nasal cartilages

Greater alar cartilage,
lateral crus

Greater alar cartilage,
medial crus

Nasomaxillary
suture

Lesser alar cartilages

Septal cartilage of nose

Fig. 825: Cartilages and Bones of the External Nose

NOTE: 1) the distal and lateral parts of the external nose mostly consist of nasal cartilages. The bony framework which forms the base of the nose consists of the nasal bones and the nasal processes of the maxillary and frontal bones.

2) the oval-shaped external openings are called the external nares (or nostrils). These lead into the nasal vestibules, which are continuous with the nasal cavities.

Sphenoid sinus

Frontal sinus

Sphenoethmoidal recess

Opening of sphenoidal sinus

Middle nasal concha

Superior nasal concha

Opening of frontal sinus

Limen nasi

Vestibule of nose

Inferior nasal concha

**Opening of
nasolacrimal duct;**
lacrimal fold

Hard palate (bony);
soft palate (muscular)

Foramen cecum of tongue

Epiglottis; entrance into larynx

Ventricle of larynx

Optic nerve;
internal carotid artery

Sella turcica;
pituitary gland

Free margin of
tentorium cerebelli

III

IV

Hiatus semilunaris;
bulla ethmoidalis

Pharyngeal tonsil

1

2

2

3

Vertebral artery

3

Torus tubarius;
pharyngeal recess

Opening of auditory tube; salpingopalatine fold

Fig. 826: Lateral Wall of the Right Nasal Cavity Showing Openings of the Paranasal Air Sinuses and the Nasopharynx

NOTE: 1)   this paramedian sagittal section of the head shows the right nasal cavity after the middle and inferior nasal conchae were removed. The nasal cavity communicates anteriorly with the exterior through the nostril and posteriorly with the nasopharynx.

2)   the following openings of the paranasal sinuses and other structures:

a)   the **sphenoid sinus**, which drains into the **sphenoethmoid recess** above the superior concha;

b)   the **frontal** and **maxillary sinuses** both of which open in a groove called the **hiatus semilunaris** in the middle meatus below the middle concha;

c)   the **nasolacrimal duct**, which opens into the inferior meatus below the inferior concha;

d)   the **auditory tube**, which opens into the nasopharynx just behind the inferior concha.

Figs. 825, 826

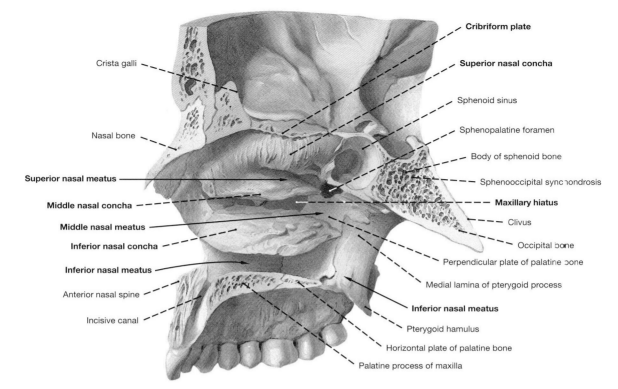

Fig. 827: Bony Lateral Wall of the Right Nasal Cavity

NOTE: 1)   the nasal septum has been removed and the mucosa stripped from the irregular lateral wall of the nasal cavity and the hard palate. Note also that in front of the nasal conchae are the **nasal bone** (gray) and the **maxilla** and behind is the **perpendicular plate** of the **palatine bone** (blue).

2)   the **crista galli**, **cribriform plate** and the **superior** and **middle nasal conchae** are all part of the **ethmoid bone** (light orange). Below these is the **inferior nasal concha**, which is a separate bone (gray). The bony floor of the nasal cavity is the hard palate, formed by the **palatine process** of the **maxilla** and the **horizontal plate** of the **palatine bone.**

3)   the arrows that follow the courses of the **superior**, **middle**, and **inferior meatuses**, each under its respective nasal concha. Note also the **sphenoid sinus,** the **sphenopalatine foramen** and the opening of the maxillary sinus **(maxillary hiatus).**

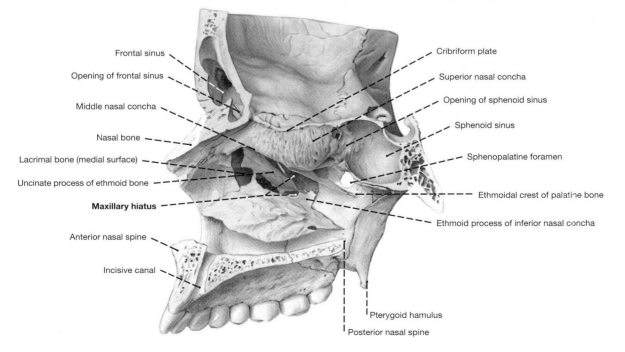

Fig. 828: Bony Lateral Wall of the Right Nasal Cavity with the Middle Nasal Concha Removed

NOTE: more complete exposure of the **maxillary hiatus** and the bony structures deep to (lateral to) the middle nasal concha. Compare with Figure 827.

PLATE 524   **Nasal Septum: Skeletal Parts, Vessels and Nerves**

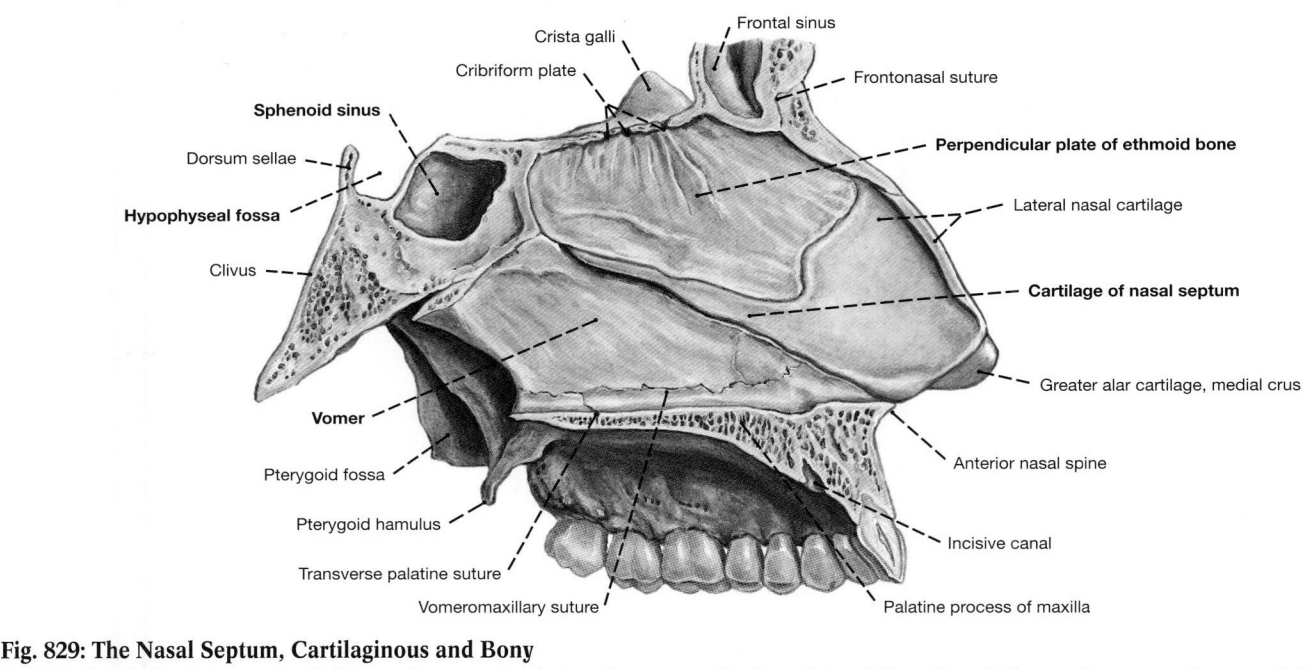

Fig. 829: The Nasal Septum, Cartilaginous and Bony

NOTE: the skeletal structure of the nasal septum includes the **perpendicular plate of the ethmoid bone,** the **vomer bone** and the **cartilage of the nasal septum.**

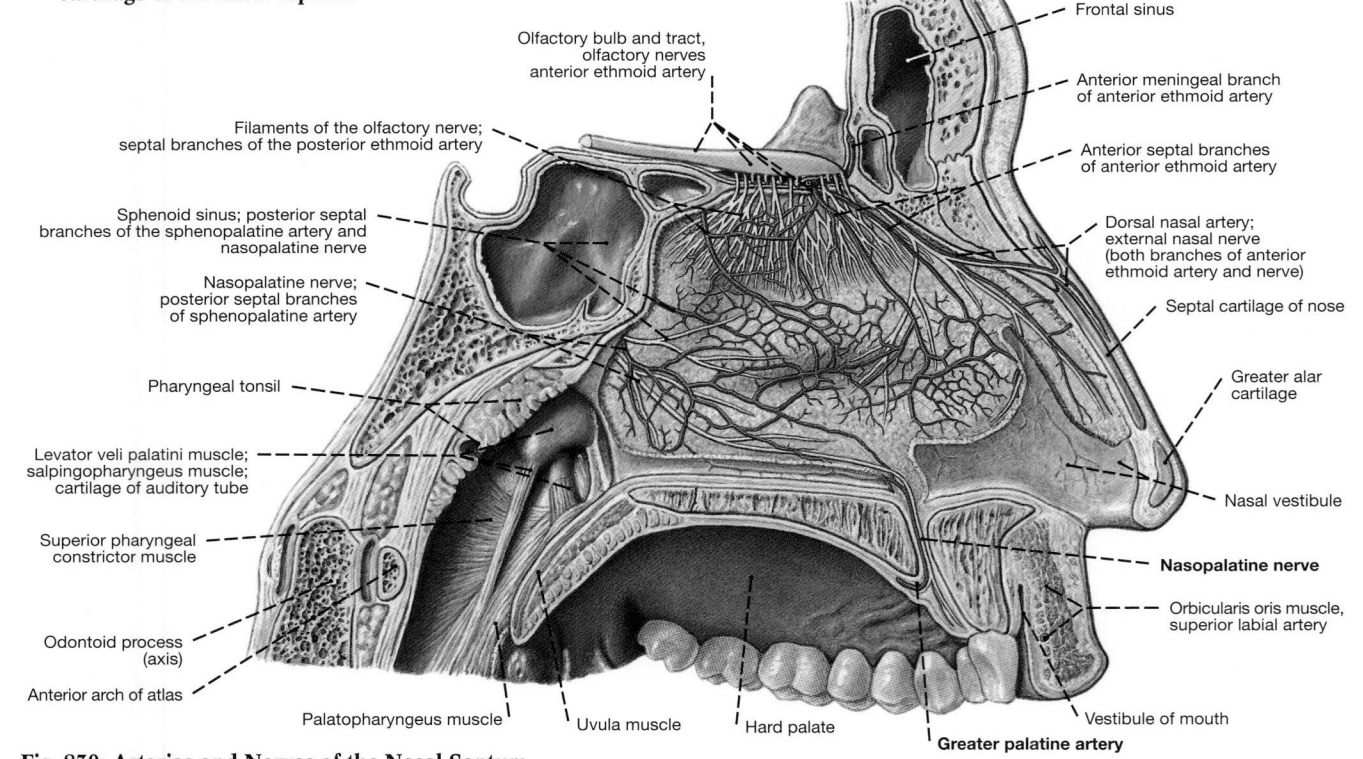

Fig. 830: Arteries and Nerves of the Nasal Septum

NOTE: 1) *from above and behind* the **arteries of the septum** include:
    a) branches of the **anterior** and **posterior ethmoid artery** and
    b) **posterior septal branches** of the **sphenopalatine artery**
    from below and in front:
    a) **septal branch** of the **superior labial artery** that enters through the nostrils (not shown in this figure) and
    b) the **septal branch** of the **greater palatine artery** that enters the nasal cavity by way of the incisive foramen
2) the **septal nerves** include:
    a) branches of the **anterior ethmoid nerve** (from the ophthalmic nerve);
    b) the **nasopalatine nerve** (from the maxillary nerve) and,
    c) the **internal nasal branches** of ske infraorbital nerves that enter the nasal cavities through the nostrils (not shown in this figure).

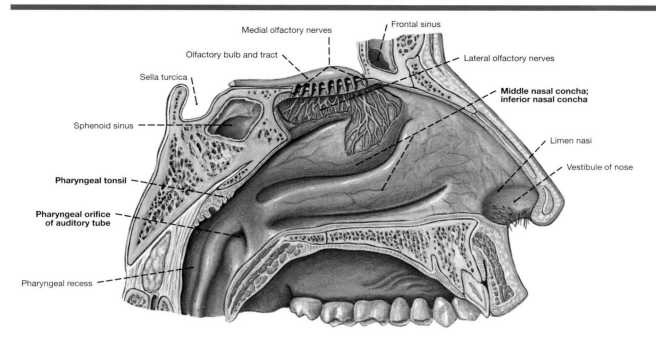

Fig. 831: Lateral Wall of the Left Nasal Cavity Showing the Olfactory Nerves

NOTE: the mucous membrane overlying the **lateral olfactory nerves** has been removed. The lateral wall of the nasal cavity is marked by the **superior**, **middle**, and **inferior nasal conchae.** Beneath each concha courses the corresponding nasal passage or **meatus.**

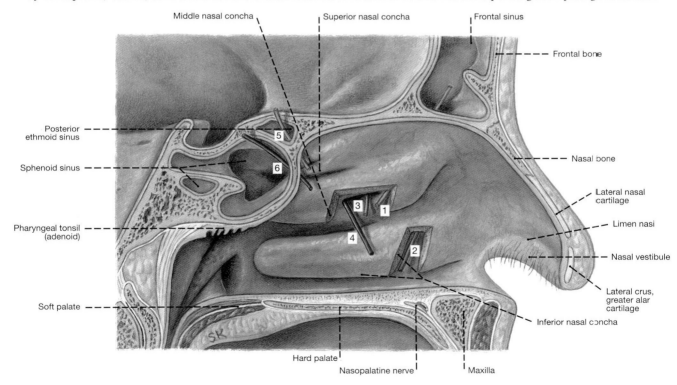

Fig. 832: Drainage Routes of the Paranasal Sinuses and the Nasolacrimal Duct

NOTE: this drawing shows the left nasal cavity and variously colored probes emerging through orifices that drain into the nasal cavity. These are numbered as follows:

1. Frontal sinus
2. Nasolacrimal duct
3. Anterior ethmoid sinus
4. Maxillary sinus
5. Posterior ethmoid sinus
6. Sphenoid sinus

PLATE 526   Nasal Cavity: Vessels and Nerves of the Lateral Wall

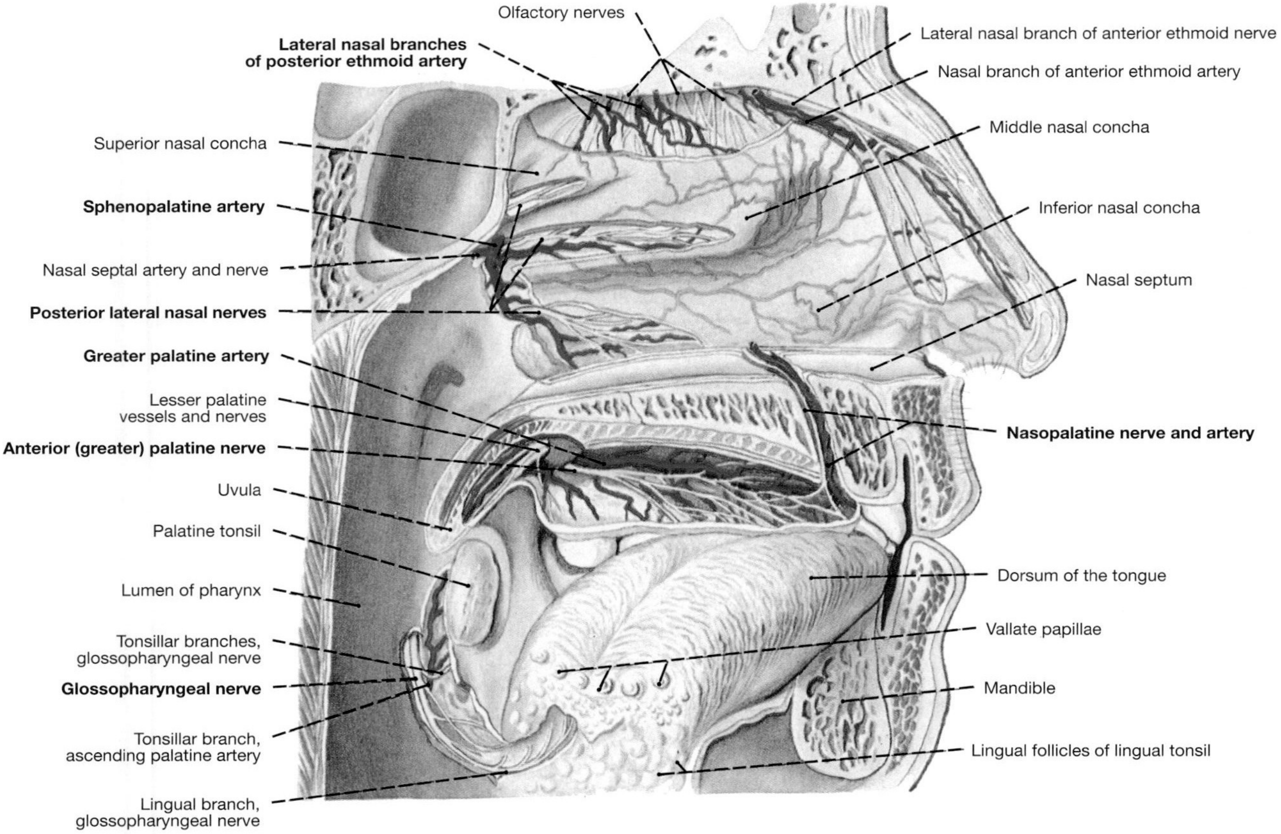

Olfactory nerves

**Lateral nasal branches
of posterior ethmoid artery**

Lateral nasal branch of anterior ethmoid nerve

Nasal branch of anterior ethmoid artery

Superior nasal concha

Middle nasal concha

Sphenopalatine artery

Inferior nasal concha

Nasal septal artery and nerve

Nasal septum

Posterior lateral nasal nerves

Greater palatine artery

Nasopalatine nerve and artery

Lesser palatine
vessels and nerves

Anterior (greater) palatine nerve

Uvula

Dorsum of the tongue

Palatine tonsil

Vallate papillae

Lumen of pharynx

Tonsillar branches,
glossopharyngeal nerve

Mandible

Glossopharyngeal nerve

Tonsillar branch,
ascending palatine artery

Lingual follicles of lingual tonsil

Lingual branch,
glossopharyngeal nerve

Fig. 833: Nerves and Arteries of the Palate and Lateral Wall of the Nasal Cavity

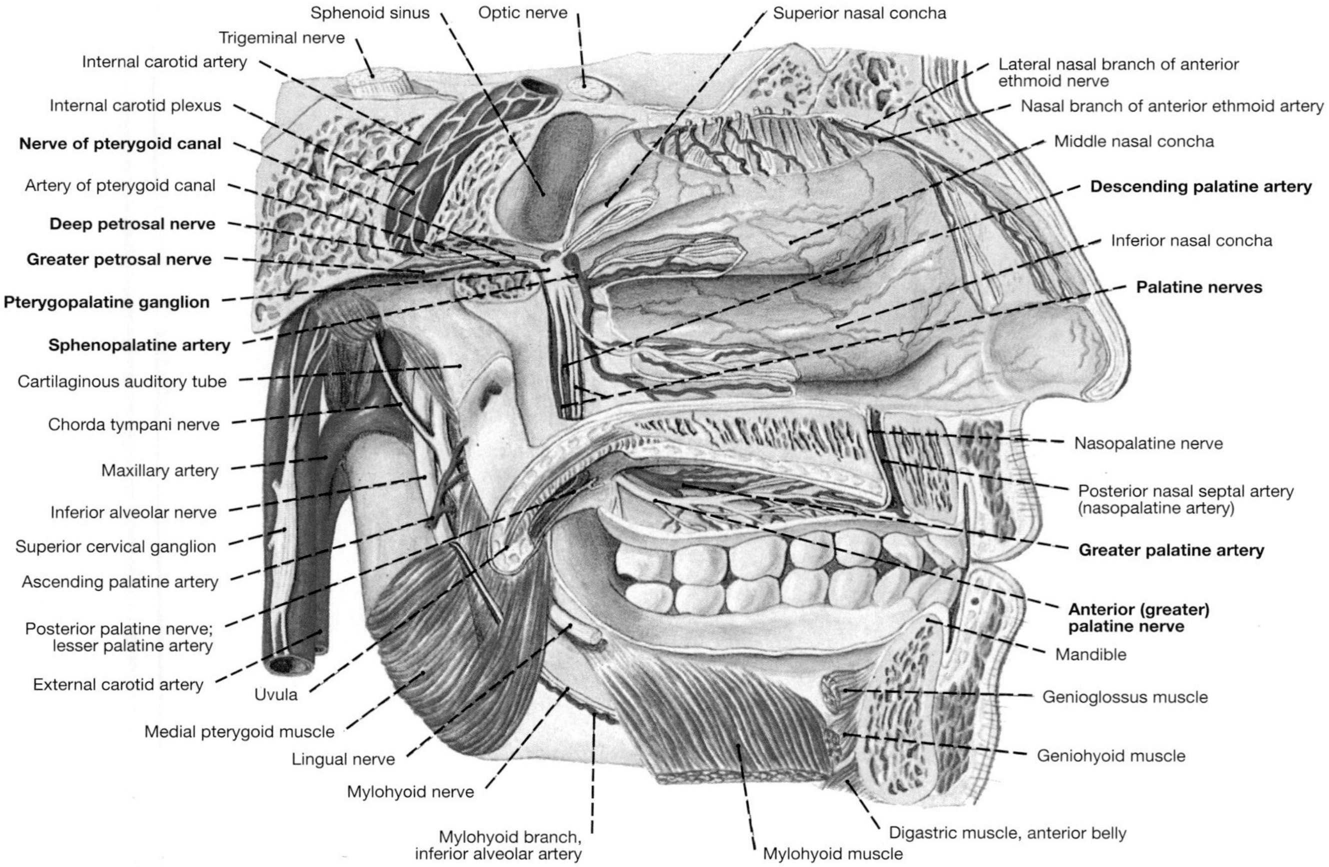

Sphenoid sinus

Optic nerve

Superior nasal concha

Trigeminal nerve

Internal carotid artery

Lateral nasal branch of anterior
ethmoid nerve

Internal carotid plexus

Nasal branch of anterior ethmoid artery

Nerve of pterygoid canal

Middle nasal concha

Artery of pterygoid canal

Descending palatine artery

Deep petrosal nerve

Inferior nasal concha

Greater petrosal nerve

Palatine nerves

Pterygopalatine ganglion

Sphenopalatine artery

Cartilaginous auditory tube

Chorda tympani nerve

Nasopalatine nerve

Maxillary artery

Posterior nasal septal artery
(nasopalatine artery)

Inferior alveolar nerve

Greater palatine artery

Superior cervical ganglion

Ascending palatine artery

**Anterior (greater)
palatine nerve**

Posterior palatine nerve;
lesser palatine artery

Mandible

External carotid artery

Uvula

Genioglossus muscle

Medial pterygoid muscle

Geniohyoid muscle

Lingual nerve

Mylohyoid nerve

Digastric muscle, anterior belly

Mylohyoid branch,
inferior alveolar artery

Mylohyoid muscle

Fig. 834: Pterygopalatine Ganglion and Its Branches

Figs. 833, 834

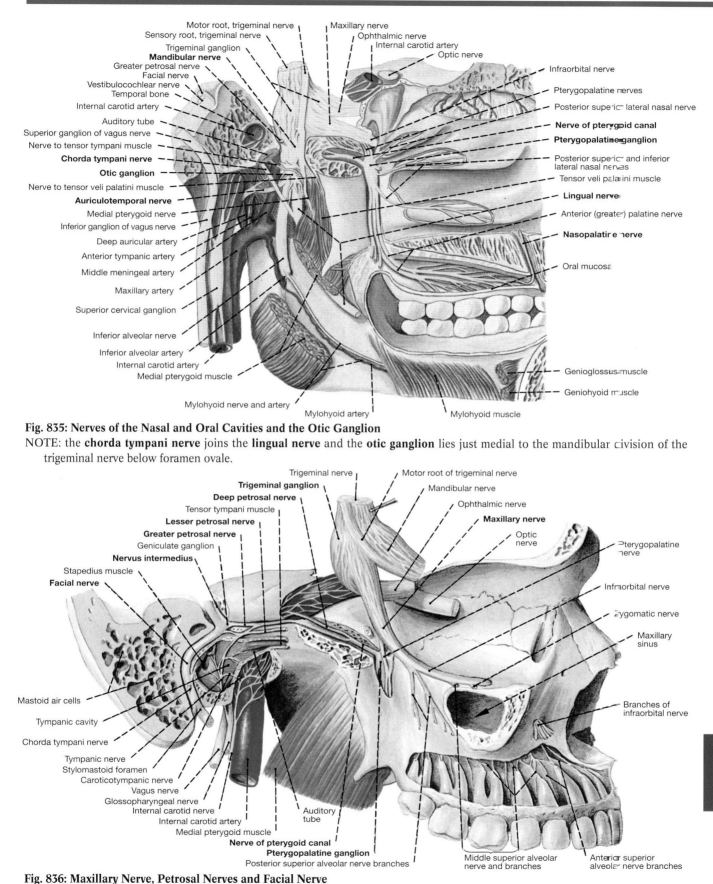

Fig. 835: Nerves of the Nasal and Oral Cavities and the Otic Ganglion

NOTE: the **chorda tympani nerve** joins the **lingual nerve** and the **otic ganglion** lies just medial to the mandibular division of the trigeminal nerve below foramen ovale.

Fig. 836: Maxillary Nerve, Petrosal Nerves and Facial Nerve

NOTE: the **nerve of the pterygoid canal** is formed by the union of the **deep petrosal nerve** (postganglionic sympathetic) and the **greater petrosal nerve** (sensory and preganglionic, **VII**, parasympathetic fibers). The **lesser petrosal nerve** carries preganglionic, **IX**, parasympathetic fibers to the **otic ganglion**.

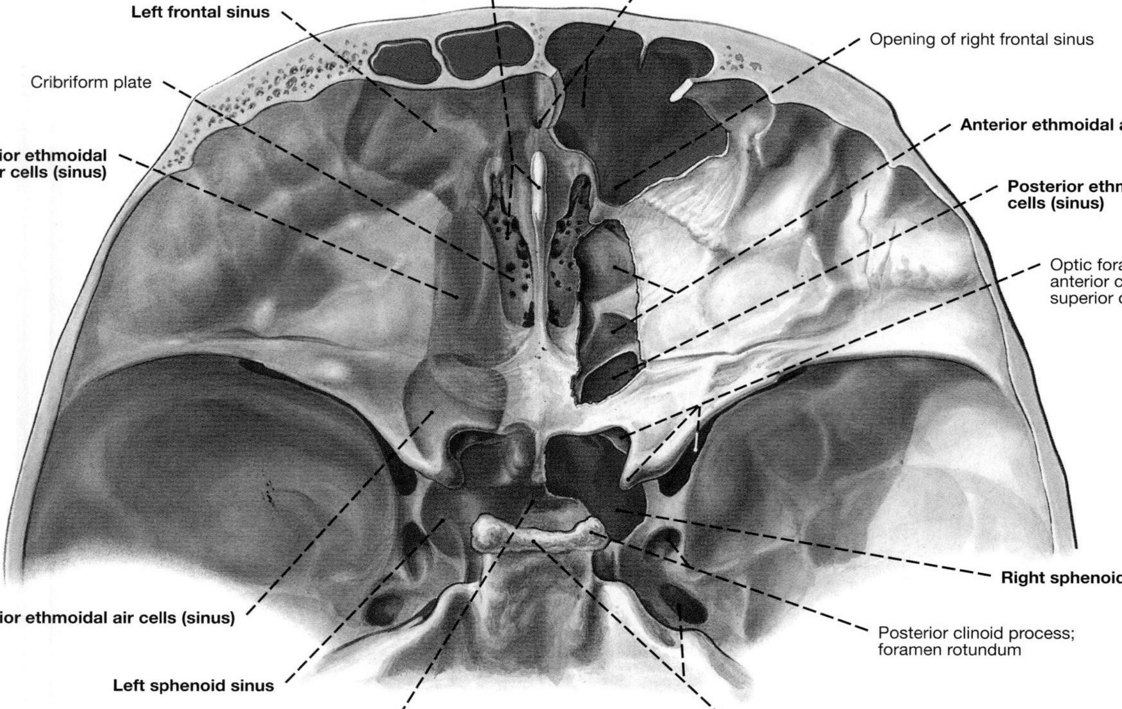

PLATE 528   Paranasal Sinuses and Ethmoid Bone

Crista galli;
cribriform plate

Foramen cecum; right frontal sinus

Left frontal sinus

Opening of right frontal sinus

Cribriform plate

Anterior ethmoidal air cells (sinus)

**Left anterior ethmoidal
air cells (sinus)**

**Posterior ethmoidal air
cells (sinus)**

Optic foramen;
anterior clinoid process;
superior orbital fissure

Right sphenoid sinus

Left posterior ethmoidal air cells (sinus)

Posterior clinoid process;
foramen rotundum

Left sphenoid sinus

Hypophyseal fossa

Dorsum sellae; foramen ovale

Fig. 837: Paranasal Sinuses Viewed From Above

NOTE: 1) the *left side* of the **frontal** (reddish brown), **anterior ethmoid** (green), **posterior ethmoid** (lavender) and **sphenoid** (brown)
sinuses are projected onto the bones of the base of the skull. On the *right side* portions of the frontal, ethmoid and sphenoid bones
have been removed to bring the sinuses into view from above.

2) each of these sinuses drain into the nasal cavity, as shown in Figures 826 and 832. There is some variation in the size and
the geometry of the sinuses but all are lined by a delicate mucosa and an underlying connective tissue layer containing many
mucous glands.

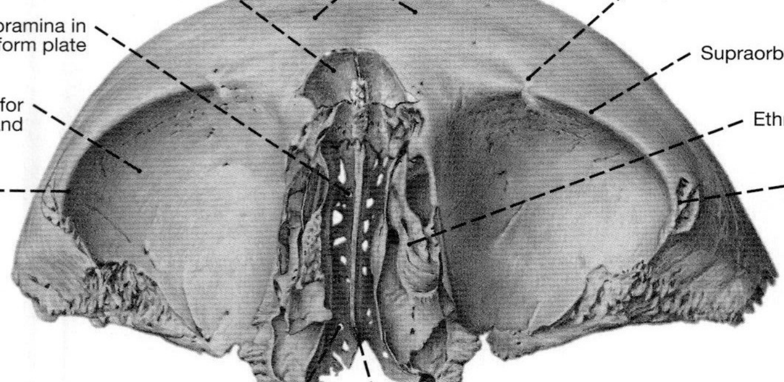

Frontal bone, squamous part

Nasal bone

Supraorbital notch

Foramina in
cribriform plate

Supraorbital margin

Fossa for
lacrimal gland

Ethmoidal labyrinth

Lateral
margin

Zygomatic process
of frontal bone

Cribriform plate of ethmoid bone

Perpendicular plate of
ethmoid bone

Fig. 838: Frontal, Ethmoid and Nasal Bones Viewed From Below ◄

NOTE: the cribriform plate of the ethmoid bone (orange), which
extends laterally from the midline on both sides, is perforated
by many foramina. Through these foramina course the nerve
fibers of the primary olfactory receptor cells.

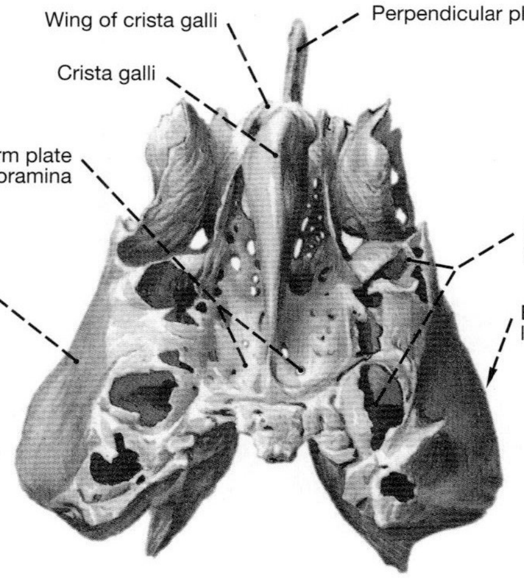

Wing of crista galli

Perpendicular plate

Crista galli

Cribriform plate
and foramina

Ethmoidal
air cells

Orbital plate
(lamina
papyracea)

Ethmoidal
labyrinth

Fig. 839: Ethmoid Bone: Superior Surface, Viewed from Above ▶

NOTE: this bone is in the same orientation as Figure 837.

Figs. 837, 838, 839

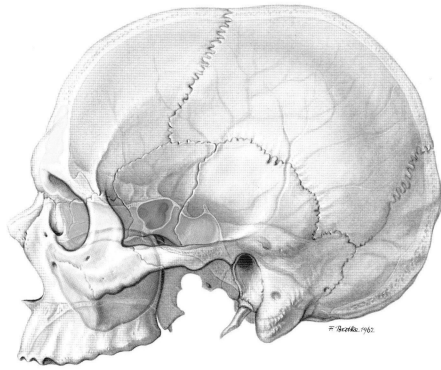

Fig. 840: Paranasal Sinuses, Lateral Projection on Skull ◄

For both Figures 840 and 841:
Yellow = Frontal sinus
Green   = Ethmoid sinus
Blue   = Sphenoid sinus
Red   = Maxillary sinus

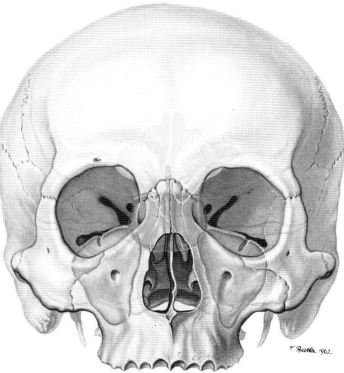

Fig. 841: Paranasal Sinuses, Frontal Projection on Skull ▶

Fig. 842: Ethmoid Bone, Left Lateral View ▼

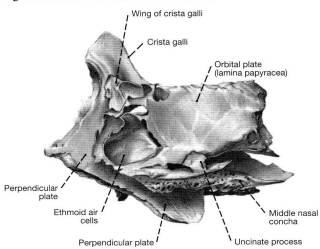

Wing of crista galli

Crista galli

Orbital plate
(lamina papyracea)

Perpendicular
plate

Ethmoid air
cells

Perpendicular plate

Middle nasal
concha

Uncinate process

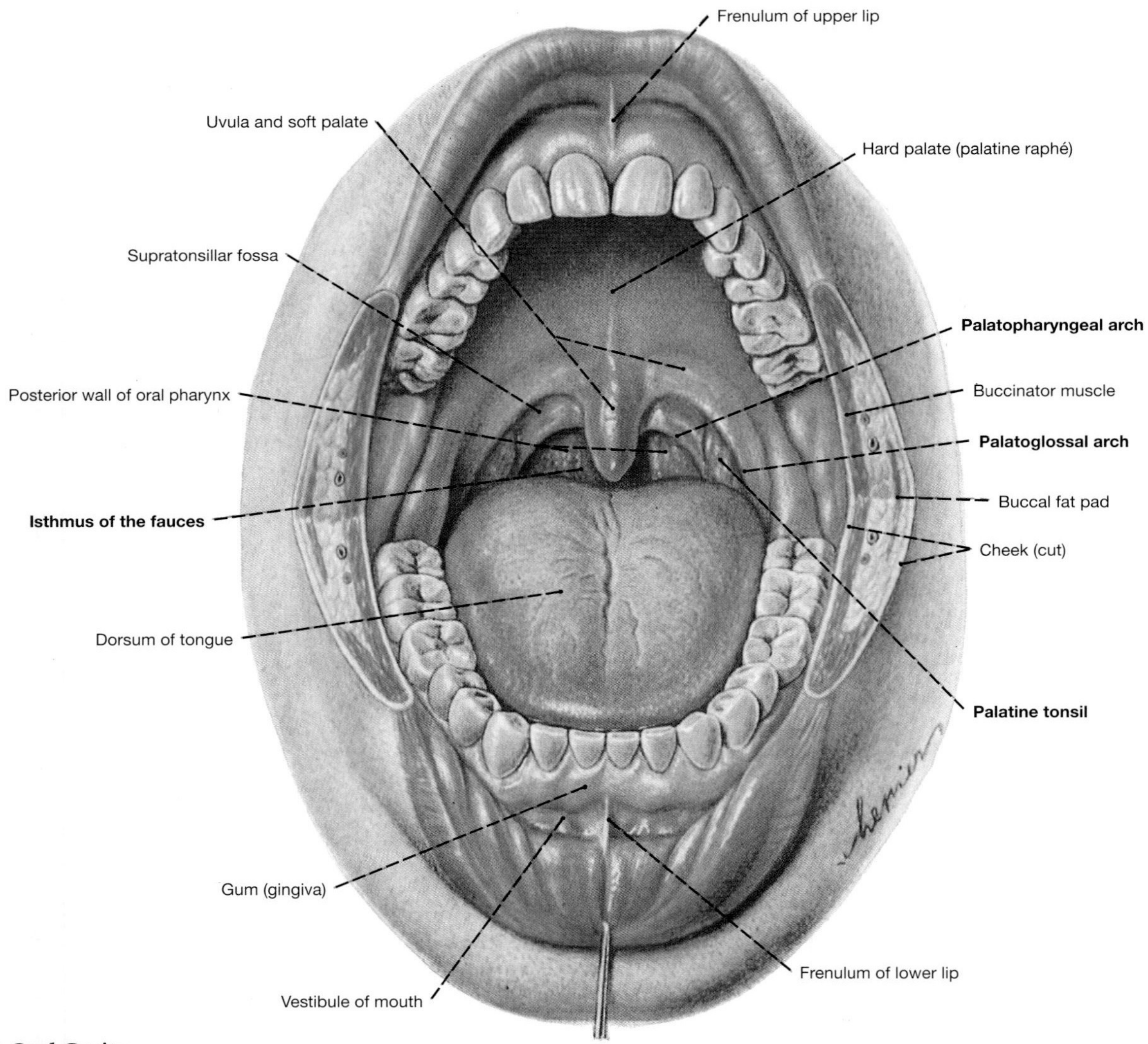

PLATE 530   Oral Cavity: Palate and Tongue, Anterior View; Oral Muscles

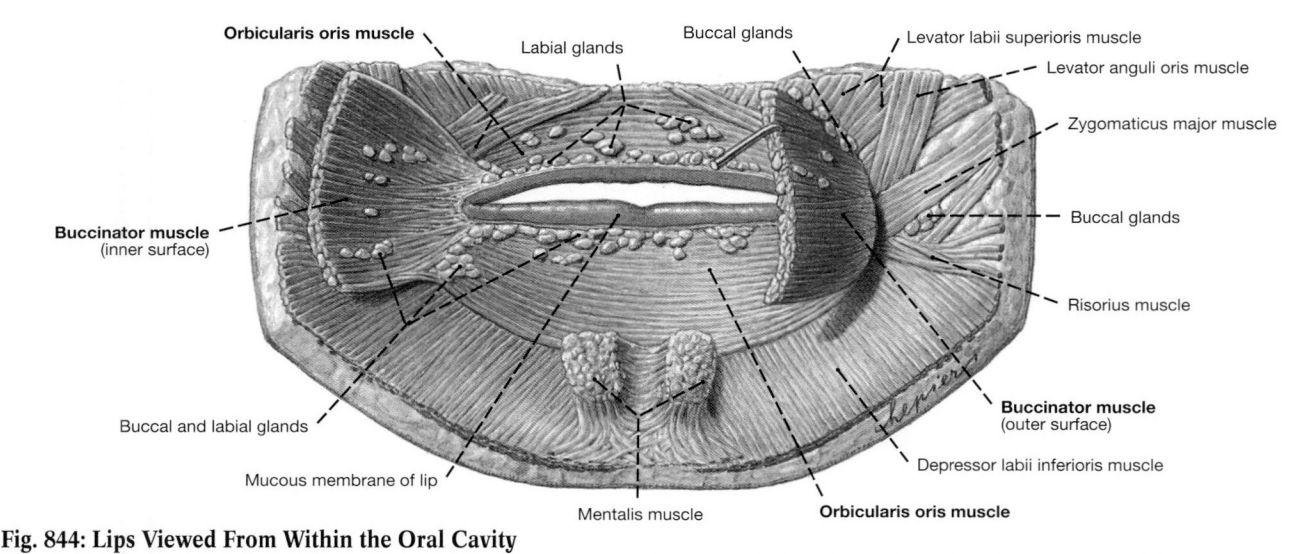

Frenulum of upper lip

Uvula and soft palate

Hard palate (palatine raphé)

Supratonsillar fossa

Palatopharyngeal arch

Buccinator muscle

Posterior wall of oral pharynx

Palatoglossal arch

Buccal fat pad

Isthmus of the fauces

Cheek (cut)

Dorsum of tongue

Palatine tonsil

Gum (gingiva)

Frenulum of lower lip

Vestibule of mouth

Fig. 843: Oral Cavity

NOTE: 1)   the position of the **palatine tonsils** located on each side of the oral cavity within fossae between the **palatoglossal** and **palatopharyngeal folds (or arches).**

2)   the passage between the oral cavity and the oral pharynx is called the **fauces.** This aperture or isthmus commences anteriorly at the palatoglossal arches on each side and is also bounded by the soft palate superiorly and the dorsum of the tongue inferiorly.

Orbicularis oris muscle

Labial glands

Buccal glands

Levator labii superioris muscle

Levator anguli oris muscle

Zygomaticus major muscle

Buccal glands

Buccinator muscle
(inner surface)

Risorius muscle

Buccinator muscle
(outer surface)

Buccal and labial glands

Depressor labii inferioris muscle

Mucous membrane of lip

Mentalis muscle

Orbicularis oris muscle

Fig. 844: Lips Viewed From Within the Oral Cavity

NOTE: the contour of the lips depends on the arrangement of the muscular bundles, which interlace at the labial margins. These include the elevators and depressors of the lips and their angles along with the **orbicularis oris** and **buccinator muscles.**

Figs. 843, 844

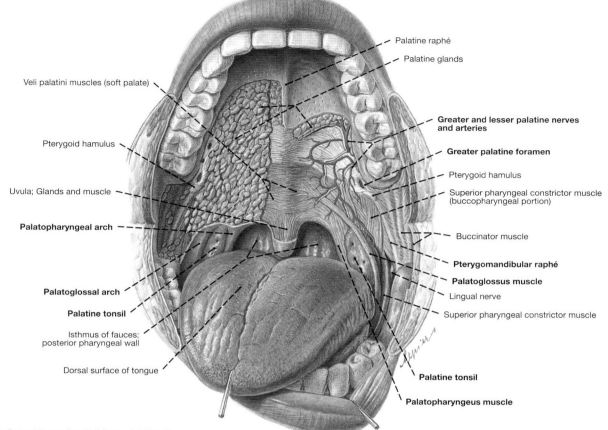

Palatine raphé

Palatine glands

Veli palatini muscles (soft palate)

Pterygoid hamulus

Uvula; Glands and muscle

Palatopharyngeal arch

Palatoglossal arch

Palatine tonsil

Isthmus of fauces;
posterior pharyngeal wall

Dorsal surface of tongue

**Greater and lesser palatine nerves
and arteries**

Greater palatine foramen

Pterygoid hamulus

Superior pharyngeal constrictor muscle
(buccopharyngeal portion)

Buccinator muscle

Pterygomandibular raphé

Palatoglossus muscle

Lingual nerve

Superior pharyngeal constrictor muscle

Palatine tonsil

Palatopharyngeus muscle

Fig. 845: Palate: Muscular Folds and Glands
NOTE: the oral mucosa has been removed from both the hard and soft palate revealing the palatal musculature, vessels, and glands.
Observe the **palatoglossus** and **palatopharyngeus muscles** along with the **greater** and **lesser palatine nerves** and **vessels**.

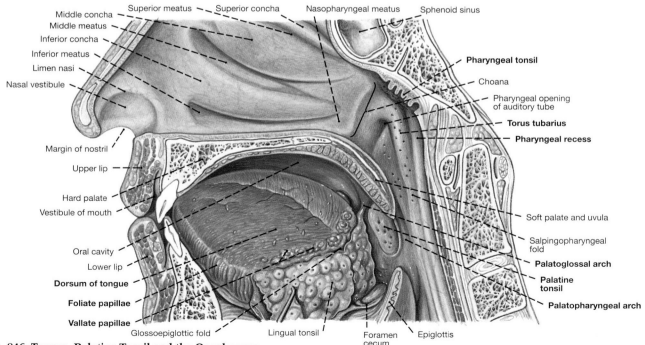

Superior meatus   Superior concha   Nasopharyngeal meatus   Sphenoid sinus

Middle concha
Middle meatus
Inferior concha
Inferior meatus
Limen nasi
Nasal vestibule

Margin of nostril

Upper lip

Hard palate
Vestibule of mouth

Oral cavity
Lower lip
Dorsum of tongue
Foliate papillae
Vallate papillae

Glossoepiglottic fold   Lingual tonsil   Foramen   Epiglottis
cecum

Pharyngeal tonsil

Choana

Pharyngeal opening
of auditory tube

Torus tubarius

Pharyngeal recess

Soft palate and uvula

Salpingopharyngeal
fold

Palatoglossal arch

**Palatine
tonsil**

Palatopharyngeal arch

Fig. 846: Tongue, Palatine Tonsil and the Oropharynx
NOTE: 1) in this sagittal view, the tongue has been deviated to demonstrate the right palatoglossal arch and right palatine tonsil. Observe
the large **vallate papillae.**

2) the opening of the **auditory tube** in the nasopharynx behind which is a cartilaginous elevation of the tube called the **torus
tubarius.** Note also the **pharyngeal tonsil (adenoid).**

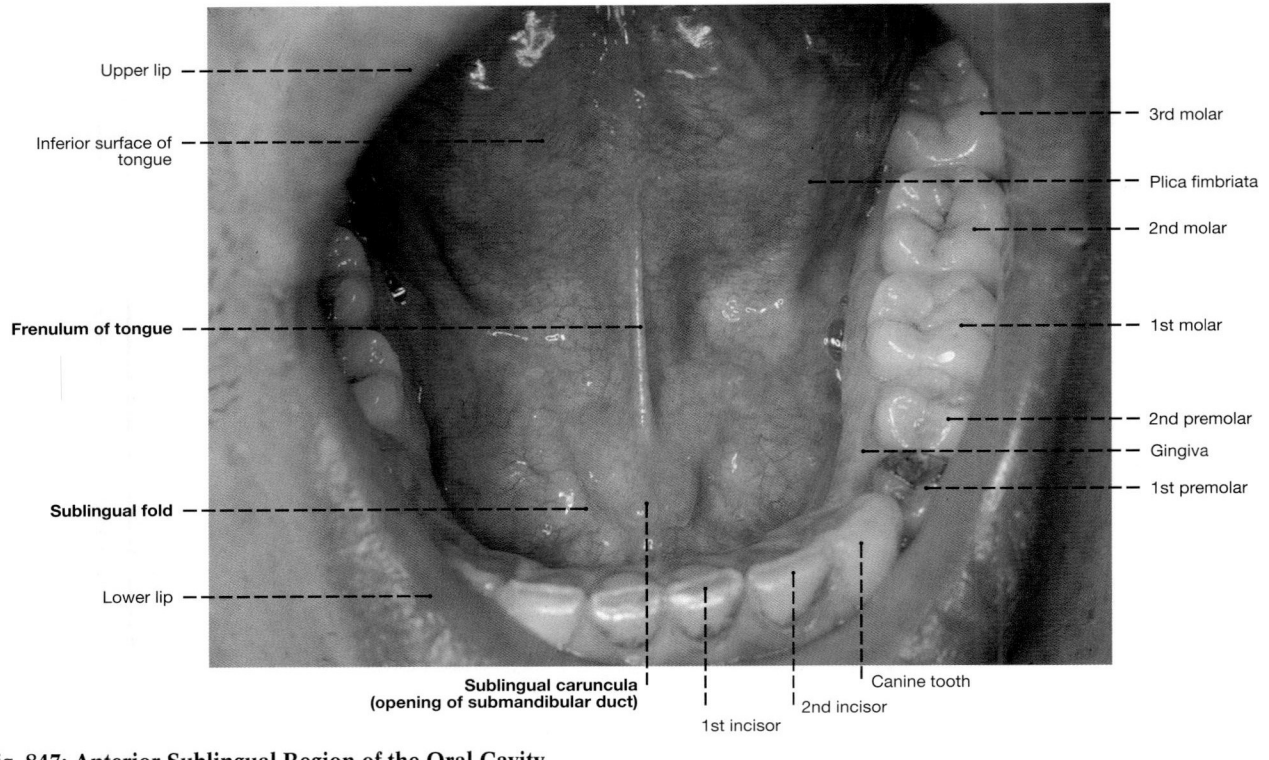

Upper lip

Inferior surface of tongue

Frenulum of tongue

Sublingual fold

Lower lip

3rd molar

Plica fimbriata

2nd molar

1st molar

2nd premolar

Gingiva

1st premolar

Sublingual caruncula (opening of submandibular duct)

1st incisor

2nd incisor

Canine tooth

Fig. 847: Anterior Sublingual Region of the Oral Cavity

NOTE: 1)   the mucous membrane covering the floor of the oral cavity continues over the inferior surface of the tongue and meets at the midline as an elevated fold called the **frenulum of the tongue.**

2)   the **sublingual folds.** Along these open the **ducts of the sublingual glands,** and at their anterior end on each side is an orifice for the **submandibular duct** called the **sublingual caruncula.**

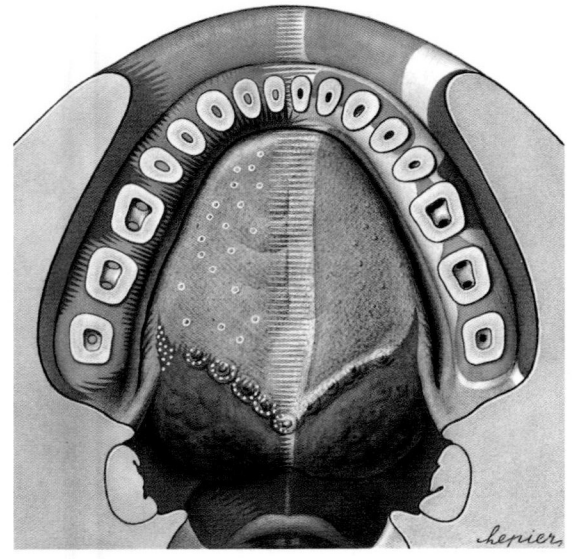

Fig. 848: Sensory Innervation of the Tongue, Cheeks and Floor of the Oral Cavity

NOTE: on the **right side** are indicated areas of distribution, while on the **left side** the overlapping fields of the peripheral nerves. **White circles:** taste zone of **chorda tympani nerve; white dots:** taste zone of **glossopharyngeal nerve.**

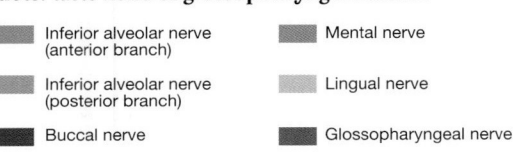

Inferior alveolar nerve (anterior branch)

Inferior alveolar nerve (posterior branch)

Buccal nerve

Mental nerve

Lingual nerve

Glossopharyngeal nerve

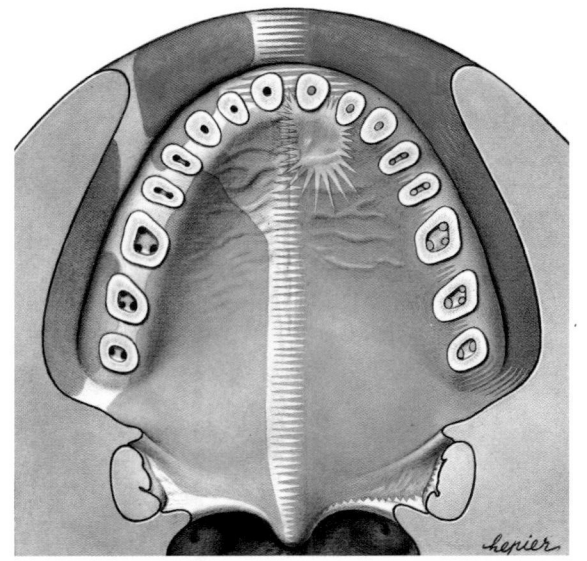

Fig. 849: Sensory Innervation of the Palate, Cheeks and Upper Gums of the Oral Cavity

NOTE: on the (reader's) **left side** are shown specific fields of distribution of the individual sensory nerves, while on the **right side** the overlapping fields of innervation are shown.

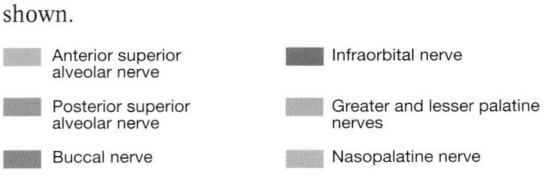

Anterior superior alveolar nerve

Posterior superior alveolar nerve

Buccal nerve

Infraorbital nerve

Greater and lesser palatine nerves

Nasopalatine nerve

Figs. 847, 848, 849

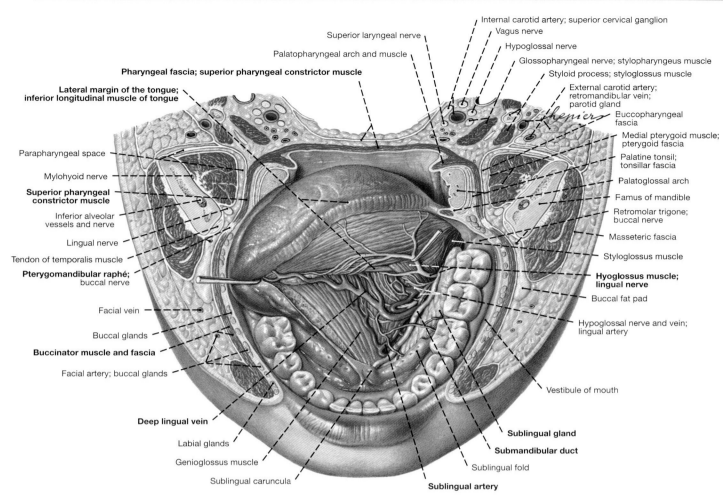

Superior laryngeal nerve

Internal carotid artery; superior cervical ganglion
Vagus nerve

Palatopharyngeal arch and muscle

Hypoglossal nerve

Glossopharyngeal nerve; stylopharyngeus muscle

Pharyngeal fascia; superior pharyngeal constrictor muscle

Styloid process; styloglossus muscle

External carotid artery; retromandibular vein; parotid gland

Lateral margin of the tongue; inferior longitudinal muscle of tongue

Buccopharyngeal fascia

Parapharyngeal space

Medial pterygoid muscle; pterygoid fascia

Mylohyoid nerve

Palatine tonsil; tonsillar fascia

Superior pharyngeal constrictor muscle

Palatoglossal arch

Inferior alveolar vessels and nerve

Ramus of mandible

Lingual nerve

Retromolar trigone; buccal nerve

Tendon of temporalis muscle

Masseteric fascia

Pterygomandibular raphé; buccal nerve

Styloglossus muscle

Hyoglossus muscle; lingual nerve

Facial vein

Buccal fat pad

Buccal glands

Hypoglossal nerve and vein; lingual artery

Buccinator muscle and fascia

Facial artery; buccal glands

Vestibule of mouth

Deep lingual vein

Sublingual gland

Labial glands

Submandibular duct

Genioglossus muscle

Sublingual fold

Sublingual caruncula

Sublingual artery

Fig. 850: Vessels and Nerves in the Floor of the Oral Cavity, Viewed From Above and Anteriorly With Salivary Glands in Place
NOTE: 1) the tongue has been deflected to the (specimen's) right, and the left **lingual nerve** and vessels and the **hypoglossal nerve, sublingual gland** and **submandibular duct** exposed in the floor of the oral cavity.

   2) the lateral walls of the oral cavity and the oropharynx have been cut in frontal section, showing the muscles of mastication laterally, the buccinator muscle medially and the superior pharyngeal constrictor posteriorly.

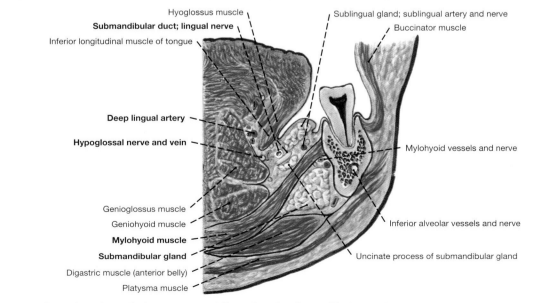

Hyoglossus muscle

Sublingual gland; sublingual artery and nerve

Submandibular duct; lingual nerve

Buccinator muscle

Inferior longitudinal muscle of tongue

Deep lingual artery

Hypoglossal nerve and vein

Mylohyoid vessels and nerve

Genioglossus muscle

Geniohyoid muscle

Mylohyoid muscle

Inferior alveolar vessels and nerve

Submandibular gland

Digastric muscle (anterior belly)

Uncinate process of submandibular gland

Platysma muscle

Fig. 851: Frontal Section Through the Tongue, Sublingual and Submandibular Regions
NOTE: the locations of the **lingual nerve, submandibular duct,** and **hypoglossal nerve** and its vein. The mylohyoid muscle separates the sublingual and submandibular regions.

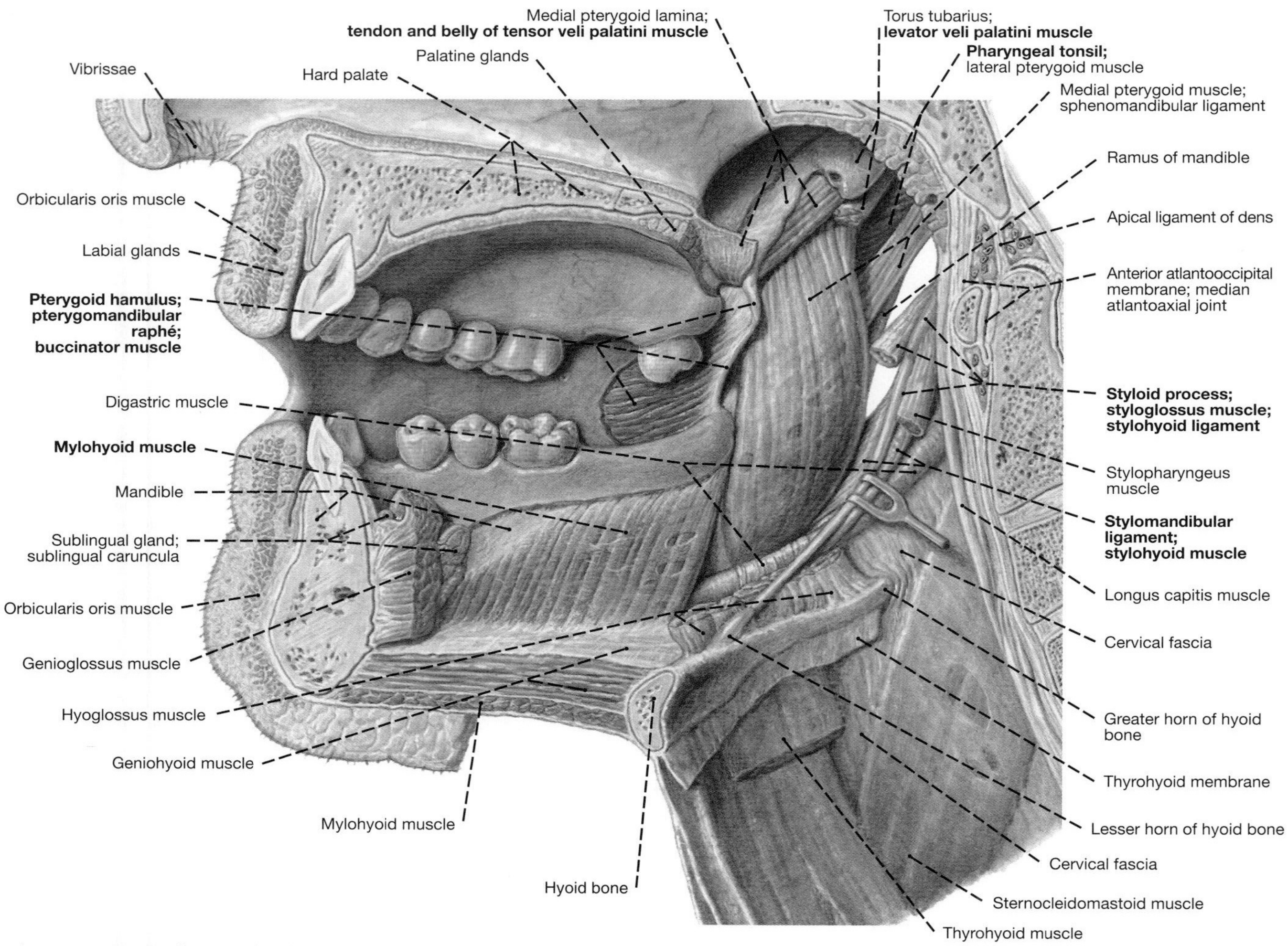

PLATE 534   Oral Cavity: Muscular Floor From Above

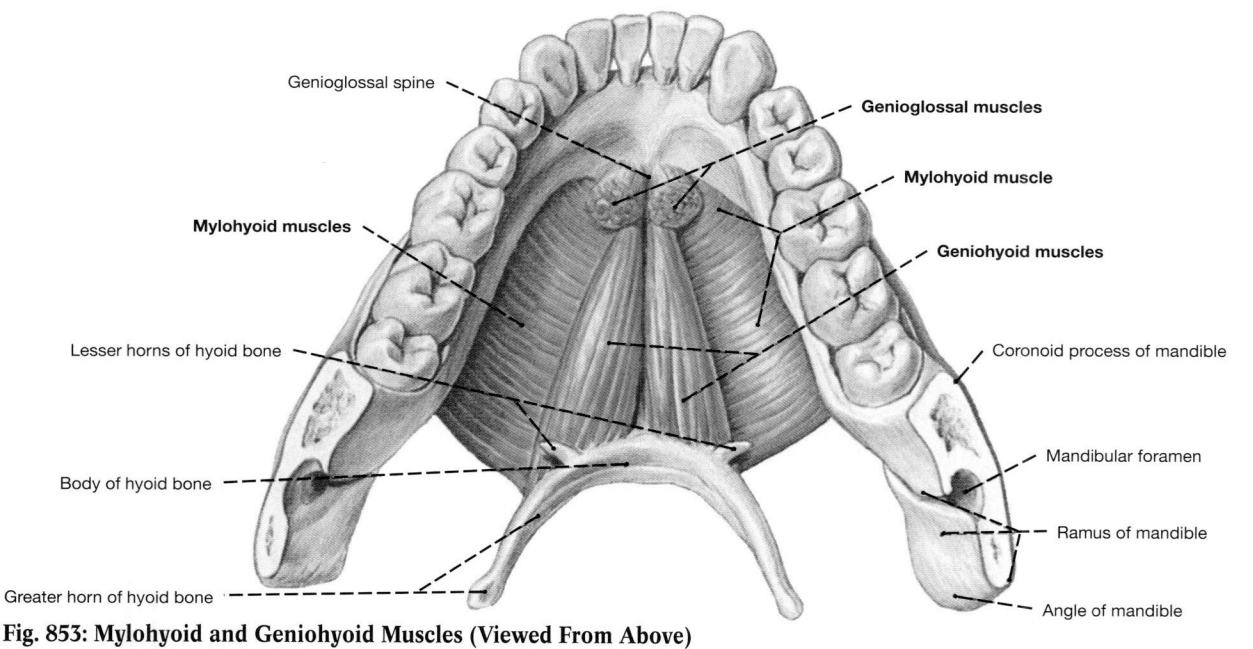

Vibrissae

Orbicularis oris muscle

Labial glands

Pterygoid hamulus; pterygomandibular raphé; buccinator muscle

Digastric muscle

Mylohyoid muscle

Mandible

Sublingual gland; sublingual caruncula

Orbicularis oris muscle

Genioglossus muscle

Hyoglossus muscle

Geniohyoid muscle

Mylohyoid muscle

Hyoid bone

Hard palate

Palatine glands

Medial pterygoid lamina; **tendon and belly of tensor veli palatini muscle**

Torus tubarius; **levator veli palatini muscle**

Pharyngeal tonsil; lateral pterygoid muscle

Medial pterygoid muscle; sphenomandibular ligament

Ramus of mandible

Apical ligament of dens

Anterior atlantooccipital membrane; median atlantoaxial joint

Styloid process; styloglossus muscle; stylohyoid ligament

Stylopharyngeus muscle

Stylomandibular ligament; stylohyoid muscle

Longus capitis muscle

Cervical fascia

Greater horn of hyoid bone

Thyrohyoid membrane

Lesser horn of hyoid bone

Cervical fascia

Sternocleidomastoid muscle

Thyrohyoid muscle

Fig. 852: Paramedian Sagittal View of the Interior of the Right Oral Cavity and the Upper Neck (Muscles and Ligaments)
NOTE: in this dissection, the right half of the oral cavity was exposed and the mucous membrane removed from the floor of the mouth to reveal the **mylohyoid muscle.** Observe also the **pterygomandibular raphé** and **buccinator muscle.**

Genioglossal spine

Mylohyoid muscles

Lesser horns of hyoid bone

Body of hyoid bone

Greater horn of hyoid bone

Genioglossal muscles

Mylohyoid muscle

Geniohyoid muscles

Coronoid process of mandible

Mandibular foramen

Ramus of mandible

Angle of mandible

Fig. 853: Mylohyoid and Geniohyoid Muscles (Viewed From Above)
NOTE: the **mylohyoid** and **geniohyoid muscles** form the floor of the oral cavity. The mylohyoids arise along the mylohyoid lines of the mandible and insert into the median raphé, which extends from the hyoid bone to the symphysis menti. The genioglossal muscles have been severed near their origin.

Figs. 852, 853

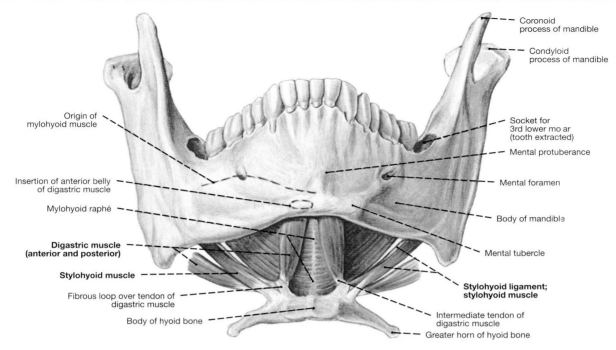

Fig. 854: Suprahyoid Muscles and Floor of the Mouth (Viewed From Below)
NOTE: indicated on the mandible are the inner attachments of the **mylohyoid muscle** (broken line) and the **anterior belly of the digastric muscle** (circle). Observe the attachments of the **mylohyoid, digastric,** and **stylohyoid muscles** and the **stylohyoid ligament** on the hyoid bone.

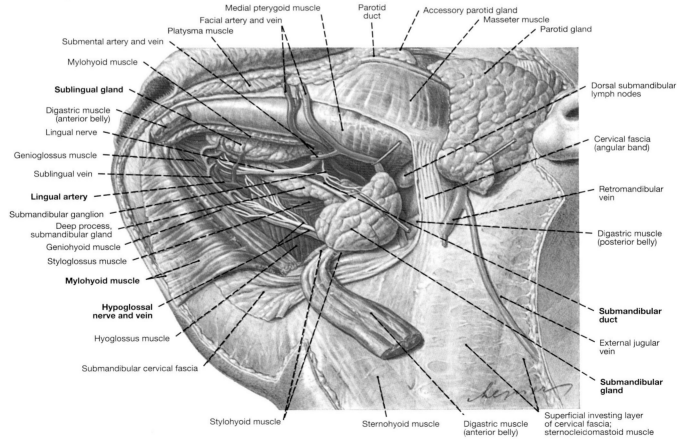

Fig. 855: Suprahyoid Muscles and Floor of the Mouth (Viewed From Below)
NOTE: 1)   the anterior belly of the digastric and mylohyoid muscles have been reflected to reveal: the **sublingual gland, lingual nerve, submandibular ganglion** and **duct, hypoglossal nerve** and **vein** and the **lingual artery.**

    2)   the hypoglossal nerve is the motor nerve to all tongue muscles **except** the palatoglossus. The lingual nerve supplies the anterior 2/3rds of the tongue with general sensation.

PLATE 536   Oral Cavity: Salivary Glands

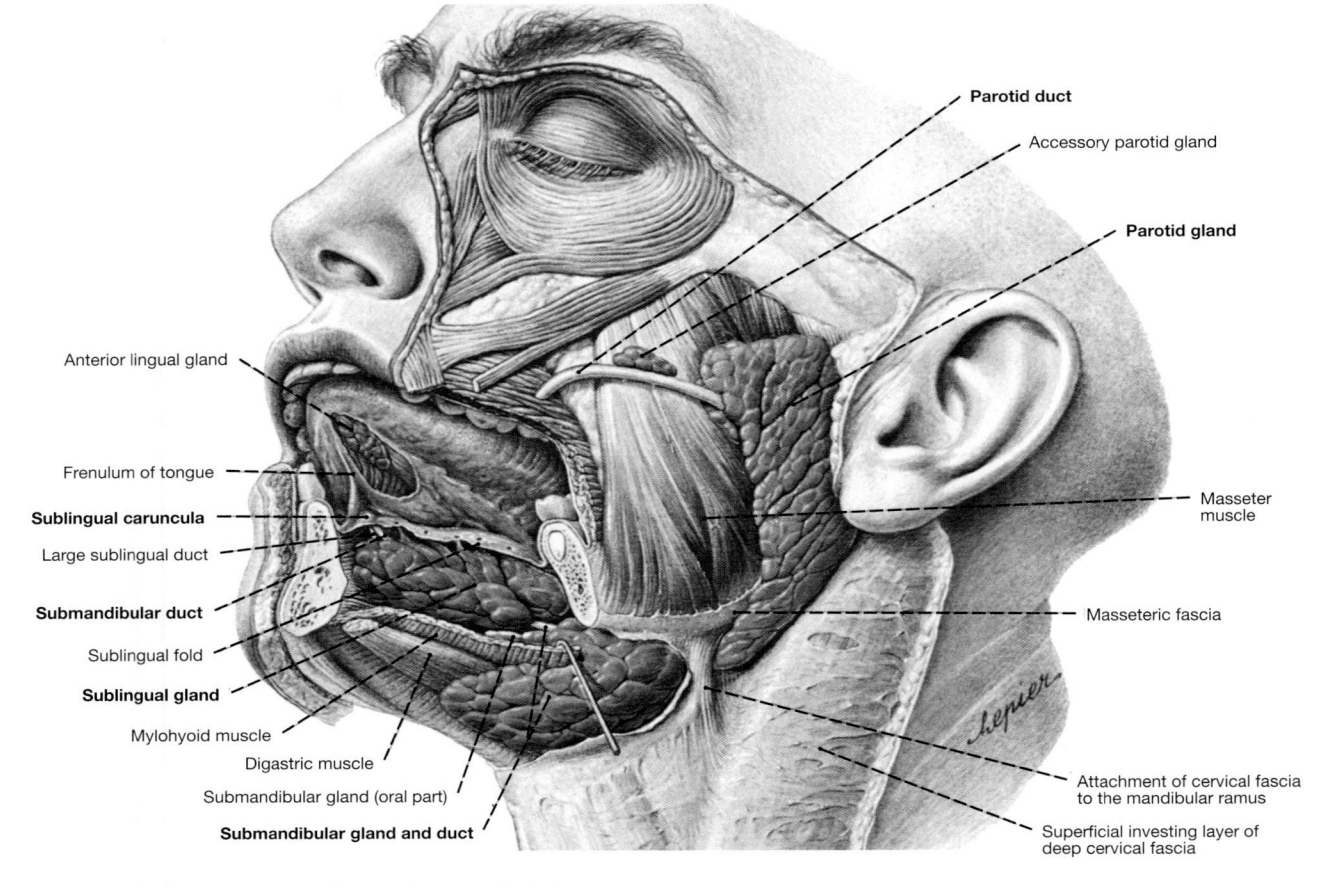

Parotid duct

Accessory parotid gland

Parotid gland

Anterior lingual gland

Frenulum of tongue

Sublingual caruncula

Large sublingual duct

Submandibular duct

Sublingual fold

Sublingual gland

Mylohyoid muscle

Digastric muscle

Submandibular gland (oral part)

Submandibular gland and duct

Masseter muscle

Masseteric fascia

Attachment of cervical fascia to the mandibular ramus

Superficial investing layer of deep cervical fascia

Fig. 856: Lateral View of the Salivary Glands and Their Ducts

PAROTID GLAND

DEVELOPMENT: Arises during the 6th week as an epithelial outgrowth from the mouth and forms a tube that grows backward toward the ear. The posterior part of the tube branches into lobes that become the gland, and it enmeshes the facial nerve. The tube remains as the **parotid duct** which opens into the mouth opposite the 2nd upper molar tooth.

ADULT GLAND: A serous gland weighing about 25 grams on either side of the face in front of the ear. Located between the mandible and the sternocleidomastoid muscle.

ARTERIES: Branches of the external carotid artery as it passes behind the gland.

VEINS: Empty into the external jugular vein.

INNERVATION: *Sympathetic:* Postganglionic vasomotor fibers come from the superior cervical ganglion by way of the external carotid plexus. *Parasympathetic:* Preganglionic secretomotor fibers course in the **glossopharyngeal nerve** and then the **lesser petrosal nerve** to the **otic ganglion** where they synapse. Postganglionic fibers course to the parotid gland by way of the **auriculotemporal nerve (V).**

LYMPH DRAINAGE: Superficial and deep parotid nodes drain into cervical lymph nodes.

SUBMANDIBULAR GLAND

DEVELOPMENT: Arises during the 6th week from an epithelial ridge in a groove between the tongue and the lower jaw. The caudal end of the ridge forms numerous branches that extend backward and ventrally beneath the mandible as glandular lobules. The main stalk, connected to the deep part of the gland persists as the **submandibular duct.**

ADULT GLAND: A seromucous gland of about 8 grams on each side. **Superficial part,** the size of a walnut, located in the digastric triangle of the upper neck. The **deep part** extends above the mylohyoid muscle into the oral cavity. The **submandibular duct** extends forward from the deep part and opens at the **sublingual caruncula** at the side of the frenulum below the tongue.

ARTERIES: Submental branches of the **facial artery** in neck and of **lingual artery** in oral cavity.

VEINS: Drain into the facial and lingual veins and then into the **internal jugular vein.**

INNERVATION: *Sympathetic:* Postganglionic vasomotor fibers come from the superior cervical ganglion by way of the external carotid plexus. *Parasympathetic:* Preganglionic fibers course in the **nervus intermedius** part of the **facial nerve.** They travel to the **submandibular ganglion** by way of the **chorda tympani nerve** and then the **lingual nerve.** Postganglionic fibers from the ganglion course directly to the gland.

LYMPH DRAINAGE: Into submandibular nodes and then into upper and lower deep cervical nodes.

Fig. 856

Fig. 857: Submandibular and Sublingual Glands

NOTE: 1) with the tongue removed and the genioglossus and geniohyoid
muscles cut, the submandibular and sublingual glands are exposed and their
relationship to the inner aspect of the mandible demonstrated.

2) the submandibular duct measures about 5 cm and courses anteriorly
between the sublingual gland and genioglossus muscle (cut). It opens in the
floor of the mouth at the sublingual caruncle.

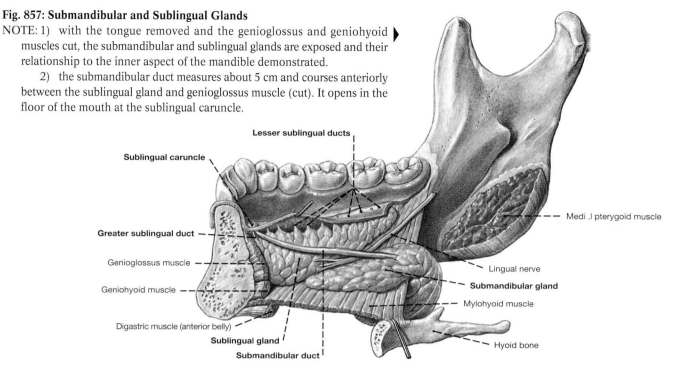

SUBLINGUAL GLAND

DEVELOPMENT: Appears as a series of epithelial buds along the groove between the lower jaw and tongue during the
8th week, just lateral to the submandibular primordium. The buds enlarge and some of the more anterior ones join to form a
duct that opens near the submandibular duct. The remaining buds open by separate ducts (8 to 10) in the floor of the mouth
above the sublingual fold.

ADULT GLAND: A seromucous gland on each side (30% serous, 70% mucous) weighing about 4 grams. It is narrow and flattened
and located deep to the mucous membrane in the floor of the mouth. Its ducts (10 to 20) open in a line along the surface of the
sublingual fold. Several anterior ducts join to form the main sublingual duct. This opens near the caruncula of the submandibular
duct.

ARTERIES: **Sublingual branch** of the **lingual artery** which anastomoses with the **submental branch** of the **facial artery.**

VEINS: Drain into lingual vein and then into internal jugular vein.

INNERVATION: Same as for the submandibular gland.

LYMPH DRAINAGE: Superficial and deep submandibular nodes and then into deep cervical nodes.

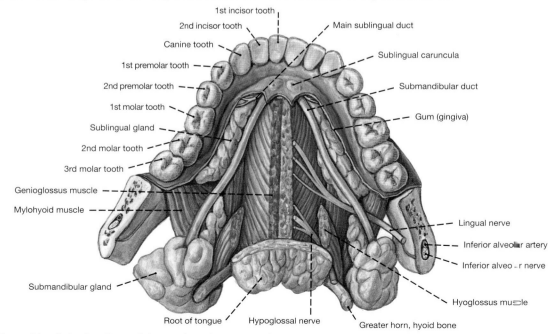

Fig. 858: Salivary Glands in the Floor of the Oral Cavity (From Above)

PLATE 538   Oral Cavity: Muscles of Tongue and Pharynx

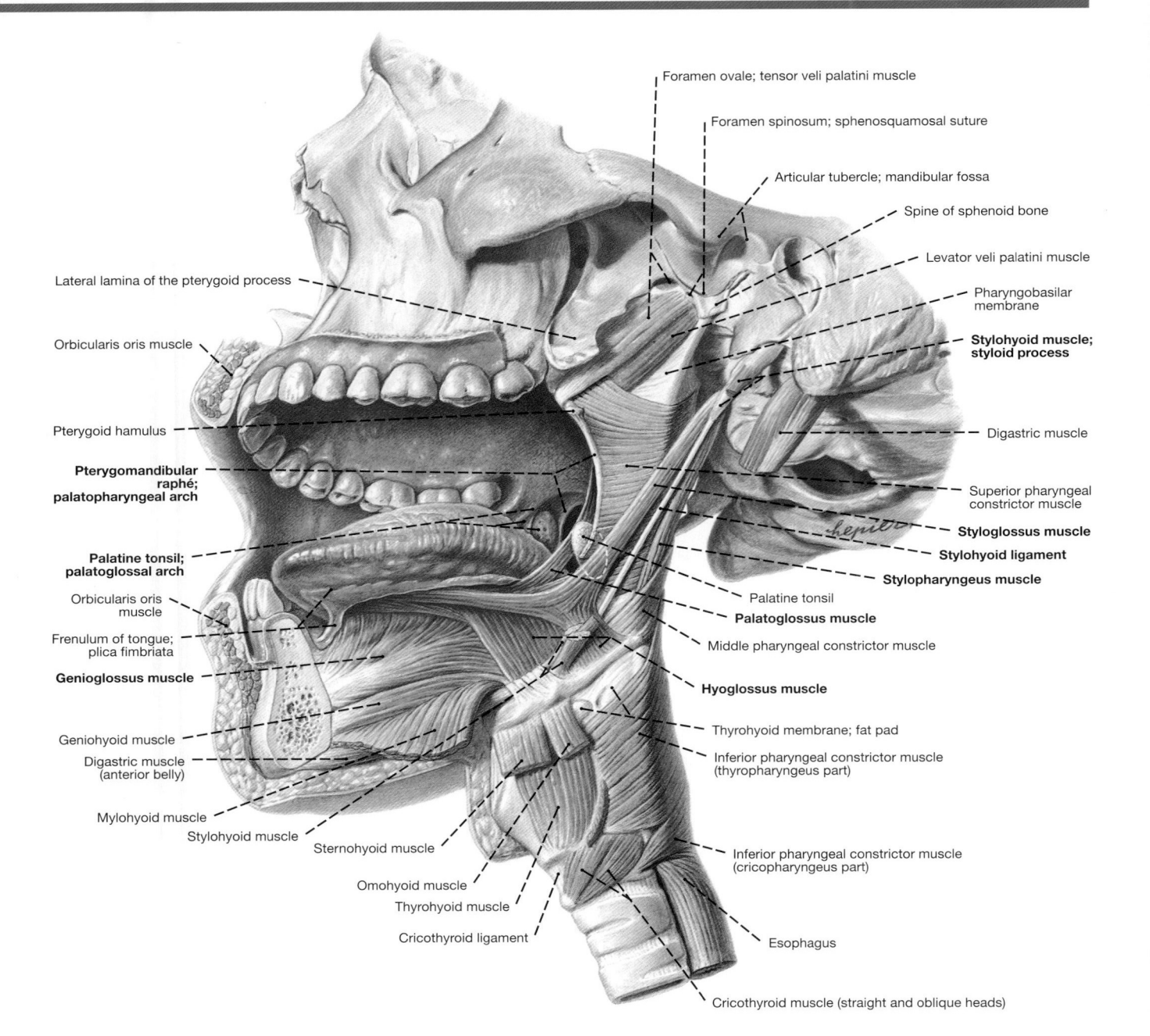

Foramen ovale; tensor veli palatini muscle

Foramen spinosum; sphenosquamosal suture

Articular tubercle; mandibular fossa

Spine of sphenoid bone

Levator veli palatini muscle

Pharyngobasilar membrane

Stylohyoid muscle; styloid process

Digastric muscle

Superior pharyngeal constrictor muscle

Styloglossus muscle

Stylohyoid ligament

Stylopharyngeus muscle

Palatine tonsil

Palatoglossus muscle

Middle pharyngeal constrictor muscle

Hyoglossus muscle

Thyrohyoid membrane; fat pad

Inferior pharyngeal constrictor muscle (thyropharyngeus part)

Inferior pharyngeal constrictor muscle (cricopharyngeus part)

Esophagus

Cricothyroid muscle (straight and oblique heads)

Lateral lamina of the pterygoid process

Orbicularis oris muscle

Pterygoid hamulus

Pterygomandibular raphé; palatopharyngeal arch

Palatine tonsil; palatoglossal arch

Orbicularis oris muscle

Frenulum of tongue; plica fimbriata

Genioglossus muscle

Geniohyoid muscle

Digastric muscle (anterior belly)

Mylohyoid muscle

Stylohyoid muscle

Sternohyoid muscle

Omohyoid muscle

Thyrohyoid muscle

Cricothyroid ligament

Fig. 859: Lingual Musculature and Pharyngeal Constrictors, Lateral View

NOTE: 1) the superficial and deep facial structures on the left side have been removed, as has the left half of the mandible to expose the lingual muscles and the pharyngeal constrictors. The buccinator muscle has been removed but the superior pharyngeal constrictor is still attached to the pterygomandibular raphé.

  2) the stylohyoid muscle has been cut, but the stylohyoid ligament and the stylopharyngeus and styloglossus muscles are still intact. Observe the hyoglossus, geniohyoid and genioglossus muscles, and that the palatoglossus descends into the tongue from the soft palate.

Fig. 859

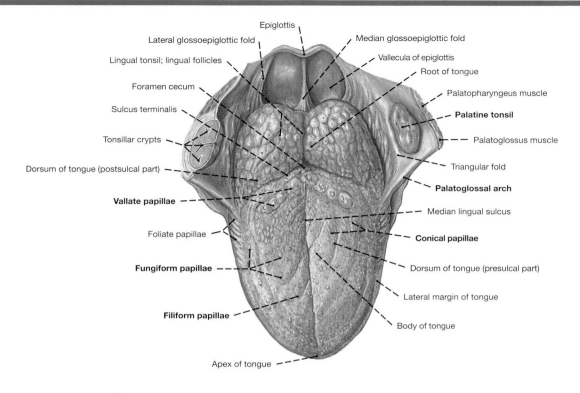

Fig. 860: Dorsal Surface of the Tongue

NOTE: 1) the dorsum of the tongue is marked by numerous elevations called papillae. These serve as location sites of receptors for the special sense of **taste.** Observe the inverted V-shaped group of large **vallate papillae.**

2) the **fungiform papillae,** which are found principally at the sides and apex of the tongue. These are large and round and are deep red.

3) the **filiform** (conical) **papillae.** These are small and arranged in rows that course parallel to the vallate papillae.

4) the parallel vertical folds (about five in number) called the **foliate papillae** on the lateral border of the tongue just anterior to the palatoglossal arch. These are studded with taste receptors.

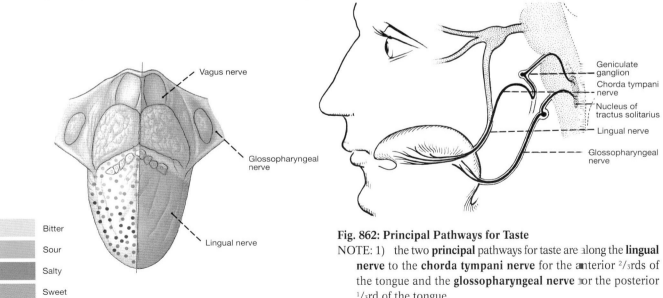

Fig. 861: Innervation and Location of Taste Qualities on the Dorsum of the Tongue

NOTE: *On the right:* fields of innervation by the **lingual, glosso-pharyngeal** and **vagus nerves.** *On the left:* Receptors for the basic tastes of **salt** and **sweet** are clustered anterior to those for **bitter** and **sour.**

Fig. 862: Principal Pathways for Taste

NOTE: 1) the two **principal** pathways for taste are along the **lingual nerve** to the **chorda tympani nerve** for the anterior ²/₃rds of the tongue and the **glossopharyngeal nerve** for the posterior ¹/₃rd of the tongue.

2) two lesser pathways (not shown) are:

a) from the epiglottis along the **internal laryngeal branch** of the **vagus** and,

b) from the palate along the **palatine nerves** and the **nerve of the pterygoid canal** to the **greater petrosal nerve** and then the **nervus intermedius part** of the facial nerve.

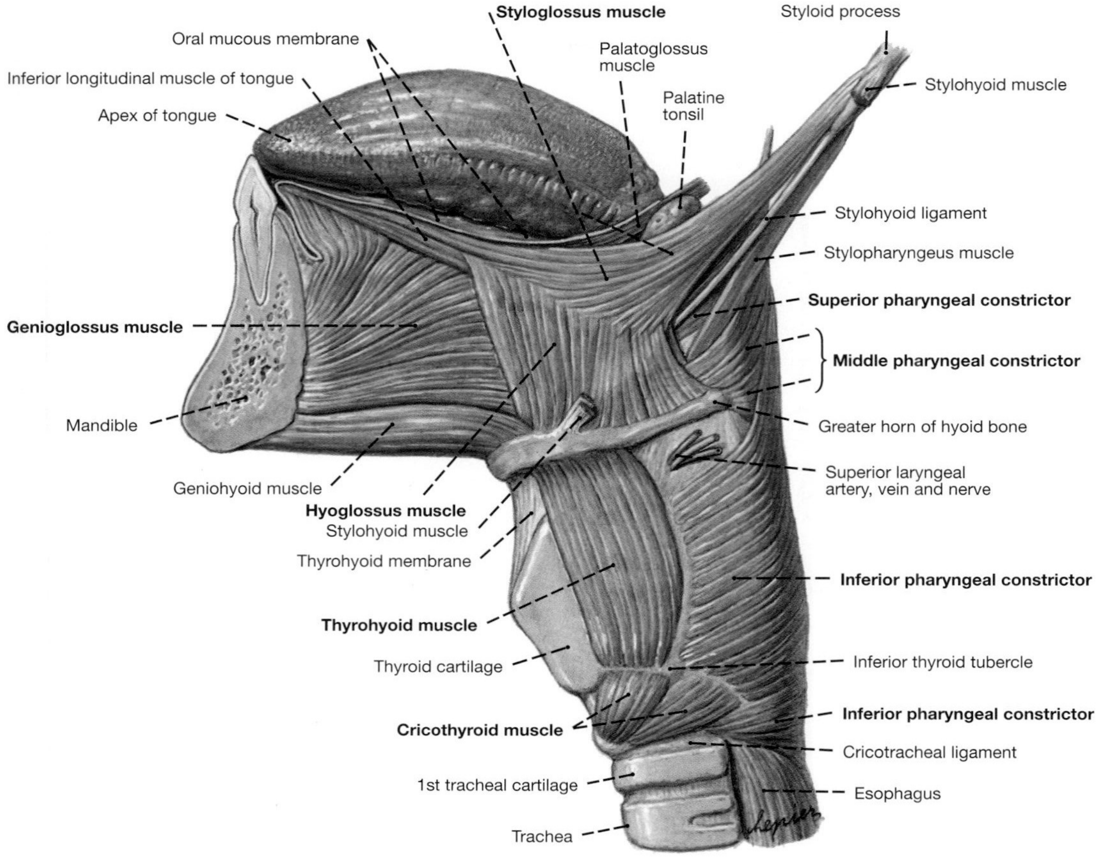

PLATE 540   **Muscles of the Tongue and Pharynx**

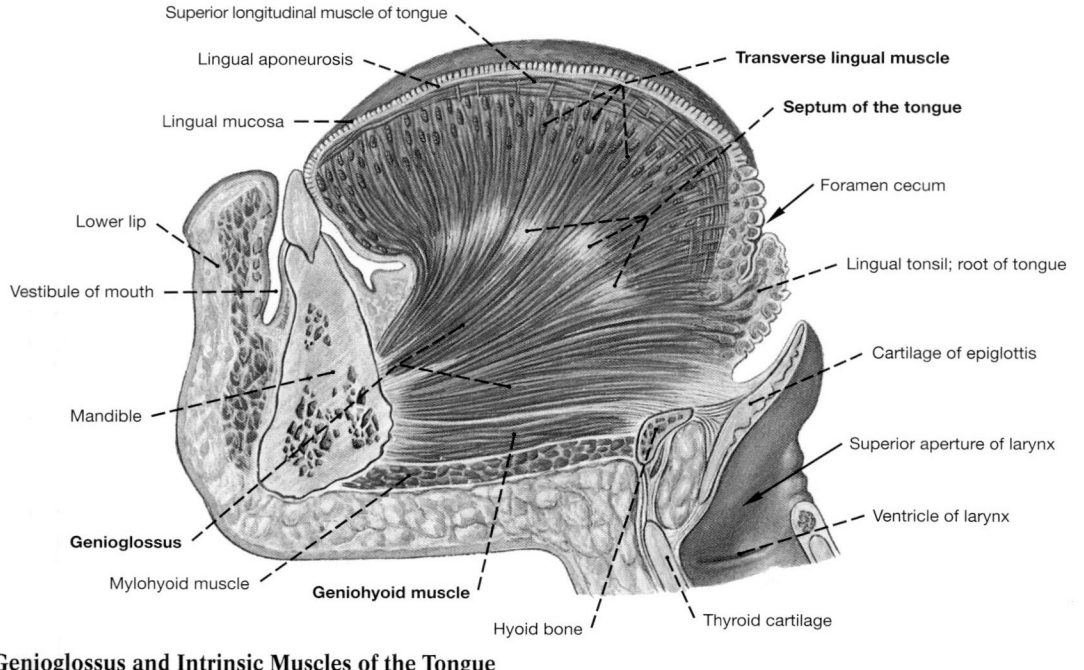

Oral mucous membrane
Inferior longitudinal muscle of tongue
Apex of tongue
Genioglossus muscle
Mandible
Geniohyoid muscle
Hyoglossus muscle
Stylohyoid muscle
Thyrohyoid membrane
Thyrohyoid muscle
Thyroid cartilage
Cricothyroid muscle
1st tracheal cartilage
Trachea

Styloglossus muscle
Palatoglossus muscle
Palatine tonsil
Styloid process
Stylohyoid muscle
Stylohyoid ligament
Stylopharyngeus muscle
Superior pharyngeal constrictor
Middle pharyngeal constrictor
Greater horn of hyoid bone
Superior laryngeal artery, vein and nerve
Inferior pharyngeal constrictor
Inferior thyroid tubercle
Inferior pharyngeal constrictor
Cricotracheal ligament
Esophagus

Fig. 863: Extrinsic Tongue Muscles; External Larynx and Pharynx (Lateral View 1)
NOTE: the tongue is attached to the hyoid bone, the mandible, the styloid process, the soft palate and the pharyngeal wall.

Superior longitudinal muscle of tongue
Lingual aponeurosis
Lingual mucosa
Lower lip
Vestibule of mouth
Mandible
Genioglossus
Mylohyoid muscle
Geniohyoid muscle
Hyoid bone

Transverse lingual muscle
Septum of the tongue
Foramen cecum
Lingual tonsil; root of tongue
Cartilage of epiglottis
Superior aperture of larynx
Ventricle of larynx
Thyroid cartilage

Fig. 864: Genioglossus and Intrinsic Muscles of the Tongue
NOTE: 1) in this midsagittal section can be seen the median fibrous septum of the tongue and the **intrinsic** tongue musculature, which
    includes the longitudinal, transverse and vertical muscles of the tongue.

    2) the **genioglossus** constitutes most of the tongue musculature and its fibers radiate backward and upward in a fan-like manner
from the uppermost of the mental spines (genial tubercles) on the inner surface of the mandible, just above the origin of the geniohyoid
muscle.

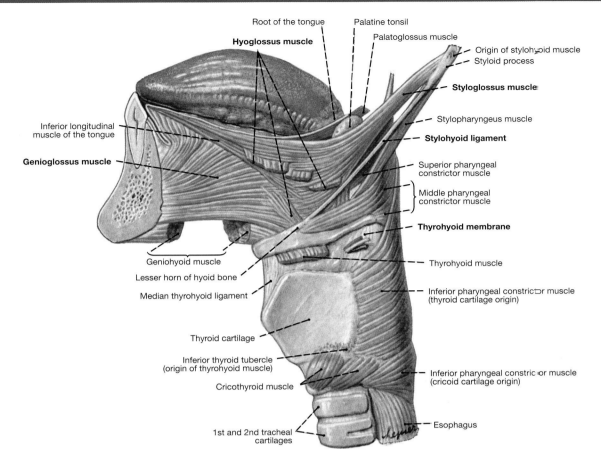

Fig. 865: Extrinsic Tongue Muscles; External Larynx and Pharynx (Lateral View 2)

NOTE: 1) in this dissection the hyoglossus muscle has been removed, revealing the attachments of the **stylohyoid ligament** and the **middle pharyngeal constrictor muscle** along the hyoid bone. The geniohyoid muscle has been cut and the thyrohyoid muscle removed.

2) the blending of the fibers of the styloglossus, hyoglossus and genioglossus at the base of the tongue.

3) the penetration through the **thyrohyoid membrane** by the **internal laryngeal vessels** and **nerve.**

EXTRINSIC MUSCLES OF THE TONGUE

Muscle	Origin	Insertion	Innervation	Action
Genioglossus Muscle	Upper part of the mental spine of mandible	In a fan-like manner along the ventral surface of tongue; anterior surface of body of hyoid bone	Hypoglossal nerve	Draws the tongue forward and protrudes the apex of the tongue
Hyoglossus Muscle	Entire length of the greater horn of hyoid bone and lateral part of body of hyoid bone	Into the side of tongue	Hypoglossal nerve	Depresses the tongue
Styloglossus Muscle	Styloid process of temporal bone and the stylohyoid ligament	Side and inferior aspect of the tongue	Hypoglossal nerve	Draws the tongue upward and backward
Palatoglossus Muscle	Oral surface of the palatine aponeurosis	Side and dorsum of the tongue	Pharyngeal branch of the vagus nerve (fibers emerge from brain in cranial part of accessory nerve i.e., XI via X)	Elevates the posterior part of the tongue

Additionally, the tongue contains longitudinal, transverse, and vertical muscles whose fibers commence and terminate within the tongue itself and, hence, are considered **intrinsic tongue muscles.** These are all supplied by the **hypoglossal nerve.**

Fig. 865   **VII**

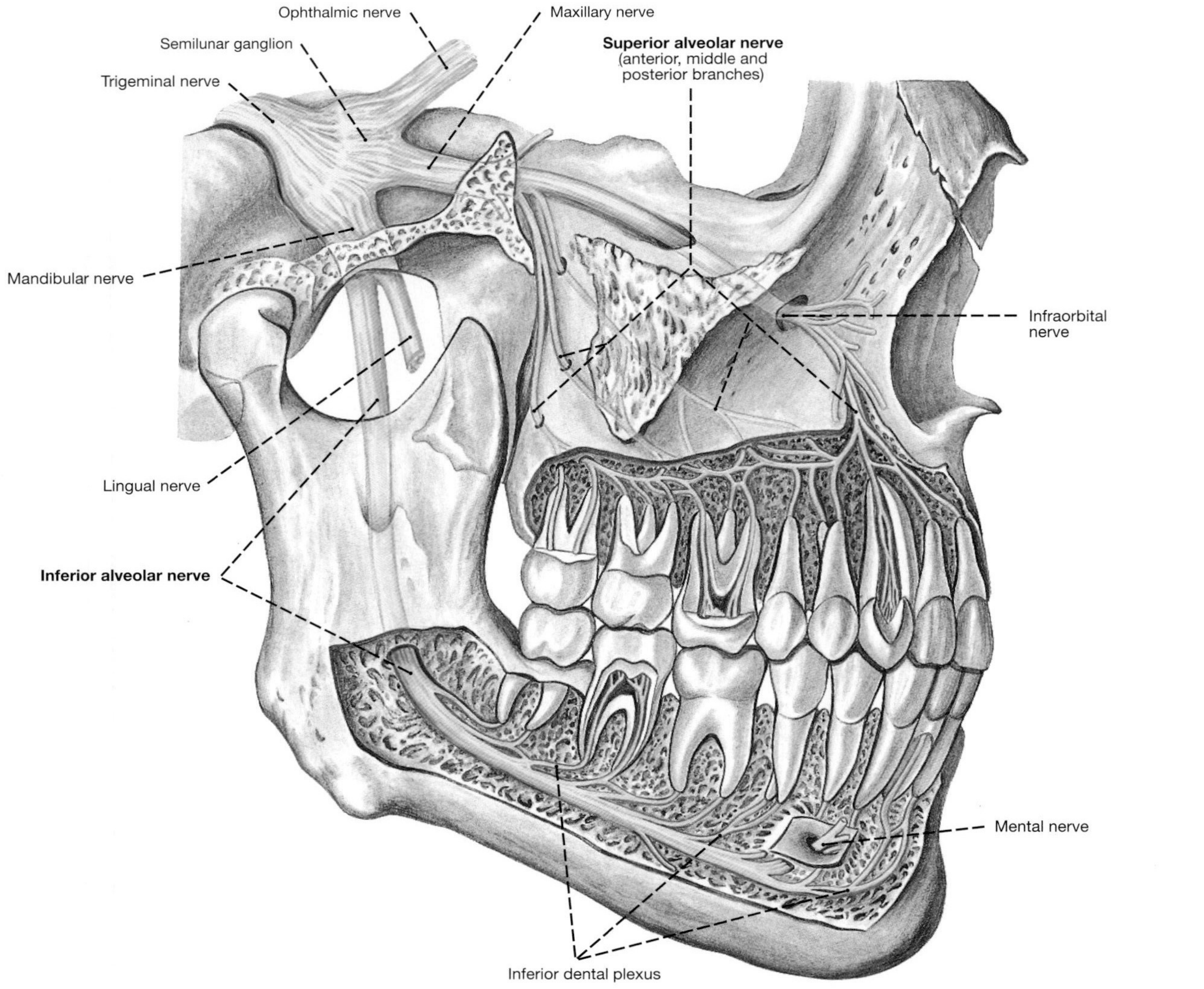

PLATE 542   Teeth: Innervation of Upper and Lower Teeth; Mandible

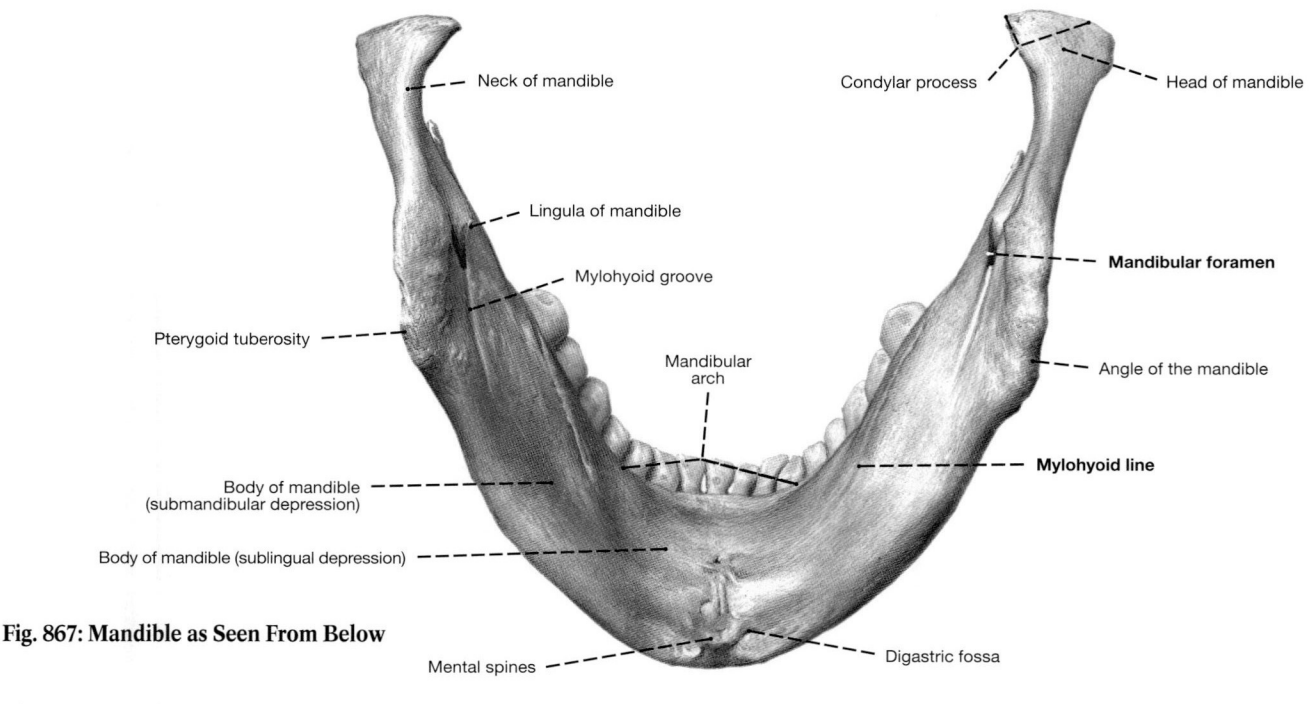

Ophthalmic nerve

Maxillary nerve

Semilunar ganglion

Superior alveolar nerve
(anterior, middle and
posterior branches)

Trigeminal nerve

Mandibular nerve

Infraorbital
nerve

Lingual nerve

Inferior alveolar nerve

Mental nerve

Inferior dental plexus

Fig. 866: Superior Alveolar Nerve (Maxillary) and Inferior Alveolar Nerve (Mandibular) and Their Branches to the Upper and Lower Teeth

Neck of mandible

Condylar process

Head of mandible

Lingula of mandible

Mylohyoid groove

Mandibular foramen

Pterygoid tuberosity

Mandibular
arch

Angle of the mandible

Body of mandible
(submandibular depression)

Mylohyoid line

Body of mandible (sublingual depression)

Mental spines

Digastric fossa

Fig. 867: Mandible as Seen From Below

Figs. 866, 867

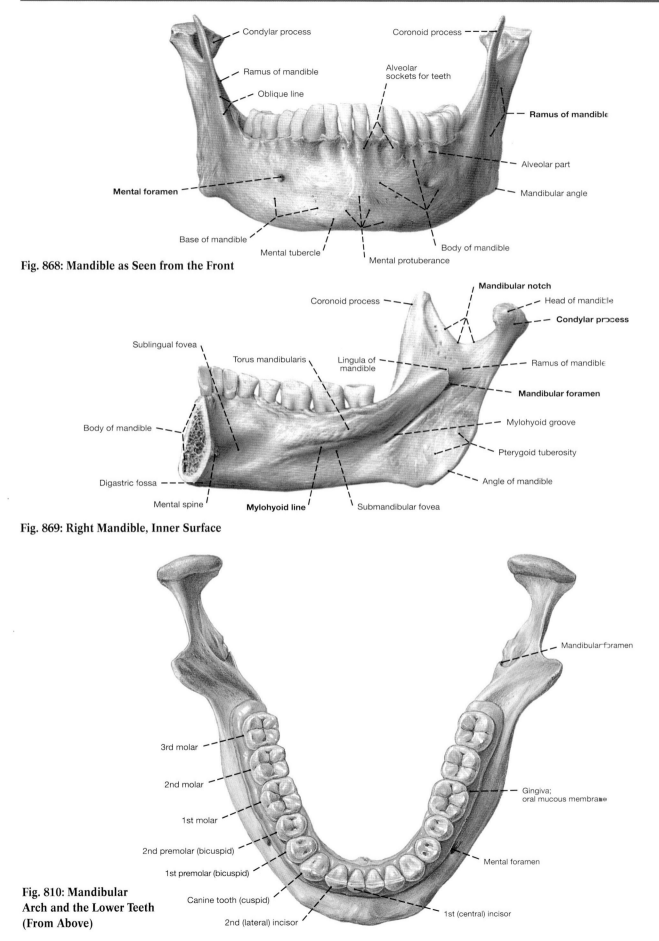

Fig. 868: Mandible as Seen from the Front

Fig. 869: Right Mandible, Inner Surface

Fig. 810: Mandibular
Arch and the Lower Teeth
(From Above)

PLATE 544   Upper Teeth and Palate From Below

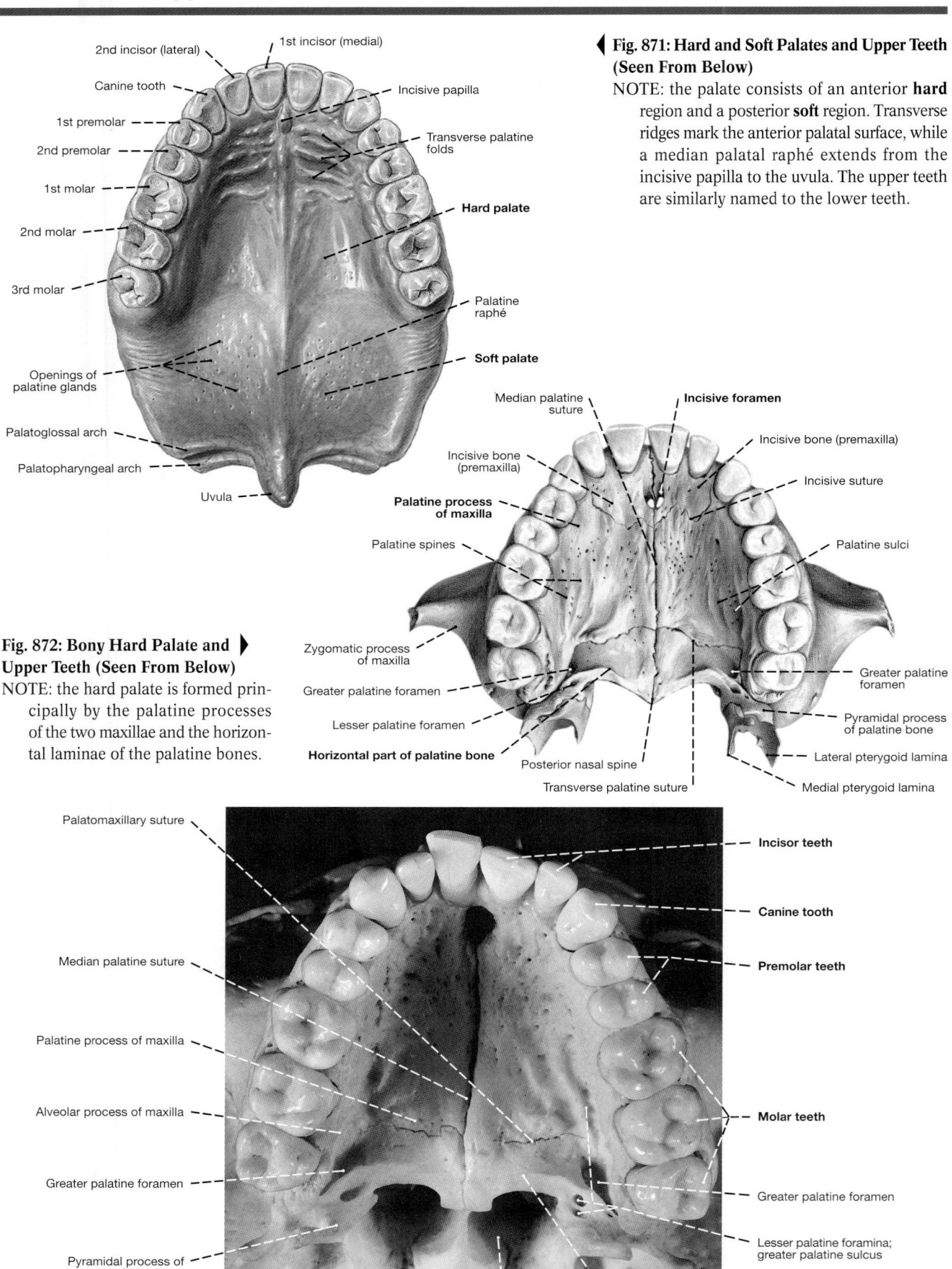

2nd incisor (lateral)
1st incisor (medial)
Canine tooth
Incisive papilla
1st premolar
2nd premolar
Transverse palatine folds
1st molar
Hard palate
2nd molar
3rd molar
Palatine raphé
Soft palate
Openings of palatine glands
Palatoglossal arch
Palatopharyngeal arch
Uvula

Fig. 871: Hard and Soft Palates and Upper Teeth (Seen From Below)
NOTE: the palate consists of an anterior **hard** region and a posterior **soft** region. Transverse ridges mark the anterior palatal surface, while a median palatal raphé extends from the incisive papilla to the uvula. The upper teeth are similarly named to the lower teeth.

Median palatine suture
Incisive foramen
Incisive bone (premaxilla)
Incisive bone (premaxilla)
Incisive suture
Palatine process of maxilla
Palatine spines
Palatine sulci
Zygomatic process of maxilla
Greater palatine foramen
Greater palatine foramen
Lesser palatine foramen
Pyramidal process of palatine bone
Horizontal part of palatine bone
Lateral pterygoid lamina
Posterior nasal spine
Medial pterygoid lamina
Transverse palatine suture

Fig. 872: Bony Hard Palate and Upper Teeth (Seen From Below)
NOTE: the hard palate is formed principally by the palatine processes of the two maxillae and the horizontal laminae of the palatine bones.

Palatomaxillary suture
Incisor teeth
Canine tooth
Median palatine suture
Premolar teeth
Palatine process of maxilla
Alveolar process of maxilla
Molar teeth
Greater palatine foramen
Greater palatine foramen
Lesser palatine foramina; greater palatine sulcus
Pyramidal process of palatine bone
Choana
Horizontal plate of palatine bone

Fig. 873: Photograph of the Bony Palate Showing the Maxillary Arch and Upper Teeth

Figs. 871, 872, 873

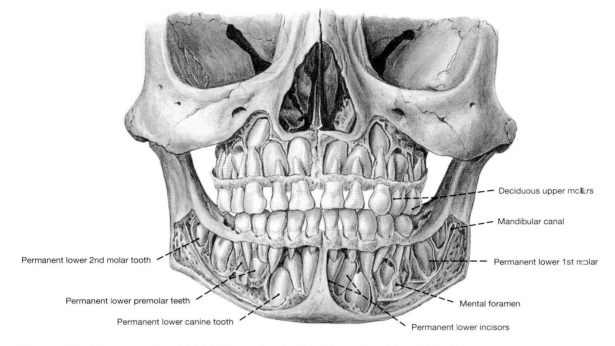

Labels (Fig. 874):
- Deciduous upper molars
- Mandibular canal
- Permanent lower 1st molar
- Mental foramen
- Permanent lower incisors
- Permanent lower canine tooth
- Permanent lower premolar teeth
- Permanent lower 2nd molar tooth

Fig. 874: Facial Skeleton of a 5-Year-Old Child Showing Full Deciduous Dentition (20 Teeth)

NOTE: 1) the **deciduous teeth** are shown as white, whereas the rudiments of the **permanent teeth,** shown in blue, have been exposed by removing the outer walls of the alveolar processes of both maxillae and the mandible.

2) all 20 deciduous teeth have erupted: 8 incisors, 4 canines, and 8 molars. Normally all deciduous teeth are replaced by the 12th year.

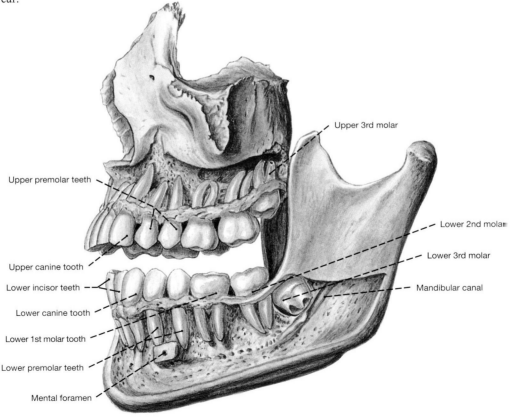

Labels (Fig. 875):
- Upper 3rd molar
- Upper premolar teeth
- Lower 2nd molar
- Lower 3rd molar
- Mandibular canal
- Upper canine tooth
- Lower incisor teeth
- Lower canine tooth
- Lower 1st molar tooth
- Lower premolar teeth
- Mental foramen

Fig. 875: Dentition of a 20-Year-Old Person, Seen From the Left Side

NOTE: 1) the roots of the permanent teeth have been exposed by removal of the alveolar walls. All of the permanent teeth have erupted through the gums with the exception of the lower 3rd molar.

2) the canines and incisors have but one root, as generally do the premolars, although the latter may have two roots. The 1st and 2nd molars usually have three roots, whereas the smaller 3rd molar may have less than three and may even be single rooted.

UPPER TEETH

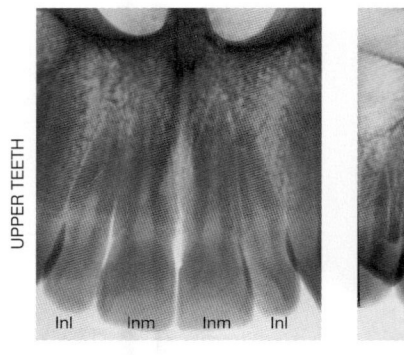

Fig. 876: Four Incisors

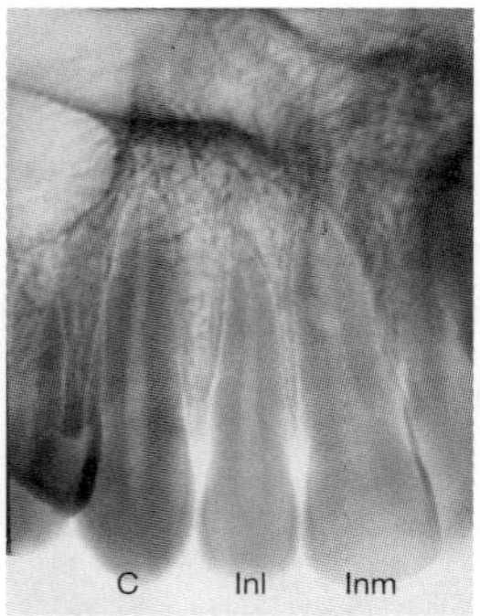

Fig. 877: Two Right Incisors and Canine Teeth

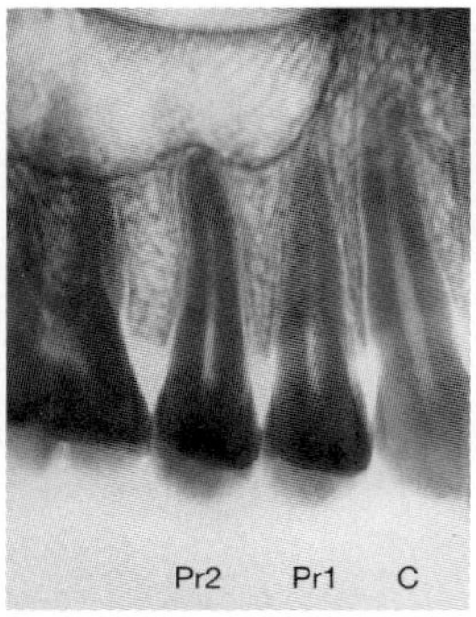

Fig. 878: Right Canine Tooth and Two Premolars

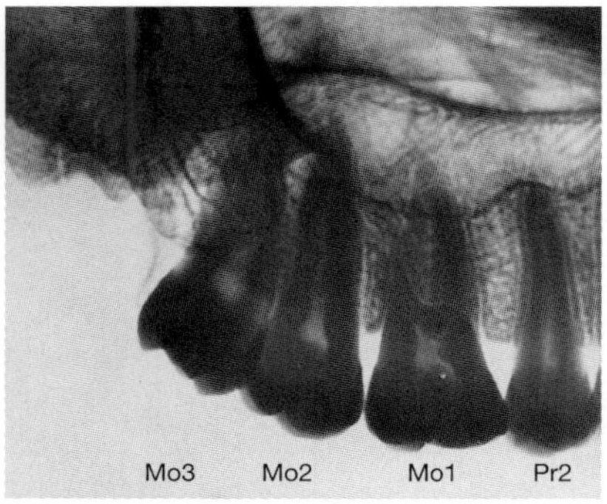

Fig. 879: Right Second Premolar and Three Molars

LOWER TEETH

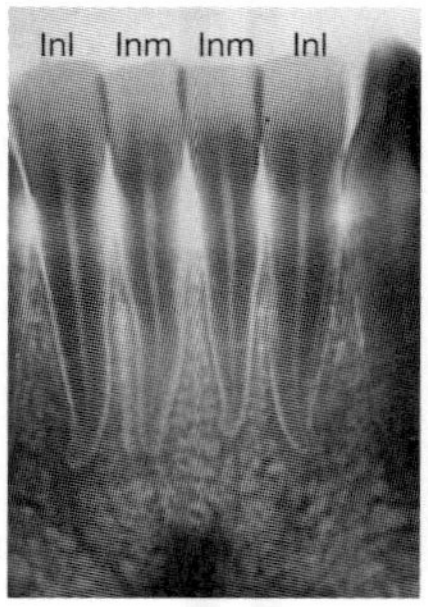

Fig. 880: Four Incisors

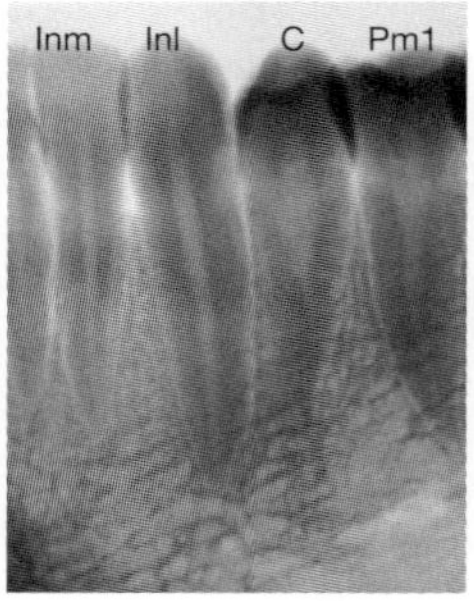

Fig. 881: Two Incisors, Canine and First Premolar

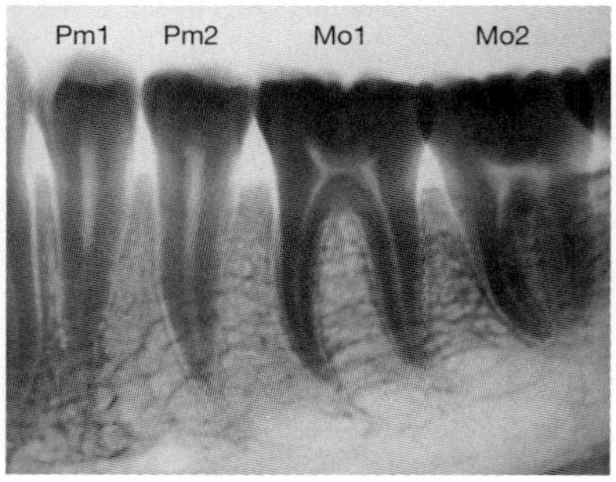

Fig. 882: Two Premolars and First Two Molar Teeth

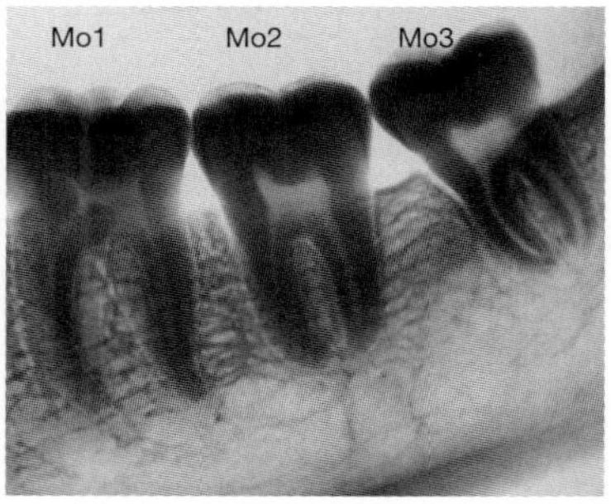

Fig. 883: Three Molar Teeth

Figs. 876–879: X-rays of the Permanent Upper Teeth
Figs. 880–883: X-rays of the Permanent Lower Teeth

Inl	= Lateral incisor	Pr2	= 2nd premolar
Inm	= Medial incisor	Mo1	= 1st molar
C	= Canine tooth	Mo2	= 2nd molar
Pr1	= 1st premolar	Mo3	= 3rd molar

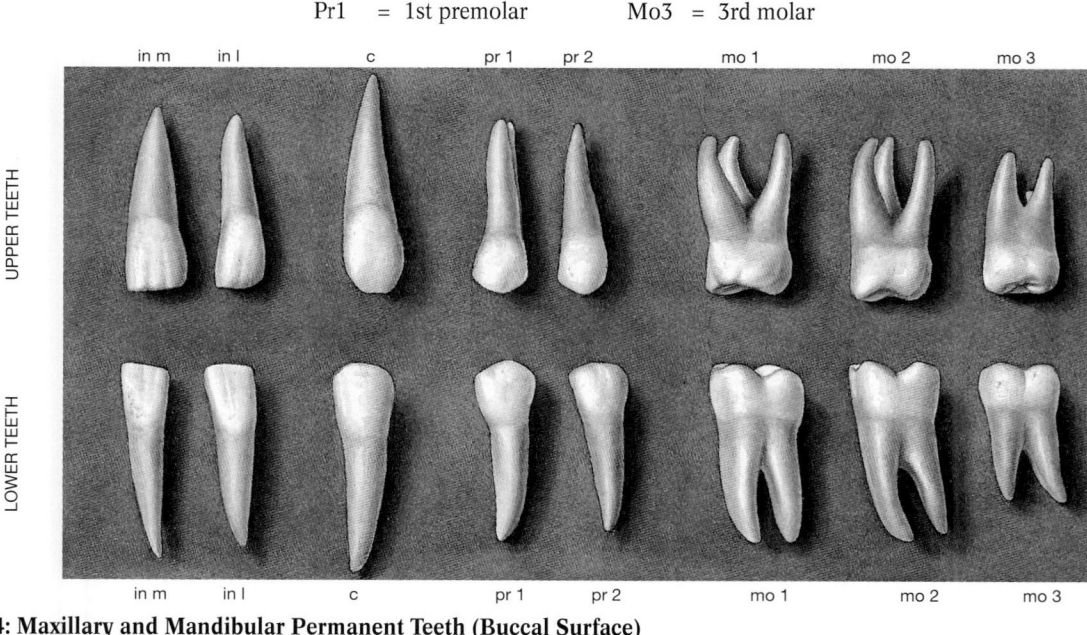

Fig. 884: Maxillary and Mandibular Permanent Teeth (Buccal Surface)

in m	= Medial incisor	pr 2	= 2nd premolar
in l	= Lateral incisor	mo 1	= 1st molar
c	= Canine	mo 2	= 2nd molar
pr 1	= 1st premolar	mo 3	= 3rd molar

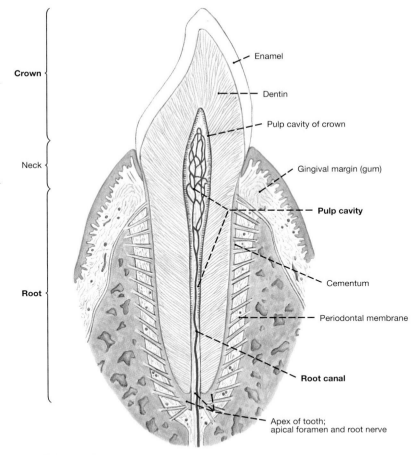

Fig. 885: Longitudinal Section of the Tooth

NOTE: the crown of the tooth is covered with **enamel** and projects from the **gingiva** or gum. The **root** is embedded within the alveolar bony **socket** and covered by a thin layer of **cementum.** The main portion of the tooth consists of **dentin,** which surrounds the **root canal** and **pulp cavity** containing the **dental artery** and **nerve.**

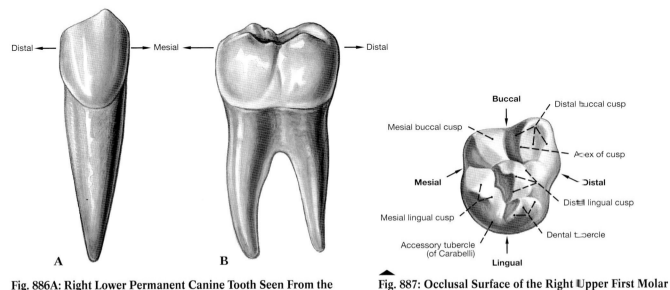

Fig. 886A: Right Lower Permanent Canine Tooth Seen From the Vestibular Surface

Fig. 886B: Left Lower 2nd Molar Tooth Seen From the Vestibular Surface

Fig. 887: Occlusal Surface of the Right Upper First Molar

NOTE: the upper 1st molar may have a 5th cusp, the tubercle of Carabelli on the mesiolingual surface of its crown.

PLATE 548   Pharynx: External Muscles, Lateral View

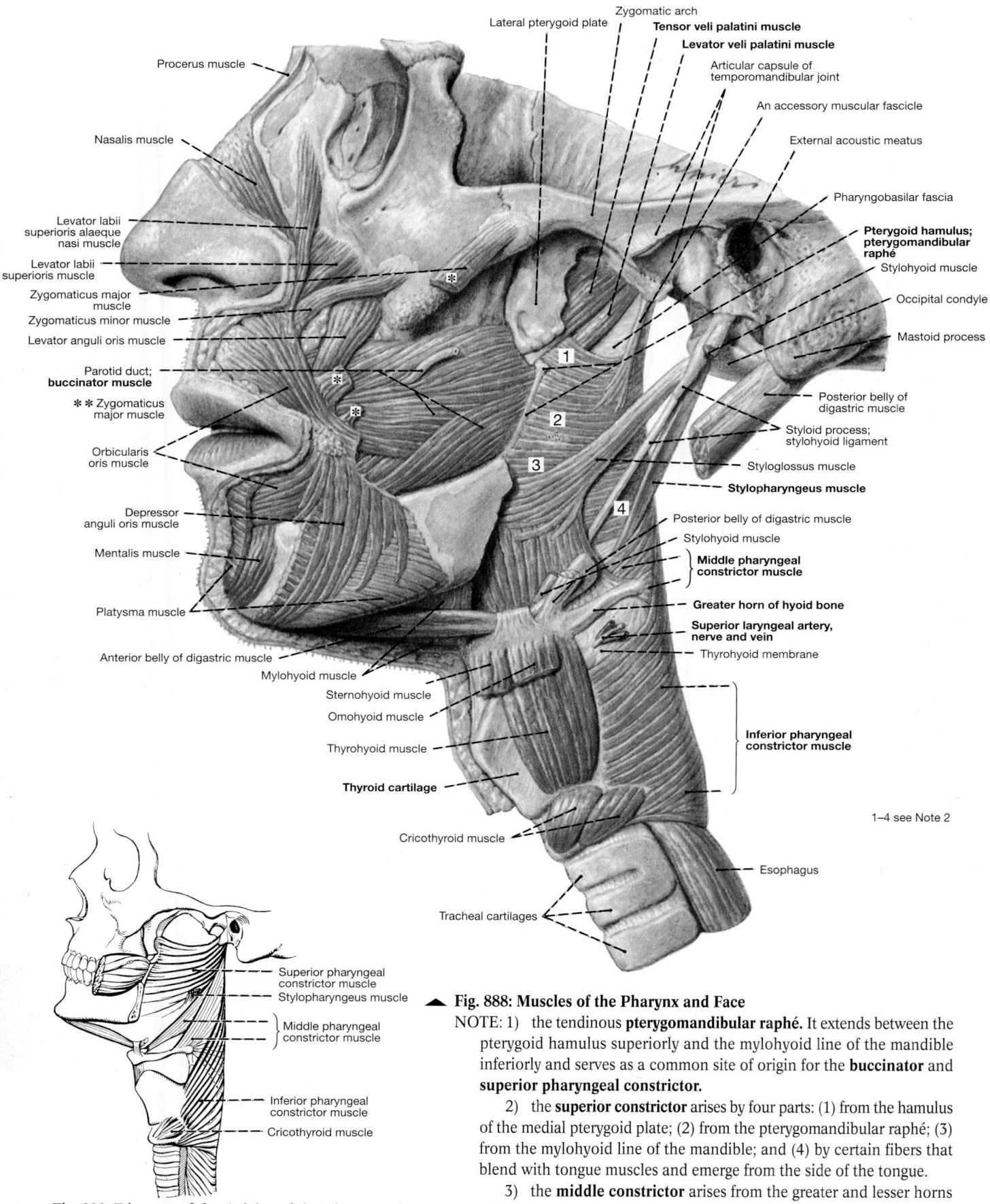

Procerus muscle

Nasalis muscle

Levator labii superioris alaeque nasi muscle

Levator labii superioris muscle

Zygomaticus major muscle

Zygomaticus minor muscle

Levator anguli oris muscle

Parotid duct; **buccinator muscle**

✱✱ Zygomaticus major muscle

Orbicularis oris muscle

Depressor anguli oris muscle

Mentalis muscle

Platysma muscle

Anterior belly of digastric muscle

Mylohyoid muscle

Sternohyoid muscle

Omohyoid muscle

Thyrohyoid muscle

Thyroid cartilage

Cricothyroid muscle

Tracheal cartilages

Lateral pterygoid plate

Zygomatic arch

Tensor veli palatini muscle

Levator veli palatini muscle

Articular capsule of temporomandibular joint

An accessory muscular fascicle

External acoustic meatus

Pharyngobasilar fascia

Pterygoid hamulus; pterygomandibular raphé

Stylohyoid muscle

Occipital condyle

Mastoid process

Posterior belly of digastric muscle

Styloid process; stylohyoid ligament

Styloglossus muscle

Stylopharyngeus muscle

Posterior belly of digastric muscle

Stylohyoid muscle

Middle pharyngeal constrictor muscle

Greater horn of hyoid bone

Superior laryngeal artery, nerve and vein

Thyrohyoid membrane

Inferior pharyngeal constrictor muscle

1–4 see Note 2

Esophagus

Superior pharyngeal constrictor muscle

Stylopharyngeus muscle

Middle pharyngeal constrictor muscle

Inferior pharyngeal constrictor muscle

Cricothyroid muscle

Fig. 889: Diagram of the Origins of the Pharyngeal ◀
Constrictor Muscles

◀ **Fig. 888: Muscles of the Pharynx and Face**
NOTE: 1) the tendinous **pterygomandibular raphé.** It extends between the pterygoid hamulus superiorly and the mylohyoid line of the mandible inferiorly and serves as a common site of origin for the **buccinator** and **superior pharyngeal constrictor.**

2) the **superior constrictor** arises by four parts: (1) from the hamulus of the medial pterygoid plate; (2) from the pterygomandibular raphé; (3) from the mylohyoid line of the mandible; and (4) by certain fibers that blend with tongue muscles and emerge from the side of the tongue.

3) the **middle constrictor** arises from the greater and lesser horns of the hyoid bone, while the larger and thicker **inferior constrictor** arises from the thyroid and cricoid cartilages.

Figs. 888, 889

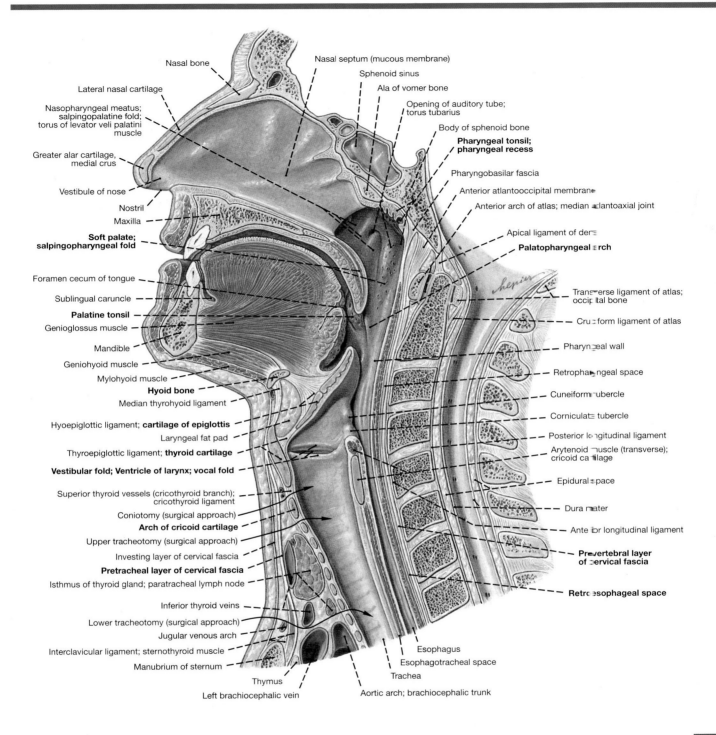

Nasal bone

Lateral nasal cartilage

Nasopharyngeal meatus;
salpingopalatine fold;
torus of levator veli palatini
muscle

Greater alar cartilage,
medial crus

Vestibule of nose

Nostril

Maxilla

**Soft palate;
salpingopharyngeal fold**

Foramen cecum of tongue

Sublingual caruncle

Palatine tonsil

Genioglossus muscle

Mandible

Geniohyoid muscle

Mylohyoid muscle

Hyoid bone

Median thyrohyoid ligament

Hyoepiglottic ligament; **cartilage of epiglottis**

Laryngeal fat pad

Thyroepiglottic ligament; **thyroid cartilage**

Vestibular fold; Ventricle of larynx; vocal fold

Superior thyroid vessels (cricothyroid branch);
cricothyroid ligament

Coniotomy (surgical approach)

Arch of cricoid cartilage

Upper tracheotomy (surgical approach)

Investing layer of cervical fascia

Pretracheal layer of cervical fascia

Isthmus of thyroid gland; paratracheal lymph node

Inferior thyroid veins

Lower tracheotomy (surgical approach)

Jugular venous arch

Interclavicular ligament; sternothyroid muscle

Manubrium of sternum

Thymus

Left brachiocephalic vein

Nasal septum (mucous membrane)

Sphenoid sinus

Ala of vomer bone

Opening of auditory tube;
torus tubarius

Body of sphenoid bone

**Pharyngeal tonsil;
pharyngeal recess**

Pharyngobasilar fascia

Anterior atlantooccipital membrane

Anterior arch of atlas; median atlantoaxial joint

Apical ligament of dens

Palatopharyngeal arch

Transverse ligament of atlas;
occipital bone

Cruciform ligament of atlas

Pharyngeal wall

Retropharyngeal space

Cuneiform tubercle

Corniculate tubercle

Posterior longitudinal ligament

Arytenoid muscle (transverse);
cricoid cartilage

Epidural space

Dura mater

Anterior longitudinal ligament

**Prevertebral layer
of cervical fascia**

Retroesophageal space

Esophagus

Esophagotracheal space

Trachea

Aortic arch; brachiocephalic trunk

Fig. 890: Midsagittal Section of the Mouth, Pharynx, Larynx and Other Head and Neck Viscera

NOTE: 1) the closed oral cavity is occupied principally by the tongue. The posterior end of the oral cavity opens into the **oropharynx.** Superiorly, the posterior nasal cavities are continuous with the **nasopharynx,** whereas inferiorly the **laryngeal part of the pharynx** (between the levels of the epiglottis and cricoid cartilages) communicates with the larynx.

2) the pharynx continues inferiorly as the **esophagus,** while the larynx becomes the **trachea** below the level of the cricoid cartilage.

3) during **deglutition** (swallowing) food gets directed toward the posterior part of the oral cavity. The soft palate is then elevated and tensed (levator and tensor veli palatini muscles) thereby closing off the nasopharynx so that food enters the oropharynx. At the same time the larynx is drawn upward toward the epiglottis and the pharynx ascends as well. This action closes off the laryngeal orifice (aditus) and prevents food from entering the larynx.

4) the arrows indicate surgical approaches to the airway (larynx and trachea).

Fig. 390   **VII**

PLATE 550   Pharynx From Behind: Muscles

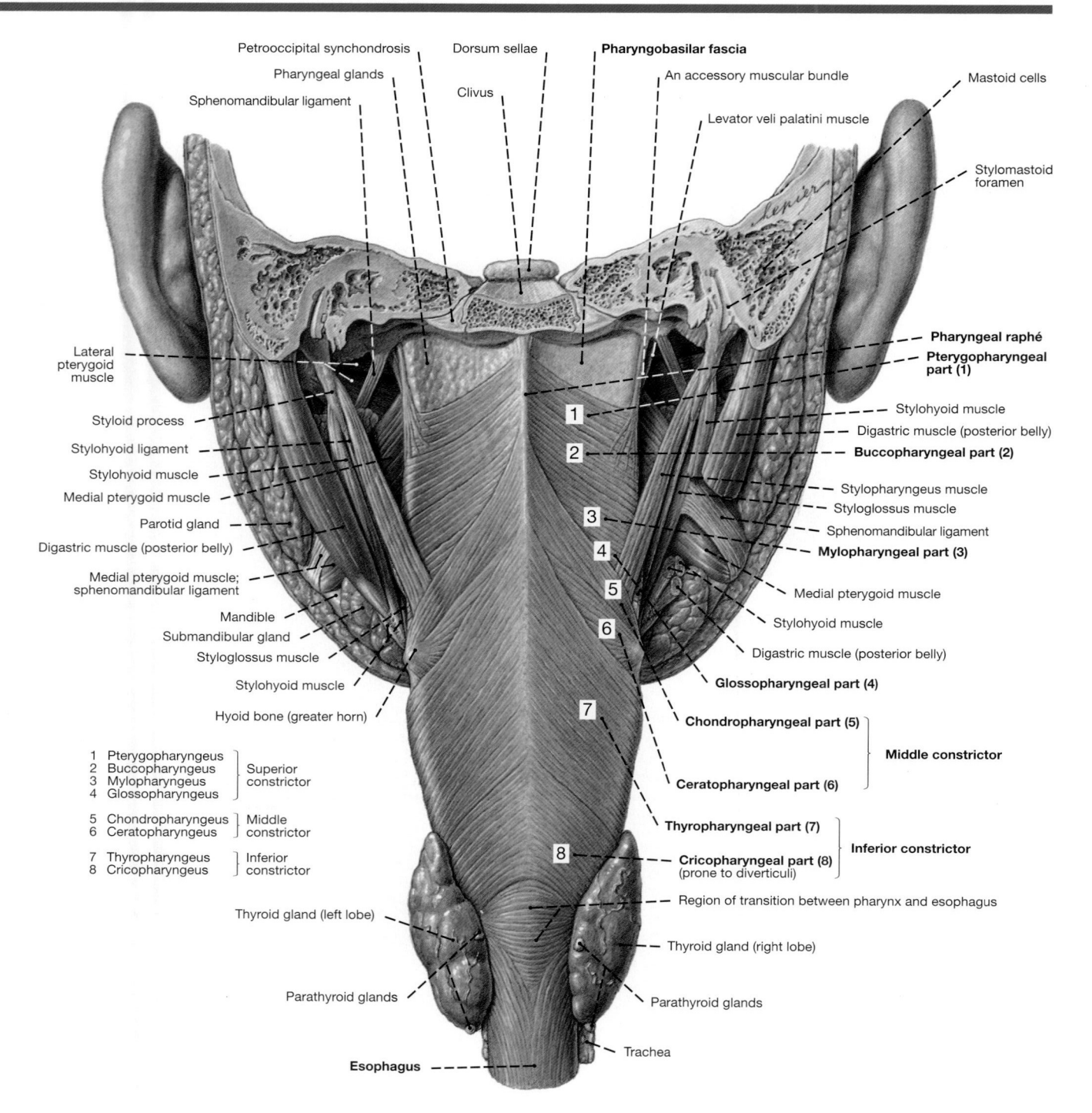

Petrooccipital synchondrosis
Pharyngeal glands
Sphenomandibular ligament
Dorsum sellae
Clivus
Pharyngobasilar fascia
An accessory muscular bundle
Levator veli palatini muscle
Mastoid cells
Stylomastoid foramen

Pharyngeal raphé
Pterygopharyngeal part (1)

Lateral pterygoid muscle
Styloid process
Stylohyoid ligament
Stylohyoid muscle
Medial pterygoid muscle
Parotid gland
Digastric muscle (posterior belly)
Medial pterygoid muscle; sphenomandibular ligament
Mandible
Submandibular gland
Styloglossus muscle
Stylohyoid muscle
Hyoid bone (greater horn)

Stylohyoid muscle
Digastric muscle (posterior belly)
Buccopharyngeal part (2)
Stylopharyngeus muscle
Styloglossus muscle
Sphenomandibular ligament
Mylopharyngeal part (3)
Medial pterygoid muscle
Stylohyoid muscle
Digastric muscle (posterior belly)
Glossopharyngeal part (4)
Chondropharyngeal part (5)
Ceratopharyngeal part (6)
Middle constrictor
Thyropharyngeal part (7)
Cricopharyngeal part (8) (prone to diverticuli)
Inferior constrictor
Region of transition between pharynx and esophagus
Thyroid gland (right lobe)
Parathyroid glands
Trachea

1 Pterygopharyngeus
2 Buccopharyngeus   Superior
3 Mylopharyngeus   constrictor
4 Glossopharyngeus

5 Chondropharyngeus   Middle
6 Ceratopharyngeus   constrictor

7 Thyropharyngeus   Inferior
8 Cricopharyngeus   constrictor

Thyroid gland (left lobe)
Parathyroid glands
Esophagus

Fig. 891: Dorsal View of the Pharyngeal Muscles

NOTE: 1) this posterior view of the pharynx was achieved by making a frontal transection through the petrous and mastoid parts of the temporal bone and through the body of the occipital bone. The styloid processes and their muscular attachments are left intact.

2) the divisions of the **pharyngeal constrictors.** Their muscle fibers arise laterally to insert in a posterior raphé in the midline. The **superior constrictor** is divisible into four parts, while the **middle and inferior constrictors** are each divisible into two.

3) above the superior constrictor is found the fibrous **pharyngobasilar fascia,** which attaches to the basal portion of the occipital bone and to the temporal bones. Below the inferior constrictor, the pharynx is continuous with the muscular esophagus.

4) the superior and middle constrictor muscles and the thyropharyngeal part of the inferior constrictor are innervated by the **pharyngeal branch of the vagus nerve.** These fibers have their cell bodies in the nucleus ambiguus in the medulla oblongata, they emerge from the brain in the rootlets of the bulbar part of the accessory nerve and then, by a communicating branch, join the vagus nerve.

5) the cricopharyngeal part of the inferior constrictor is supplied by the recurrent laryngeal branch of the vagus nerve.

Fig. 891

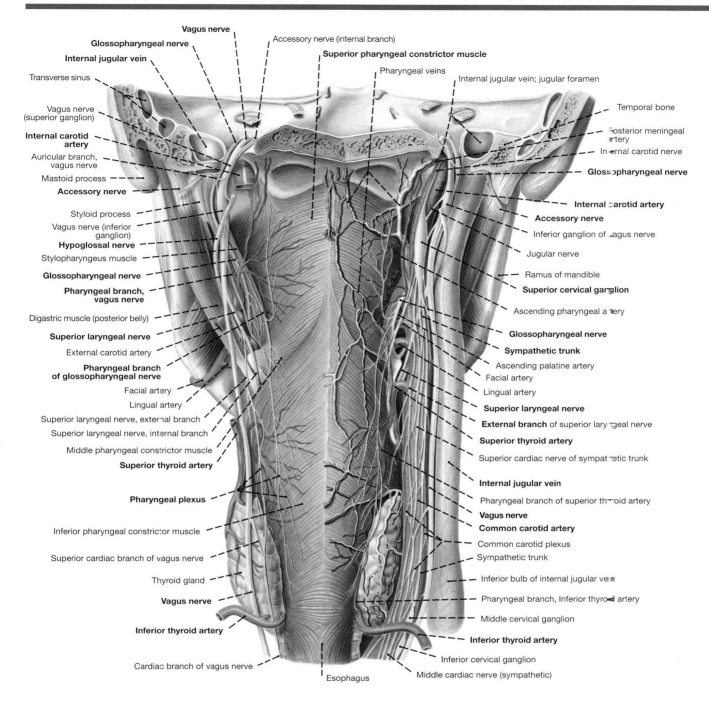

Fig. 892: Nerves and Vessels on the Dorsal and Lateral Walls of the Pharynx

NOTE: 1) the head has been split longitudinally. The pharynx, larynx, and facial structures were separated from the vertebral column and its associated muscles. This posterior view of pharynx also shows the large nerves and blood vessels which course through the neck. On the right side, observe the **carotid artery, internal jugular vein, vagus nerve** and the **sympathetic trunk.**

   2) on the left side are the **glossopharyngeal** and **hypoglossal nerves** which were exposed by the removal of the carotid arteries and internal jugular vein. In addition to the jugular vein, the **jugular foramen** transmits the 9th, 10th and 11th cranial nerves.

   3) the **thyroid gland** and its **superior and inferior thyroid arteries.** The superior and middle thyroid veins drain into the internal jugular vein, while the inferior thyroid veins (not shown) usually drain into the left brachiocephalic vein.

Fig. 892   **VII**

PLATE 552   **Pharynx, Opened From Behind; Lymphatic Ring**

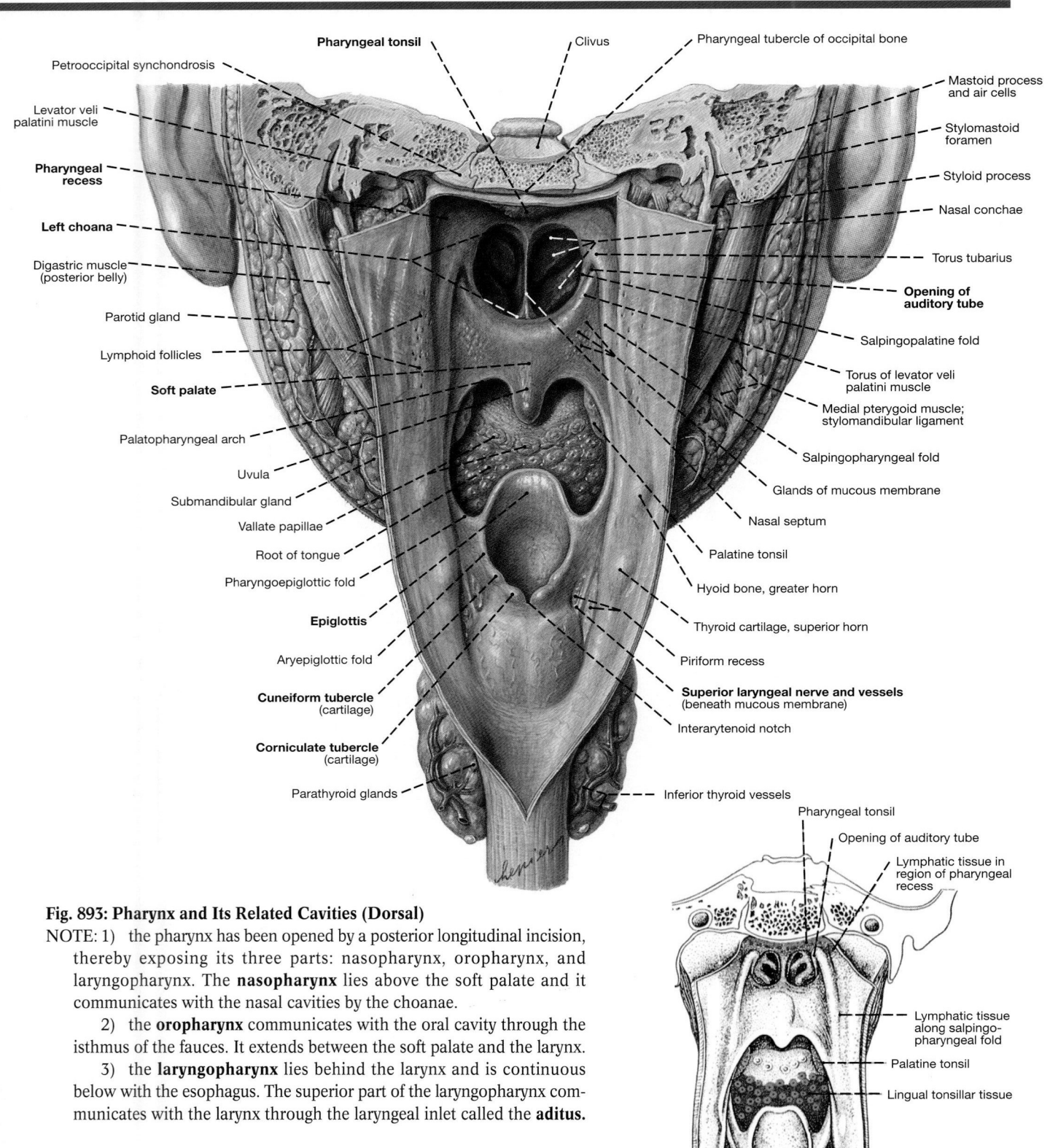

Pharyngeal tonsil
Clivus
Pharyngeal tubercle of occipital bone
Petrooccipital synchondrosis
Mastoid process and air cells
Levator veli palatini muscle
Stylomastoid foramen
Pharyngeal recess
Styloid process
Left choana
Nasal conchae
Digastric muscle (posterior belly)
Torus tubarius
Parotid gland
Opening of auditory tube
Lymphoid follicles
Salpingopalatine fold
Soft palate
Torus of levator veli palatini muscle
Palatopharyngeal arch
Medial pterygoid muscle; stylomandibular ligament
Uvula
Salpingopharyngeal fold
Submandibular gland
Glands of mucous membrane
Vallate papillae
Nasal septum
Root of tongue
Palatine tonsil
Pharyngoepiglottic fold
Hyoid bone, greater horn
Epiglottis
Thyroid cartilage, superior horn
Aryepiglottic fold
Piriform recess
Cuneiform tubercle (cartilage)
Superior laryngeal nerve and vessels (beneath mucous membrane)
Corniculate tubercle (cartilage)
Interarytenoid notch
Parathyroid glands
Inferior thyroid vessels

Pharyngeal tonsil
Opening of auditory tube
Lymphatic tissue in region of pharyngeal recess
Lymphatic tissue along salpingopharyngeal fold
Palatine tonsil
Lingual tonsillar tissue

Fig. 893: Pharynx and Its Related Cavities (Dorsal)

NOTE: 1) the pharynx has been opened by a posterior longitudinal incision, thereby exposing its three parts: nasopharynx, oropharynx, and laryngopharynx. The **nasopharynx** lies above the soft palate and it communicates with the nasal cavities by the choanae.

  2) the **oropharynx** communicates with the oral cavity through the isthmus of the fauces. It extends between the soft palate and the larynx.

  3) the **laryngopharynx** lies behind the larynx and is continuous below with the esophagus. The superior part of the laryngopharynx communicates with the larynx through the laryngeal inlet called the **aditus.**

Fig. 894: Oro-naso-pharyngeal Lymphatic Ring ▶

NOTE: the lymphatic ring is shown in red. This circular accumulation of lymphatic tissue includes the lingual tonsil (which consists of lymphoid follicles on the posterior one third of the tongue), the palatine tonsils, the pharyngeal tonsil and more diffuse lymphoid tissue in the wall of Lyme nasopharynx along the salpingopharyngeal fold.

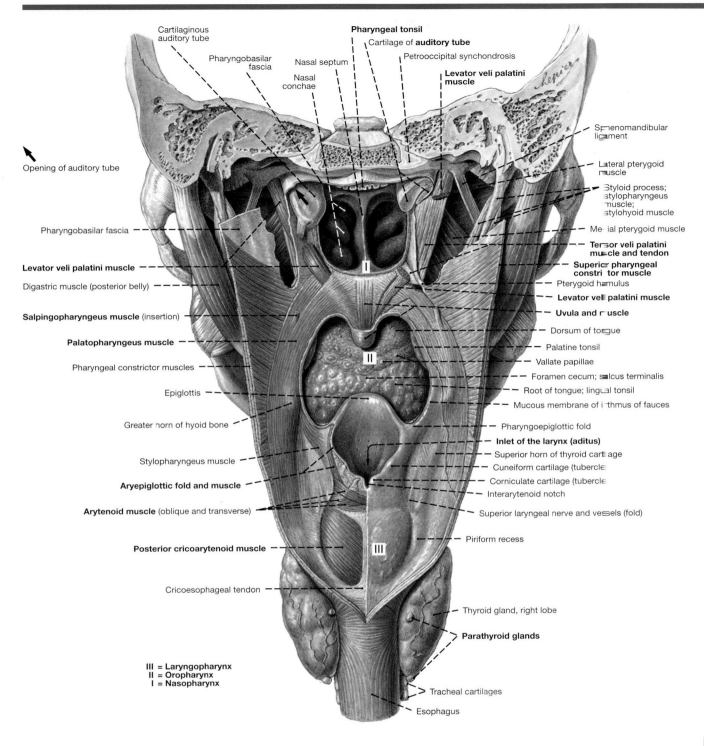

Cartilaginous auditory tube

Pharyngobasilar fascia

Nasal septum

Nasal conchae

Pharyngeal tonsil

Cartilage of **auditory tube**

Petrooccipital synchondrosis

Levator veli palatini muscle

Opening of auditory tube

Sphenomandibular ligament

Lateral pterygoid muscle

Styloid process; stylopharyngeus muscle; stylohyoid muscle

Medial pterygoid muscle

Pharyngobasilar fascia

Tensor veli palatini muscle and tendon

Levator veli palatini muscle

Superior pharyngeal constrictor muscle

Digastric muscle (posterior belly)

Pterygoid hamulus

Levator veli palatini muscle

Salpingopharyngeus muscle (insertion)

Uvula and muscle

Palatopharyngeus muscle

Dorsum of tongue

Palatine tonsil

Pharyngeal constrictor muscles

Vallate papillae

Foramen cecum; sulcus terminalis

Epiglottis

Root of tongue; lingual tonsil

Mucous membrane of isthmus of fauces

Greater horn of hyoid bone

Pharyngoepiglottic fold

Inlet of the larynx (aditus)

Superior horn of thyroid cartilage

Stylopharyngeus muscle

Cuneiform cartilage (tubercle)

Aryepiglottic fold and muscle

Corniculate cartilage (tubercle)

Interarytenoid notch

Arytenoid muscle (oblique and transverse)

Superior laryngeal nerve and vessels (fold)

Piriform recess

Posterior cricoarytenoid muscle

Cricoesophageal tendon

Thyroid gland, right lobe

Parathyroid glands

III = Laryngopharynx
II = Oropharynx
I = Nasopharynx

Tracheal cartilages

Esophagus

Fig. 895: Muscles of the Soft Palate, Pharynx, and Posterior Larynx

NOTE: 1) this dissection is similar to that in Figure 893. The pharynx has been opened dorsally by a midline incision and the mucous membrane has been removed from the soft palate, pharynx and the left posterior larynx. On the right, a part of the **levator veli palatini muscle** has been removed to expose the adjacent **tensor veli palatini muscle.**

2) the **muscles of the soft palate.** Both the muscle of the uvula and the levator veli palatini muscle are innervated by the pharyngeal branch of the vagus nerve, whereas the tensor veli palatini is supplied by the mandibular division of the trigeminal nerve.

3) the **palatopharyngeus muscle** arises by two fascicles from the soft palate. The muscle fibers of these fascicles arise posterior and anterior to the insertion of the levator veli palatini muscle. The fascicles descend and merge and then insert into the posterior border of the thyroid cartilage and onto the adjacent pharyngeal wall.

Fig. 895   **VII**

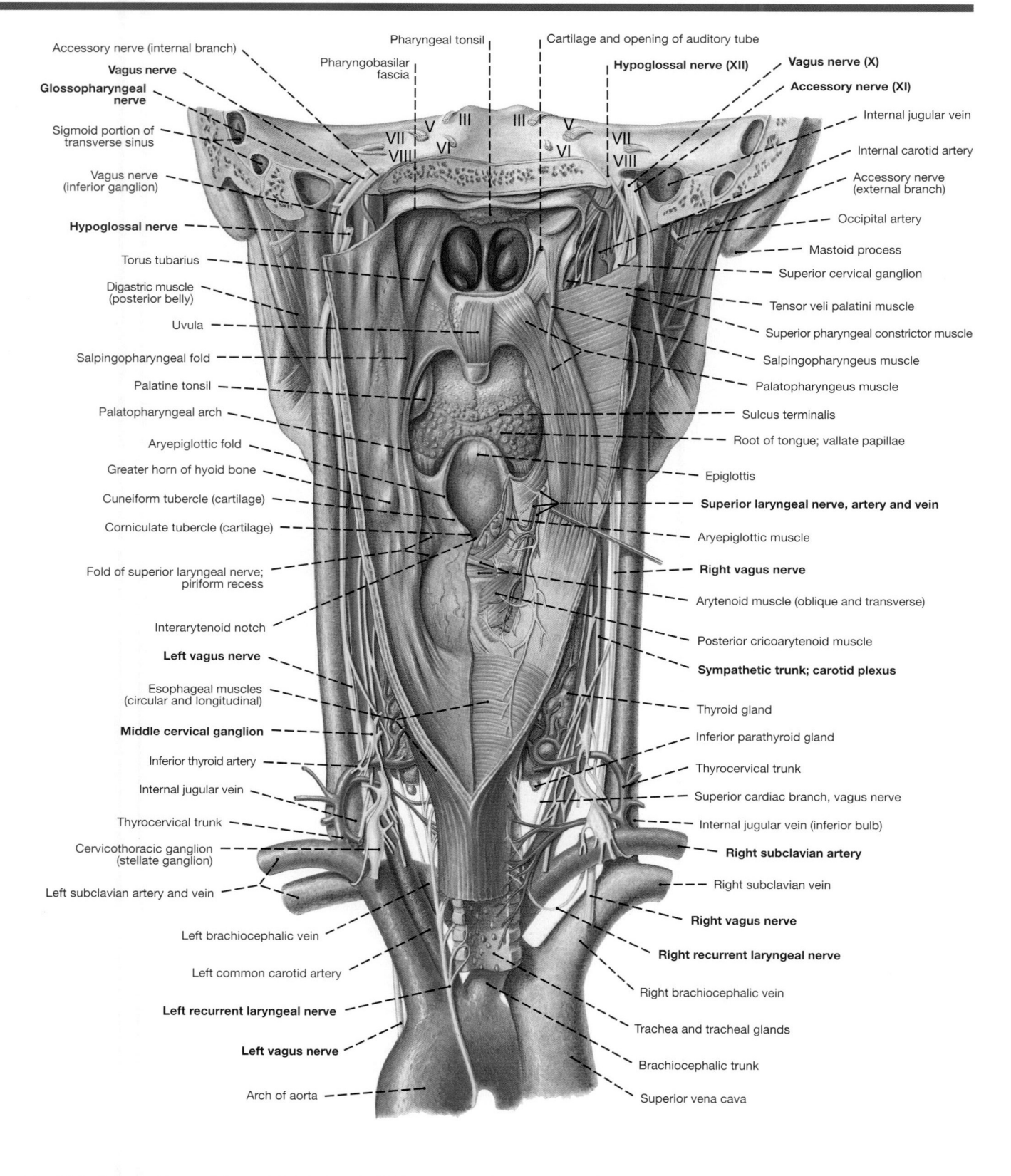

Accessory nerve (internal branch)
Vagus nerve
Glossopharyngeal nerve
Sigmoid portion of transverse sinus
Vagus nerve (inferior ganglion)
Hypoglossal nerve
Torus tubarius
Digastric muscle (posterior belly)
Uvula
Salpingopharyngeal fold
Palatine tonsil
Palatopharyngeal arch
Aryepiglottic fold
Greater horn of hyoid bone
Cuneiform tubercle (cartilage)
Corniculate tubercle (cartilage)
Fold of superior laryngeal nerve; piriform recess
Interarytenoid notch
Left vagus nerve
Esophageal muscles (circular and longitudinal)
Middle cervical ganglion
Inferior thyroid artery
Internal jugular vein
Thyrocervical trunk
Cervicothoracic ganglion (stellate ganglion)
Left subclavian artery and vein
Left brachiocephalic vein
Left common carotid artery
Left recurrent laryngeal nerve
Left vagus nerve
Arch of aorta

Pharyngeal tonsil
Pharyngobasilar fascia
Cartilage and opening of auditory tube
Hypoglossal nerve (XII)
Vagus nerve (X)
Accessory nerve (XI)
Internal jugular vein
Internal carotid artery
Accessory nerve (external branch)
Occipital artery
Mastoid process
Superior cervical ganglion
Tensor veli palatini muscle
Superior pharyngeal constrictor muscle
Salpingopharyngeus muscle
Palatopharyngeus muscle
Sulcus terminalis
Root of tongue; vallate papillae
Epiglottis
Superior laryngeal nerve, artery and vein
Aryepiglottic muscle
Right vagus nerve
Arytenoid muscle (oblique and transverse)
Posterior cricoarytenoid muscle
Sympathetic trunk; carotid plexus
Thyroid gland
Inferior parathyroid gland
Thyrocervical trunk
Superior cardiac branch, vagus nerve
Internal jugular vein (inferior bulb)
Right subclavian artery
Right subclavian vein
Right vagus nerve
Right recurrent laryngeal nerve
Right brachiocephalic vein
Trachea and tracheal glands
Brachiocephalic trunk
Superior vena cava

V III III V
VII VI VI VII
VIII VIII

Fig. 896: Pharynx Opened From Behind: Cervical Viscera, Muscles, Vessels and Nerves

NOTE: 1) the nasal, oral, and laryngeal orifices which communicate with the pharynx. Observe the **superior laryngeal artery, vein and nerve** entering the larynx from above.

    2) the **recurrent laryngeal nerves** ascending to the larynx from the thorax. The **left** nerve courses around the arch of the aorta, while on the **right** side the recurrent laryngeal nerve curves around the subclavian artery.

    3) the **inferior cervical ganglion** at the level of the 7th cervical vertebra is fused with the 1st thoracic ganglion (in about 80% of cases). When fused, the joint ganglion is called the **stellate ganglion.**

Fig. 896

MUSCLES OF THE PALATE

Muscle	Origin	Insertion	Innervation	Action
Muscle of Uvula	Posterior nasal spine (palatine bone); palatine aponeurosis	Descends into the mucous membrane of the uvula	Pharyngeal branch of the vagus nerve	Pulls the uvula up and contracts the uvula on its own side
Tensor Veli Palatini Muscle	Scaphoid fossa of pterygoid process; cartilaginous part of auditory tube; spine of sphenoid	Tendon courses around the pterygoid hamulus and then inserts into the palatine aponeurosis	Branch of the mandibular division of the trigeminal nerve	Tenses the soft palate; acting singly, it pulls the soft palate to one side
Levator Veli Palatini Muscle	Inferior surface of temporal bone; cartilaginous part of auditory tube	Upper surface of the palatine aponeurosis	Pharyngeal branch of the vagus nerve	Elevates the soft palate
Palatoglossus Muscle	Oral surface of the palatine aponeurosis	Into the side of the tongue	Pharyngeal branch of the vagus nerve	Elevates root of tongue; two muscles together close off oral cavity from oropharynx
Palatopharyngeus Muscle	Posterior border of the hard palate; palatine aponeurosis	Posterior border of thyroid cartilage; lateral wall of pharynx	Pharyngeal branch of the vagus nerve	Pulls the pharynx upward during swallowing

MUSCLES OF THE PHARYNX

Muscle	Origin	Insertion	Innervation	Action
Superior Pharyngeal Constrictor	PTERYGOPHARYNGEAL PART Pterygoid hamulus of sphenoid bone	Pharyngobasilar fascia and the midline raphé	*Motor fibers:* Pharyngeal branch of vagus nerve (fibers originating in the medullary part of accessory nerve)	The constrictor muscles act as sphincters of the pharynx and induce peristaltic waves during swallowing
	BUCCOPHARYNGEAL PART Pterygomandibular raphé	Posterior midline pharyngeal raphé		
	MYLOPHARYNGEAL PART Mylohyoid line of mandible	Posterior midline pharyngeal raphé		
	GLOSSOPHARYNGEAL PART A few fibers arise from the side of tongue	Posterior midline pharyngeal raphé	*Sensory fibers of mucosa:* Glossopharyngeal nerve and some trigeminal nerve fibers	
Middle pharyngeal Constrictor	CHONDROPHARYNGEAL PART Lesser horn of hyoid bone	Posterior midline pharyngeal raphé		
	CERATOPHARYNGEAL PART Greater horn of hyoid bone	Posterior midline pharyngeal raphé		
Inferior Pharyngeal Constrictor	THYROPHARYNGEAL PART Oblique line on the lamina of thyroid cartilage	Posterior midline pharyngeal raphé		
	CRICOPHARYNGEAL PART Side of the cricoid cartilage	Posterior midline pharyngeal raphé	Cricopharyngeus: Recurrent laryngeal branch of vagus	
Stylopharyngeus Muscle	Medial side of base of styloid process	Lateral wall of pharynx between the superior and middle constrictors	Glossopharyngeal nerve	Elevates the lateral wall of the pharynx during swallowing and speech
Salpingopharyngeus Muscle	Inferior part of the cartilage of the auditory tube	Blends with the palatopharyngeus on the lateral wall of the pharynx	Pharyngeal branch of vagus nerve	Raises upper part lateral wall of the pharynx
Palatopharyngeus Muscle	Described with the palatal muscles above			

PLATE 556   **Larynx: Anterior Relationships, Vessels and Nerves**

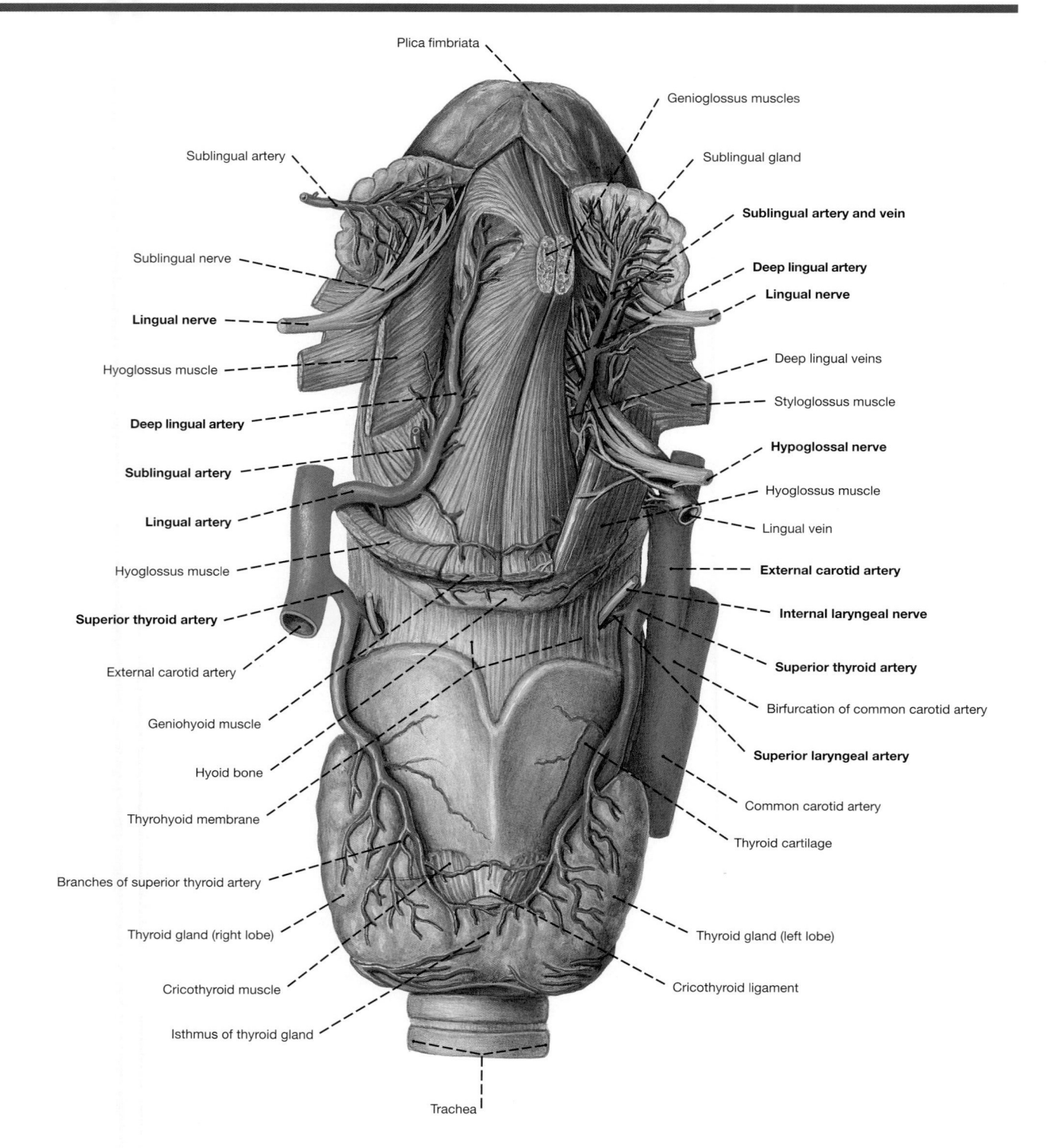

Plica fimbriata

Genioglossus muscles

Sublingual artery

Sublingual gland

Sublingual artery and vein

Sublingual nerve

Deep lingual artery

Lingual nerve

Lingual nerve

Hyoglossus muscle

Deep lingual veins

Styloglossus muscle

Deep lingual artery

Hypoglossal nerve

Sublingual artery

Hyoglossus muscle

Lingual artery

Lingual vein

Hyoglossus muscle

External carotid artery

Superior thyroid artery

Internal laryngeal nerve

External carotid artery

Superior thyroid artery

Geniohyoid muscle

Birfurcation of common carotid artery

Hyoid bone

Superior laryngeal artery

Thyrohyoid membrane

Common carotid artery

Thyroid cartilage

Branches of superior thyroid artery

Thyroid gland (right lobe)

Thyroid gland (left lobe)

Cricothyroid muscle

Cricothyroid ligament

Isthmus of thyroid gland

Trachea

Fig. 897: Anterior View of Larynx, Tongue and Thyroid Gland, Vessels and Nerves

NOTE: 1)   the **superior thyroid arteries** descending to the thyroid gland. In their course they give off the **superior laryngeal arteries** which penetrate the thyrohyoid membrane to enter the interior of the larynx. They are accompanied by the **internal laryngeal branch** of the **superior laryngeal nerve.**

   2)   the cranial and medial course of the **lingual artery** deep to the hyoglossus muscle and its suprahyoid (not labelled), sublingual and deep lingual branches.

   3)   the **lingual nerves** as they enter the tongue to supply its anterior ²/₃rds with general sensation. The motor nerve to the tongue is the **hypoglossal,** seen coursing along with its accompanying veins. It enters the base of the tongue just above the hyoid bone, passing anteriorly across the external carotid and lingual arteries.

   4)   the **common carotid artery** bifurcates at about the level of vese upper border of the thyroid cartilage. The lingual artery branches from the external carotid above the hyoid bone, while the superior laryngeal arises at the level of the thyrohyoid membrane.

Fig. 897

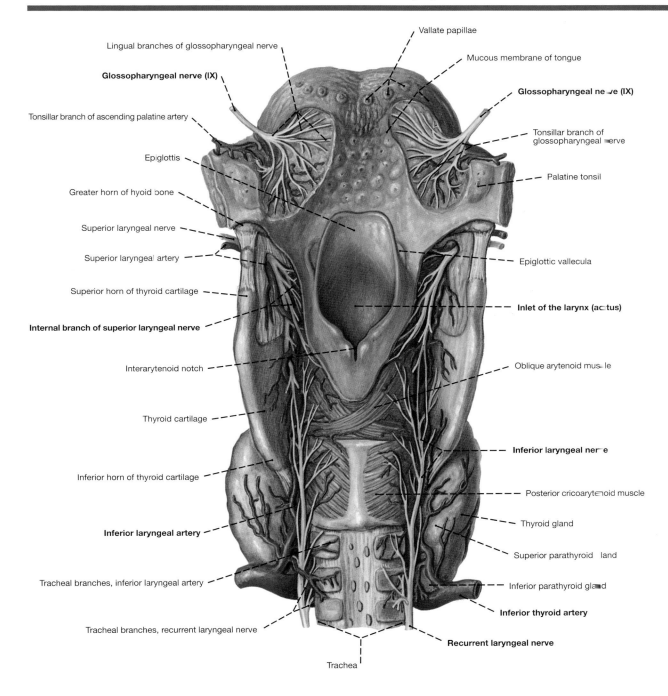

Vallate papillae

Lingual branches of glossopharyngeal nerve

Mucous membrane of tongue

Glossopharyngeal nerve (IX)

Glossopharyngeal nerve (IX)

Tonsillar branch of ascending palatine artery

Tonsillar branch of glossopharyngeal nerve

Epiglottis

Palatine tonsil

Greater horn of hyoid bone

Superior laryngeal nerve

Superior laryngeal artery

Epiglottic vallecula

Superior horn of thyroid cartilage

Inlet of the larynx (aditus)

Internal branch of superior laryngeal nerve

Interarytenoid notch

Oblique arytenoid muscle

Thyroid cartilage

Inferior laryngeal nerve

Inferior horn of thyroid cartilage

Posterior cricoarytenoid muscle

Thyroid gland

Inferior laryngeal artery

Superior parathyroid gland

Inferior parathyroid gland

Tracheal branches, inferior laryngeal artery

Inferior thyroid artery

Tracheal branches, recurrent laryngeal nerve

Recurrent laryngeal nerve

Trachea

Fig. 898: Posterior View of the Larynx, Tongue and Thyroid Gland, Vessels and Nerves

NOTE: 1)   the **glossopharyngeal nerves (IX)** as they enter the root or pharyngeal part of the tongue to supply the posterior 1/3rd of the surface of the tongue with both general sensation and the special sense of taste. Note also the **tonsillar branch** of the **ascending palatine artery** (from facial artery) supplying the palatine tonsil.

2)   the course of the **internal branch** of the **superior laryngeal nerve.** It is sensory to the laryngeal mucous membrane on the interior of the larynx as far down as the vocal folds.

3)   the **recurrent laryngeal nerve** which is the principal motor nerve to the larynx, and supplies all of the laryngeal muscles *except* the cricothyroid muscle (supplied by the external branch of the superior laryngeal nerve). Additionally, the recurrent laryngeal nerve supplies sensory innervation to the interior of the larynx below the vocal folds.

4)   the **important relationship** of the recurrent laryngeal nerves to the inferior thyroid artery and its inferior laryngeal branches. Observe also the proximity of the recurrent laryngeal nerves to the posterior aspect of the thyroid glands.

Fig. 898   **VII**

PLATE 558   Larynx: Cartilages and Membranes

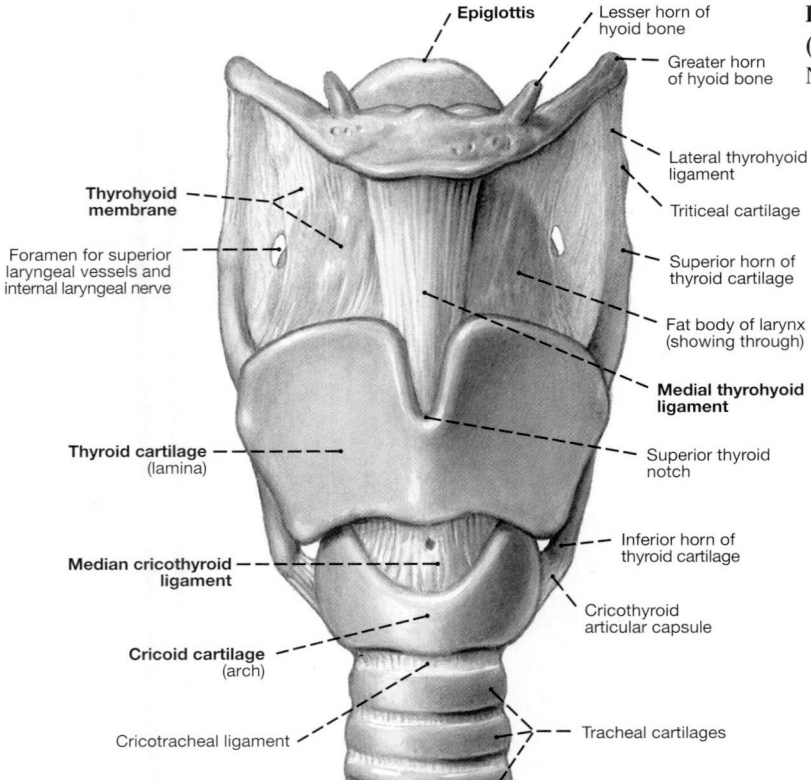

Epiglottis

Lesser horn of hyoid bone

Greater horn of hyoid bone

Lateral thyrohyoid ligament

Triticeal cartilage

Thyrohyoid membrane

Foramen for superior laryngeal vessels and internal laryngeal nerve

Superior horn of thyroid cartilage

Fat body of larynx (showing through)

Medial thyrohyoid ligament

Thyroid cartilage (lamina)

Superior thyroid notch

Inferior horn of thyroid cartilage

Median cricothyroid ligament

Cricothyroid articular capsule

Cricoid cartilage (arch)

Cricotracheal ligament

Tracheal cartilages

Fig. 899: Cartilages and Ligaments of the Larynx (Ventral View)

NOTE: 1) the laryngeal cartilages form the skeleton of the larynx and they are interconnected by ligaments and membranes. There are three larger **unpaired** cartilages **(cricoid, thyroid and epiglottis)** and three sets of **paired** cartilages **(arytenoid, corniculate and cuneiform).** In this anterior view, the unpaired cricoid, thyroid, and epiglottis are all visible.

2) the **thyrohyoid membrane** and the centrally located thyrohyoid ligament. Attached to the upper border of the thyroid cartilage, this membrane stretches across the posterior surfaces of the greater horns of the hyoid bone. The medial thyrohyoid ligament extends from the thyroid notch to the body of the hyoid bone. The membrane is pierced by the **superior laryngeal vessels** and the **internal laryngeal nerve.**

3) the **cricothyroid ligament** attaching the apposing margins of the cricoid and thyroid cartilages. This ligament underlies the cricothyroid muscles.

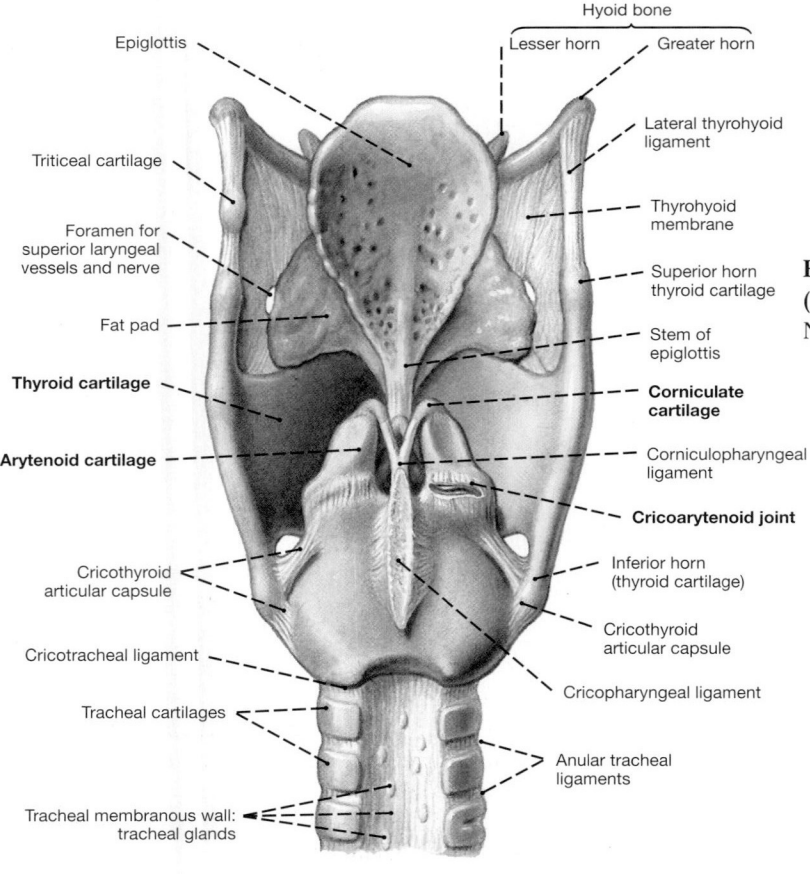

Epiglottis

Hyoid bone

Lesser horn   Greater horn

Lateral thyrohyoid ligament

Triticeal cartilage

Thyrohyoid membrane

Foramen for superior laryngeal vessels and nerve

Superior horn thyroid cartilage

Fat pad

Stem of epiglottis

Thyroid cartilage

Corniculate cartilage

Arytenoid cartilage

Corniculopharyngeal ligament

Cricoarytenoid joint

Cricothyroid articular capsule

Inferior horn (thyroid cartilage)

Cricothyroid articular capsule

Cricotracheal ligament

Cricopharyngeal ligament

Tracheal cartilages

Anular tracheal ligaments

Tracheal membranous wall: tracheal glands

Fig. 900: Cartilages and Ligaments of the Larynx (Dorsal View)

NOTE: 1) the articulation of the paired arytenoid cartilages with the cricoid cartilage below. These synovial cricoarytenoid joints are surrounded by articular capsules and strengthened by the posterior cricoarytenoid ligaments.

2) the cricoarytenoid joints allow for a) **rotation of the arytenoid cartilage** on an axis that is nearly vertical and b) **the horizontal gliding movement** of the arytenoid cartilages.

3) rotation of the arytenoid cartilages results in medial or lateral displacement of the vocal folds, thereby increasing or decreasing the size of the opening between the folds, the **rima glottis.**

4) horizontal gliding of the arytenoid cartilages permits the bases of these cartilages to be approximated or moved apart. Medial rotation and medial gliding of the arytenoid cartilages occur simultaneously as do the two lateral movements.

Figs. 899, 900

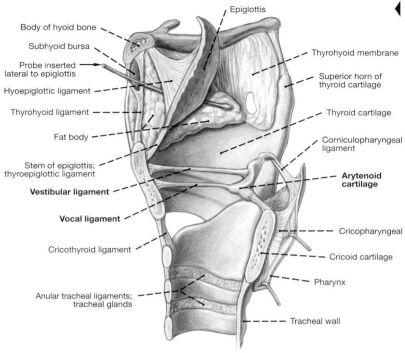

Body of hyoid bone
Subhyoid bursa
Probe inserted lateral to epiglottis
Hyoepiglottic ligament
Thyrohyoid ligament
Fat body
Stem of epiglottis; thyroepiglottic ligament
Vestibular ligament
Vocal ligament
Cricothyroid ligament
Anular tracheal ligaments; tracheal glands

Epiglottis
Thyrohyoid membrane
Superior horn of thyroid cartilage
Thyroid cartilage
Corniculopharyngeal ligament
Arytenoid cartilage
Cricopharyngeal
Cricoid cartilage
Pharynx
Tracheal wall

Fig. 901: Right Half of the Larynx Showing the Cartilages and Vestibular and Vocal Ligaments

NOTE: 1) the **vestibular ligament** is a compact band of fibrous tissue attached anteriorly to the thyroid cartilage and posteriorly to the anterior and lateral surface of the arytenoid cartilage. It is enclosed by mucous membrane to form the vestibular fold (or false vocal fold).

2) the **vocal ligament** consists of elastic tissue and is attached anteriorly to the thyroid cartilage and posteriorly to the vocal process of the arytenoid cartilage. It, too, is surrounded by mucous membrane which, along with the vocalis muscle forms the vocal fold. Laryngeal sounds are producted by oscillations of the vocal folds initiated by puffs of air.

Fig. 902: Vocal Ligaments and Conus Elasticus From Above

NOTE: 1) the **conus elasticus** is a membrane consisting principally of yellow elastic fibers and it interconnects the thyroid, cricoid and arytenoid cartilages. It underlies the mucous membrane below the vocal folds and is overlain to some extent by the cricothyroid muscle on the exterior of the larynx.

2) the symmetry of the arytenoid cartilages and their related vocal ligaments.

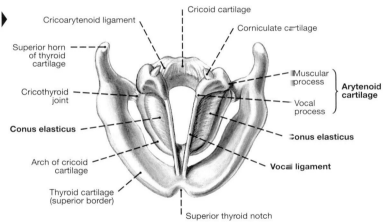

Cricoarytenoid ligament
Superior horn of thyroid cartilage
Cricothyroid joint
Conus elasticus
Arch of cricoid cartilage
Thyroid cartilage (superior border)

Cricoid cartilage
Corniculate cartilage
Muscular process
Vocal process
Arytenoid cartilage
Conus elasticus
Vocal ligament
Superior thyroid notch

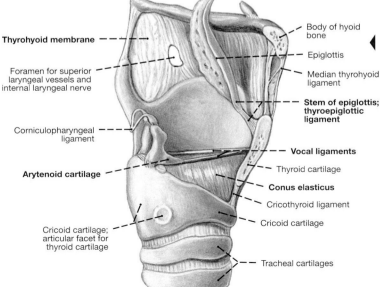

Thyrohyoid membrane
Foramen for superior laryngeal vessels and internal laryngeal nerve
Corniculopharyngeal ligament
Arytenoid cartilage
Cricoid cartilage; articular facet for thyroid cartilage

Body of hyoid bone
Epiglottis
Median thyrohyoid ligament
Stem of epiglottis; thyroepiglottic ligament
Vocal ligaments
Thyroid cartilage
Conus elasticus
Cricothyroid ligament
Cricoid cartilage
Tracheal cartilages

Fig. 903: Upper Left Part of the Larynx

NOTE: 1) the right halves of the hyoid bone, epiglottis and thyroid cartilage have been removed to open the upper left portion of the larynx. The two vocal ligaments, the arytenoid cartilages and the conus elasticus are also displayed.

2) the attachment of the stem of the epiglottis to the thyroid cartilage by means of the thyroepiglottic ligament.

3) the conus elasticus as it attaches to the vocal fold and the arytenoid, thyroid and cricoid cartilages.

4) although sounds are initiated at the vocal folds, the pitch, range, quality, volume tone and overtones of the human voice incorporate also structures in the mouth (tongue, teeth, and palate), the nasal sinuses, the pharynx, the rest of the larynx the lungs, diaphragm and abdominal muscles.

PLATE 560   Larynx: Muscles

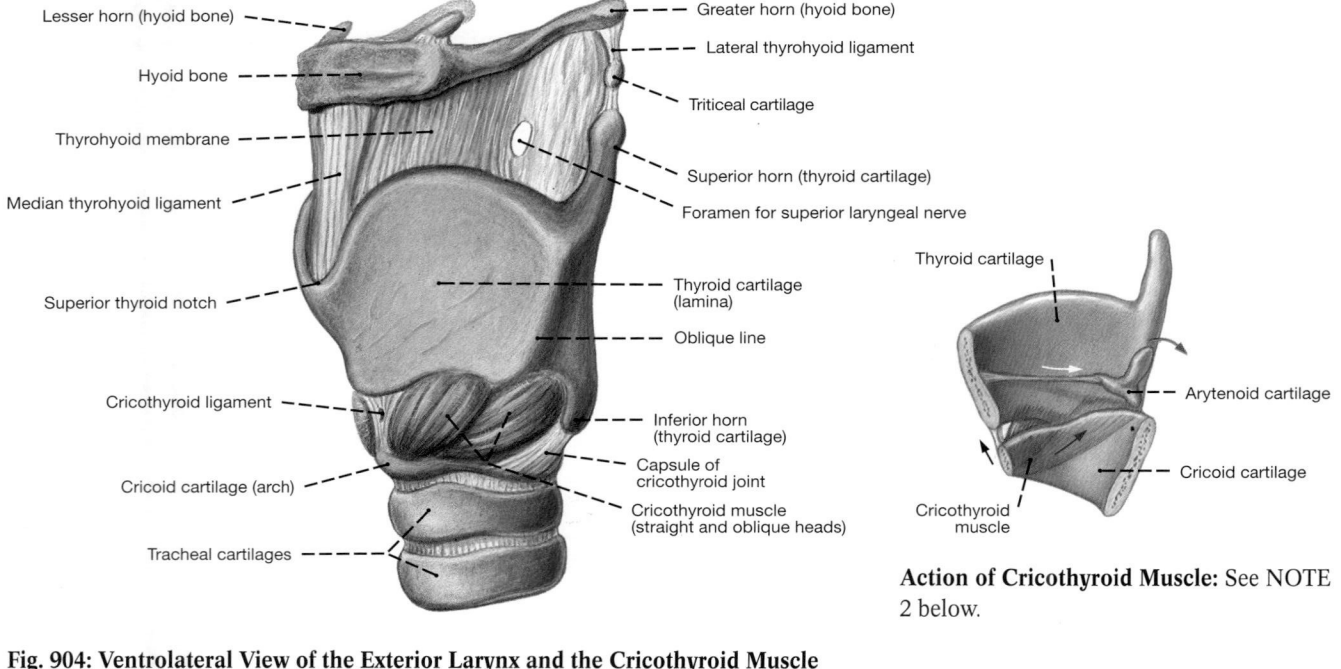

Fig. 904: Ventrolateral View of the Exterior Larynx and the Cricothyroid Muscle

NOTE: 1)   the **cricothyroid muscle** consists of *straight* and *oblique* heads. The straight head is more vertical and inserts onto the lower border of the lamina of the thyroid cartilage, while the oblique head is more horizontal and inserts onto the inferior horn of the thyroid cartilage.

2)   the cricothyroid muscle tilts the anterior part of the cricoid cartilage upward. In so doing, the arytenoid cartilages (which are attached to the cricoid) are pulled dorsally. In addition, the thyroid cartilage is pulled forward and downward. These actions increase the distance between the arytenoid and thyroid cartilages, thereby increasing the tension of and elongating the vocal folds (see insert diagram above).

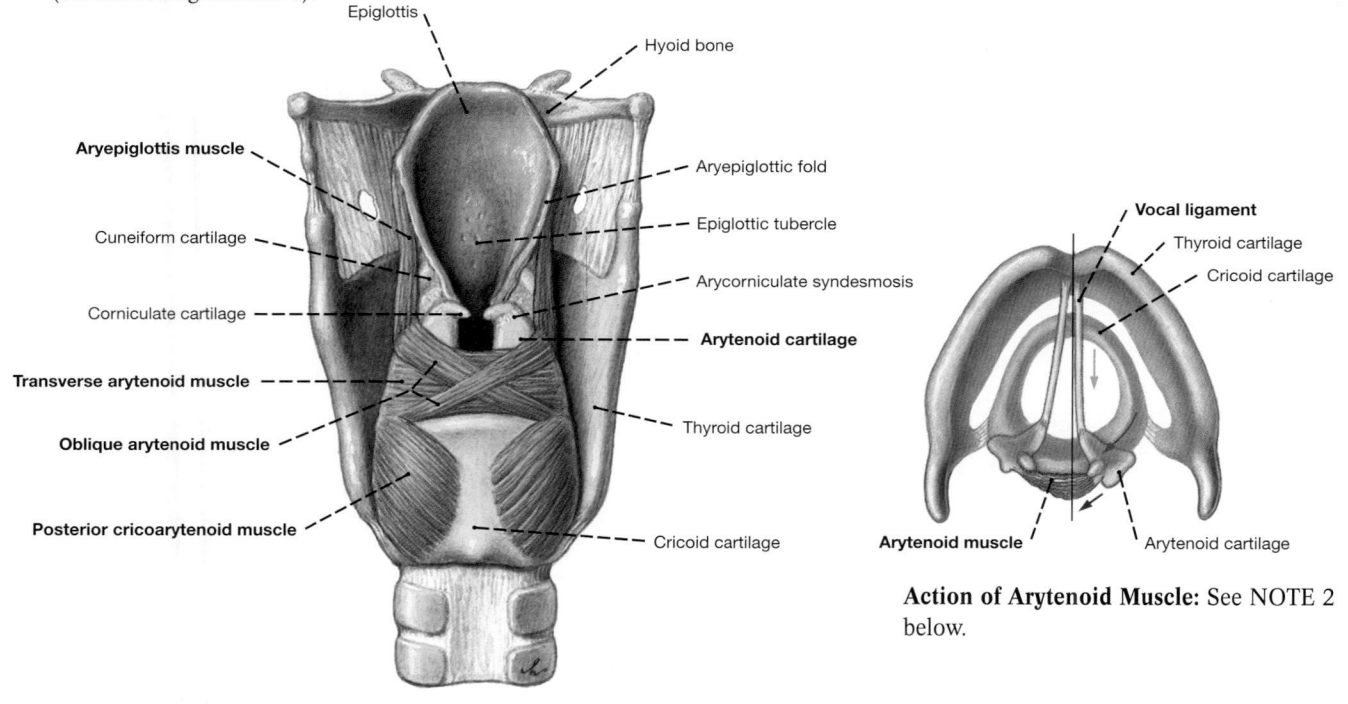

Fig. 905: Posterior View of the Larynx: Muscles

NOTE: 1)   the **arytenoid muscle** consists of a **transverse portion** that spans the zone between the arytenoid cartilages, and an **oblique portion** that consists of muscular fascicles that cross. Each of the fascicles of the oblique part extends from the base of the one arytenoid cartilage to the apex of the other cartilage. Some oblique fibers continue to the epiglottis as the **aryepiglottis muscle.**

2)   the transverse arytenoid approximates the arytenoid cartilages closing the posterior part of the rima glottis. The oblique arytenoid and the aryepiglottis muscles tend to close the inlet into the larynx by pulling the aryepiglottic folds together and approximating the arytenoid cartilages and epiglottis.

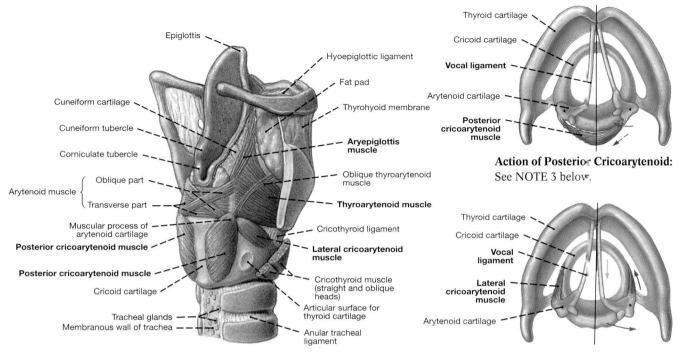

Fig. 906: Posterolateral View of the Laryngeal Muscles

Action of Posterior Cricoarytenoid: See NOTE 3 below.

Action of Lateral Cricoarytenoid: See NOTE 3 below

NOTE: 1) the right lamina of the thyroid cartilage and the thyrohyoid membrane have been partially cut away to expose the lateral cricoarytenoid and thyroarytenoid muscles.

2) the **posterior cricoarytenoid muscle** extends from the lamina of the cricoid cartilage to the muscular process of the arytenoid cartilage, while the **lateral cricoarytenoid muscle** arises laterally from the arch of the cricoid cartilage and inserts with the posterior cricoarytenoid muscle onto the arytenoid cartilage.

3) the posterior cricoarytenoids are the only **abductors** of the vocal folds, while the lateral cricoarytenoids act as antagonists and **adduct** the vocal folds. The posterior muscle abducts by pulling the base of the arytenoid cartilages medially and posteriorly, while the lateral muscle adducts by pulling these same cartilages anteriorly and laterally.

4) the **thyroarytenoid muscle** is a thin sheet of muscle radiating from the thyroid cartilage backward toward the arytenoid cartilage. Its upper fibers continue to the epiglottis and, joining the aryepiglottic fibers, become the **thyroepiglottic muscle.** Its deepest and most medial fibers form the **vocalis muscle** which is attached to the lateral aspect of the vocal fold. The thyroarytenoid muscles draw the arytenoid cartilages toward the thyroid cartilage and, thus shorten (relax) the vocal folds.

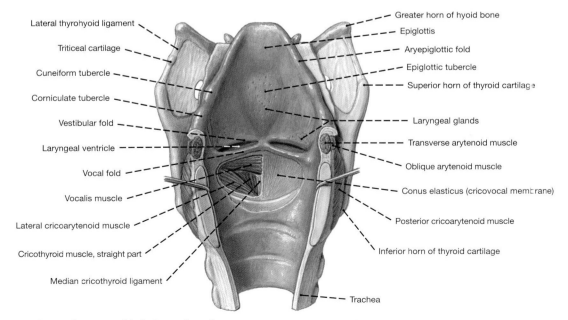

Fig. 907: Larynx Opened From Behind, Posterior View
NOTE: the lateral walls of the larynx have been opened widely and the left part of the conus elasticus has been removed.

PLATE 562   Larynx: Frontal and Midsagittal Sections

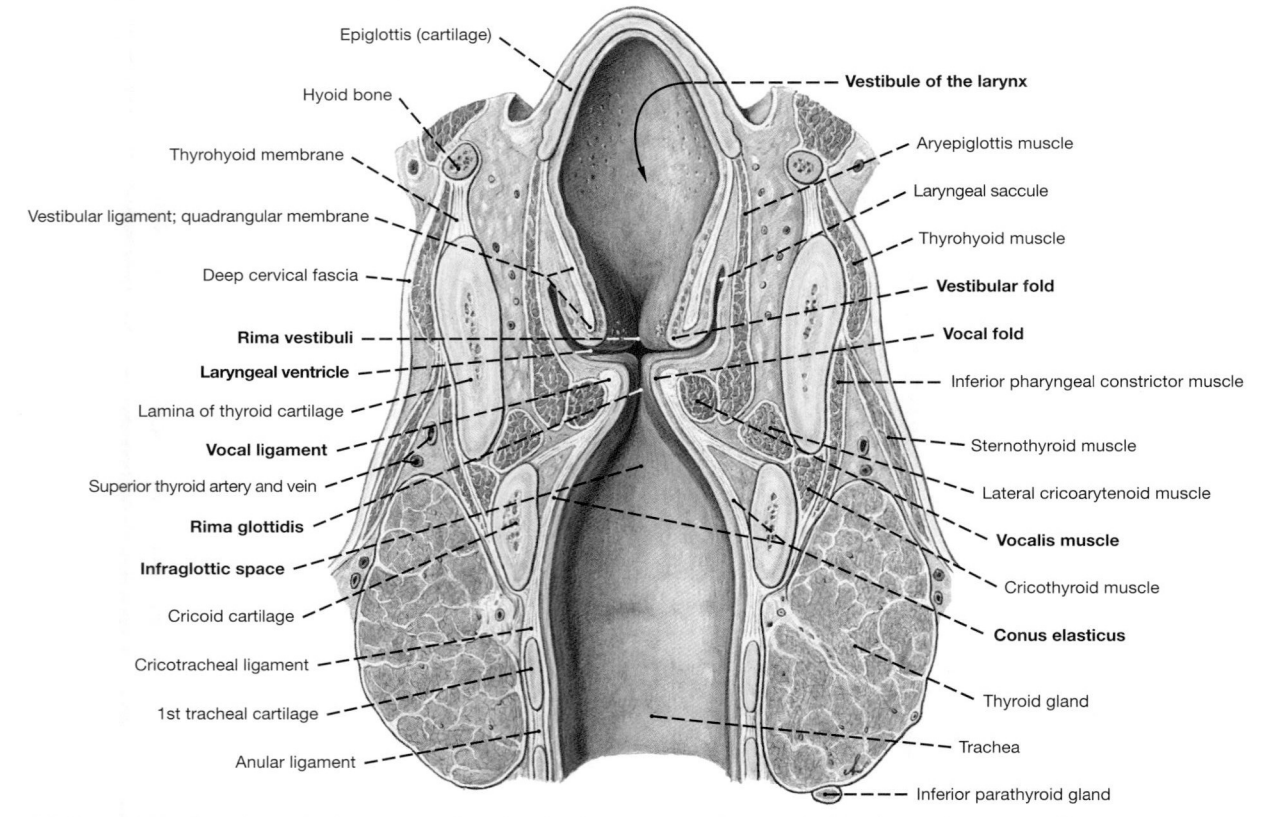

Epiglottis (cartilage)

Hyoid bone

Thyrohyoid membrane

Vestibular ligament; quadrangular membrane

Deep cervical fascia

Rima vestibuli

Laryngeal ventricle

Lamina of thyroid cartilage

Vocal ligament

Superior thyroid artery and vein

Rima glottidis

Infraglottic space

Cricoid cartilage

Cricotracheal ligament

1st tracheal cartilage

Anular ligament

Vestibule of the larynx

Aryepiglottis muscle

Laryngeal saccule

Thyrohyoid muscle

Vestibular fold

Vocal fold

Inferior pharyngeal constrictor muscle

Sternothyroid muscle

Lateral cricoarytenoid muscle

Vocalis muscle

Cricothyroid muscle

Conus elasticus

Thyroid gland

Trachea

Inferior parathyroid gland

Fig. 908: Frontal Section Through the Larynx Showing the Laryngeal Folds and Cavities in Its Anterior Half

NOTE: 1)   the paired **vocal folds** consist of mucous membrane overlying the **vocal ligaments** and **vocalis muscles.** Just superior to the vocal folds observe the **vestibular folds,** which are separated from the vocal folds by a recess called the **laryngeal ventricle** (or sinus).

2)   above the vestibular folds is the **vestibule** of the larynx which lies just below the laryngeal inlet. Below the vocal folds is the **infraglottic space** which communicates with the trachea below and is limited above by the **rima glottis** between the two vocal folds.

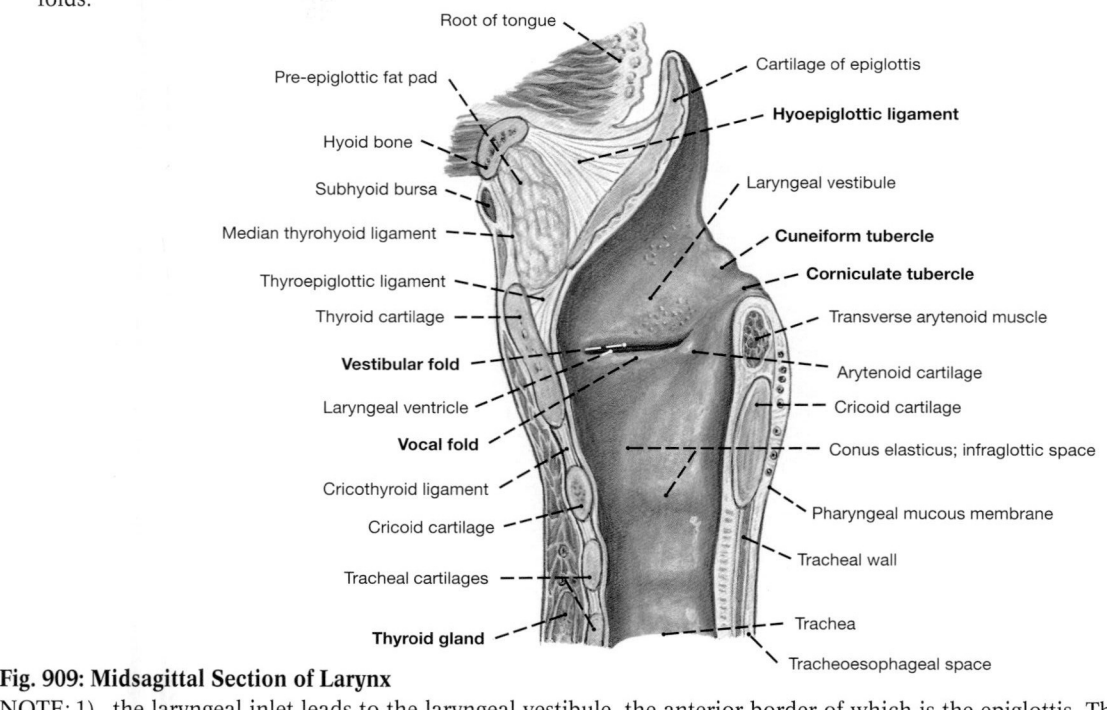

Root of tongue

Pre-epiglottic fat pad

Hyoid bone

Subhyoid bursa

Median thyrohyoid ligament

Thyroepiglottic ligament

Thyroid cartilage

Vestibular fold

Laryngeal ventricle

Vocal fold

Cricothyroid ligament

Cricoid cartilage

Tracheal cartilages

Thyroid gland

Cartilage of epiglottis

Hyoepiglottic ligament

Laryngeal vestibule

Cuneiform tubercle

Corniculate tubercle

Transverse arytenoid muscle

Arytenoid cartilage

Cricoid cartilage

Conus elasticus; infraglottic space

Pharyngeal mucous membrane

Tracheal wall

Trachea

Tracheoesophageal space

Fig. 909: Midsagittal Section of Larynx

NOTE: 1)   the laryngeal inlet leads to the laryngeal vestibule, the anterior border of which is the epiglottis. The **aryepiglottic folds,** marked by oval elevations (cuneiform and corniculate cartilages), define the borders of the laryngeal inlet.

2)   the epiglottis attaches **superiorly** to the hyoid bone (by the hyoepiglottic ligament); **inferiorly** to the thyroid cartilage (by the thyroepiglottic ligament); and **laterally** to the arytenoid cartilages (by the aryepiglottic folds).

Fig. 910: Cross-section of Larynx at the Vocal Folds ▶

NOTE: 1)   the orientation of the arytenoid cartilages and their articulations with the cricoid cartilage.

2) the vocal folds consist of mucous membrane over the vocal ligaments, lateral to which extend the deeper part of the thyroarytenoid muscle.

3) by drawing the arytenoid cartilages forward, the thyroarytenoids shorten and relax the vocal folds. At the same time, they medially rotate the arytenoid cartilages and, thus, approximate the vocal folds.

I = intermembranous part of the rima glottis
II = intercartilaginous part of the rima glottis

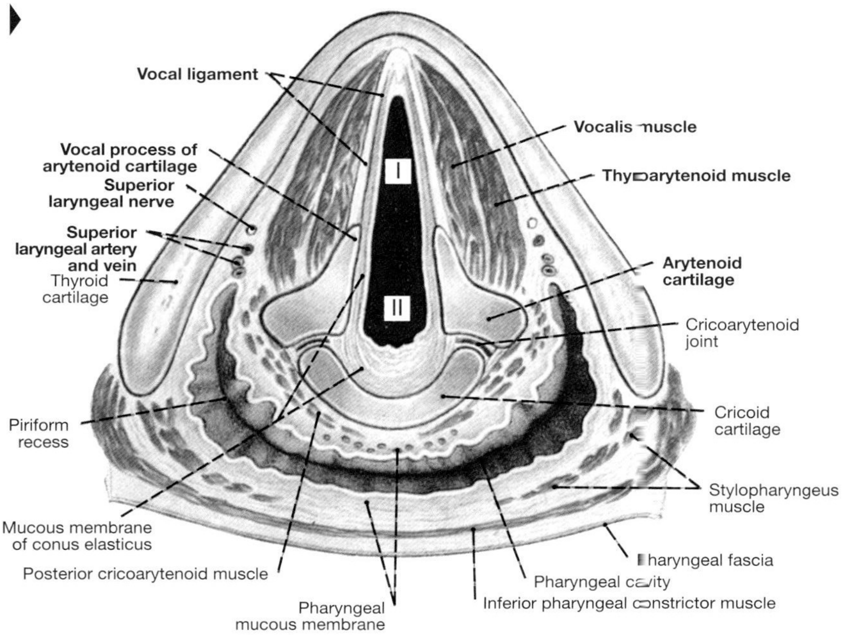

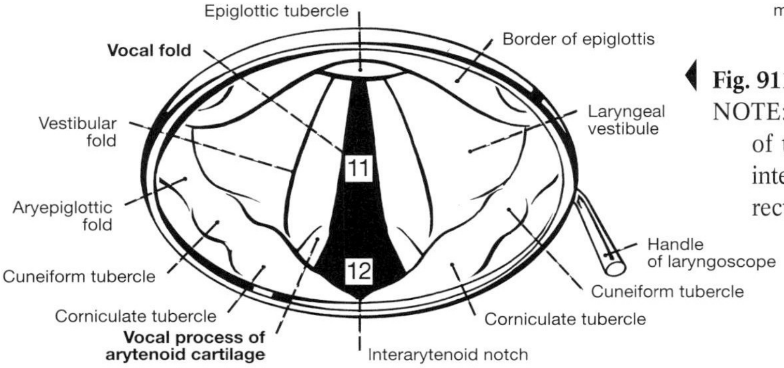

Fig. 911: Rima Glottidis During Normal Respiration

NOTE: during quiet respiration, the intermembranous portion of the rima glottidis (11) is triangular in shape while the intercartilaginous portion of the rima glottidis (12) is somewhat rectangular in shape.

Fig. 912: Rima Glottidis During Forced or Deep Inspiration ▶

NOTE: during forced inspiration, both the membranous and intercartilaginous parts of the rima glottidis present triangular shapes and the entire rima glottidis is rhomboid in shape. The muscular processes of the arytenoid cartilages are fully abducted, while the vocal processes are laterally rotated and retracted (principally by the posterior cricoarytenoids).

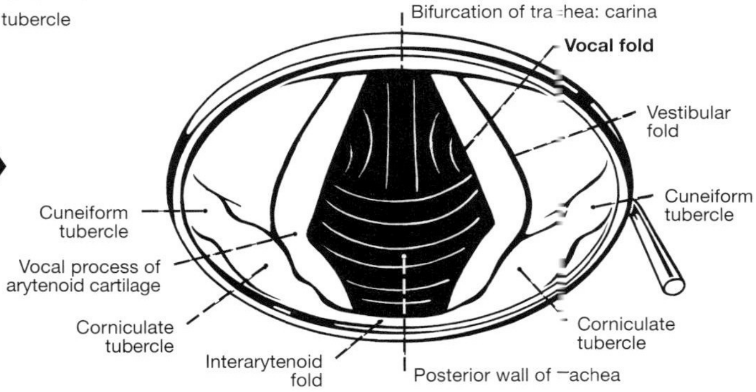

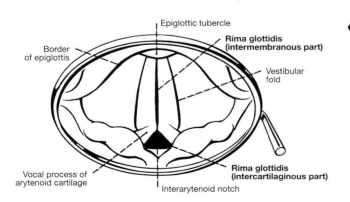

Fig. 913: Rima Glottidis During Whispering ◀

NOTE: in whispering, the intermembranous parts of the vocal folds are approximated, while the intercartilaginous parts are separated. The anterior part of the rima glottidis is slit-like and the posterior, intercartilaginous part remains open.

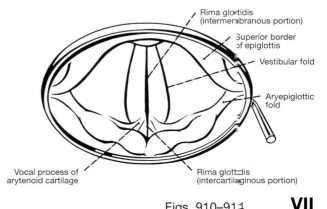

Fig. 914: Rima Glottidis During Phonation (Shrill Tones) ▶

NOTE: during the emission of shrill tones, the vocal folds are approximated and the vocal ligaments tensed. This results in a narrowing of the rima glottidis to a thin slit.

PLATE 564   **External Ear: Surface Anatomy, Cartilage and Muscles**

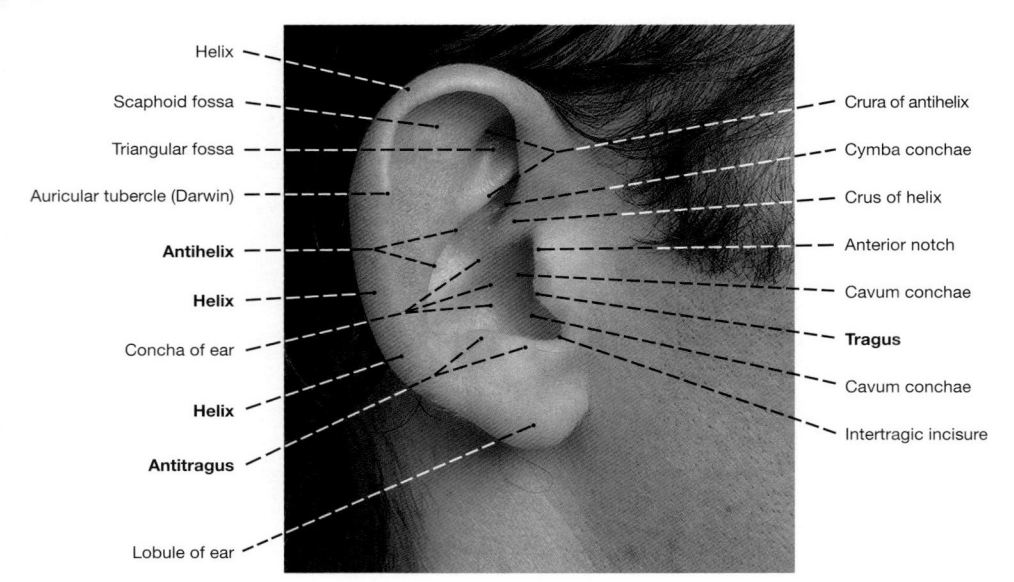

Helix
Scaphoid fossa
Triangular fossa
Auricular tubercle (Darwin)
Antihelix
Helix
Concha of ear
Helix
Antitragus
Lobule of ear

Crura of antihelix
Cymba conchae
Crus of helix
Anterior notch
Cavum conchae
Tragus
Cavum conchae
Intertragic incisure

Fig. 915: Right External Ear (Lateral View)

NOTE: 1)   the external ear (or auricle) consists of skin overlying an irregularly shaped elastic fibrocartilage. The ear lobe or lobule does not contain cartilage, but is soft and contains connective tissue and fat.

2)   the **external acoustic meatus** courses through the auricle to the tympanic membrane. It is an oval canal that extends for about 2.5 cm in an **S**-shaped curve to the tympanic membrane. It consists of an outer cartilaginous part (1 cm) and a narrower more medial part that is osseous (1.5 cm).

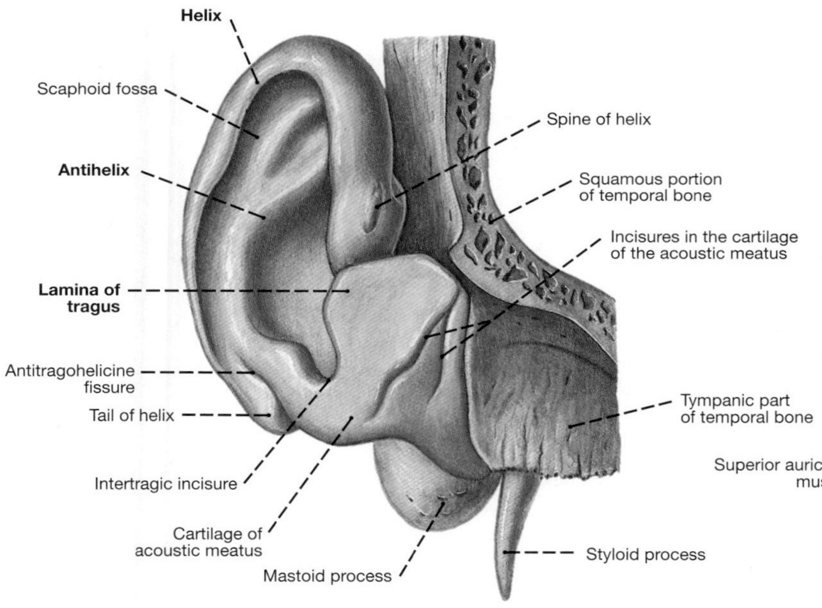

Helix
Scaphoid fossa
Antihelix
Lamina of tragus
Antitragohelicine fissure
Tail of helix
Intertragic incisure
Cartilage of acoustic meatus
Mastoid process

Spine of helix
Squamous portion of temporal bone
Incisures in the cartilage of the acoustic meatus
Tympanic part of temporal bone
Styloid process

Fig. 916: Cartilage of the Right External Ear (Seen From Front)

NOTE: 1)   with the skin of the external ear removed, the contours of the single cartilage conform generally with those of the intact auricle. The cartilage is seen to be absent inferiorly at the site of the ear lobe.

2)   The external rim of the auricle is called the **helix.** Another curved prominence anterior to the helix is the **antihelix.** A notch inferiorly (intertragic incisure) separates the **tragus** anteriorly from the **antitragus** posteriorly.

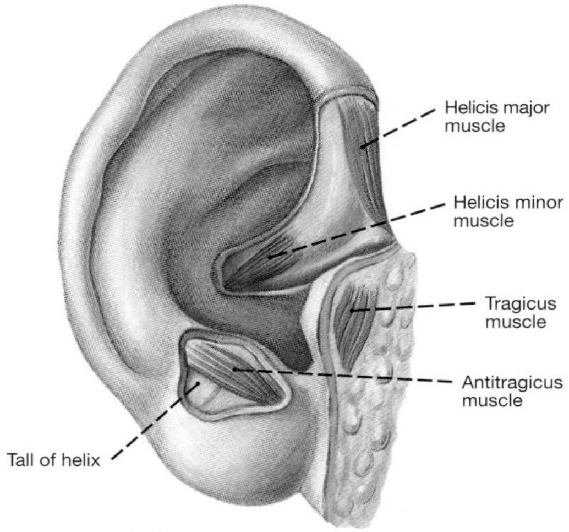

Helicis major muscle
Helicis minor muscle
Tragicus muscle
Antitragicus muscle
Tail of helix

Fig. 917: Intrinsic Muscles of External Ear (Lateral Surface)

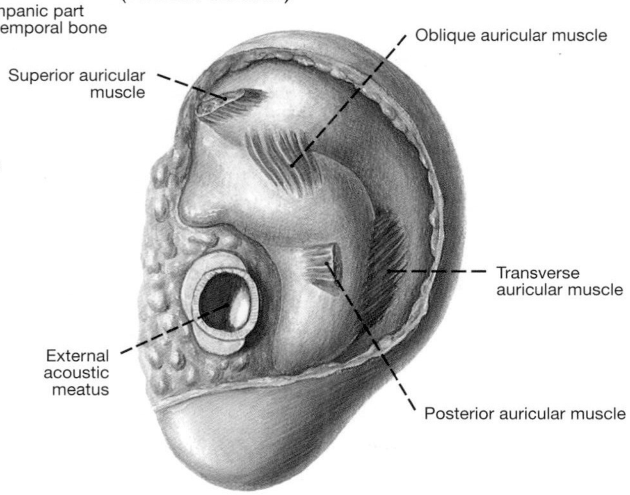

Superior auricular muscle
Oblique auricular muscle
Transverse auricular muscle
External acoustic meatus
Posterior auricular muscle

Fig. 918: Muscles Attaching to the Medial Surface of External Ear

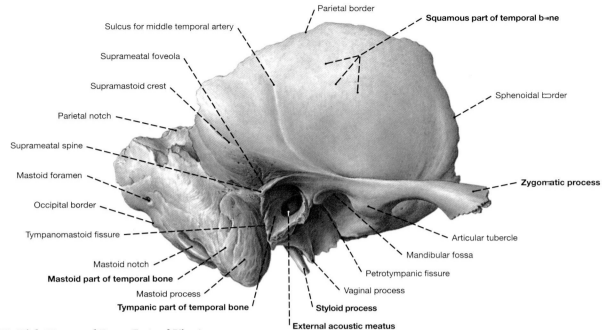

Parietal border

Squamous part of temporal bone

Sulcus for middle temporal artery

Suprameatal foveola

Supramastoid crest

Parietal notch

Sphenoidal border

Suprameatal spine

Mastoid foramen

Occipital border

Zygomatic process

Tympanomastoid fissure

Mastoid notch

Articular tubercle

Mandibular fossa

Mastoid part of temporal bone

Petrotympanic fissure

Mastoid process

Vaginal process

Tympanic part of temporal bone

Styloid process

External acoustic meatus

Fig. 919: Right Temporal Bone (Lateral View)

NOTE: 1)   the temporal bone which forms the osseous encasement for the middle and internal ear consists of three parts: **squamous, tympanic,** and **petrous.**

2)   the **squamous part** is broad in shape and it is thin and flat. From it extends the zygomatic process. The **tympanic part** is interposed below the squamous and anterior to the petrous parts. The external acoustic meatus, which leads to the tympanic membrane, is surrounded by the tympanic part of the temporal bone.

3)   the hard **petrous part** contains the organ of hearing and the vestibular canals. Its mastoid process is not solid but contains many air cells, and its external surface affords attachment to several muscles.

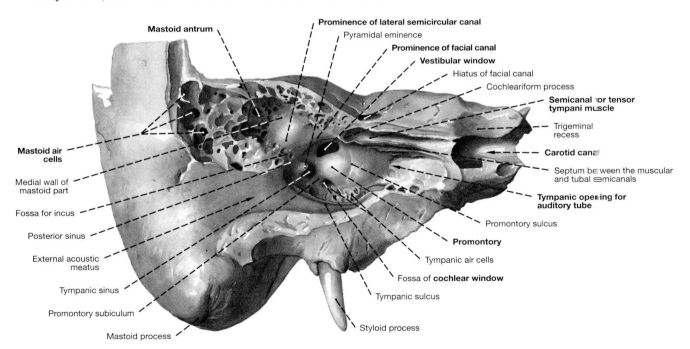

Mastoid antrum

Prominence of lateral semicircular canal

Pyramidal eminence

Prominence of facial canal

Vestibular window

Hiatus of facial canal

Cochleariform process

Semicanal for tensor tympani muscle

Trigeminal recess

Carotid canal

Mastoid air cells

Septum between the muscular and tubal semicanals

Medial wall of mastoid part

Tympanic opening for auditory tube

Fossa for incus

Promontory sulcus

Posterior sinus

Promontory

External acoustic meatus

Tympanic air cells

Fossa of **cochlear window**

Tympanic sinus

Tympanic sulcus

Promontory subiculum

Styloid process

Mastoid process

Fig. 920: Lateral Dissection of the Right Temporal Bone Showing the Tympanic Cavity

NOTE: 1)   the tympanic cavity (middle ear) communicates posteriorly with the mastoid antrum and, in turn, with the mastoid air cells. It also is in communication with the nasopharynx by way of the auditory tube.

2)   the **lateral wall** of the tympanic cavity is formed by the tympanic membrane (not shown), while the **medial wall** (or labyrinthine wall) presents the following important structures: the **promontory** (projection of the 1st turn of the cochlea); the **vestibular window** (oval window); the **cochlear window** (round window); the bony prominence of the **facial canal;** and posteriorly, the prominence of the **lateral semicircular canal.**

PLATE 566   **Ear: External and Middle Ear, Fronal Sections**

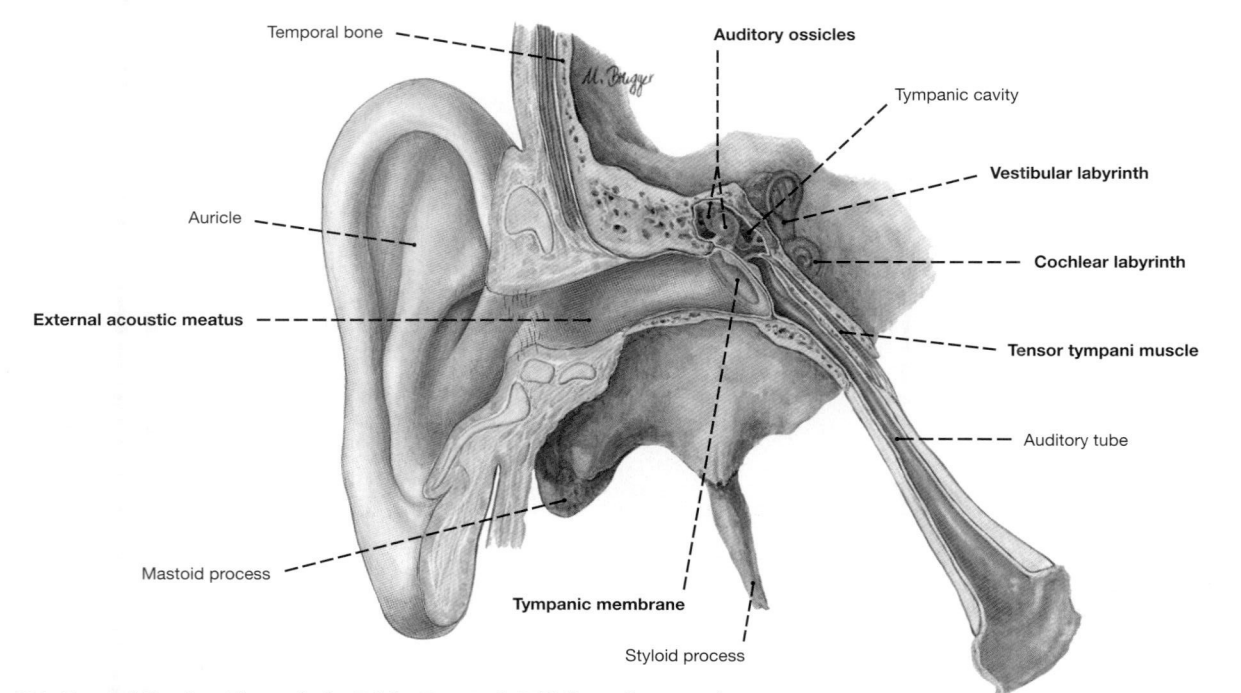

Fig. 921: Frontal Section Through the Right External, Middle and Internal Ear

NOTE: 1) the external acoustic meatus commences at the auricle and leads to the external surface of the tympanic membrane. Through the meatus course the sound waves which cause vibration of the tympanum.

   2) the *middle ear* (or tympanic cavity) contains three ossicles (malleus, incus and stapes) and two muscles (tensor tympani and stapedius, the latter is not shown).

   3) the cavity of the middle ear communicates with the *mastoid antrum* and *mastoid air cells* posteriorly, and the nasopharynx by way of the *auditory tube.* This tube courses downward, forward and medially from the middle ear.

   4) the ossicles interconnect the tympanic membrane with the inner ear. The inner ear contains the coiled *cochlea* (or organ of hearing) and the three *semicircular canals* (the vestibular organ) and their associated vessels and nerves.

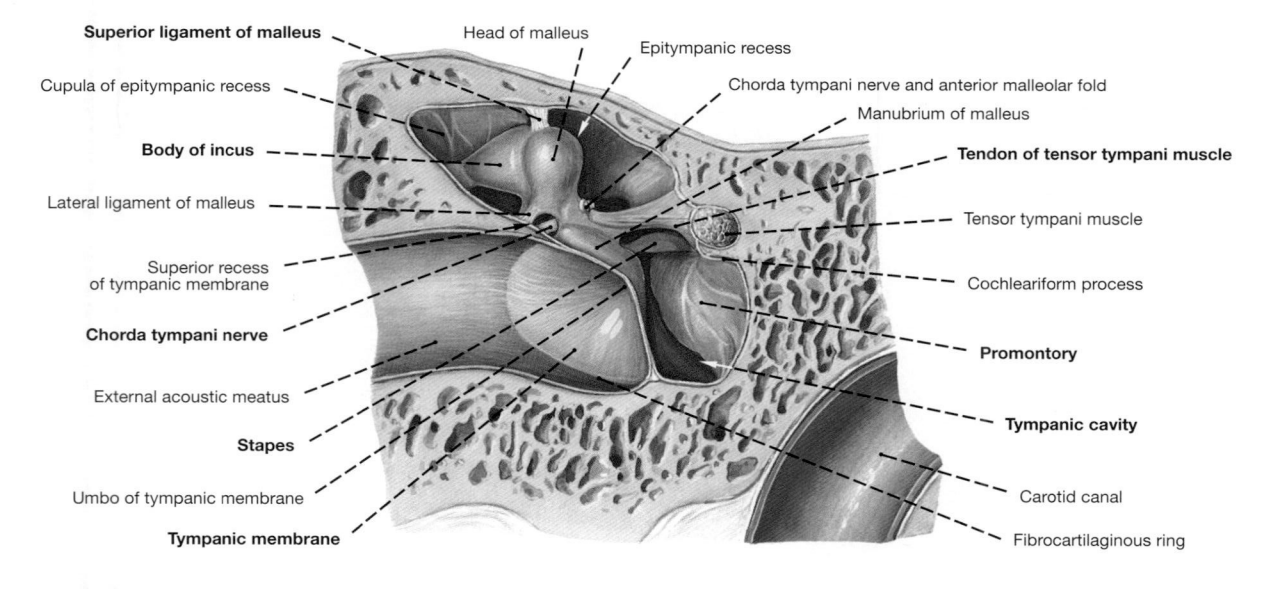

Fig. 922: Frontal Section Through the Right External and Middle Ear

NOTE: 1) the slender tendon of the *tensor tympani muscle* as it turns sharply upon reaching the tympanic cavity to terminate on the manubrium of the malleus.

   2) the tympanic cavity is extended superiorly by the epitympanic recess located above the level of the tympanic membrane. On the medial wall of the middle ear observe the promontory which protrudes into the tympanic cavity. This bony prominence is formed by the spiral cochlea of the internal ear.

   3) the lateral and superior ligaments attaching to the head of the malleus. The anterior ligament of the malleus which interconnects the neck of the malleus to the anterior wall of the tympanic cavity is not shown.

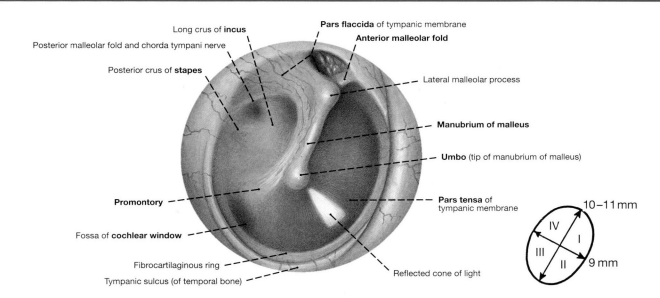

Fig. 923: Right Tympanic Membrane as Seen with an Otoscope in a Living Person

NOTE: 1)   the tympanic membrane is oval and measures about 9 mm across and from 10 to 11 mm vertically; it often is described as consisting of four quadrants (see lower inset diagram).

     2)   the **anterior** and **posterior malleolar folds.** The more lax part (pars flaccida) of the tympanic membrane lies above and between these folds, while the rest is more tightly stretched (pars tensa).

     3)   the blood supply of the membrane is derived from the **deep auricular** and **anterior tympanic branches** of the maxillary artery and the **stylomastoid branch** of the posterior auricular artery.

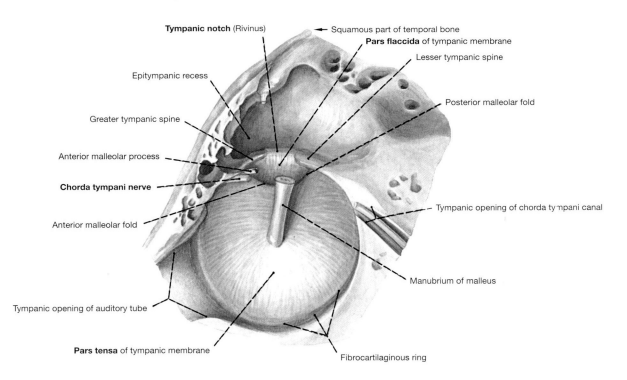

Fig. 924: Lateral Wall of the Right Middle Ear (Tympanic Membrane Viewed from within the Tympanic Cavity)

NOTE: 1)   the **manubrium** of the **malleus** has been severed from the remainder of the ossicle and left attached to the tympanic membrane. The fibrocartilaginous tympanic ring is deficient superiorly, forming the **tympanic notch** (of Rivinus). The looser portion of the tympanic membrane **(pars flaccida)** covers this zone.

     2)   the tympanic membrane below the malleolar folds is the **pars tensa.** This portion is made taut by the **tensor tympani muscle** which attaches to the manubrium of the malleus.

     3)   the external surface of the tympanic membrane is innervated by the **auriculotemporal branch** of the mandibular nerve (V) and the **auricular branch** of the vagus nerve (X). The internal surface of the membrane is supplied by the **tympanic branch** of the glossopharyngeal nerve (IX).

PLATE 568   Ear: Lateral Wall of Tympanic Cavity; Middle Ear Ossicles

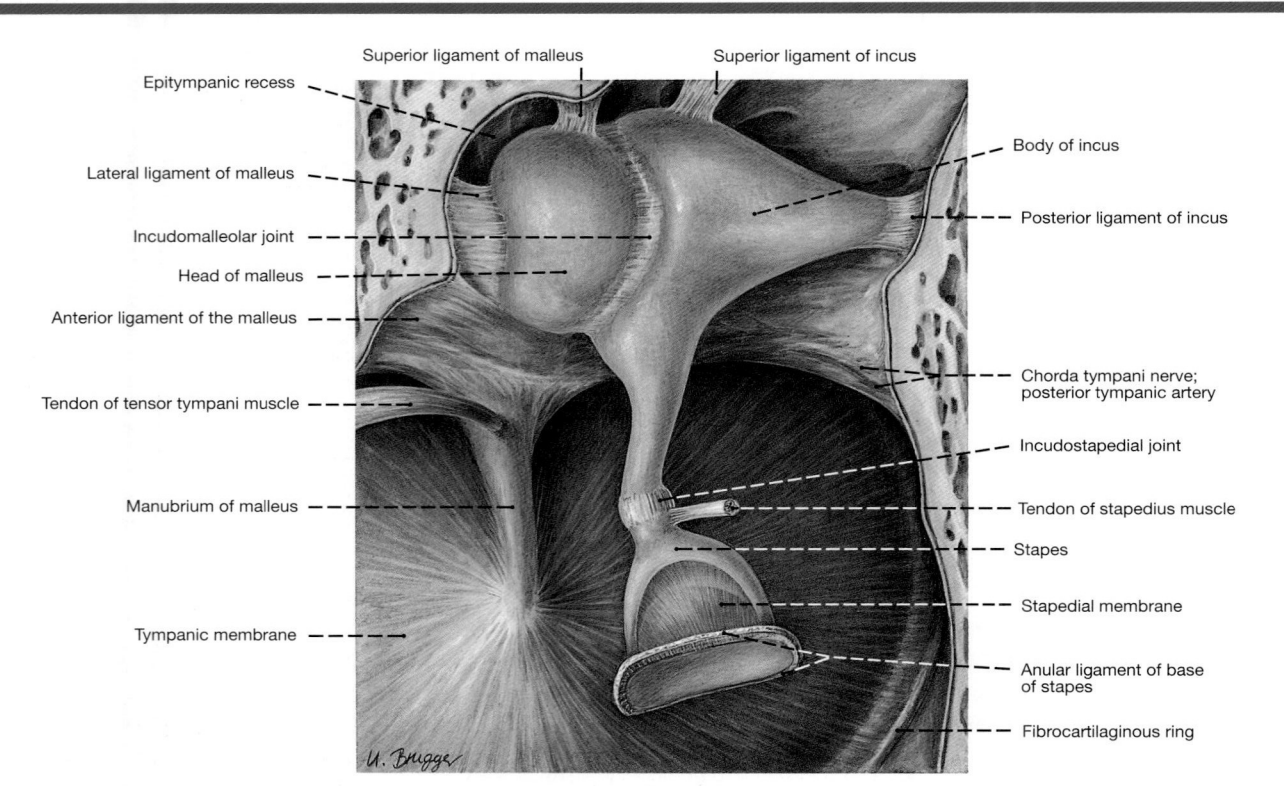

Superior ligament of malleus

Superior ligament of incus

Epitympanic recess

Lateral ligament of malleus

Incudomalleolar joint

Head of malleus

Anterior ligament of the malleus

Tendon of tensor tympani muscle

Manubrium of malleus

Tympanic membrane

Body of incus

Posterior ligament of incus

Chorda tympani nerve; posterior tympanic artery

Incudostapedial joint

Tendon of stapedius muscle

Stapes

Stapedial membrane

Anular ligament of base of stapes

Fibrocartilaginous ring

U. Brugge

Fig. 925: Middle Ear Ossicles and Attachment of Muscle Tendons, Right Side

NOTE: 1) the tendon of the **tensor tympani muscle** inserts on the manubrium of the malleus and the short tendon of the **stapedius muscle** inserts onto the neck of the stapes close to its articulation with the incus.

2) the tensor tympani draws the manubrium medially, thereby making the tympanic membrane taut. At the same time its action pushes the base of the stapes more securely into the vestibular window. The tensor is innervated by the mandibular division of the **trigeminal nerve.**

3) the stapedius opposes the action of the tensor at the vestibular window, tilting the head of the stapes away from the window. Its denervation results in hyperacusis, a condition in which sounds are perceived as unduly loud. The stapedius is supplied by the **facial nerve.**

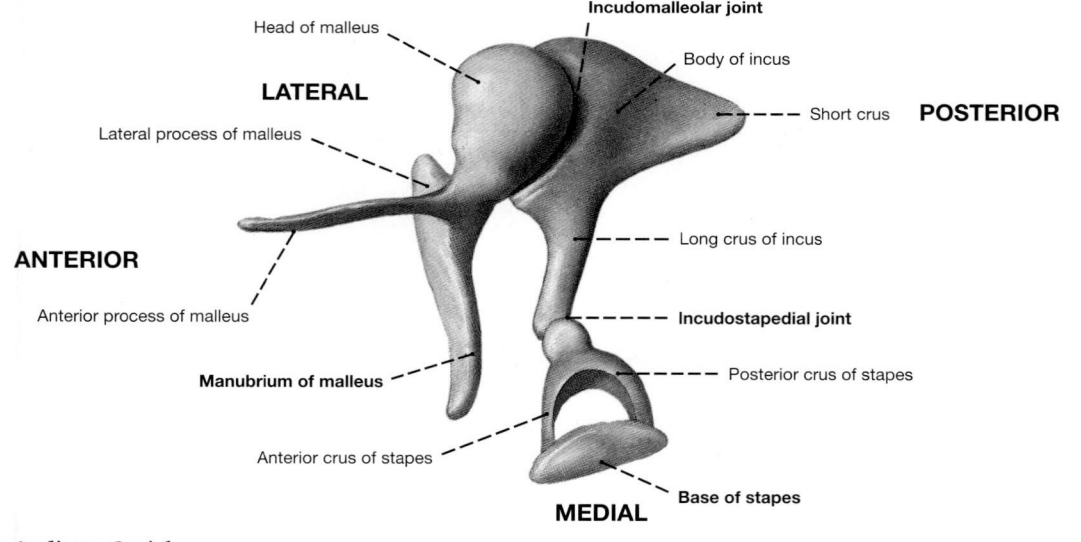

Incudomalleolar joint

Head of malleus

Body of incus

LATERAL

Short crus   **POSTERIOR**

Lateral process of malleus

Long crus of incus

ANTERIOR

Incudostapedial joint

Anterior process of malleus

Posterior crus of stapes

Manubrium of malleus

Anterior crus of stapes

Base of stapes

MEDIAL

Fig. 926: Right Auditory Ossicles

NOTE: 1) when sound waves are received at the tympanic membrane, they cause a **medial** displacement of the manubrium of the malleus. The head of the malleus is then tilted **laterally,** pulling with it the body of the incus. At the same time the long process of incus is displaced **medially,** as is the articulation between the incus and stapes.

2) the base of the stapes rocks as if it were on a fulcrum at the vestibular window, thereby establishing waves in the perilymph. These waves stimulate the auditory receptors and become dissipated at the secondary tympanic membrane covering the cochlear window.

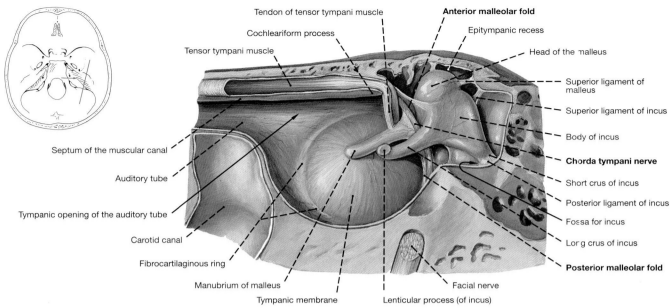

Tendon of tensor tympani muscle
Cochleariform process
Tensor tympani muscle
Anterior malleolar fold
Epitympanic recess
Head of the malleus
Superior ligament of malleus
Superior ligament of incus
Body of incus
Chorda tympani nerve
Short crus of incus
Posterior ligament of incus
Fossa for incus
Long crus of incus
Posterior malleolar fold

Septum of the muscular canal
Auditory tube
Tympanic opening of the auditory tube
Carotid canal
Fibrocartilaginous ring
Manubrium of malleus
Tympanic membrane
Facial nerve
Lenticular process (of incus)

Fig. 927: Lateral Wall of the Right Tympanic Cavity (Viewed From the Medial Aspect)

NOTE: 1) the tympanic cavity is completely lined with a mucous membrane that attaches onto the surface of all the structures of the middle ear. This tympanic mucosa is continuous with that lining the mastoid air cells posteriorly and the auditory tube anteriorly.

2) reflections of the tympanic mucous membrane form the **anterior** and **posterior malleolar folds.** These are also reflected around the **chorda tympani nerve** as it curves along the medial side of the manubrium of the malleus.

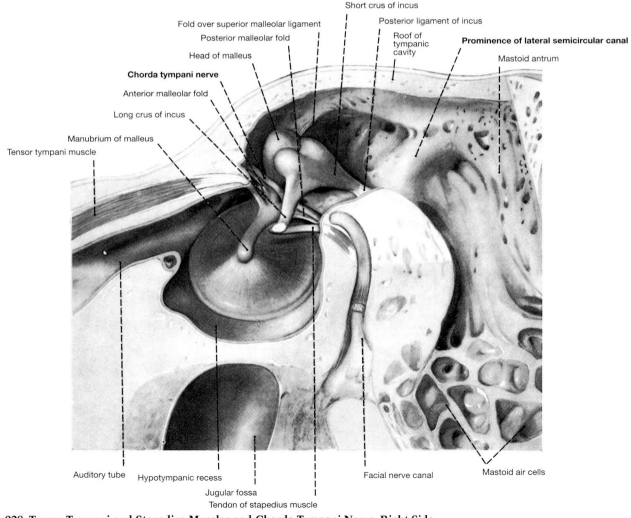

Short crus of incus
Fold over superior malleolar ligament
Posterior malleolar fold
Posterior ligament of incus
Roof of tympanic cavity
Prominence of lateral semicircular canal
Mastoid antrum
Head of malleus
Chorda tympani nerve
Anterior malleolar fold
Long crus of incus
Manubrium of malleus
Tensor tympani muscle

Auditory tube   Hypotympanic recess
Jugular fossa
Tendon of stapedius muscle
Facial nerve canal
Mastoid air cells

Fig. 928: Tensor Tympani and Stapedius Muscles and Chorda Tympani Nerve, Right Side

PLATE 570   Ear: Medial Wall of the Tympanic Cavity

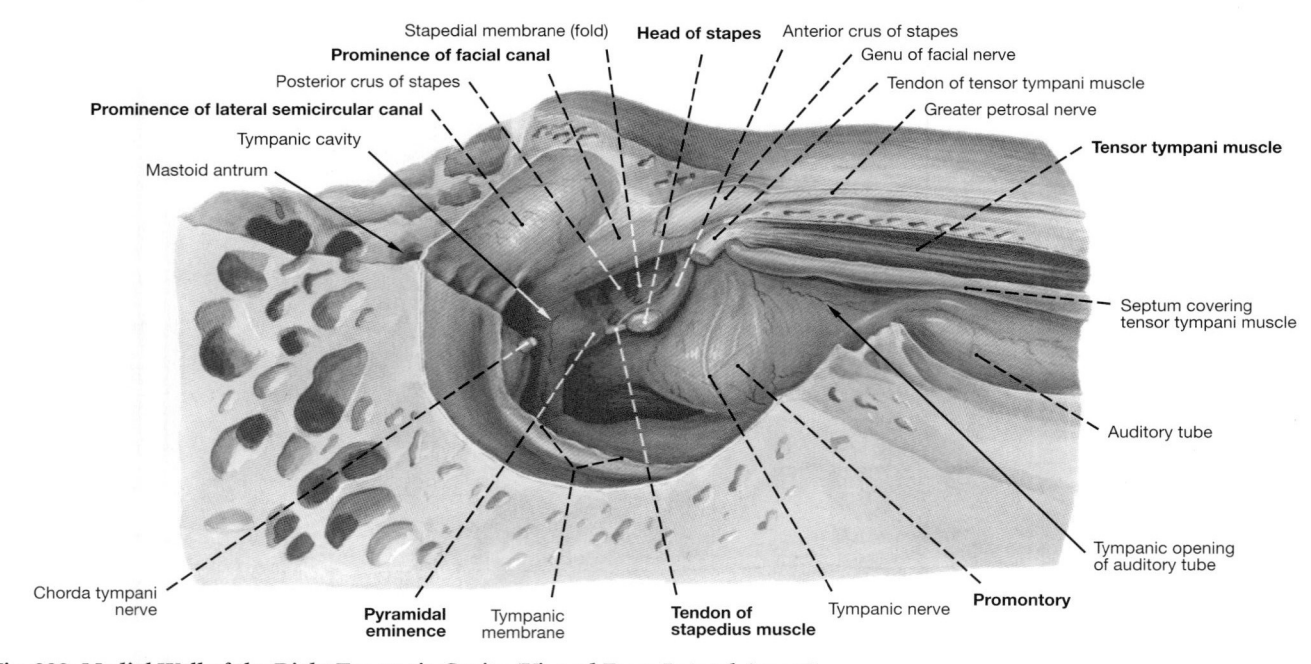

Fig. 929: Medial Wall of the Right Tympanic Cavity (Viewed From Lateral Aspect)

NOTE: 1)   the tympanic membrane has been removed along with the bony roof of the tympanic cavity. The malleus and incus have also been removed and the tendon of the tensor tympani severed. Observe the **stapes** with its base directed toward the vestibular window and the **stapedius muscle** still attached to its neck.

2)   several bony markings: a) the prominence containing the **lateral semicircular canal,** b) the curved prominence of the **facial canal** with its facial nerve, c) the **promontory,** which is a rounded thin bony covering over the **cochlea,** and d) the hollow **pyramidal eminence** from which arises the **stapedius muscle.**

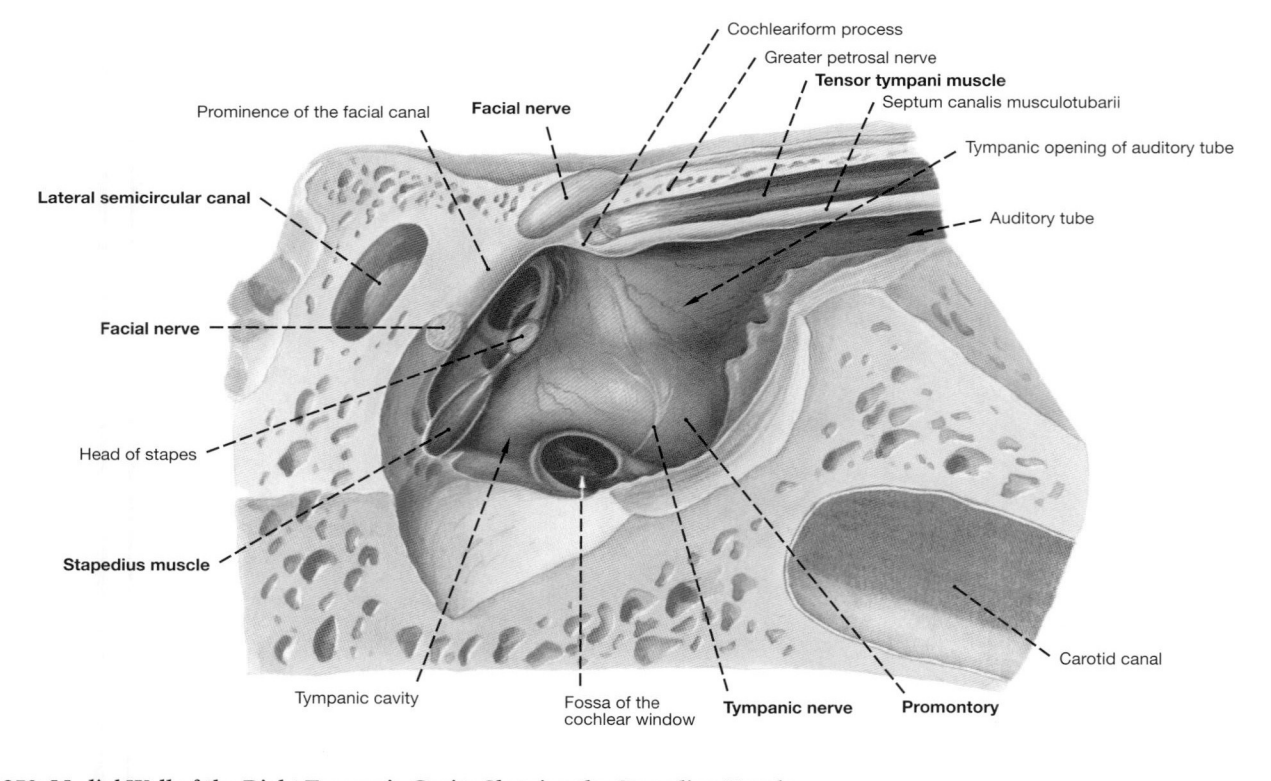

Fig. 930: Medial Wall of the Right Tympanic Cavity Showing the Stapedius Muscle

NOTE: 1)   the stapedius muscle emerges through the apex of the pyramidal eminence and it is about 4 mm in length. It pulls the base of the stapes laterally and protects the inner ear from damage caused by loud sounds.

2)   the **tympanic branch** of the **glossopharyngeal nerve** (IX) coursing along the promontory. This nerve is sensory to the mucous membrane of the middle ear, and is also known as the nerve of Jacobson. Its fibers are joined by sympathetic fibers to form the **tympanic plexus.**

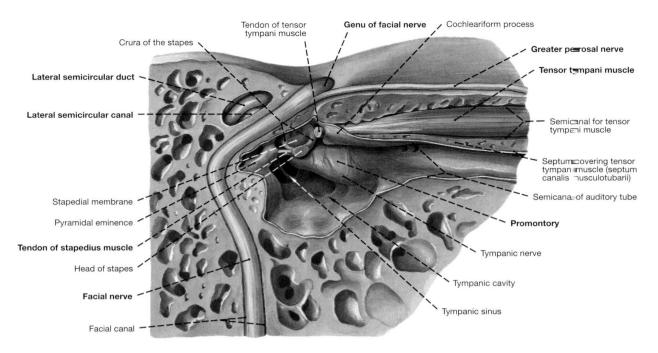

Crura of the stapes
Tendon of tensor tympani muscle
Genu of facial nerve
Cochleariform process
Lateral semicircular duct
Greater petrosal nerve
Lateral semicircular canal
Tensor tympani muscle
Semicanal for tensor tympani muscle
Septum covering tensor tympani muscle (septum canalis musculotubarii)
Stapedial membrane
Semicanal of auditory tube
Pyramidal eminence
Promontory
Tendon of stapedius muscle
Tympanic nerve
Head of stapes
Tympanic cavity
Facial nerve
Tympanic sinus
Facial canal

Fig. 931: Medial Wall of Right Tympanic Cavity (Lateral View)
NOTE: 1) the bone forming the prominences of the **lateral semicircular canal** and the **facial canal** has been removed to reveal their internal structures.

2) the **greater petrosal nerve,** which carries preganglionic parasympathetic fibers from the facial nerve to the pterygopalatine ganglion as well as many taste fibers from the soft palate.

3) coursing along the surface of the promontory can be seen the **tympanic branch** of the **glossopharyngeal nerve** and the tympanic vessels along with sympathetic fibers from the carotid plexus (caroticotympanic nerves).

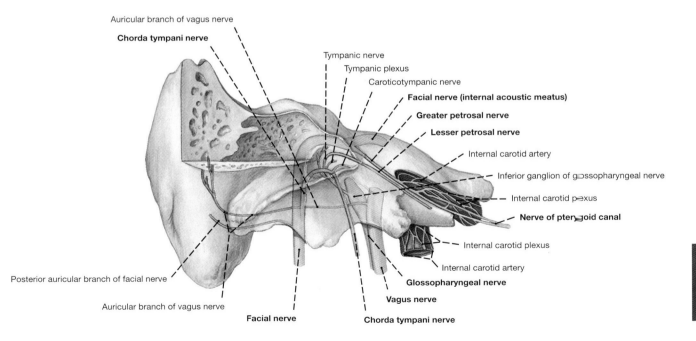

Auricular branch of vagus nerve
Chorda tympani nerve
Tympanic nerve
Tympanic plexus
Caroticotympanic nerve
Facial nerve (internal acoustic meatus)
Greater petrosal nerve
Lesser petrosal nerve
Internal carotid artery
Inferior ganglion of glossopharyngeal nerve
Internal carotid plexus
Nerve of pterygoid canal
Internal carotid plexus
Internal carotid artery
Glossopharyngeal nerve
Posterior auricular branch of facial nerve
Vagus nerve
Auricular branch of vagus nerve
Facial nerve
Chorda tympani nerve

Fig. 932: Facial, Glossopharyngeal and Vagus Nerves Projected on Temporal Bone
NOTE: 1) from the tympanic plexus (see Note 3, Fig. 931) emerges the **lesser petrosal nerve,** which courses to the **otic ganglion.**

2) the **greater petrosal nerve** joins with sympathetic branches of the internal carotid plexus (actually the **deep petrosal nerve**) to form the **nerve of the pterygoid canal.**

3) the **auricular branch** of the **vagus nerve,** which is distributed to the upper surface of the external auricle, to the posterior wall and floor of the external acoustic meatus and part of the lateral (outer) surface of the tympanic membrane.

PLATE 572   Ear: Facial Nerve Dissections 1 and 2

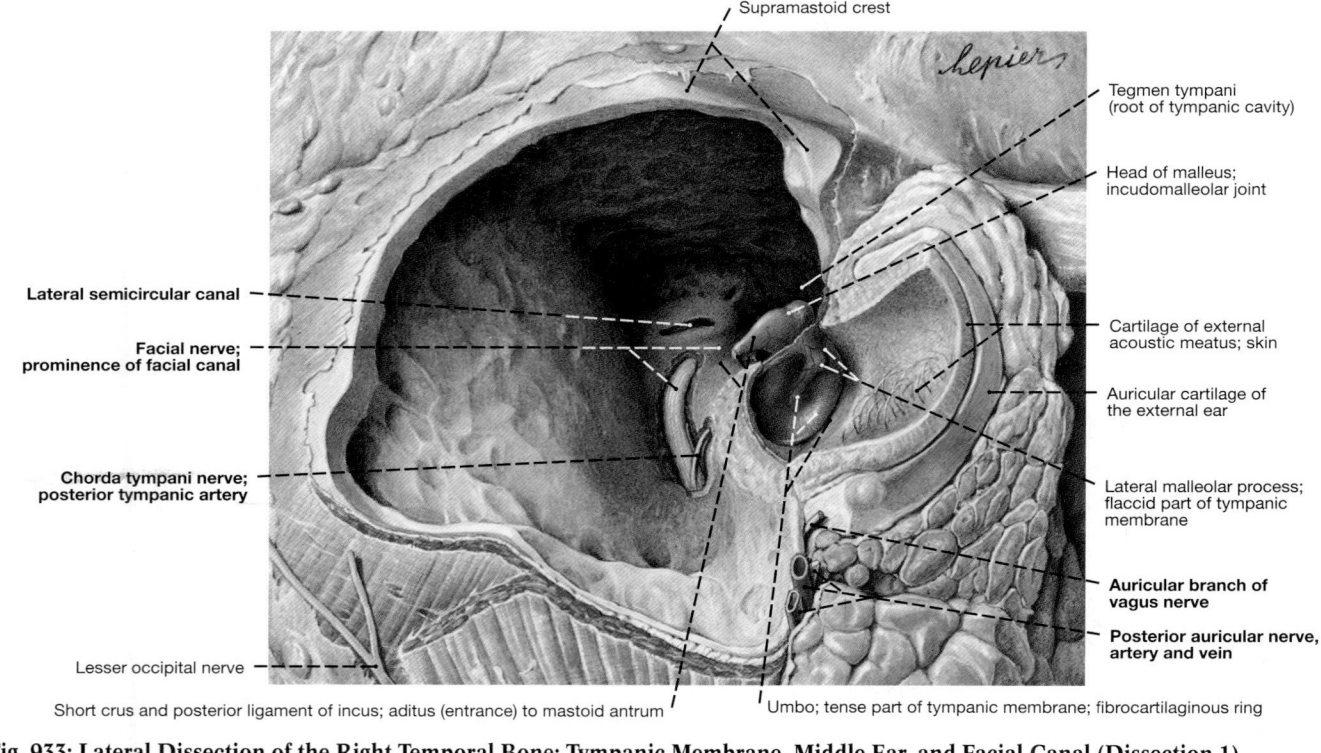

Supramastoid crest

Tegmen tympani
(root of tympanic cavity)

Head of malleus;
incudomalleolar joint

Lateral semicircular canal

Facial nerve;
prominence of facial canal

Cartilage of external
acoustic meatus; skin

Auricular cartilage of
the external ear

Chorda tympani nerve;
posterior tympanic artery

Lateral malleolar process;
flaccid part of tympanic
membrane

**Auricular branch of
vagus nerve**

**Posterior auricular nerve,
artery and vein**

Lesser occipital nerve

Short crus and posterior ligament of incus; aditus (entrance) to mastoid antrum

Umbo; tense part of tympanic membrane; fibrocartilaginous ring

Fig. 933: Lateral Dissection of the Right Temporal Bone: Tympanic Membrane, Middle Ear, and Facial Canal (Dissection 1)
NOTE: 1) this dissection has proceeded through the mastoid region of the temporal bone with the posterior wall of the external acoustic meatus removed. The descending part of the facial canal and the lateral semicircular canal have been opened.

2) the lateral surface of the tympanic membrane. Observe the manubrium of the malleus on the inner surface of the membrane and the head of the malleus, the incus, and the incudomalleolar joint within the tympanic cavity. Also note the junctions of the chorda tympani nerve with the facial nerve.

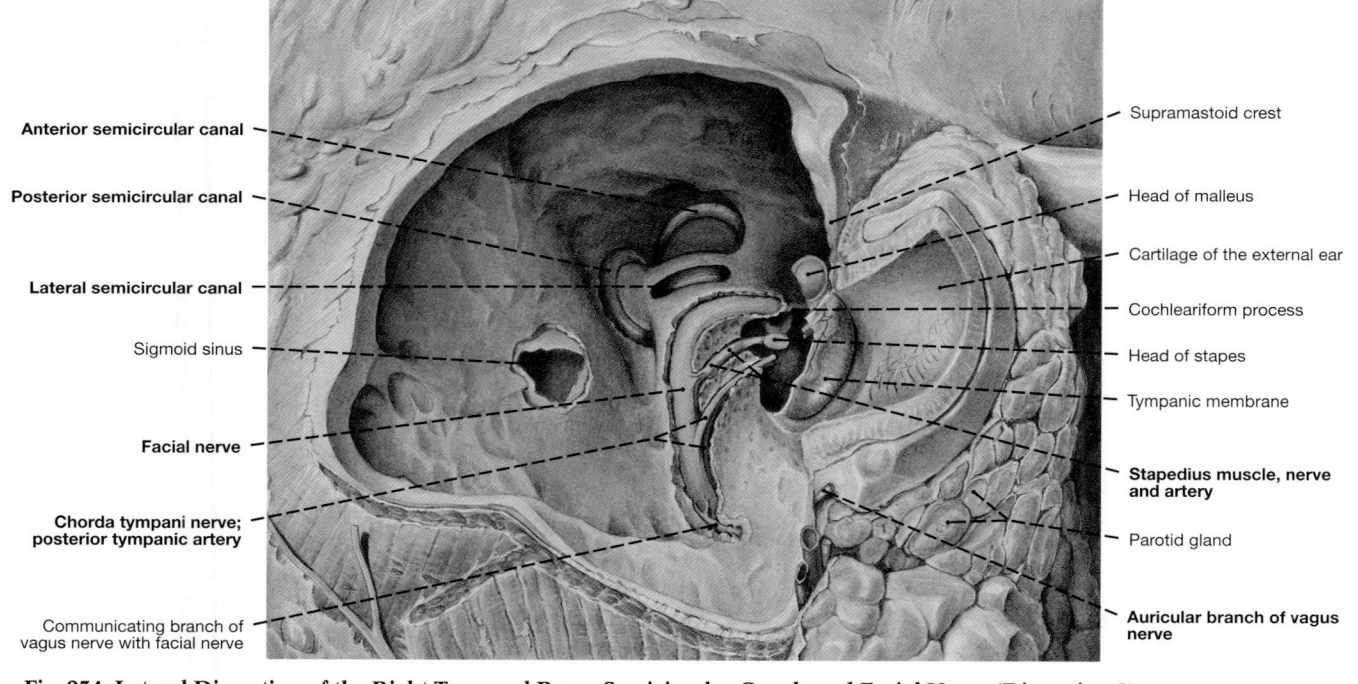

Anterior semicircular canal

Supramastoid crest

Posterior semicircular canal

Head of malleus

Cartilage of the external ear

Lateral semicircular canal

Cochleariform process

Sigmoid sinus

Head of stapes

Tympanic membrane

Facial nerve

**Stapedius muscle, nerve
and artery**

Parotid gland

**Chorda tympani nerve;
posterior tympanic artery**

Communicating branch of
vagus nerve with facial nerve

**Auricular branch of vagus
nerve**

Fig. 934: Lateral Dissection of the Right Temporal Bone: Semicircular Canals and Facial Nerve (Dissection 2)
NOTE: 1) Further opening of the facial canal exposes more completely the chorda tympani nerve and the posterior tympanic branch of the stylomastoid artery which helps supply the internal surface of the tympanic membrane. Also note the stapedius muscle and artery.

2) the anterior, posterior, and lateral semicircular canals. These become exposed after removal of the bony prominence over the lateral canal and additional bone above and behind that prominence.

Figs. 933, 934

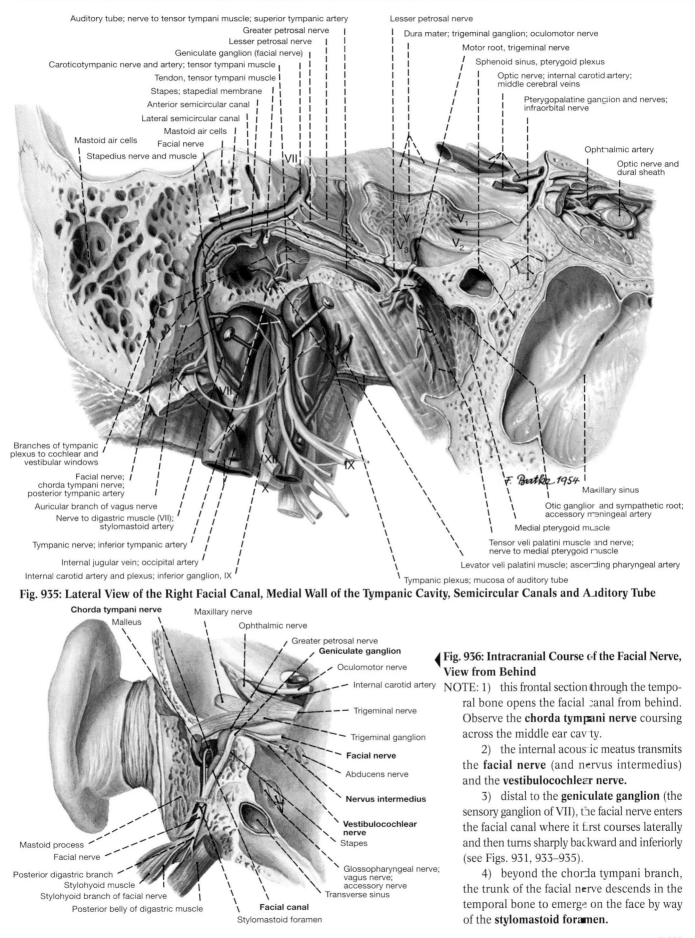

Auditory tube; nerve to tensor tympani muscle; superior tympanic artery
Greater petrosal nerve
Lesser petrosal nerve
Geniculate ganglion (facial nerve)
Caroticotympanic nerve and artery; tensor tympani muscle
Tendon, tensor tympani muscle
Stapes; stapedial membrane
Anterior semicircular canal
Lateral semicircular canal
Mastoid air cells
Mastoid air cells
Facial nerve
Stapedius nerve and muscle

Lesser petrosal nerve
Dura mater; trigeminal ganglion; oculomotor nerve
Motor root, trigeminal nerve
Sphenoid sinus, pterygoid plexus
Optic nerve; internal carotid artery; middle cerebral veins
Pterygopalatine ganglion and nerves; infraorbital nerve
Ophthalmic artery
Optic nerve and dural sheath

V
V_1
V_3
V_2

Branches of tympanic plexus to cochlear and vestibular windows
Facial nerve; chorda tympani nerve; posterior tympanic artery
Auricular branch of vagus nerve
Nerve to digastric muscle (VII); stylomastoid artery
Tympanic nerve; inferior tympanic artery
Internal jugular vein; occipital artery
Internal carotid artery and plexus; inferior ganglion, IX

F. Bathe 1954

Maxillary sinus
Otic ganglion and sympathetic root; accessory meningeal artery
Medial pterygoid muscle
Tensor veli palatini muscle and nerve; nerve to medial pterygoid muscle
Levator veli palatini muscle; ascending pharyngeal artery
Tympanic plexus; mucosa of auditory tube

Fig. 935: Lateral View of the Right Facial Canal, Medial Wall of the Tympanic Cavity, Semicircular Canals and Auditory Tube

Chorda tympani nerve
Malleus
Maxillary nerve
Ophthalmic nerve
Greater petrosal nerve
Geniculate ganglion
Oculomotor nerve
Internal carotid artery
Trigeminal nerve
Trigeminal ganglion
Facial nerve
Abducens nerve
Nervus intermedius
Vestibulocochlear nerve
Stapes

Mastoid process
Facial nerve
Posterior digastric branch
Stylohyoid muscle
Stylohyoid branch of facial nerve
Posterior belly of digastric muscle
Facial canal
Stylomastoid foramen
Glossopharyngeal nerve; vagus nerve; accessory nerve
Transverse sinus

Fig. 936: Intracranial Course of the Facial Nerve, View from Behind

NOTE: 1) this frontal section through the temporal bone opens the facial canal from behind. Observe the **chorda tympani nerve** coursing across the middle ear cavity.

2) the internal acoustic meatus transmits the **facial nerve** (and nervus intermedius) and the **vestibulocochlear nerve.**

3) distal to the **geniculate ganglion** (the sensory ganglion of VII), the facial nerve enters the facial canal where it first courses laterally and then turns sharply backward and inferiorly (see Figs. 931, 933–935).

4) beyond the chorda tympani branch, the trunk of the facial nerve descends in the temporal bone to emerge on the face by way of the **stylomastoid foramen.**

PLATE 574   Ear: Tympanic Cavity From Above; Nerves III to XII

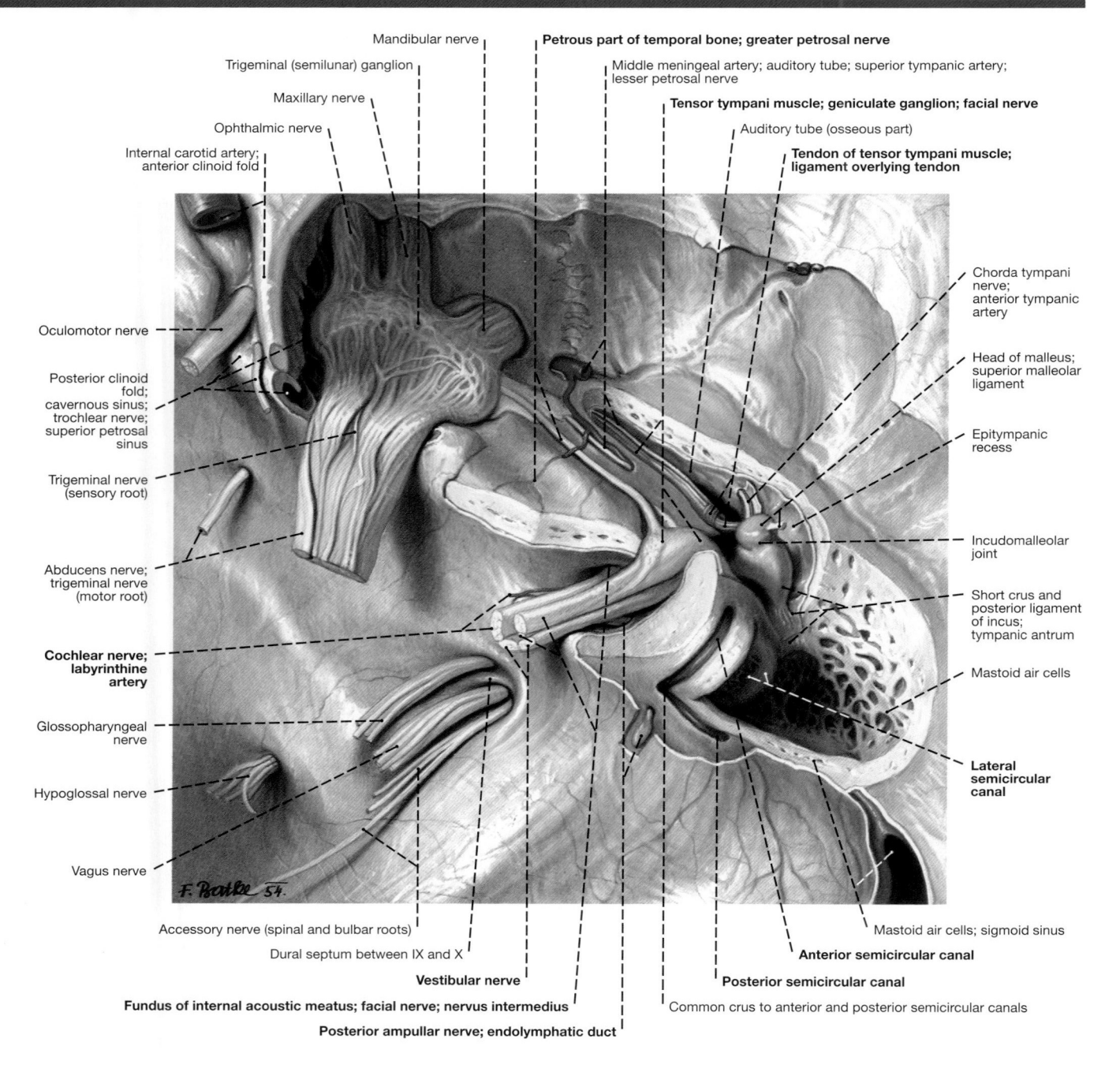

Mandibular nerve

Trigeminal (semilunar) ganglion

Maxillary nerve

Ophthalmic nerve

Internal carotid artery; anterior clinoid fold

Petrous part of temporal bone; greater petrosal nerve

Middle meningeal artery; auditory tube; superior tympanic artery; lesser petrosal nerve

Tensor tympani muscle; geniculate ganglion; facial nerve

Auditory tube (osseous part)

Tendon of tensor tympani muscle; ligament overlying tendon

Oculomotor nerve

Posterior clinoid fold; cavernous sinus; trochlear nerve; superior petrosal sinus

Trigeminal nerve (sensory root)

Abducens nerve; trigeminal nerve (motor root)

Cochlear nerve; labyrinthine artery

Glossopharyngeal nerve

Hypoglossal nerve

Vagus nerve

Chorda tympani nerve; anterior tympanic artery

Head of malleus; superior malleolar ligament

Epitympanic recess

Incudomalleolar joint

Short crus and posterior ligament of incus; tympanic antrum

Mastoid air cells

Lateral semicircular canal

F. Boatke 54.

Accessory nerve (spinal and bulbar roots)

Dural septum between IX and X

Vestibular nerve

Fundus of internal acoustic meatus; facial nerve; nervus intermedius

Posterior ampullar nerve; endolymphatic duct

Posterior semicircular canal

Anterior semicircular canal

Mastoid air cells; sigmoid sinus

Common crus to anterior and posterior semicircular canals

Fig. 937: Right Tympanic Cavity, Auditory Tube, and Semicircular Canals Opened From the Floor of the Cranial Cavity and Viewed From Above

NOTE: 1) the orientation of this dissection is similar to that in Figure 938. The petrous and mastoid parts of the temporal bone have been dissected from the floor of the cranial cavity. The internal acoustic meatus was also opened exposing the **facial nerve** and its **nervus intermedius,** the **cochlear,** and **vestibular** divisions of **VIII** and the **labyrinthine artery.**

2) the **geniculate ganglion** at the lateral end of the internal acoustic meatus. This sensory ganglion of the facial nerve contains the cell bodies of the afferent neurons (both general sensory and special sense of taste) that course in the facial nerve.

3) attached to the facial ganglion are: a) the main trunk of the facial nerve which descends into the facial canal behind the tympanic cavity (see Figs. 931–936), and b) the **greater petrosal nerve** which courses along a shallow groove (the hiatus of the facial canal) that extends to the **foramen lacerum,** through which this nerve reaches the pterygoid canal (see Fig. 771).

4) the **auditory tube** and its tympanic opening. The tensor tympani muscle lies in a thin bony canal just above the tube and its tendon bends around the **cochleariform process** to attach to the handle of the malleus. This muscle is supplied by a small branch from the mandibular division of the trigeminal nerve (see Fig. 935).

5) the **anterior** and **posterior semicircular canals** have been opened, but the bone that forms the **lateral semicircular canal** is still intact. Behind these canals is found an opening for the small **endolymphatic sac** called the aqueduct of the vestibule. Also note the communication between the tympanic cavity, its antrum, and the mastoid air cells.

Fig. 937

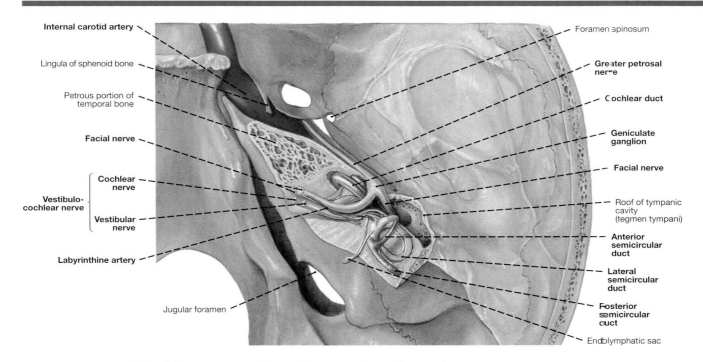

Fig. 938: Structures of the Right Inner Ear and the Facial Nerve, Dissected From Above

NOTE: 1) the upper part of the petrous portion of the temporal bone has been removed to expose the membranous labyrinth, the cochlear duct, the facial and vestibulocochlear nerves and the labyrinthine artery.

   2) the orientation of the cochlea and semicircular ducts is similar to that in Figure 939. Note also the geniculate ganglion from which extends the greater petrosal nerve inferomedially toward the pterygoid canal.

   3) the facial nerve entering the facial canal lateral and posterior to the ganglion.

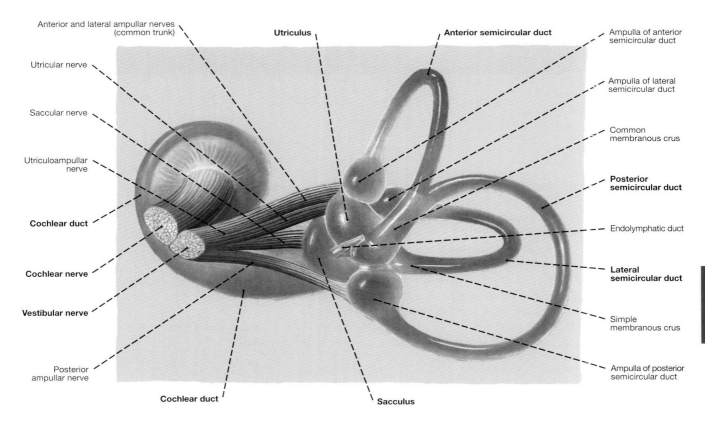

Fig. 939: Right Membranous Labyrinth (Medial View)

NOTE: the ampullae of the three semicircular ducts, the sacculus, the utriculus and cochlear duct, and the connections of the endolymphatic duct to the utriculus and sacculus.

PLATE 576   Ear: Nerves and Vessels of Internal Ear

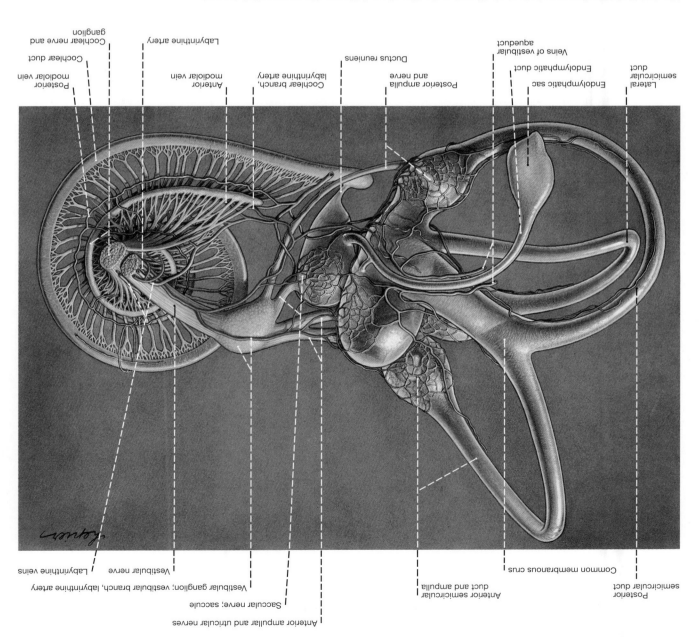

Fig. 940: Left Membranous Labyrinth Showing the Vessels and Nerves (Posteromedial Aspect)

NOTE: 1) the nerve branches from each of the ampullae of the semicircular ducts and from the utriculus and saccule join to form the **vestibular division** of the **vestibulocochlear nerve**. The ganglion containing the sensory nerve cell bodies for this division is the **vestibular (Scarpa's) ganglion**.

2) the **cochlear division** of the **vestibulocochlear nerve** serves the cochlear duct, and its ganglion, the **spiral ganglion**, is long and coiled and its cell bodies course with the cochlear nerve fibers in the spiral canal of the modiolus.

3) the arterial supply to the labyrinth comes by way of the **labyrinthine artery** which may branch directly from the basilar artery or more frequently from the anterior inferior cerebellar artery. It enters the internal auditory meatus and at the distal end of this meatus it divides into **cochlear and vestibular branches** as shown above.

4) the cochlear branch courses along the cochlea and divides into 10 to 15 branches as it traverses the turns of the cochlea. The vestibular branch is distributed to the utriculus, saccule and the semicircular ducts.

Labels (clockwise):
- Posterior modiolar vein
- Cochlear duct
- Cochlear nerve and ganglion
- Labyrinthine artery
- Anterior modiolar vein
- Cochlear branch, labyrinthine artery
- Ductus reuniens
- Posterior ampulla and nerve
- Veins of vestibular aqueduct
- Endolymphatic duct
- Endolymphatic sac
- Lateral semicircular duct
- Posterior semicircular duct
- Common membranous crus
- Anterior semicircular duct and ampulla
- Saccular nerve; saccule
- Anterior ampullar and utricular nerves
- Vestibular ganglion; vestibular branch, labyrinthine artery
- Vestibular nerve
- Labyrinthine veins

Fig. 940